Gross Morphology of Common Diseases

Gross Morphology of Common Diseases

Editor: Zu-hua Gao, MD, PhD, FRCPC

Assistant editor: Yu Shi, MD, PhD, FCAP

Supported by the Montreal General Hospital Foundation

Brush
Education Inc.

20 21 22 23 24 5 4 3 2 1

Brush Education Inc.
www.brusheducation.ca
contact@brusheducation.ca

Editorial: Kay Rollans
Index: François Trahern
Cover design: Dean Pickup
Interior design and layout: Carol Dragich, Dragich Design

Printed and manufactured in Canada

Library and Archives Canada Cataloguing in Publication

Title: Gross morphology of common diseases / editor, Zu-hua Gao, MD, PhD, FRCPC ; assistant editor, Yu Shi, MD, PhD, FCAP.
Names: Gao, Zu-hua, 1962- editor.

Description: Includes bibliographical references and index.
Identifiers: Canadiana (print) 20190095709 | Canadiana (ebook) 20190095784 | ISBN 9781550596854 (softcover) | ISBN 9781550596861 (PDF) | ISBN 9781550596878 (Kindle) | ISBN 9781550596885 (EPUB)

Subjects: LCSH: Diseases. | LCSH: Morphology.
Classification: LCC RC46 .G76 2020 | DDC 616—dc23

We acknowledge the support of the Government of Canada
Nous reconnaissons l'appui du gouvernement du Canada | Canada

Contents

Preface

This book presents a systematic compilation of macroscopic images of common human diseases. For each image, we provide a gross description and the most relevant clinical and pathological information. The goal is to provide a comprehensive guide of macropathology to undergraduate medical students and pathology trainees. However, the images and information provided will also help clinicians in formulating differential diagnoses, and help readers from the general public in visualizing particular diseases of their interest.

In keeping with most medical textbooks, we have organized disease entities by organ system. We have strived to make the collection as complete as possible, but there are gaps. As it stands now, this collection covers the most commonly encountered entities. I am confident that — with more than 100 000 surgical cases going through the McGill pathology department each year — future editions will see any gaps filled, and the collection as a whole enriched with more entities and more representative images.

The images in this book come from historical collections of teaching materials from the departments of pathology at McGill University, the University of Ottawa, the University of Calgary, and Dalhousie University, as well as from recent surgical and autopsy specimens from McGill University Health Centre, and from the personal collections of contributing authors. This book would not be possible without these contributions, which in turn relied on the hard diagnostic work of pathologists, pathology residents and pathologists' assistants involved in the cases these pages present.

Montreal, Canada — where I, and many of the authors of this book, live and work — is home to an enormous wealth of resources in the field of pathology. This book would not have been possible without the financial support of the Montreal General Hospital Foundation, the time and expertise of all the contributing authors, and access to the invaluable collections of the McGill Department of Pathology. In addition, we were kindly allowed to use 25 images from the collections of the Maude Abbott Medical Museum, home of the world-class McGill Pathology Museum Osler Collection established by Sir William Osler and Dr. Maude Abbott in the late 1800s and early 1900s. We are privileged and honored to serve as a conduit to transfer the precious teaching materials contained in these pages to the current and future generations of practitioners, medical students, and pathology trainees.

Disclaimer

1

Diseases of the Skull, Brain, Pituitary Gland, Spinal Cord, and Peripheral Nerves

AMAL AL-ODAINI, LINNEA DUKE, JUDY WANG,
JEFFERY T. JOSEPH, JASON KARAMCHANDANI

Skull

Basal skull fracture

Basal skull fractures involve 1 or more of the 5 bones of the base of the skull: the occipital bone; sphenoid bone; petrous and squamous portions of the temporal bone; orbital plate of the frontal bone; and cribriform plate of the ethmoid bone. Leaks of cerebral spinal fluid (CSF), which present as otorrhea or rhinorrhea, are pathognomonic for basal skull fractures. Other classic clinical signs are periorbital ecchymoses ("raccoon eyes"), retroauricular ecchymoses (Battle sign), and hemotympanum.

FIGURE 1.1. This image shows a superior view of a skull opened to expose the base of the skull, revealing a linear fracture extending between the 2 temporal bones (arrows).

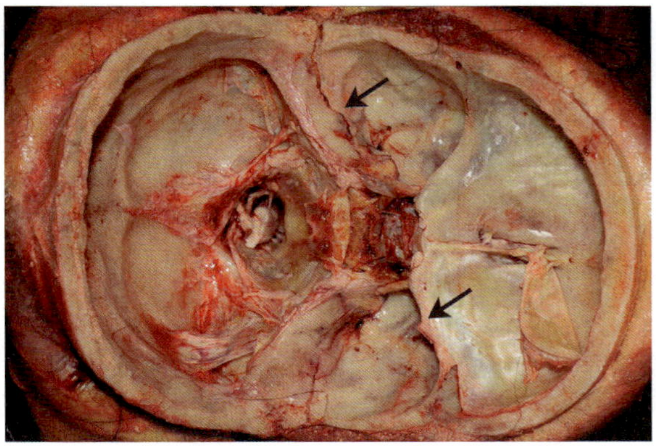

Intracranial hemorrhage

EPIDURAL HEMORRHAGE (EDH) VERSUS SUBDURAL HEMORRHAGE (SDH)

In EDH, the blood is located between the dura and the skull. By contrast, in SDH, the blood is located between the arachnoid layer and the dura. EDH is typically caused by head trauma that fractures the temporal bone and disrupts the middle meningeal artery. EDH > 100 mL in volume is typically fatal.

FIGURE 1.2. These images show superior views of 2 brain autopsies: (A) EDH and (B) SDH.

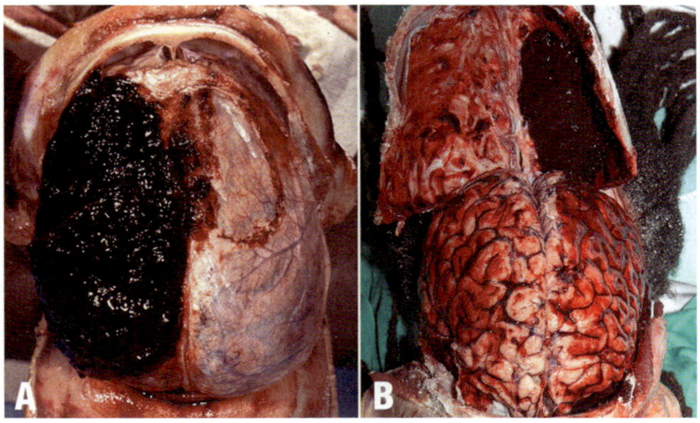

SUBDURAL HEMORRHAGE (SDH) VERSUS SUBARACHNOID HEMORRHAGE (SAH)

In SAH, the blood is located beneath the delicate arachnoid layer. On gross examination, blood from SAH does not wipe off the surface of the brain, because it is beneath the meninges. SDH can be multifocal.

FIGURE 1.3. These images show superior views of 2 brain autopsies: (A) SDH and (B) SAH.

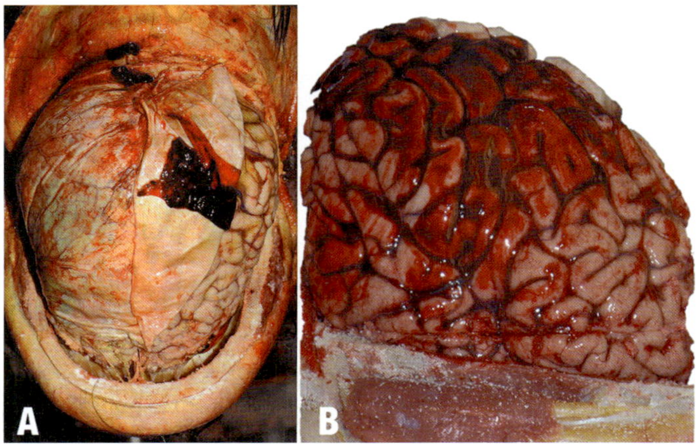

SUBARACHNOID HEMORRHAGE (SAH)

Primary SAH that results from the rupture of an intracranial saccular aneurysm may manifest as sudden, unexpected death. In most cases, the ruptured saccular aneurysm bleeds directly into the subarachnoid space. Occasionally, the arterial blood dissects through the parenchyma and into the ventricles. Saccular aneurysms are focal dilations of the arterial vessels that typically occur at arterial branch points.

FIGURE 1.4. In (A), a superior view of a fixed brain at autopsy illustrates SAH due to a ruptured aneurysm in the territory of the middle cerebral artery. In (B), an image of a formalin-fixed autopsy brain in coronal section illustrates SAH due to a ruptured aneurysm in the territory of the middle cerebral artery that dissected into the ventricular system.

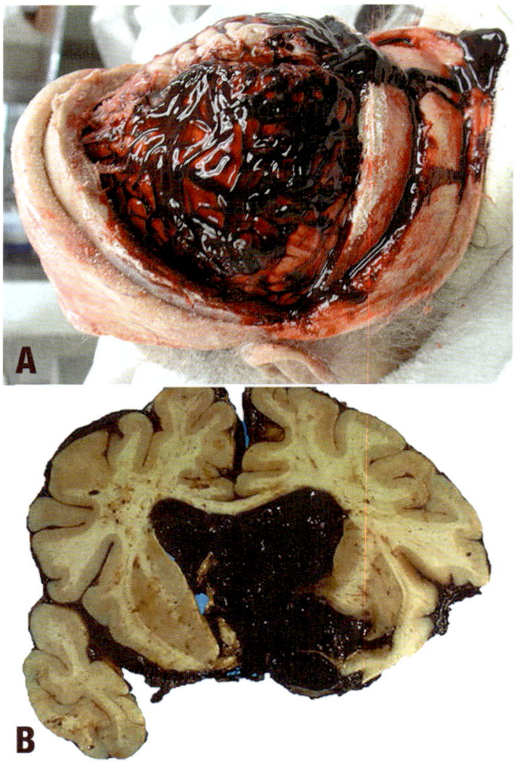

Arachnoid granulations

Arachnoid granulations are villous extensions of the arachnoid membrane into the dural sinuses that serve as a conduit for the circulation of CSF. They are commonly mistaken for pathological entities.

FIGURE 1.5. This specimen demonstrates arachnoid granulations (arrow).

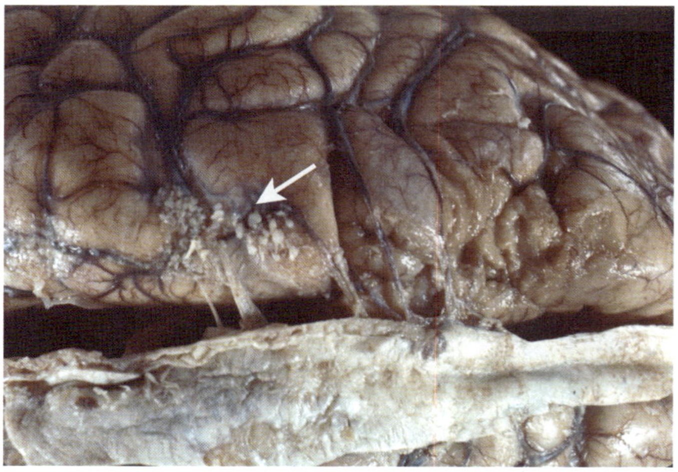

Brain

Congenital and Acquired Anomalies of the Brain

Encephalocele

An encephalocele is a type of neural tube defect (NTD) that results from the herniation of brain tissue through cranial bone defects. It most commonly affects the posterior fossa.

FIGURE 1.6. Image (A) shows a fetus with a large congested cranial lesion in the occipital area on external examination. In (B), internal examination of the same fetus reveals incomplete formation of the cranial bone at its posterior, and connection of the lesion to the parietooccipital lobes.

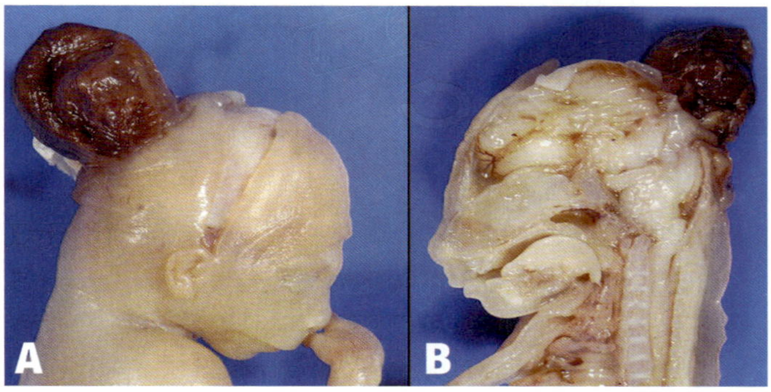

Holoprosencephaly

Holoprosencephaly is a forebrain anomaly that occurs in 0.4 per 1000 pregnancies. In holoprosencephaly, the forebrain fails to develop into 2 separate hemispheres and lateral ventricles. This results in partial or complete midline hemisphere fusion. Holoprosencephaly is mostly sporadic and of unknown etiology, but can be associated with trisomy 13.

FIGURE 1.7. Image (A) shows a fetus with dysmorphic features and complete cleft lip. In (B), internal examination of the brain of the fetus shows absent midline cleavage with loss of normal brain gyrations consistent with holoprosencephaly.

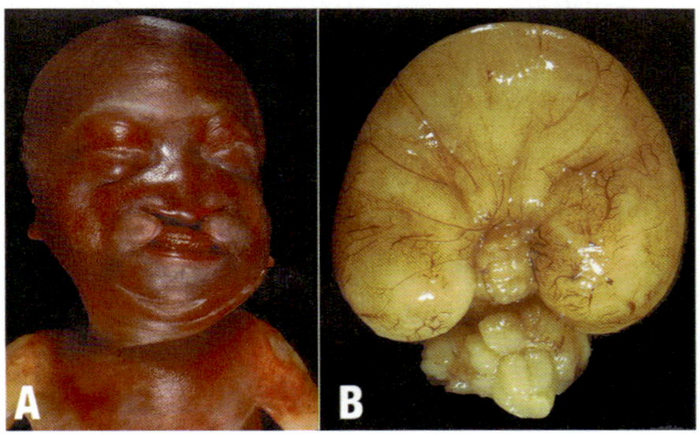

Lissencephaly

Lissencephaly is a forebrain malformation in which the normal cerebral gyri are reduced in number or totally lost (agyria). Two lissencephaly patterns exist: type 1 (smooth outer surface) and type 2 (cobblestoned surface). The anomaly is caused by abnormal neuronal migration due to a mutation in the migration-signaling enzymes.

FIGURE 1.8. In (A), a full coronal section of a cerebrum shows marked loss of normal brain folding with a smooth outer surface. In (B), a stained cerebrum (Luxol fast blue with PAS stain) shows loss of the normal gyrification.

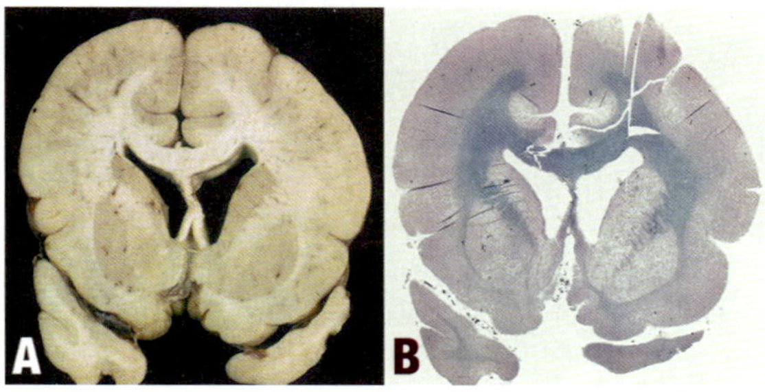

Polymicrogyria

Polymicrogyria is a forebrain anomaly and, like lissencephaly and pachygyria, is a disease in the spectrum of neuronal migration disorders.

FIGURE 1.9. The cerebral hemisphere in (A) has numerous, abnormally small and irregular cortical gyrations. Microscopically, the number of cortical neuronal layers is reduced to 4 or fewer, and the layers show meningeal tissue entrapment. Image (B) shows a stained section of the same brain (Luxol fast blue with H&E stain).

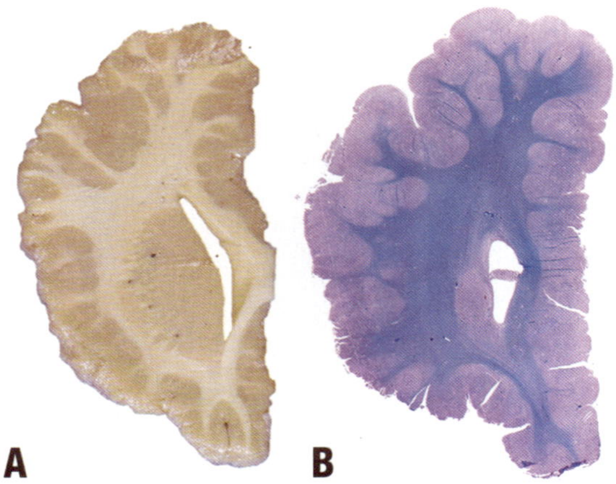

Pachygyria

Pachygyria presents as abnormally large, poorly formed gyri, and may occur focally in the cerebral cortex or with lissencephaly in other regions. This forebrain malformation, along with polymicrogyria and lissencephaly, is another type of developmental disorder within the continuum of abnormal neuronal migration. Clinically, gyral cortical defects cause developmental delay, convulsions, and motor deficits.

FIGURE 1.10. This image shows a superior view of a brain with pachygyria.

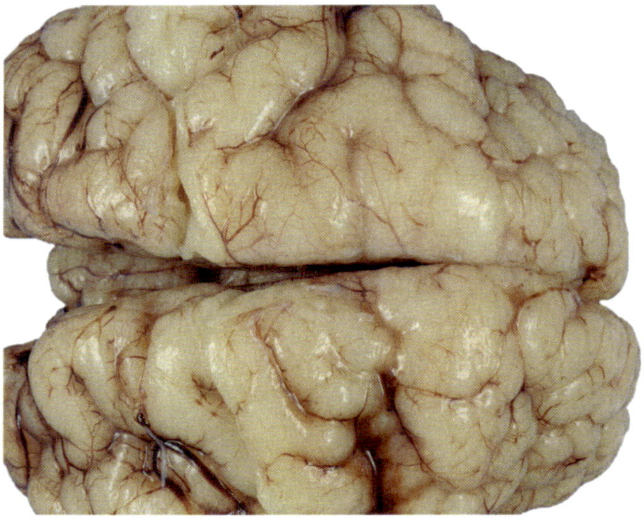

Hydrocephalus

Hydrocephalus is caused by excessive CSF, which results in dilation of the ventricles. The condition can result from either CSF outflow obstruction (noncommunicating or internal type) or impaired resorption (communicating or external type). Hydrocephalus can be congenital (e.g., CNS malformation) or acquired (e.g., infection or tumor), and in some cases it is secondary to brain atrophy.

FIGURE 1.12. In this image, a coronal section of a fixed brain shows bilaterally dilated ventricles.

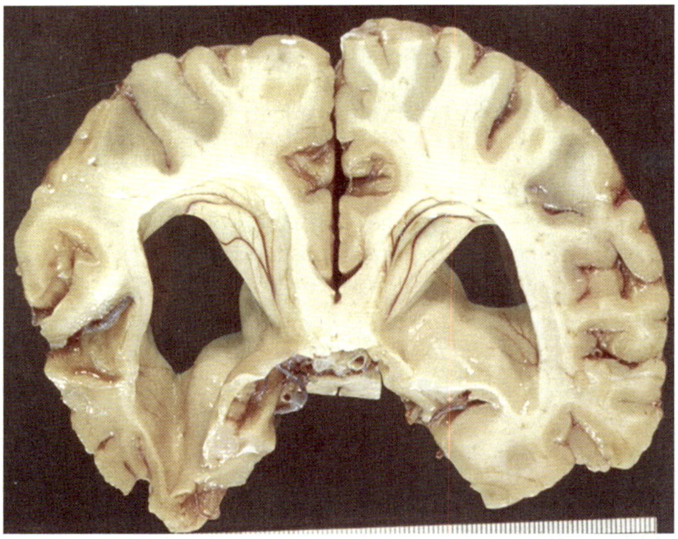

Encephalomalacia

The softening and loss of brain tissue secondary to hemorrhage or inflammation is known as encephalomalacia. It is the end result of liquefactive necrosis of brain tissue after cerebral trauma, infection, ischemia, or infarction. This condition occurs in both pediatric and adult populations. Clinically, patients demonstrate neurological dysfunction that is location dependent.

FIGURE 1.11. This image shows multiple large and honeycomb-shaped cystic areas within the cortex of the temporoparietal lobe. The gyri are shrunken and irregular with consequent widening of the lateral fissure. Note the cystic cavitation (arrows).

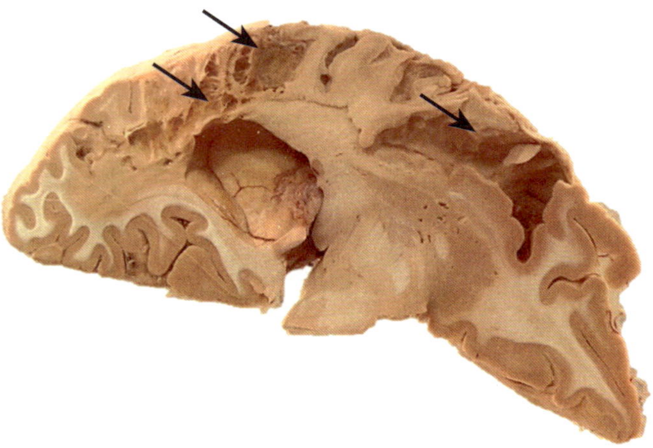

Multiple sclerosis (MS)

MS is an autoimmune demyelinating disease that preferentially involves the myelin sheath. MS affects middle-aged individuals and is most common in women. Clinically, MS manifests as intermittent episodes of neurological dysfunction.

FIGURE 1.13. This coronal section of a brain exhibits the characteristic irregular, depressed, and gray periventricular plaques (arrows) seen in MS. On palpation, these white matter lesions are firmer than the surrounding parenchyma. Plaques can also occur in the optic chiasm, brain stem, and spinal cord.

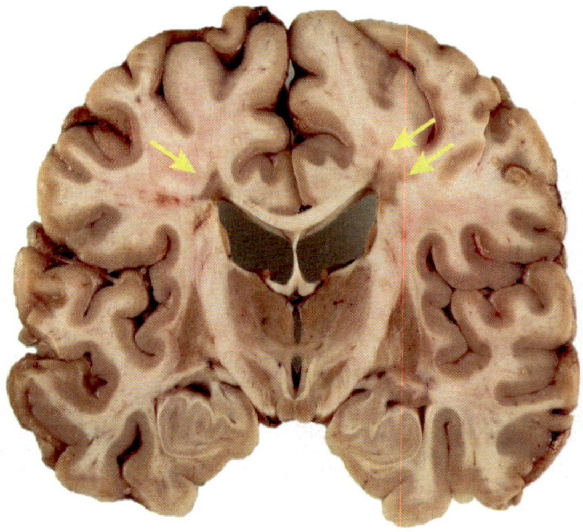

Alzheimer disease (AD)

AD is the most common cause of dementia in older individuals. This neurodegenerative disease starts insidiously, with loss of higher cognitive function over the course of many years. AD results from faulty accumulation of amyloid-α peptide and tau protein, with the consequent formation of plaques and tangles in the hippocampus, amygdala, and neocortex. In AD, the brain is small and atrophic with widened cortical sulci, which reflects the cortical atrophy most evident in the fontal, temporal, and parietal lobes.

FIGURE 1.14. This image shows the brain of a patient with advanced AD. The brain is small and atrophic with widened cortical sulci (arrows).

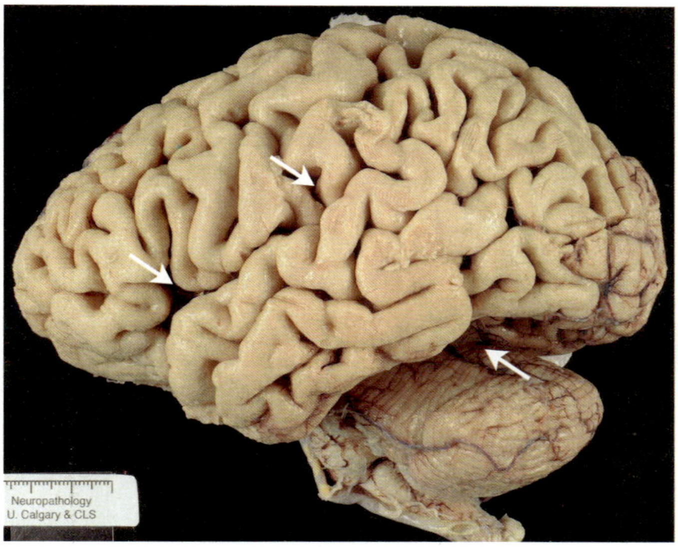

HYDROCEPHALUS EX VACUO

In advanced AD with significant atrophy, a secondary ventricular dilatation develops as a consequence of brain volume loss particularly in the temporal horns.

FIGURE 1.15. This image shows the brain of a patient with advanced AD. Note the brain volume loss particularly in the temporal horns.

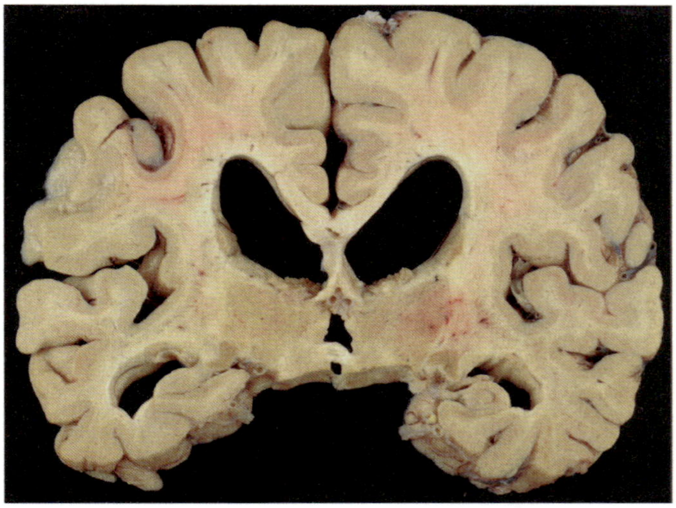

Methanol toxicity

The brain is, perhaps, the organ most likely to demonstrate "selective vulnerability." Selective vulnerability can help indicate the etiology of a pathology based on its location. The effect of methanol toxicity on the brain is an example.

FIGURE 1.16. In this image, the striking feature is of bilateral hemorrhagic necrosis of the putamen. This particular area of the basal ganglia is most affected by methanol toxicity.

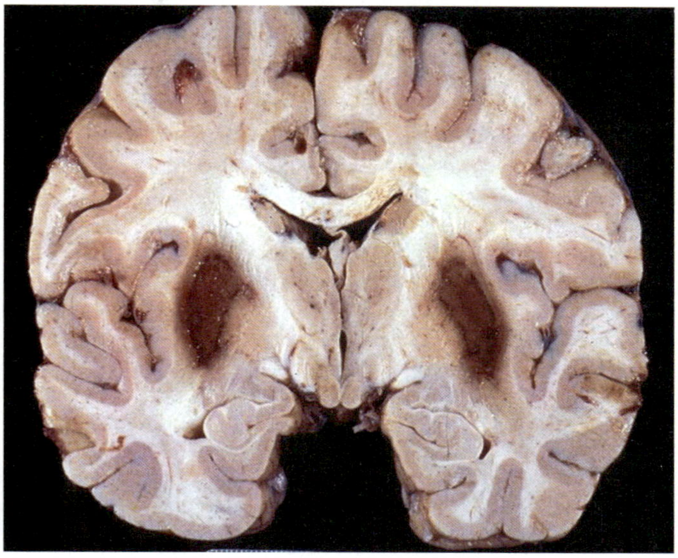

Image courtesy of Dr. Hannes Vogel.

Pick disease

Pick disease is a neurodegenerative disease of frontotemporal lobar degeneration (FTLD) and a common cause of early onset dementia. Like AD, it is associated with tau protein accumulation (called Pick bodies). Grossly, it is characterized by marked localized brain atrophy, mainly in the frontal and temporal lobes.

FIGURE 1.17. In this image, a lateral view of a left hemisphere shows asymmetric brain atrophy that markedly affects the frontal and anterior temporal lobes and spares the other lobes. Note the "knife edge" gyri in the anterior temporal lobe (arrows), another feature of Pick disease.

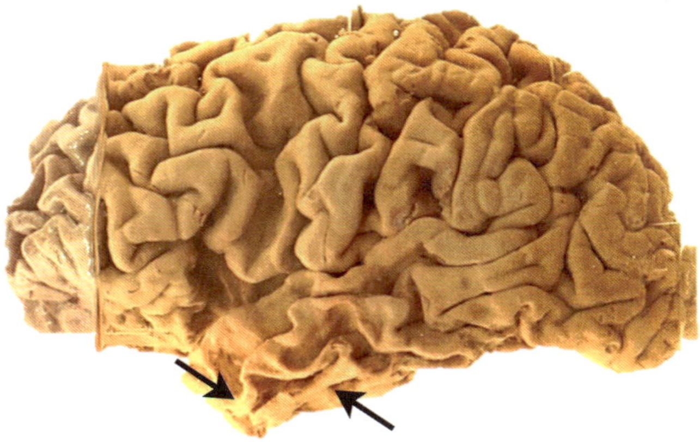

Specimen from Maude Abbott Medical Museum, McGill University

Infections and Inflammation of the Brain

Meningitis

Meningitis is an inflammatory process of the leptomeninges that is, in the vast majority of cases, caused by infection. In some cases, meningitis can be noninfectious in etiology (chemical meningitis). Infectious meningitis can be classified into 3 types: acute pyogenic, aseptic, and chronic.

FIGURE 1.18. The autopsy brains shown in (A) and (B) exhibit purulent exudate accumulating within the leptomeninges on the surface of the brain. Note in (A) the engorged meningeal blood vessels (arrows) over the parietal lobe.

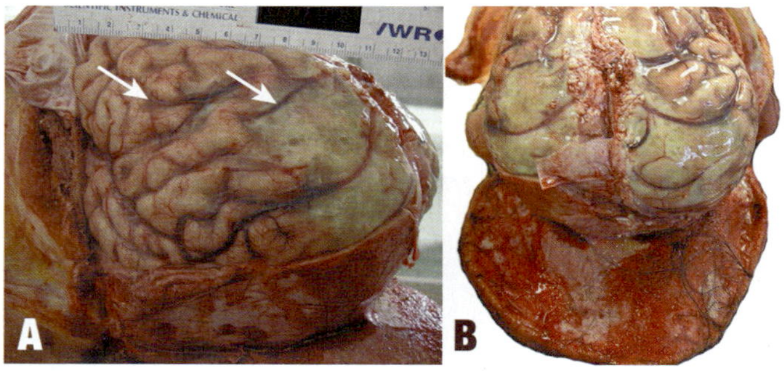

PURULENT MENINGITIS OF THE BRAIN

FIGURE 1.19. This autopsy brain shows purulent exudate accumulating within the leptomeninges on the surface of the brain and masking the normal gyrated brain surface. Note also the engorged meningeal blood vessels over the frontal lobes (arrows).

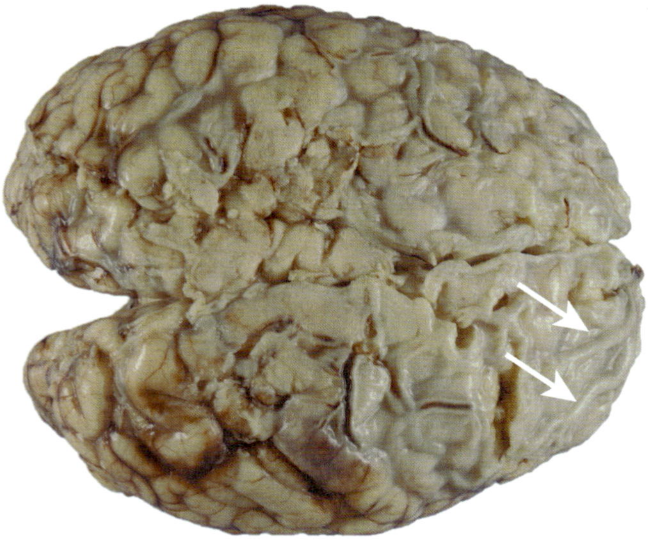

Brain abscess

Brain abscesses can result from extension of direct infection (e.g., sinusitis) or from hematogenous spread. The most common offending organisms in immunocompetent patients are streptococci and staphylococci. Complications of brain abscesses include brain herniation secondary to increased intracranial pressure; abscess rupture with ventriculitis and meningitis; and venous sinus thrombosis.

CEREBRUM ABSCESS

Cerebrum abscesses are localized brain parenchymal infections that result in necrosis and inflammation. Clinically, cerebral abscesses present with focal neurologic symptoms related to their location.

FIGURE 1.20. This macrograph of the left cerebral hemisphere shows a discrete single periventricular necrotic cavitary lesion with yellow-green discoloration (arrow).

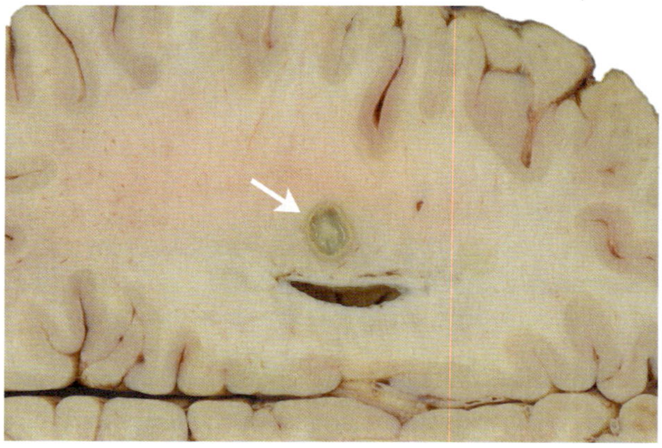

CEREBELLUM ABSCESS

FIGURE 1.21. An inferior view of a bivalved cerebellum shows a right cerebellar abscess (arrows). This patient presented with a 3 week history of headache prior to death. The patient had a remote history of surgically treated mastoiditis.

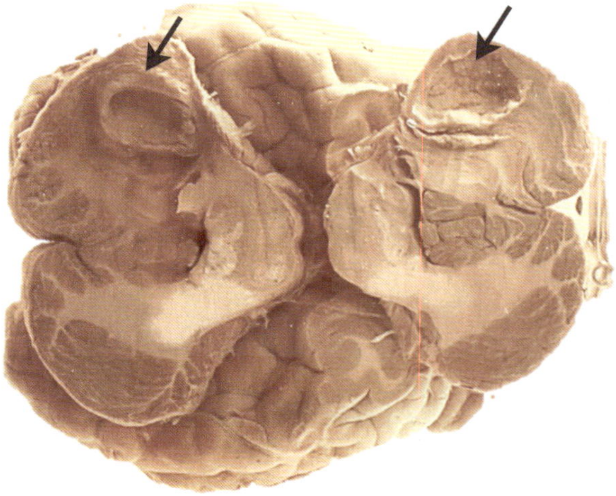

Cerebrum postmortem anaerobic bacterial growth

Anaerobic bacteria are part of normal mouth flora and are associated with otorhinolaryngeal infections. The most frequent anaerobes cultured from brain abscesses include anaerobic streptococci, and bacteria of the *Bacteroides* and *Actinomyces* genera.

FIGURE 1.22. This image shows a uniformly enlarged brain with large, irregular spaces throughout the cerebral hemispheres caused by anaerobic bacteria.

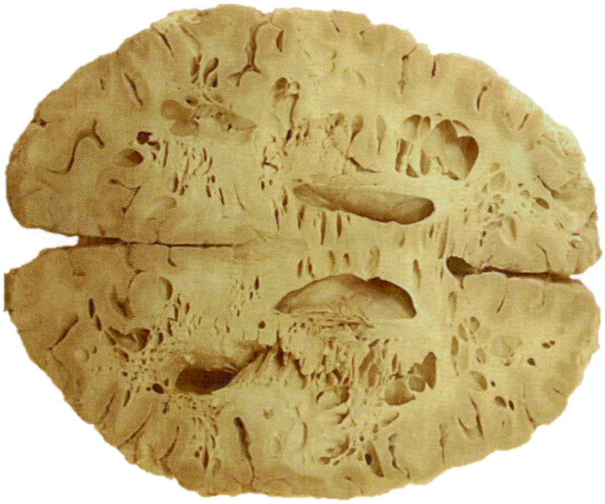

Specimen from Maude Abbott Medical Museum, McGill University

CNS tuberculosis

CNS tuberculosis can be a manifestation of an active infection elsewhere in the body, or an isolated seeding from a distant, silent site. The most common pattern of involvement is diffuse meningoencephalitis, which most frequently presents with basilar meningitis. Another pattern involves tuberculomas, which take the form of 1 or more well-circumscribed intraparenchymal caseous lesions.

FIGURE 1.23. Image (A) shows gross (although subtle) findings of a case of CNS tuberculosis: accumulation of exudate over the midbrain and cerebellum. The accumulation of this exudate can cause secondary cerebrospinal fluid outflow obstruction and subsequent hydrocephalus, which is shown in (B).

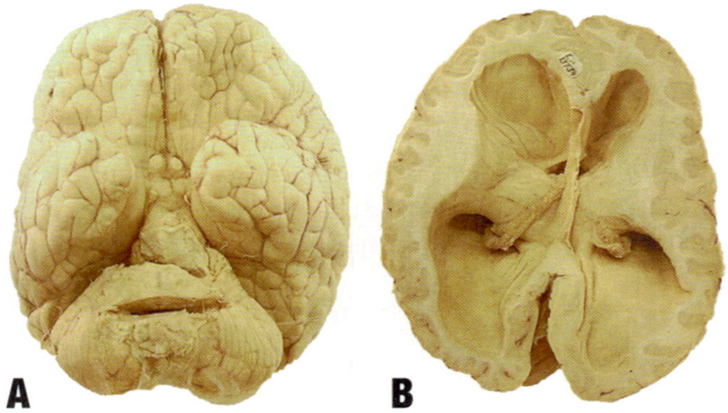

Specimen B from Maude Abbott Medical Museum, McGill University

Brain Neoplasms

Cerebrum glioblastoma

PROGRESSION OF GLIOMA TO GLIOBLASTOMA

Infiltrating astrocytomas are assigned a World Health Organization (WHO) grade. Grade II tumors are called diffuse astrocytoma; grade III tumors, anaplastic astrocytoma; grade IV tumors, glioblastoma. The majority of low-grade gliomas are characterized by either *IDH1* or *IDH2* mutation. The progression of a primary glioma of a lower WHO grade to a secondary glioblastoma is characterized by additional genetic alterations. Primary glioblastomas harbor telomerase reverse transcriptase (TERT) promoter mutations and receptor kinase amplification.

FIGURE 1.24. This image of a coronal section shows a large, heterogeneous, hemorrhagic, and necrotic frontal mass involving the 2 hemispheres with midline shift typical of glioblastoma.

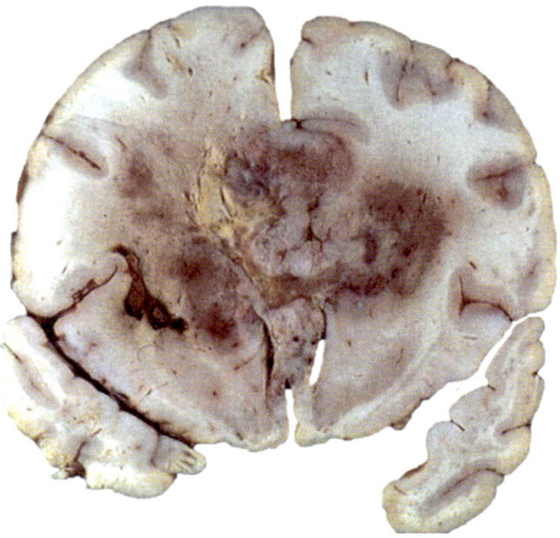

GLIOBLASTOMA (WHO GRADE IV)

Glioblastomas are typically mitotically active, pleomorphic, cellular tumors with microvascular proliferation and/or necrosis. They can develop de novo in older subjects (i.e., primary glioblastoma), or result from progression of a lower-grade glioma, as typically occurs in younger patients (i.e., secondary glioblastoma). Patients with glioblastoma have an estimated survival of less than 2 years. Some ameliorating factors include O^6-methylguanine-DNA methyltransferase methylation status (occurs in 40% to 50% of glioblastomas) and proneural gene expression.

FIGURE 1.25. Image (A) shows a brain glioblastoma at the left temporal lobe (arrow). Image (B) shows a close, lateral view of the same tumor; image (C) shows an inferior view (arrow).

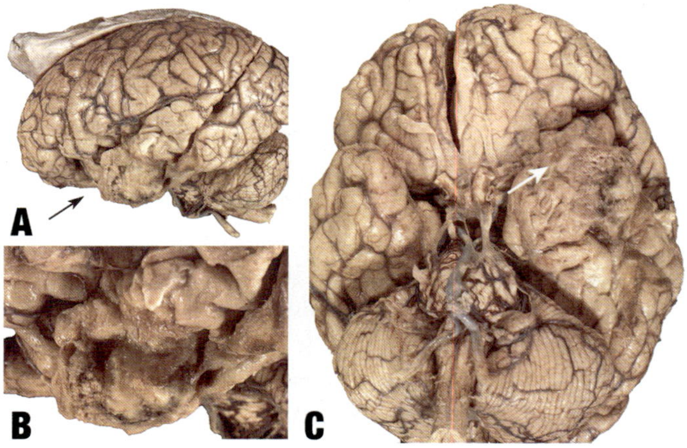

FIGURE 1.26. Image (A) shows a brain cross-section, with an infiltrative left frontal lobe glioblastoma. Image (B) shows an inferior view of a whole brain with a left frontal lobe glioblastoma.

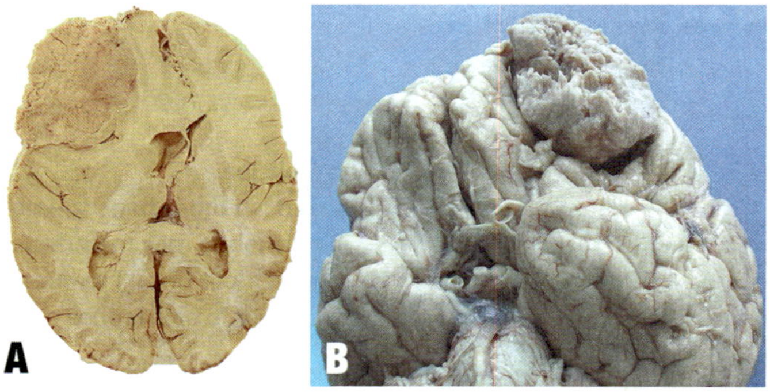

Specimen A from Maude Abbott Medical Museum, McGill University

Oligodendroglioma

Oligodendrogliomas are infiltrating gliomas with oligodendroglial morphological features. These tumors are genetically characterized by *IDH1* or *IDH2* mutations with concomitant 1p/19q codeletion. Grossly, they have a thickened cortex with well-defined borders. Histological features of oligodendrogliomas include oligodendroglial cell proliferation with perineuronal satellitosis, perivascular and subpial accumulations, and calcifications. Prognosis is variable and grade dependent.

FIGURE 1.27. Image (A) shows a right frontal lobe oligodendroglioma (arrow). Image (B) shows an enlarged view of this oligodendroglioma.

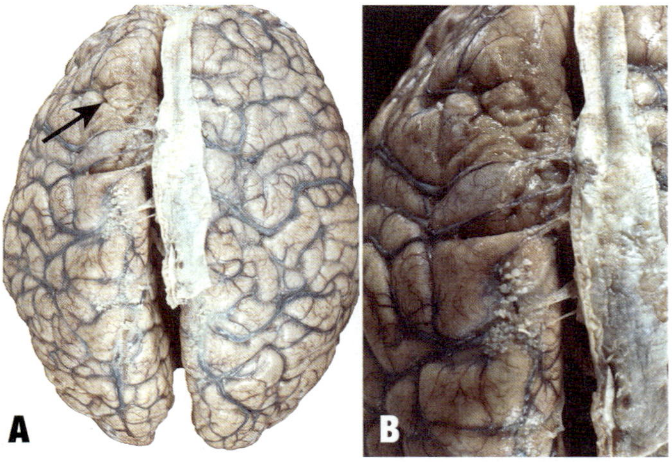

Diffuse large B-cell lymphoma (DLBCL)

Cerebral lymphomas can sometimes represent metastatic disease, most commonly in the pediatric population. Some CNS lymphomas are primary, occurring in the absence of lymphomas outside the nervous system. Primary CNS lymphomas make up to 3% of primary intracranial neoplasms; of these, 98% have a B-cell phenotype, with more than 95% being DLBCL.

FIGURE 1.28. This image shows a coronal brain section with a soft, friable, grayish-tan, gelatinous mass with central hemorrhage located in the white matter of the right frontal lobe.

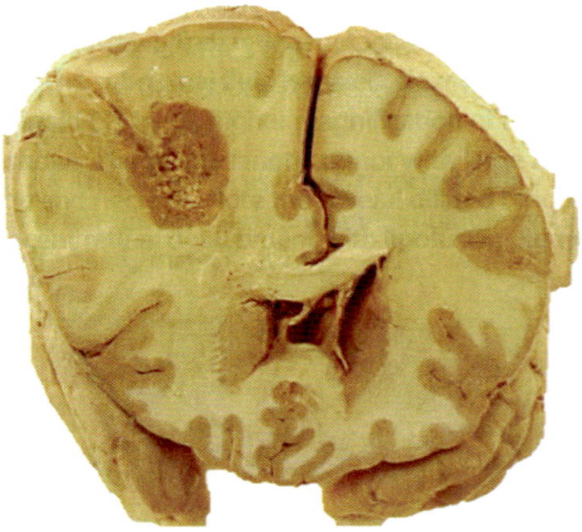

Specimen from Maude Abbott Medical Museum, McGill University

Epithelioid hemangioendothelioma

Most vascular lesions of the CNS are types of malformation. Primary CNS vascular tumors are rare. Epithelioid hemangioendothelioma is a rare, malignant vascular tumor that can arise in the skull base, dura, or brain parenchyma.

FIGURE 1.29. In this image, a superior view of the left cerebral hemisphere shows a large firm tumor (arrow) that is attached to the dura. It is significantly compressing the left occipital lobe and is on the parietal lobe.

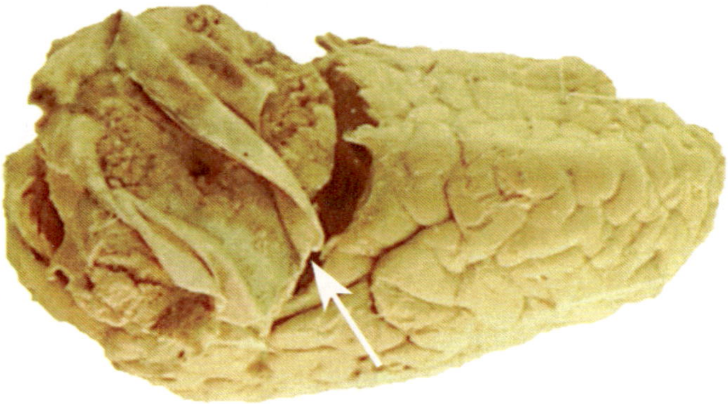

Specimen from Maude Abbott Medical Museum, McGill University

Meningioma

Meningiomas are meningothelial cell neoplasms. These are the most common primary intracranial tumors in adults, with peak occurrence in the sixth to seventh decades. Previous skull radiation and neurofibromatosis type 2 (NF2) are known risk factors, and chromosome 22 deletion is a consistent cytogenetic aberration in meningiomas. Other cytogenetic aberrations include chromosome 1p deletion and loss of chromosomes 6, 10, and 14. Meningiomas have a wide range of histologic appearances and are subdivided into 3 subgroups (WHO grades I, II, and III) based on their histologic features. Grade II tumors (atypical meningiomas) are associated with an increased likelihood of recurrence, and grade III tumors are associated with significant mortality.

FIGURE 1.30. Images (A) through (D) show examples of meningiomas.

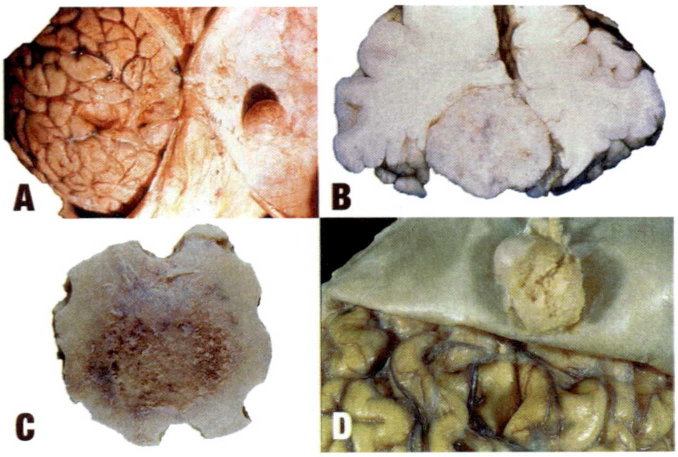

MENINGIOMA: MASS EFFECT

The mass effect of a lesion, such as a tumor, refers to the secondary pathological perturbations that are caused by the tumor as it grows and displaces the surrounding tissues.

FIGURE 1.31. This image shows a meningioma attached to the inferior surface of the dural membrane. The depression made by the mass effect of the growing lesion is visible on the left (arrow).

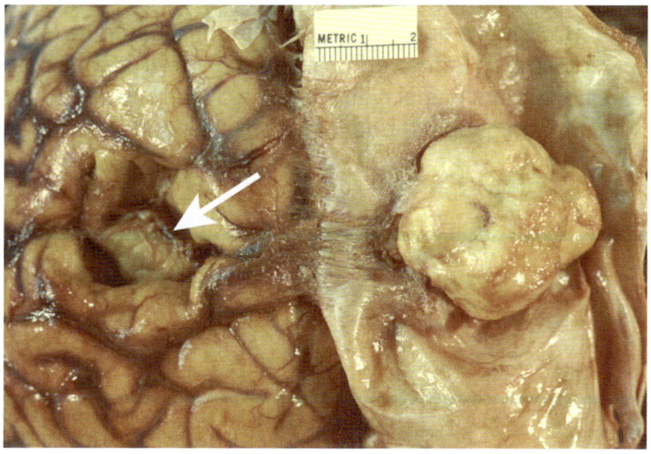

FIGURE 1.32. The meningiomas in (A) and (B), over the course of their gradual growth, compressed, and caused atrophy of, underlying brain substance. The brain in (B) has a depression in the upper end of the central fissure of Rolando on the right hemisphere that is filled with a firm fibroid tumor (arrow) that is growing from the dura. Surprisingly, the lesion in (B) was asymptomatic.

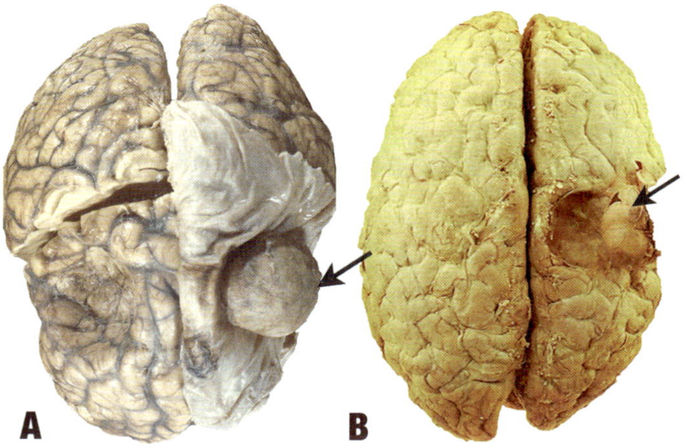

Specimen B from Maude Abbott Medical Museum, McGill University

Craniopharyngioma

Craniopharyngiomas are sellar cystic lesions that are derived from Rathke pouch epithelium and histologically correspond to WHO grade I tumors. These tumors account for 1.2% to 4.6% of all intracranial tumors. They can present with visual disturbances (around 80% of patients, especially in adults) or endocrine deficiencies (around 80% of patients, especially in children). Histologically, craniopharyngioma has 2 subtypes: adamantinomatous and papillary.

FIGURE 1.33. In (A), a craniopharyngioma compresses the optic chiasm in the sellar region (arrow). Image (B) shows a closer view of this craniopharyngioma.

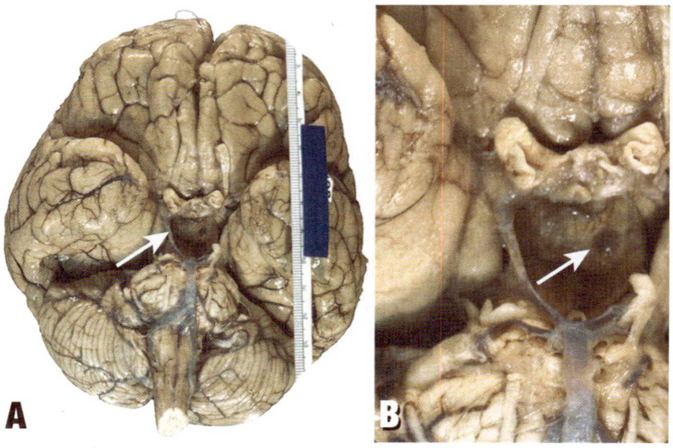

Metastasis to the Brain

Metastases are the most common CNS neoplasms. Of patients who die from cancer, 25% have brain metastasis at autopsy. The most frequent sources of brain metastases in adults, in decreasing order, are lung (mainly small cell and adenocarcinoma), breast, melanoma, renal cell carcinoma, and colon. Ten percent of brain metastases have no known primary malignancy at presentation.

Metastasis from lung cancer

FIGURE 1.34. This image shows metastatic intraventricular lung carcinoma filling the left ventricular cavity and abutting the periventricular tissues. Perilesional brain edema is also present.

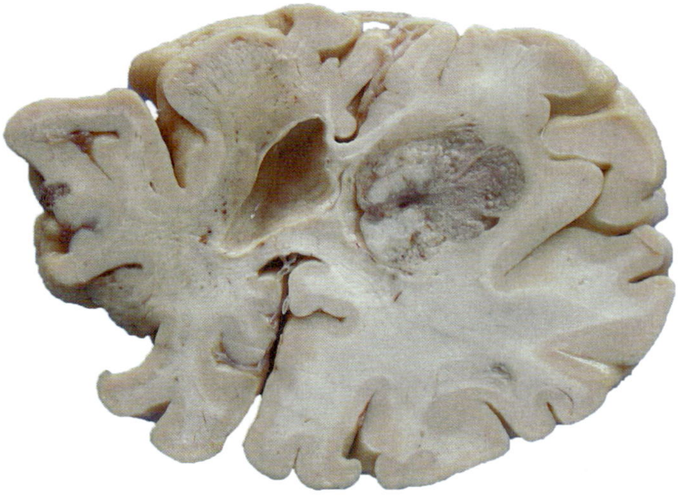

FIGURE 1.35. Image (A) shows a metastatic tumor from the lung in the right parietal lobe of the cerebrum. Image (B) shows a hemorrhagic metastatic lesion, also from the lung, in the cerebellum.

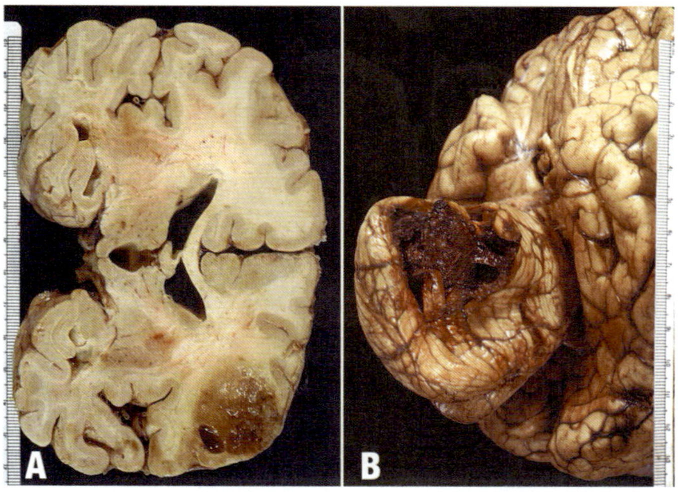

Metastasis from breast cancer

FIGURE 1.36. This image shows a cross-section of a large, well-circumscribed mass with a pushing border occupying the inferior aspect of the left frontal lobe. The brain tissue surrounding the mass appears edematous. The single lesion depicted here is a metastasis from a breast carcinoma.

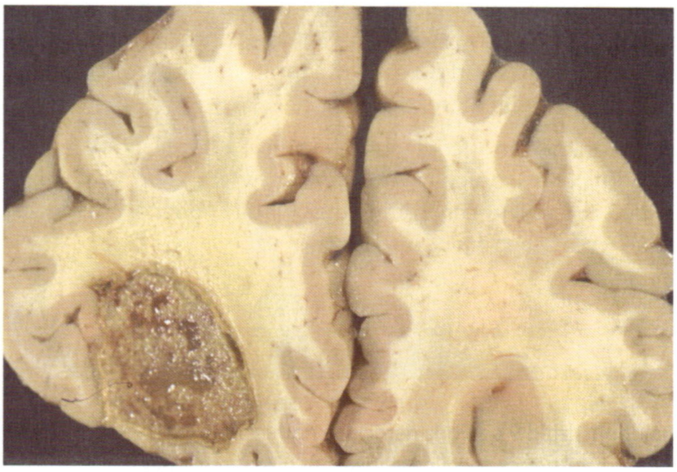

FIGURE 1.37. The brain cross-section in (A) shows a metastatic mass from a breast carcinoma. The tumor is within the optic chiasm, which is a somewhat rare location for a metastasis. Image (B) shows a close-up of the optic chiasm containing the metastasis.

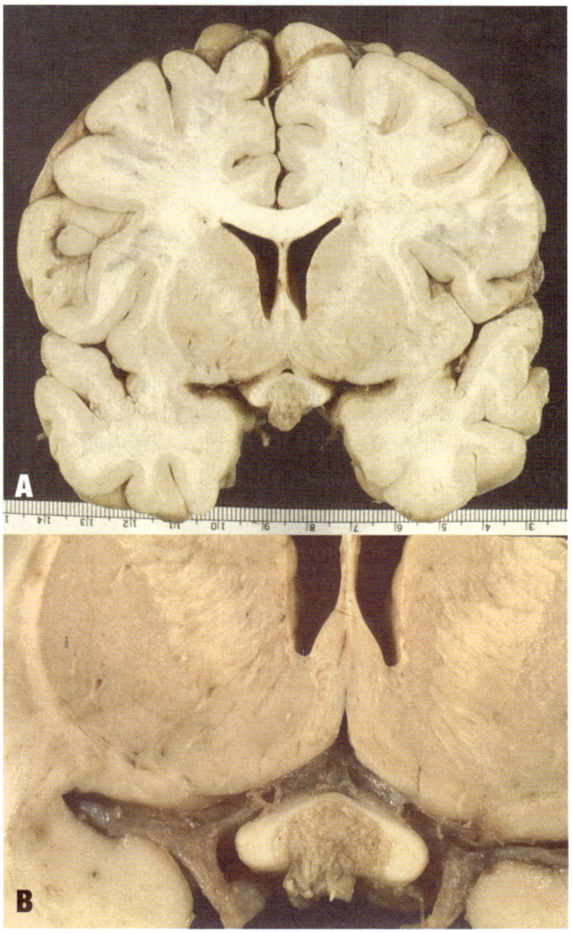

Brain Trauma

Contusion

COUP-CONTRECOUP CONTUSION

Coup-contrecoup contusions are a type of brain injury that occurs when a person falls and hits the back of their head. This typically results in extensive contusions to the inferior surfaces and poles of the temporal and frontal lobes opposite the site of impact.

FIGURE 1.38. An inferior view of a brain at autopsy shows a hemorrhagic contusion of the cerebellar surface (coup injury, white arrow), and a larger contusion in the opposite frontal and temporal lobes (contrecoup injury, black arrow).

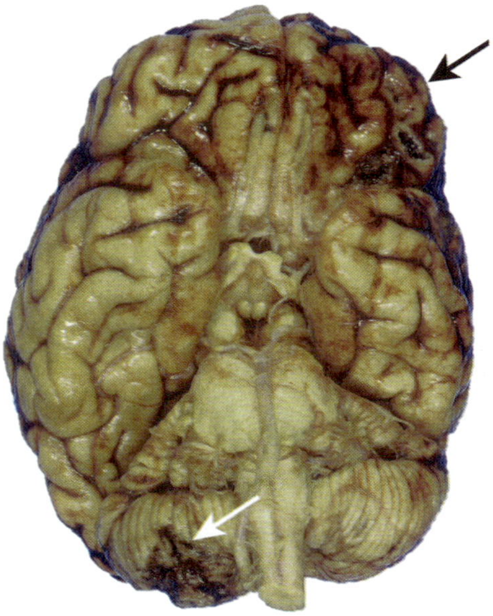

LATERAL COUP-CONTRECOUP CONTUSION

Contusions on the brain surface often appear as ragged, slightly discolored regions. Lateral coup-contrecoup contusions, as seen in this image, may also occur if the site of impact is the temporal or parietal regions of the head.

FIGURE 1.39. This image shows an inferior view of a brain at autopsy with a contrecoup lesion on the right temporal region (white arrow). The smaller coup lesion presents on the left temporal lobe (black arrow). Contrecoup lesions of the posterior brain (not shown here) due to injury of the frontal region of the head are very rare.

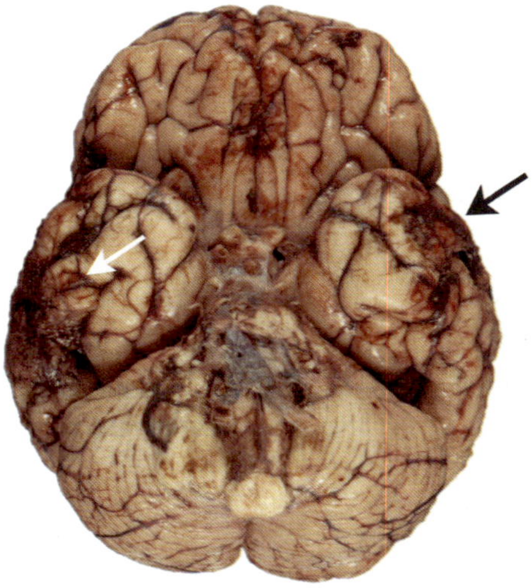

Uncal herniation

Uncal herniation is a type of brain herniation that occurs secondary to increased intracranial pressure. In uncal herniation, the uncus of the parahippocampal gyrus of the temporal lobe herniates through the tentorial notch. Clinically, this results in compression of the oculomotor nerve leading to loss of the pupillary reflex ("blown pupil"), or compression of the posterior cerebral artery leading to infarction of the occipital or temporal lobes.

FIGURE 1.40. This inferior view of a brain at autopsy shows the deeply grooved right uncus with hemorrhagic necrosis at the site of herniation (arrow).

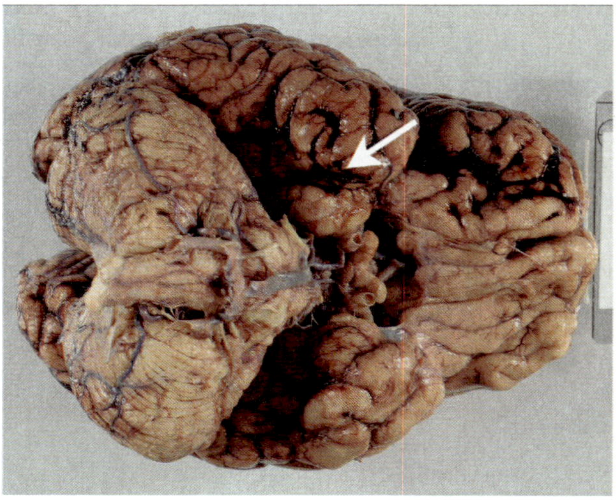

Vascular Diseases of the Brain

Infarction

In cerebral infarctions, gross alteration is not visible until 6 to 8 hours postinfarction. The earliest changes include swelling of the affected tissues, and loss of the demarcation between the gray and white matter. After 24 to 48 hours, the affected brain tissue becomes congested, dusky, and soft. Large, acute infarctions may be accompanied by herniation.

FIGURE 1.41. These images show coronal sections of different brain autopsies demonstrating: (A) recent intracerebral hemorrhage involving the right thalamus and extending to the cortex; (B) left frontal lobe infarction with herniation to the opposite side; and (C) recent right parietooccipital cerebral hemorrhagic infarction.

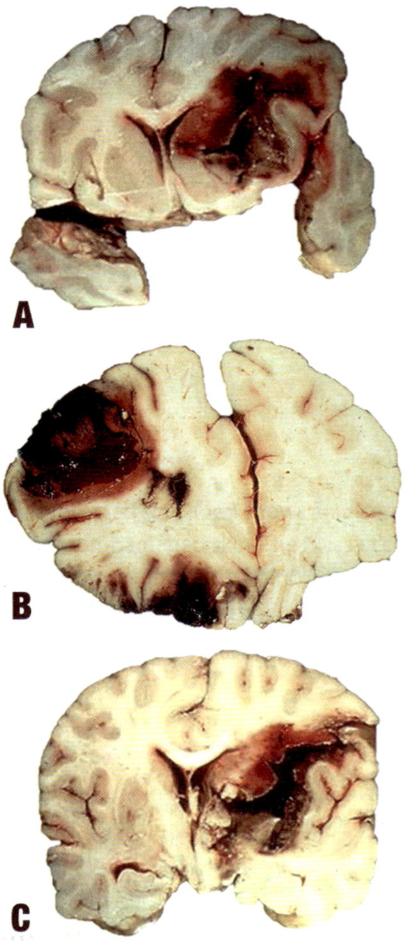

LACUNAR INFARCTION

Lacunar infarctions are classically associated with hypertension. They are typically located in the deep brain structures such as the basal ganglia (especially within the putamen), and are characterized by the formation of small cavities (< 10 mm in size) called lacunae, which form after liquefactive necrosis. Lacunar infarctions may also occur within the periventricular white matter and the cerebellum. In all cases, lacunar infarctions are caused by occlusion of the penetrating arteries that provide blood to these deep structures.

FIGURE 1.42. A coronal section of a fixed brain at the level of the basal ganglia shows a cerebral infarction as demonstrated by an area of necrosis (arrow).

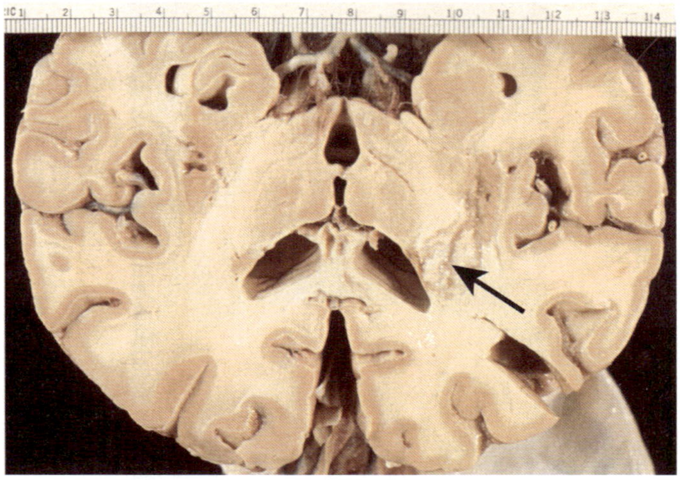

BASAL GANGLIA INFARCTION

Spontaneous (nontraumatic) intracerebral hemorrhage accounts for approximately 10% to 20% of all strokes, and 15% of deaths in chronic hypertensive patients. The peak age of presentation is 60 years and the risk is 5% to 20% higher in men than in women. The most frequently affected locations are the pontine perforators of the basilar artery and the lenticulostriate branches of the middle cerebral artery.

FIGURE 1.43. In (A), a cerebral cross-section shows a left putamen infarction (arrow) associated with parenchymal hemorrhage. In (B), a cerebral cross-section shows an infarction with liquefactive necrosis in the right putamen.

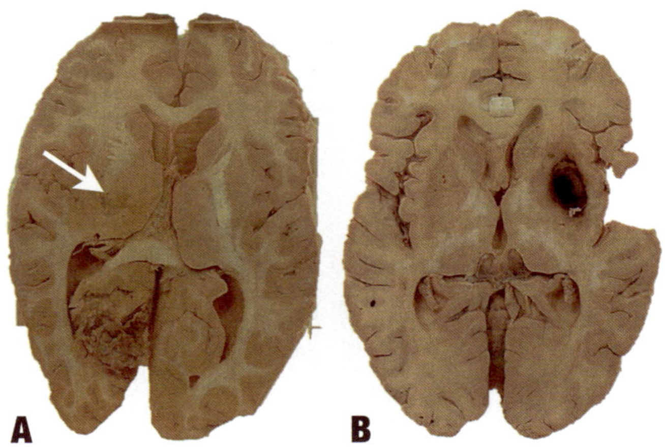

Both specimens from Maude Abbott Medical Museum, McGill University

CEREBRUM INFARCTION, MIDDLE CEREBRAL ARTERY (MCA) DISTRIBUTION

FIGURE 1.44. These coronal sections of the brain illustrate the wide distribution of the middle cerebral artery. In (A), a cross-section at the level of the mammillary bodies (arrowheads) shows a remote infarction with cavitation of the right putamen (arrow). In (B), a cross-section of the anterior brain shows the right frontal lobe with a more recent infarction. Liquefactive necrosis is also beginning to form (arrow), indicating that the infarction occurred several days prior to the patient's death.

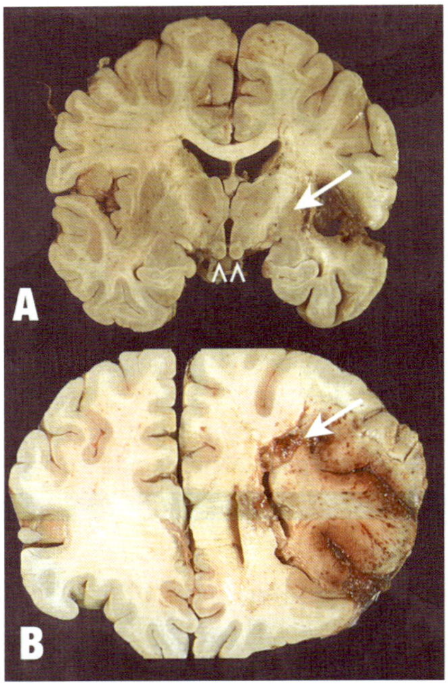

CEREBRUM INFARCTION

Brain infarctions undergo 3 overlapping stages of maturation: acute, intermediate, and cavitary. In the acute stage (the first 3 days postinfarction), hypoperfusion causes necrosis in the territory fed by the occluded blood vessel. The intermediate stage lasts between 3 days and 2 months. The cavitary stage begins with parenchymal loss and the formation of an empty space. The empty space typically contains some residual macrophages, glial strands, and newly formed capillaries.

FIGURE 1.45. Images (A) and (B) show inferior views of whole brains that have gone through the 3 stages infarction maturation, resulting in visible parenchymal loss (arrows).

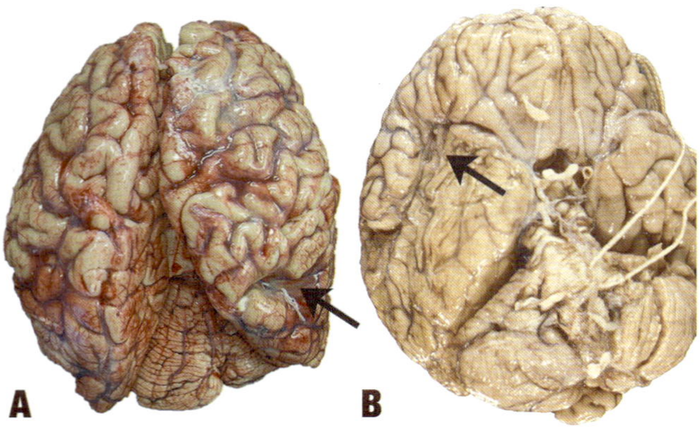

CEREBELLUM INFARCTION

Isolated cerebellar infarctions account for 3% of all ischemic strokes. Patients present with nonspecific symptoms such as dizziness, headache, nausea, and vomiting.

FIGURE 1.46. This macrograph shows a cross-section of a cerebellum. The cut surface of the right cerebellar hemisphere is irregular, heterogeneous, and necrotic, which is consistent with an infarction.

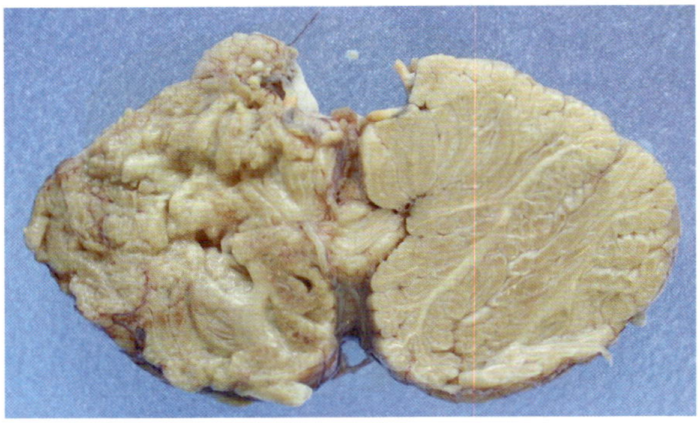

MIDDLE CEREBRAL ARTERY (MCA) REMOTE OCCLUSION AND LEFT PARIETAL LOBE INFARCTION

The MCA is the most common territory to be affected by cerebral infarction. The MCA territory is large and provides the easiest path for thromboemboli to follow, because it receives its flow directly from the internal carotid artery. Mortality after an acute ischemic MCA-territory infarction ranges between 5% and 45%.

FIGURE 1.47. This lateral view of a whole brain shows massive brain volume loss in the MCA territory. The inset image shows a coronal section of the same brain with impressive brain substance loss.

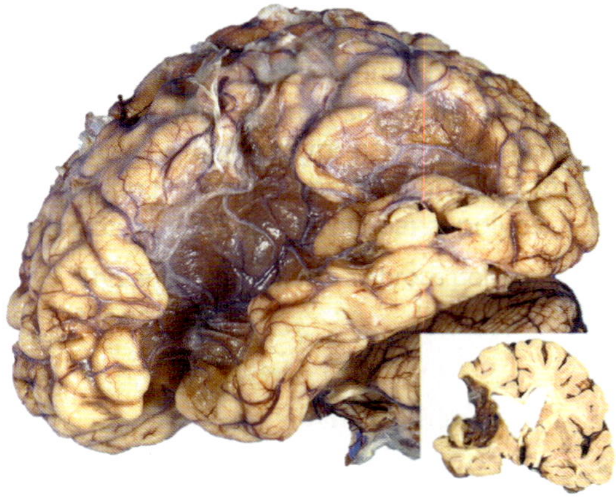

Intraventricular hemorrhage (IVH)

IVH is an unusual cause of natural, sudden death in adults. The most common sources of bleeding in spontaneous IVH include vascular abnormalities of the choroid plexus (e.g., choroidal artery aneurysm); abnormalities in the parenchyma of the periventricular brain (e.g., vascular malformations); and tumors either located within the ventricle itself or abutting the ventricle (e.g., choroid plexus papilloma/carcinoma, ependymoma, lymphoma).

FIGURE 1.48. This brain cross-section shows a left lateral intraventricular hemorrhage with extension into the left parietofrontal cortex.

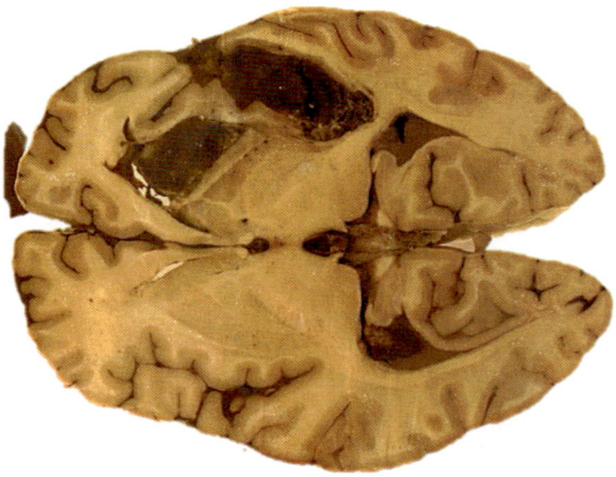

Specimen from Maude Abbott Medical Museum, McGill University

PROCEDURE: DIAGNOSIS AND GRADING OF IVH

IVH can be diagnosed by ultrasound. The grading system for IVH is divided into 4 categories based on the degree of hemorrhage present. In grade 1, blood is seen in the periventricular germinal matrix. In grade 2, blood is seen in nondilated lateral ventricles. In grade 3, the lateral ventricles are dilated due to hemorrhage. In grade 4, blood extends from the ventricular system into the parenchyma.

FIGURE 1.49. Images (A) and (B) illustrate different grades of IVH. Image (A) shows a coronal section of a neonatal brain with IVH in the lateral and third ventricles. In (B), 2 segments of a coronally sectioned neonatal brain show IVH in the lateral ventricles and extending into the inferior horn.

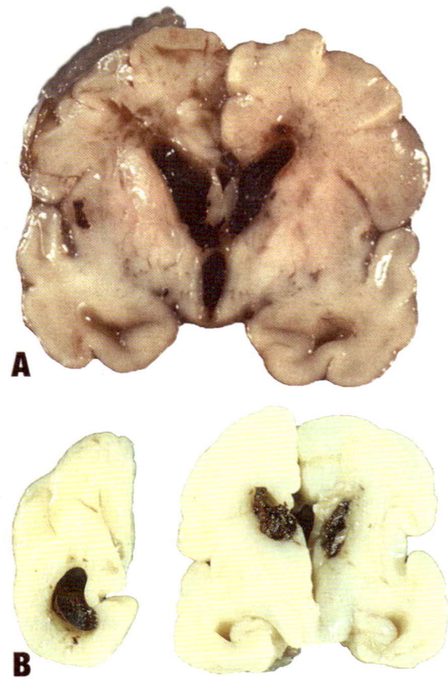

CEREBRUM AND CEREBELLUM IVH

IVH may expand and enter the subarachnoid space via the foramina of Magendie or Luschka. A basilar subarachnoid hemorrhage noted on gross examination should prompt consideration of primary IVH in the differential diagnosis.

FIGURE 1.50. Image (A) shows a cross-section of a brain with a large right intraventricular hemorrhage of the right parietal lobe that extends into the subarachnoid space. In (B), a cross-section of a cerebellum shows a massive intraventricular hemorrhage in the fourth ventricle.

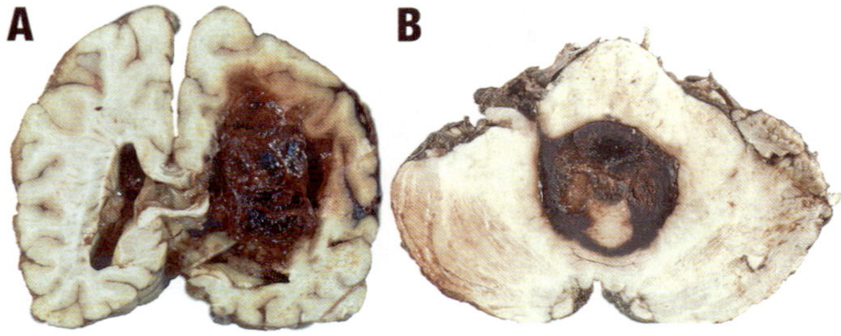

IVH AND VENTRICULOPERITONEAL (VP) SHUNT

IVH associated with the removal or revision of a ventriculoperitoneal (VP) shunt is a well-documented complication of shunt surgeries. The rate of VP shunt–associated IVH is 2% in adult populations and 2.4% in pediatric populations. Its etiology is believed to be disruption of the vascular choroid plexus that grows around and into the shunt.

FIGURE 1.51. Three coronal sections of different brain autopsies show IVH of variable sizes and locations associated with previous VP shunts.

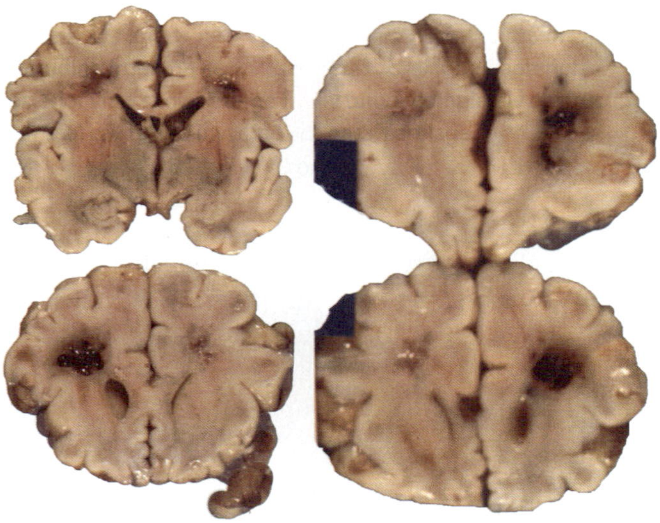

IVH IN INFANTS

In infants, 2 major risk factors for IVH are low birth weight and prematurity. IVH is common in very low birth weight (< 1500 g) and extremely low birth weight (< 1000 g) infants. The first 72 hours after birth is the most critical time in terms of development of IVH in susceptible neonates: 80% to 90% of cases occur within the first 3 days after birth. Long-term sequelae of IVH can include seizure disorders, cerebral palsy, and paralysis.

FIGURE 1.52. In (A), an inferior view of a whole neonatal brain (A) shows IVH in the central canal. Image (B) shows a cut section of a pediatric brainstem and cerebellum: IVH is present in the fourth ventricle.

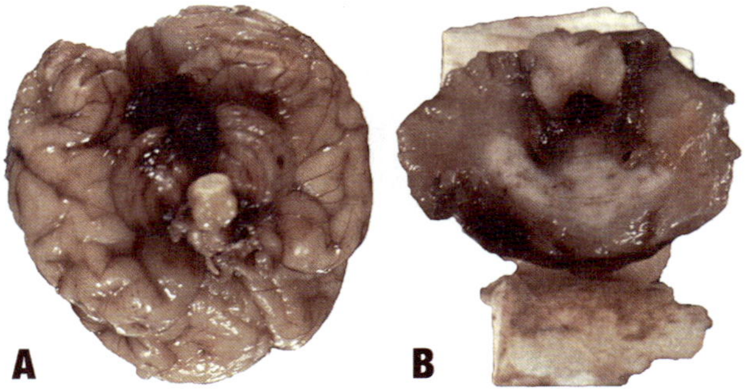

IVH IN PREMATURE BABIES

Premature babies are at risk for IVH because the cerebral autoregulation system, and the blood vessels within the periventricular germinal matrix, are not fully developed. Changes in cerebral pressures are easily transmitted to the delicate vasculature, which can result in the rupture of the veins within the periventricular germinal matrix and the subsequent development of subependymal hemorrhage (SEH). IVH develops as SEH expands into the adjacent ventricles.

FIGURE 1.53. The inferior view of the midbrain in (A) shows IVH in the aqueduct. The inferior view of the cerebellum in (B) shows IVH in the fourth ventricle.

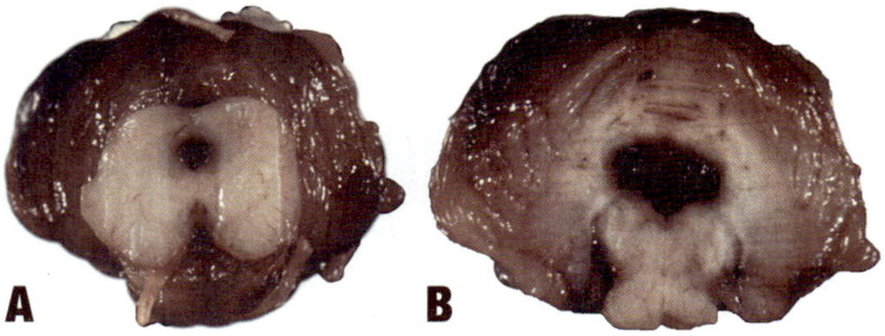

Encephalomalacia

Encephalomalacia is the end result of liquefactive necrosis of brain tissue after cerebral trauma, infection, ischemia, or infarction.

FIGURE 1.54. This image shows a left lateral view of a cerebrum from a 47-year-old woman with a large area of encephalomalacia in the left frontoparietal region. There are also smaller foci of encephalomalacia in the occipital region. The patient suffered for many years from mania and psychosis and, 6 years before her death, developed a right-sided hemiplegia.

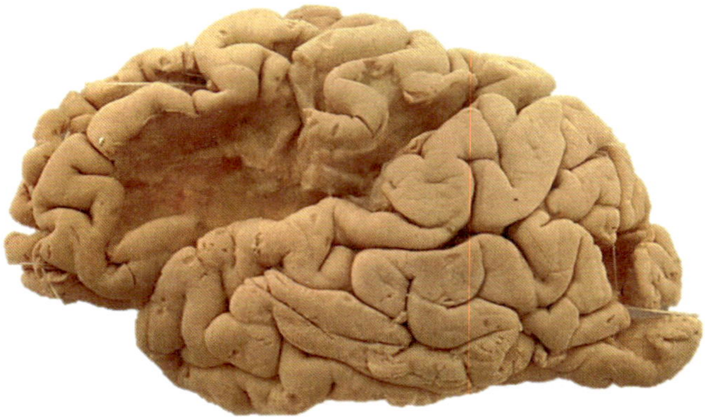

Specimen from Maude Abbott Medical Museum, McGill University

Aneurysm

CIRCLE OF WILLIS (CW) ANEURYSM

The CW is a system of connected arteries located at the base of the brain. It can demonstrate a number of anatomic variations. In a recent autopsy study of 100 brains, the posterior communicating artery was the most common site of anatomic variation. The observed variations included unilateral hypoplasia (27%), bilateral hypoplasia (19%), unilateral absence (14%), and bilateral absence (2%). Saccular aneurysms are the most frequent type of aneurysm occurring in the CW, and are commonly located between the anterior cerebral and anterior communicating arteries of the circle (40%), the M1 to M2 divisions of the middle cerebral artery (34%), the internal carotid / posterior communicating arteries (20%), the basilar artery / posterior cerebral arteries (4%), and other arterial branch points (2%).

FIGURE 1.55. This inferior-anterior view of a brain autopsy shows a ruptured left anterior communicating artery aneurysm (arrow) with congenital absence of the right posterior communicating artery (arrowhead).

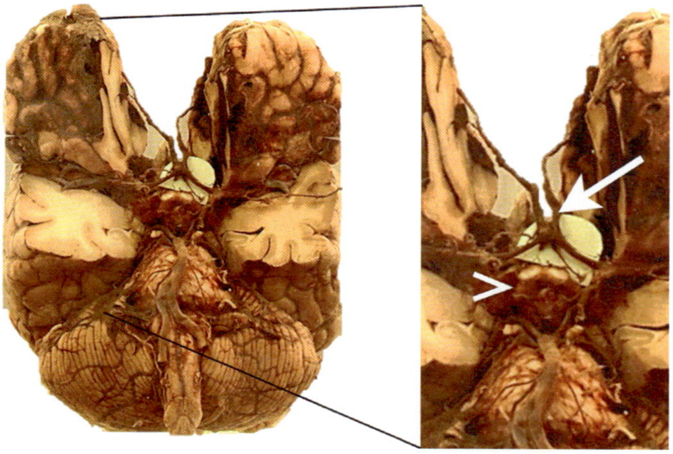

Images courtesy of Maude Abbott Medical Museum, McGill University

FIGURE 1.56. This image shows a coronal section of the cerebrum, viewed from the inferior surface, with the CW exhibiting a ruptured right anterior cerebral artery aneurysm (arrow).

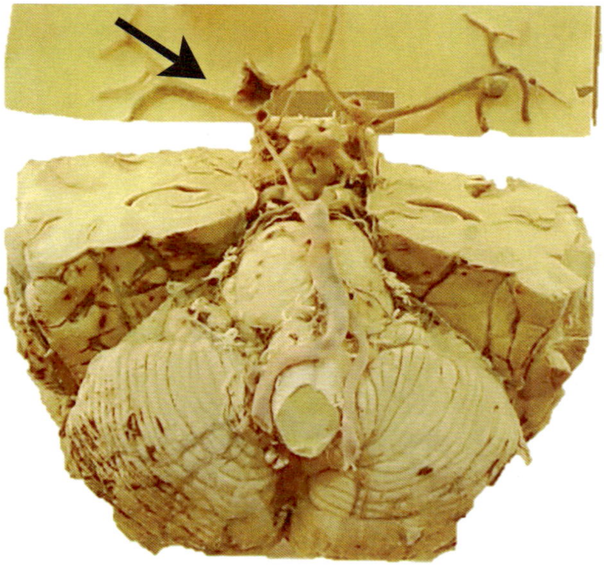

Specimen from Maude Abbott Medical Museum, McGill University

SACCULAR ANEURYSM

A saccular (berry) aneurysm consists of a sac-like, thin-walled structure that is attached to an arterial branch point by a narrow neck. The sac itself may be lobulated, oval, or spherical. The typical size of these aneurysms is 0.1 cm to 2.5 cm; saccular aneurysms measuring > 2.5 cm are "giant aneurysms." The site of rupture is typically located at the apex of the sac, and ruptured aneurysms may cut through the brain parenchyma and expand into the adjacent ventricle. Ruptured aneurysms account for 25% of all cerebrovascular deaths, and 25% of individuals with ruptured cerebral aneurysms die in the first 24 hours.

FIGURE 1.57. In (A), a saccular aneurysm of the right middle cerebral artery shows as a large mass arising from the lower part of the artery. The artery is filled with laminated clot (arrow). Image (B) shows a ruptured saccular aneurysm of the left internal carotid artery (arrow) with an associated subarachnoid hemorrhage tracking along the inferior surface of the brain.

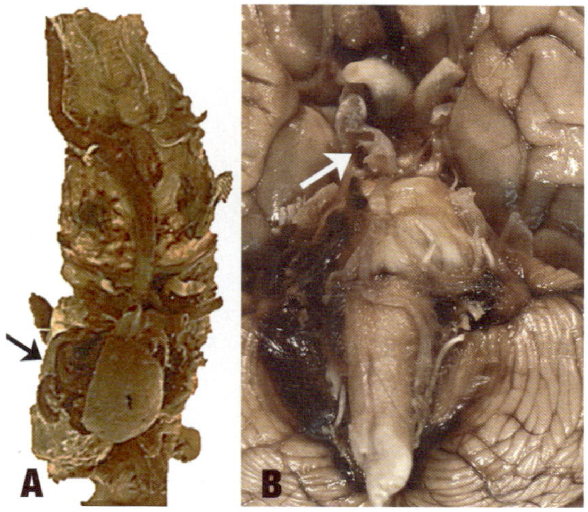

Specimen A from Maude Abbott Medical Museum, McGill University

MIDDLE CEREBRAL ARTERY ANEURYSM

FIGURE 1.58. This specimen shows an intact congenital saccular aneurysm at the bifurcation of the middle cerebral artery.

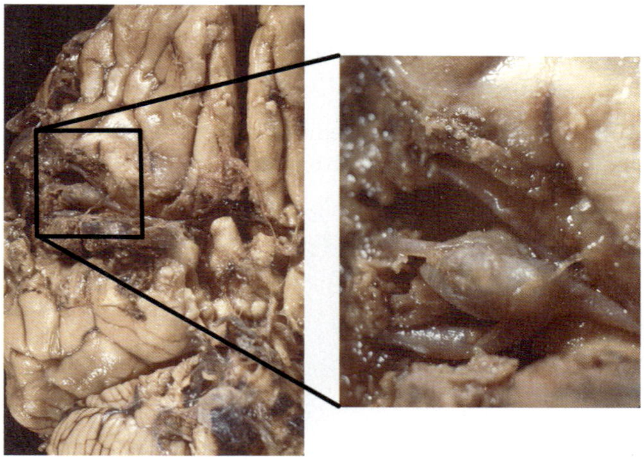

MYCOTIC ANEURYSM WITH CEREBRAL HEMORRHAGE

Mycotic aneurysms can form secondary to septic emboli from an infected mitral valve. They are rare complications of infective endocarditis (IE), seen in 2% to 3% of IE patients.

FIGURE 1.59. This coronal section of the brain from a 73-year-old man with a history of acute bacterial mitral valve endocarditis demonstrates multiple cerebral hemorrhages secondary to rupture of mycotic aneurysms. Two recent hemorrhagic areas in the left parietal and temporal lobes (arrows) and an older hemorrhage in the right temporal lobe (arrowhead) are visible.

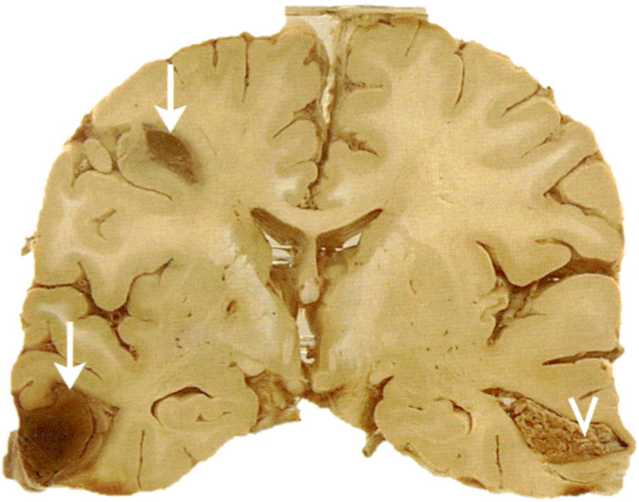

Specimen from Maude Abbott Medical Museum, McGill University

Arteriovenous malformation (AVM)

An AVM is a tangled mass of abnormal arterial and venous blood vessels without an intervening capillary bed. AVMs represent 1.5% to 4% of all brain masses. Most AVMs are supratentorial and are found within the distributions of the major cerebral vessels. AVMs are most commonly found in association with the middle cerebral artery, followed by the anterior cerebral artery and posterior cerebral artery. AVMs demonstrate no gender predilection. The peak incidence in adults is between 20 and 40 years of age. The mean age at diagnosis is 30 years.

FIGURE 1.60. This image shows a surgically removed irregular, congested vascular lesion of variable diameter.

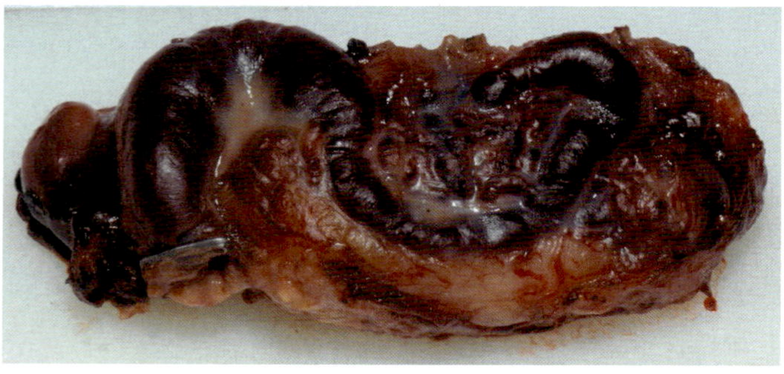

Thrombosis

INTERNAL CAROTID ARTERY EMBOLUS OR THROMBOSIS

Internal carotid artery occlusion accounts for 6.8% of patients with stroke or transient ischemic attack (TIA) involving the anterior circulation. Patients with occlusion at this location have comparatively worse clinical outcomes, with greater rates of recurrent in-hospital stroke and death, compared to patients without internal carotid artery occlusion.

FIGURE 1.61. This close-up from an inferior view of a brain focuses on the internal carotid arteries, where an embolus in the right internal carotid artery almost completely blocks the lumen (white arrow).

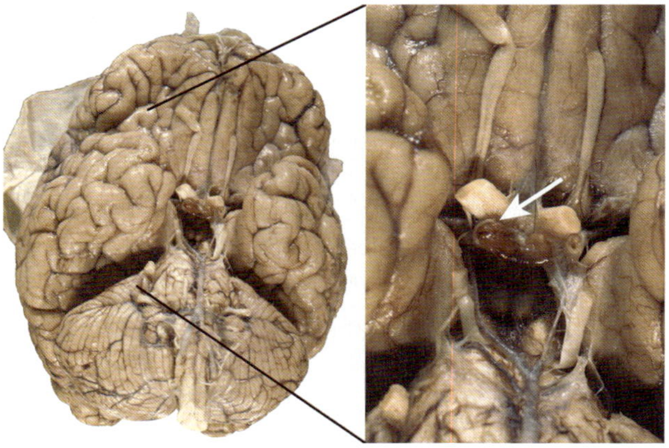

VENOUS THROMBOSIS

Cerebral venous sinus thrombosis (CVST) most commonly involves the superior sagittal sinus. Risk factors for CVST include infection, head trauma, thrombophilia, and dehydration. In the pediatric population, neonates are disproportionally affected, and in adults, young women are disproportionally affected.

FIGURE 1.62. A superior view of this cerebral hemisphere shows marked prominence of the meningeal vessels, which are filled with thrombus.

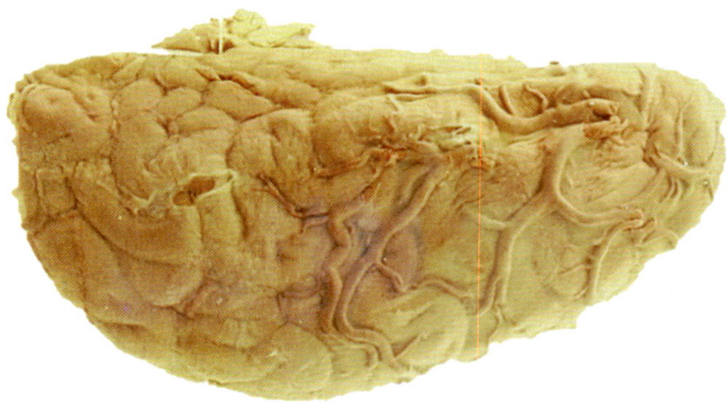

Specimen from Maude Abbott Medical Museum, McGill University

Brainstem and Cerebellum Diseases

Brainstem astrocytoma

Astrocytomas arise from astrocytes, a subtype of supporting glial cell. Histologically, astrocytomas range from WHO grade I to IV. They demonstrate increased cellularity, mitosis, necrosis, and vascular proliferation as they progress in grade. Prognosis depends on grade and location. The majority of brainstem gliomas are associated with mutations in Histone H3.

FIGURE 1.63. This image shows an ill-defined fleshy lesion with partial engulfment of the basilar artery (arrow) at the pons. Histologically, this tumor was diagnosed as an anaplastic astrocytoma, WHO grade III.

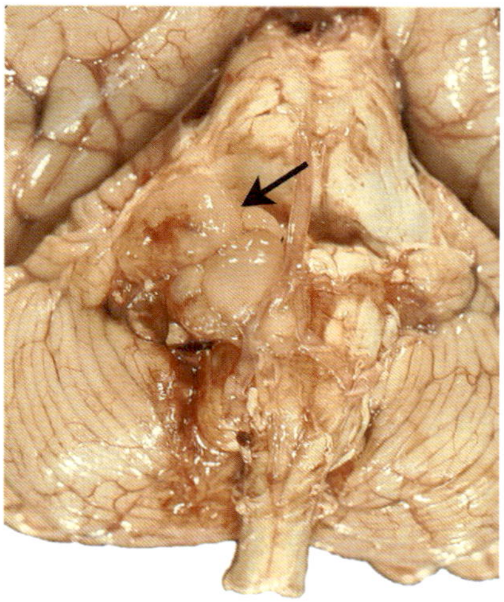

Medulloblastoma (WHO grade IV)

This tumor consists of small anaplastic embryonal cells of the cerebellum. Microscopically, these have 3 variants: classic (70%), desmoplastic or nodular (20%), and large or anaplastic (10%). Patients present with hydrocephalus-related symptoms or cerebellar dysfunction. Characteristically, these lesions disseminate through CSF.

FIGURE 1.65. This superior view of the cerebellum shows a well-demarcated, large lesion arising from the roof of the pons with a dilated fourth ventricle secondary to CFS outflow obstruction.

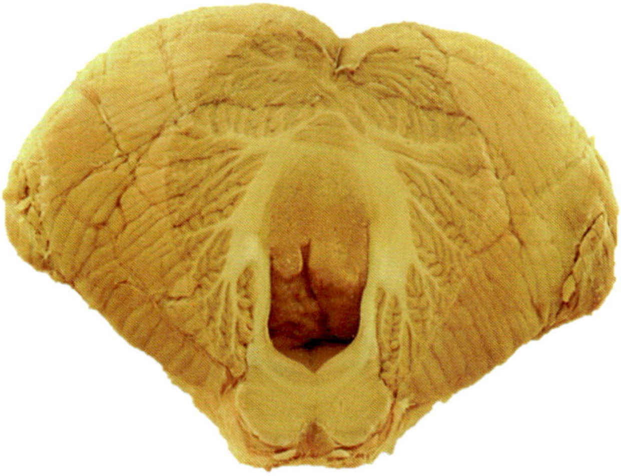

Specimen from Maude Abbott Medical Museum, McGill University

Brainstem Duret hemorrhage

A Duret hemorrhage is a secondary hemorrhage resulting from increased intracranial pressure and rapid transtentorial herniation of the medial temporal lobe. It occurs at the midline in the pons or midbrain. The basilar artery is anchored at the clivus and the rapid herniation results in secondary disruption of the perforator branches. Other causes of Duret hemorrhage include venous thrombosis and reperfusion injury after surgical intervention. A Duret hemorrhage is a sign of irreversible brain damage.

FIGURE 1.64. Images (A) and (B) show midbrain cross-sections demonstrating Duret hemorrhages.

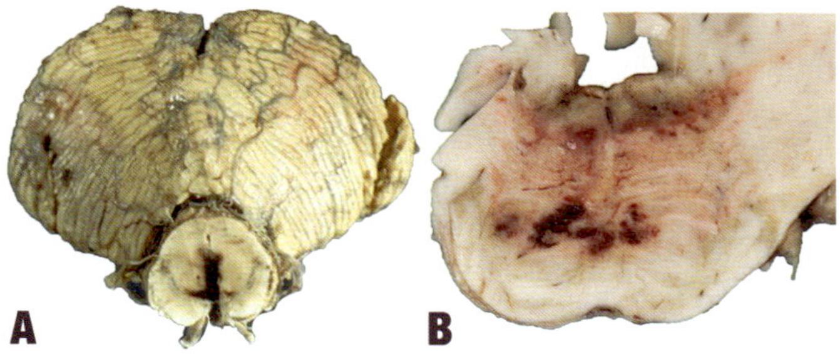

Cerebellum metastasis

The cerebellum is affected in 15% of brain metastases and the posterior fossa is a relatively common site of involvement in patients with renal cell carcinomas and colorectal carcinomas.

FIGURE 1.66. This cerebellar cross-section shows multiple metastatic mucinous adenocarcinomas (arrows) affecting the left cerebellar hemisphere.

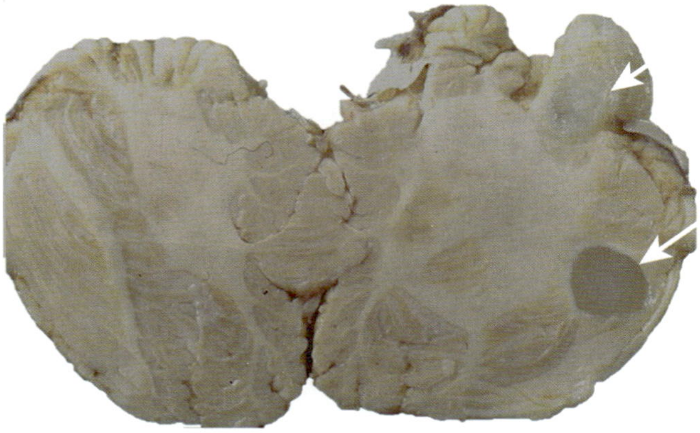

Pituitary Gland

Pituitary adenoma of the sellar region

Pituitary adenomas are neoplasms that arise from secretory cells in the adenohypophysis. Adenomas can be classified based on their size as microadenomas (< 10 mm) and macroadenomas (≥ 10 mm). Macroadenomas can cause mass effects that manifest clinically as headaches, visual disturbances, and cranial nerve palsies. Pituitary adenomas can be of 2 types: functional or nonfunctional. Clinical manifestations vary depending on the hormone that is secreted. Secreted hormones can include growth hormone, prolactin, corticotropin, thyrotropin, follicle-stimulating hormone, and luteinizing hormone.

FIGURE 1.67. This image shows a very large bulky mass within the sellar region (arrow). The cut surface of the mass has a smooth, homogeneous surface. The growing tumor caused a marked enlargement of sella turcica and compression of the brain's surrounding structures.

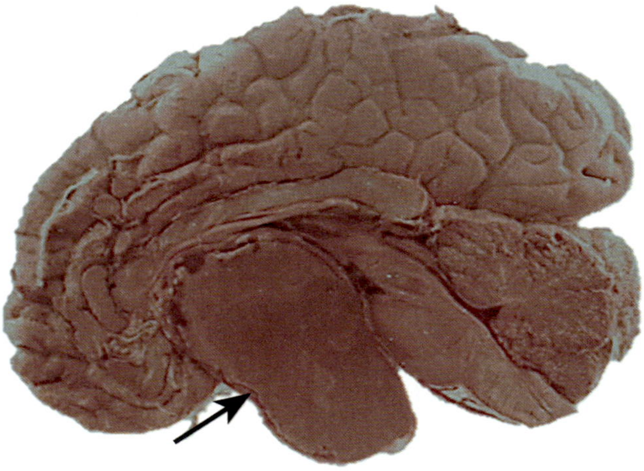

Specimen from Maude Abbott Medical Museum, McGill University

FIGURE 1.68. This gross image shows a well-circumscribed tumor located in the pituitary fossa (arrow). The cranial vault is markedly thickened. This could be a feature of acromegaly, which typically occurs with growth hormone–secreting pituitary adenomas in adults. Growth hormone–secreting adenomas are the second most common type of functional adenoma.

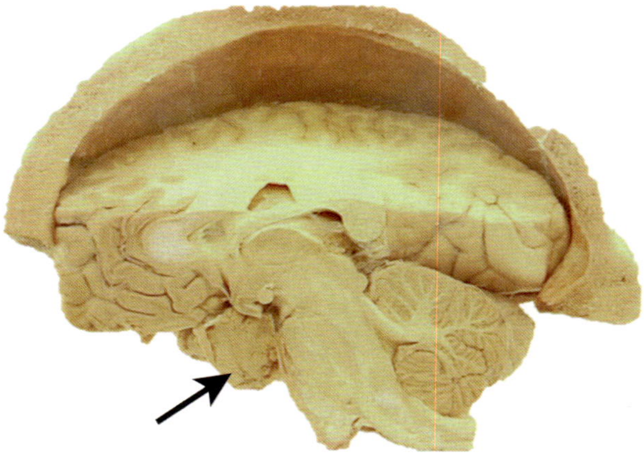

Specimen from Maude Abbott Medical Museum, McGill University

Pituitary carcinoma of the sellar region

Diagnosis of pituitary carcinoma requires at least 1 of the following: extracranial metastasis, gross brain invasion, and/or discontinuous nodule spreading within the cerebral–spinal space.

FIGURE 1.69. This sagittal brain section shows a well-circumscribed tumor filling the entire pituitary fossa and extending into the suprasellar region. Additional tumor nodules are present in the right temporal and posterior fossa (arrow).

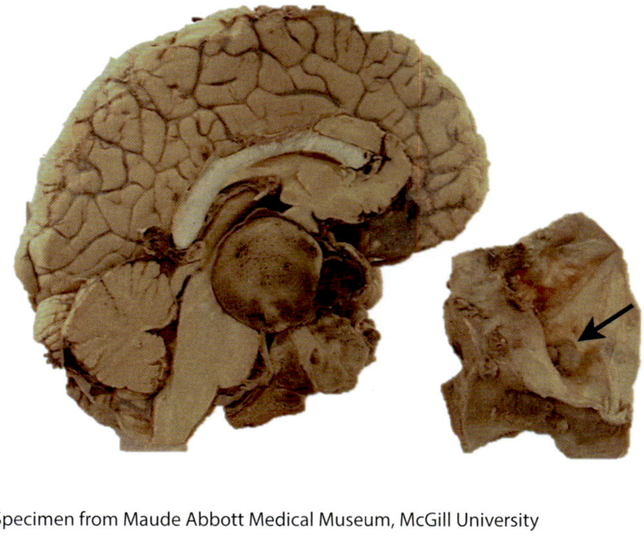

Specimen from Maude Abbott Medical Museum, McGill University

Spinal Cord

Spina bifida (spinal dysraphism)

Spina bifida is a spinal-column bone defect and neural tube defect (NTD). NTDs are considered the most common malformation of the CNS. Spina bifida occurs when a segment of the neural tube either fails to close or reopens after having closed. It can be asymptomatic (occulta) or associated with other malformations of varying severity.

FIGURE 1.70. Image (A) shows a posterior view of a fetus with open spina bifida in the lumbosacral region. Image (B) gives a closer view of this lesion.

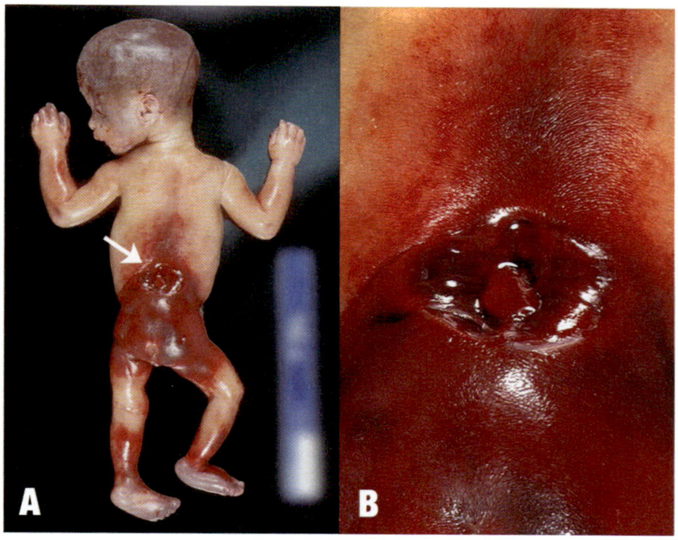

Dural calcification

Diffuse dural calcification, a common asymptomatic autopsy finding, can be an age-related condition, but may also arise from a number of diseases including hyperthyroidism and renal failure. It is different from the focal dural calcification associated with meningioma or post–subdural hemorrhage.

FIGURE 1.71. This image shows 2 dorsally opened spinal cords. The inner surface of the leptomeninges shows multiple, variably sized, white-to-brown calcified plaques (arrows).

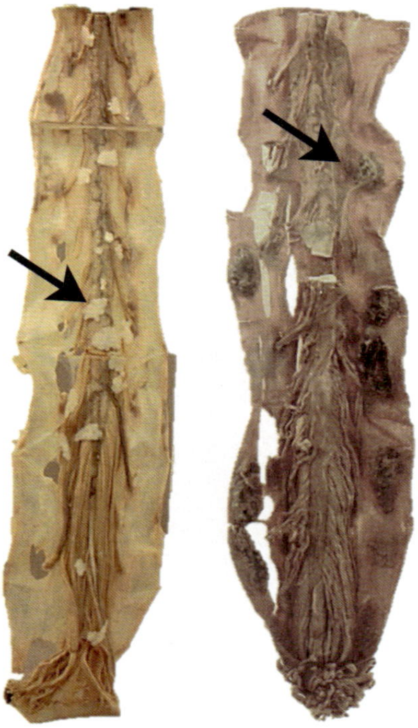

Specimens from Maude Abbott Medical Museum, McGill University

Nerves

Schwannoma

Schwannomas are benign nerve sheath tumors composed entirely of well-differentiated Schwann cells. The majority of schwannomas occur outside the CNS. Multiple schwannomas occur in patients with NF2. Schwannomas account for 8% of intracranial tumors. Most occur at the cerebellopontine angle (85%). Conventional, nonmelanocytic schwannomas are categorized as WHO grade I tumors. Ninety percent of schwannomas are sporadic; 4% are associated with NF2 inactivation. Most schwannomas present with symptoms related to nerve or adjacent structure compression.

PERIPHERAL NERVE SCHWANNOMA

Peripheral nerve schwannomas are usually gray, encapsulated, and well-circumscribed masses.

FIGURE 1.72. Images (A) through (C) show peripheral nerve schwannomas. The cystic degenerative changes (arrow) in (C) are not uncommon.

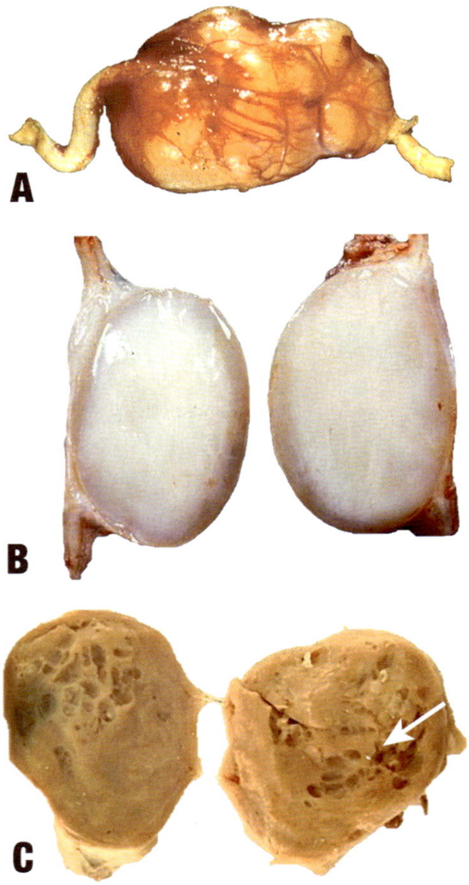

INTRACRANIAL SCHWANNOMA

Intracranial schwannomas have a strong predilection for the eighth cranial nerve at the cerebropontine angle, specifically the vestibular division.

FIGURE 1.73. A brain stem at the level of the cerebellar peduncles exhibits an intracranial schwannoma (arrow) of the eighth cranial nerve at the cerebropontine angle. Note that bilateral vestibular schwannomas are pathognomonic for NF2 mutation.

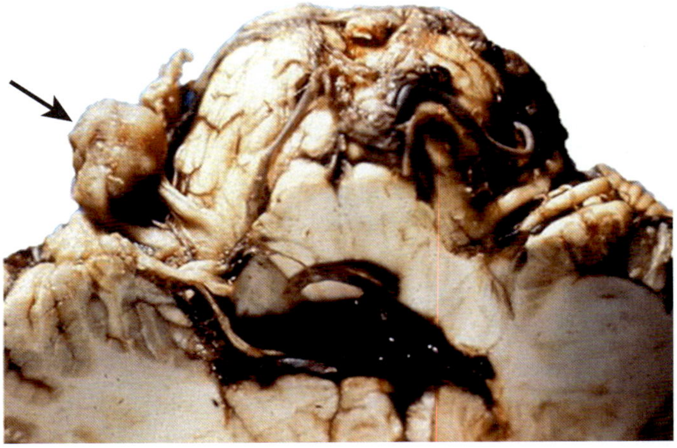

VESTIBULAR SCHWANNOMA

FIGURE 1.74. This inferior view of a whole brain shows a large hemorrhagic tumor (arrow) in the left cerebellopontine angle, compressing the pons and cerebellum. The tumor is intimately connected with the V, VI and VIII nerves.

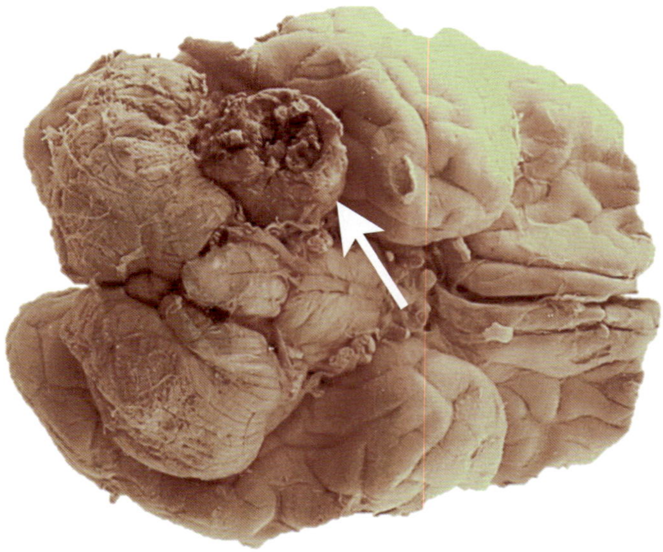

Specimen from Maude Abbott Medical Museum, McGill University

Neurofibroma

Neurofibromas are benign nerve sheath tumors composed of neoplastic Schwann cells, perineural-like cells, fibroblasts, CD34-positive spindle cells, and mast cells. They can be sporadic or associated with neurofibromatosis type 1 (NF1). They can have 1 of 3 growth patterns: nodular, diffuse, or plexiform.

FIGURE 1.75. Superficial neurofibromas, as shown in (A), are unencapsulated nodular lesions. Diffuse neurofibromas, seen in (B), usually involve the cutaneous and subcutaneous tissues. On cut surface, both types of neurofibromas are firm, glistening, and tan-gray lesions.

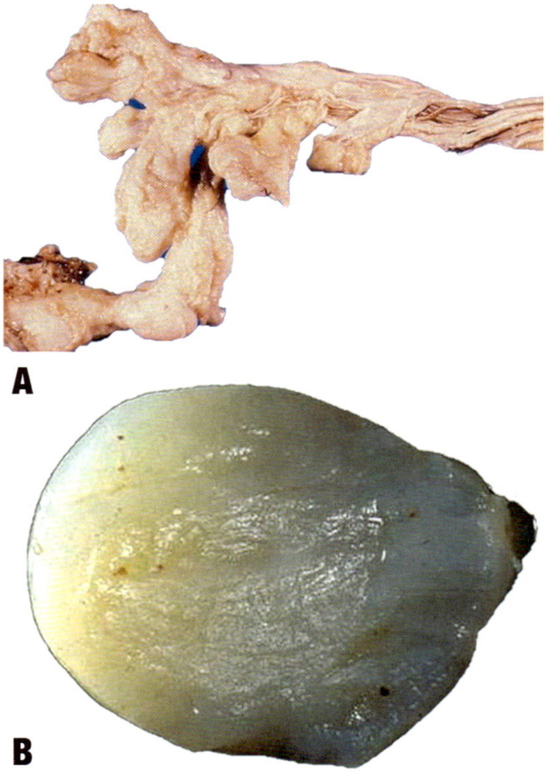

Malignant nerve sheath tumor (MPNST)

MPNSTs are rare malignant tumors with peripheral nerve sheath differentiation. Fifty percent of MPNSTs are associated with NF1. Intracranial MPNSTs are very rare and commonly arise from the vestibular and vagal cranial nerves.

FIGURE 1.76. Image (A) shows an inferior view of a brain with a trigeminal MPNST as a large irregular nodule (arrow) attached to the right vertebral artery. Image (B) shows the liver of the same patient, which revealed a white, well-demarcated nodule consistent with MPNST metastasis.

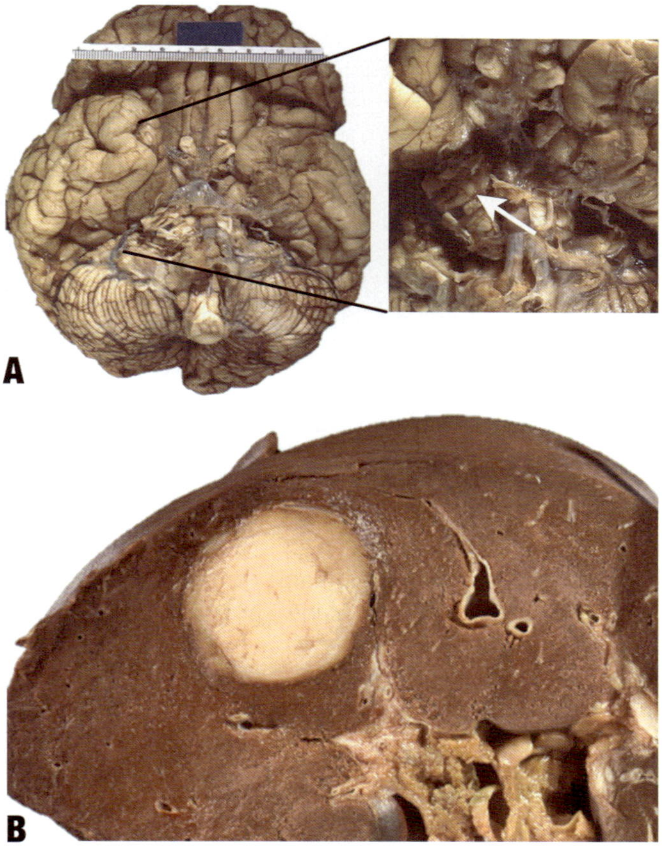

FIGURE 1.77. This example of an MPNST shows the intimate association with the parent nerve, with the tumor splaying the nerve. This tumor, arising in a patient with NF1, shows evidence on the cut section of spontaneous necrosis.

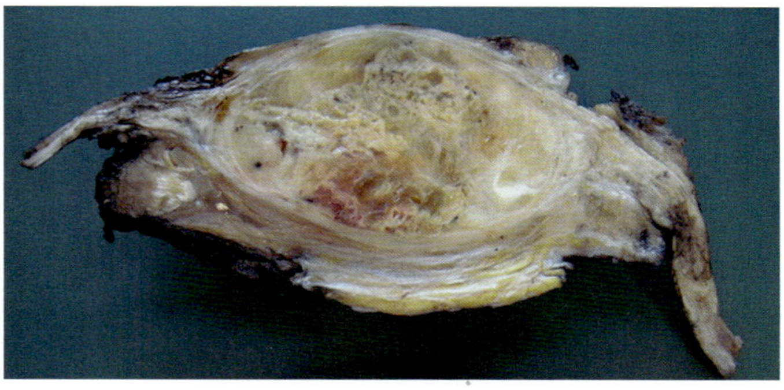

Neural fibrolipoma

Neural fibrolipoma (also called fibrolipomatosis of nerve, fibrolipomatous hamartoma of nerve, lipofibroma of nerve, lipomatosis of nerve, neural lipofibromatous hamartoma, and neurolipomatosis) is typically associated with macrodactyly.

FIGURE 1.78. The normal nerve is visible on the right-hand side of the lesion.

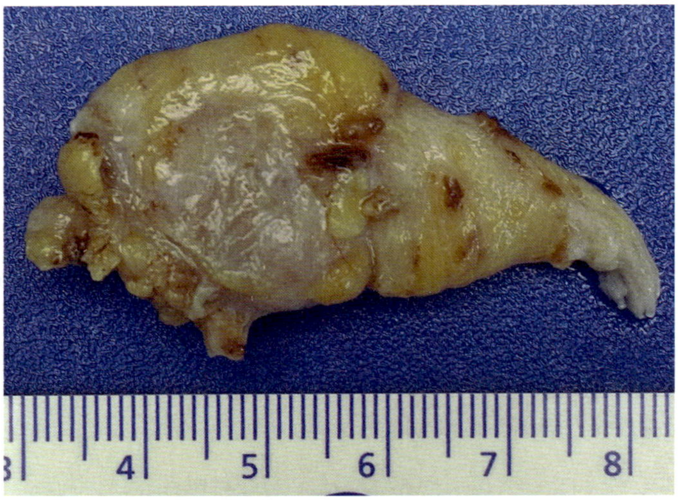

ACKNOWLEDGMENTS

We would like to thank the valuable contributions of Dr. John Richardson and Dr. Marie-Christine Guiot.

REFERENCES

Burke MJ, Vergouwen MD, Fang J, et al, and on behalf of the Investigators of the Registry of the Canadian Stroke Network. Short-term outcomes after symptomatic internal carotid artery occlusion. Stroke. 2011;42(9):2419–2424. https://doi.org/10.1161/STROKEAHA.111.615278. Medline:21757665

Calayag M, Paul AR, Adamo MA. Intraventricular hemorrhage after ventriculoperitoneal shunt revision: a retrospective review. J Neurosurg Pediatr. 2015 Jul;16(1):42–45. https://doi.org/10.3171/2014.11.PEDS14246. Medline:25860981

Ellison D, Love S, Chimelli L, et al. *Neuropathology: a reference text of CNS pathology*. 3rd Ed. New York, NY: Mosby-Elsevier; 2012.

Klimek-Piotrowska W, Rybicka M, Wojnarska A, Wójtowicz A, Koziej M, Hołda MK. A multitude of variations in the configuration of the circle of Willis: an autopsy study. Anat Sci Int. 2016 Sep;91(4):325–333. https://doi.org/10.1007/s12565-015-0301-2. Medline:26439730

Krebs C. *Neuroanatomy of the brain: web atlas [Internet]*. Vancouver (Canada) University of British Columbia, Med Ed Media; c2006–2018 [cited 2017 Jan 3]. Available from: http://www.neuroanatomy.ca/index.html.

Kurul S, Cakmakçi H, Dirik E. Agyria-pachygyria complex: MR findings and correlation with clinical features. Pediatr Neurol. 2004;30(1):16–23. https://doi.org/10.1016/S0887-8994(03)00312-6. Medline:14738944

Louis DN, Ohgaki H, Wiestler OD, et al. *WHO classification of tumors of the central nervous system*. Revised 4th Edition. Lyon Cedex, France: International Agency for Research on Cancer; 2016.

Prayson RA. *Neuropathology*. 2nd ed. Philadelphia, PA: Elsevier/Saunders; 2012.

Sangha N, Albright KC, Peng H, et al. Misdiagnosis of cerebellar infarctions. Can J Neurol Sci. 2014;41(5):568–571. https://doi.org/10.1017/cjn.2014.4. Medline:25373805

Treadwell SD, Thanvi B. Malignant middle cerebral artery (MCA) infarction: pathophysiology, diagnosis and management. Postgrad Med J. 2010;86(1014):235–242. Medline:20354047

Troncoso JC, Rubio A, Fowler DR. *Essential forensic neuropathology*. Philadelphia, PA: Wolters Kluwer Health/Lippincott Williams & Wilkins; 2010.

Wijdicks CA, Williams JM. Spinal arachnoid calcifications. Clin Anat. 2007;20(5):521–523. https://doi.org/10.1002/ca.20455. Medline:17149734

2

Eye Diseases

SABRINA BERGERON, PABLO ZOROQUIAIN, EVANGELINA ESPOSITO, SONIA CORREDOR CASAS, PATRICK LOGAN, ALEXANDRE ODASHIRO, MIGUEL N. BURNIER JR.

Eye

PROCEDURE: MACROSCOPIC EVALUATION OF OCULAR STRUCTURES

Enucleation

Enucleation consists of the removal of the ocular globe and a section of the optic nerve, conjunctiva, and muscle insertion points. Several landmarks — such as the cornea, the muscle insertion points, the ciliary artery, and vortex veins — can help orient the specimen correctly.

FIGURE 2.1. All images show the right eye. In (A), an anterior view shows the cornea — which is ovoid in shape with a longer horizontal length (dotted lines) — and the insertion points of the 4 rectus muscles (arrowheads). Note in (B) that the distance between the insertion of the rectus muscle and the limbus increases in a clockwise fashion (nasal, inferior, temporal, superior). The posterior aspect of the globe in (C) shows the ciliary arteries marking the horizontal plane and the thick muscular insertion of the inferior oblique muscle (arrowhead), indicating the inferotemporal quadrant.

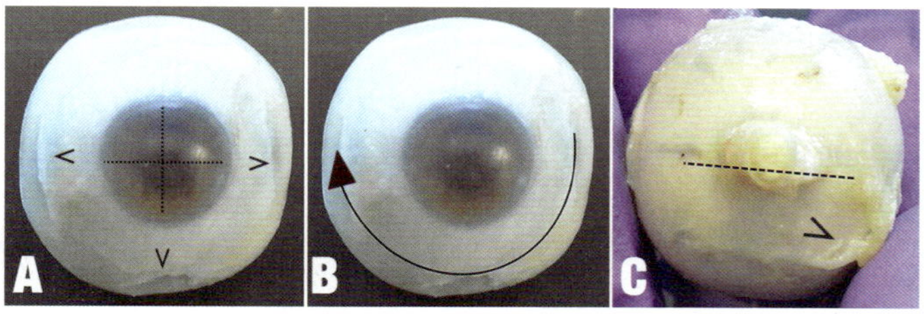

ENUCLEATION SPECIMEN: CROSS-SECTION

The eye is an organ with 3 layers (from the outermost to the innermost): fibrous layer (sclera and cornea), uveal tract (iris, ciliary body, and choroid), and retina. The lens divides the eye into the aqueous chamber (filled with aqueous humor) and vitreous chamber (filled with vitreous humor). The iris divides the aqueous chamber into anterior and posterior chambers.

FIGURE 2.2. This image illustrates the aqueous chamber (1), posterior chamber (2), and vitreous chamber (3).

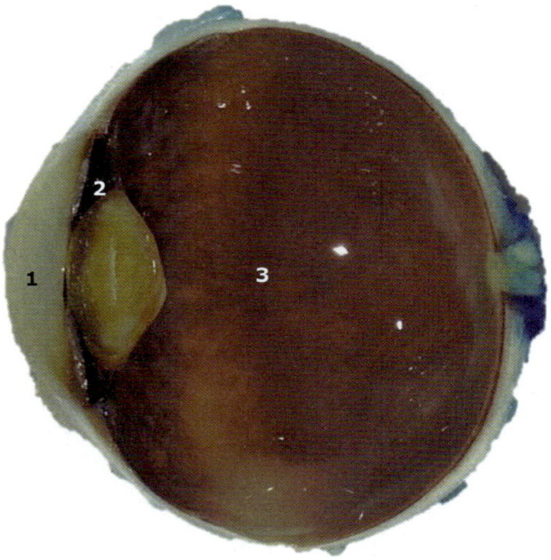

FIGURE 2.3. In (A), the cornea is transparent and thin. The lens is cataractous. The ora serrata (arrow) demarcates a transition zone in the uveal tract between the pars plana of the ciliary body and the retina. Image (B) shows a higher magnification of the iridocorneal angle of the same specimen. The anterior chamber (1) is separated from the posterior chamber (2) by the iris. The zonulae (3) hold the lens in place. Note the pars plicata of the ciliary body (arrow).

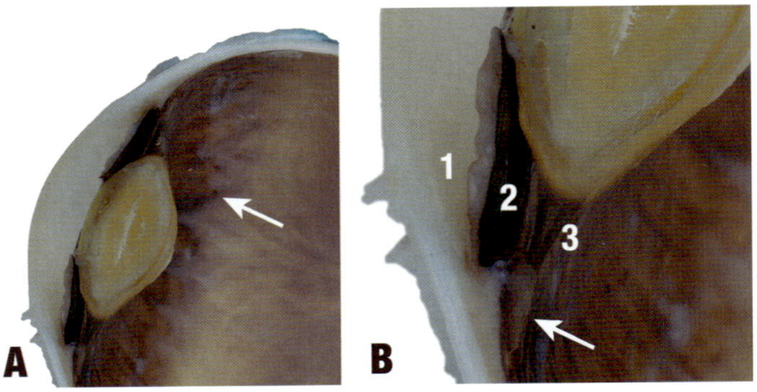

FIGURE 2.4. In (A), note the central retinal artery (arrow) in the optic nerve. The meningeal sheets surround the nerve (*). In the magnification of the eye wall in (B), note the neurosensory retina (1), the retinal pigment epithelium (arrow), a thin layer overlying the choroid (2), and the sclera (3).

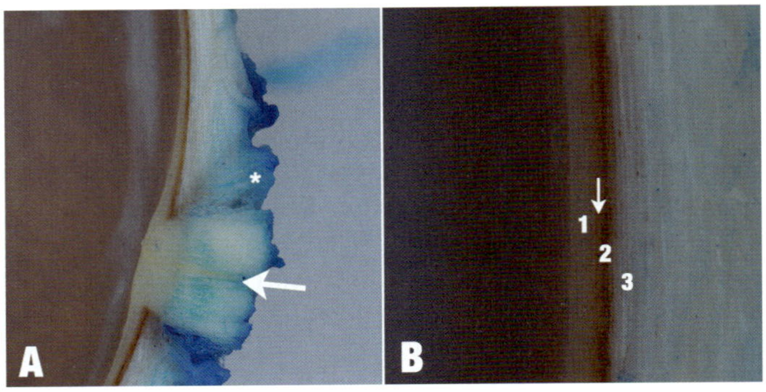

ENUCLEATION SPECIMEN: PHTHISIS BULBI

Phthisis bulbi is the designation for an enucleation specimen that is shrunken, and usually refers to an eye at the end stage of disease. Phthisis bulbi leads to a blind, painful eye.

FIGURE 2.5. The enucleation specimen in (A) shows an atrophic eye (< 16 mm in its largest dimension) with complete disorganization of the posterior structures. In (B), higher magnification reveals bone spicules (arrow) corresponding to ossification due to metaplastic changes of the retinal pigmented epithelium (RPE) cells toward osteoblasts.

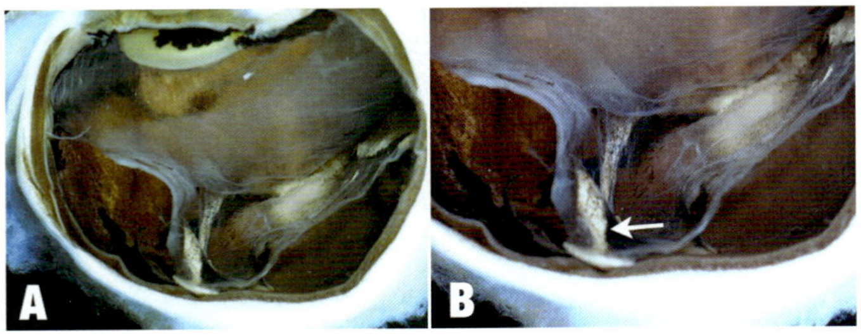

ENUCLEATION SPECIMEN: INTRAOCULAR TUMOR

Transillumination is always useful to detect the presence of an intraocular mass prior to sectioning of the globe. Transillumination causes the intraocular tumor to appear as a dark area inside the ocular globe. The neoplastic process is demarcated on the globe with a felt tip pen; the anatomical location is reported in clock hours, and in distance from the limbus or the optic nerve.

The outer surface of the globe in fixed specimens tends to become more rigid and opaque. Transillumination of these specimens requires a dark chamber with an isolated, direct source of light. For fresh tissue, if a chamber is not readily available, the globe can be carefully transilluminated with a direct source of light.

FIGURE 2.6. Image (A) shows an example of a transillumination chamber with a unique source of light and an opening on the side to manipulate the glove. Image (B) shows transillumination of a fresh enucleation specimen using a light microscope; the tumor is located between 2 and 5 o'clock (dotted circle), extending 8 mm past the limbus.

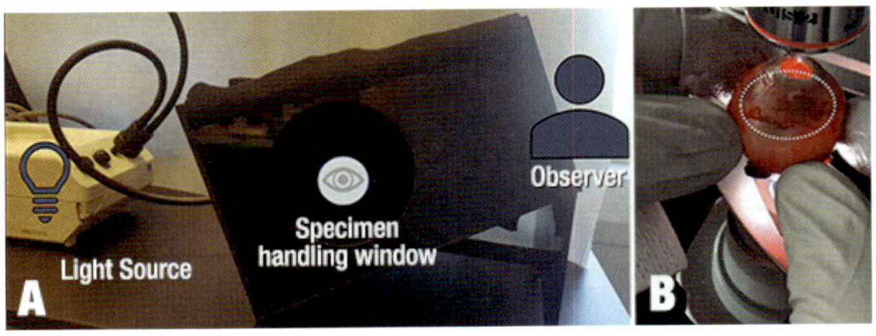

FIGURE 2.7. The anterior view in (A) shows a cataractous lens seen through the pupil. The posterior view of the same specimen in (B) shows the extraocular extension of an intraocular tumor and extensive areas of hemorrhage, including a subdural hemorrhage.

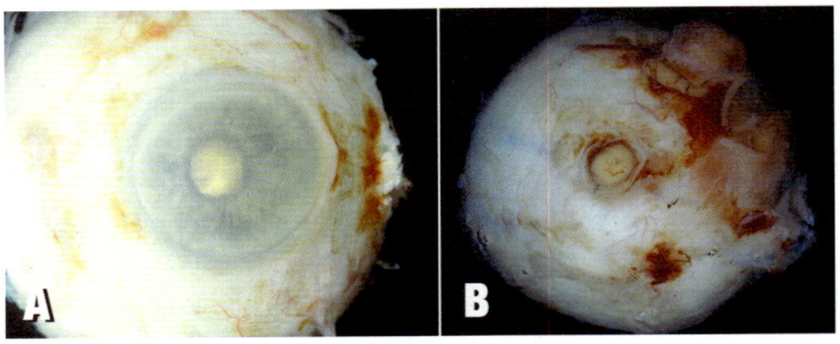

SCHEME FOR MACROSCOPIC EVALUATION OF AN ENUCLEATION SPECIMEN

FIGURE 2.8. The enucleated eye is transilluminated through the pupil, and the shadow (which corresponds to the clinical tumor location) is measured and inked from the exterior of the globe. The location and size of the tumor is recorded. Next, 2 parallel cuts are made, 1 on either side of the tumor, generating a pupil–optic nerve section in which the pupil, the tumor, and the optic nerve are on the same plane. Note that, for retinoblastoma cases, both calottes must also be cut perpendicular to the sclera and submitted.

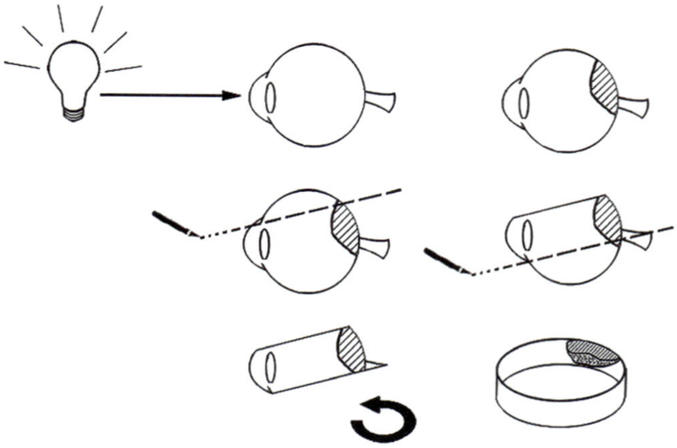

Evisceration

Evisceration involves removal of the intraocular contents, leaving the scleral calotte and muscles intact.

FIGURE 2.9. This sample was retrieved from a patient with a blind, painful eye. Blind, painful eye may be the end stage of several conditions including glaucoma, retinal detachment, and endophthalmitis, among others. Evisceration specimens are generally submitted in fragments. Different intraocular structures are identifiable: retina (A), cornea and capsular bag (B), choroidal tissue (C), and hematic material (D).

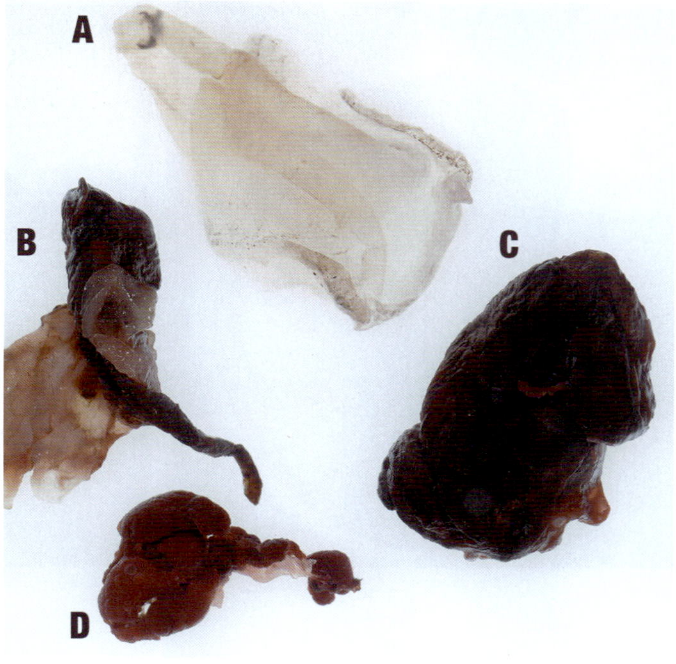

Common artifacts in macroscopic ocular globe evaluation

PSEUDO–RETINAL DETACHMENT AND PSEUDO-CHOROIDAL DETACHMENT

Pseudo–retinal detachment is created when the eye is sectioned. To minimize this artifact, cut the eye from posterior to anterior using a sharp blade; avoid back-and-forth sawing movements and avoid applying pressure to the eyeball. The causative mechanism of pseudo–choroidal detachment is similar to pseudo–retinal detachment; in addition, it is associated with extended enucleation-to-fixation delays.

FIGURE 2.10. In (A), a pupil–optic view of an enucleation specimen shows pseudo–retinal detachment. Note the absence of fluid beneath the retina (arrow). In (B), high magnification of a pseudo–choroidal detachment shows the bare sclera separate from the choroid and retinal pigmented epithelium.

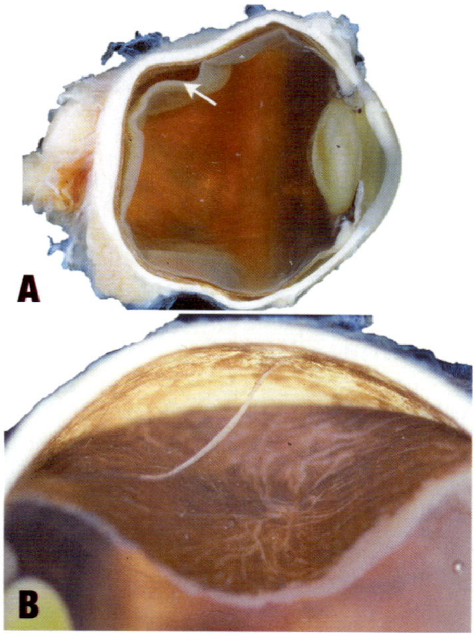

NEUROSENSORIAL RETINAL DETACHMENT WITH PIGMENT RETINAL EPITHELIUM STILL IN PLACE

A true retinal detachment always involves accumulation of subretinal fluid.

FIGURE 2.11. In this specimen, note the retinal vessels exiting the optic nerve (arrow).

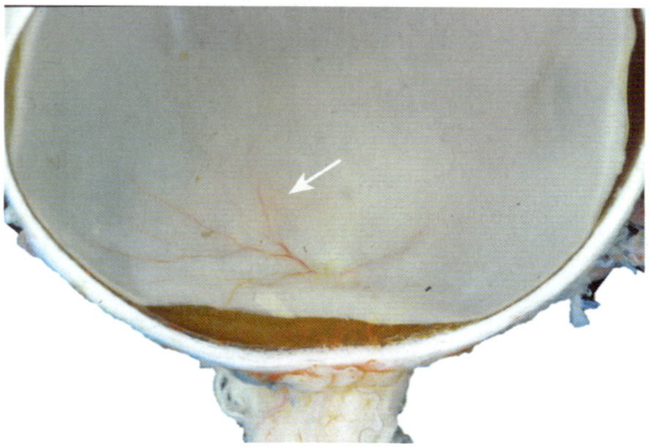

Macroscopic Manifestation of Retinal Disease

Optic nerve cupping

Optic nerve cupping describes an increase in cup-to-disc ratio, which leads to progressive and irreversible vision loss. The most common cause of this condition is glaucoma. Glaucoma is the second leading cause of blindness globally after cataracts.

FIGURE 2.12. This case of iridocorneal endothelial syndrome shows cupping of the optic nerve consistent with glaucoma (arrow).

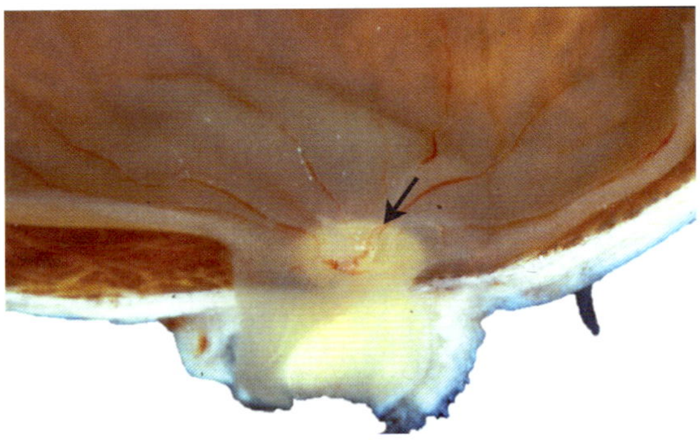

Macular edema

FIGURE 2.13. In (A), an ophthalmoscopic-like view of an enucleation specimen shows macular edema. Note the folds surrounding the foveal area (arrow). Image (B) shows a specimen with irregular pigmentation of the macular area, which suggests age-related macular degeneration. The white, rounded shapes (arrows) may correspond to laser treatment. Note the air inside the retinal vessels.

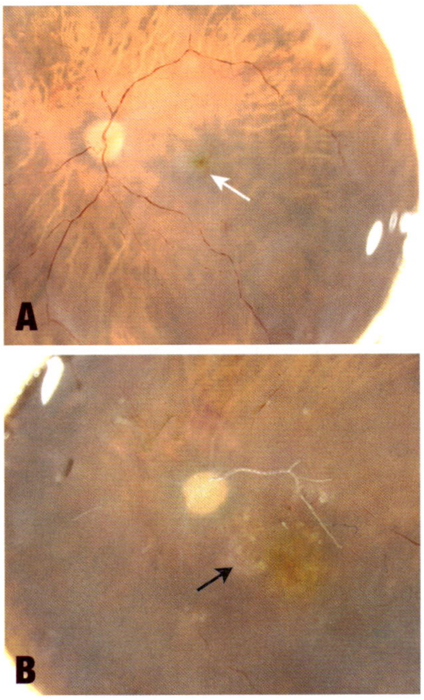

Subretinal hematoma (hemorrhage)

A subretinal hematoma consists of an accumulation of blood between the neurosensory retina and the retinal pigmented epithelium (RPE) overlying the choroid. The choroidal blood supply is generally the source of the hemorrhage. The hemorrhage can arise from angiogenic diseases such as age-related macular degeneration (AMD) or from trauma.

FIGURE 2.14. This enucleation specimen shows a subretinal hematoma (arrow). In addition, a diffuse, flat retinal detachment artifact is present. The lens is cataractous.

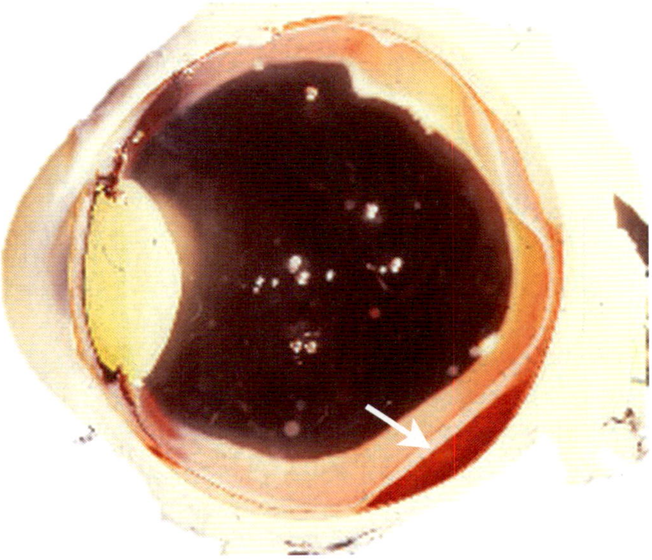

FIGURE 2.15. This enucleation specimen shows a diffuse and extended choroidal hemorrhage (*). Note the detached retina and extraocular hemorrhage (arrow).

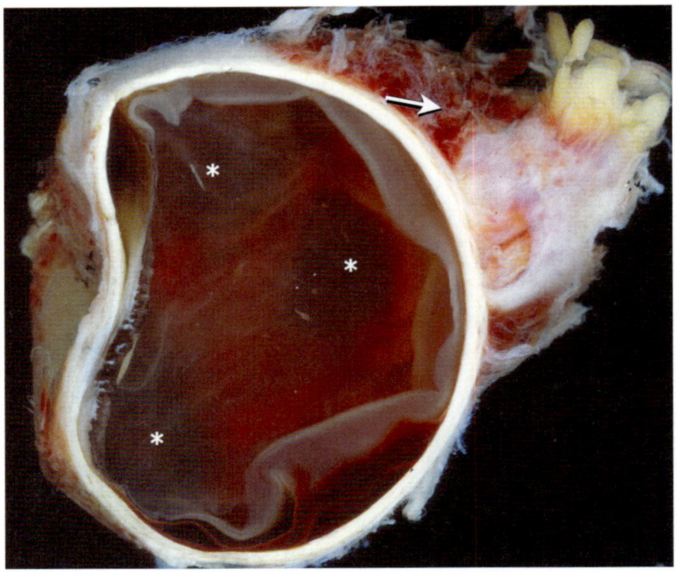

Retinitis pigmentosa

Retinitis pigmentosa refers to a group of inheritable degenerative diseases of the retina characterized by photoreceptor damage and retinal atrophy. The estimated incidence is 1 per 5000 worldwide. Retinitis pigmentosa follows classic monogenic inheritance patterns such as X-linked autosomal-recessive or autosomal-dominant inheritance. More than 75 causal genes have been identified.

FIGURE 2.16. This image illustrates marked retinal atrophy with several bone-spicule-shaped pigment deposits in the peripheral retina. The macular area is preserved but has a rim of depigmentation (arrowheads). Note the thin blood vessels and the pallor of the optic nerve (arrow).

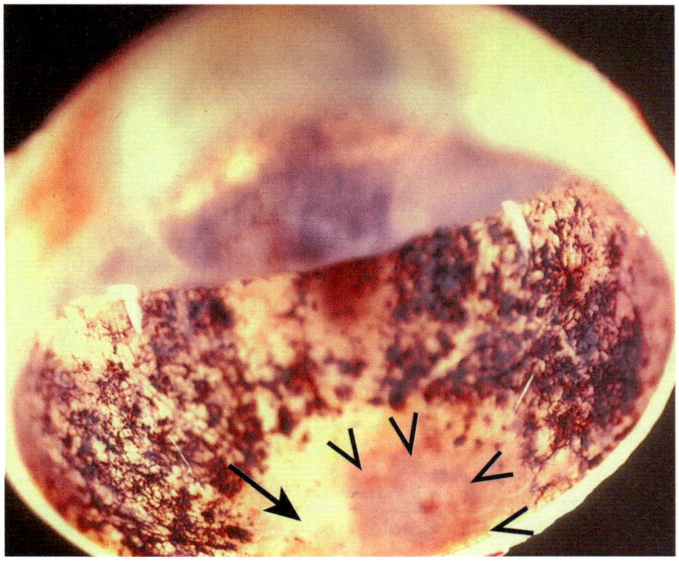

Retinal atrophy and vitreomacular traction

Macular traction occurs when the gel-like liquid (vitreous) that fills the globe begins to detach from the posterior part of the globe, and the remaining anchor points form strong adhesions to the retina, which pull on the retina.

FIGURE 2.17. This enucleation specimen shows areas of retinal atrophy (*) and areas of vitreomacular traction (arrow). This specimen also demonstrates keratoconus: a degenerative disorder of the eye in which the cornea thins and distorts into a pronounced conical shape (arrowhead). The keratoconus and vitreomacular tractions are unrelated.

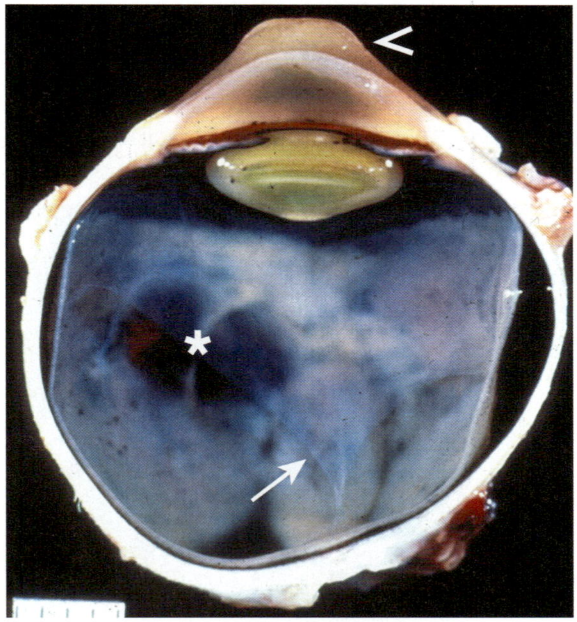

Uveitis

Uveitis is inflammation of the uvea, the pigmented layer that lies between the inner retina and the outer fibrous layer composed of the sclera and cornea. The uvea consists of the middle layer of pigmented vascular structures of the eye and includes the iris, ciliary body, and choroid. Uveitis can be classified as either nongranulomatous or granulomatous.

Nongranulomatous uveitis

Nongranulomatous uveitis is a group of diseases often related to systemic autoimmune diseases such as arthritis.

FIGURE 2.18. In this enucleation specimen, the choroid is diffusely thickened (arrow) and a choroidal detachment is present (*). The retina is opaque and the lens is cataractous.

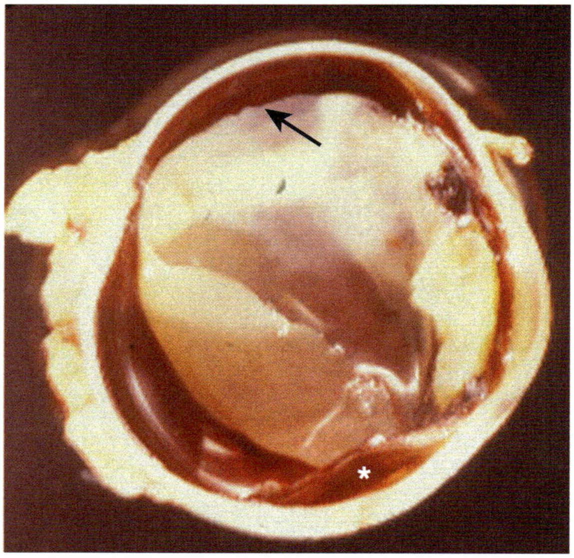

FIGURE 2.19. This image shows a thickened uveal track (arrows) and a complete, long-standing retinal detachment (*). The lens is cataractous and the iris, ciliary body, and parts of the retina are attached to it. A scleral buckle is present (arrowheads).

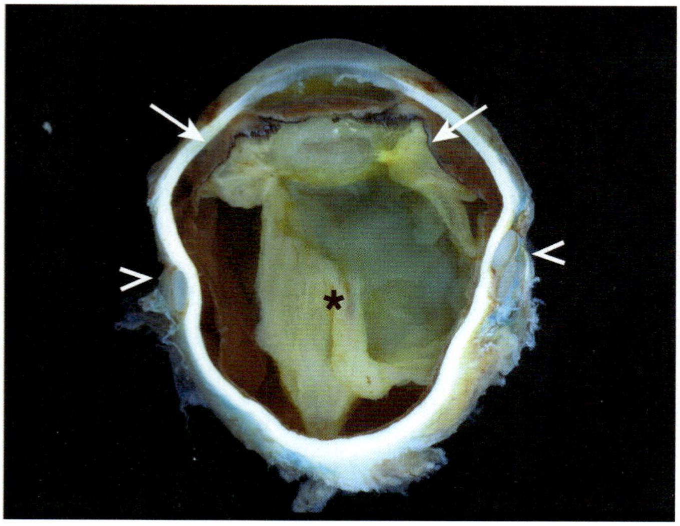

INTERMEDIATE UVEITIS

FIGURE 2.20. This enucleation specimen shows "snowballs" or localized inflammatory foci (arrow); and a "snow bank" or inflammation at the ora serrata, the anterior-most limit of the retina (arrowheads). These are caused by a reaction to the subjacent uveitis.

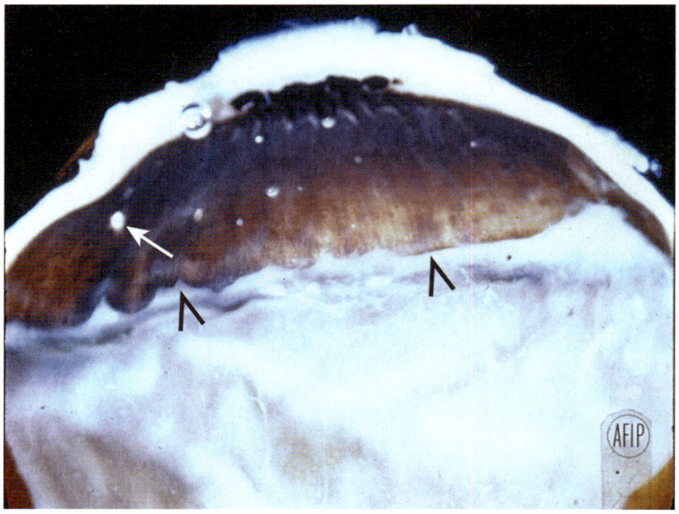

DIFFUSE UVEITIS

FIGURE 2.21. In this enucleation specimen, the uveal tract is completely replaced by purulent material (*). There is a subretinal hemorrhage underlying the detached retina and fibrous material in the vitreous cavity (arrowhead). The lens is cataractous and is surrounded by fibrinoid membranes (arrow).

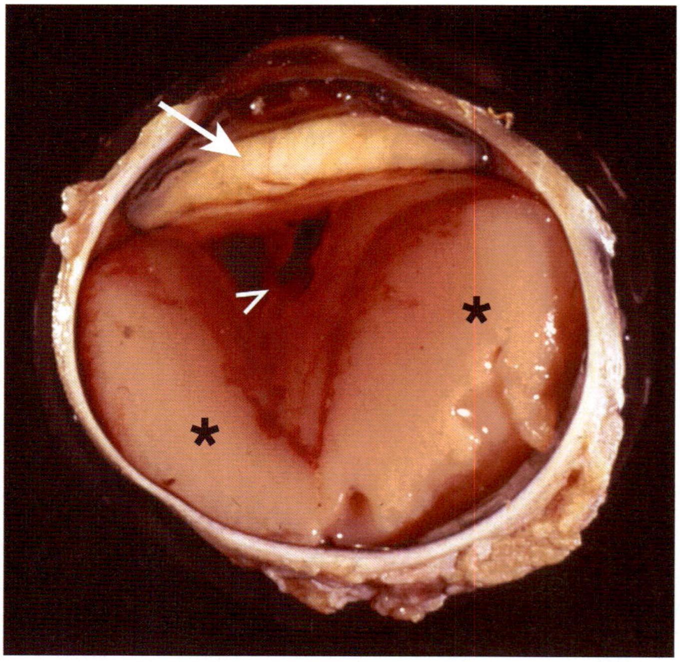

Granulomatous uveitis

Granulomatous uveitis is found in many inflammatory diseases, and is generally characterized by a predominant histiocytic infiltrate forming a "wall" (granuloma) around a pathogen or foreign body.

FIGURE 2.22. This is an example of granulomatous uveitis. The eye is aphakic; the uveal track is thickened; and a granuloma is present and attached to the endothelium of the cornea (arrow). The anterior chamber is filled with a hazy material (arrowhead). The vitreous is fibrotic and tractional bands are also present (*).

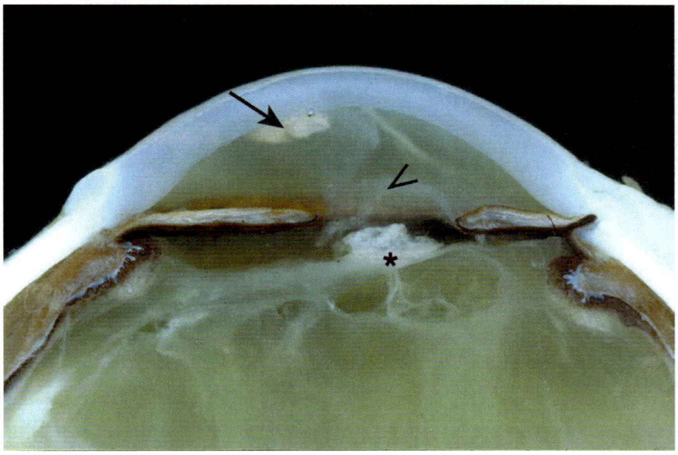

SARCOIDOSIS

Sarcoidosis is a disease involving abnormal collections of inflammatory cells (granulomas) that can form as nodules in multiple organs, including the eye.

FIGURE 2.23. This image shows an enucleation specimen with multifocal retinal detachment and subretinal fluid (*). Note the granulomatous reaction in the choroid (arrow). In the cornea, neovascularization is present (arrowheads).

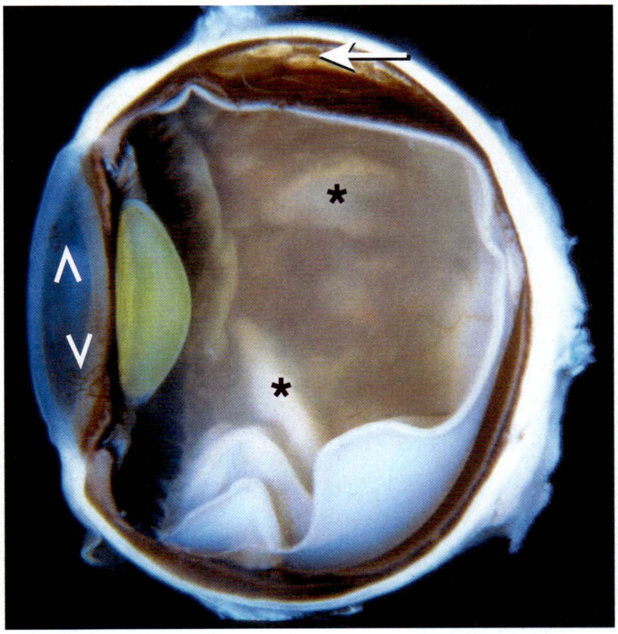

LENS-INDUCED UVEITIS

In lens-induced uveitis, lens protein in the anterior chamber causes a zonal granulomatous response, which occurs usually 1 day to 3 weeks after capsule rupture. This may be associated with sympathetic ophthalmia.

FIGURE 2.24. This enucleation specimen shows an indented cornea, accompanied by complete hypopyon occupying the anterior chamber with intense vitreitis. Note that the translucent vitreous has become whitish, and the lens surface is irregular with decoloration of the peripheral areas (arrowheads).

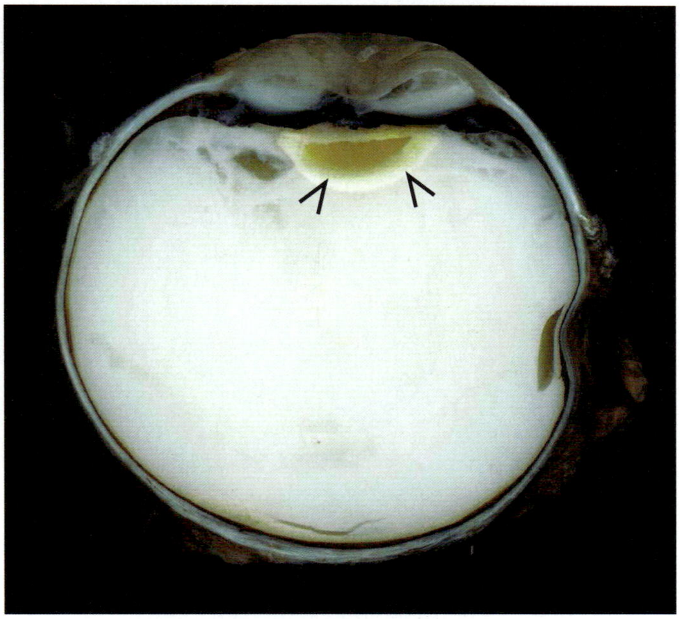

SUBRETINAL FIBROSIS AND UVEITIS SYNDROME

Uveitis syndrome is a rare posterior uveitis that usually begins as a multifocal choroiditis and then progresses to subretinal fibrosis. Recurrences are not uncommon and the visual prognosis is generally poor.

FIGURE 2.25. In this enucleation specimen, a thickened choroid is clearly observed (arrow). The retina is detached and a fibrovascular subretinal membrane is present (arrowhead).

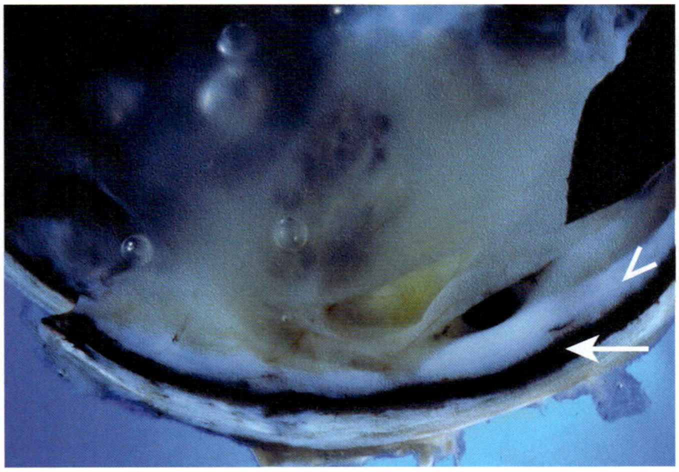

SYMPATHETIC OPHTHALMIA

Sympathetic ophthalmia is characterized by bilateral diffuse granulomatous uveitis that occurs 2 weeks to many years after traumatic penetration or perforation of the eye. It threatens the sight of the uninjured (sympathizing) eye.

FIGURE 2.26. In this enucleation specimen, thickening of the uveal tract is evident (arrows). Complete proteinaceous retinal detachment (*) is also present, along with posterior synechia (adhesion of the iris to the anterior capsule of the lens).

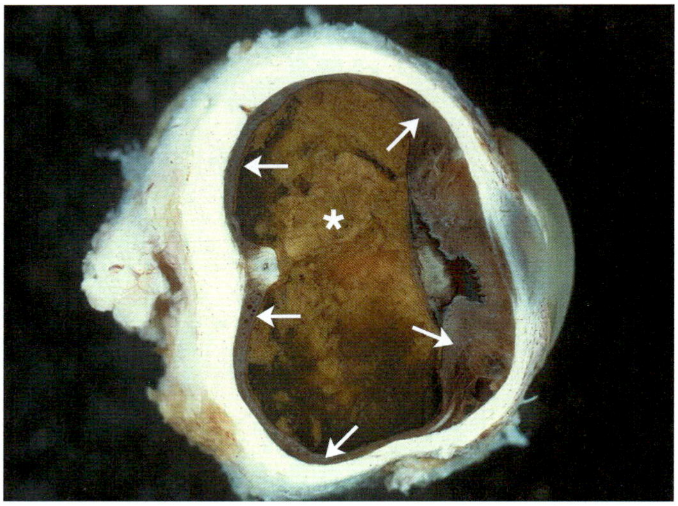

VOGT–KOYANAGI-HARADA (VKH) DISEASE

VKH disease is an autoimmune condition that causes bilateral chronic granulomatous panuveitis, and extraocular manifestations in the central nervous system, auditory system, and integument. VKH disease is twice as prevalent in women than men, and is believed to be associated with specific human leukocyte antigen (HLA) types, suggesting a possible hereditary component. The exact cause of VKH disease, however, remains unclear.

FIGURE 2.27. In (A), an enucleation specimen shows a retinal detachment and a scleral buckle (*). Image (B) shows several aggregate RPE cells and histiocytes, called Dalen–Fuchs nodules (arrowheads).

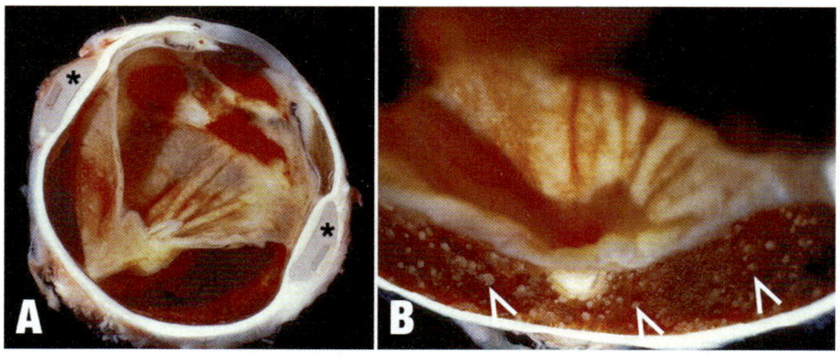

CHRONIC VKH DISEASE

FIGURE 2.28. This enucleation specimen shows complete distortion of the anterior chamber. Image (A) is the gross specimen and image (B) is a histopathological section of the same specimen. The iris and the chamber are completely replaced by a mass (arrow) corresponding to inflammatory exudate. The eye is aphakic and the retina is completely detached from the choroid, although it is attached anteriorly to the mass. Note the proteinaceous exudate beneath the retina (arrowheads).

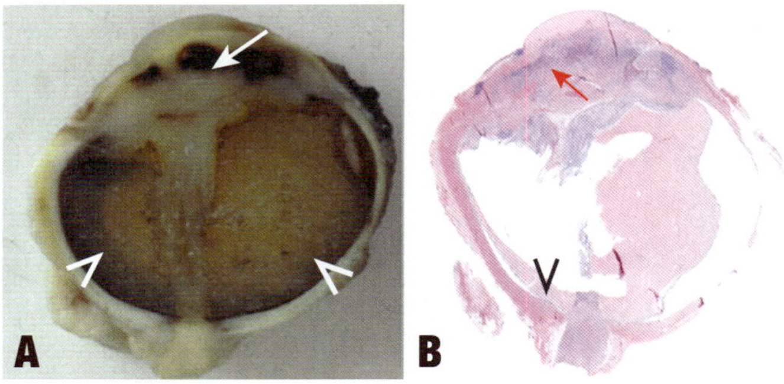

Granulomatous uveitis caused by viral or microorganism infection

OCULAR TUBERCULOSIS

Ocular tuberculosis refers to necrotizing granulomatous uveitis caused by *Mycobacterium tuberculosis* infection. The mechanism of infection of ocular structures is via hematogenous dissemination of the bacteria during the primary infection.

FIGURE 2.29. In this enucleation specimen, the anterior chamber and vitreous cavity are filled by caseous exudate. The iris is also replaced by a whitish material, and the retina is completely detached. Note the whitish thickening of the posterior choroid (arrow).

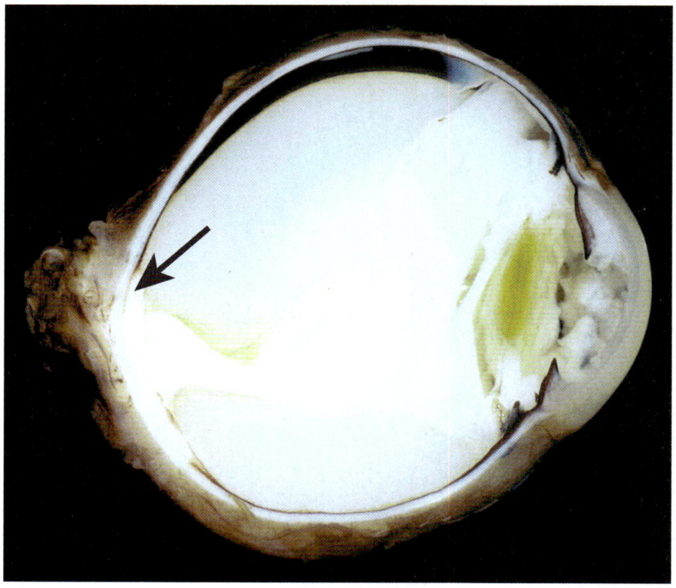

RETINAL CYTOMEGALOVIRUS INFECTION IN AN AIDS PATIENT

Cytomegalovirus is a genus of viruses in the *Herpesviridae* family. Humans, in particular immunosuppressed patients, are natural hosts to this virus. AIDS patients have poor immunity and massive retinal infections are common.

FIGURE 2.30. Image (A) shows a posterior view of an enucleation specimen with a calotte of the eye removed. Notice the whitish exudates overlying the retina (*). In (B), higher magnification of the same specimen shows that the retinal pigment epithelium is preserved.

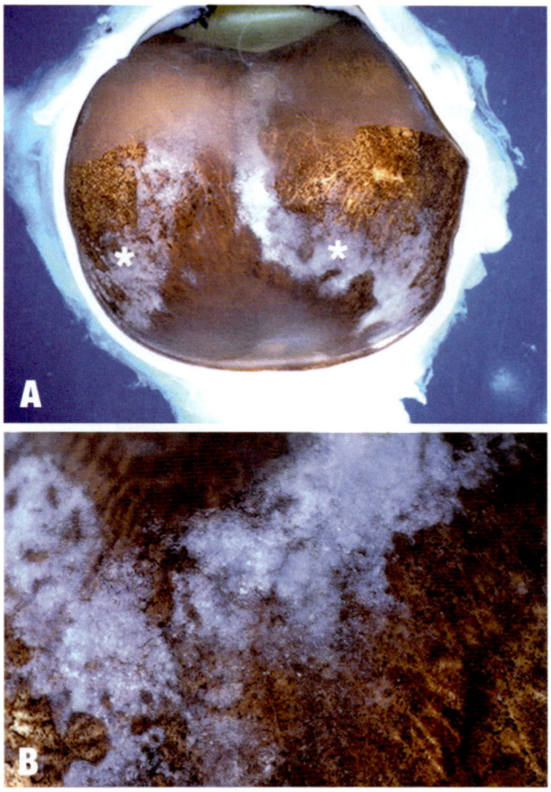

FIGURE 2.31. In this evisceration specimen, only the retina and the choroid are present. Note the necrotic whitish retina (arrow). The choroid is thickened and is tan-yellowish in appearance (arrowheads).

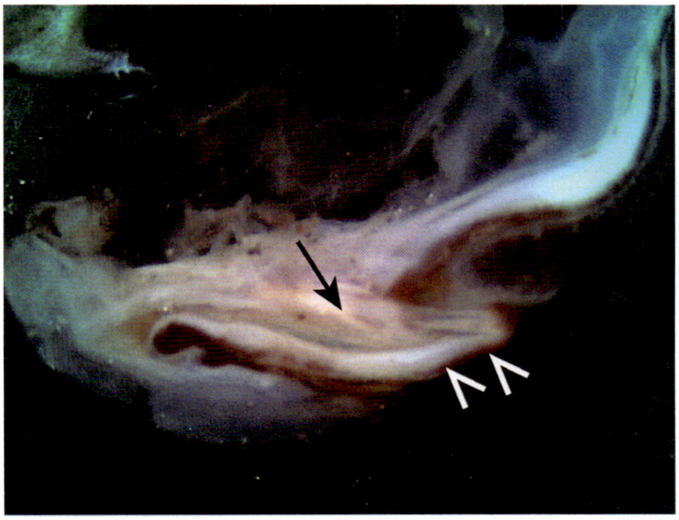

TOXOPLASMIC CHORIORETINITIS

Toxoplasmic chorioretinitis is caused by parasitic infection from *Toxoplasma gondii*. Two forms are recognized: congenital and acquired. Congenital toxoplasmic chorioretinitis occurs because the infection is transplacental: *T. gondii* is among infections that cause TORCH syndrome. Acquired toxoplasmic chorioretinitis is produced by parasite ingestion, usually from raw or undercooked food. After parasitemia, the parasite directly invades the photoreceptors in the retina.

FIGURE 2.32. In this enucleation specimen, chronic and subacute lesions coexist. In the active lesion located in the macula (arrow), the retina is necrotic, and reactive RPE cell hyperplasia surrounds the lesion. The chronic lesion (arrowhead) demonstrates atrophy of the retina and RPE in the center; in the periphery, RPE proliferation is present.

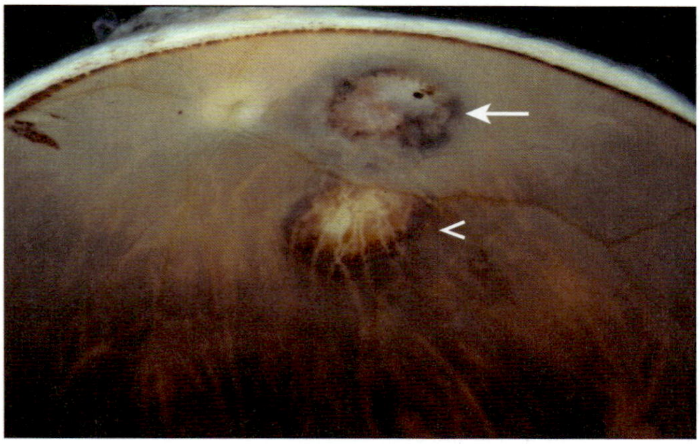

TOXOPLASMIC UVEITIS

FIGURE 2.33. This enucleation specimen shows multiple irregular chorioretinal scars, surrounded by hyperplastic retinal pigment epithelium (arrowheads). Some adherent membranes are present in the vitreous cavity (arrow). The lens has a total cataract and the anterior chamber is filled with whitish material that corresponds to hypopyon.

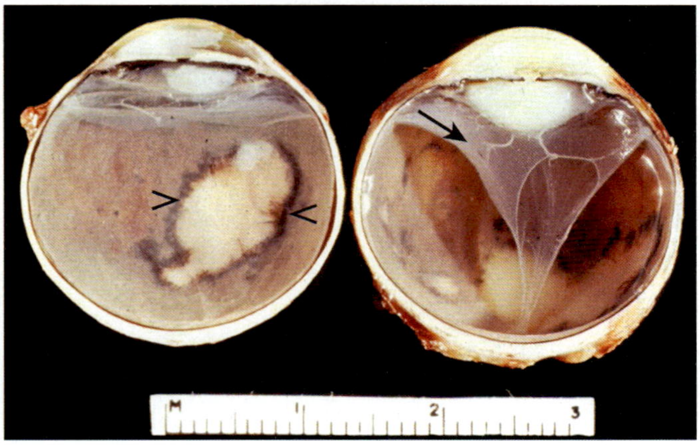

TOXOPLASMIC ACUTE RETINAL NECROSIS

Toxoplasmosis can have several manifestations in the eye, of which toxoplasmic acute retinal necrosis has the worst prognosis.

FIGURE 2.34. This enucleation specimen shows extensive retinal necrosis with multiple coalescent foci. The vitreous is hazy (*).

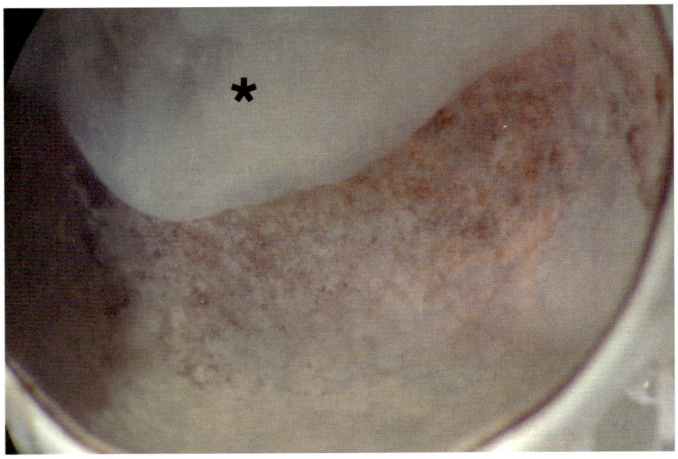

CYSTICERCOSIS

Ocular cysticercosis is a disease that is caused by the encystment of cysticercus larvae from certain tapeworms in the eye.

FIGURE 2.35. In this enucleation specimen, a choroidal cyst (arrow) containing a larva (*) is clearly visible. Note the retinal detachment overlying the cyst.

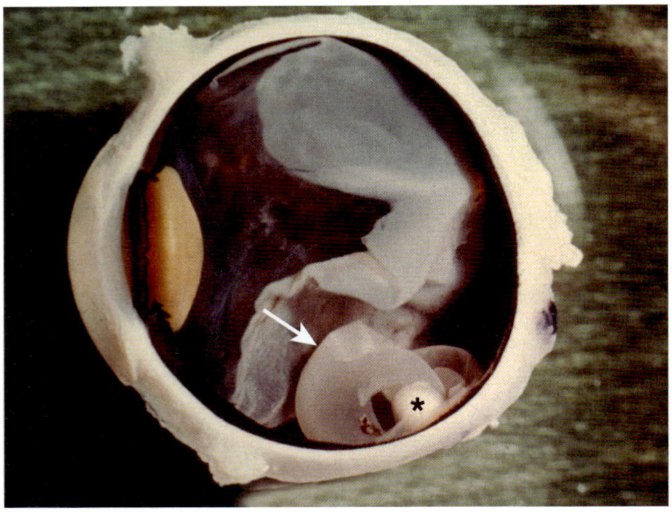

GNATHOSTOMIASIS

Gnathostomiasis is a parasitic infection caused by the ingestion of larvae from *Gnathostoma* species. The intermediate host is freshwater fish. When larvae affect the eye, the uveitic process begins.

FIGURE 2.36. Image (A) shows a scolex surrounded by 4 rows of hooks, which have an open base and a sharper end. Image (B) shows a higher magnification of hooks in the body of a worm that have a similar morphology to those in (A).

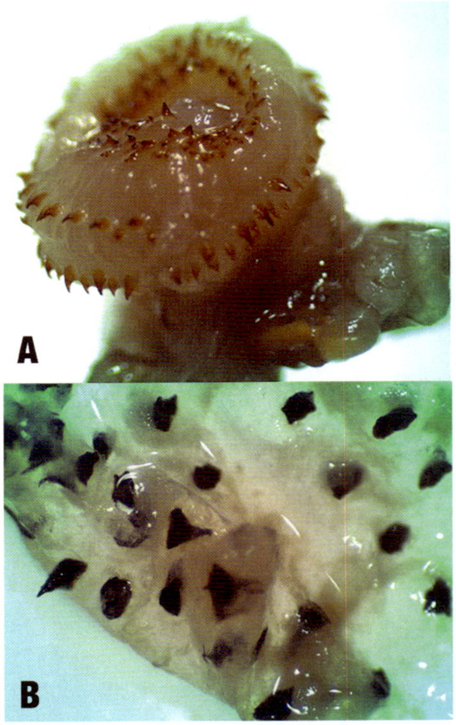

MOOREN ULCER

A Mooren ulcer is a rapidly progressive ulcerative keratitis that first affects the periphery of the cornea before spreading circumferentially toward its center. Mooren ulcer is a diagnosis of exclusion: it can only be diagnosed after ruling out infectious and systemic causes.

FIGURE 2.37. In this enucleation specimen, the periphery of the cornea is circumferentially ulcerated (arrow) and the cornea is thinning. There is also scarring of the corneoscleral junction.

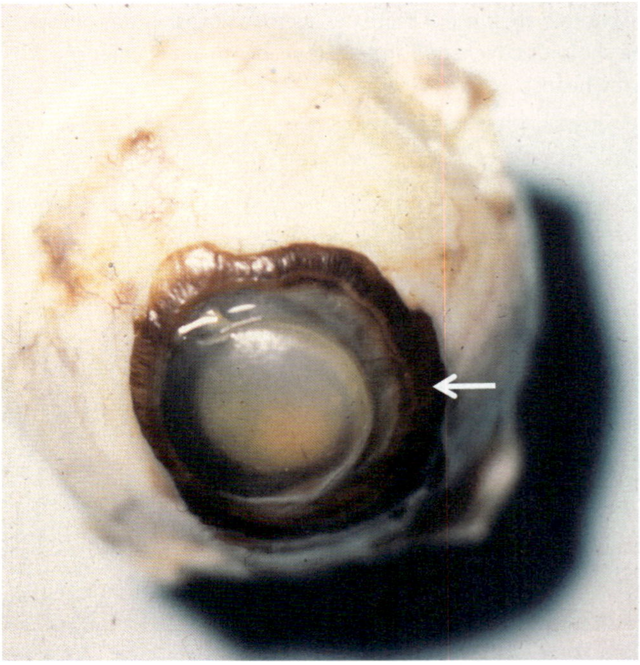

Ocular Neoplasia

Leiomyoma

Leiomyoma is a benign, smooth muscle tumor. Ninety percent of cases occur in women. The differential diagnosis includes amelanotic melanoma and nerve sheath tumors.

FIGURE 2.38. This transversal pupil–optic nerve (PO) section of an enucleation specimen shows a nodular, well-delineated, whitish tumor in the ciliary body. The cut surface shows small foci of hemorrhage without necrosis. The retina partially covers the inner surface of the tumor, and the sclera is not infiltrated. Note the slightly displaced (subluxated) cataractous lens and the choroidal detachment artifact in the right inferior corner.

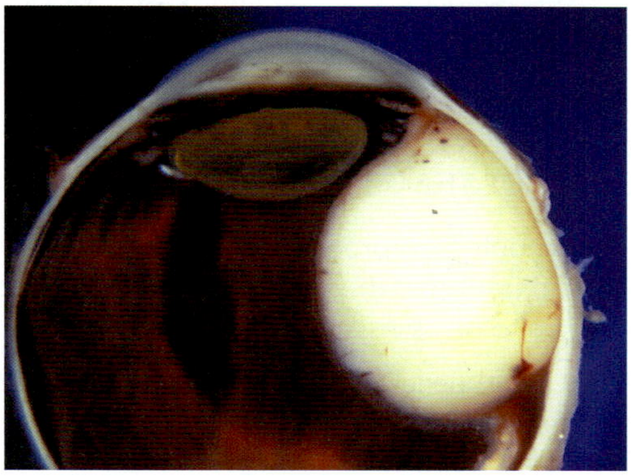

Lymphoma

PRIMARY RETINAL AND VITREOUS LARGE B-CELL LYMPHOMA

These tumors are associated with intracranial nervous system lymphomas.

FIGURE 2.39. Image (A) shows an enucleation specimen with a multifocal, necrotic, and hemorrhagic whitish retinal tumor (arrows). Note the thickened, opaque cornea; the cataractous lens; the diffuse, flat retinal detachment; and the retinal hemorrhages overlying the tumor (arrowhead). In (B), magnification of a nodule from the same specimen shows thickening of the sensory retina. Note the infiltration of the subretinal pigment epithelium area (arrows).

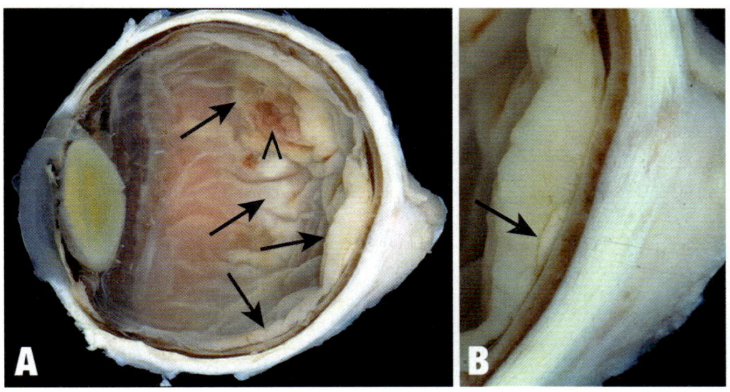

UVEAL TRACT LYMPHOMA

Uveal tract lymphoma most frequently occurs as a secondary location of a systemic disease. The presence of a tumor in the choroid and ciliary body with an extensive orbital component may indicate a primary lymphoma or metastatic disease.

FIGURE 2.40. In (A), gross examination of a specimen shows a whitish, solid, and homogeneous tumor located at the posterior pole of the choroid and at the entire posterior orbit. Note that the tumor is also present in the ciliary body. In (B), the tumor surrounds the optic nerve, mimicking a meningioma. In this patient, histopathological examination with immunohistochemistry confirmed the diagnosis of large B-cell lymphoma.

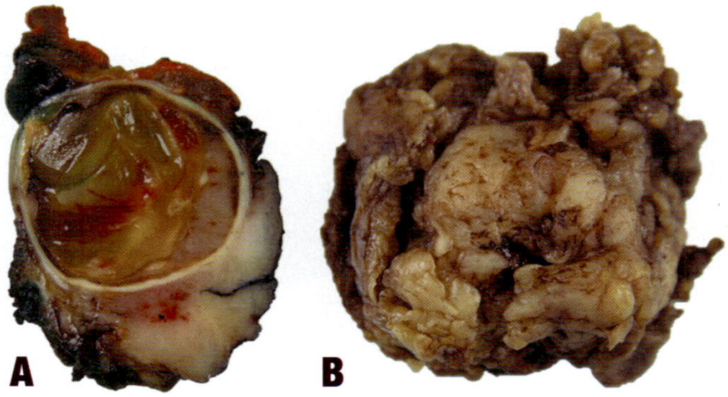

Metastatic adenocarcinoma

Metastatic disease is the most frequent intraocular malignant tumor. In women, the most common origin is breast cancer. In men, the most common origin is lung cancer.

FIGURE 2.41. This pupil–optic nerve section shows a whitish tumor with several foci of necrosis (*) occupying the posterior aspect of the choroid. Note the pigment epithelium over the inner surface of the tumor. A serous retinal detachment is present (arrow) with a retinal detachment artifact overlying the tumor and normal choroid. Note the air bubble artifacts in the vitreous cavity. Another artifact, the compression of the eyeball, is present on the right side.

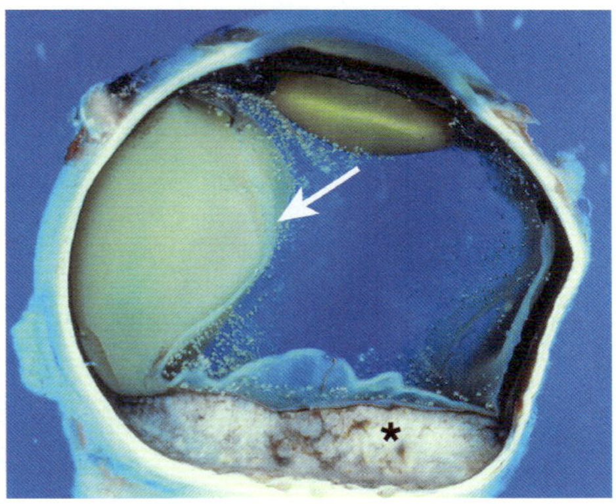

CARCINOID

These are usually secondary tumor foci, arising most frequently from a primary tumor in the gastrointestinal tract or lung. Melanoma should be considered as part of the differential diagnosis, because neither carcinoid nor melanoma tumors have a necrotic component.

FIGURE 2.42. This enucleation specimen shows a well-differentiated neuroendocrine tumor in the choroid. The overlying pigment is caused by proliferation of the retinal pigment epithelium (arrowhead). Focal microhemorrhages are visible on the surface of the retina (arrows).

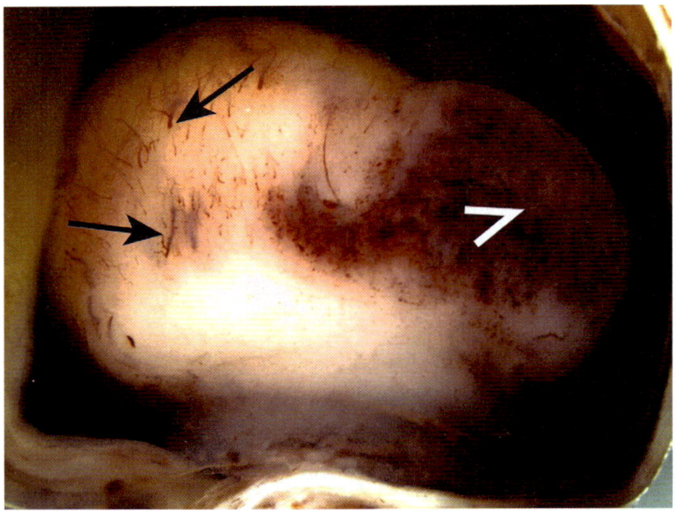

Retinoblastoma

Retinoblastoma is the most frequent intraocular tumor in children. It usually affects patients younger than 2 years. Leukocoria is the major clinical sign. The tumor arises in the sensory retina, and can be endophytic, exophytic, or diffuse. The molecular signature is the inactivation of both copies of the retinoblastoma gene on chromosome 13.

FIGURE 2.43. In this enucleation specimen, the eye is sectioned to show the posterior pole and above the optic nerve, revealing an endophytic tumor; the rest of the retina is diffusely infiltrated. Note the retinal vessels overlying the area of the tumor.

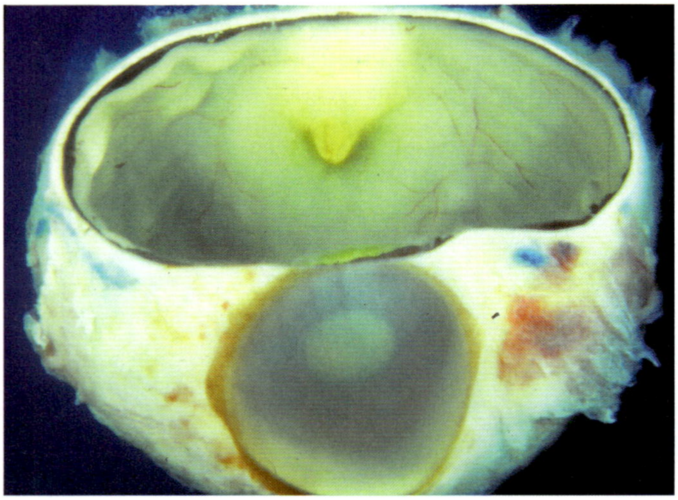

MIXED RETINOBLASTOMA

FIGURE 2.44. This enucleation specimen shows a whitish, thickened area of the neurosensory retina over the head of the optic nerve, corresponding to a mixed retinoblastoma. Snowball-like structures are present in the vitreous chamber overlying the tumor, corresponding to vitreous seeding. A retinal detachment artifact is present.

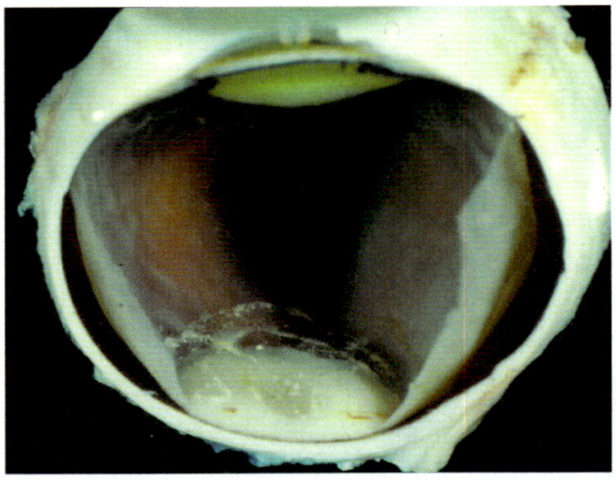

INFILTRATION OF THE OPTIC NERVE

The main morphological prognostic factor for retinoblastoma is infiltration of the optic nerve. The invasion of the optic nerve has to be assessed by a pathologist in all cases.

FIGURE 2.45. The superior calotte is removed in this enucleation specimen to show an extensively exophytic necrotic tumor occupying the vitreous chamber with severe infiltration of the optic nerve (arrowhead). Intratumoral calcification is a hallmark of this tumor and can be seen in the chalky white areas (arrow).

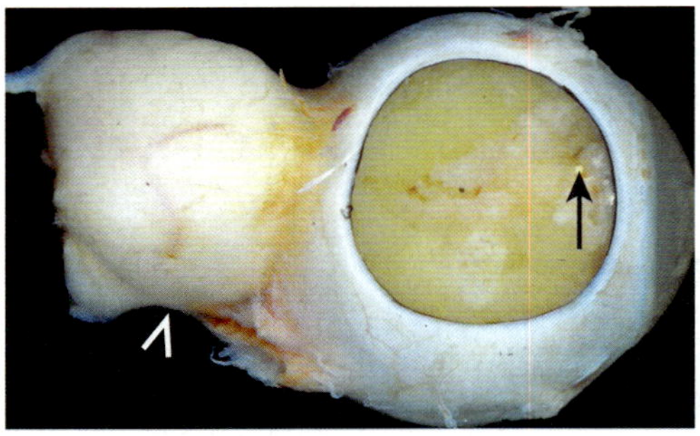

EXO-ENDOPHYTIC RETINOBLASTOMA

FIGURE 2.46. An exo-endophytic tumor is located on the optic nerve head and has produced a retinal detachment. Note the proteinaceous subretinal fluid. The optic nerve is thickened due to retinoblastoma infiltration.

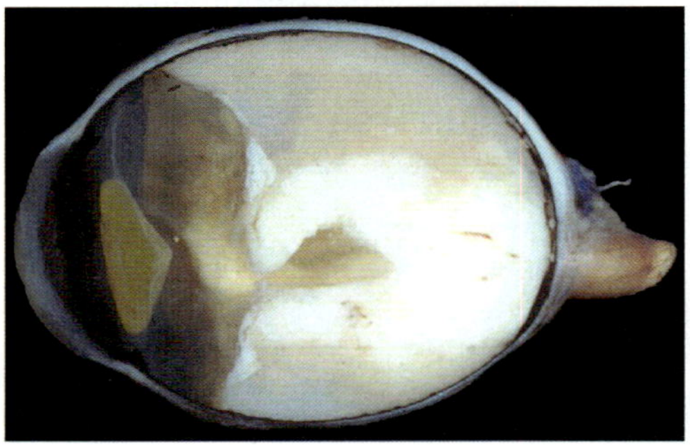

EXOPHYTIC RETINOBLASTOMA

This type of tumor grows from the retina toward the choroid.

FIGURE 2.47. In this enucleation specimen, the retina is completely detached, and the tumor is growing inside the subretinal proteinaceous fluid. Note the distance between the tumor and the optic nerve head.

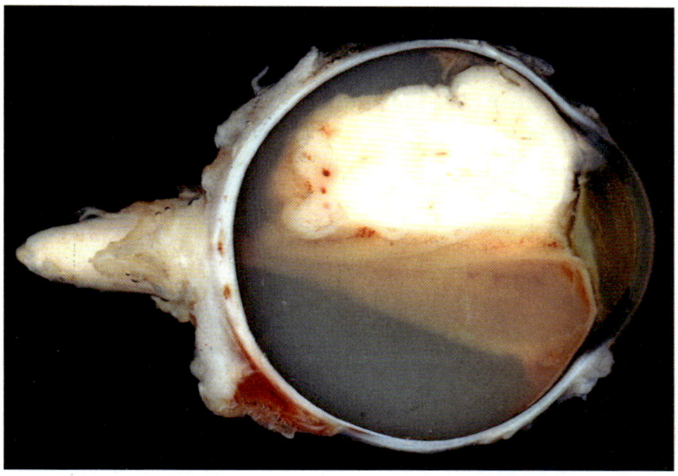

ENDOPHYTIC RETINOBLASTOMA

FIGURE 2.48. Image (A) shows an endophytic grayish tumor located on the retina of this enucleation specimen (arrow). Higher magnification of the same specimen (B) shows small hemorrhagic areas (arrow). The choroidal layer is not compromised.

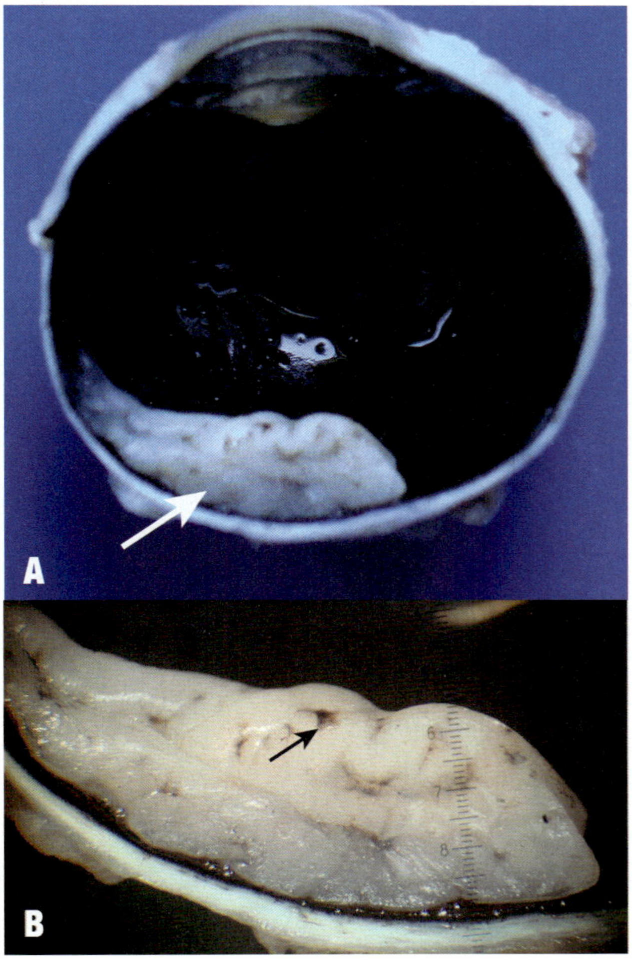

Melanocytic Ocular Neoplasia

Melanocytoma

Melanocytoma (magnocellular nevus) is a rare lesion of unknown etiology. It is a benign tumor arising from intraocular melanocytes and it is much less common than its malignant counterpart, melanoma.

MELANOCYTOMA OF THE CILIARY BODY AND CHOROID

This type of melanocytoma, which tends to undergo spontaneous necrosis, is a variant of melanocytic nevi of the uveal tract. Follow-up is recommended due to the possibility of malignant transformation (melanoma), which occurs in up to 2% of cases. Gross examination reveals a very pigmented, solid, homogeneous tumor located in the ciliary body and choroid. Tumor thickness and pigmentation suggests uveal melanoma on gross examination; however, the heavy pigmentation can indicate melanocytoma. Diagnosis is confirmed by microscopic examination.

FIGURE 2.49. This image shows a transverse section of an enucleation specimen. A thick melanocytic tumor is present in the uveal tract, at the retina and near the ciliary bodies

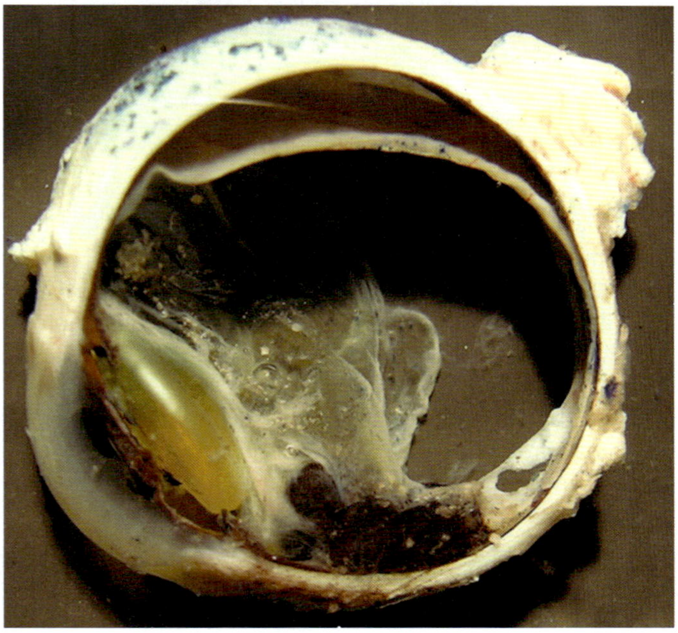

OPTIC DISC MELANOCYTOMA

Similar to ciliary body and choroidal melanocytomas, optic disc melanocytomas are pigmented variants of melanocytic nevi.

FIGURE 2.50. This image shows a posterior view of an enucleation specimen in which a calotte of the eye has been removed. Note the nodular pigmented tumor in the optic nerve parenchyma. No meningeal extension is observed.

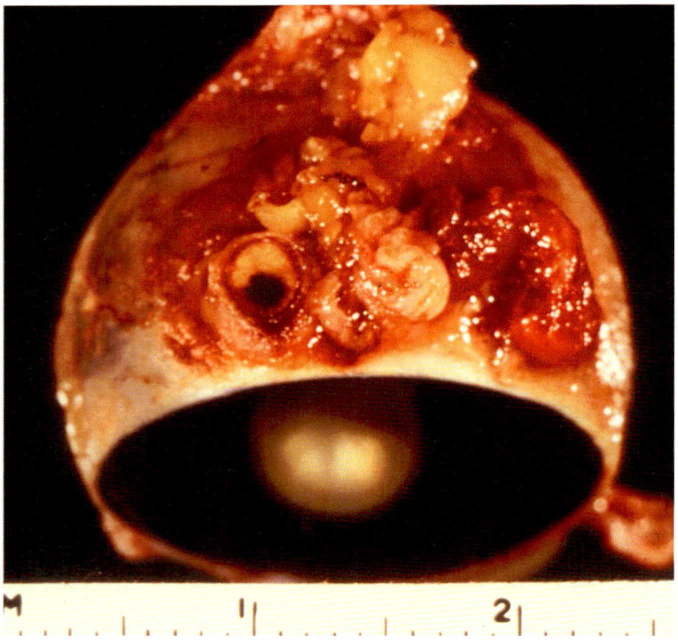

Uveal melanoma

Uveal melanoma is the most common primary eye malignancy in adulthood, occurring mainly after age 60. The uveal tract — composed of the iris, ciliary body, and choroid — can be affected by uveal melanoma. Despite advances in treatment of the primary tumor, metastatic disease occurs in almost half of patients, generally affecting the liver and lungs via hematogenous dissemination of the primary tumor. Tumors have different levels of pigmentation, and some are amelanocytic (nonpigmented). The differential diagnosis for amelanotic choroidal melanoma is metastatic disease.

IRIS AND CILIARY BODY MELANOMA

Large tumors displace the lens. Of the 3 locations in the uveal tract, tumors of the ciliary body have the worst prognosis.

FIGURE 2.51. The enucleation specimen in (A) shows a firm, dome-shaped, deeply pigmented tumor arising from the ciliary body (arrow). The lens has been removed, and a diffuse retinal detachment artifact is present. The enucleation specimen in (B) shows a large, dome-shaped, mixed melanotic and amelanotic choroidal melanoma. The anterior chamber is closed, and the angle is infiltrated (arrow). Total secondary retinal detachment with subretinal serous fluid and some subretinal hemorrhages are present (arrowhead). The lens is cataractous.

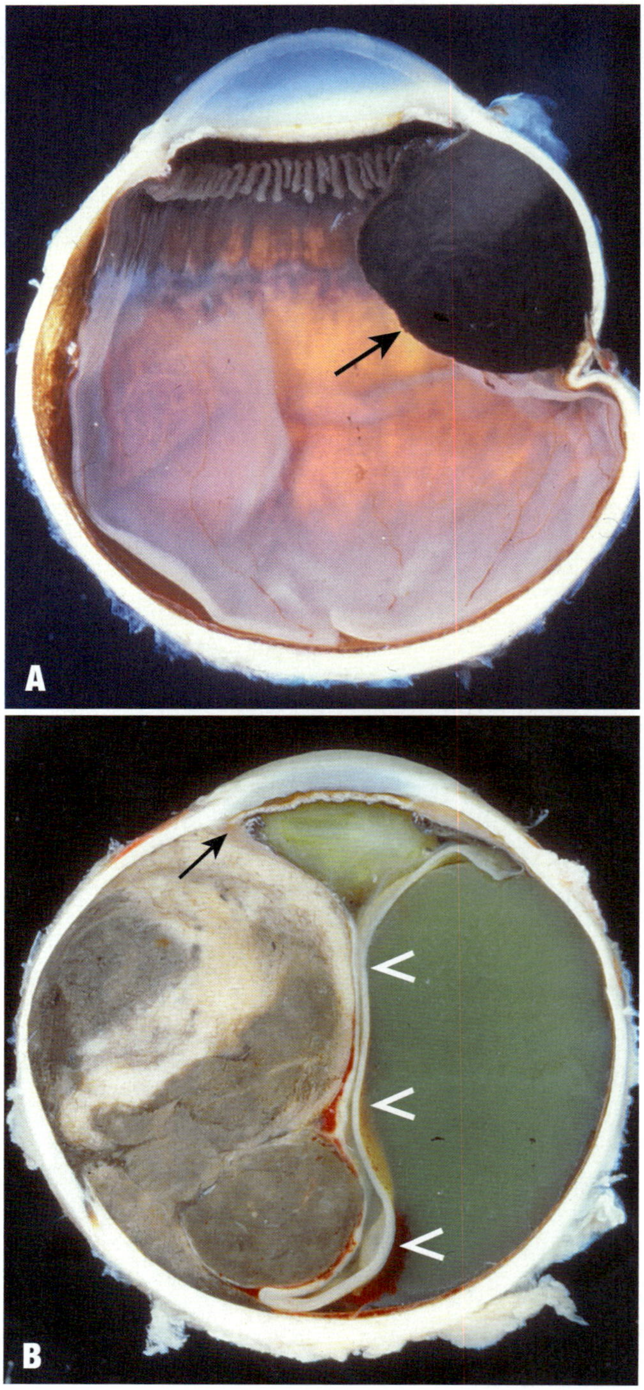

FIGURE 2.52. This enucleation specimen shows a pigmented, nodular-shaped ciliary body melanoma (arrow) with extensive necrosis (*). A retinal detachment is present with subretinal fluid (arrowhead), and the retina is folded (•).

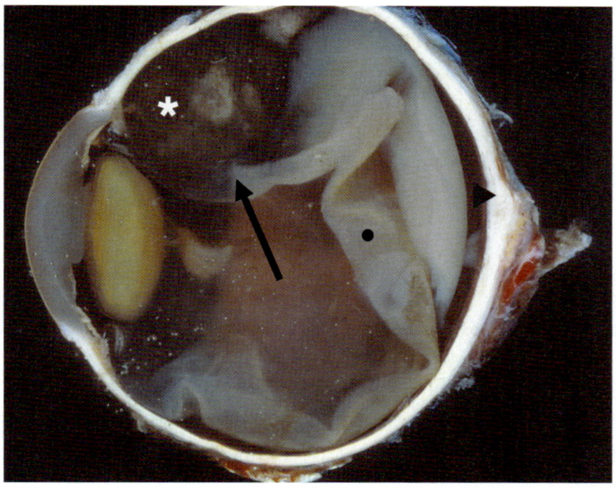

FIGURE 2.53. This enucleation specimen shows a pigmented, bilobed, dome-shaped tumor arising from the ciliary body (arrows). The lens has been removed, and a diffuse, flat retinal detachment artifact is present.

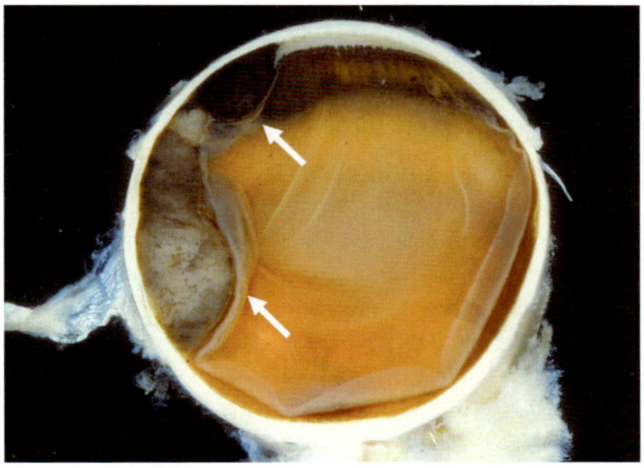

FIGURE 2.54. This enucleation specimen shows a heavily pigmented, solid tumor infiltrating the ciliary body. The tumor infiltrates the left angle, producing secondary glaucoma. Note the dislocation of the lens and the choroidal detachment artifact on the right bottom angle of the image.

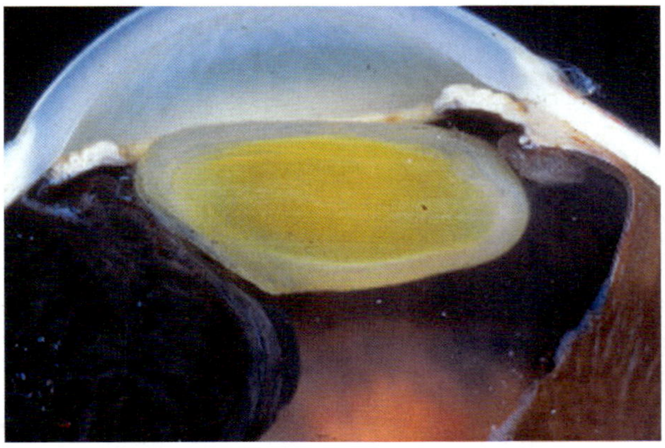

CHOROIDAL MELANOMA

Choroidal melanoma is often asymptomatic and diagnosis is incidental. The tumors may grow beneath the retina, or may break through the Bruch membrane and disrupt the retina. Tumors breaking through the Bruch membrane and disrupting the retina have a characteristic "mushroom" shape.

FIGURE 2.55. This enucleation specimen shows an aphakic eye with a large, solid choroidal tumor. The tumor is heavily pigmented; it shows different shades in some areas. The tumor reaches the ciliary body.

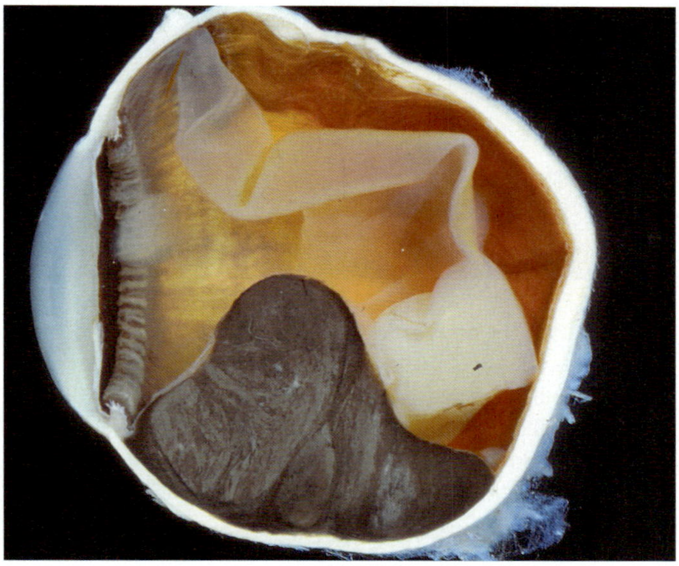

FIGURE 2.56. This enucleation specimen shows a pigmented, dome-shaped choroidal melanoma (arrow) with serous retinal detachment (*). Note the deeply pigmented area in the retina, which corresponds to hyperplastic pigment epithelium proliferation (arrowheads). In general, this proliferation is congenital and not related to the tumor.

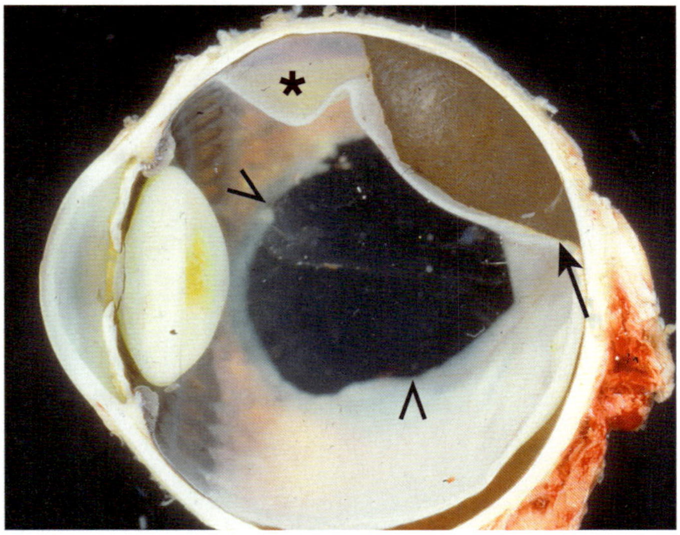

FIGURE 2.57. This enucleation specimen shows a pigmented dome-shaped choroidal melanoma (arrow). The cataractous lens is dislocated (*) and the retina is folded (•).

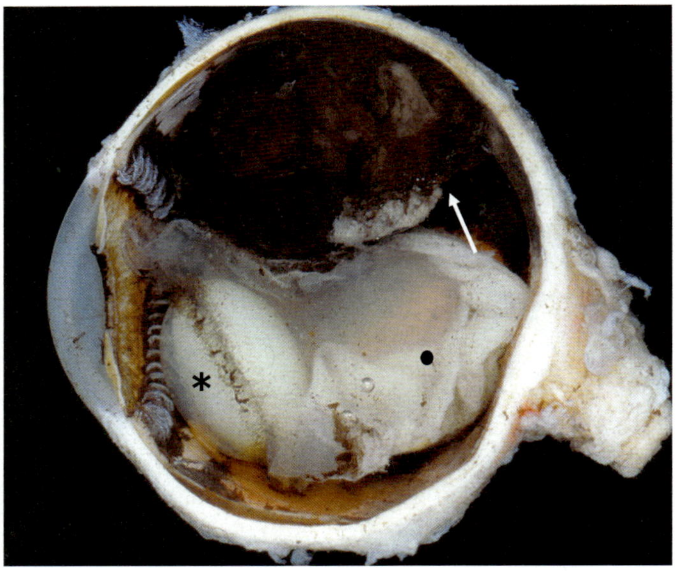

FIGURE 2.58. The enucleation specimen in (A) shows a 2-lobed melanotic (arrow) and amelanotic (arrowhead) tumor in the posterior pole of the eye overlying the optic nerve head. In (B), higher magnification shows the optic nerve head and a feeder tumor vessel (arrow). Necrosis is present in the amelanotic tumor (arrowheads).

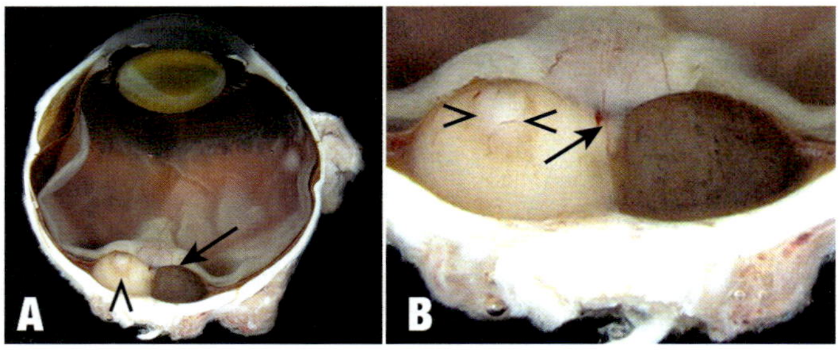

FIGURE 2.59. This enucleation specimen shows an amelanotic, dome-shaped choroidal tumor with several dilated blood vessels. The tumor has not infiltrated the sclera, ciliary body, or optic nerve. Note the retinal detachment next to the tumor (arrow).

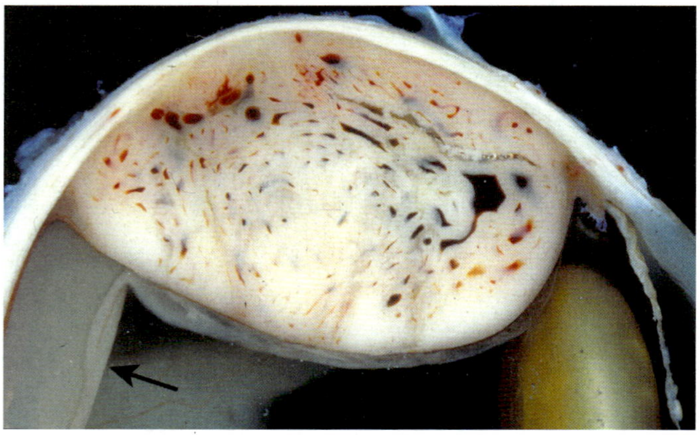

FIGURE 2.60. The enucleation specimen in (A) shows a whitish, nodular choroidal tumor at the posterior pole (*). Note the retinal detachment overlying the tumor. In (B), higher magnification of the same specimen shows the pushing borders of the lesions.

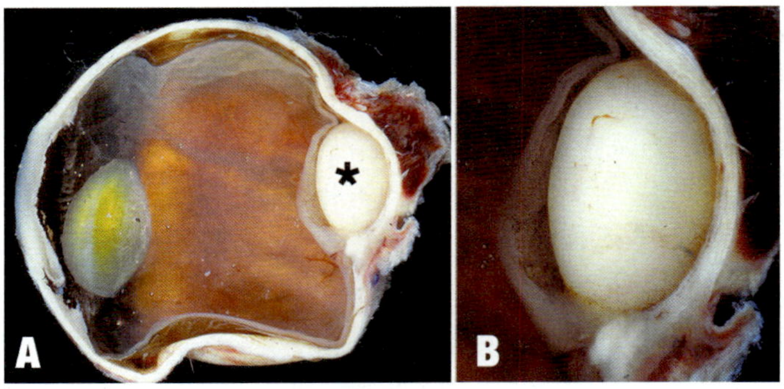

FIGURE 2.61. This enucleation specimen shows a partially pigmented choroidal tumor. The tumor reaches the optic nerve. Note the proteinaceous retinal detachment overlying and adjacent to the tumor (arrows).

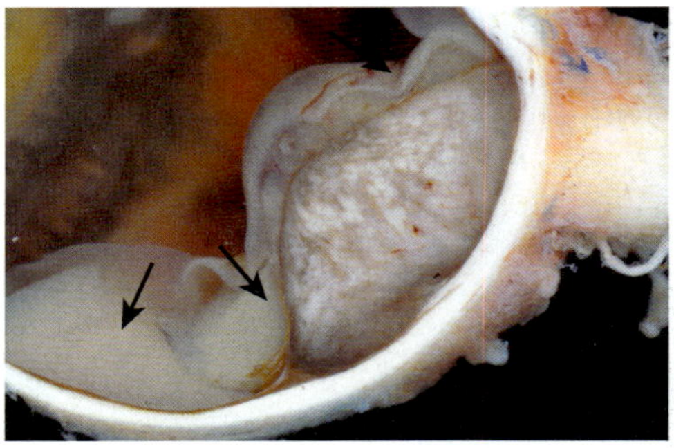

FIGURE 2.62. This enucleation specimen shows a melanotic, dome-shaped choroidal tumor (arrow). There is partial retinal detachment with underlying subretinal fluid in the area opposite the tumor (*) and slight macular edema in the posterior pole (seen in the central area of the image).

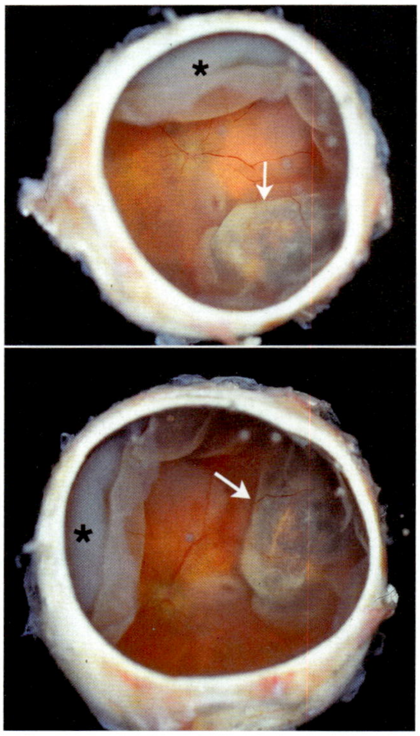

MUSHROOM-SHAPED CHOROIDAL MELANOMA

FIGURE 2.63. The enucleation specimen in (A) shows a diffuse melanoma infiltrating the choroid and ciliary body. In the center, a large area of necrosis and hemorrhage is present (*) and the retina is infiltrated (arrows). Note hypopyon in the anterior chamber and the cataractous lens. The enucleation specimen in (B) shows an amelanotic, mushroom-shaped, slightly hemorrhagic tumor near the optic nerve (arrow). The shape is due to infiltration of the retina by a rupture of the Bruch membrane. A retinal detachment artifact is present.

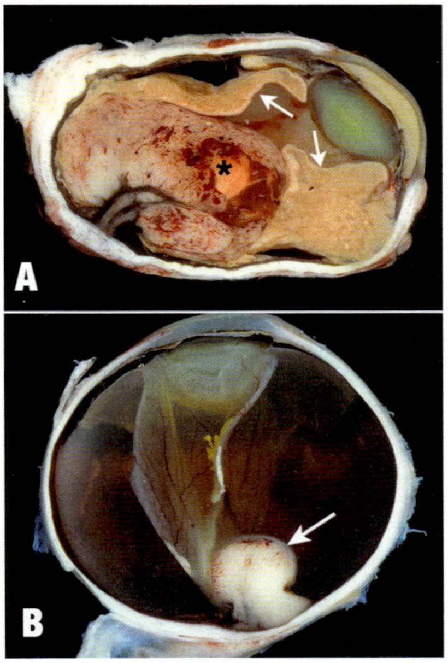

FIGURE 2.64. The enucleation specimen in (A) shows an amelanotic, mushroom-shaped tumor arising from the choroid. Microhemorrhages are present within the tumor and also surround the tumor base (arrow). True retinal detachment is present (arrowhead). The subretinal fluid is mixed: clear (1), hemorrhagic (2), and fibrinoid (3). In (B), higher magnification of the same specimen shows a large amelanotic tumor with large areas of hemorrhage and necrosis. Note the several dilated blood vessels and an adjacent retinal detachment with lipofuscin pigment on its surface (arrow).

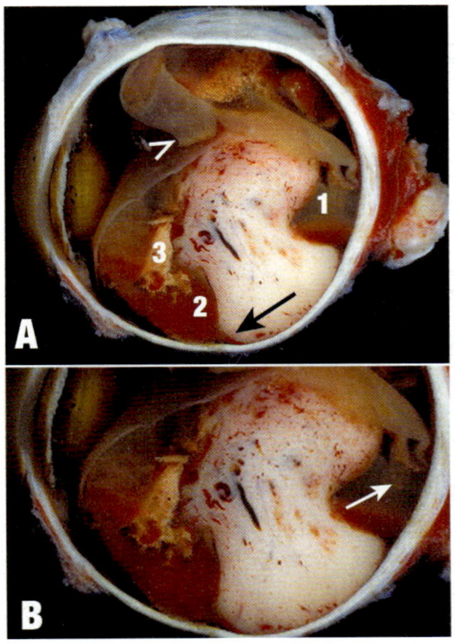

FIGURE 2.65. This enucleation specimen demonstrates an amelanotic, mushroom-shaped, slightly hemorrhagic tumor near the optic nerve (arrow). True retinal detachment is present, and the retina is folded (arrowhead). The subretinal fluid is hazy (*).

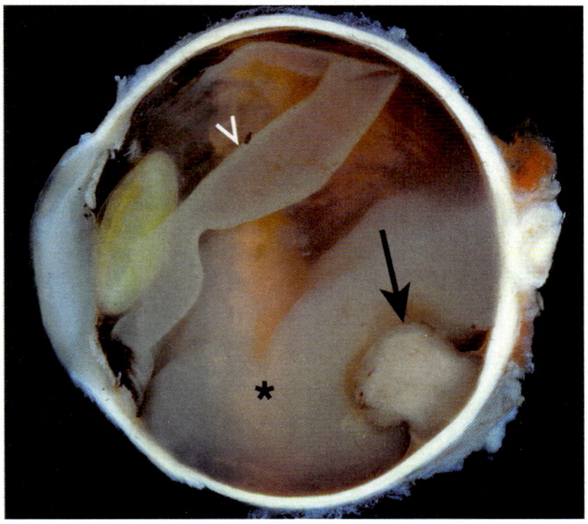

CHOROIDAL MELANOMA WITH EXTRAOCULAR EXTENSION

FIGURE 2.66. This enucleation specimen demonstrates a section of a choroidal melanoma showing an intraocular tumor with an extraocular extension (arrow).

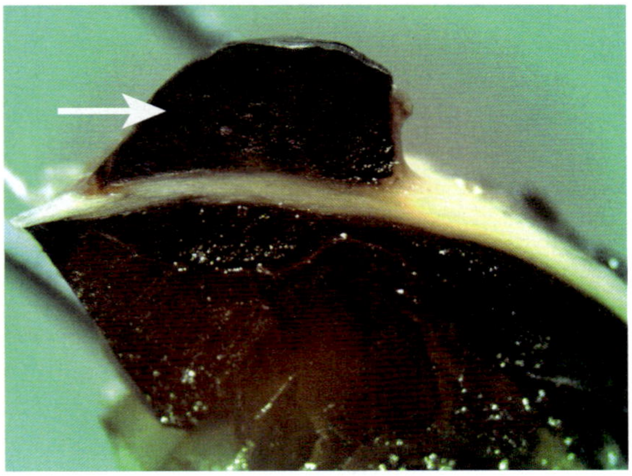

FIGURE 2.67. The diffuse melanoma seen in this enucleation specimen is infiltrating the choroid. Extensive areas of necrosis and hemorrhage are present (arrowhead). The extraocular involvement is large and surrounded by hemorrhage (*). The retina is folded (arrow).

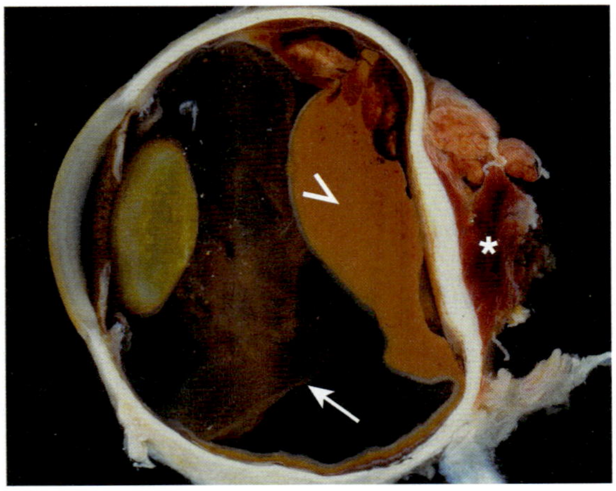

Eyelid

PROCEDURE: SPECIMEN PREPARATION

When a specimen is received, the margins should be painted. The tumor should be cut as illustrated, and the lateral and medial margins are embedded *en face* with the inked surface as the cut surface. The central fragment is embedded with the cut surface on a lateral margin to assess the distance between the tumor and the deep margin.

FIGURE 2.68. This image shows the lateral (1 and 3) and medial (2) margins.

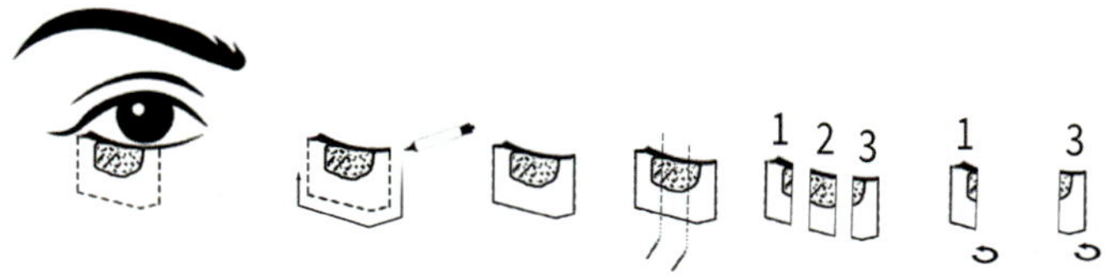

Eyelid Tumors

Epitheloid hemangioma

FIGURE 2.69. This image shows the cut surface of an orbital tumor. The tumor is nonencapsulated, pale yellow in color, and has several areas of hemorrhage and dilated blood vessels.

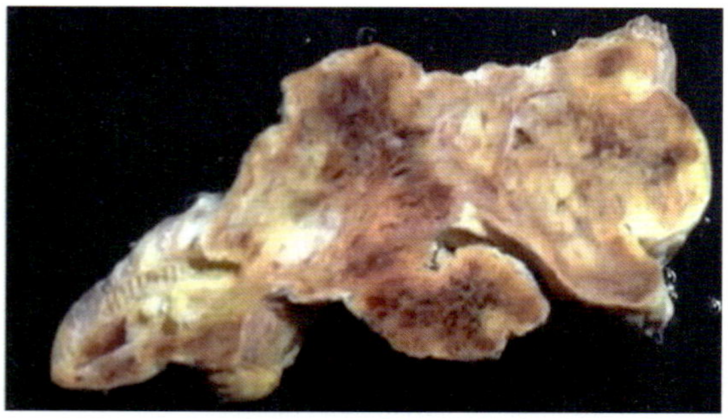

Sebaceous carcinoma

Sebaceous carcinoma is a rare tumor that is frequently misdiagnosed as a chalazion or blepharoconjunctivitis. Misdiagnosis negatively affects prognosis, because sebaceous carcinoma tends to be highly invasive. Look for pagetoid spread of the tumor to the conjunctiva, which is a hallmark of this tumor.

FIGURE 2.70. The exenteration specimen in (A) shows an extensive ulcerated tumor located mostly in the inferior eyelid. In (B), a cross-section of the same specimen shows a whitish tumor involving the inferior and superior eyelids, and the posterior orbit.

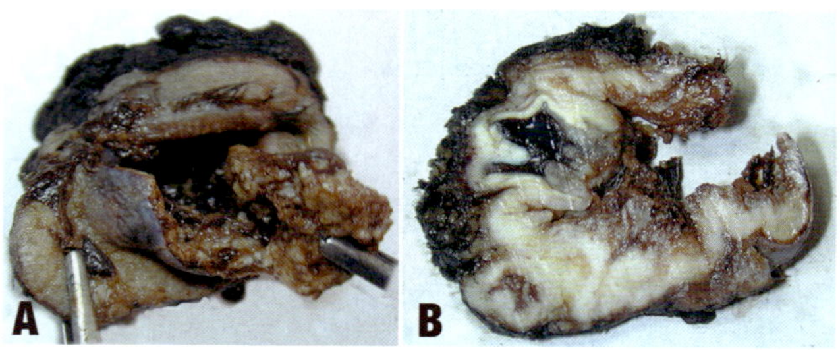

SEBACEOUS CARCINOMA AND SOLITARY EYELID NODULE PRESENTATION

FIGURE 2.71. The conjunctival surface of an eyelid shows a yellowish, slightly nodular tumor extending into the skin surface. The ciliary margin is involved (*).

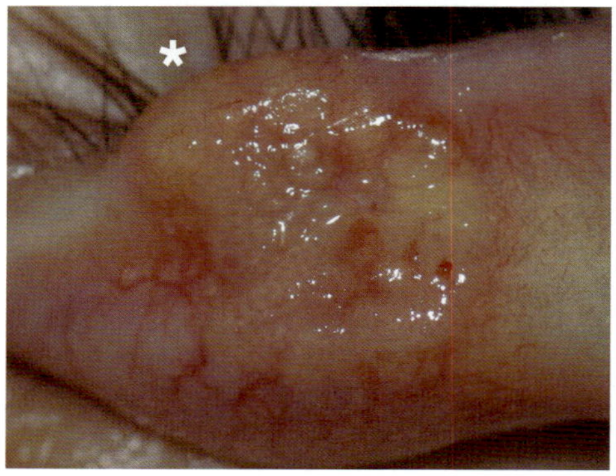

SEBACEOUS CARCINOMA AND DIFFUSE EYELID THICKENING

FIGURE 2.72. This exenteration specimen shows a large, yellowish diffuse tumor invading the periocular fatty tissue of the orbit surrounding the eye (*). The superior and inferior eyelid is thickened by the presence of a whitish tissue (arrows). Cataractous lens and retinal detachment artifacts are also present.

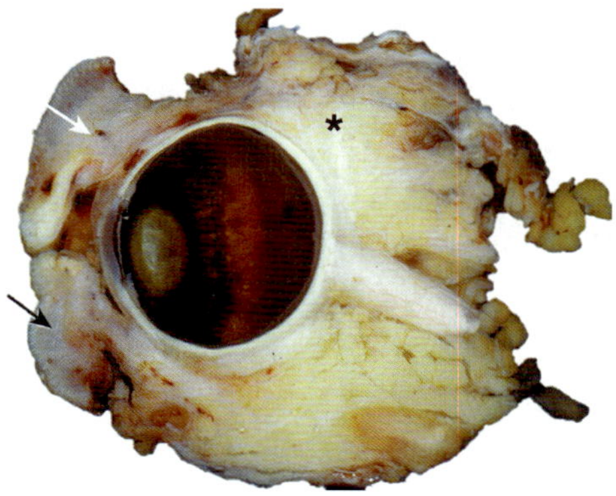

Histiocytoid carcinoma of the eyelid

FIGURE 2.73. Histiocytoid carcinoma is a rare variant of conjunctival carcinoma in which isolated cells with histiocytoid appearance invade the stroma. In this specimen, an extensive, whitish, diffuse, and homogeneous tumor in the superior eyelid extends through the orbit surrounding the eyeball. The tumor is also present in the inferior eyelid.

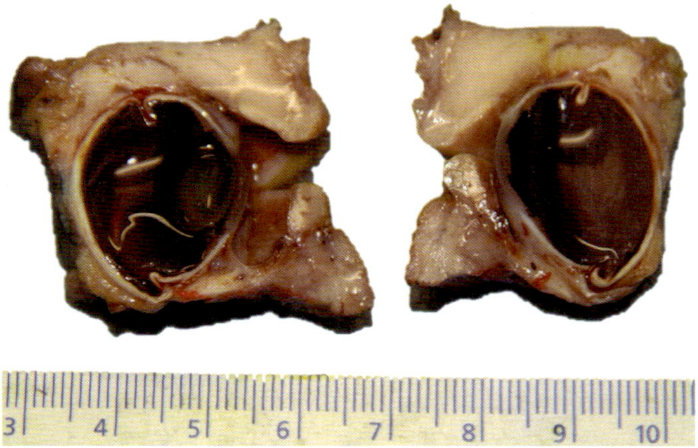

Conjunctival Tumors

Papilloma of the conjunctiva

Papillomas of the conjunctiva are benign tumors arising from the squamous epithelium. They can be sessile or pedunculated.

FIGURE 2.74. In (A), a sessile papilloma shows excretion of the mucosa with a wide implantation base. In (B), a pedunculated papilloma grows in an exophytic manner with a thin fibrovascular stem.

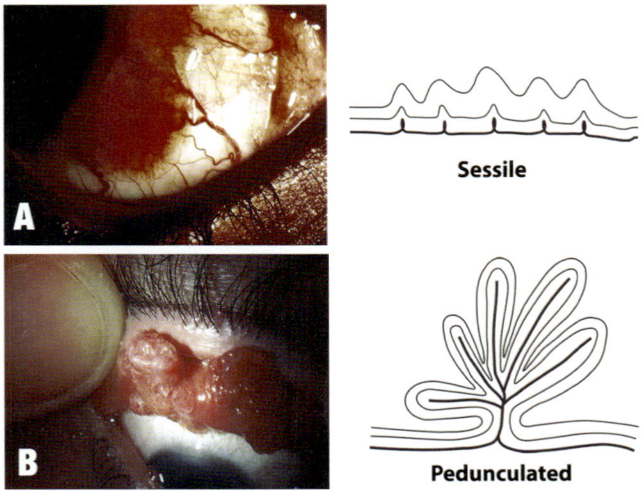

Squamous cell carcinoma of the conjunctiva (SCC)

SCC is the most common conjunctival malignancy. It arises more frequently in the limbal area, has a male predominance, and occurs during the seventh to eighth decades.

FIGURE 2.75. The enucleation specimen in (A) shows a flat, whitish, small tumor in the perilimbal conjunctiva (arrow). Note the yellowish cataractous lens, the hazy vitreous, and the diffuse retinal detachment artifact still attached to the optic nerve head. In (B), magnification of the anterior segment reveals infiltration of the superficial layers of the cornea up to the midline (arrowhead).

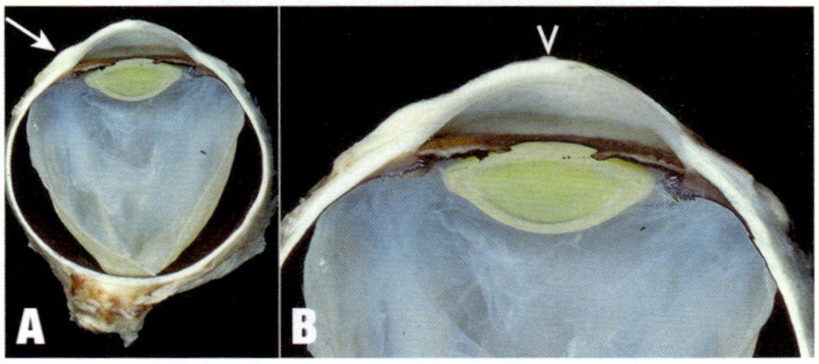

FIGURE 2.76. This enucleation specimen shows a whitish, nodular conjunctival tumor present in the perilimbal conjunctiva (arrow). Note the invasion of the iridocorneal angle, and the hazy aqueous humor (*) and vitreous (•). The lens (arrowhead) is cataractous.

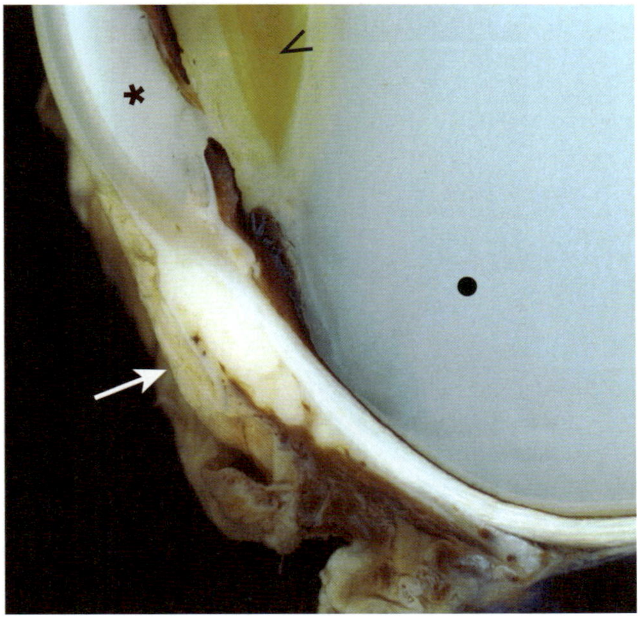

Conjunctival melanoma

Melanomas of the conjunctiva tend to behave much more like cutaneous melanoma than intraocular melanoma. Histopathological analysis of lesions is necessary to differentiate conjunctival melanoma from benign melanocytic lesions of the conjunctiva, such melanosis and nevus.

FIGURE 2.77. In the exenteration specimen in (A), a sagittal cut reveals a 13-mm inferior eyelid tumor infiltrating in the orbit (arrow). At higher magnification in (B), the tumor is amelanotic and has a slightly nodular appearance.

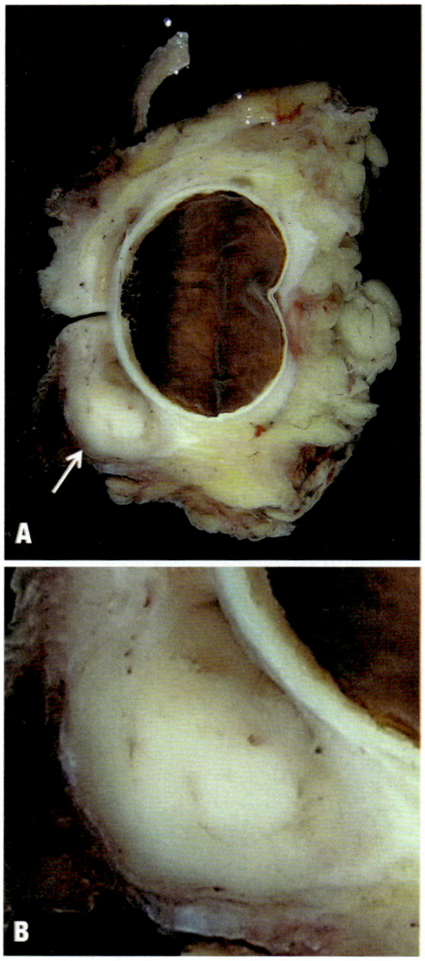

REFERENCES

Eagle RC. *Eye pathology: an atlas and text*. Wolters Kluwer Health; 2012.

Kingman S. Glaucoma is second leading cause of blindness globally. Bulletin of the World Health Organization. 2004;82(11):887-888.

Lavezzo MM, Sakata VM, Morita C, et al. Vogt-Koyanagi-Harada disease: review of a rare autoimmune disease targeting antigens of melanocytes. Orphanet Journ Rare Dis. 2016;11:29-29.

Rivolta C, Sharon D, DeAngelis MM, Dryja TP. Retinitis pigmentosa and allied diseases: numerous diseases, genes, and inheritance patterns. Hum Molec Genet. 2002;11(10):1219-1227.

Roberts F, Thum CK. *Lee's ophthalmic histopathology*. 3rd ed. London: Springer-Verlag London; 2014.

Singh AD, Damato BE, Pe'er J, Murphree AL, Perry J, editors. *Clinical ophthalmic oncology*. Edinburgh: W.B. Saunders; 2007.

3

Diseases of the Ear, Nose, Throat, and Related Structures

DERIN CAGLAR, HUI JUN WANG, JULIE GUILMETTE

Ear

Squamous cell carcinoma (SCC)

SCC is the most common type of cancer of the outer ear. Other types include basal cell carcinoma and melanoma. High-risk factors for cutaneous SCC include location on the ear, depth of invasion, primary ear site, perineural invasion, and poorly differentiated, sarcomatoid, or undifferentiated tumors.

FIGURE 3.1. This resected specimen shows an ulcerating mass on a background of sun-damaged skin. The mass occupies the triangular fossa and scaphoid fossa, and involves the helix and concha.

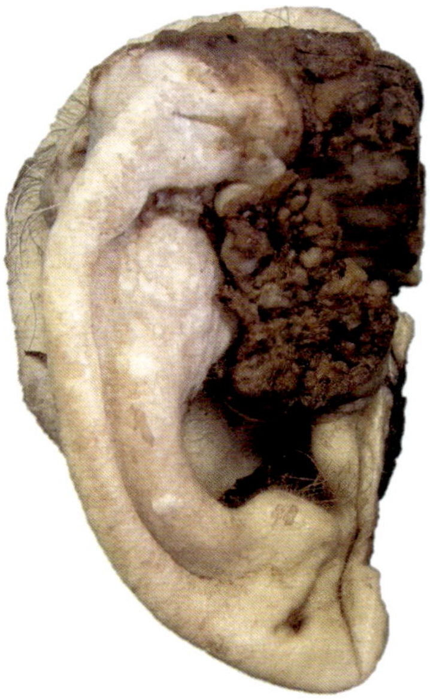

PROCEDURE: STAGING SCC

The staging system for cancers of the outer ear is the same as for skin cancer.

FIGURE 3.2. This image shows an example of a T2 tumor involving the helix and antihelix. T2 tumors are > 2 cm and < 4 cm at their greatest dimension.

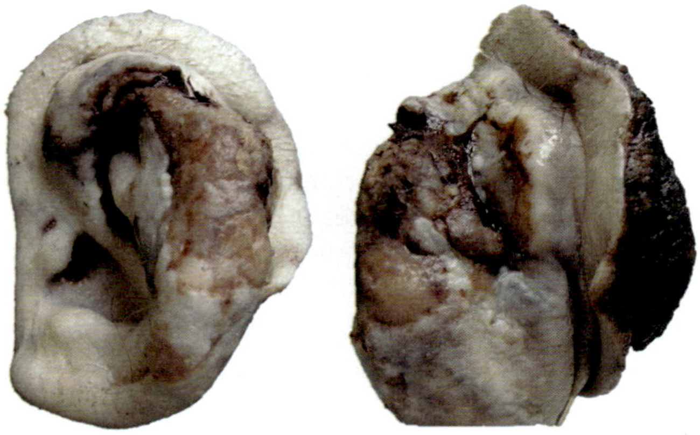

ULCERATING SCC

FIGURE 3.3. The ulcerating tumor in (A) occupies the acoustic meatus, concha, antihelix, antitragus, and tragus. It has destroyed ear cartilage and invaded the external auditory canal. In (B), serial sections show a white, fleshy tumor with fungating and endophytic invasive growth patterns.

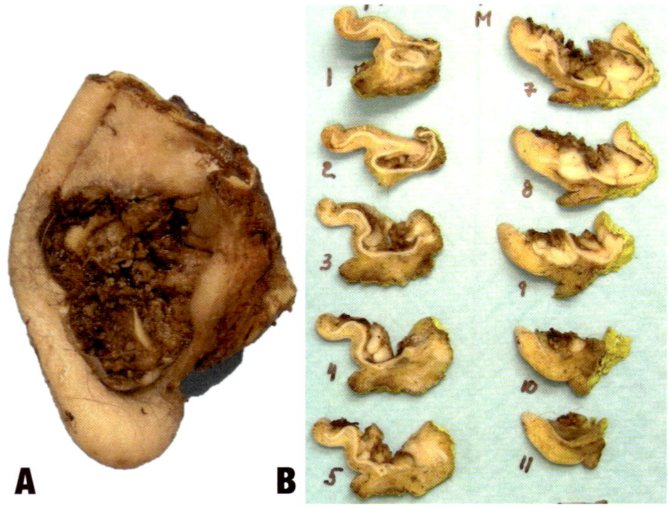

Nose

Sinonasal inflammatory polyp

Sinonasal inflammatory polyps have multifactorial etiology including allergy, infection, aspirin hypersensitivity, asthma, cystic fibrosis, and diabetes that results in lamina propria expansion filled by fluid, protein, and fibrosis. These polyps commonly occur in nose and paranasal sinuses, and are most often seen in adults older than age 20, with the exception of patients with cystic fibrosis who develop them in their first and second decades. Patients present with rhinorrhea, nasal stuffiness, obstruction, and headache. The treatment is conservative endoscopic removal.

FIGURE 3.4. In (A), an endoscopic view shows a pedunculated edematous polyp with visible fine vessels on the surface. In (B), the resected polyp shows a characteristic "teardrop" appearance.

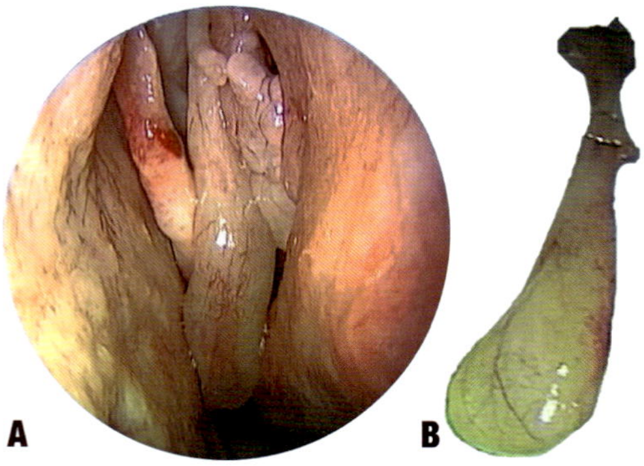

Specimen B courtesy of Dr. Marc Tewfik

Antrochoanal polyp

Antrochoanal polyps represent 4% to 6% of nasal polyps and are frequently seen in children. They arise from the wall of the maxillary antrum, extending through the large primary or secondary maxillary ostium into the nasal cavity. They usually have a long, narrow stalk with a firm, fibrous body. Histologically, these polyps have fewer glands and less inflammation than inflammatory polyps. Prominent eosinophils occur in 20% of antrochoanal polyps.

FIGURE 3.5. This endoscopy shows a fibrous polyp with a stalk connected to the wall of the maxillary antrum.

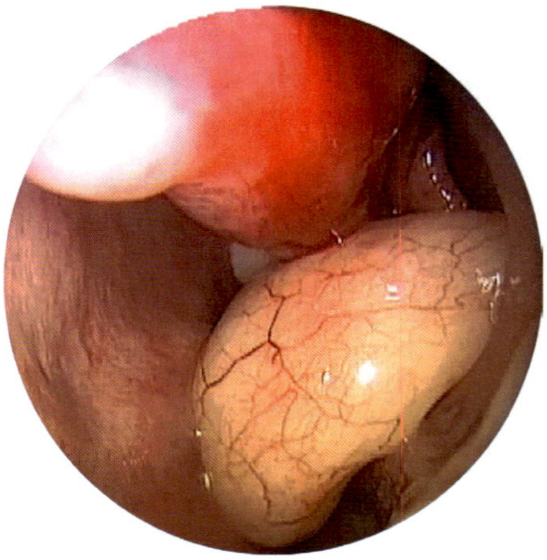

Courtesy of Dr. Marc Tewfik

Fungus ball

A fungus ball is a mass formed by continuous growth of fungal organisms in a sinus, usually the maxillary sinus. Special stains for fungal organisms show tightly packed fungal hyphae.

FIGURE 3.6. This image shows an endoscopic view of a fungus ball resembling gelatinous peanut butter.

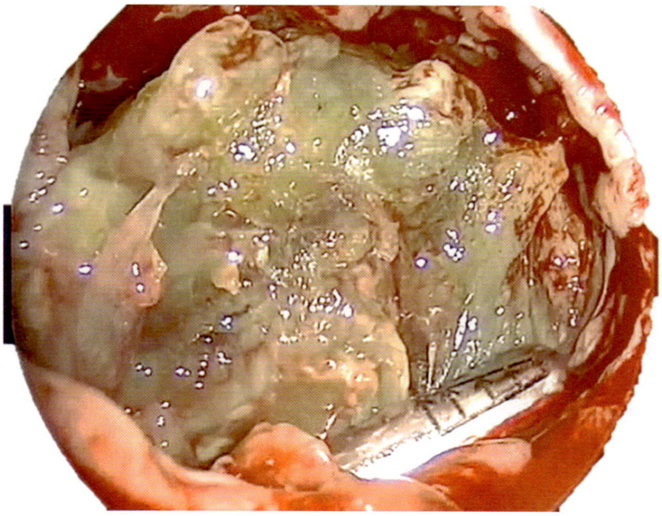

Courtesy of Dr. Marc Tewfik

Inverting sinonasal papilloma

Inverting sinonasal papillomas show a downward growth pattern and arise from the lateral nasal wall in older age groups. In younger adults, an exophytic type commonly arises from the nasal septum. Mixed inverting and exophytic patterns are not uncommon. They have the potential to grow locally into adjacent structures.

FIGURE 3.7. This endoscopic view shows a large papilloma. In contrast to nasal polyps, the lesion does not have a stalk. Microscopic examination showed an inverting papilloma.

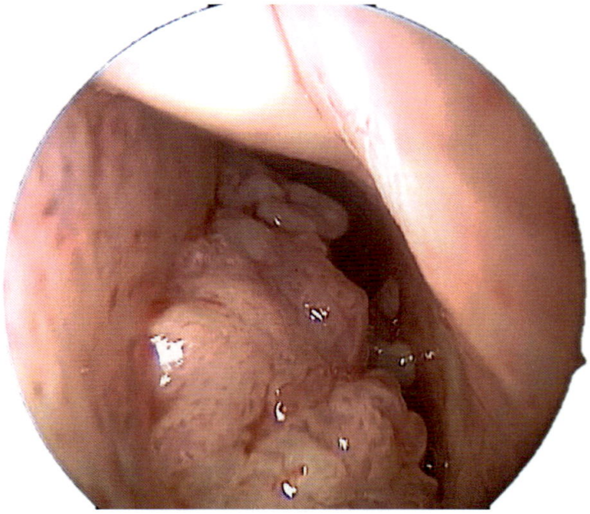

Courtesy of Dr. Marc Tewfik

Juvenile angiofibroma

Angiofibroma is a highly cellular and vascularized benign mesenchymal tumor that can be locally aggressive. It is exclusively seen in males, often in teenagers and young adults.

FIGURE 3.8. An endoscopic view (A) shows an oval, beefy-red mass. The red color and spongy consistency are due to rich blood supply. Image (B) shows a juvenile angiofibroma postembolization. The whitish discoloration corresponds to ischemic necrosis.

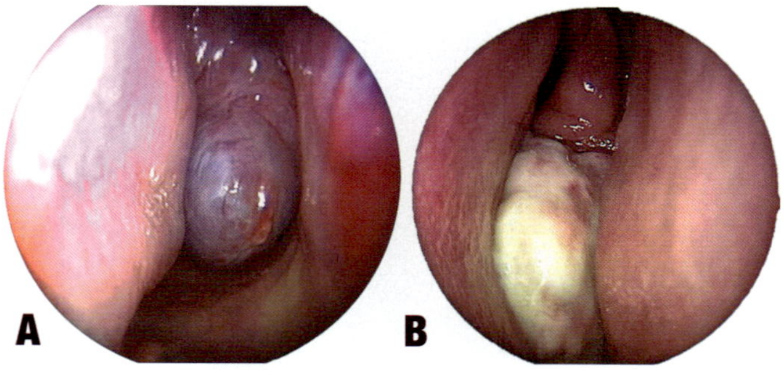

A and B courtesy of Dr. Marc Tewfik

Squamous cell carcinoma (SCC)

SCC is the most common malignant neoplasm found in the lateral nasal wall, nasal septa, and sinonasal tract. The prognosis is better for tumors arising from the nose than those in the paranasal sinuses. Tumors found in the paranasal sinuses are associated with higher recurrence, frequent extension to the cranial vault, and metastasis to cervical lymph nodes.

FIGURE 3.9. In (A), inferior views show a polypoid tumor protruding from the right nasal vestibule. In (B), an anterior-posterior view shows a large fleshy tumor completely obstructing the nasal cavity and invading the nasal cartilage.

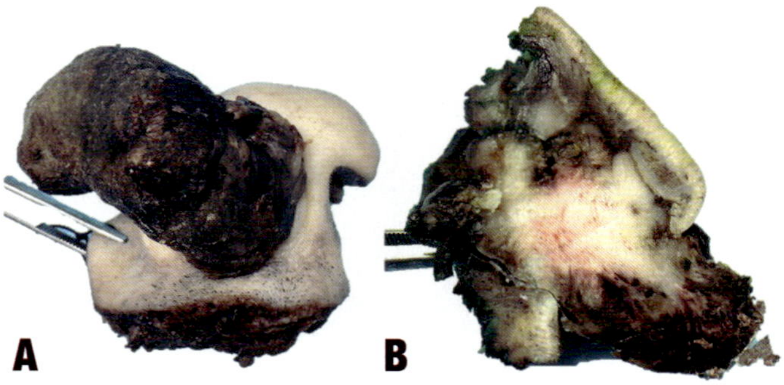

NASAL MUCOSA SCC

FIGURE 3.10. This image shows a nasal mucosa SCC invading the nasal cartilage.

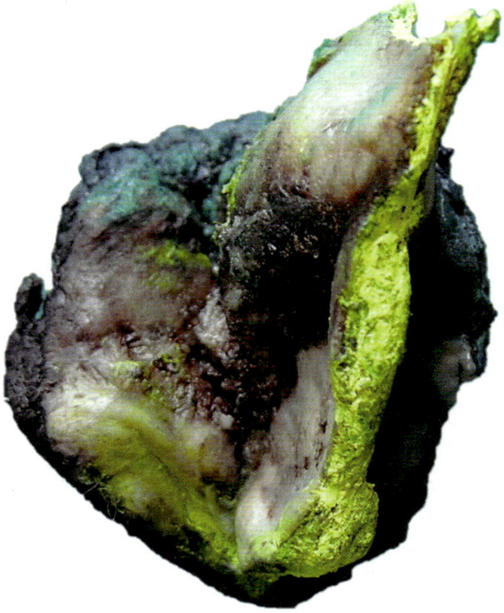

Rhinoscleroma

Rhinoscleroma is a chronic granulomatous inflammation of the upper respiratory tract caused by *Klebsiella rhinoscleromatis*. It occurs more frequently in lower socioeconomic classes. Silver stain can be used to identify the gram-negative bacteria within macrophages (Mikulicz cells).

FIGURE 3.11. The overall size of this nodular nasal mass was > 10 cm, causing significant facial deformity. The mass was removed in multiple pieces. Image (A) shows a piece of the rhinoscleroma at proliferative stage. Image (B) shows characteristic yellow cut surfaces.

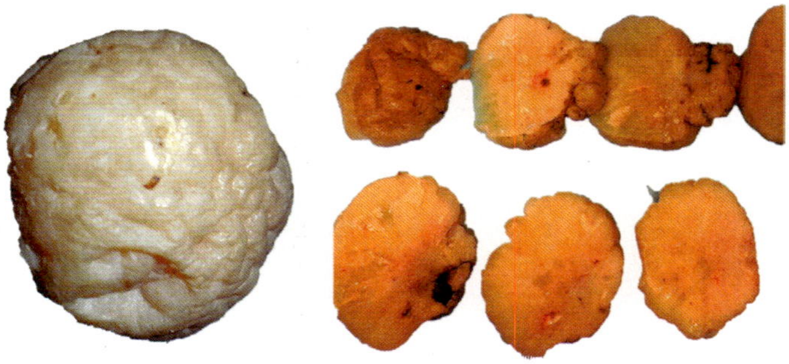

Salivary Gland

Pleomorphic adenoma

Pleomorphic adenoma is the most common type of salivary gland tumor and the most common tumor of the parotid gland. Histologically, it is characterized by proliferation of glandular cells and myoepithelial cells that typically melt into chondroid, chondromyxoid, or myxoid stroma.

FIGURE 3.12. This resected parotid gland tumor shows a characteristic gelatinous, chondroid, gritty cut surface.

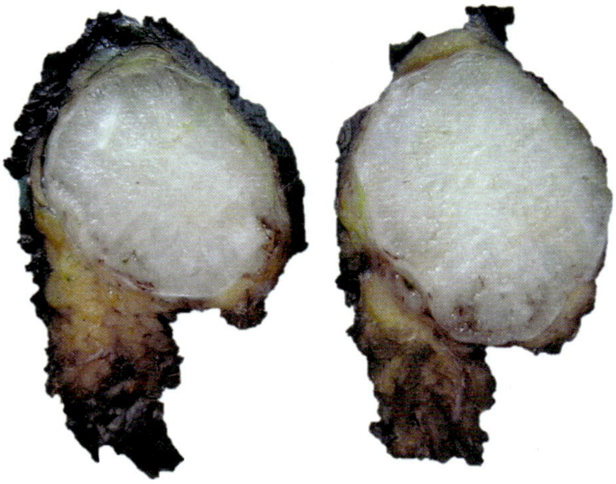

INFARCTION AND MALIGNANT TRANSFORMATION

Pleomorphic adenomas can undergo infarction or malignant transformation. The most common carcinomas arising from pleomorphic adenomas are adenocarcinomas (not otherwise specified) and salivary duct carcinomas.

FIGURE 3.13. This resected tumor shows predominant gelatinous cut surfaces that are consistent with myxoid, stroma-rich, pleomorphic adenoma. The center part of the tumor appears infarcted.

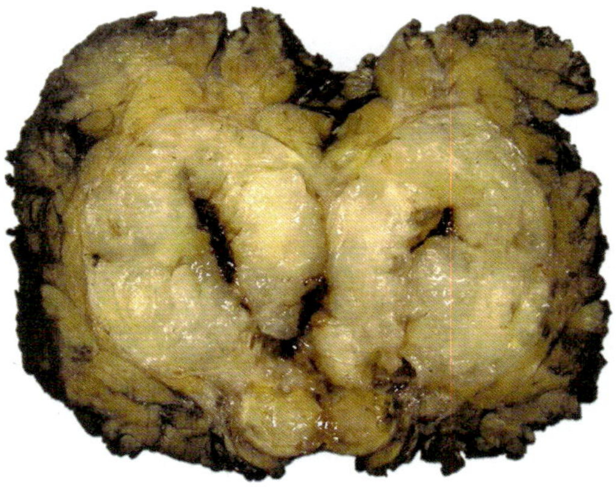

CELLULAR PLEOMORPHIC ADENOMA

Detection of early carcinoma ex pleomorphic adenoma requires thorough sampling and careful microscopic examination. The cut surfaces of cellular pleomorphic adenomas are firmer than hypocellular types. They lack histologic features of malignancy, such as significant cytological atypia, atypical mitosis, tumor necrosis, and invasion. Cellular pleomorphic adenomas can pose diagnostic difficulties on fine needle aspiration cytology examination.

FIGURE 3.14. This resected tumor appears firmer than usual pleomorphic adenomas and has a dense, tan-white cut surface.

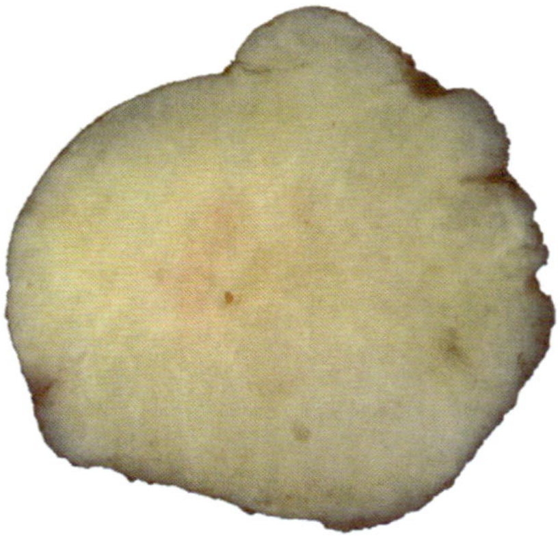

Warthin tumor

Warthin tumor is the second most common benign tumor of the major salivary glands. It is strongly associated with cigarette smoking and can be bilateral. Histologically, it is composed of cystic cavities and papillary structures lined by bilayer epithelium (inner oncocytic, outer basaloid cells) and mature lymphoid stroma.

FIGURE 3.15. The cut surfaces of this resected tumor show an encapsulated, tan-brown mass containing multiple cysts (cyst fluid has solidified after formalin fixation).

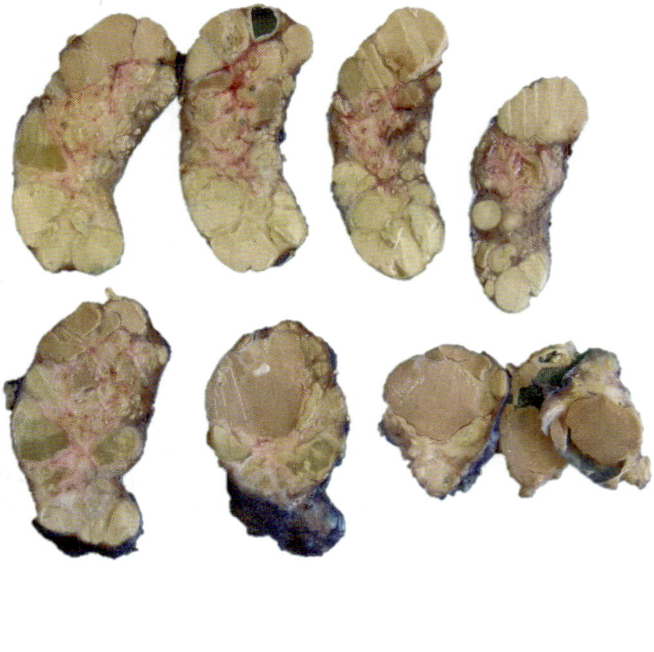

Oncocytoma

Oncocytomas are rare, benign, well-circumscribed tumors exclusively composed of oncocytes, and are usually found in patients in their fifth and seventh decades of life. Malignant transformation is rare. Oncocytomas are susceptible to central hemorrhage and infarction.

FIGURE 3.16. This specimen illustrates the typical mahogany brown cut surface of oncocytoma. Focal cystic change is visible.

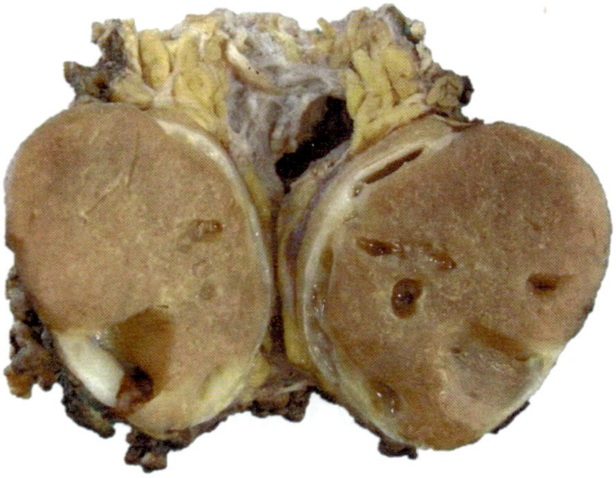

FIGURE 3.17. This freshly resected oncocytoma of the parotid gland shows a typical homogeneous, solid, and light brown tumor.

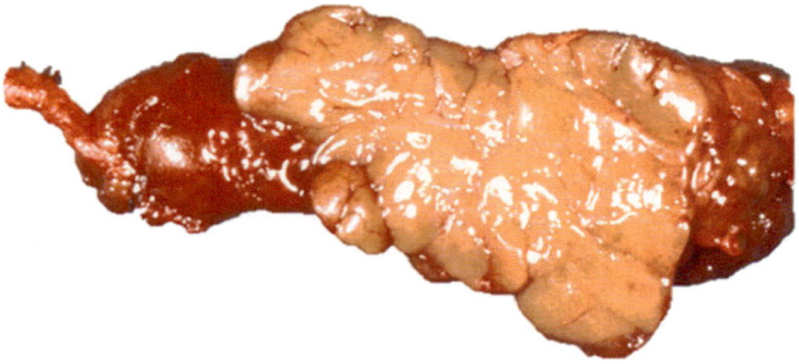

FIGURE 3.18. These images show an oncocytoma with central hemorrhage and infarction.

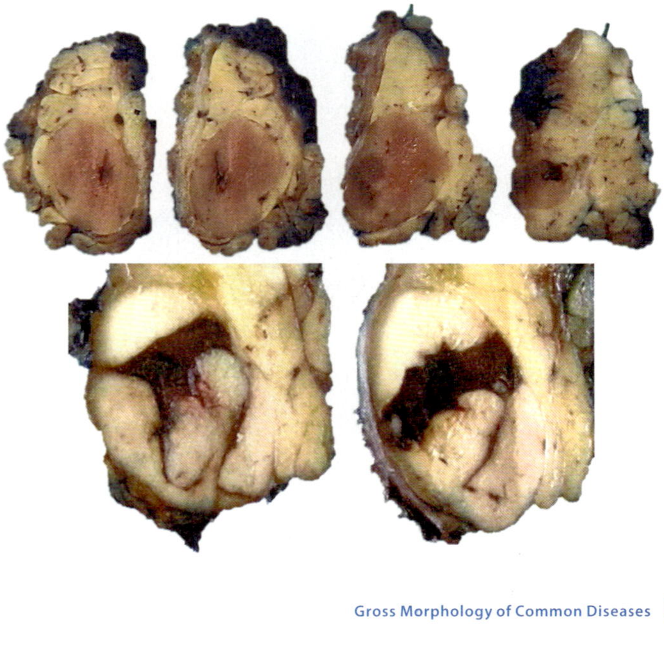

Myoepithelioma

Myoepitheliomas are rare, benign salivary gland tumors composed entirely of myoepithelial cells. They are commonly seen in patients in their third or fourth decade, and have no sex predilection. The most common site of involvement is the parotid gland, followed by the palate.

FIGURE 3.19. This resected specimen shows an encapsulated tumor with a characteristic tan-yellow cut surface.

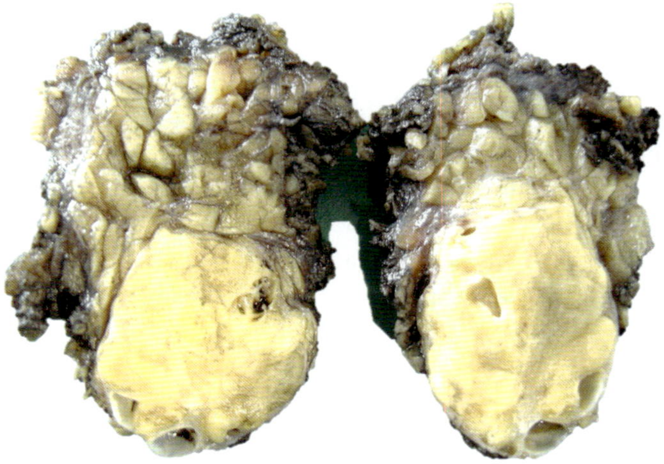

Salivary Gland Cancers

Mucoepidermoid carcinoma (MEC)

MEC is considered the most common malignant tumor of the major and minor salivary glands. Histologically, it consists of a mixture of mucus-secreting cells, squamous cells, and intermediate-type cells.

FIGURE 3.20. This MEC is located in the submucosa of the soft palate (arrows) without involvement of the overlying mucosa tissue. Low-grade tumors are often < 2 cm in their greatest dimension.

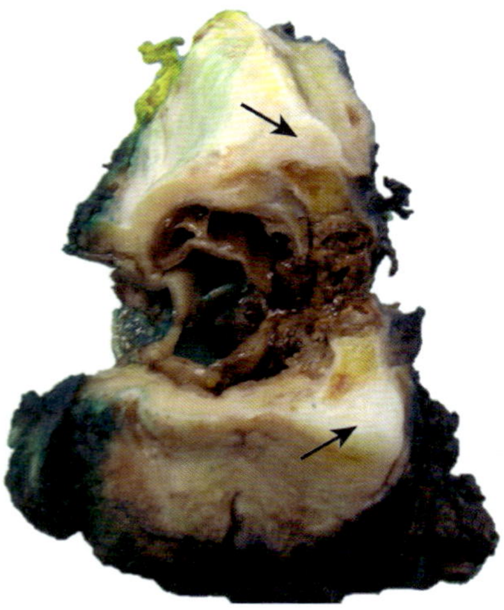

Adenoid cystic carcinoma (ACC)

ACC is a malignant neoplasm that mostly involves the major and minor salivary glands of the head and neck. Other sites of origin include the trachea, lacrimal gland, breast, skin, and vulva. ACC is slow growing with frequent perineural invasion and a rate of distant metastasis (to lung, bone, brain, liver) of more than 50% in late stages.

FIGURE 3.21. This resected tumor of the tongue demonstrates a gray-white, firm cut surface (arrows). This tumor did not show necrosis. (Presence of necrosis indicates high-grade transformation.)

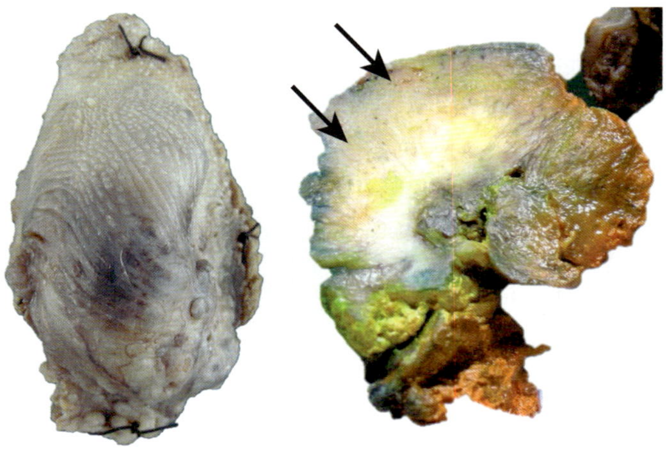

Clear cell carcinoma (CCC)

CCC is a low-grade salivary gland carcinoma most frequently arising from the intraoral salivary glands.

FIGURE 3.22. The cut surfaces of this resected tumor of the soft palate appear gray-white and solid.

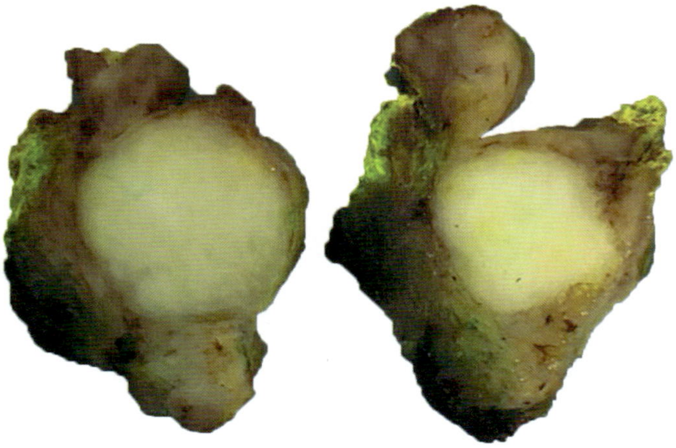

Acinic cell carcinoma

Acinic cell carcinoma represents 2% of all salivary tumors and is commonly found in the parotid gland.

FIGURE 3.23. This resected parotid-gland tumor is pseudoencapsulated, and shows necrosis and hemorrhage.

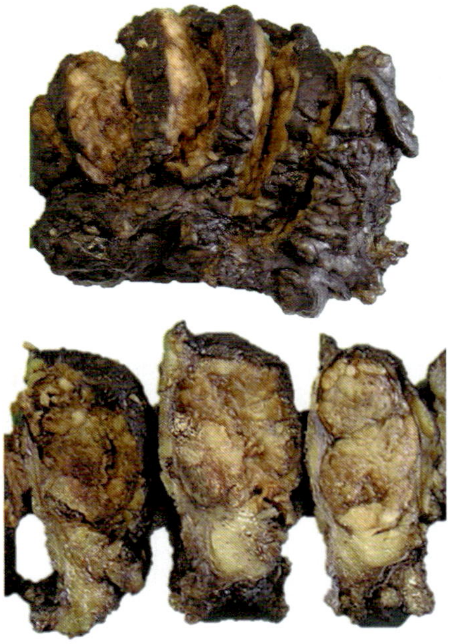

Primary lymphoepithelial-like carcinoma

This rare tumor shows strong predilection for people of Inuit and Southeast Asian decent, and is associated with Epstein–Barr virus (EBV). Parotid and submandibular glands are the most commonly affected salivary glands.

FIGURE 3.24. This image shows the cut surface of a parotid gland containing a poorly demarcated, fleshy tumor.

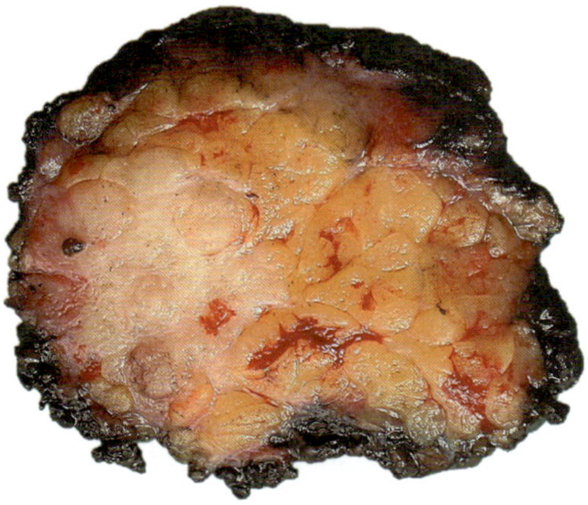

Epithelial-myoepithelial carcinoma (EMC)

EMC is a rare, low-grade malignant tumor that commonly occurs in the parotid gland.

FIGURE 3.25. This resected tumor of the parotid gland shows nodular protrusions (indicating invasive growth) and a fibrous pseudocapsule. Histologically, it consisted of distinct malignant epithelial and myoepithelial components.

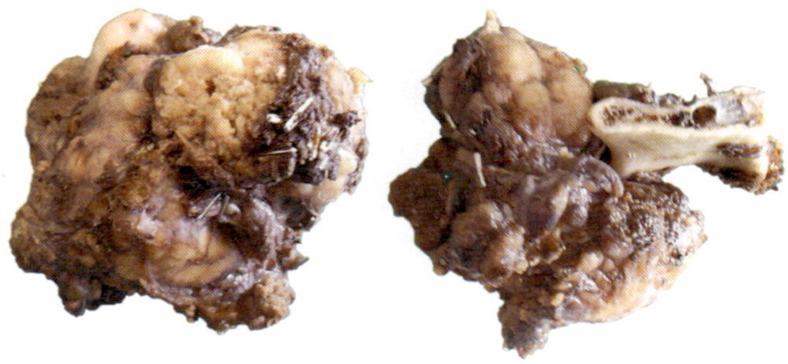

Merkel cell carcinoma

Merkel cell carcinoma is a neuroendocrine carcinoma of the skin with a predilection for the head-and-neck region, extremities, and buttocks. The location of this tumor on the head and neck is associated with frequent nodal metastasis.

FIGURE 3.26. This image shows dome-shaped nodular lesions with purple tinge, which is typical of Merkel cell carcinoma. The recurrent tumor in this image had deep extension into the parotid gland.

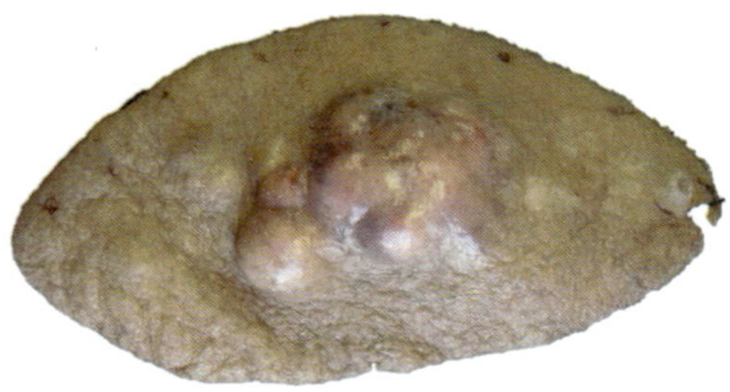

Oral Cavity

Nonneoplastic Diseases and Benign Neoplasms of the Oral Cavity

Leukoplakia

Leukoplakia is a clinical term. Histologically, leukoplakia is hyperkeratosis with or without dysplasia. Lesions > 4 cm are associated with malignant transformation and should be extensively sampled to rule out invasive carcinoma. The presence of firm nodules or unhealed ulcers should alert clinicians to the possibility of malignancy.

FIGURE 3.27. These resected specimens show characteristic irregularly shaped white patches with focal nodular appearance.

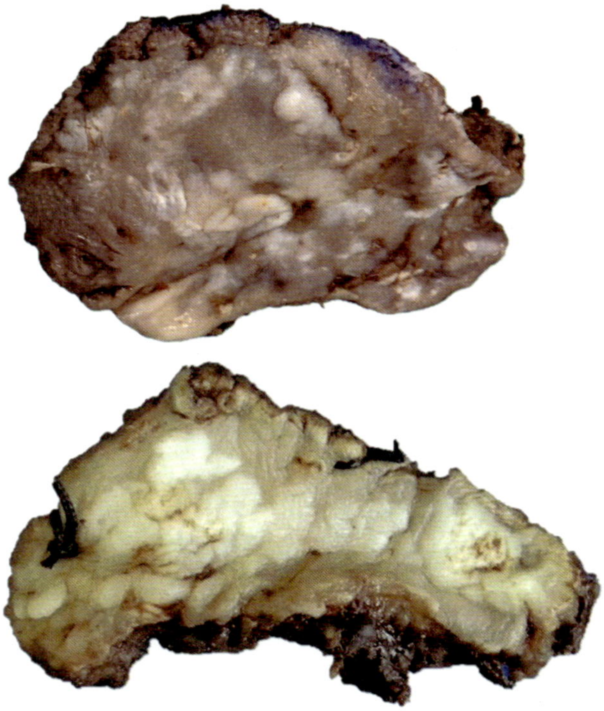

Odontogenic keratocyst

This type of tumor may present as a sporadic tumor, or it may be associated with nevoid basal cell carcinoma syndrome (also called Gorlin syndrome). The sporadic form usually occurs as a solitary lesion that develops in the second or third decade of life. Patients with Gorlin syndrome exhibit multiple lesions that generally occur at a younger age. The most common site for odontogenic keratocyst is the posterior mandible.

FIGURE 3.28. This posterior mandible is irregularly thickened by an odontogenic keratocyst (arrow).

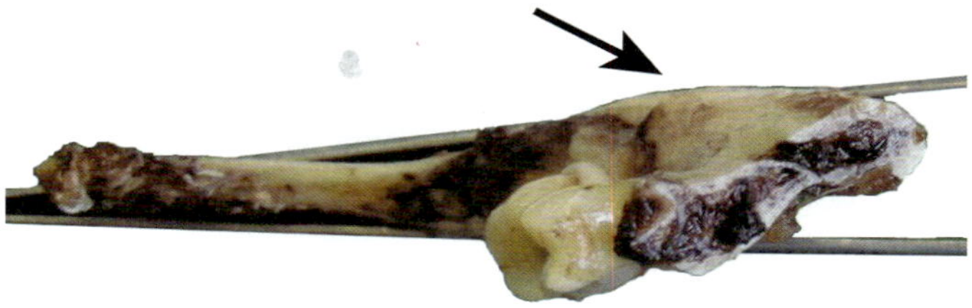

FIGURE 3.29. This image shows a distorted mandible secondary to an intraosseous odontogenic keratocyst.

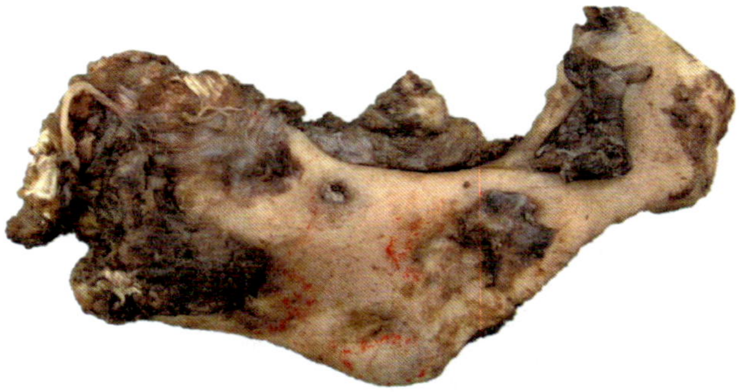

Ameloblastoma

Ameloblastoma is a benign, locally aggressive tumor of the odontogenic epithelium. It is commonly found in the mandible, especially the posterior mandible. Due to high recurrence rates (25% to 35% of cases recur), wide local excision is recommended. Grossly, the tumor can be solid or multicystic, intraosseous or extraosseous.

FIGURE 3.30. This resected tumor shows multicystic intraosseous growth.

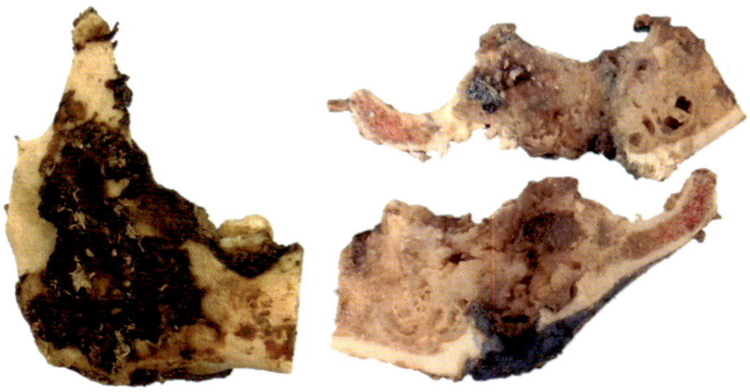

FIGURE 3.31. This ameloblastoma shows a cystic mass with a solid component.

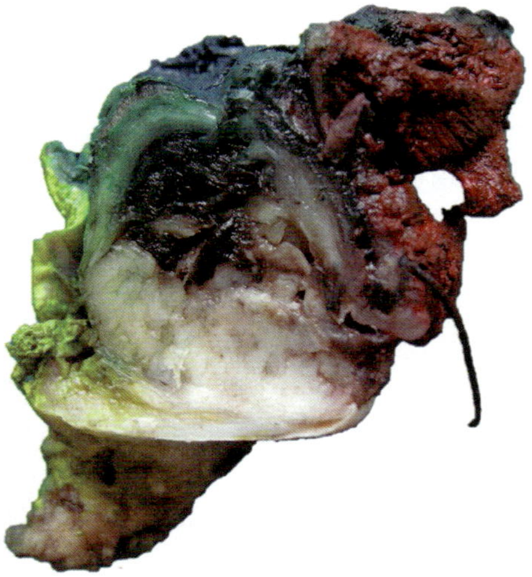

UNICYSTIC AMELOBLASTOMA

The unicystic variant of ameloblastoma is usually found in the third molar and is associated with an unerupted tooth.

FIGURE 3.32. This image shows a largely cystic mass from the mandible with a minor solid component.

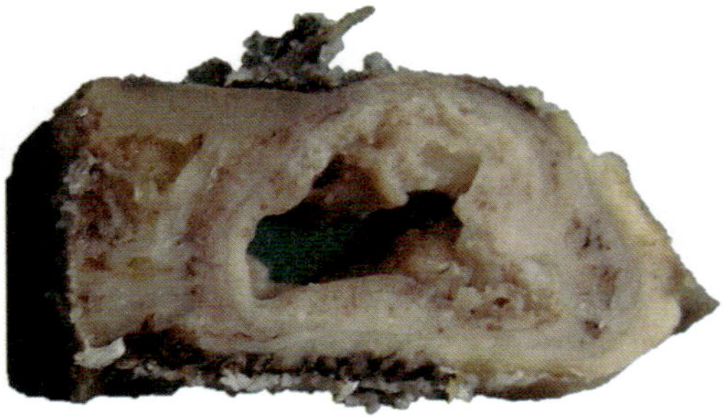

Gingival cysts

Gingival cysts are benign cysts lined by the odontogenic epithelium. They can occur in middle-aged adults as solitary cysts on the gingiva, or in newborn babies as white papules on the gingiva.

FIGURE 3.33. Image (A) shows a solitary cyst on the gingiva of a middle-aged adult. Image (B) shows white gingival papules in a newborn baby.

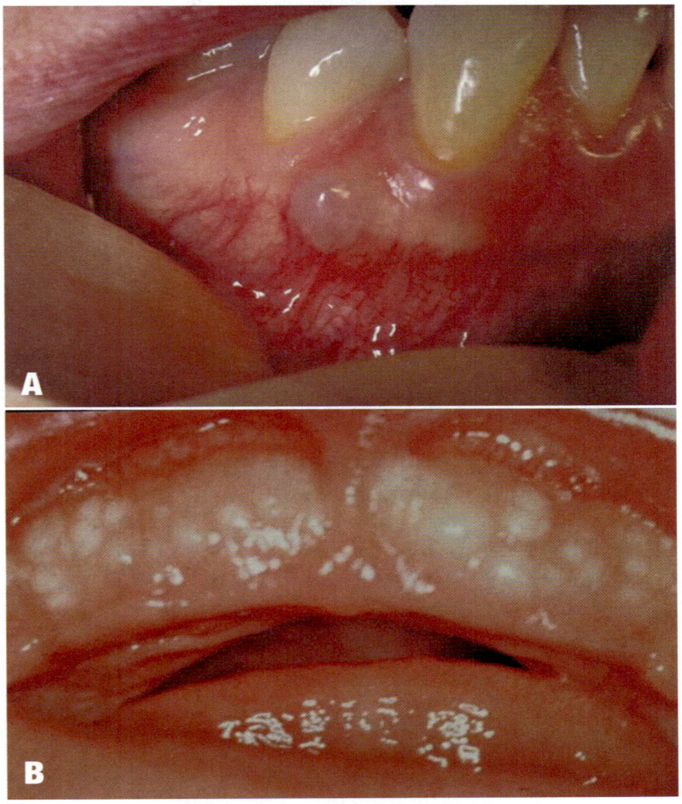

Cancers of the Oral Cavity

Squamous cell carcinoma (SCC)

SCC accounts for approximately 95% of all oral cavity malignancies. Tumor thickness should be measured by microscopy and correlated with macroscopic findings. Fifty percent of oral SCC occurs in the tongue. Risk factors for SCC include tobacco use, alcohol consumption, radiation, immunosuppression, and betel nut chewing. Submucosal spread is common and contributes to higher SCC recurrence rates in the oral cavity.

FIGURE 3.34. This superficially invasive SCC from the lateral side of the tongue is centrally depressed with slightly raised borders.

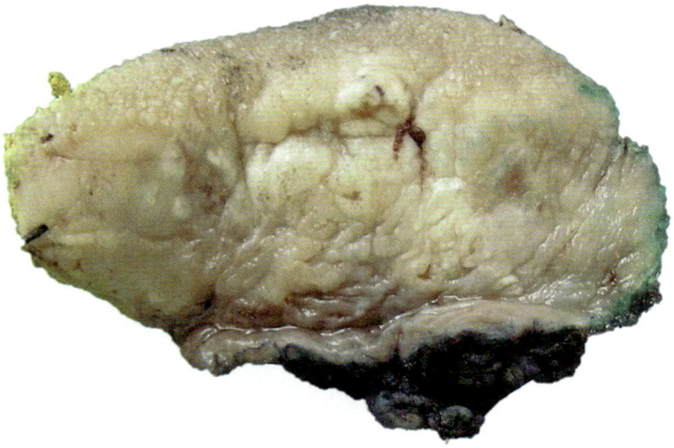

FIGURE 3.35. This centrally ulcerated tumor of the lateral tongue shows an endophytic growth pattern. The tumor size is larger on cut surfaces than the mucosal lesion, which is a common phenomenon in oral SCC.

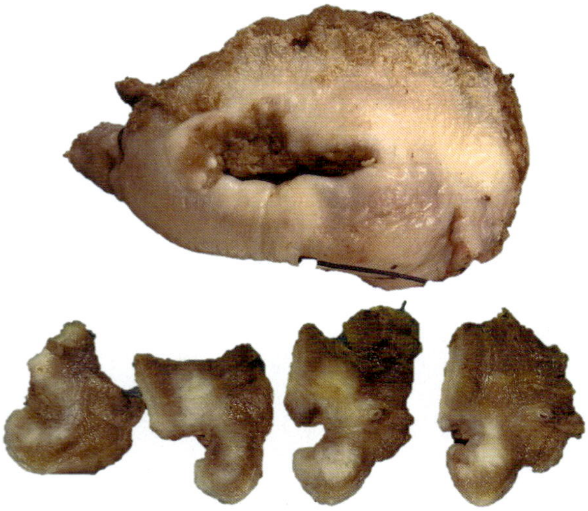

FIGURE 3.36. This image shows an endophytic SCC of the tongue. Note the whitish color of the tumor in contrast to the brownish nonneoplastic tissue. In this type of case, the tumor-size measurement will be more accurate when measured from the cut surface.

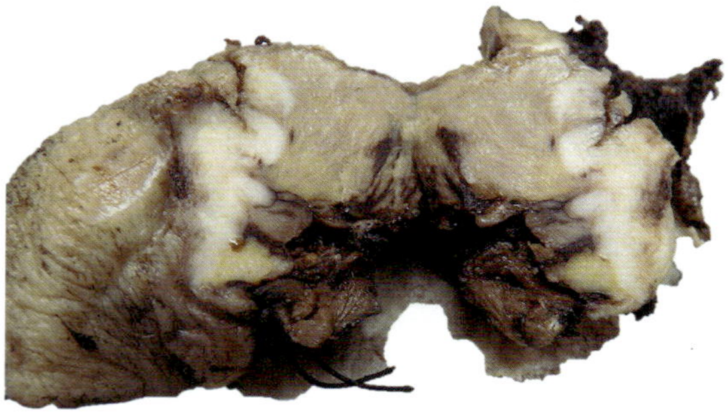

RETROMOLAR SCC

Retromolar tumors are often diagnosed at a later stage due to nonspecific symptoms and close proximity to bone.

FIGURE 3.37. This image shows an ulcerated endophytic retromolar SCC. This case presented as an ulcer in the retromolar region.

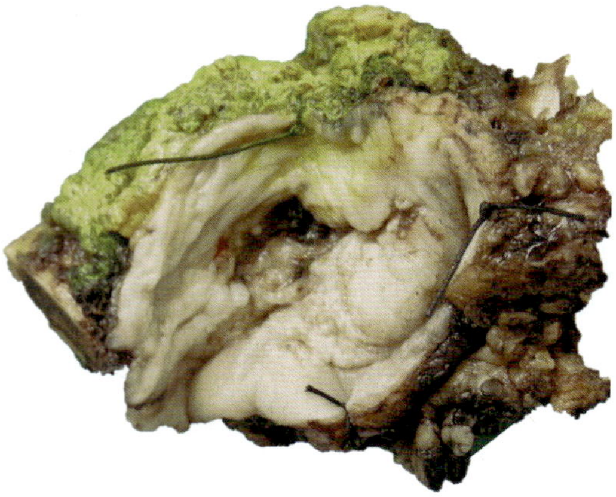

EXOPHYTIC SCC

Exophytic SCC is noticeable on clinical examination, which may facilitate early detection. Exophytic growth and deep, invasive growth can present in the same tumor. Careful sampling of underlying mandibular bone is required to identify bone invasion for proper tumor staging.

FIGURE 3.38. This tumor of the lateral tongue shows exophytic growth.

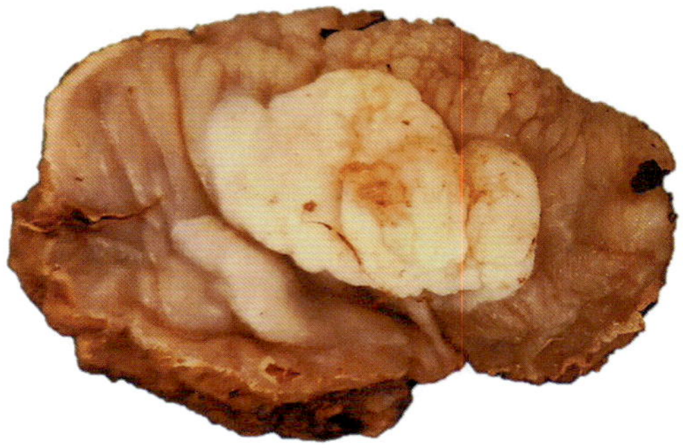

FIGURE 3.39. This carcinoma of the right mandible shows prominent exophytic growth.

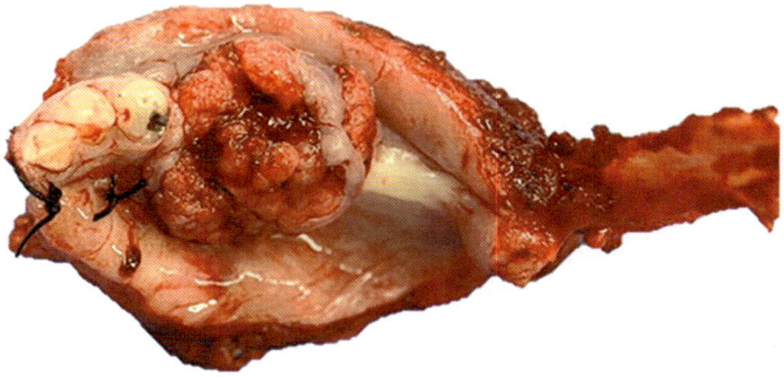

Courtesy of Dr. M. El-Hakim and Dr. O. Alghamdi

GINGIVAL SCC

FIGURE 3.40. This ulcerating tumor invades the bone where the roots of teeth are planted. The teeth around this invasive tumor are loose.

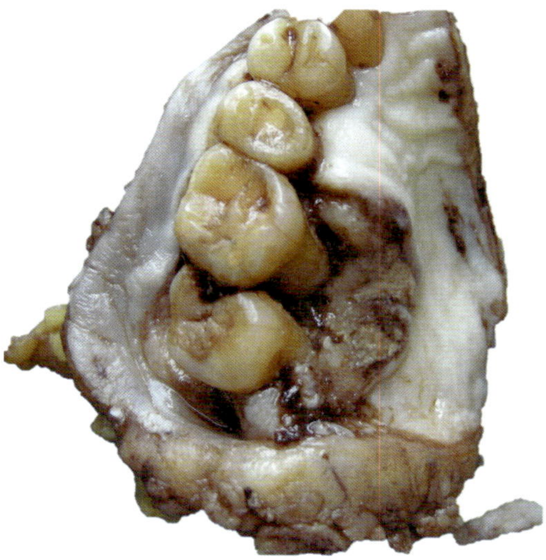

FLOOR OF MOUTH SCC

FIGURE 3.41. This tumor presented as an irregular ulcer with variegated base. The teeth are absent in this case.

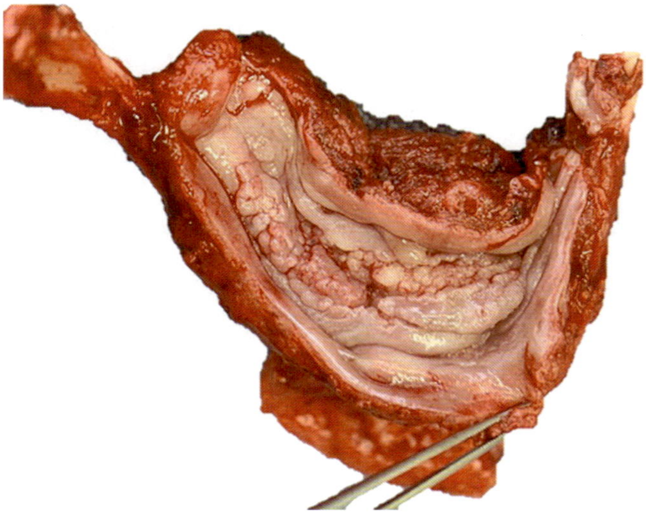

HUMAN PAPILLOMAVIRUS–RELATED SCC

SCCs related to human papillomavirus (HPV) are nonkeratinizing SCCs, often with basaloid or papillary features, that arise from the base of crypts and grow submucosally. In 90% of cases, the high-risk HPV virus type 16 is identified. Strong and diffuse staining with p16 immunostain is a reliable surrogate marker for diagnosis. The primary tumor is often small or difficult to identify; the metastatic focus can be quite large. The vast majority of metastatic SCC in the neck of unknown primary origin is associated with HPV-positive oropharyngeal carcinoma.

FIGURE 3.42. This image shows a submucosal nodular tumor of the tongue with foci of ulceration.

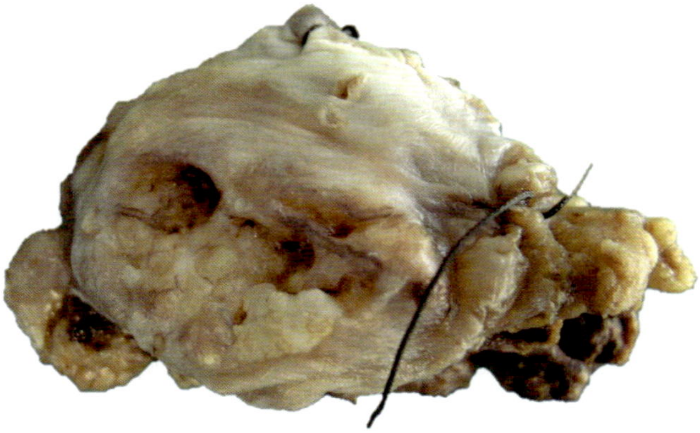

FIGURE 3.43. This tumor is an HPV-related SCC involving the left tonsil and extending to left base of the tongue. The tumor extends from the medial to lateral end. While nearly half of the mucosa was spared, the entire submucosal tissues of this resection specimen were involved by carcinoma. P16 immunostain is routinely obtained on all SCCs of the oropharynx.

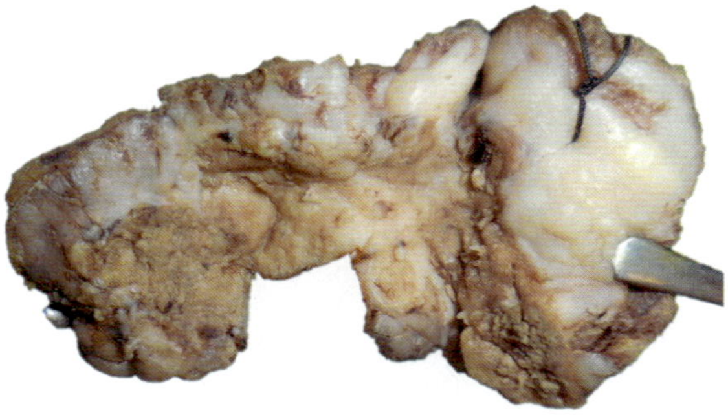

RADIOTHERAPY-RELATED SCC

FIGURE 3.44. This exophytic SCC of the maxilla shows spindle cell morphology and was clinically caused by previous radiotherapy. The teeth are missing due to previous treatment.

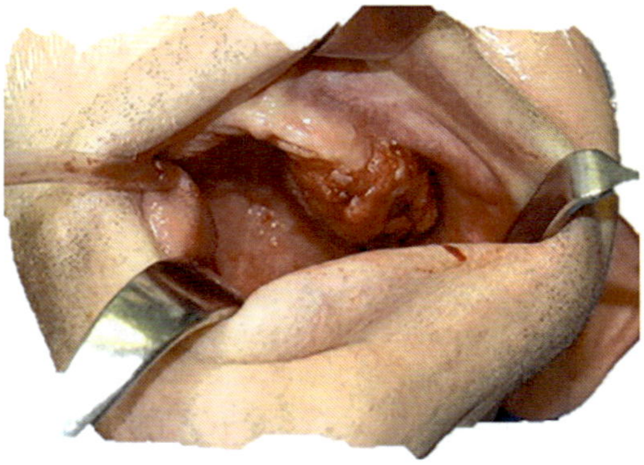

Courtesy of Dr. M. El-Hakim and Dr. O. Alghamdi

SPINDLE CELL SCC

The spindle cell (sarcomatoid) variant is a fast-growing type of SCC with worse prognosis when compared to conventional SCC. These tumors are typically polypoid.

FIGURE 3.45. This image shows a polypoid spindle cell–type SCC of the buccal mucosa.

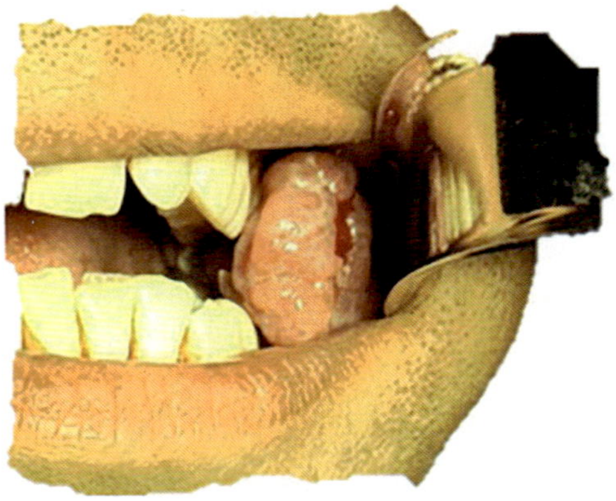

Courtesy of Dr. Nicholas Mahkoul

Verrucous carcinoma

Verrucous carcinoma is a well-differentiated, locally invasive carcinoma associated with cigarette smoking. It does not metastasize to the lymph nodes and there is no definite association with HPV.

FIGURE 3.46. This image shows a verrucous carcinoma of the buccal mucosa with a characteristic broad base and warty appearance.

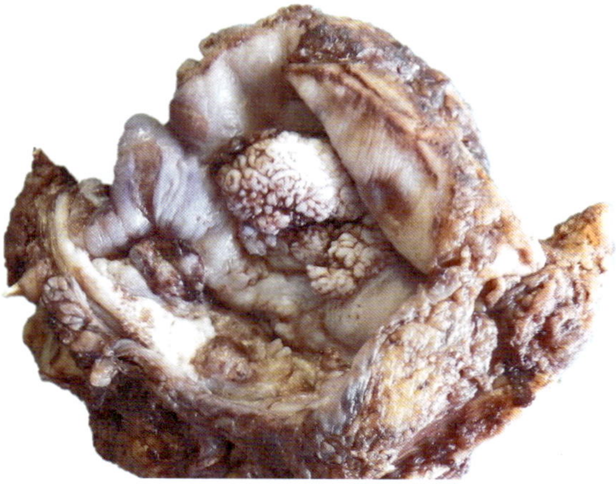

Melanoma of the oral cavity

MUCOSAL MELANOMA

Mucosal melanoma is a rare form of melanoma arising from melanocytes in the mucosal surfaces of the body lining the sinuses, nasal passages, oral cavity, vagina, anus, and other areas. It has a high recurrence rate after resection. Palate and gingiva are the most common sites.

FIGURE 3.47. This mucosa melanoma of the retromolar trigone shows dark, blackish discoloration (circled area).

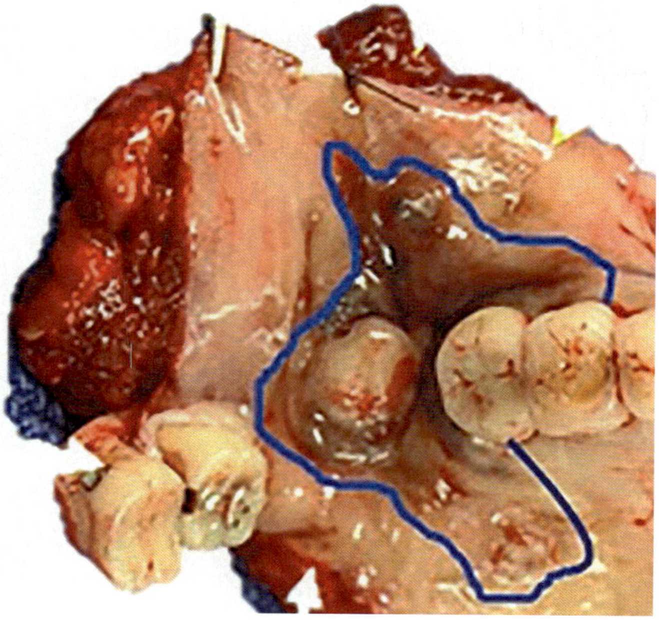

FIGURE 3.48. This brown-black tumor of the maxillary gingiva (arrows) has a nodular appearance.

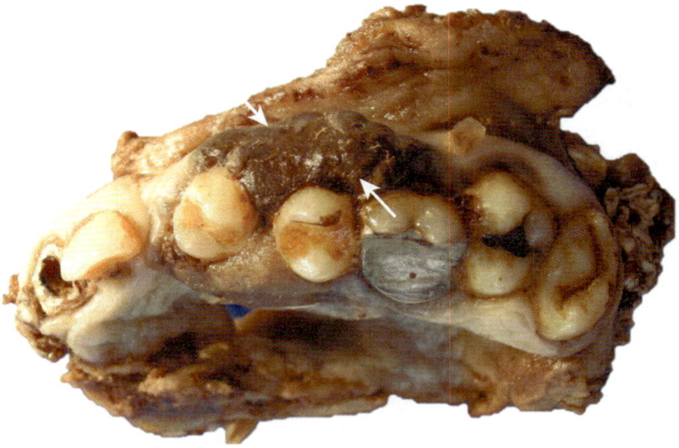

Intraosseous chondrosarcoma

FIGURE 3.49. This white cartilaginous tumor has replaced the left temporal mandibular bone and invaded into adjacent tissue.

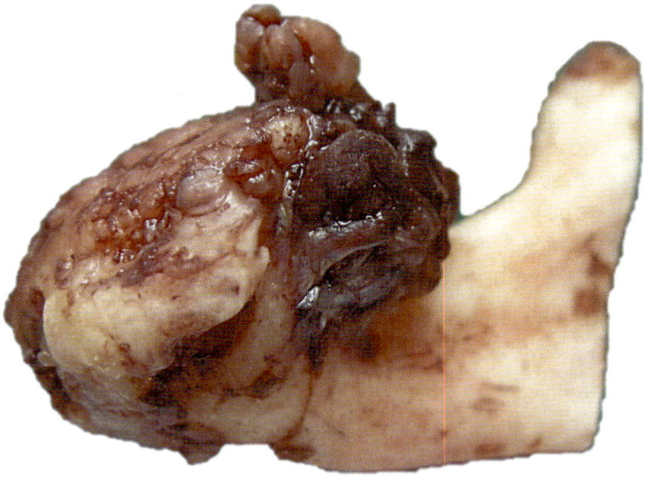

Larynx

Nonneoplastic Diseases and Benign Neoplasms of the Larynx

Nodule or polyps of the vocal cord

Vocal cord nodules and polyps are caused by stromal reactions to trauma or inflammation.

FIGURE 3.50. Vocal cord nodules are bilateral and typically located at the junction of the anterior third and middle third of the vocal cords. Note the fusiform appearance of the bilateral vocal cord in this image.

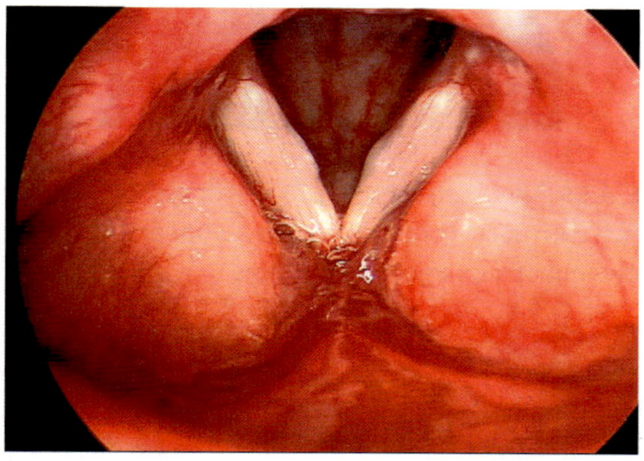

Courtesy of Dr. Jonathan Young

FIGURE 3.51. These images show a wide-based, translucent polyp (arrows) in the middle portion of the left vocal cord, shown during phonation (A) and respiration (B).

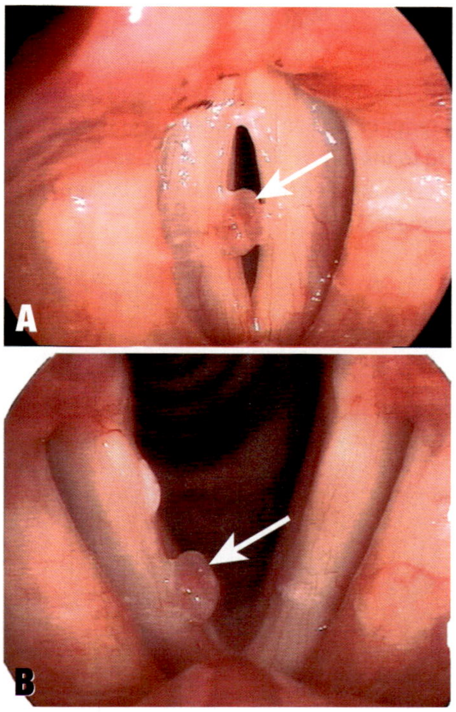

Courtesy of Dr. Jonathan Young

Thyroglossal duct cyst

Thyroglossal duct cysts are the most common cause of midline neck masses derived from a persistent thyroglossal duct. They are generally located below the hyoid bone but can occur anywhere along the path of the thyroglossal duct, from the base of the tongue to the suprasternal notch.

FIGURE 3.52. Image (A) shows a thyroglossal duct cyst causing a midtongue lump. In (B), a resected thyroglossal duct cyst shows a smooth mucosa and fibrous wall.

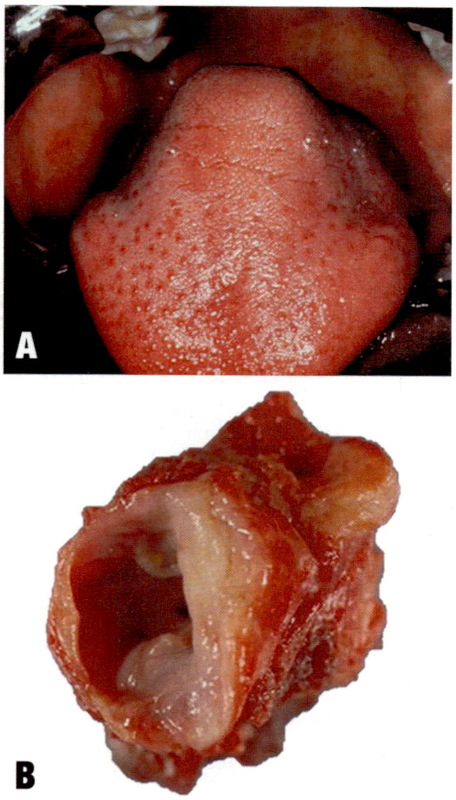

Cancers of the Larynx

SCC of the larynx

More than 95% of laryngeal tumors are SCCs. For staging purposes, the larynx is divided into 3 anatomical regions: the glottis (true vocal cords, anterior and posterior commissures); the supraglottis (epiglottis, arytenoids and aryepiglottic folds, and false cords); and the subglottis. Less common variants of laryngeal SCC include verrucous, spindle cell, and basaloid SCC. Each variant has a different biological course than conventional SCC. Neck metastases are more common in supraglottic cancers, due to the rich lymphatic network of the supraglottis. The poor lymphatic network of the true vocal cords means glottic tumors rarely present with regional neck metastases at the time of diagnosis.

SUPRAGLOTTIC SCC

FIGURE 3.53. The ulcerating tumor pictured here is above the vocal cord and involves the epiglottis; therefore, it is a supraglottic SCC.

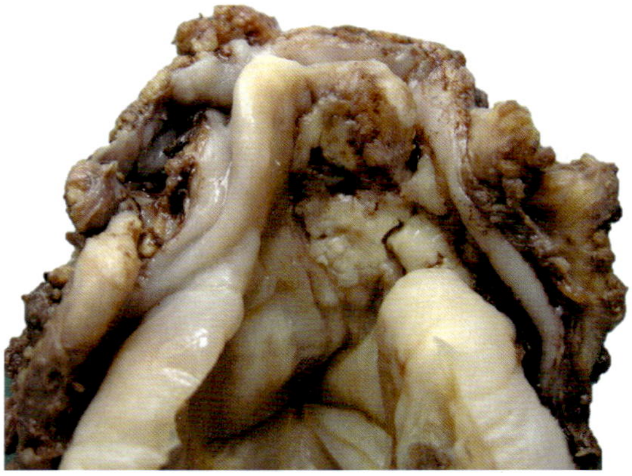

GLOTTIC AND SUBGLOTTIC SCC

FIGURE 3.54. In this image, the vocal cords (arrows) are invaded by a subglottic ulcerating tumor.

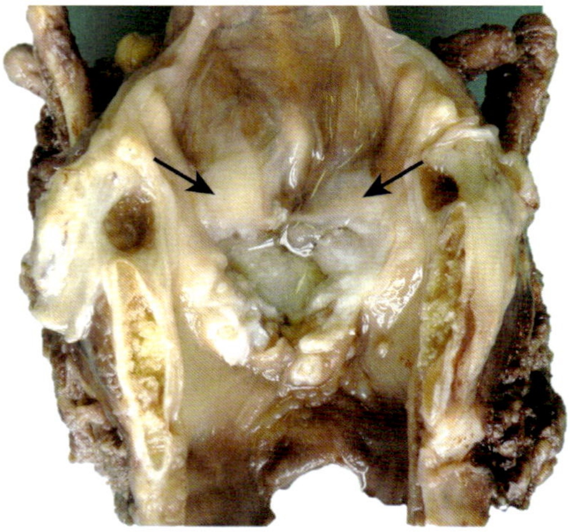

FIGURE 3.55. This image shows an anterior subglottic and glottic SCC. This tumor presented as a poorly defined ulcer in the anterior midline (arrow).

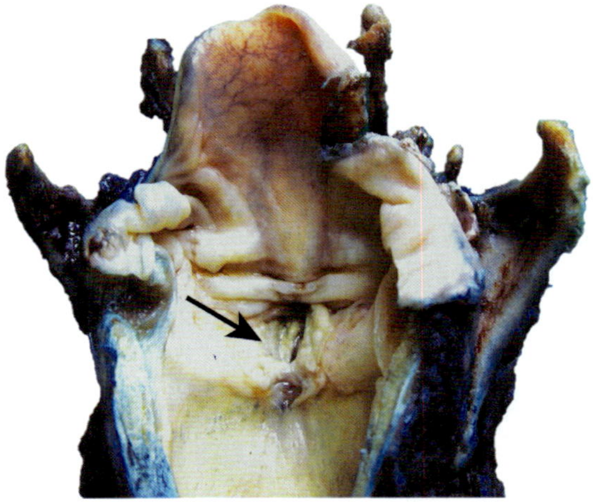

FIGURE 3.56. This image shows a T3 glottic tumor invading the vocal cords with vocal cord fixation. The tumor on the right vocal cord shows minor supraglottic extension.

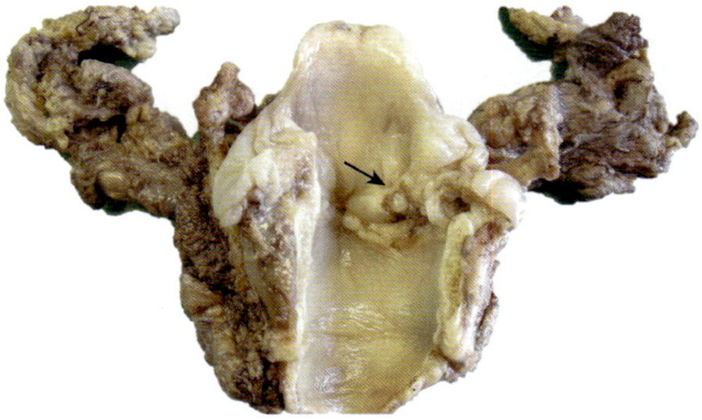

FIGURE 3.57. This image shows a glottic and subglottic SCC with right anterior extension. The deep, ulcerating tumor is fixing the vocal cord to the larynx. Fixation of the vocal cords signifies a deeply invasive lesion. Regardless of the initial tumor location, such lesions are graded T3.

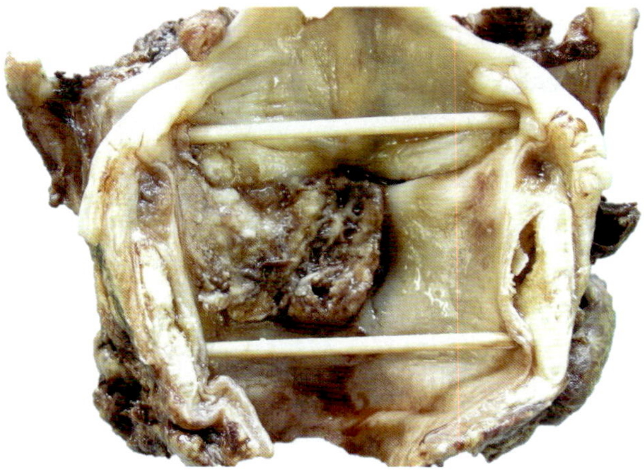

TRANSGLOTTIC SCC

Transglottic tumors cross the laryngeal ventricles vertically to involve the supraglottis, the glottis, and often the subglottis.

FIGURE 3.58. The tumor in this image extends from the supraglottic to subglottic region and involves the vocal cords; it is therefore considered a transglottic carcinoma.

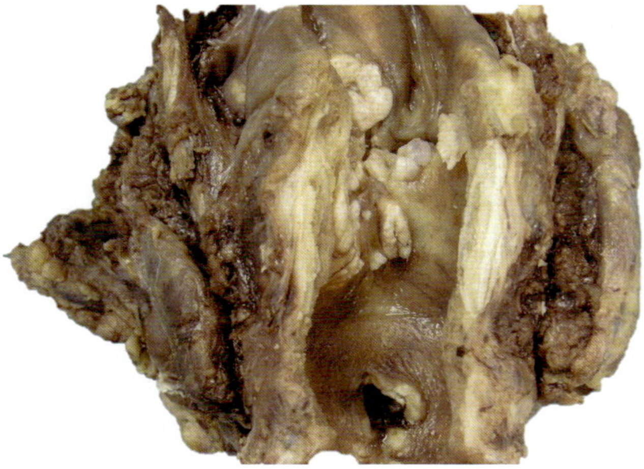

SPINDLE CELL SCC

Spindle cell SCC is a rare variant of SCC, representing less than 3% of all head and neck malignancies of epithelial origin. It usually presents as a polypoid mass and has been reported to be more aggressive than conventional SCC. Histologically, spindle cell SCC can be differentiated from sarcoma by positive cytokeratin or p40 staining, and the presence of carcinoma in-situ or identification of conventional SCC components.

FIGURE 3.59. These images of a spindle cell SCC of the posterior larynx show a characteristic polypoid mass with surface ulceration.

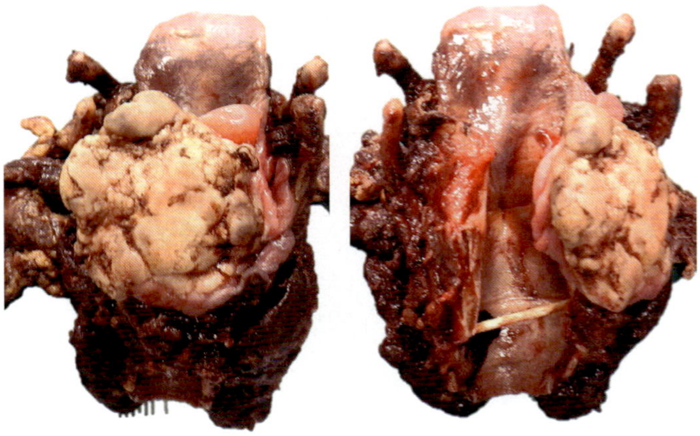

FIGURE 3.60. This image shows a spindle cell SCC of the left aryepiglottic fold and pyriform sinus. It illustrates the characteristic polypoid growth of spindle cell SCC.

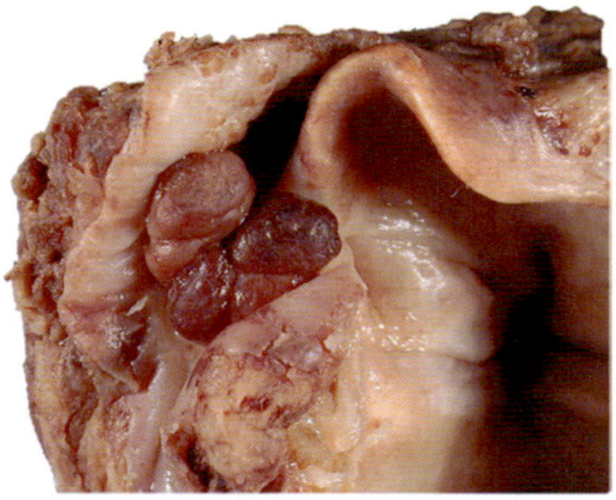

INVASIVE SCC WITH INVASION OF PERILARYNGEAL SOFT TISSUES

SCCs that invade perilaryngeal soft tissues are designated as pT4 tumors.

FIGURE 3.61. This image shows SCC invading perilaryngeal soft tissue.

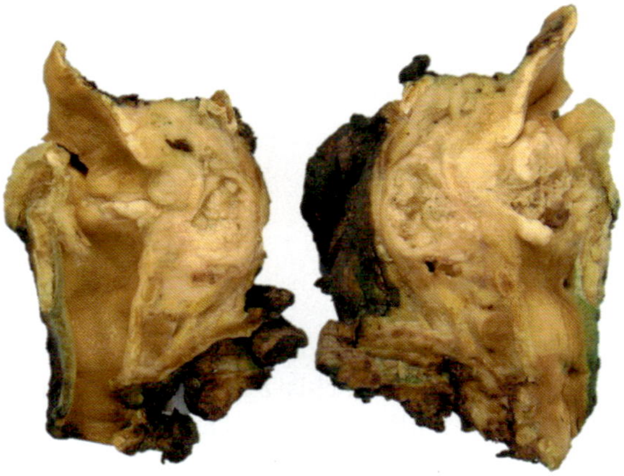

RECURRENT LARYNGEAL SCC WITH SKIN INVASION

FIGURE 3.62. This recurrent tumor measures 12 cm. The image shows a focal skin ulceration, while the tumor occupied the entire subcutaneous tissues.

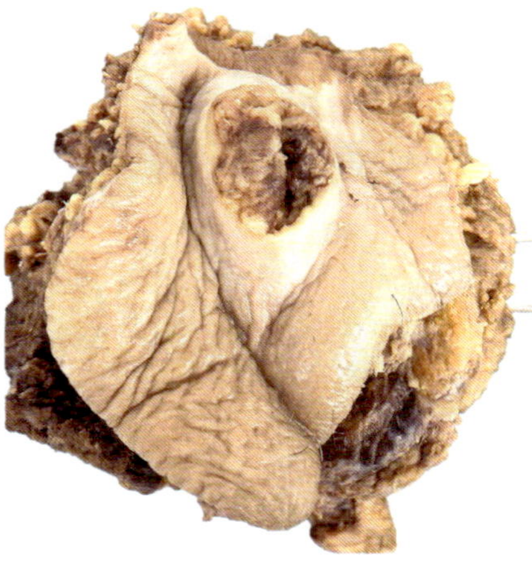

Liposarcoma of larynx

Liposarcoma of the head-and-neck region is very rare. The most common sites of involvement are pharynx, mouth, larynx, and neck. The mainstay of treatment for liposarcoma is surgical excision, and the prognosis is determined by the histological grade and clinical stage.

FIGURE 3.63. This image shows a large, yellow, submucosal mass bulging from the left side of the larynx.

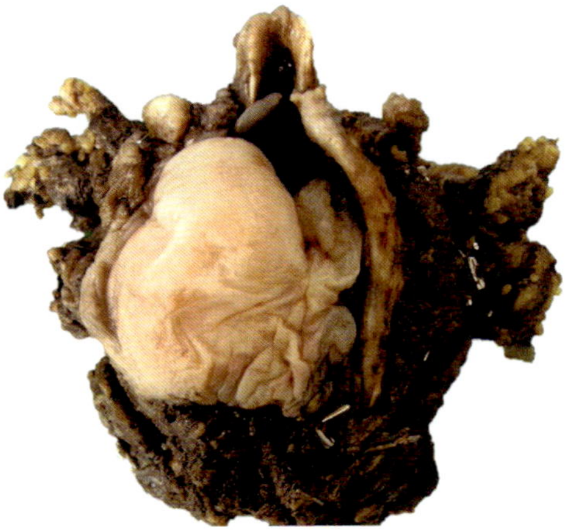

FIGURE 3.64. In this image, the yellow areas (double arrow) correspond to well-differentiated areas that constituted the majority of the cut surfaces. The white and firm area (single arrow) is a site of dedifferentiation.

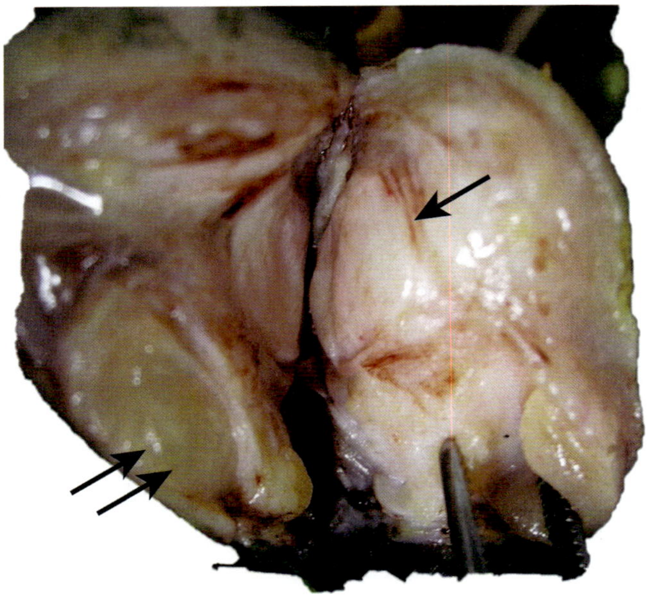

Neck

Branchial cleft cyst

The vast majority of branchial cleft cysts arise from remnants of the second branchial arch, which commonly occurs in the third to fifth decades of life. These benign, painless cysts usually appear on the anterior border of the sternocleidomastoid muscle. The contents of brachial cleft cysts may be clear, watery, or mucinous, and may contain desquamated, granular cellular debris.

FIGURE 3.65. Grossly, branchial cleft cyst is well-circumscribed and 2 cm to 5 cm in diameter, as illustrated in this image. Histologically, it is lined by stratified squamous or pseudostratified columnar epithelium.

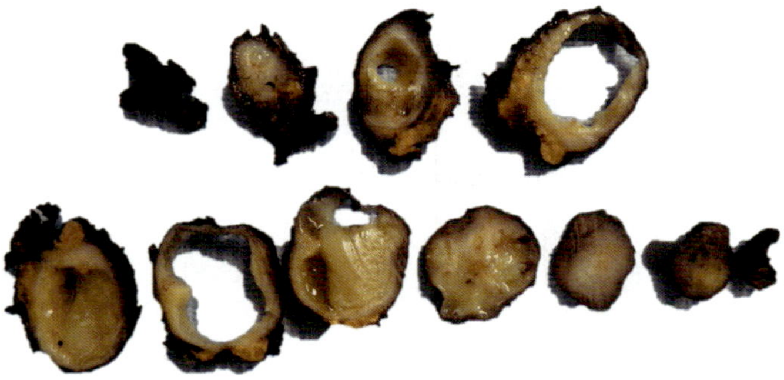

FIGURE 3.66. In this image, note how the cystic wall on the right has partially shrunk due to drainage of cyst fluid in the operating room.

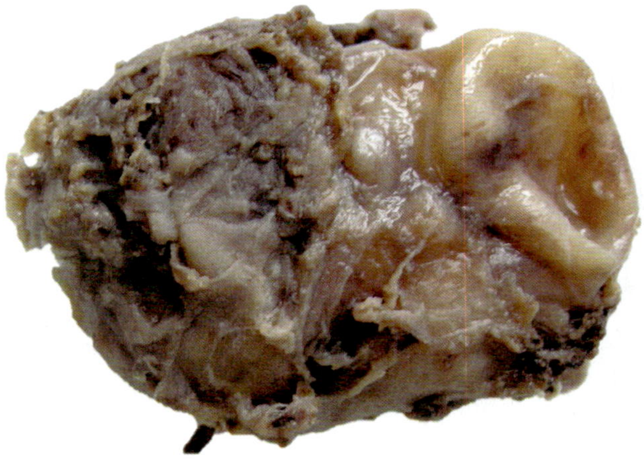

FIGURE 3.67. The inner surface of this cyst shows some nodularity. In this case, the cyst contents had been drained.

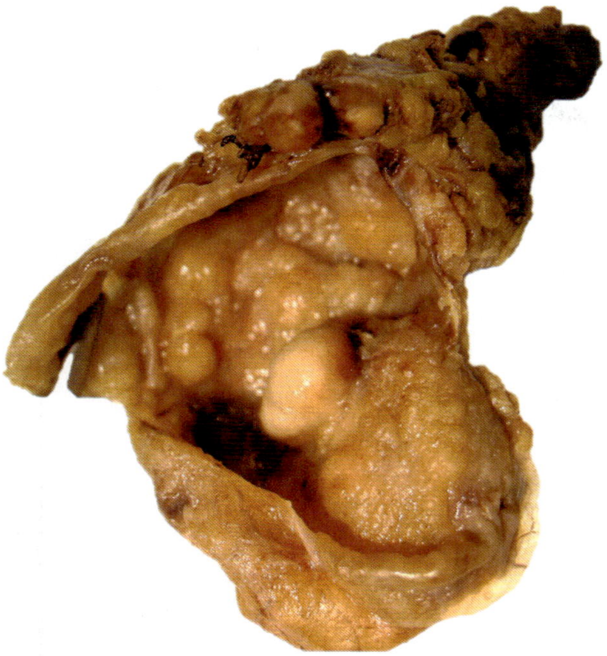

Arteriovenous malformation (AVM)

AVM is a benign condition in which the artery is directly connected to the vein without capillaries. The head-and-neck region is a common region for AVM. Clinically, AVM presents as a warm, bluish lesion. The diagnosis of AVM requires radiologic or clinical correlation.

FIGURE 3.68. This image shows an AVM of the right neck. AVMs are nonencapsulated lesions that consist of closely aggregated, thin- and thick-walled vessels.

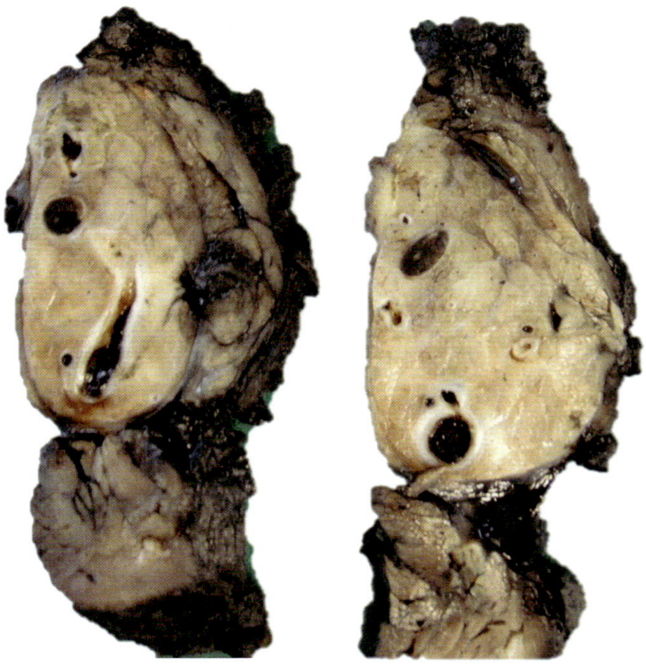

PROCEDURE: NECK DISSECTION

Neck dissection is an en bloc resection of multiple lymph nodes for control of neck lymph node metastasis. Lymph nodes in the neck are divided into 6 areas, called levels, and numbered from head (I) to chest (VI) using roman numerals.

Lymph node levels

FIGURE 3.69. This image shows the upper 4 levels (I–IV) of dissected neck lymph nodes.

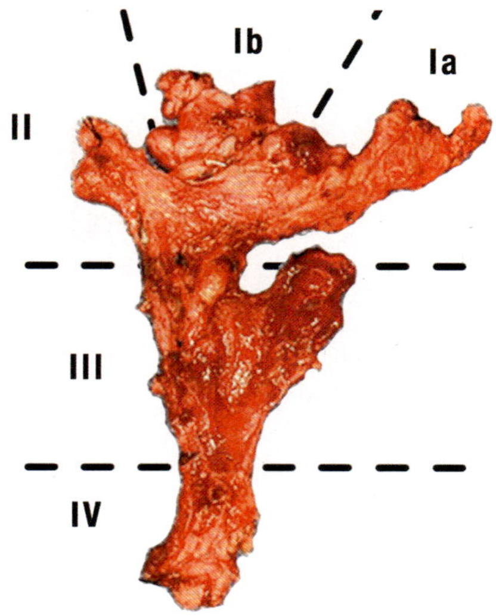

Courtesy of Dr. Nicholas Makhoul and Dr. Osama Alghamdi

LEVEL II, III, IV NECK DISSECTION OF METASTATIC PAPILLARY THYROID CARCINOMA

FIGURE 3.70. This image shows metastatic papillary thyroid carcinoma, with significantly enlarged, cystic, and colloid rich nodules in level III compared to levels II and IV. SCC and papillary thyroid carcinoma are the main carcinomas than can present with cystic metastasis in the neck. This specimen was oriented by the surgeon.

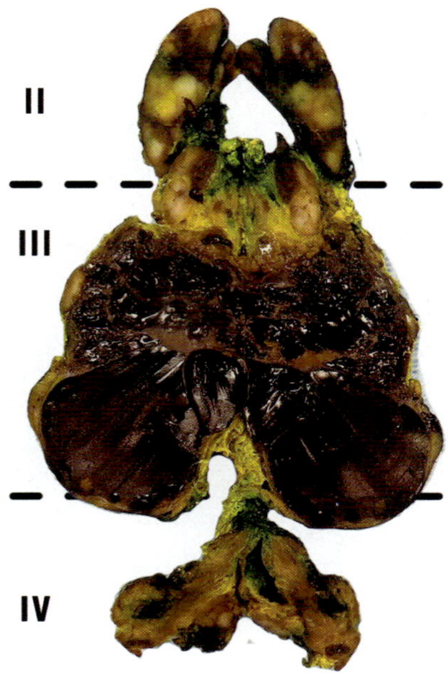

Courtesy of Dr. Nader Sadeghi

LEVEL II METASTATIC SCC

FIGURE 3.71. This right dissection shows significant enlargement in level II from massive metastatic SCC. This specimen was oriented by the surgeon.

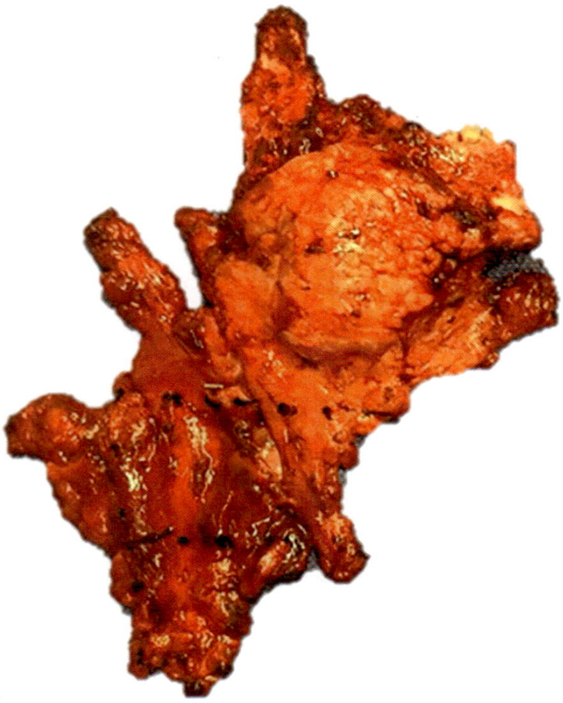

Courtesy of Dr. Nicholas Makhoul and Dr. Osama Alghandi

Neck lipoma

A lipoma is a benign tumor of the adipose tissue that can be found anywhere in the body. Lipomas located in the neck, back, and shoulder region tend to have spindle cell or pleomorphic cell histology.

FIGURE 3.72. This image shows an encapsulated mass containing yellow-tan adipose tissue.

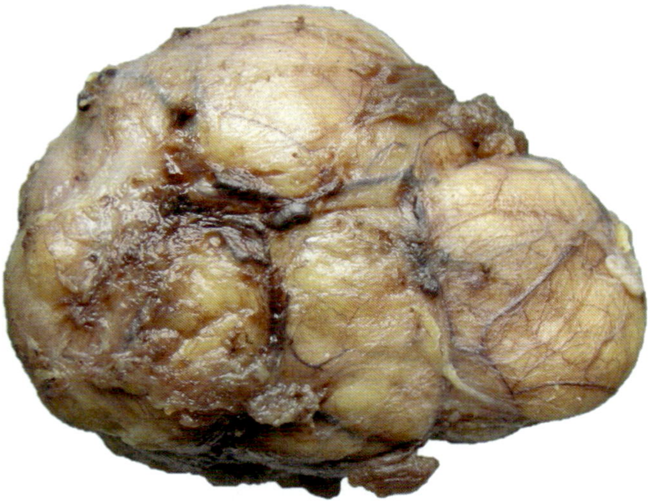

Carotid body paraganglioma

The carotid body is the most common location for head and neck paragangliomas. They are well-circumscribed, firm, rubbery tumors with yellow, tan-to-pink, red, or brown cut surfaces. They can measure from 2 cm to 8 cm.

FIGURE 3.73. Paragangliomas are often removed along with a vessel; notice the vessels at the periphery of the tumor.

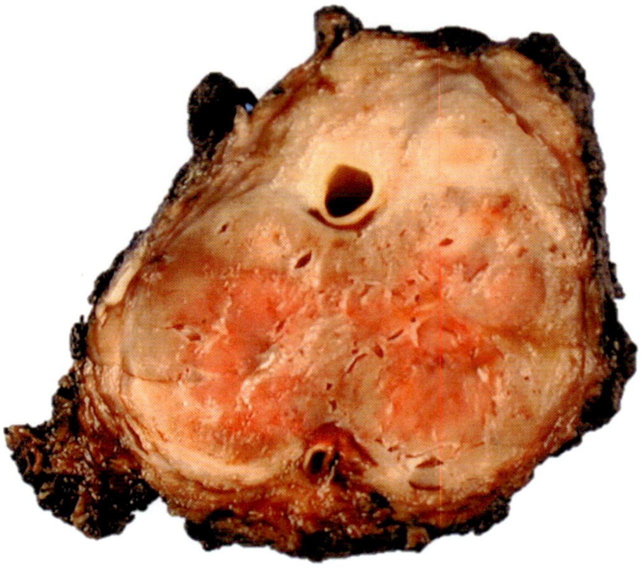

ACKNOWLEDGMENTS

We would like to thank the valuable contributions Dr. P. Chauvin and the technical help of R. Gilot, E. Griss, A. Hossain, L. Korneichyuk Pasyuk, M. Mikhael, and E. Yaney.

REFERENCES

Amin MB, Edge SB, editors. *AJCC cancer staging manual*. 8th ed. Chicago: Springer; 2018.

Barnes L. *Surgical pathology of the head and neck*. 3rd ed. New York: Informa Healthcare; 2009.

Barnes L, Chiosea S, Seethala R. *Head and neck pathology*. Demos Medical Pub; 2010. (Consultant pathology series, vol. 3).

El-Naggar AK, Chan JKC, Grandis JR, Takata T, Slootweg PJ. *WHO classification of head and neck tumours*. 4th ed. Geneva, Switzerland: IARC Press; 2017.

Wenig BM. *Atlas of head and neck pathology*. 3rd ed. Philadelphia: Saunders/Elsevier; 2015.

4

Diseases of the Thyroid, Parathyroid, and Adrenal Glands

DERIN CAGLAR, JULIE GUILMETTE

Thyroid Gland

REFERENCE: NORMAL THYROID GLAND

The thyroid gland consists of 2 lobes connected by an isthmus. Occasionally, a pyramidal lobe is found. The thyroid gland is located in the lower anterior region of the neck, below the Adam's apple. On average, it weighs 18 g in adult males and 13 g in adult females.

FIGURE 4.1. Image (A) shows a normal thyroid gland, anterior view. Image (B) shows a rear view of the same specimen.

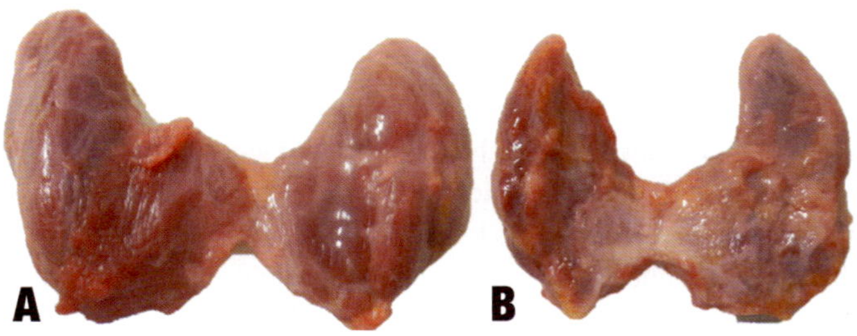

PROCEDURE: SECTIONING OF A TOTAL THYROIDECTOMY SPECIMEN

Most resections are oriented by the surgeon with a suture, which marks a pole of a lobe. Unoriented thyroidectomy specimens can be oriented by identifying the concave posterior surface, convex anterior and lateral surfaces, and the tapered and longer superior poles of the lateral lobes. Transverse sectioning of the thyroid in 2-mm to 3-mm intervals (with the exception of vertical sectioning of the isthmus, and upper and lower poles of the right and left lobe) helps to identify even the smallest nodules. Color-coding of lobes and photographing of slices in anatomic position can aid in solving human errors of dictation at the grossing station and can help identify the resection surface. Tumors that are ≤ 2 cm in size are submitted in their entirety. For follicular neoplasms, entire tumor capsule sampling with 2 mm to 3 mm of tumor tissue is required. Sections should also include any involved margins, possible extrathyroidal extension sites, and tumor and/or uninvolved parenchyma sections. For nontumoral cases, 1 section per 5 grams of thyroid tissue is recommended. Specimens should be examined for parathyroids (often found in the posterior surface) and lymph nodes (frequently found around the isthmus) prior to inking.

FIGURE 4.2. This image shows color-coded lobes in anatomical position.

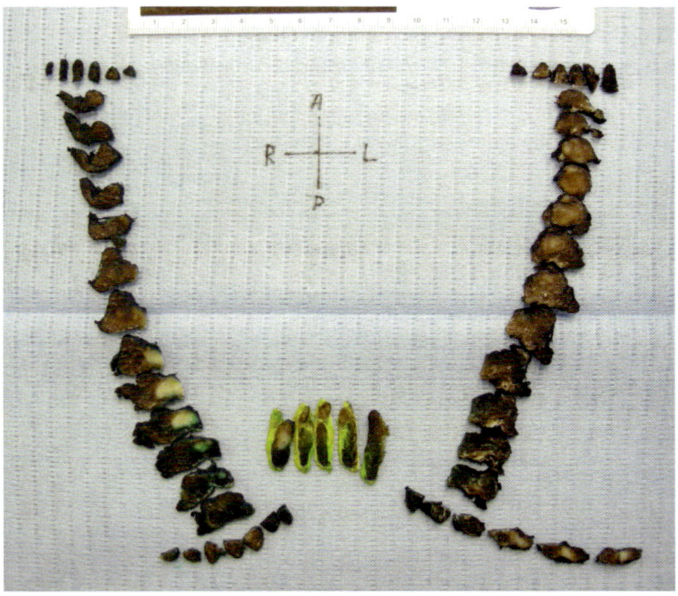

Multinodular goiter

Multinodular goiters occur more often in individuals from iodine-deficient areas, older individuals, and women.

FIGURE 4.3. The cut surfaces of this massively enlarged thyroid shows numerous colloid-rich nodules of varying sizes separated by thin, fibrous septa replacing the entire thyroid parenchyma. The white specks are due to the drying out of the colloid, seen more prominently in the left lower slice. A focus of secondary calcification (white, measuring a few millimeters) is also seen. The occasional brown-black discolorations in the upper slice are hemorrhagic sites.

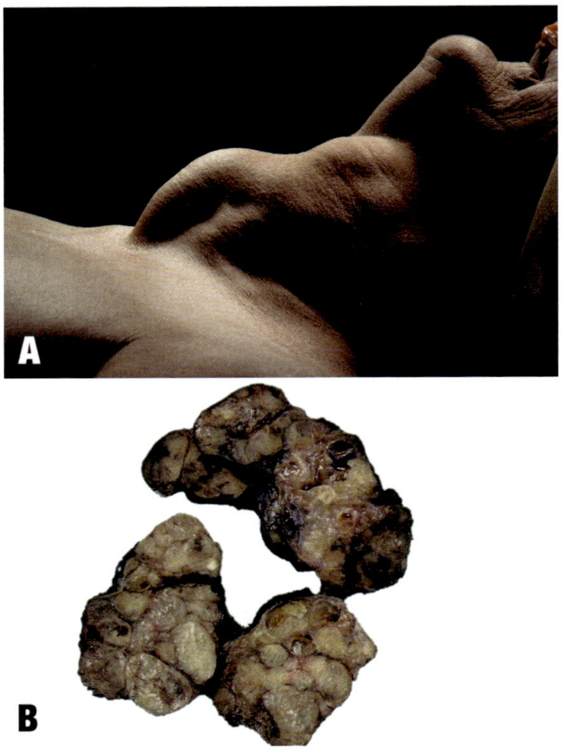

(B) courtesy of Dr. Roger Tabah

ASYMMETRICAL GOITER

A neoplastic lesion needs to be excluded whenever there is an asymmetric enlargement or a dominant nodule.

FIGURE 4.4. These thyroid specimens are distorted due to an asymmetrically enlarged lobe.

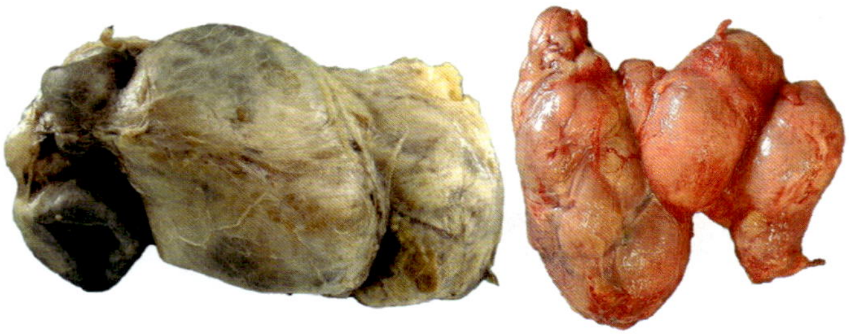

FOLLICULAR NODULAR HYPERPLASIA

FIGURE 4.5. These sections show multiple, semitranslucent, colloid-rich nodules separated by thin, fibrous septa. The capsule of the largest nodule is partial and very thin (< 1 mm).

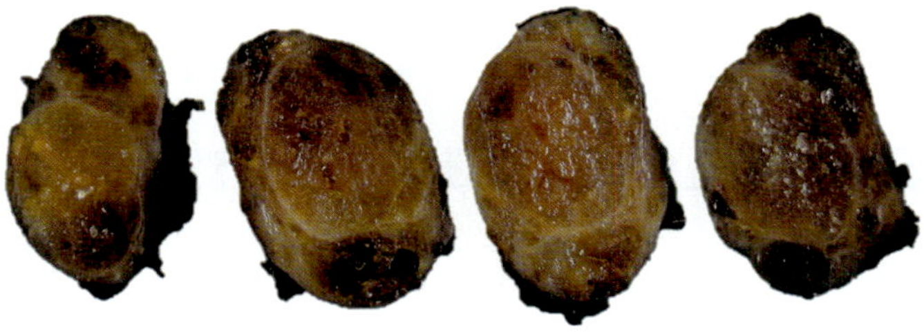

FOLLICULAR NODULAR HYPERPLASIA WITH DEGENERATIVE CHANGE

Degenerative change is common, especially in large nodules of long duration.

FIGURE 4.6. This nodule is remarkable for its prominent fibrous bands of varying thickness, and for the hemorrhage present in otherwise glistening, colloid-rich cut surfaces.

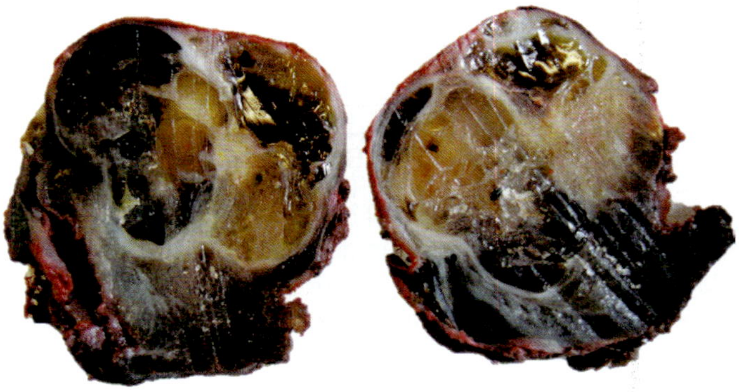

COLLOID NODULE

Colloid nodules are benign thyroid nodules containing abundant colloid.

FIGURE 4.7. These images show a specimen measuring 4.8 cm in its greatest dimension. Image (A) shows glistening, sticky cut surfaces. In (B), the section is held against a light to better show the translucent nature of the amber-color colloid and its few thin vascular structures. A central space was formed secondary to draining of colloid prior to photographing.

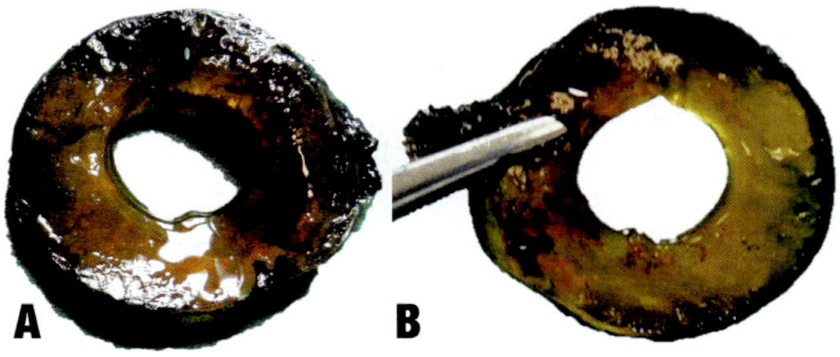

HEMORRHAGIC CYSTIC BENIGN FOLLICULAR NODULE

Sometimes, benign follicular nodules can have a secondary hemorrhage resulting in a cystic appearance.

FIGURE 4.8. Note the dark brown, soft, and cystic cut surface resulting from extensive hemorrhage.

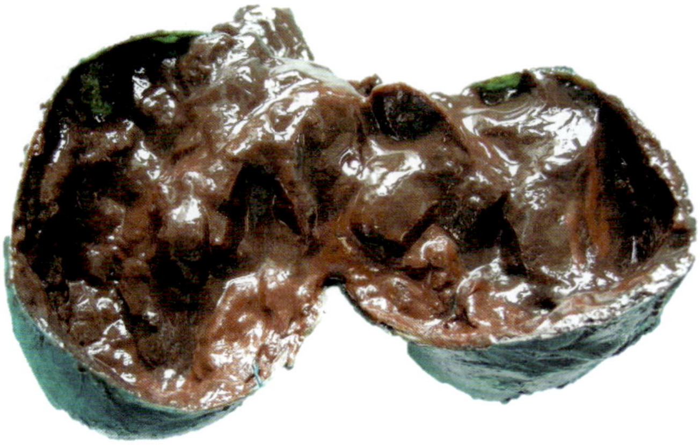

FIGURE 4.9. After the removal of the hemorrhagic fluid, this cystic lesion shows a thin and translucent capsule. No malignant follicular cells were found within the nodule.

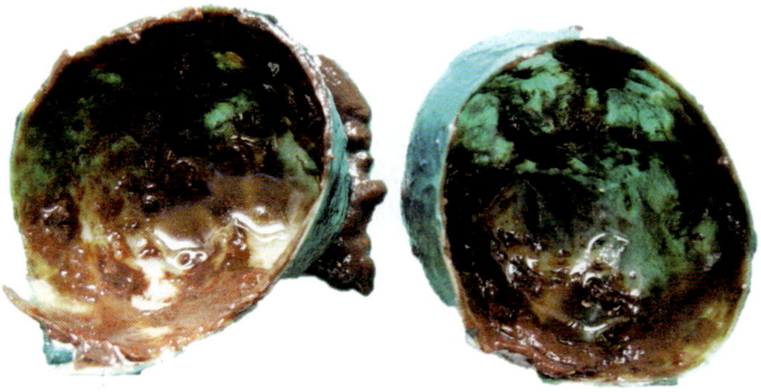

DOMINANT HYPERPLASIC NODULE WITH CENTRAL HYALINIZATION

FIGURE 4.10. This hyperplastic nodule is still translucent, indicating the presence of colloid. The central hyalinization may be caused by fine needle aspiration; it is also commonly found in oncocytic follicular tumors. In this case, the nodule was surrounded with an incomplete capsule.

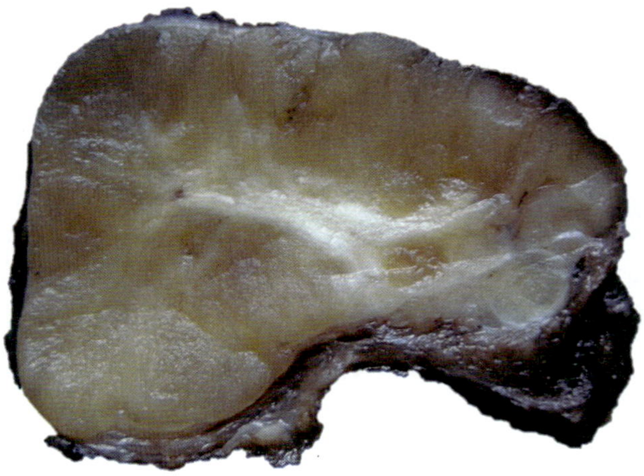

Chronic lymphocytic thyroiditis (Hashimoto thyroiditis)

Chronic lymphocytic thyroiditis, also called Hashimoto thyroiditis, is an autoimmune disorder in which antibodies attack follicular cells. Occurrence of this disorder peaks in the fifth decade of life and is more common in women. In cases of chronic lymphocytic thyroiditis, the thyroid gland is often symmetrically enlarged with less prominent nodularity. When lymphoid tissue is florid, the normal thyroid parenchyma can be very hard to identify. On macroscopy, such cases can be confused with tumor.

FIGURE 4.11. These images illustrate characteristic nodular, "fish flesh," tan cut surfaces resembling a lymph node.

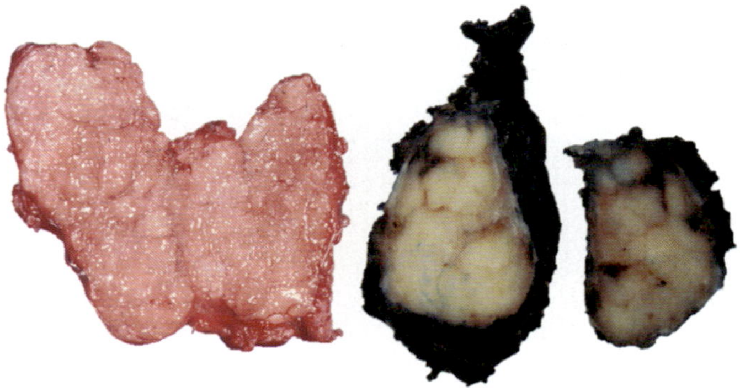

Image on left courtesy of Dr. Roger Tabah

FIGURE 4.12. In this image, the blue ink on cut surfaces is methylene blue, injected intraoperatively by the surgeon for sentinel lymph node sampling.

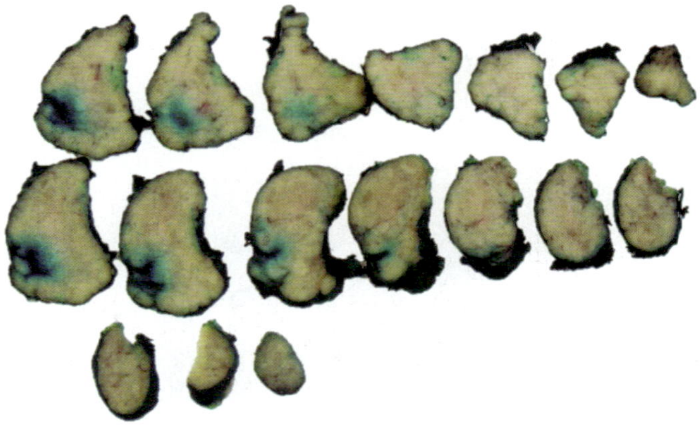

FIGURE 4.13. In this specimen, a tan-white nodule in the upper half of right lobe (arrow) indicates papillary thyroid microcarcinoma. The left lobe is paler than the right lobe due to the denser and more diffuse lymphocytic thyroiditis in the left lobe. The vague white nodules in the right lobe represent patchy lymphoid follicles; the more red-brown areas are normal thyroid parenchyma.

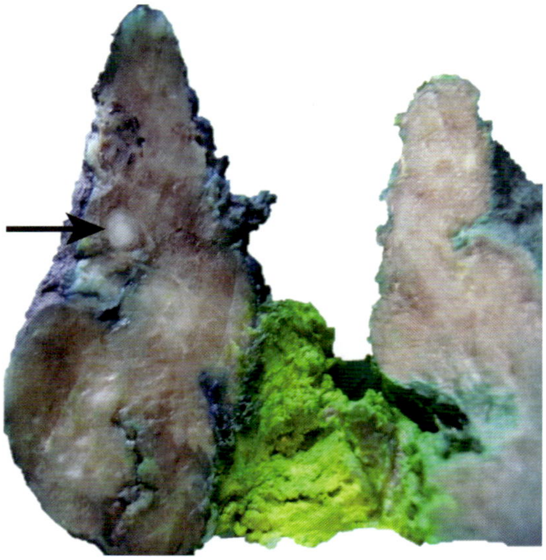

Graves disease

Graves disease, also called toxic diffuse goiter, is an autoimmune thyroid disease that often results in hyperthyroidism.

FIGURE 4.14. The resected specimen from this patient with known clinical Graves disease shows diffuse, beefy-red enlargement of the thyroid gland.

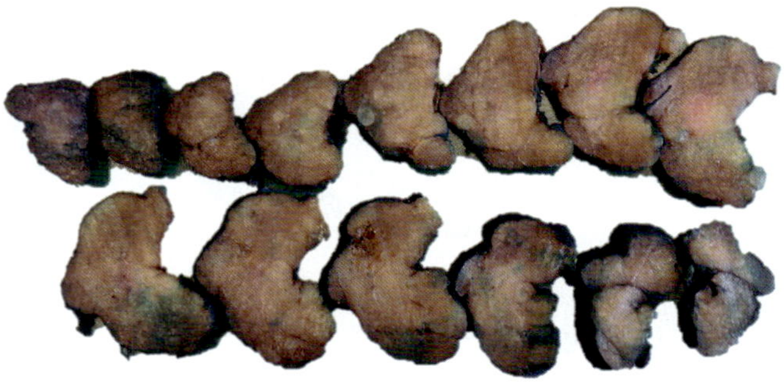

Follicular adenoma

Follicular adenoma is a common, benign neoplasm of the thyroid gland, often present clinically or on routine physical exam as a solitary, painless nodule. The entire tumor capsule should be submitted for microscopic examination. Tumors that are ≤ 2 cm can be submitted *in toto*. For larger tumors, the tumor capsule with a rim of tumor can be carved in order to fit multiple sections in 1 cassette. Sections should also include resection surface and uninvolved thyroid parenchyma.

FIGURE 4.15. Image (A) shows a solitary thyroid nodule. Image (B) shows the nodule's cut surface, which is homogeneous.

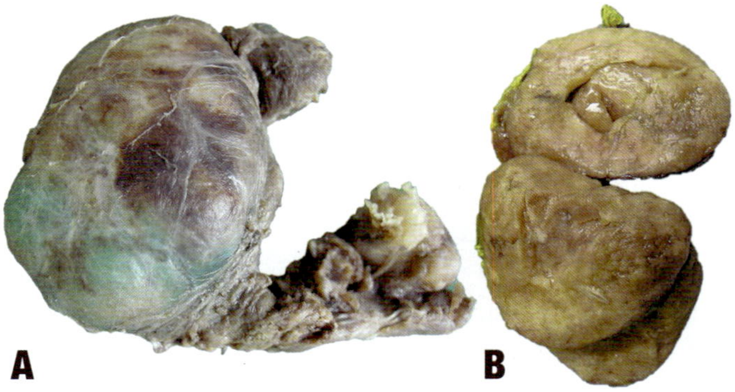

FIGURE 4.16. This thyroidectomy specimen shows an asymmetrically enlarged left lobe due to a follicular adenoma. The adenoma is well delineated, surrounded by a complete capsule. It shows no definite capsular invasion on either macroscopic or microscopic examination.

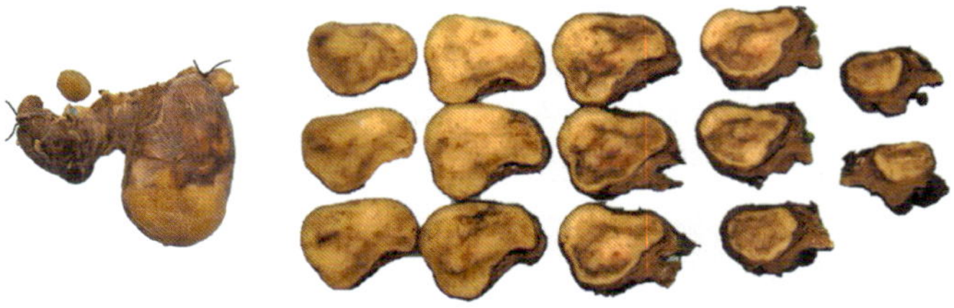

FIGURE 4.17. The mahogany brown–like color of this specimen indicates oncocytic cell change. Note that the tumor capsule is well delineated and complete. Follicular adenomas have rubbery and solid cut surfaces.

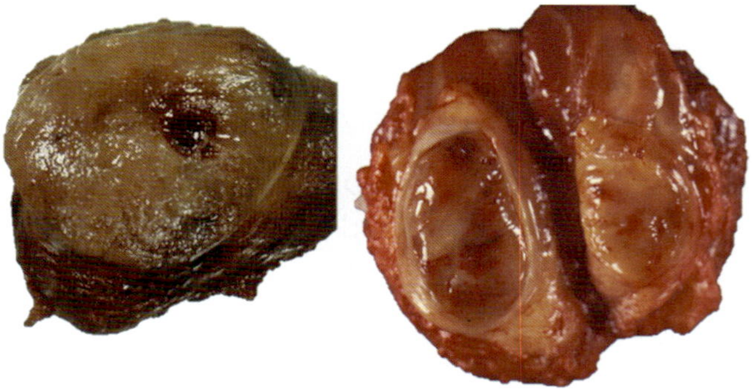

Intraoperative images courtesy of Dr. Roger Tabah

FIGURE 4.18. A tumor is visible in the left 3 slices of this specimen. Its paler color is due to higher cellularity. There is a secondary calcification at the edge of the tumor; however, no definite capsular invasion or vascular invasion is present.

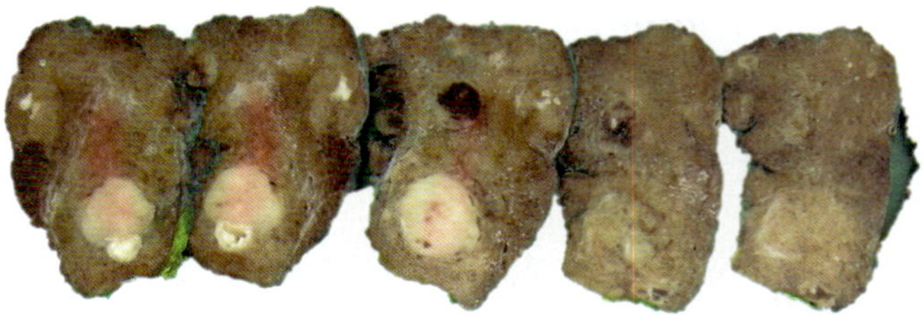

Papillary thyroid carcinoma

Papillary thyroid carcinoma is the most common type of thyroid cancer (75% to 85% of cases), and is more frequently seen in women aged 20 to 55 years. Previous radiation to the head and neck is a known risk factor for papillary thyroid carcinoma. The tumor is often well differentiated and slow growing. Classic papillary thyroid carcinoma is the most frequent variant; other variants include microcarcinoma and follicular, tall cell, columnar cell, diffuse sclerosing, and hobnail carcinoma, among others. Carcinomas are staged according to the American Joint Committee on Cancer (AJCC) staging manual (8th edition).

FIGURE 4.19. These images show a papillary thyroid carcinoma with cystic change. Note the typical papillary projections of variably sized cysts on the wall.

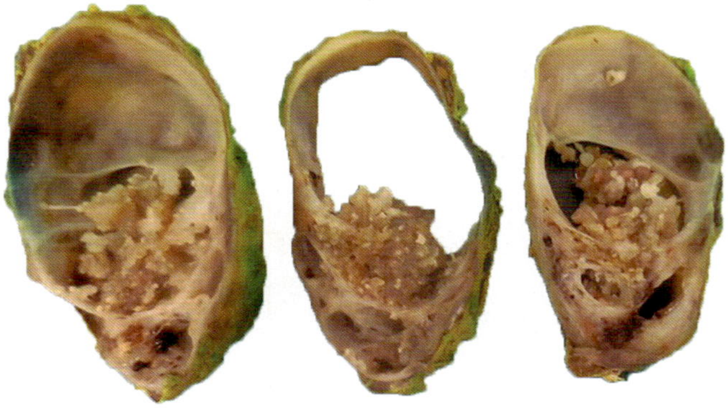

FOLLICULAR VARIANT OF PAPILLARY THYROID CARCINOMA

FIGURE 4.20. Note the areas of gritty white surface. The paler tan areas represent more cellular areas. Histology showed the follicular pattern of growth with nuclear features of papillary carcinoma.

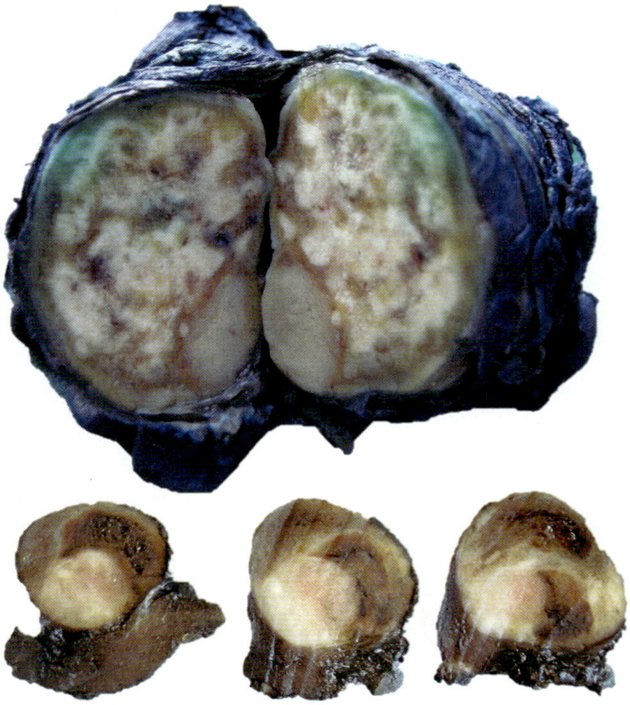

FIGURE 4.21. The macroscopic differential diagnosis of this thyroid tumor included follicular adenoma, follicular carcinoma, and the follicular variant of papillary thyroid carcinoma. The final diagnosis was follicular variant of papillary carcinoma.

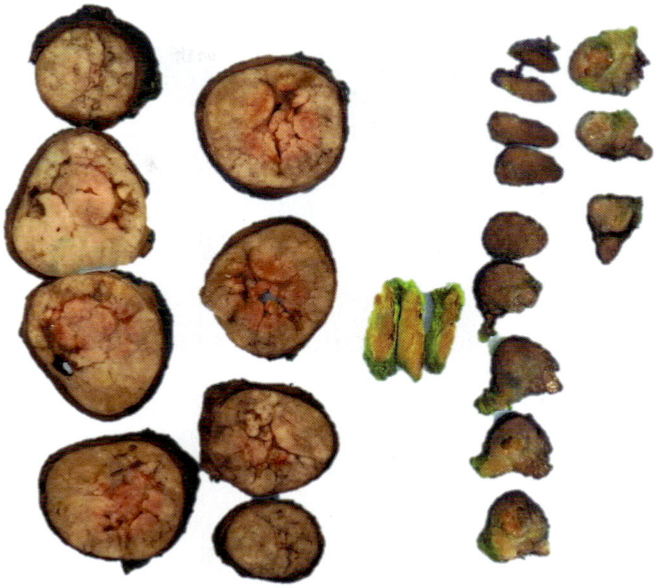

NONINVASIVE FOLLICULAR THYROID NEOPLASM WITH PAPILLARY-LIKE NUCLEAR FEATURES

Noninvasive follicular thyroid neoplasm with papillary-like nuclear features is an indolent thyroid tumor that was previously classified as an encapsulated follicular variant of papillary thyroid carcinoma. The new terminology was adopted for the purposes of 1) recognizing that encapsulated tumors without invasion have indolent behavior; and 2) avoiding overtreatment. The diagnosis relies on microscopic findings.

FIGURE 4.22. The resected lesion in this image is completely encapsulated with a smooth, round border and homogeneous cut surface.

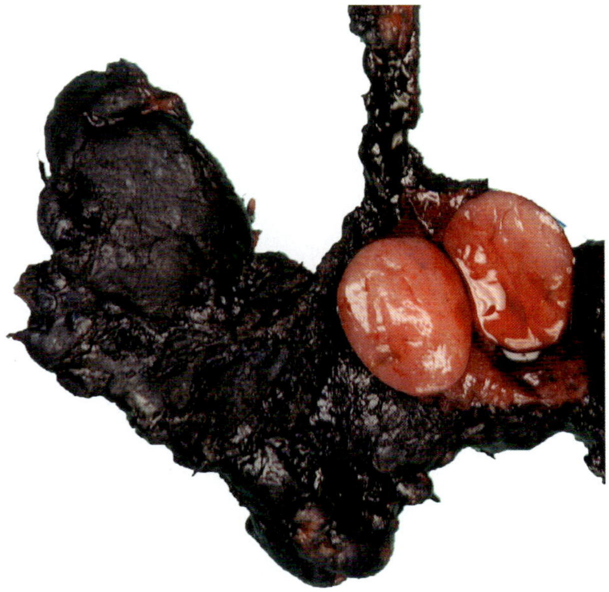

Courtesy of Dr. Moosa Khalil

SOLID VARIANT OF PAPILLARY THYROID CARCINOMA

FIGURE 4.23. This tumor shows a tan-white and solid cut surface.

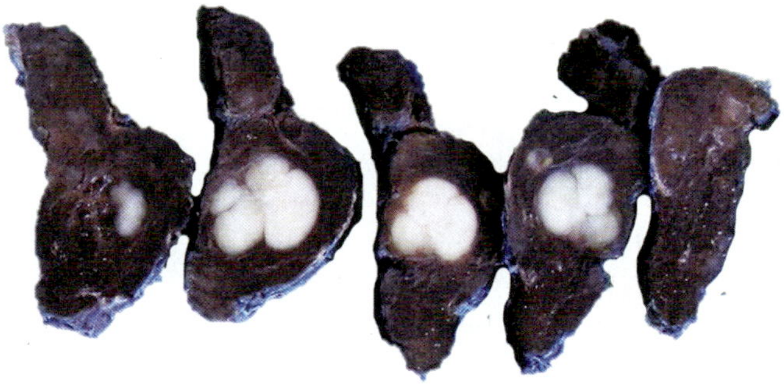

PAPILLARY THYROID CARCINOMA IN A PATIENT WITH GRAVES DISEASE

FIGURE 4.24. The invasive borders of the carcinoma are evident in this image. The beefy-red background thyroid parenchyma is characteristic of Graves disease.

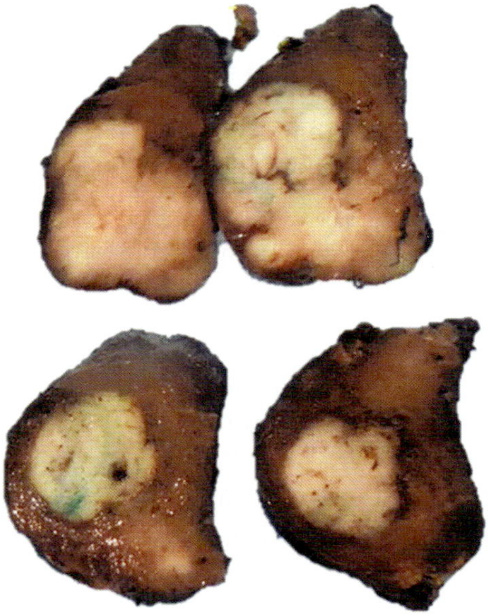

TALL CELL–VARIANT (TCV) OF PAPILLARY THYROID CARCINOMA

TCV of papillary thyroid carcinoma is among the aggressive variants. Compared to other variants, lymph node metastasis and extrathyroidal extension are more common at the time of presentation.

METASTATIC TCV OF PAPILLARY THYROID CARCINOMA

FIGURE 4.25. This image from the right jugular shows multiple enlarged lymph nodes that are partially cystic. The largest metastatic lymph node in this case was 5 cm in its largest dimension. The location of the metastatic lymph nodes at levels II, III, and IV warrants the pN1b nodal stage.

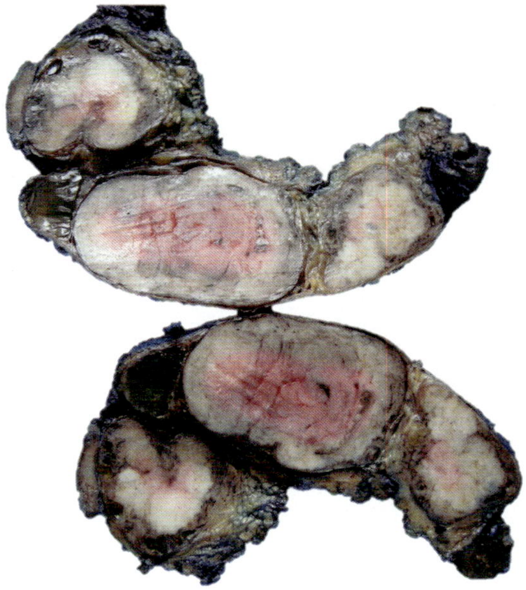

TCV OF PAPILLARY THYROID CARCINOMA WITH EXTRATHYROIDAL EXTENSION

FIGURE 4.26. The tumor in this image is invading the extrathyroidal soft tissues and is near skeletal muscle (arrows). Note the partial cystic change of the tumor.

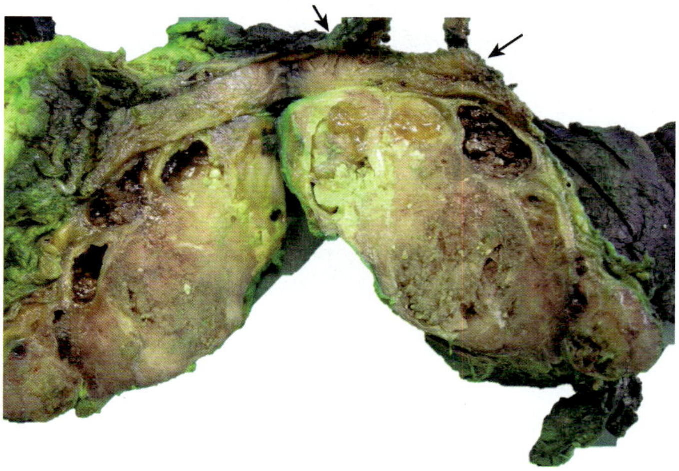

FIGURE 4.27. This recurrent tumor shows extensive invasion into tracheal cartilage and mucosa, subcutaneous tissues, and parapharyngeal soft tissues.

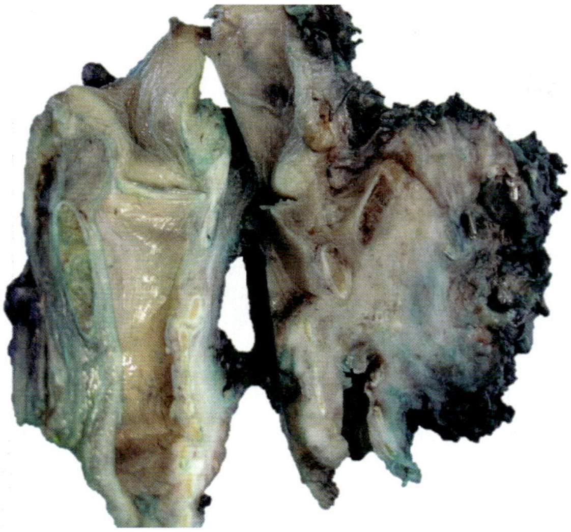

Follicular neoplasm with equivocal vascular invasion

Equivocal vascular invasion should be an uncommon diagnosis. It can only be made when suspicion for vascular invasion still exists after all efforts to rule it out.

FIGURE 4.28. This mahogany brown (oncocytic), well-delineated, single thyroid nodule was extensively sampled. On macroscopy, this neoplasm is indistinguishable from oncocytic follicular adenoma.

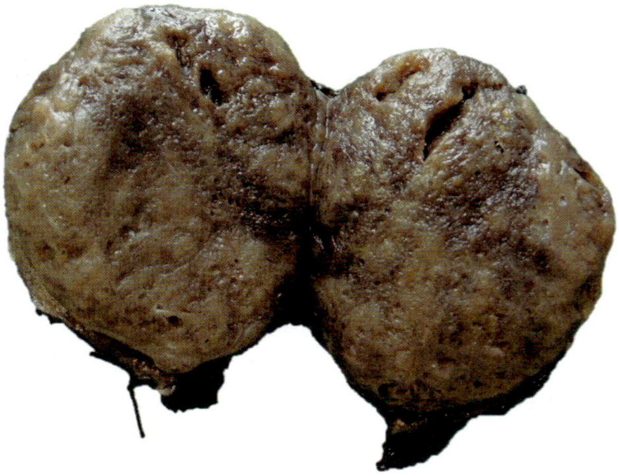

Follicular carcinoma

Follicular carcinoma is the second most common thyroid cancer (6% to 10% of cases). The highest annual incidence rate is in women over 70 years of age. If follicular neoplasm is suggested on fine needle aspiration cytology, thyroid lobectomy should be performed to establish the histopathological diagnosis. Capsular invasion and vascular invasion by tumor cells are the diagnostic features of malignancy. In contrast to cervical lymph node metastasis commonly seen in papillary thyroid carcinoma, lung and bone metastasis (via the bloodstream) is common in follicular carcinoma. Invasive follicular carcinomas are subclassified into minimally invasive, angioinvasive, and widely invasive categories, which are based on histologic findings (e.g., capsular invasion, limited or extensive vascular invasion).

FIGURE 4.29. This tumor shows suspicious areas for capsular invasion.

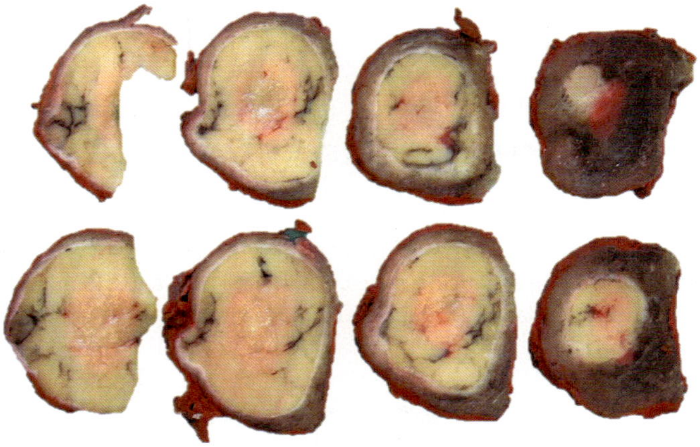

FIGURE 4.30. The tumor slice in (A) shows an area of probable capsule invasion (arrow). In (B), a tumor slice shows a more definite area of capsular invasion in which the white tumor capsule is absent (arrow).

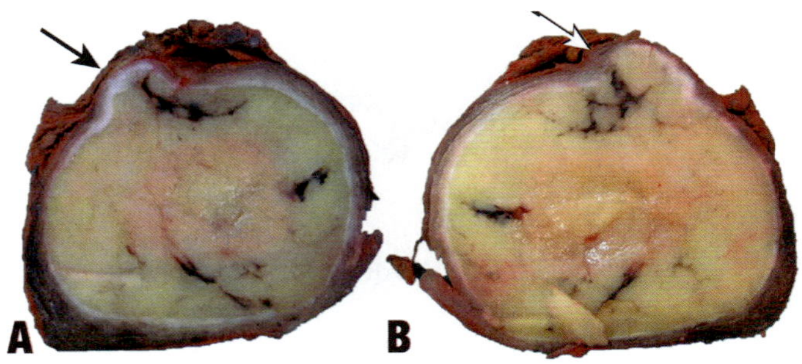

FOLLICULAR CARCINOMA WITH CAPSULAR INVASION (MINIMALLY INVASIVE FOLLICULAR CARCINOMA)

FIGURE 4.31. Notice how the fleshy tumor in this image invades out of the capsule (arrow).

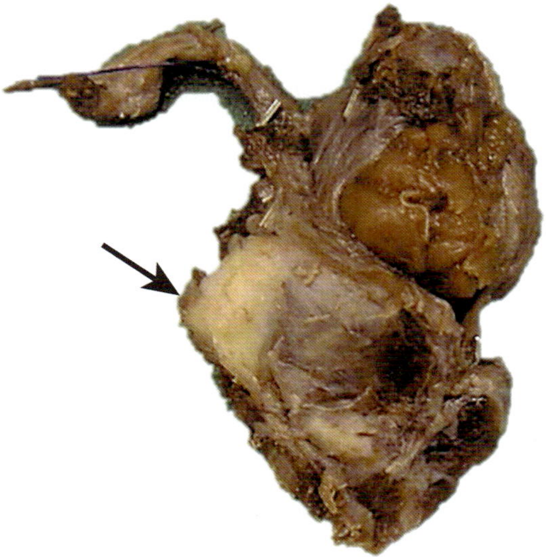

FOLLICULAR CARCINOMA WITH EXTRATHYROIDAL EXTENSION

FIGURE 4.32. Note the absence of any normal thyroid tissue or soft tissue at the advancing edge of the carcinoma in this image. The extrathyroidal extension was diagnosed by both macroscopy and microscopy.

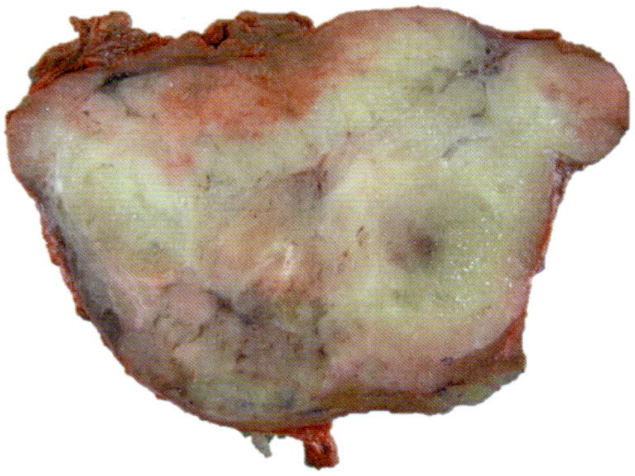

WIDELY INVASIVE FOLLICULAR CARCINOMA

FIGURE 4.33. In this case, the thyroid parenchyma was completely replaced by the infiltrating nodules. The tumor is invading the adjacent muscle in a pushing pattern.

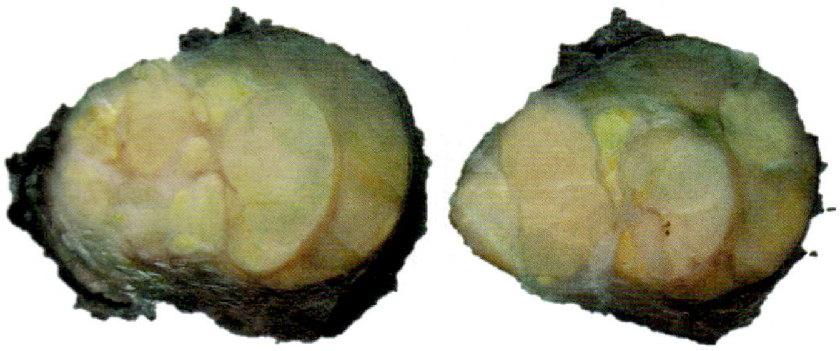

FIGURE 4.34. In this case, the dark tissue at the edge is skeletal muscle invaded by the tumor. The yellowish area is necrotic tumor tissue.

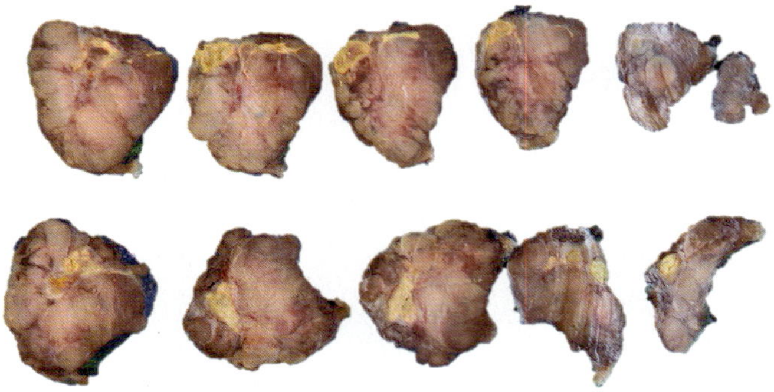

Anaplastic carcinoma

Anaplastic carcinoma is the least common but most aggressive type of thyroid cancer (occurring in 1% of cases). It is a fast growing, large (often > 5 cm), rock hard tumor with frequent wide invasion into surrounding soft tissues and skeletal muscle at the time of presentation. It can occasionally contain cartilage and bone, and necrosis may be present. Three histological patterns are recognized: sarcomatoid, epithelial, and giant cell. Distant metastasis (to lung, bone, etc.) occurs in nearly half of patients.

FIGURE 4.35. This image shows a solid, white, and firm cut surface with invasive edge.

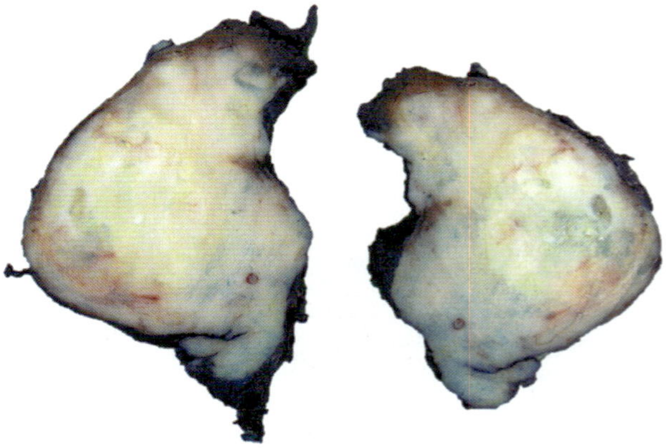

FIGURE 4.36. The white fleshy tumor in this image is invading into adipose tissue (yellow).

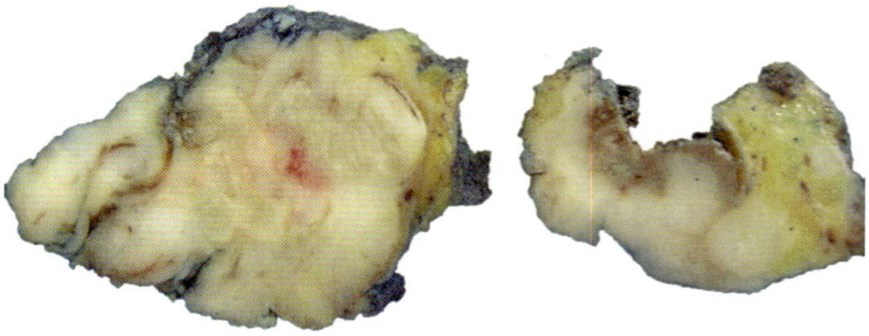

FIGURE 4.37. The tumor in (A) shows a variegated outer surface, which indicates a wide invasion front. The tumor in (B) shows a homogeneous whitish cut surface. On the lower pole of this specimen, a small portion of brownish, glistening, nonneoplastic thyroid tissue is visible (arrow).

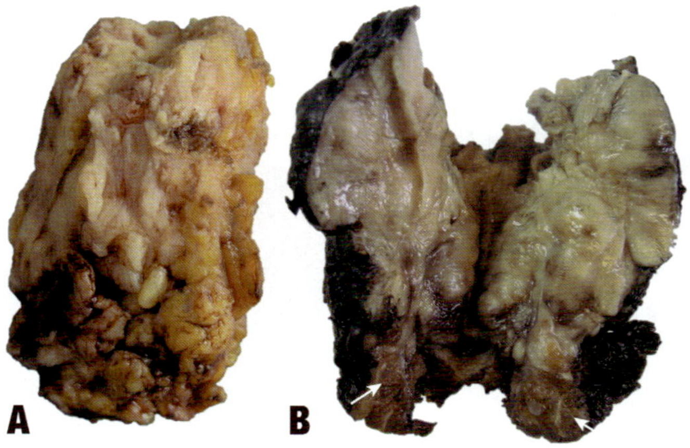

Medullary thyroid carcinoma

Medullary thyroid carcinoma originates from the parafollicular C cells that produce the hormone calcitonin. Medullary carcinoma is the third most common type of thyroid cancer (occurring in 3% of cases). It can be sporadic, familial, or associated with multiple endocrine neoplasia type 2. Medullary carcinomas arise in the upper third to upper half of lateral lobes where the C cells are commonly found. They are well delineated but lack capsule. Hereditary cases can be multifocal or bilateral; sporadic cases have poorer prognosis.

FIGURE 4.38. The color of the tumor cut surface can range from tan-white to yellow-pink. This image shows a tan-white tumor arising in the upper third of the right lobe.

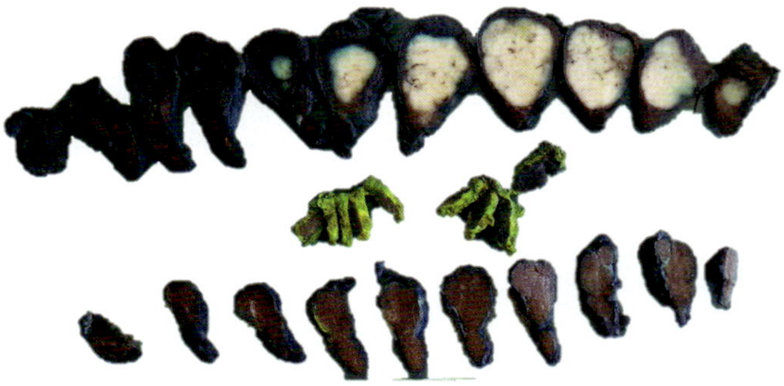

FIGURE 4.39. The tumor in this specimen has a yellow-pink color and rubbery cut surfaces.

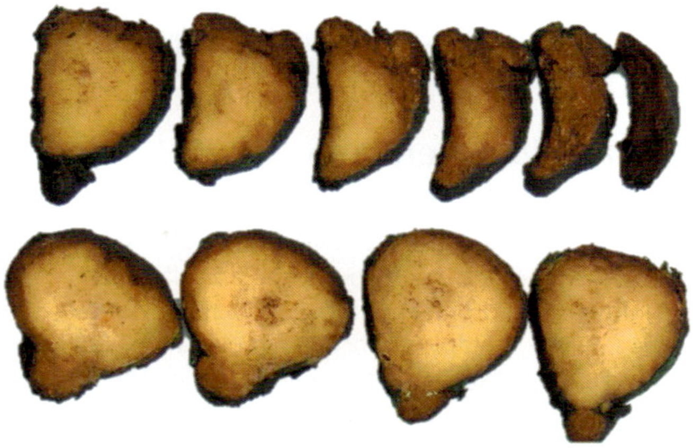

SPORADIC MEDULLARY THYROID CARCINOMA

FIGURE 4.40. This image shows a sporadic medullary carcinoma replacing the left lobe. The tumor was very vascular with intratumoral hemorrhage.

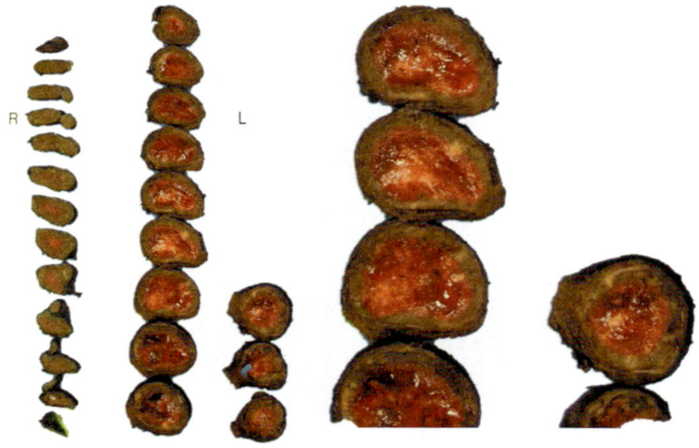

METASTATIC MEDULLARY THYROID CARCINOMA

FIGURE 4.41. In contrast to the red-brown lymph node tissue, this tumor shows a tan fleshy cut surface.

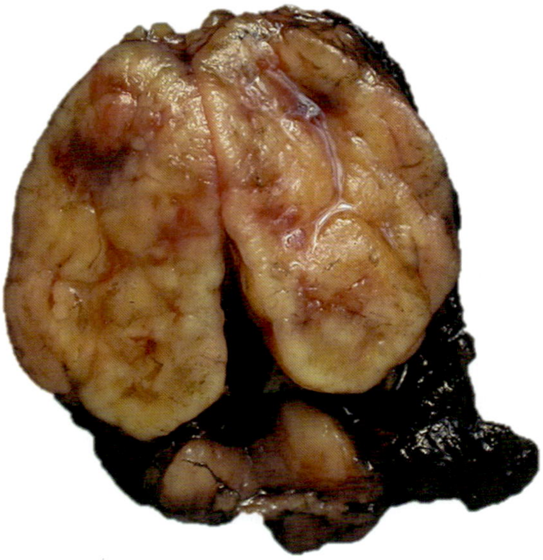

Parathyroid Glands

Parathyroid hyperplasia

Parathyroid hyperplasia is the enlargement of the parathyroid glands. It usually involves all 4 glands, but it can also be asymmetrical. It may occur sporadically or as part of 3 inherited syndromes: multiple endocrine neoplasia type 1 (MEN 1), multiple endocrine neoplasia type 2A (MEN 2A), and isolated familial hyperparathyroidism. The average weight of a normal parathyroid gland is 30 mg to 40 mg.

FIGURE 4.42. Image (A) shows 2 hyperplastic parathyroid glands. Image (B) shows asymmetrical parathyroid hyperplasia.

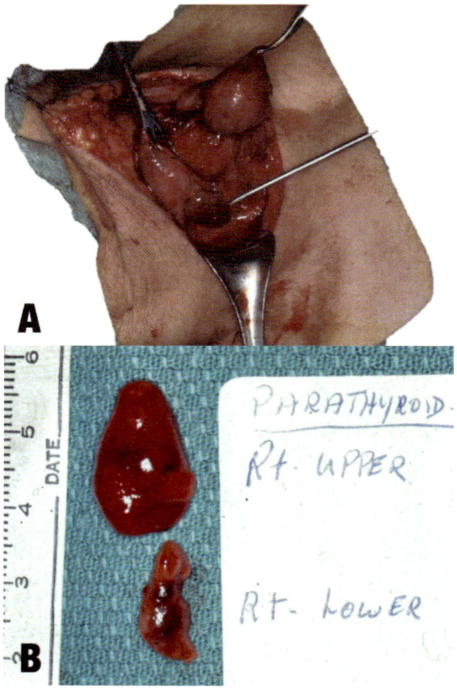

Intraoperative images courtesy of Dr. Roger Tabah

Parathyroid adenoma

Parathyroid adenoma is a benign tumor that causes hyperparathyroidism. The diagnosis of parathyroid adenoma requires a combination of clinical, laboratory, and histologic findings. The following intraoperative findings confirm the diagnosis of adenoma: presence of a single enlarged parathyroid; a drop in intraoperative parathormone levels immediately after resection of the single enlarged parathyroid; and the presence of a rim of normal parathyroid tissue at the edge of the hypercellular parathyroid neoplasm on histological examination.

FIGURE 4.43. These images show an intraoperative single enlarged parathyroid preresection (A) and postresection (B).

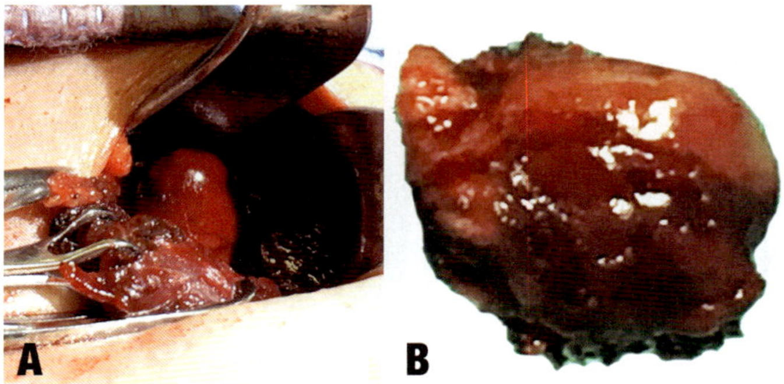

Intraoperative photos courtesy of Dr. Richard Payne

INTRATHYROIDAL PARATHYROID ADENOMA

FIGURE 4.44. Parathyroid adenoma can grow inside the thyroid gland. It has a finer texture on the cut surface that can differentiate it from the thyroid parenchyma.

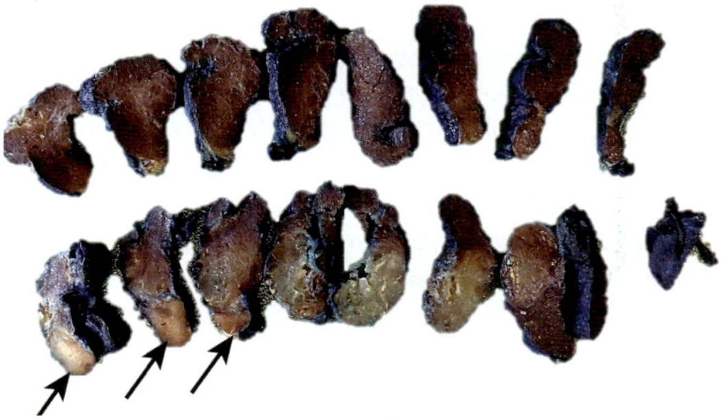

MEDIASTINAL PARATHYROID ADENOMA

Approximately 10% to 20% of patients with primary hyperparathyroidism have mediastinal parathyroid adenoma.

FIGURE 4.45. This image shows a mediastinal parathyroid adenoma (arrow) and adjacent normal thymus and thyroid tissue.

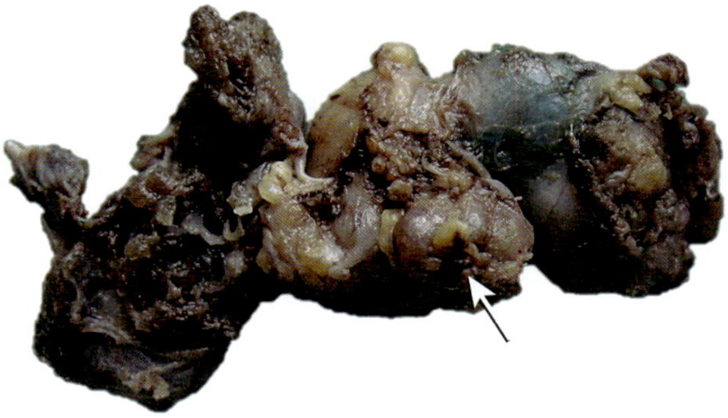

Adrenal Glands

The adrenal glands are located above and slightly medial to the kidneys. The right adrenal gland is pyramidal, the left semilunar in shape. The glands appear yellowish in color. Functionally, the adrenal cortex produces mineralocorticoids, glucocorticoids, and androgens. The adrenal medulla produces the catecholamines adrenaline and noradrenaline.

REFERENCE: NORMAL ADRENAL GLANDS

FIGURE 4.46. Image (A) shows the normal adrenal glands and kidneys of an adult. Image (B) shows the normal adrenal glands of a 1-month-old infant.

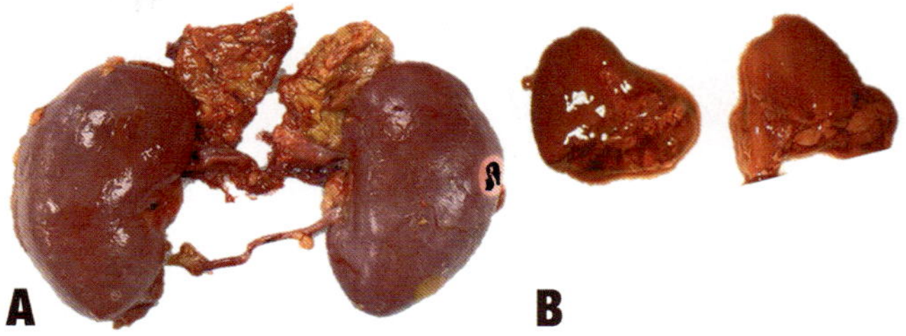

Waterhouse–Friderichsen syndrome

Waterhouse–Friderichsen syndrome is defined as adrenal gland failure due to massive hemorrhage into the adrenal glands caused by severe bacterial infection, typically by meningococcus *Neisseria meningitidis*. Patients usually progress very rapidly to multiorgan failure, disseminated intravascular coagulation, and death.

FIGURE 4.47. These images show extensive hemorrhage into the adrenal gland.

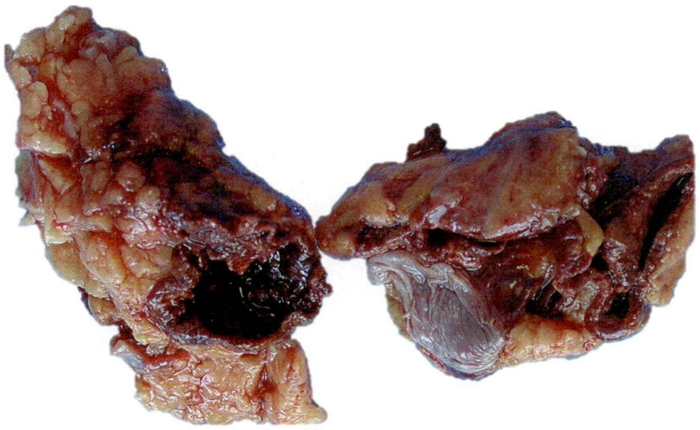

Adrenal cortical hyperplasia

Adrenal cortical hyperplasia is a nonneoplastic increase in adrenal cortical cells. It can be diffuse (62% of cases) or nodular (20% of cases).

FIGURE 4.48. The sections in the middle of this image show a thickened cortex when compared to the rest of the sections. The cortical mass is increased in response to increased adrenocorticotropin hormone (ACTH) secretion from the pituitary gland or ectopic sites.

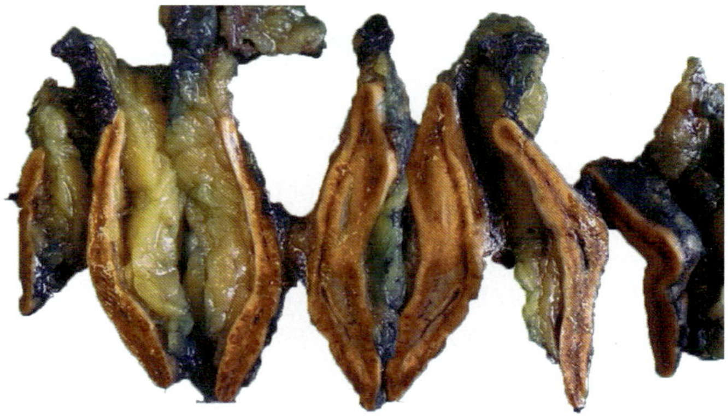

ADRENAL DIFFUSE CORTICAL HYPERPLASIA

Diffuse cases are usually bilateral and associated with elevated ACTH produced either by the pituitary gland or an ACTH-producing tumor.

FIGURE 4.49. This image shows diffuse thickening of the adrenal cortex.

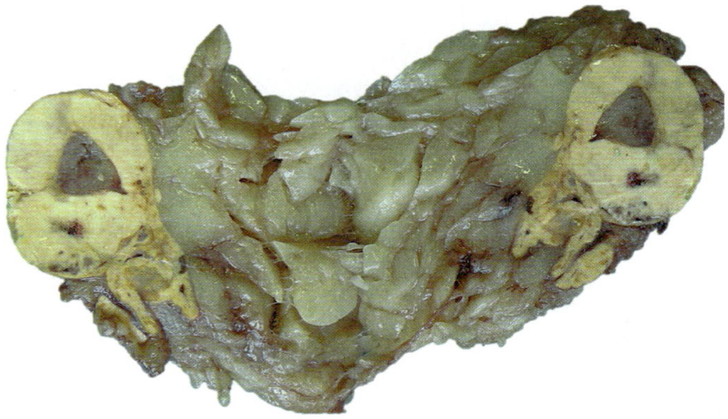

ADRENAL NODULAR CORTICAL HYPERPLASIA

FIGURE 4.50. This enlarged adrenal gland contains multiple nodules of variable size.

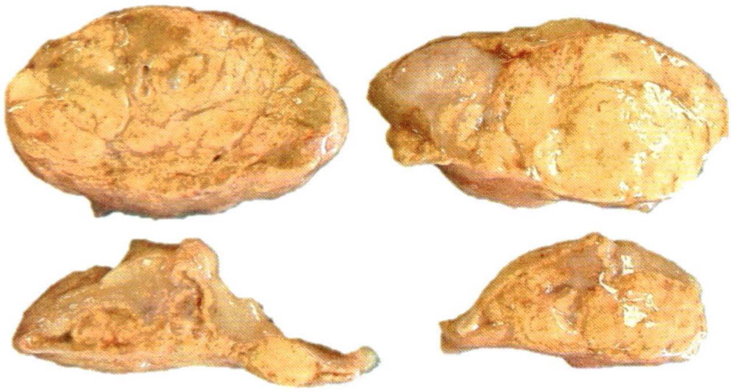

Adrenocortical adenoma

Adrenal tumors can be functional or nonfunctional. When functional, they produce in excess the hormones normally produced by the adrenal gland. Adrenocortical adenoma can be functionally heterogeneous. Aldosterone-producing adenomas are usually yellow; glucocorticoid-secreting adenomas can be either yellow or pigmented/black. Virilizing tumors are usually red-brown. Cystic change may be found in all cases, but necrosis is uncommon. When large, these adenomas can nearly replace the adrenal glands.

FIGURE 4.51. This adrenal cortical adenoma is functional, and the patient clinically presented with hyperaldosteronism.

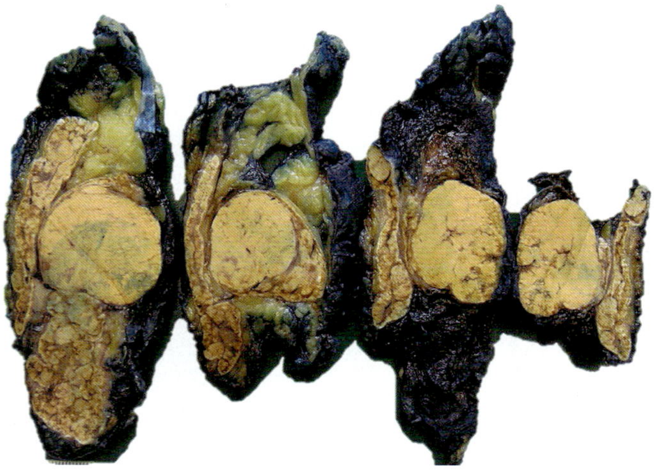

FIGURE 4.52. This image shows a single, well-delineated nodule with pushing border and hemorrhage.

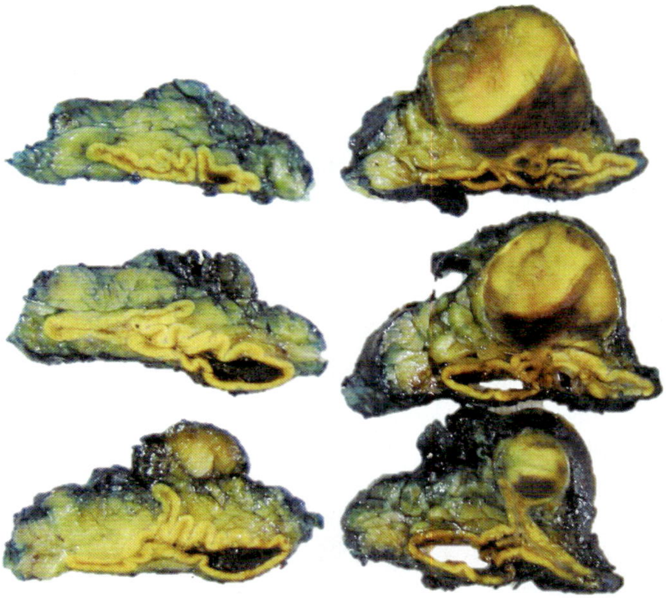

FIGURE 4.53. This large adenoma shows focal areas of hemorrhage and minor cystic change. Normal adrenal gland tissue is visible (arrow).

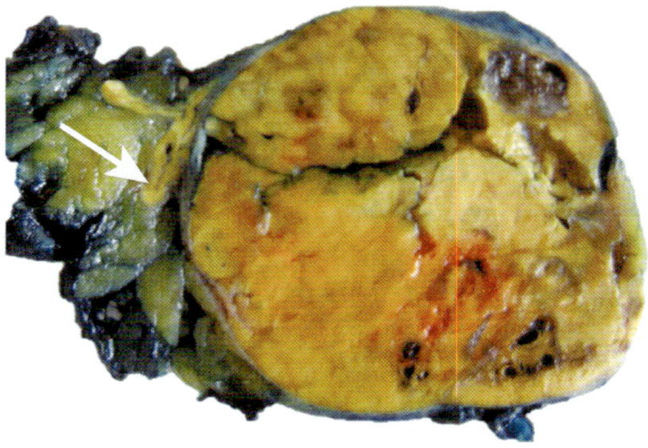

FIGURE 4.54. This adrenocortical adenoma shows central hemorrhage, giving the tumor a pseudocystic appearance.

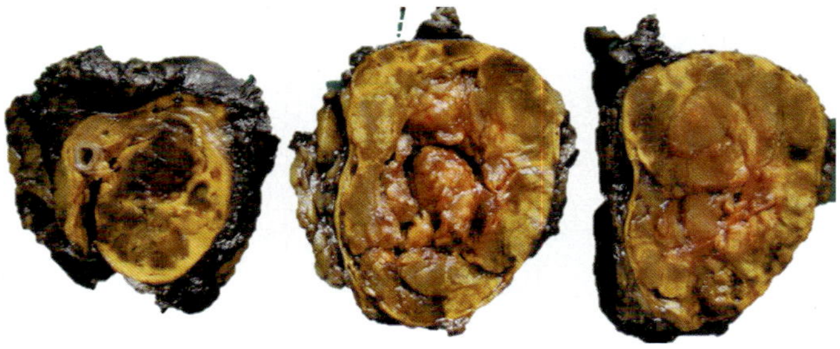

Adrenocortical carcinoma

Adrenocortical carcinoma is an aggressive cancer of the adrenal cortex. It is rare (1 to 2 cases per million). These carcinomas can be functional (steroid hormone–producing) or nonfunctional. If functional, they can cause Cushing syndrome, Conn syndrome, virilization, or feminization. They are typically very large with frequent necrosis and hemorrhage. At the time of diagnosis, they have often invaded nearby tissues or metastasized to distant organs. Only 20% to 35% of patients survive 5 years or more.

FIGURE 4.55. This image shows a tumor in the adrenal bed, growing in multiple yellow nodules and invading into periadrenal soft tissues.

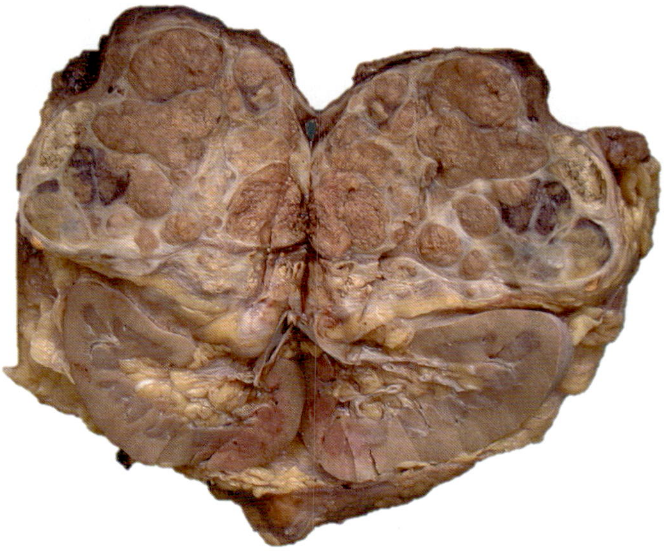

Pheochromocytoma

Pheochromocytomas, also called intraadrenal paragangliomas, are an uncommon neuroendocrine tumor arising in the medulla of the adrenal glands. They can be sporadic or associated with 3 syndromes: von Hippel–Lindau syndrome, MEN 2, and neurofibromatosis type 1. Sporadic tumors are usually unilateral; familial tumors are commonly bilateral or multicentric. High blood pressure is the most important symptom. The tumors are malignant in 10% of cases but may be cured completely by surgical removal.

FIGURE 4.56. Although adrenal pheochromocytomas are usually yellow, this color darkens when exposed to air during sectioning, as seen in this image.

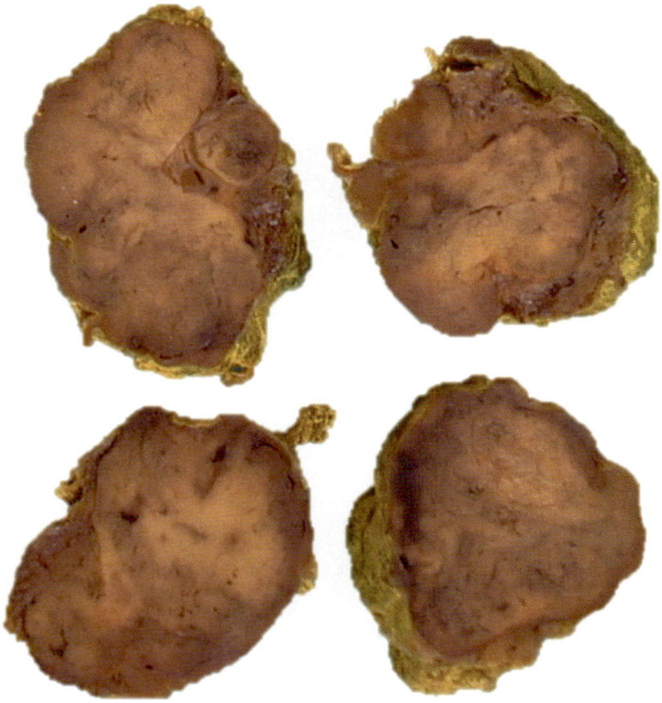

FIGURE 4.57. This tumor appears dark brownish in contrast to the yellow color of normal adrenal gland tissue.

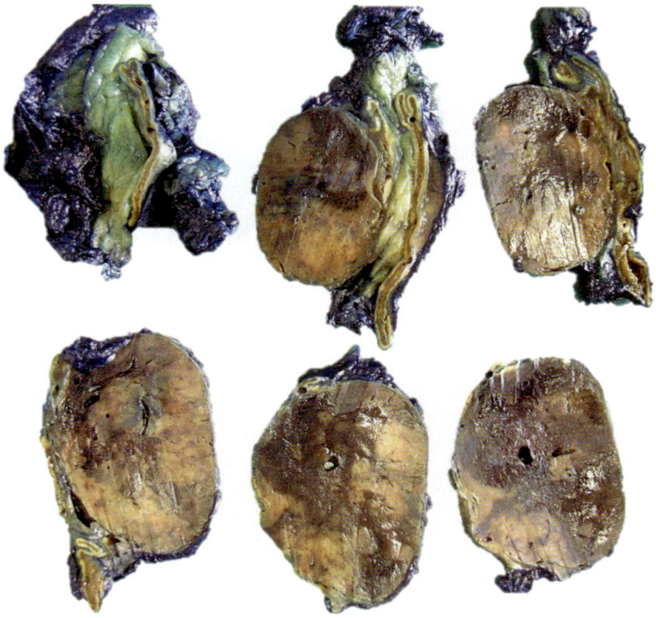

PHEOCHROMOCYTOMA WITH CYSTIC CHANGE

Cystic change is common in larger-sized pheochromocytomas.

FIGURE 4.58. This image shows pseudocysts caused by intratumoral hemorrhage and necrosis.

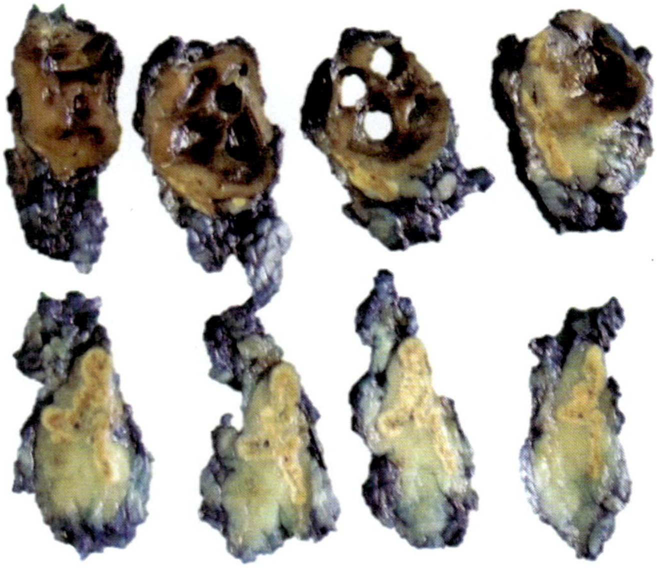

FIGURE 4.59. This pheochromocytoma presented as a cystic adrenal mass.

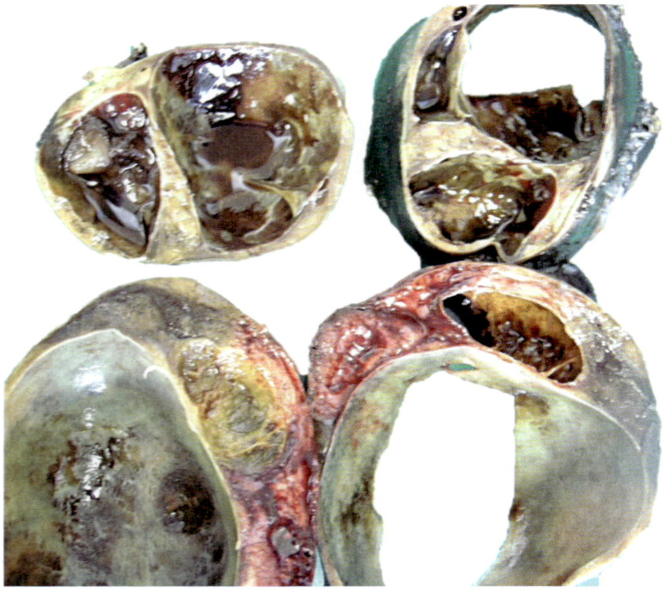

MALIGNANT PHEOCHROMOCYTOMA

All pheochromocytomas have some potential to metastasize. The definite diagnosis of malignant pheochromocytoma requires presence of lymph node metastasis or distant metastasis.

FIGURE 4.60. This large tumor showed high vascularization, necrosis, and lymph node metastasis (arrow).

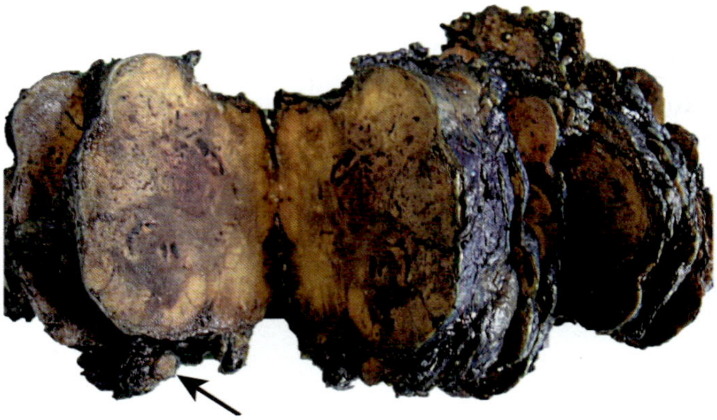

Adrenal neuroblastoma

Neuroblastoma is an aggressive and common adrenal malignancy in young children (the median age is 2 years).

FIGURE 4.61. Image (A) shows a large, lobulated adrenal mass. In (B), the cut section of the tumor shows areas of hemorrhage and necrosis.

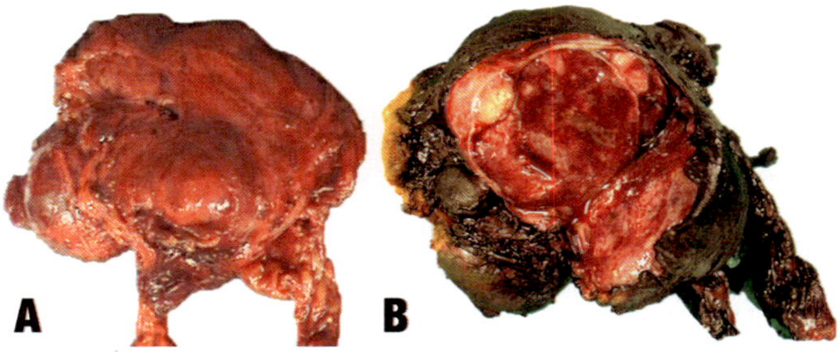

Adrenal gland hemangioma

Adrenal gland hemangioma is a rare, nonfunctioning, benign neoplasm characterized by the presence of blood-filled, dilated vascular spaces lined with mature endothelial cells. Hemangiomas in the adrenal gland are often of the cavernous type.

FIGURE 4.62. Dark red blood is filling multiloculated cavernous spaces.

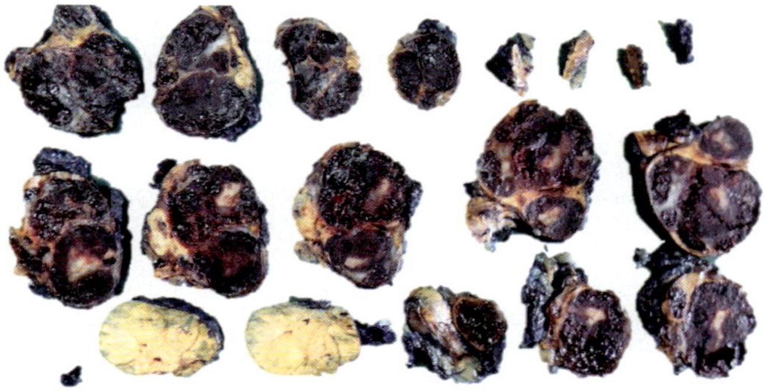

High-grade primary leiomyosarcoma of the adrenal gland bed

Primary adrenal leiomyosarcoma is extremely rare. It is believed to originate from the smooth muscle wall of the central adrenal vein and its branches. Metastasis from other sites such as the uterus must be excluded before making this diagnosis.

FIGURE 4.63. This image shows a firm, rubbery tumor with a white cut surface.

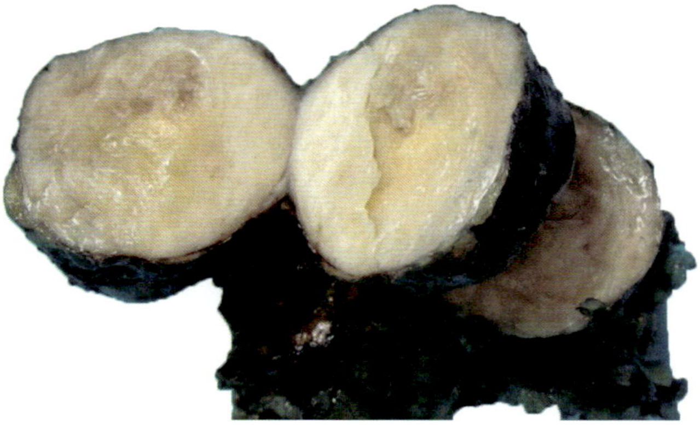

High-grade undifferentiated sarcoma of the adrenal gland

FIGURE 4.64. This large, high-grade sarcoma (16 cm in size) shows extensive necrosis. Clinically, it was thought to originate from the right adrenal bed. The final diagnosis for this case was undifferentiated sarcoma. The remnants of the adrenal gland were found embedded within the tumor. The liver and pleura were also involved.

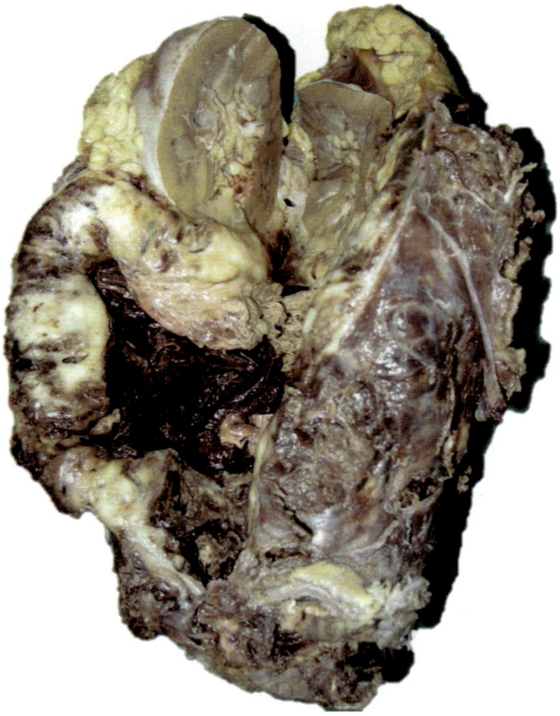

Metastasis to the adrenal gland

Lung, breast, kidney, pancreas, stomach, and liver are among the most common primary sites of metastasis.

METASTATIC RENAL CELL CARCINOMA (RCC)

FIGURE 4.65. This image shows a metastatic renal cell carcinoma with adjacent normal adrenal gland tissue.

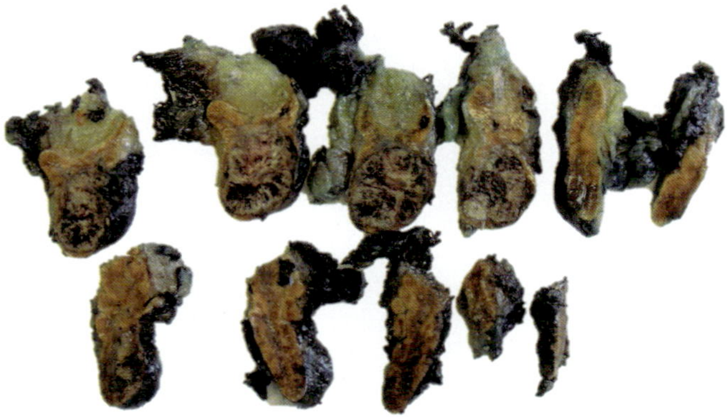

METASTATIC HEPATOCELLULAR CARCINOMA

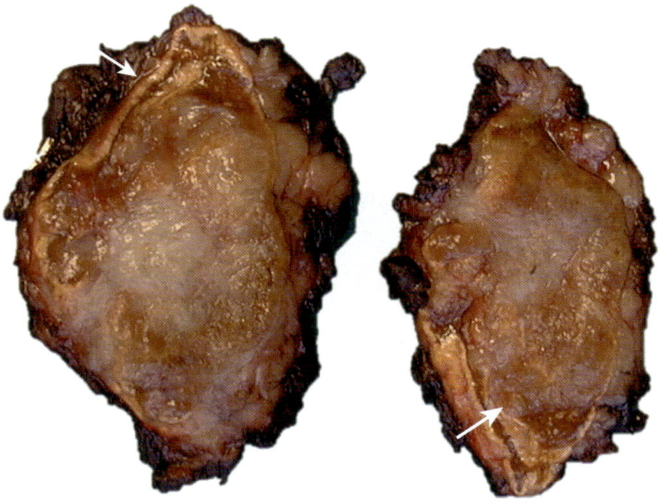

FIGURE 4.66. Note the normal adrenal gland tissue at the edge (arrows).

REFERENCES

Allolio B, Fassnacht M. Clinical review: adrenocortical carcinoma: clinical update. J Clin Endocrinol Metab. 2006;91(6):2027–2037. https://doi.org/10.1210/jc.2005-2639. Medline:16551738

Amin MB, Edge SB, editors. *AJCC cancer staging manual*. 8th ed. Chicago: Springer; 2018.

Barnes L. *Surgical pathology of the head and neck*. 3rd ed. New York: CRC Press; 2008.

Eisenhofer G, Bornstein SR, Brouwers FM, Cheung NK, Dahia PL, de Krijger RR, Giordano TJ, Greene LA, Goldstein DS, Lehnert H, Manger WM, Maris JM, Neumann HP, Pacak K, Shulkin BL, Smith DI, Tischler AS, Young WF. Malignant pheochromocytoma: current status and initiatives for future progress. Endocr Relat Cancer. 2004;11(3):423–436. https://doi.org/10.1677/erc.1.00829. Medline:15369446

Fletcher CDM. *Diagnostic histopathology of tumors*. 4th ed. Philadelphia: Saunders/Elsevier; 2013.

Ganly I, Wang L, Tuttle RM, Katabi N, Ceballos GA, Garach HR, Ghossein R. Invasion rather than nuclear features correlates with outcome in encapsulated follicular tumors: further evidence for the reclassification of the encapsulated papillary thyroid carcinoma follicular variant. Hum Pathol. 2015;46(5):657–664. https://doi.org/10.1016/j.humpath.2015.01.010. Medline:25721865

Goldman L, Schafer AI. *Goldman-Cecil medicine*. 25th ed. Philadelphia: Saunders/Elsevier; 2016.

Kumar V, Abbas AK, Fausto N, Aster J. *Robbins and Cotran pathologic basis of disease*. 9th ed. Philadelphia: Saunders/Elsevier; 2015.

Liu AH, Juan LY, Yang AH, Chen HS, Lin HD. Anaplastic thyroid cancer with uncommon long-term survival. J Chin Med Assoc. 2006;69(10):489–491. https://doi.org/10.1016/S1726-4901(09)70314-4. Medline:17098674

Lloyd RV, Osamura RY, Gunter K, Rosai J. WHO classification of tumours of endocrine organs. 4th ed. Lyon : International Agency for Research on Cancer (IARC); 2018.

Matsuda D, Iwamura M, Baba S. Cavernous hemangioma of the adrenal gland. Int J Urol. 2009;16(4):424. https://doi.org/10.1111/j.1442-2042.2009.02260.x. Medline:19416406

Menconi F, Marcocci C, Marinò M. Diagnosis and classification of Graves' disease. Autoimmun Rev. 2014;13(4-5):398–402. https://doi.org/10.1016/j.autrev.2014.01.013. Medline:24424182

Mills SE, Carter D, Greenson JK, Hornick JL, Longacre TA, Reuter VE, editors. *Sternberg's diagnostic surgical pathology*. 6th ed. Philadelphia: Wolters Kluwer Health; 2015.

Nikiforov Y, Biddinger PW, Thompson LDR. *Diagnostic pathology and molecular genetics of the thyroid*. 2nd ed. Philadelphia: Lippincott Williams & Wilkins; 2012.

Thakker RV. The parathyroid glands, hypercalcemia and hypocalcemia. In: Goldman L, Schafer AI, editors. *Goldman-Cecil medicine*. 25th ed. Philadelphia: Saunders/Elsevier; 2016: chap 245.

Wenig, BM. *Atlas of head and neck pathology*. 3rd ed. Philadelphia: Saunders/Elsevier; 2015.

Zhou Y, Tang Y, Tang J, Deng F, Gong G, Dai Y. Primary adrenal leiomyosarcoma: a case report and review of literature. Int J Clin Exp Pathol. 2015;8(4):4258–4263. Medline:26097622

5

Breast Diseases

ZARI DASTANI, ERIK NOHR, LARA RICHER, WENQIAN CHEN, HUA YANG

REFERENCE: NORMAL BREAST TISSUE

Normal breast tissue is mostly composed of fibrous and adipose tissue. Embedded in the whitish fibrous tissue are the ducts and glands that are important for lactation. Different surgeries can be performed on the breast (mastectomy, resection, lumpectomy, etc.). Prior to surgery, surgical margins are inked. Postsurgery, but prior to processing, specimens are fixed in formalin, which can alter their coloration.

FIGURE 5.1. Normal breast tissue is mostly composed of fibrous (white) and adipose (yellow) tissue.

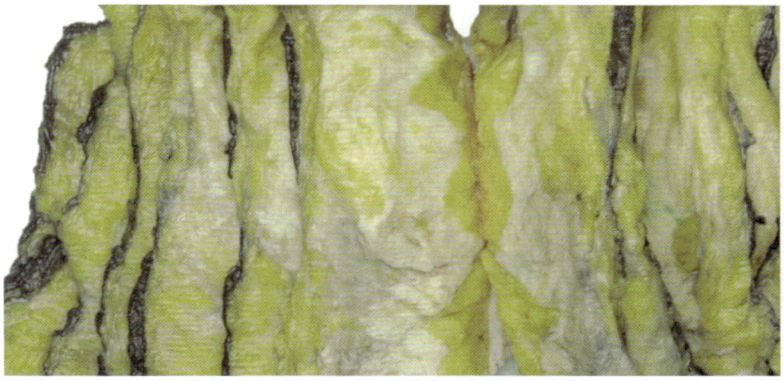

Nonneoplastic Diseases of the Breast

Breast implant

Breast implants are prosthetic devices that generally contain saline or silicone gel. They are often used for breast augmentation or reconstruction after mastectomy. In reconstruction, the surgical technique and timeline for reconstruction are chosen based on factors such as body habitus, previous breast size, desired breast size, and future planned treatments.

FIGURE 5.2. Breast implants are often used for breast augmentation or reconstruction after mastectomy.

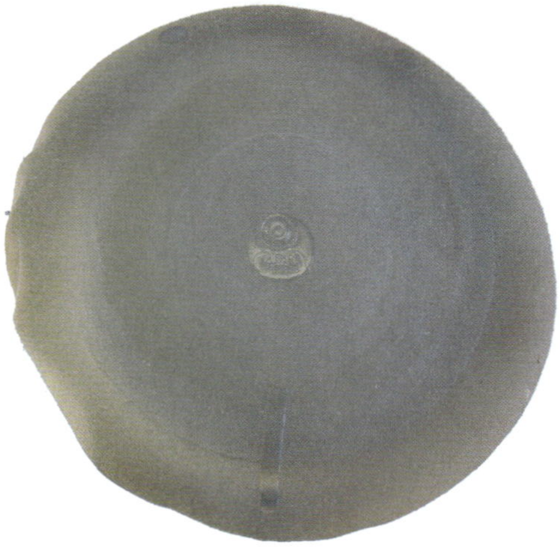

RUPTURED IMPLANT

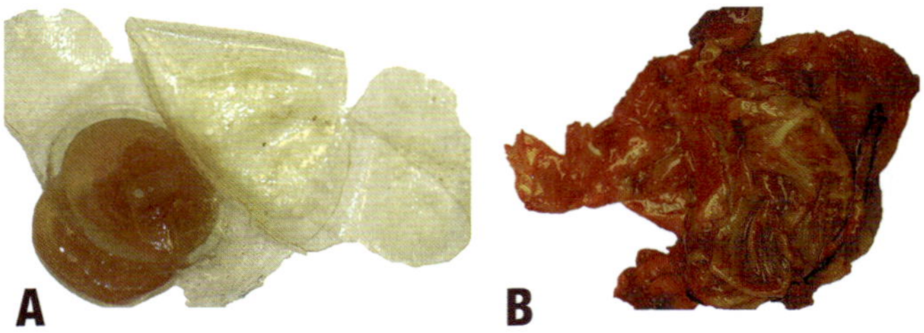

FIGURE 5.3. In (A), the implant is partially intact. Image (B) shows an implant surrounded by thick, fibrous, reactive tissue with focal calcification.

Chronic fat necrosis

Fat necrosis is a common benign inflammatory reaction in breast tissue secondary to injury. In the acute phase, necrosis of the adipose, hemorrhage, and inflammatory cell infiltration occur. In the chronic phase, fibrosis and calcification may occur resulting in a firm, ill-defined lesion that can mimic carcinoma.

FIGURE 5.4. This lumpectomy specimen shows an ill-defined sclerotic yellow-gray lesion. This is from a patient who developed a mass at a previous surgical scar. Multiple core biopsies and the final excision showed fat necrosis, inflammatory cell infiltration, and fibrosis. Immunohistochemistry for IgG4 was negative.

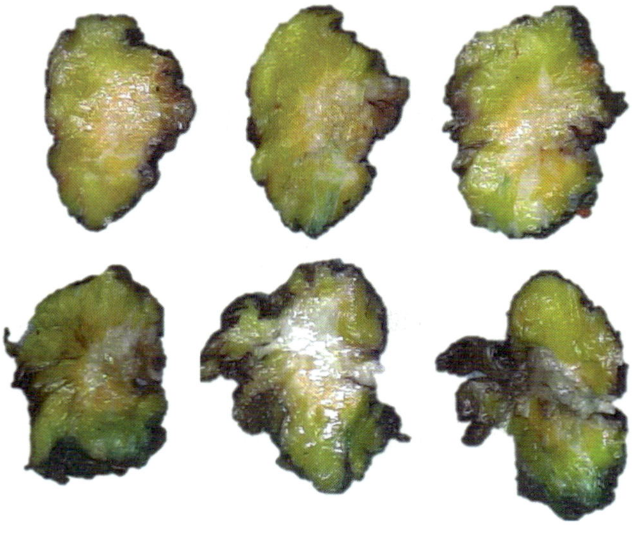

Diabetic mastopathy

Diabetic mastopathy, also called lymphocytic mastopathy, is a chronic inflammation of breast tissue in patients with long-standing diabetes mellitus or other autoimmune diseases. Clinically and radiologically, it presents as a hard, palpable mass mimicking carcinoma.

FIGURE 5.5. This excision specimen shows an ill-defined, firm, white-tan mass with no necrosis or hemorrhage.

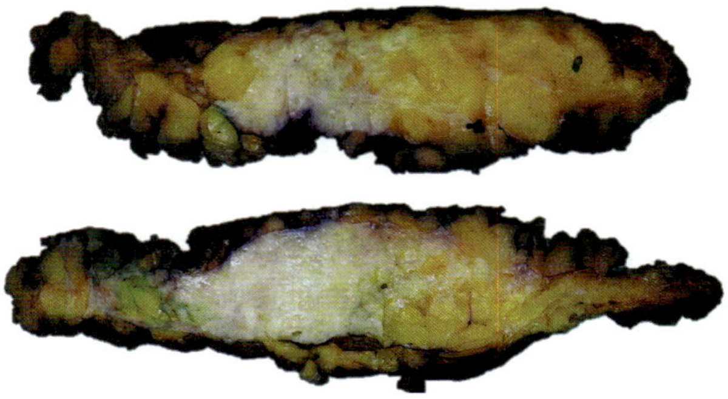

Fibrocystic change

Fibrocystic change is a common benign breast condition. It confers no increased risk of developing breast cancer despite having a characteristic "lumpy bumpy" quality on palpation. Small, clear or blue-domed cysts may be present.

FIGURE 5.6. Serial sections of this mastectomy specimen show glistening adipose tissue, fibrous tissue, and small cysts.

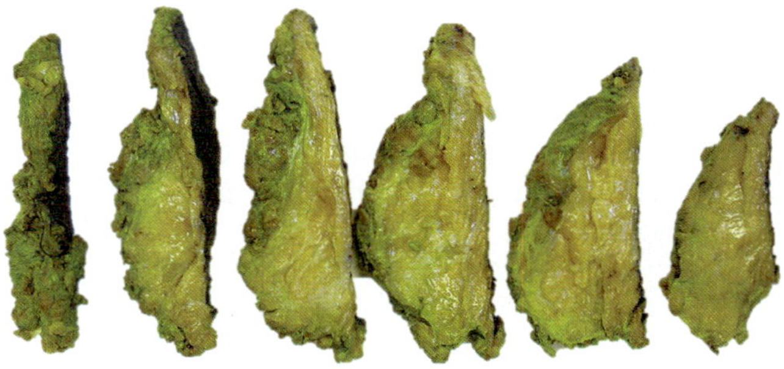

Complex sclerosing lesion

These benign lesions, similar to radial scars, show histological features of elastosis, sclerosis, and a distortion of the ductal and lobular architecture. They are often multifocal and involve both breasts. Grossly and microscopically, they are difficult to differentiate from invasive carcinoma.

FIGURE 5.7. In this resection specimen, a poorly defined, firm area mimicking invasive carcinoma is present.

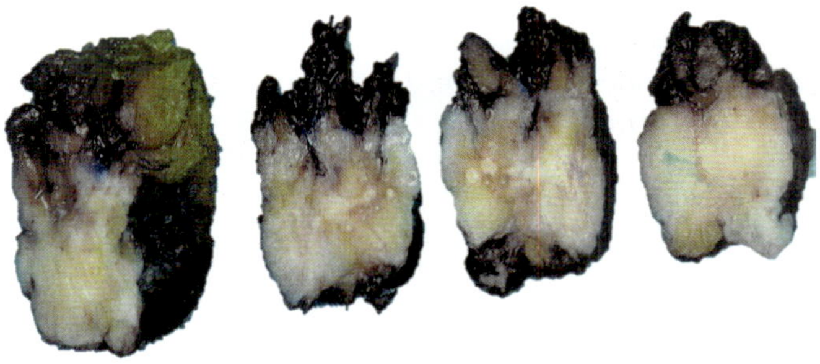

Neoplasms of the Breast

Breast adenoma

NIPPLE ADENOMA

This rare benign tumor results from a proliferation of small tubules lined by epithelial and myoepithelial cells at the nipple. Patients often present with nipple discharge and a mass on palpation.

FIGURE 5.8. This resection specimen shows a poorly defined, skin-colored nodule with a polypoid appearance at the nipple.

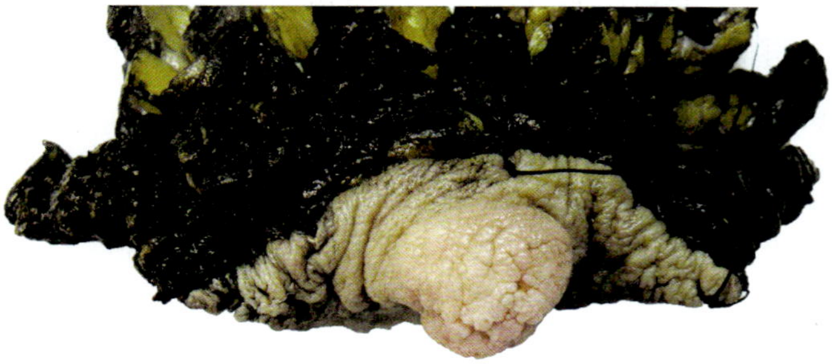

TUBULAR ADENOMA

Tubular adenomas are benign tumors mostly seen in young women. Histologically, the tumor is defined by increased tubules surrounded by epithelial and myoepithelial cells.

FIGURE 5.9. This lumpectomy specimen shows a well-circumscribed, homogeneous, tan mass with a somewhat granular cut surface.

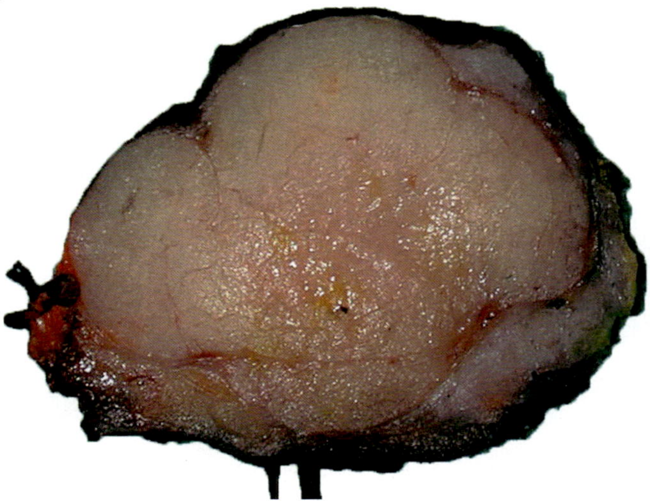

Atypical ductal hyperplasia

Atypical ductal hyperplasia results from atypical proliferation of cells within a ductal unit. It confers an increased risk of breast cancer.

FIGURE 5.10. These sections from a lesional area present as poorly defined, thick, fibrous tissue.

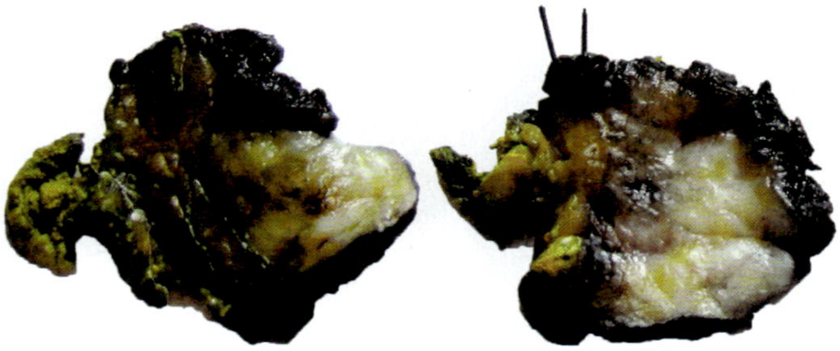

Breast papilloma

SCLEROSING PAPILLOMA

Papilloma is a benign, proliferative lesion characterized by papillary ingrowth of large central or small peripheral ducts in the breast. When involving large ducts, it can be associated with nipple discharge. The ducts are often dilated. Grossly, it appears as a soft, tan-pink, circumscribed nodule protruding to the dilated duct. Cystic spaces and hemorrhage are present. The lesion can undergo sclerosis with a firm cut surface.

FIGURE 5.11. This image shows a well-circumscribed firm tan nodule with an area of hemorrhage.

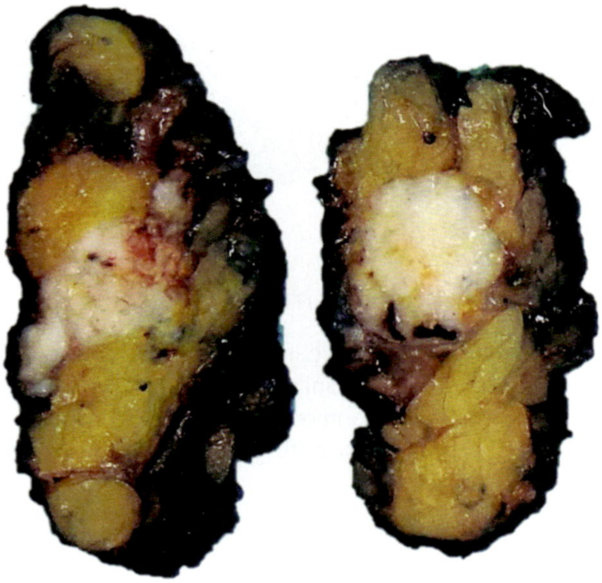

PAPILLOMATOSIS

Papillomatosis is a term applied when multiple ducts are involved by papilloma.

FIGURE 5.12. This image shows multiple small, well-circumscribed, soft, tan nodules that are papillomas on histology.

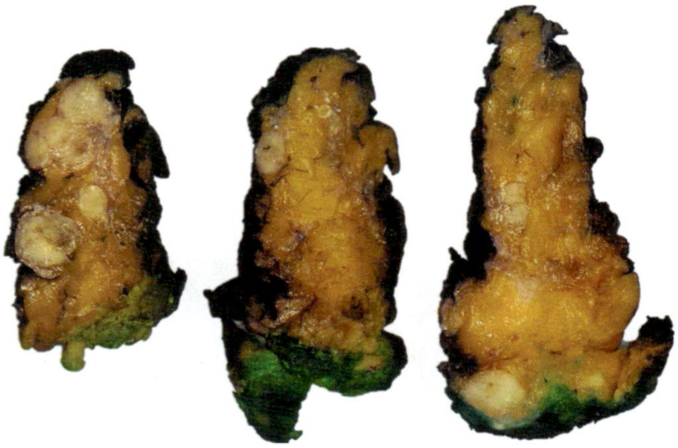

Breast carcinoma

DUCTAL CARCINOMA IN SITU (DCIS)

DCIS is an epithelial proliferation that is considered premalignant. It may present as calcifications on mammography. The incidence of this diagnosis has increased with screening programs. Grossly, extensive DCIS may form a gritty mass.

FIGURE 5.13. This excisional biopsy specimen shows poorly defined areas of firm fibrosis and punctuating necrosis.

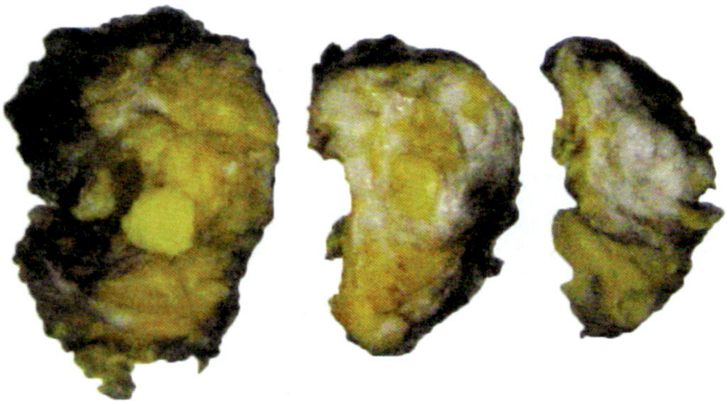

LOBULAR CARCINOMA IN SITU (LCIS)

LCIS is defined by a clonal proliferation of dyscohesive cells affecting at least half the acini within the terminal ductal lobular unit. The lesion confers an increased risk of cancer in both breasts. LCIS has no specific gross features and usually does not form a mass.

FIGURE 5.14. In this resection specimen, serial sections show fibrous areas similar to normal breast tissue.

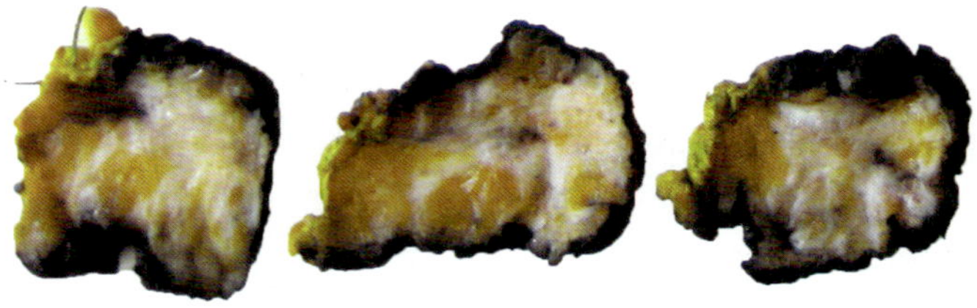

INVASIVE CARCINOMA OF NO SPECIAL TYPE (NST)

Also known as infiltrating ductal carcinoma, invasive carcinoma NST is now the favored term for the most commonly diagnosed breast cancer (representing 70% to 80% of all breast cancer diagnoses). These tumors are classically firm masses that feel gritty upon sectioning. Risk factors include old age, early menarche, late or no pregnancy, and family history, among others. Patients who test positive for *BRCA* gene mutations are 10 to 30 times more likely to develop breast cancer than those without mutations.

FIGURE 5.15. In this lumpectomy specimen, the cut surface shows an ill-defined, firm area with hemorrhage from a previous biopsy.

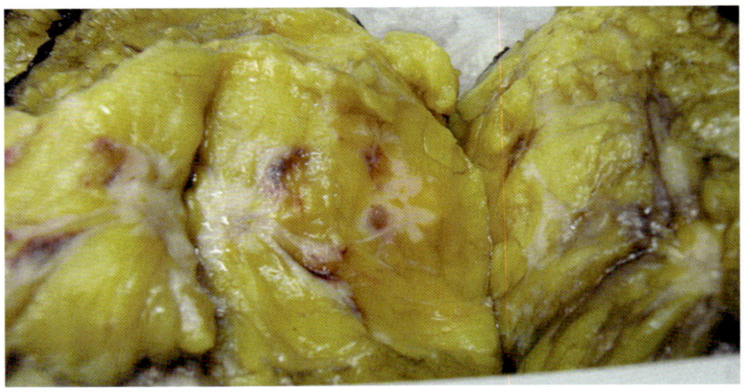

FIGURE 5.16. In this lumpectomy specimen, the cut surface shows a mass with infiltrating edges, hemorrhage, and necrosis.

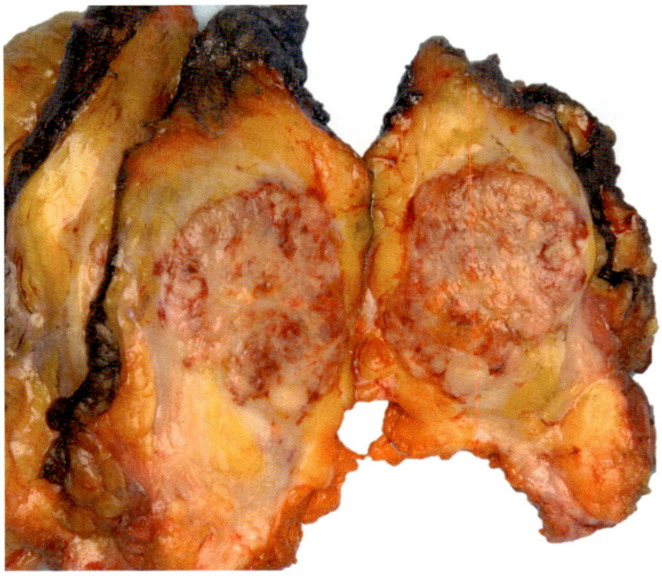

FIGURE 5.17. The cut surface of this resected tumor shows a typical white, infiltrative, scar-like lesion with firm consistency and poorly defined borders.

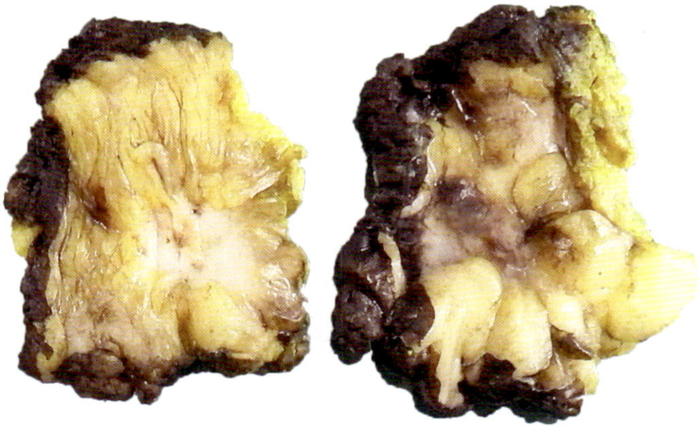

FIGURE 5.18. In this resection specimen, the tumor shows typical whitish discoloration, firm consistency, and poorly defined borders.

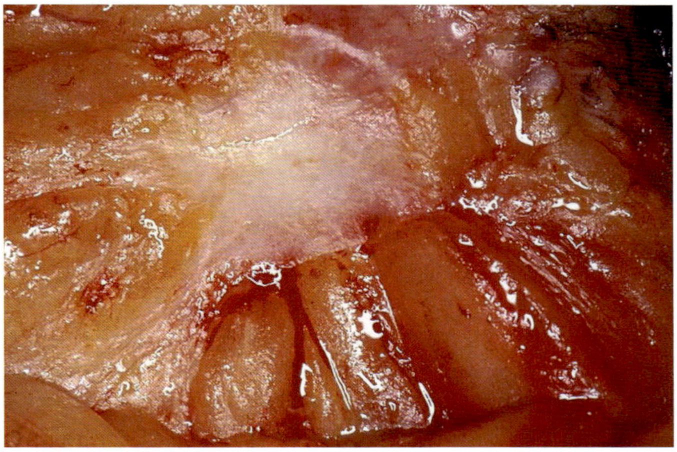

FIGURE 5.19. This cross-section demonstrates a large gray-white-yellow tumor with foci of necrosis invading directly into the skin.

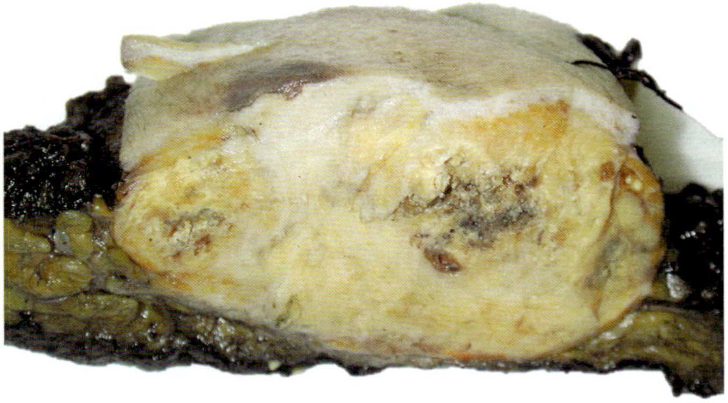

FIGURE 5.20. In this mastectomy specimen, the tumor is invading the overlying skin, causing skin necrosis and ulceration. Epidermal invasion with ulceration indicates a stage T4b tumor regardless of tumor size. Staging is based on the American Joint Committee on Cancer (AJCC) staging manual (8th edition).

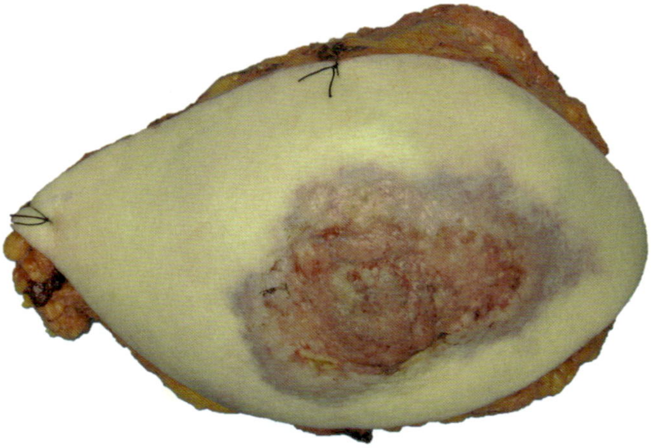

INVASIVE CARCINOMA NST POST–NEOADJUVANT CHEMOTHERAPY

It can be difficult to grossly identify residual tumor tissue or to distinguish it from scar tissue.

FIGURE 5.21. In this resection specimen, the cut surface appears yellow-white, lobulated, and fibrotic with punctate foci of hemorrhage.

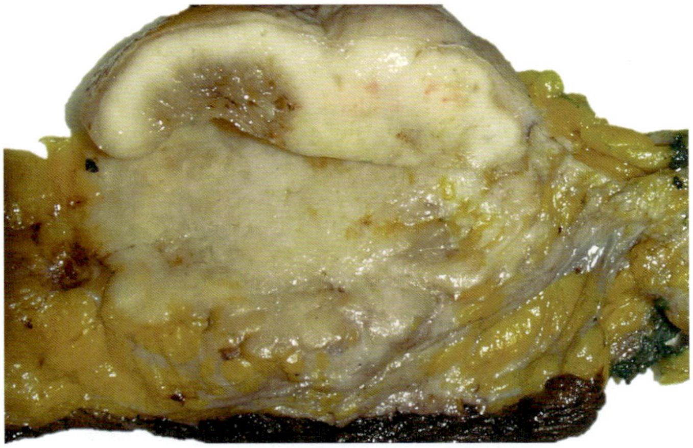

PROCEDURE: GRADING INVASIVE DUCTAL CARCINOMA

Breast cancers are classified as well differentiated (low grade), moderately differentiated (intermediate grade), and poorly differentiated (high grade), with the grades reflecting progressively worsening prognosis. The Nottingham modification of the Scarff-Bloom-Richardson grading system is used to grade breast carcinomas by adding up scores for tubule formation, nuclear pleomorphism, and mitotic count, each of which is given 1 to 3 points. The scores for each of these 3 criteria are then added together to give an overall final score and corresponding grade.

FIGURE 5.22. This specimen demonstrates a large, moderately well-defined, tan-pink mass with an infiltrative border. The tumor approaches the skin but the overlying epidermis is intact.

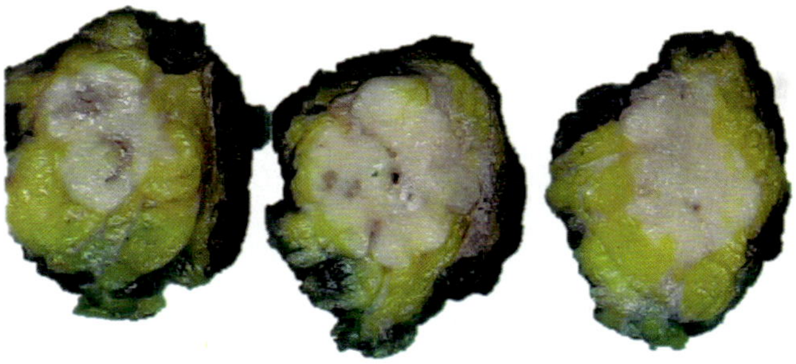

FIGURE 5.23. This lumpectomy specimen shows an irregularly shaped, firm, gray-white tumor mass that is close to the inked resection margin. This tumor was high grade on histologic examination.

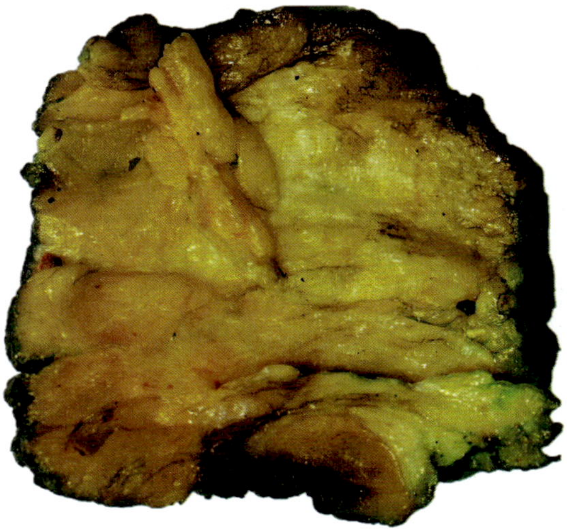

INVASIVE LOBULAR CARCINOMA

Invasive lobular carcinoma is the second most common form of breast cancer after invasive carcinoma NST. It represents 5% to 15% of breast cancer cases. It metastasizes to different organs than invasive carcinoma NST. Histologically, it is characterized by single or linear groupings of neoplastic cells infiltrating the stroma and adipose tissue. These tumors can be grossly imperceptible or they may form a mass. Unlike invasive ductal carcinomas, many invasive lobular carcinomas have subtle or vague gross appearances, and it is often difficult to define the tumor borders. Therefore, on gross examination the actual size is often underestimated.

FIGURE 5.24. In this resection specimen, there is ill-defined patchy fibrosis within the adipose tissue.

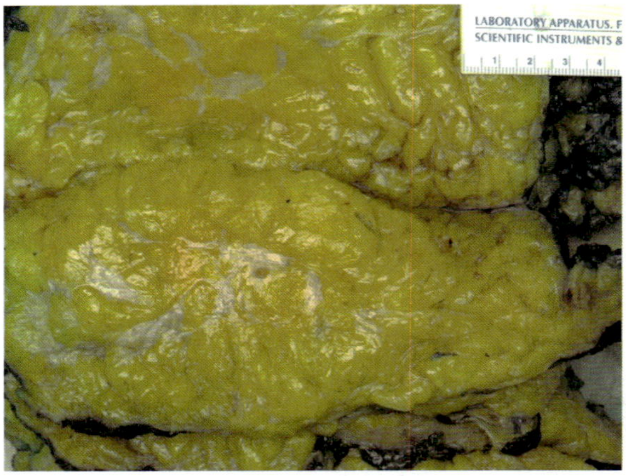

FIGURE 5.25. In the resection specimen in (A), multiple firm, poorly defined, white lesions are present throughout the breast. The ill-defined tumor in this image is difficult to distinguish from the background fibrous stroma. In (B), a small lumpectomy specimen contains an invasive lobular carcinoma. The central part of the whitish tumor can be seen, but it is difficult to define its borders by gross examination.

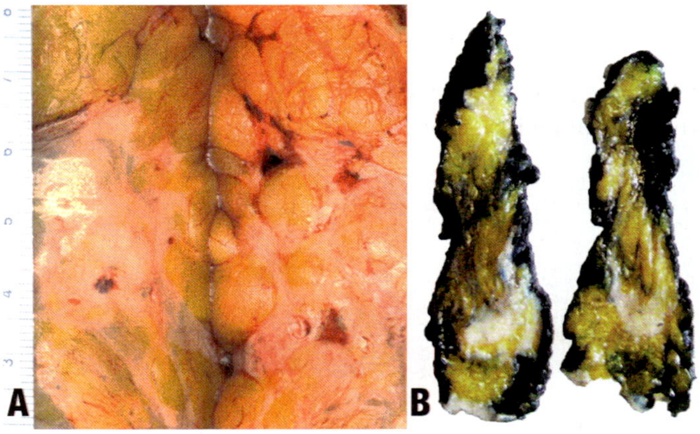

FIGURE 5.26. This ill-defined tumor extends to the breast parenchyma as fibrous bands that are difficult to differentiate from the background nonneoplastic fibrous tissue. Thorough sampling is recommended to accurately estimate tumor size.

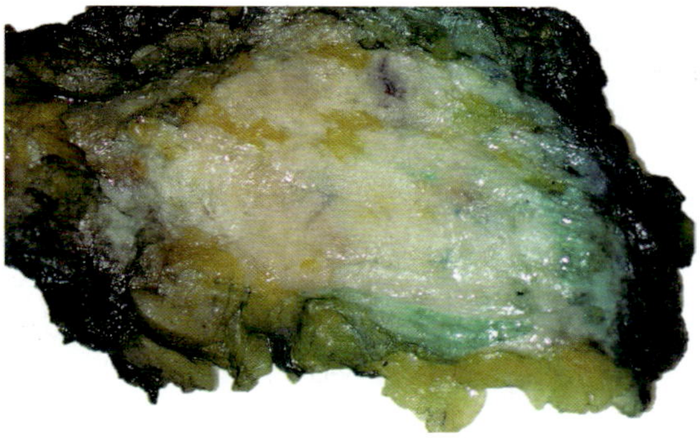

INVASIVE LOBULAR CARCINOMA — INVASIVE DUCTAL CARCINOMA MIMIC

FIGURE 5.27. Sometimes lobular carcinoma can form a mass mimicking an invasive ductal carcinoma. In this lumpectomy specimen, an ill-defined tan-pink, firm, and solid mass appears grossly akin to an invasive ductal carcinoma.

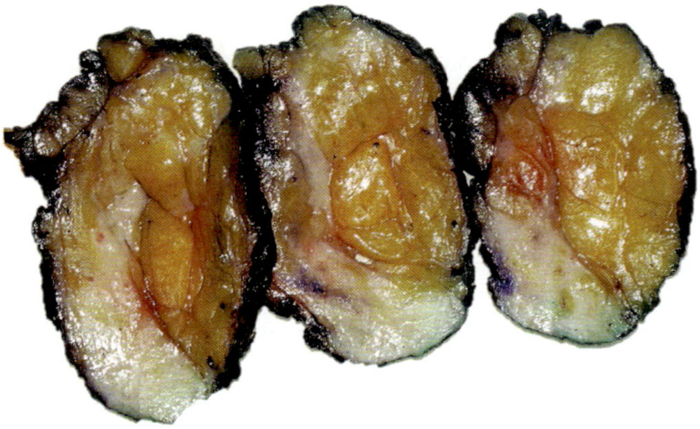

MIXED DUCTAL AND LOBULAR CARCINOMA

Diagnosis of mixed ductal and lobular carcinoma implies that the tumor has distinct ductal and lobular components.

FIGURE 5.28. In this lumpectomy specimen, there is a firm white-gray lesion with an irregular and ill-defined border.

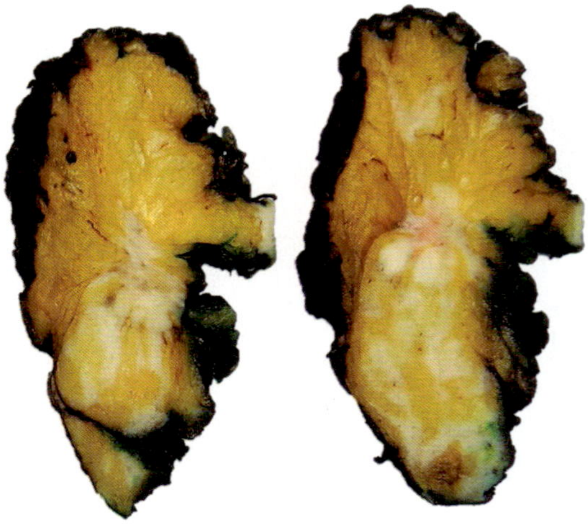

MUCINOUS CARCINOMA

This type of tumor consists of clusters of small uniform cells within extracellular mucin that is divided by fibrous septa. By definition, these features must involve at least 90% of the tumor mass. Representing 2% of all breast carcinomas, mucinous carcinomas generally have good prognoses.

FIGURE 5.29. In this lumpectomy specimen, the cut surface shows a well-demarcated, glistening, and soft tumor with focal hemorrhage.

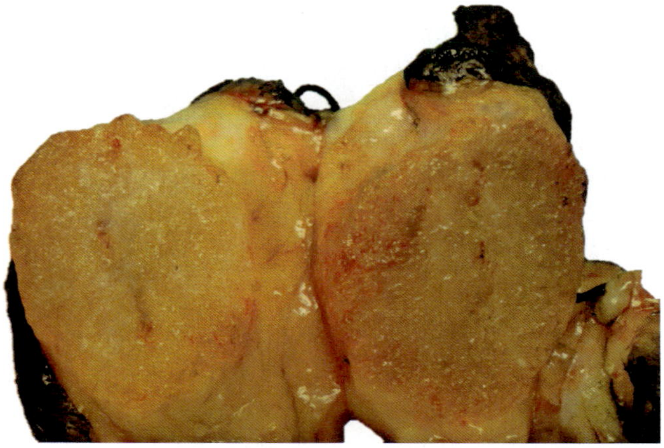

FIGURE 5.30. The cut surface of the resection specimen in (A) demonstrates a poorly demarcated, white-gray, glistening lesion. In (B), a cut surface shows a relatively well-demarcated, glistening, gelatinous tumor with areas of hemorrhage.

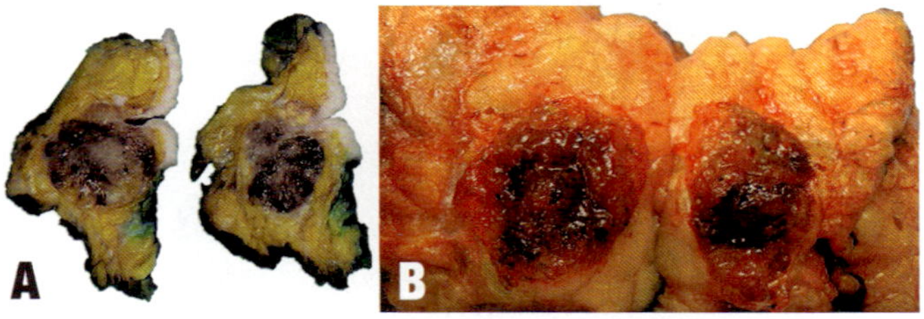

INVASIVE CARCINOMA WITH MUCINOUS CARCINOMA FEATURES

When invasive carcinoma is composed of both mucinous and other conventional types, the diagnostic term *invasive carcinoma with mucinous carcinoma features* is preferred.

FIGURE 5.31. In this specimen, despite extensive hemorrhage, the glistening appearance of the viable tumor suggests that this is a mucinous lesion.

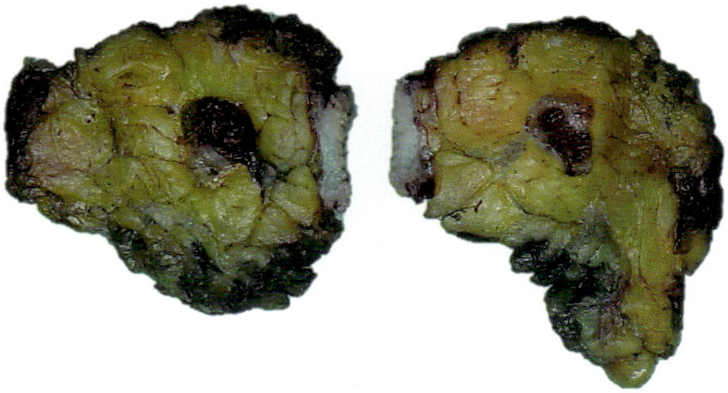

FIGURE 5.32. This specimen demonstrates a large, relatively well–circumscribed, tan-gray tumor with a mucoid appearance and prominent hemorrhage and cystic spaces. Punctate yellowish foci of necrosis or microcalcifications are present. Conventional invasive ductal carcinoma components were also present on microscopic examination.

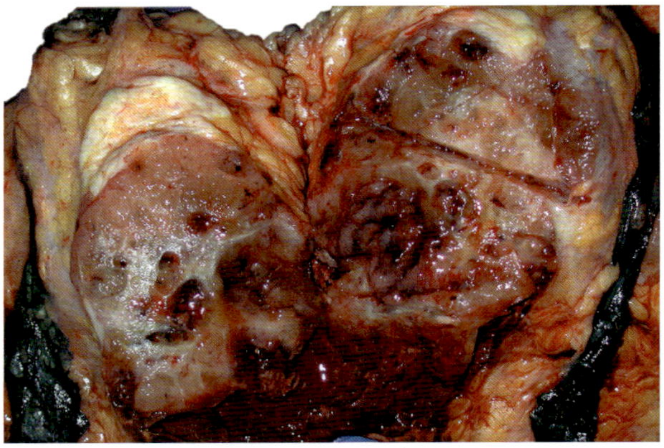

MUCINOUS CARCINOMA WITH MICROPAPILLARY COMPONENT

This is a rare variant of mucinous carcinoma.

FIGURE 5.33. In this lumpectomy specimen, the cut surface shows a well-circumscribed and tan lesion with foci of hemorrhage and fibrosis.

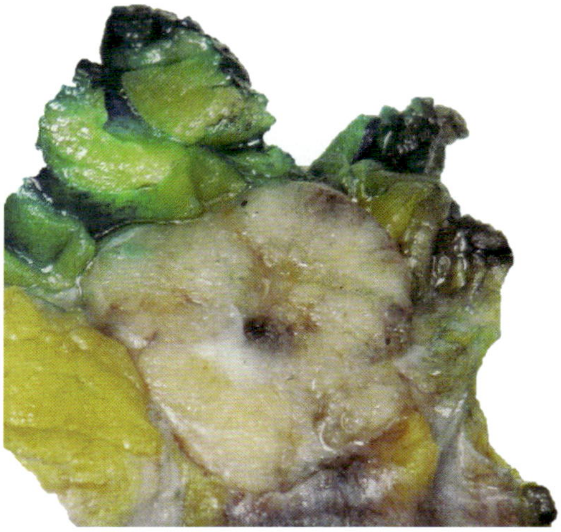

INVASIVE PAPILLARY CARCINOMA

Invasive papillary carcinoma of the breast represents approximately 0.5% of breast cancers. Some of these tumors present with bloody nipple discharge.

FIGURE 5.34. The cut section of this resected tumor demonstrates an ill-defined mass with a cut surface that is variegated, yellow-tan, hemorrhagic, and friable. Microscopic examination showed frank invasive components.

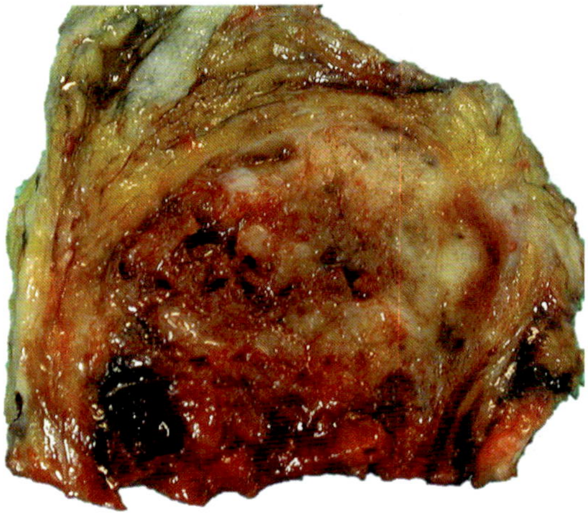

ENCAPSULATED PAPILLARY CARCINOMA OR INTRACYSTIC PAPILLARY CARCINOMA

Intracystic papillary carcinoma is now considered synonymous with encapsulated papillary carcinoma. Current literature suggests that encapsulated papillary carcinoma and solid papillary carcinoma are indolent disease when conventional invasive carcinoma is absent. Frankly invasive papillary carcinoma or micropapillary carcinoma, on the other hand, should be managed as invasive disease. Encapsulated papillary carcinoma has a fibrous capsule and lacks a myoepithelial layer at the periphery. It represents less than 1% of breast carcinomas. Grossly, it may present as a cyst with papillary excrescences and necrosis.

FIGURE 5.35. This resection shows a well-delineated, red, and friable tumor within a cystic cavity.

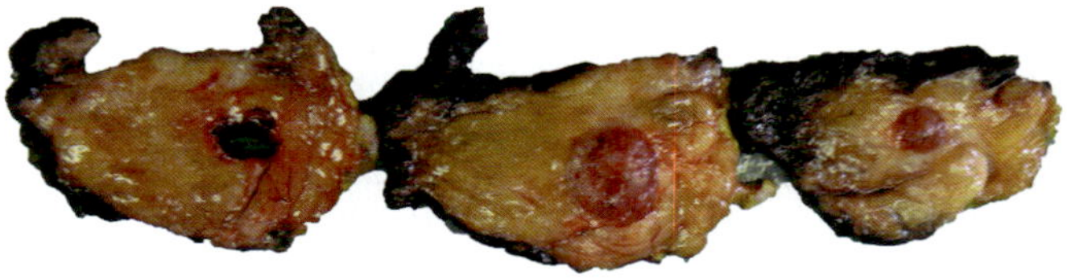

FIGURE 5.36. In this resection specimen, the tumor appears as a well-circumscribed mass with extensive hemorrhage and necrosis.

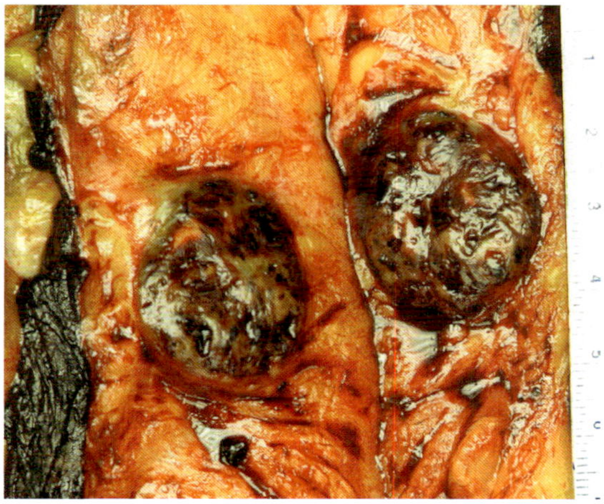

SOLID PAPILLARY CARCINOMA

Solid papillary carcinoma is an uncommon papillary carcinoma of the breast. Grossly, it commonly presents as a well-circumscribed, firm, fleshy nodule. Histologically, it has solid growth pattern with closely apposed cells forming papillary structures. The cells have neuroendocrine differentiation. Obvious invasive growth pattern may coexist.

FIGURE 5.37. This image shows a well-demarcated lesion with areas of cystic space and solid nodule, and with a fleshy cut surface. No obvious invasion into surrounding tissue is visible.

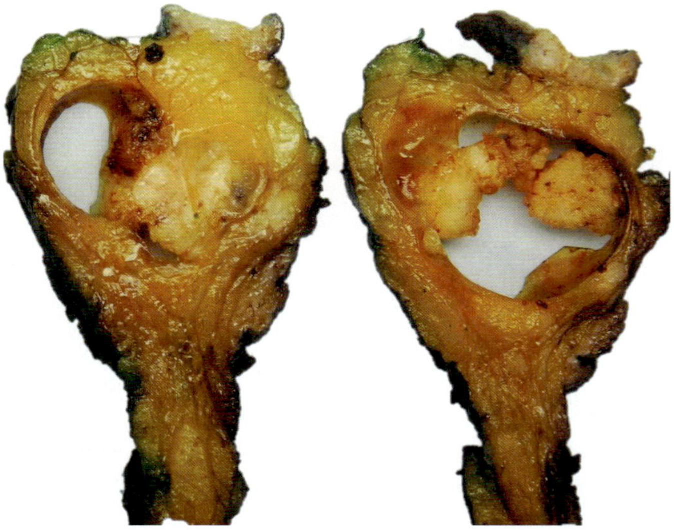

BASAL-LIKE INVASIVE CARCINOMA

At the molecular level, invasive carcinomas can be divided into 5 subtypes: luminal A, luminal B, HER2-enriched, normal breast-like, and basal-like. Though they are less likely to metastasize to lymph nodes, basal-like tumors confer a poor prognosis.

FIGURE 5.38. This resection specimen shows a basal-like carcinoma. A poorly circumscribed, rubbery, tan-white mass with focal hemorrhage is present on its cut surface.

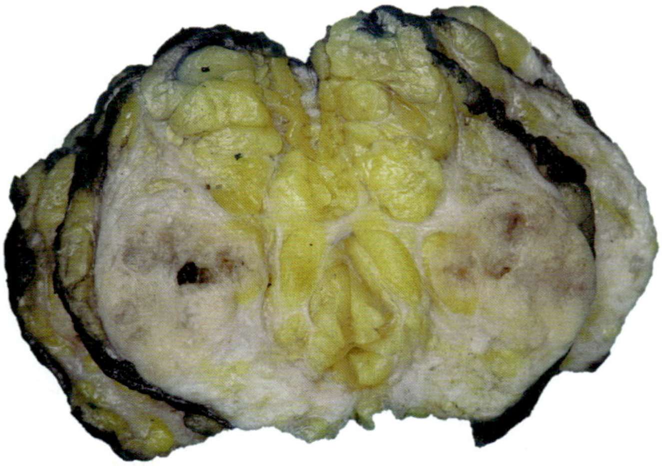

INVASIVE CRIBRIFORM CARCINOMA

Invasive cribriform carcinoma is a rare type of breast carcinoma (1% to 3% of breast cancers). It often confers an excellent prognosis.

FIGURE 5.39. This resection specimen shows an ill-defined firm tumor with central hemorrhage. The hemorrhage is due to previous core biopsy.

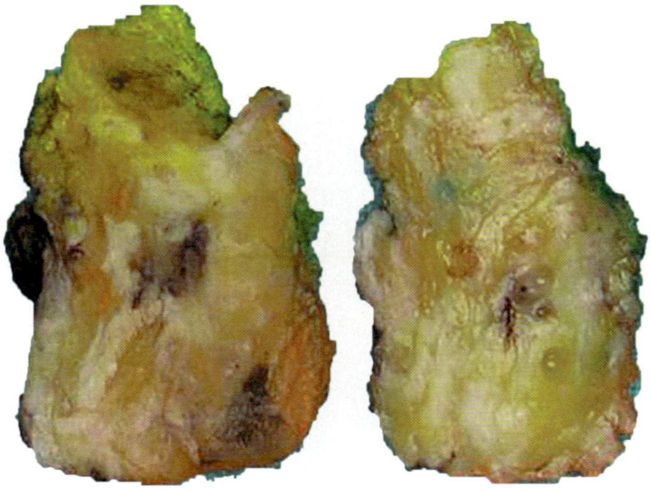

PURE INVASIVE CRIBRIFORM CARCINOMA

If more than 90% of a lesion consists of a cribriform pattern, it is considered a pure invasive cribriform carcinoma.

FIGURE 5.40. This specimen demonstrates a firm, tan, well-circumscribed spherical mass. Under microscopic examination, more than 90% of the tumor showed a cribriform pattern.

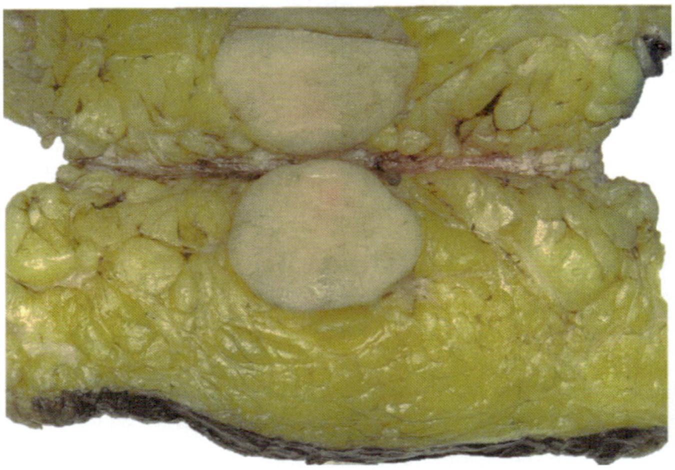

MEDULLARY CARCINOMA

Medullary carcinoma represents 3% to 5% of breast cancers. The word *medullary* comes from the texture of this tumor: it is so soft that it resembles the brain medulla. Medullary carcinoma is more common in women who have *BRCA1* mutation. Histologically, the tumor is defined by its smooth border, syncytial growth pattern, lymphocytic infiltrate, and high-grade nuclei.

FIGURE 5.41. This resection specimen shows a well-circumscribed soft tumor with a fleshy cut surface.

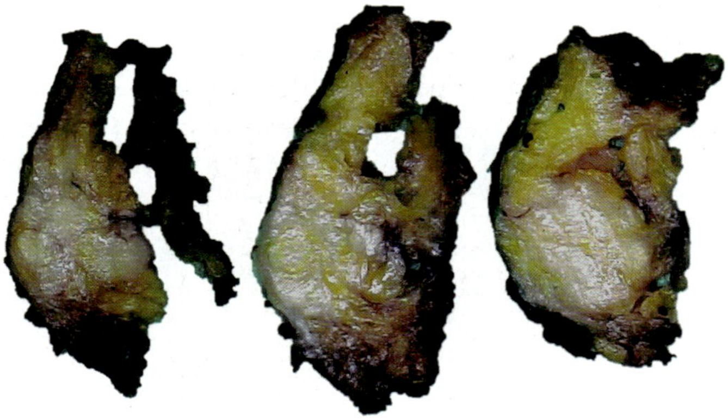

INFLAMMATORY CARCINOMA

This rare but aggressive presentation of breast carcinoma results from a blockage of the lymphatic channels in the skin by neoplastic cells.

FIGURE 5.42. Image (A) comes from a patient who presented with erythematous and thickened skin similar to the peel of an orange. A strip of orange skin on the right in (B) serves as a contrast.

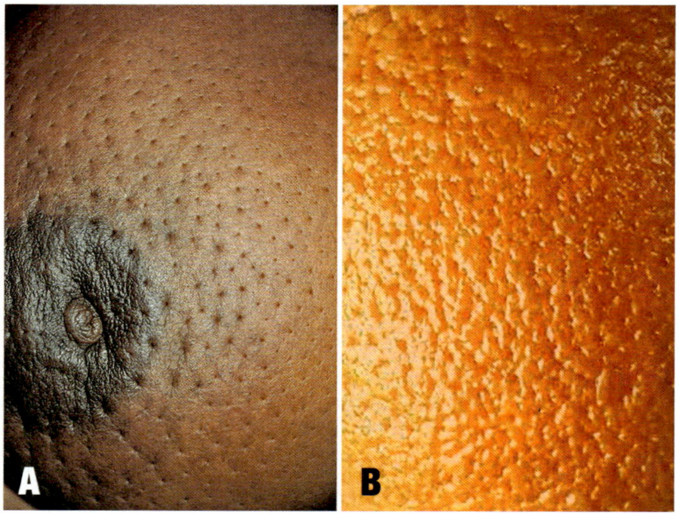

ADENOID CYSTIC CARCINOMA (ACC)

These rare tumors are typically found in the subareolar area, and are composed of epithelial and myoepithelial cells with distinct architectural patterns. Most of them involve a translocation between chromosomes 6 and 9. Despite the fact that tumor cells display a triple-negative, basal-like phenotype, they are usually low grade and confer a good prognosis.

FIGURE 5.43. In this resection specimen, the cut surface shows a firm and moderately circumscribed yellow-white mass with no hemorrhage or necrosis.

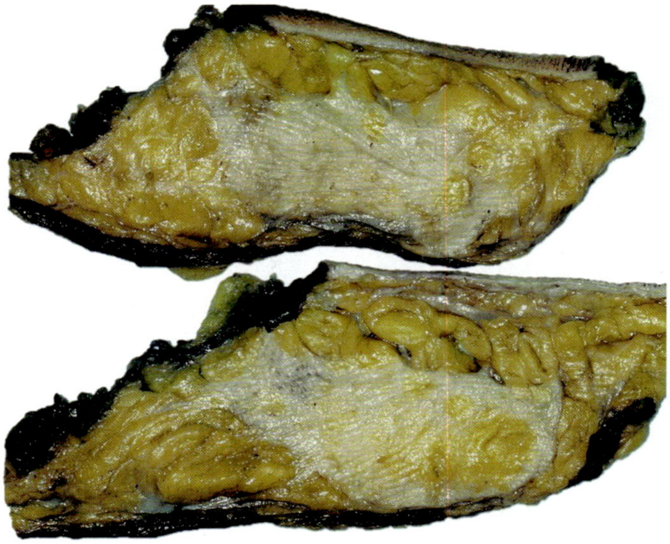

SOLID VARIANT OF ACC

According to the grading criteria for ACC of the salivary gland, tumors without solid elements are grade I, tumors consisting of no more than 30% solid growth are grade II, and tumors consisting of more than 30% solid growth are grade III. However, the AJCC staging manual (7th edition) recommends that the Nottingham modification of the Scarff-Bloom-Richardson grading system be provided uniformly for all breast carcinomas. Based on this grading scheme, most ACCs would be low-grade tumors.

FIGURE 5.44. The cut sections of this resected tumor demonstrate an ill-defined, infiltrative, firm, tan mass.

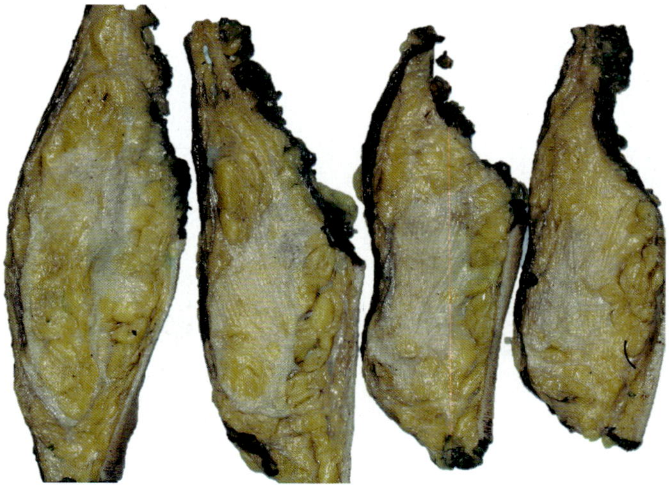

INVASIVE NEUROENDOCRINE CARCINOMA

Invasive neuroendocrine carcinomas represent less than 1% of breast cancers. Currently, the presence of neuroendocrine cells in conventional breast carcinomas does not change the clinical management. Grossly, these tumors can be fleshy, soft, and gelatinous.

FIGURE 5.45. In this resection specimen, the tumor appears well circumscribed with a tan and lobulated cut surface.

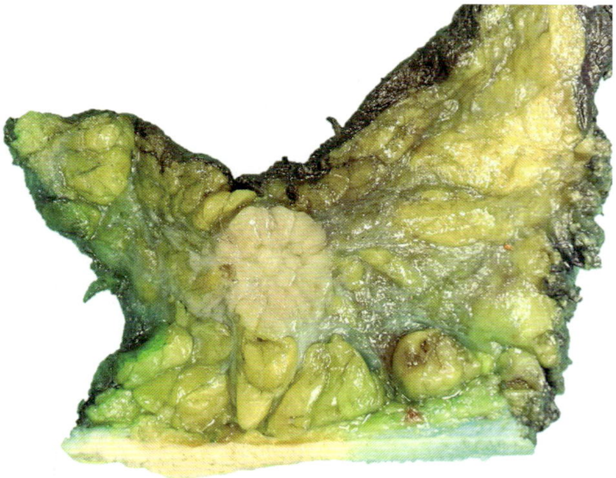

FIGURE 5.46. The cut surface of this specimen demonstrates a spheroid, fairly well-circumscribed, firm tumor with a tan-yellow cut surface. Neuroendocrine markers are positive in this case.

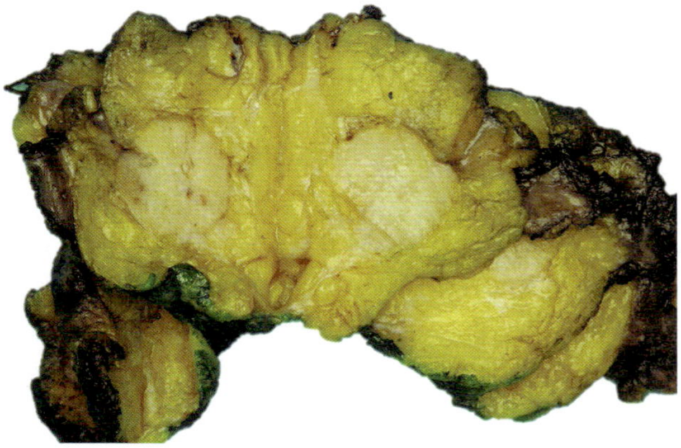

ADENOMYOEPITHELIAL CARCINOMA

These rare lesions are predominantly composed of both malignant epithelial and myoepithelial cells. They have been reported to metastasize to bone and other organs.

FIGURE 5.47. In this resection specimen, the tumor appears white, fleshy, and rubbery with well-defined borders.

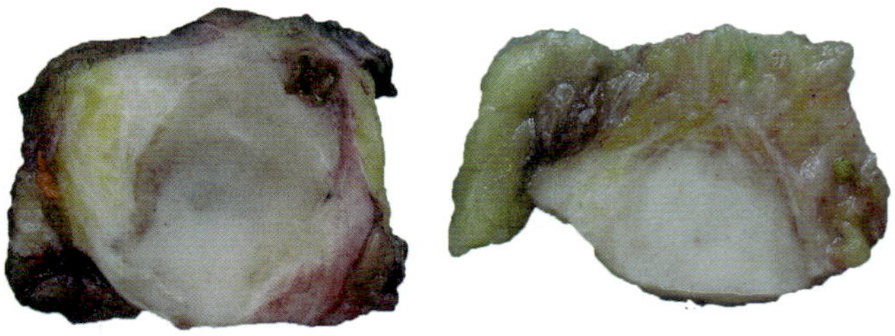

METAPLASTIC CARCINOMA

Metaplastic carcinomas represent less than 5% of breast carcinomas. Clinically, these tumors are more aggressive than invasive ductal carcinoma NST due to larger tumor size and higher histological grade. They tend to metastasize via blood circulation rather than to regional lymph nodes. Invasive metaplastic carcinoma is defined by its differentiation, in whole or in part, into squamous- or mesenchymal-like cells. It has many subtypes, which affect the gross appearance.

FIGURE 5.48. In this resection specimen of invasive metaplastic carcinoma, the tumor appears as a poorly defined, firm mass with areas of yellow discoloration and hemorrhage.

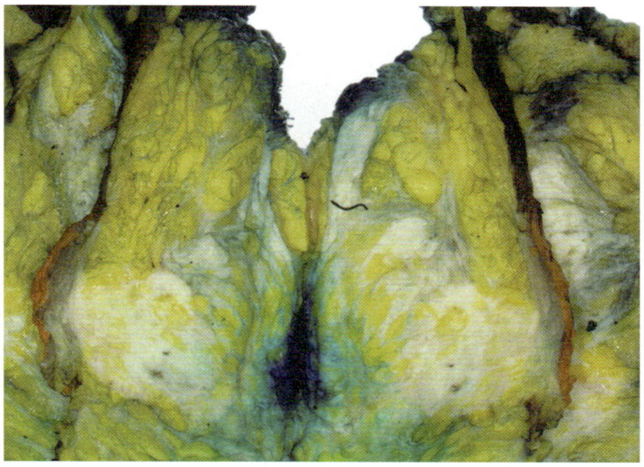

FIGURE 5.49. The mastectomy specimen in (A) shows a large, hemorrhagic, and necrotic tumor with skin ulceration. In (B), the cut surface shows a well-circumscribed, tan-white, and firm mass with small areas of hemorrhage invading through the skin at the superior margin.

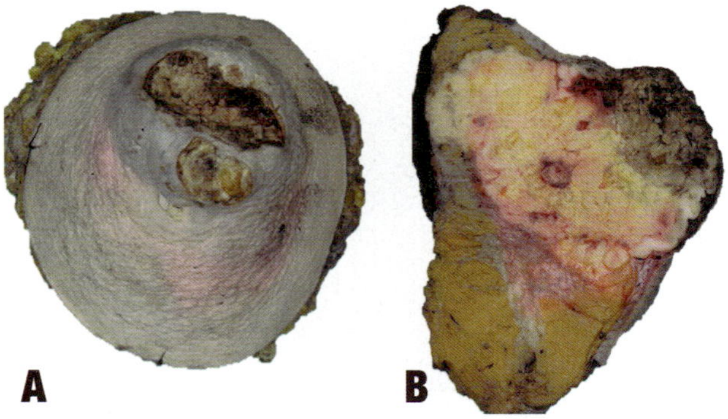

FIGURE 5.50. This image shows a large mass protruding from breast parenchyma with skin ulceration. Cut sections of the mass demonstrate mixed cystic and solid areas. Extensive hemorrhage and necrosis are present. Histologically, the yellow areas correspond to heterogenic adipose tissue with necrosis.

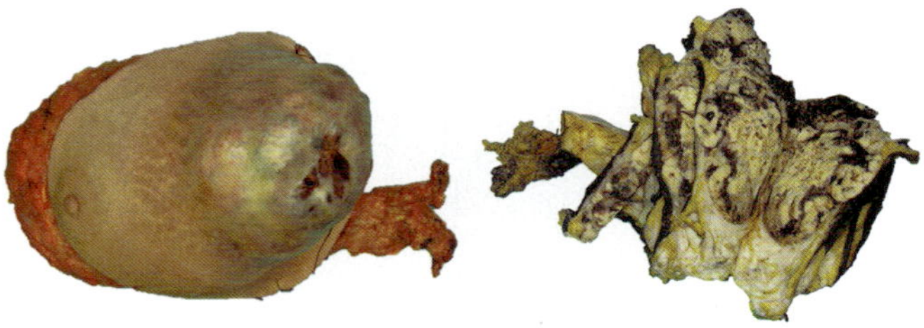

FIGURE 5.51. In this resection specimen, the tumor appears as a large and firm mass with a gritty and hemorrhagic cut surface.

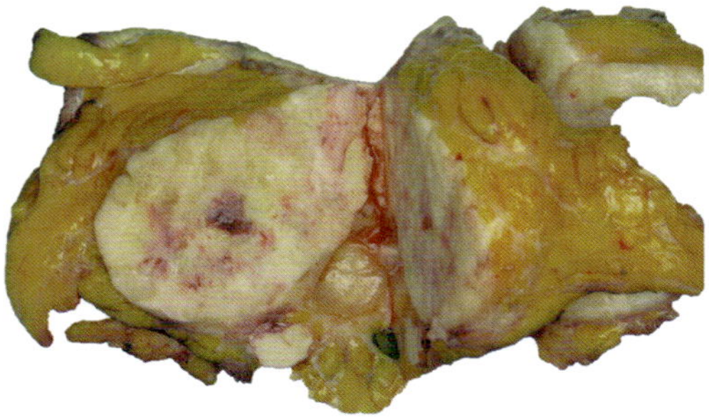

FIGURE 5.52. This image shows a circumscribed mass with a glistening cut surface, histologically corresponding to chondroid components.

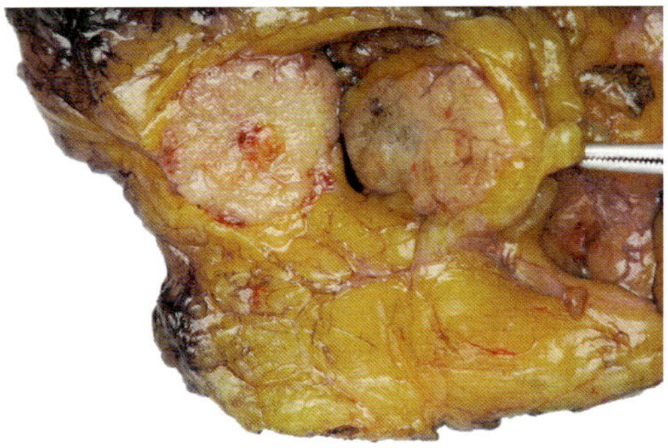

FIGURE 5.53. This image shows a relatively well-circumscribed mass with a fleshy cut surface. Microscopic examination reveals matrix-like stromal components.

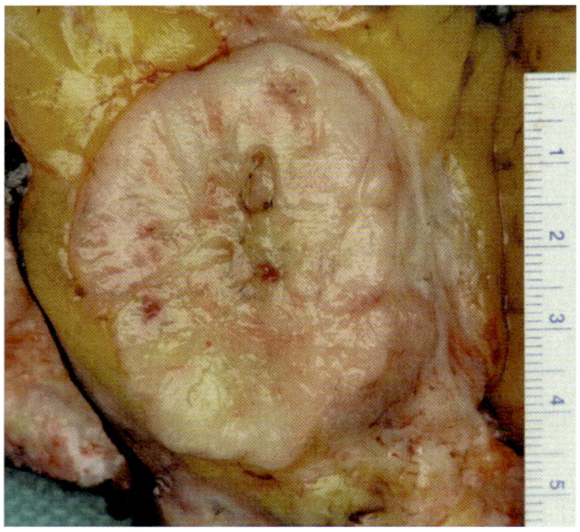

FIGURE 5.54. A large, partially cystic mass showed adenosquamous carcinoma components under microscopic examination.

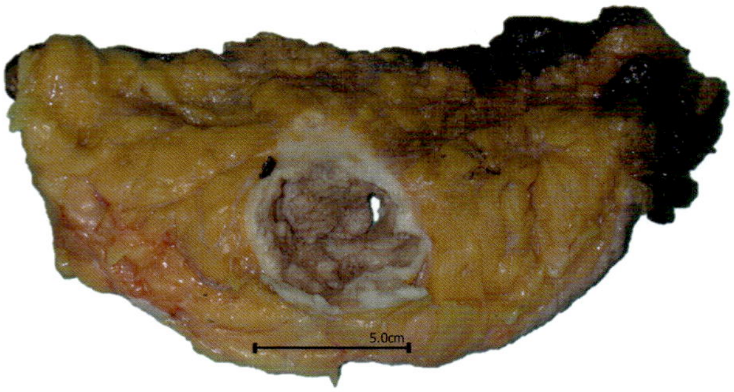

Malignant transformation of pleomorphic adenoma

Pleomorphic adenoma is a benign neoplasm that commonly occurs in salivary glands and occasionally in the breast. Malignant transformation of pleomorphic adenoma, commonly seen in salivary glands, has also been reported in the breast. Grossly, it is usually a circumscribed mass. In histology, it has a component of benign pleomorphic adenoma and a component of high-grade malignant carcinoma that can sometimes have metaplastic features.

FIGURE 5.55. This specimen shows a well-demarcated, solid-cystic, firm tan mass with an area of necrosis.

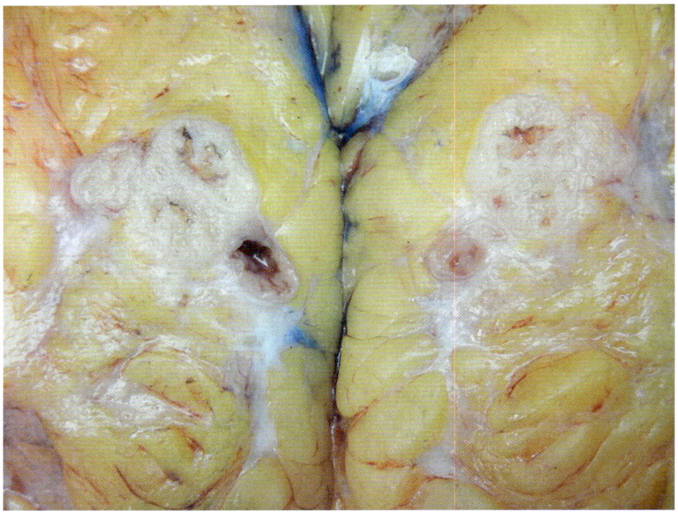

Paget disease of the nipple

These malignancies found in the epidermis of the nipple constitute less than 4% of all breast cancers. Changes in the nipple may include erythema, eczema, ulceration, discharge, and inversion.

FIGURE 5.56. In this mastectomy specimen, the nipple shows marked induration with crusty excoriation.

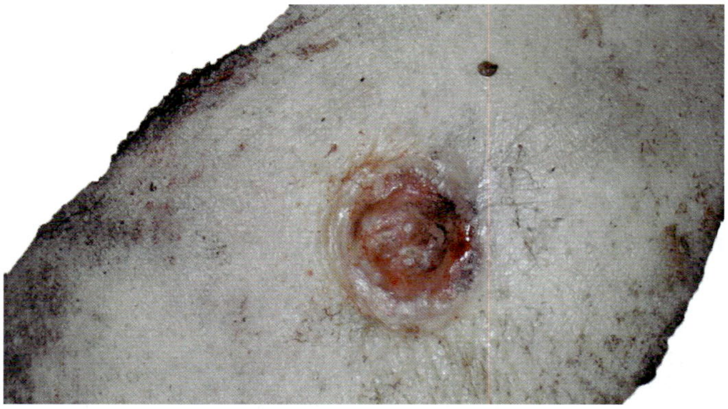

Fibroadenoma

Fibroadenomas are common and benign tumors of the breast and are often found in women of reproductive age.

FIGURE 5.57. This lumpectomy specimen shows a well-demarcated nodule (A) with a white homogenous cut surface (B).

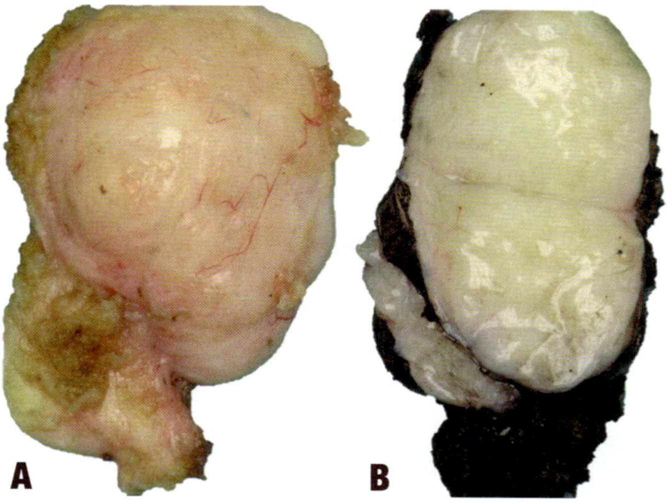

FIGURE 5.58. This resected fibroadenoma appears lobulated with a white homogeneous cut surface. It is firm and is clearly demarcated from the adjacent breast tissue.

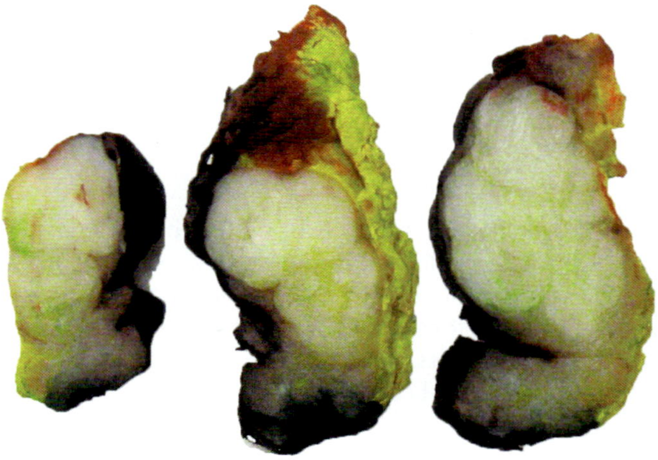

FIGURE 5.59. In this lumpectomy specimen, the fibroadenoma bulges to the cut surface in contrast to the retraction of adjacent soft tissue. It is a well-demarcated tumor with a firm consistency and white homogenous texture.

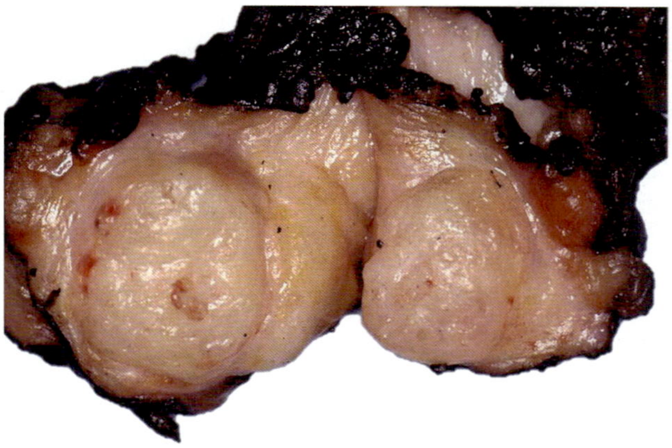

GIANT FIBROADENOMA

Fibroadenomas can range in size from < 1 cm to several centimeters in diameter, and can be single or multiple. Affected by hormonal status, the tumor size can change during the menstrual cycle, pregnancy, and breast-feeding, or due to hormone replacement therapy or oral contraceptives.

FIGURE 5.60. This image shows a 12-cm, 250-g mass with a smooth external surface.

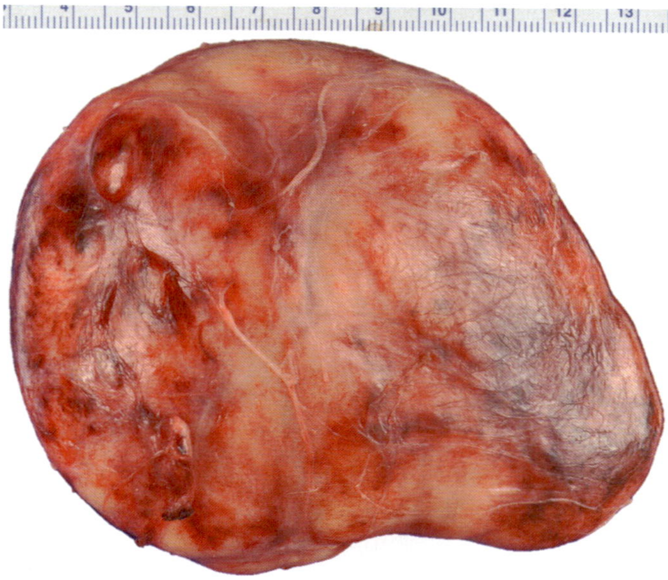

JUVENILE FIBROADENOMA

Juvenile fibroadenoma is a fibroadenoma subtype that usually occurs in adolescents. These tumors have distinct histological features and, grossly, can be quite large.

FIGURE 5.61. These images show a lumpectomy with a lobulated, thinly encapsulated mass (A) and a tan-white glistening cut surface (B).

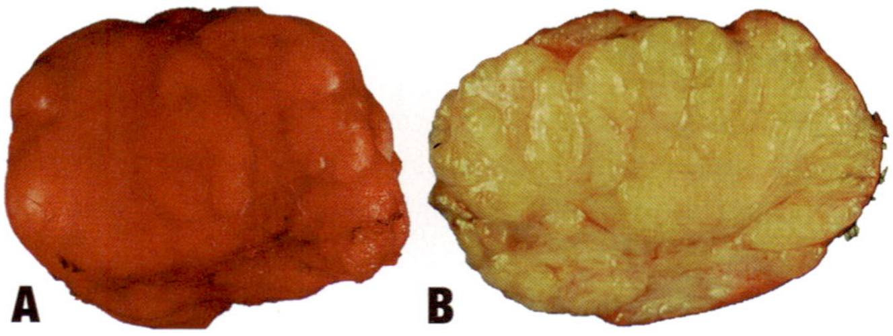

Fibromatosis

Fibromatosis represents less than 0.2% of breast tumors. It is associated with trauma, surgery, familial adenomatous polyposis, hereditary desmoid syndrome, and Gardner syndrome. Clinically, it presents as a mass with skin dimpling or nipple retraction, both of which mimic invasive carcinoma on imaging and gross examination. It can infiltrate adjacent skin and muscle.

FIGURE 5.62. This lumpectomy shows a poorly demarcated, white-pale, fibrous mass mixed with adipose tissue.

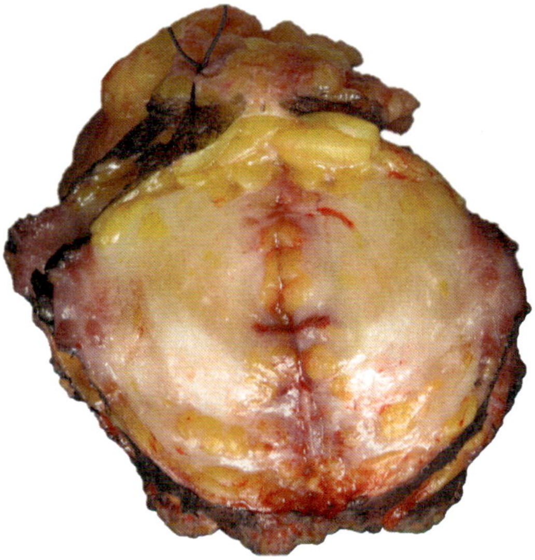

FIBROADENOMA WITH LACTATIONAL CHANGE

FIGURE 5.64. The multilocular cystic and solid mass in this resection specimen has cheesy or milk-like material within the cysts.

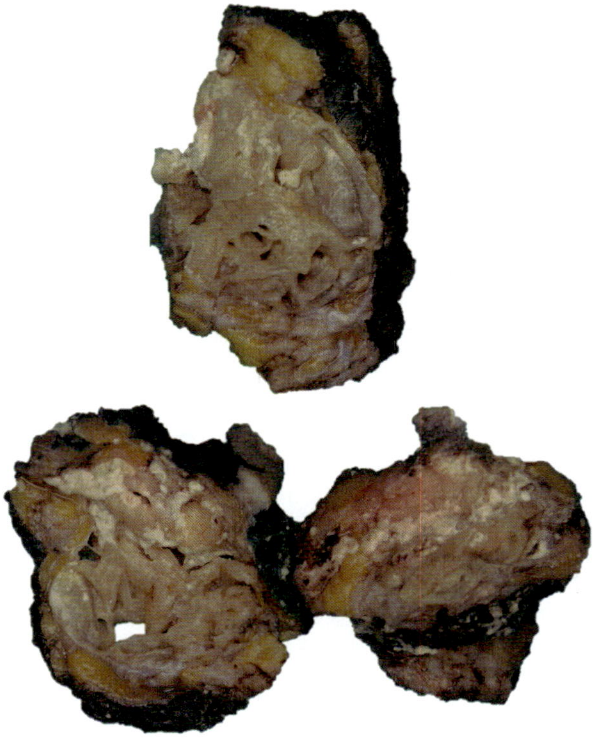

Lactating adenoma

The World Health Organization (WHO) defines lactating adenomas as nodular areas of hyperplastic lobules with secretory or lactational changes. These lesions may be fibroadenomas or tubular adenomas. They can give breasts a firm consistency. In rare instances, they can occur simultaneously with breast carcinoma, so they must be carefully evaluated.

FIGURE 5.63. In this resection specimen, the cut surface demonstrates a multilobular, well-circumscribed, and tan mass. The yellow streaks correlate with proteinaceous secretions visible on microscopy.

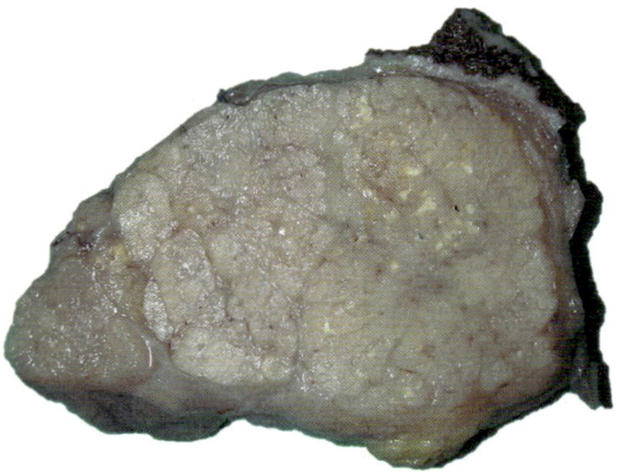

Phyllodes tumor

These fibroepithelial lesions can be benign, borderline, or malignant depending on histologic features including stromal cellularity, infiltration at the tumor edge, and mitotic activity. Together, these tumors represent less than 1% of primary breast tumors. Grossly, they show cleft-like spaces within a lobulated or bosselated mass.

FIGURE 5.65. This resection specimen shows a well-circumscribed, slightly lobulated, benign mass with a solid white-tan cut surface. There is no hemorrhage or necrosis.

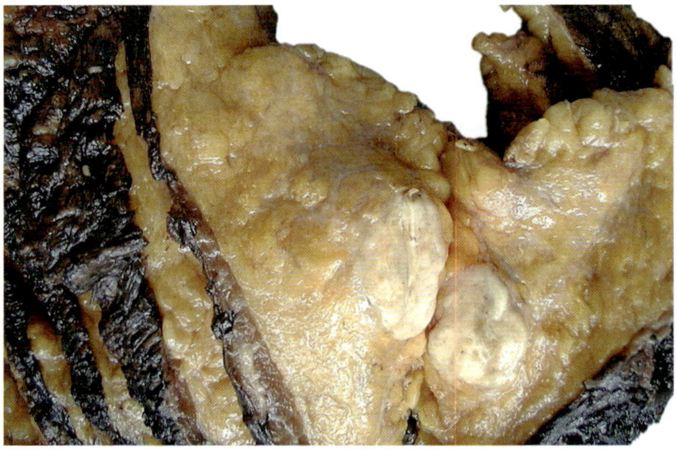

BENIGN PHYLLODES TUMOR

Phyllodes tumors are generally well circumscribed if benign. Histologically, benign phyllodes tumors have no adverse features (i.e., stromal overgrowth, stromal high cellularity, stromal nuclear pleomorphism and atypia, infiltrative margin, or increased mitosis).

FIGURE 5.66. This lumpectomy specimen shows a well-circumscribed, slightly lobulated mass with a solid white-tan cut surface. There is no hemorrhage or necrosis.

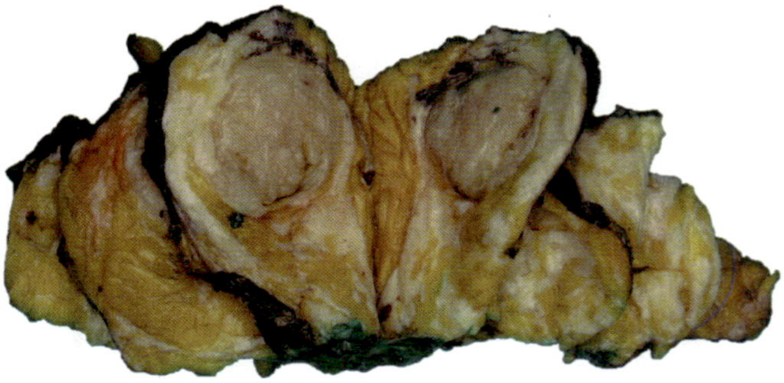

FIGURE 5.67. This resected specimen shows a well-circumscribed mass with a homogeneous, gelatinous, rubbery cut surface. There is no hemorrhage or necrosis.

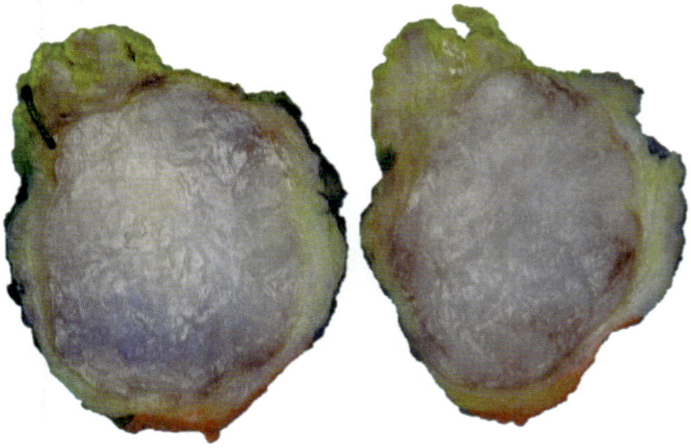

BORDERLINE PHYLLODES TUMOR

The majority of phyllodes tumors are benign. Borderline tumors have 1 or more adverse features, but are not considered malignant.

FIGURE 5.68. This lumpectomy specimen shows a well-circumscribed, solid tumor with a pushing edge and focal infiltration to the adjacent breast tissue.

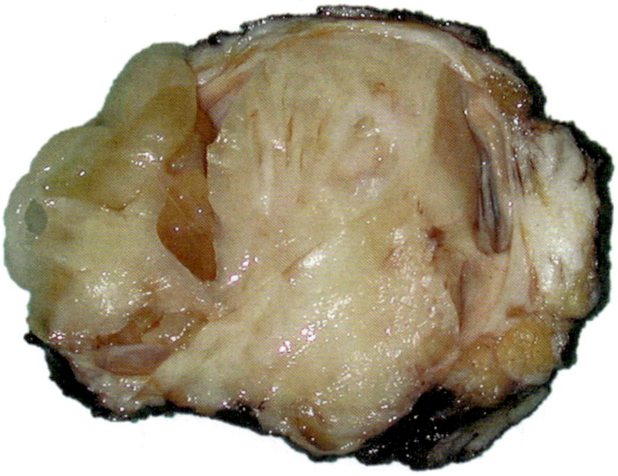

FIGURE 5.69. This resected 9-cm circumscribed and encapsulated mass shows a partially solid and partially cystic cut surface, and variegated focal hemorrhagic areas.

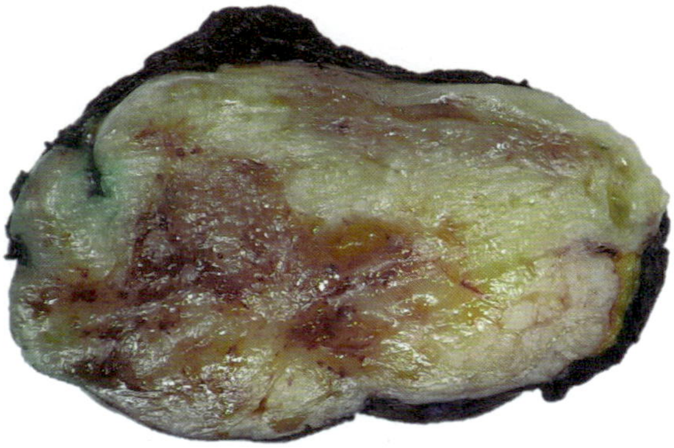

FIGURE 5.70. This resected specimen shows a relatively well-circumscribed mass with a variegated nodular or leaf-like cut surface. There is no hemorrhage or necrosis.

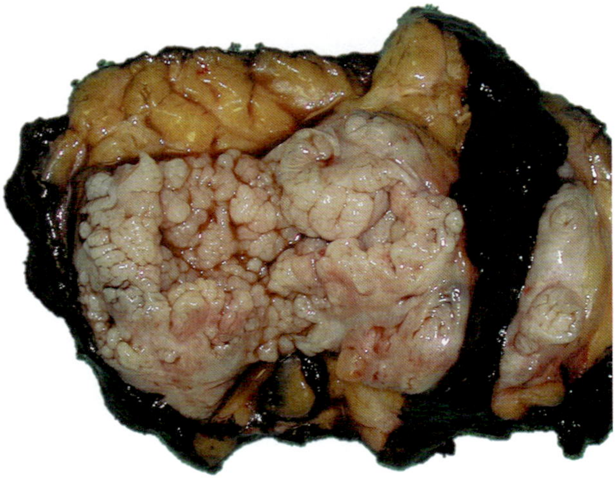

MALIGNANT PHYLLODES TUMOR

Grossly malignant tumors are not as well circumscribed as benign tumors, and they are more friable masses that tend to have areas of hemorrhage and necrosis. Malignant phyllodes tumors have adverse features: stromal overgrowth, stromal high cellularity, stromal nuclear pleomorphism and atypia, infiltrative margins, and increased mitosis. They may behave like sarcomas and metastasize via blood circulation. The most common sites for distant metastases are the lungs, bones, and abdominal viscera. A major concern for phyllodes tumors is local recurrence; therefore, resection with clear margins is recommended. As well, malignant components may be sporadically present within phyllodes tumors: thorough sampling of lesions is important.

FIGURE 5.71. This mastectomy specimen shows a lobulated mass with an irregular border and a variegated, fleshy cut surface with hemorrhagic foci.

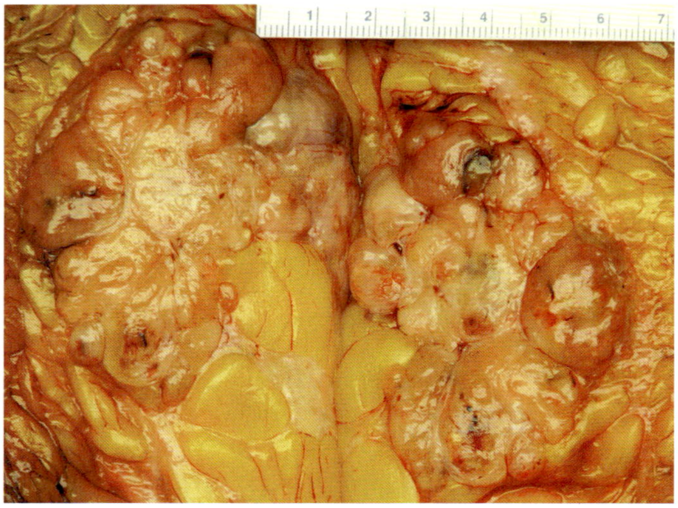

FIGURE 5.72. Malignant progression may correspond to gains in chromosome 1 and losses in chromosome 13. In this mastectomy specimen, a large solid mass with a variegated, fleshy cut surface shows areas of hemorrhage and necrosis.

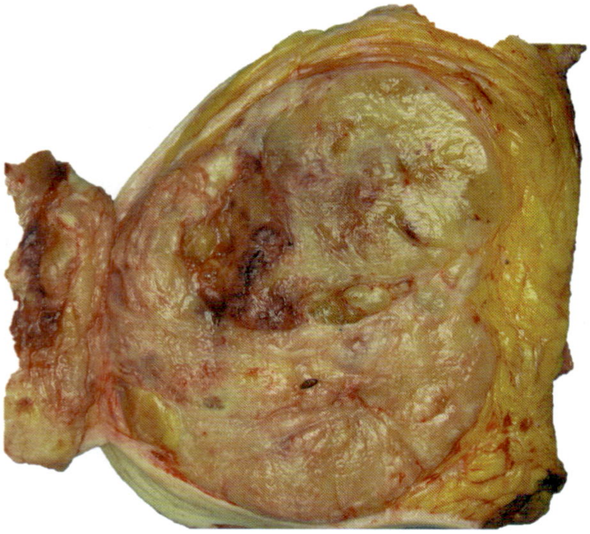

FIGURE 5.73. This resected specimen shows a 5-cm mass with irregular borders, and a variegated cut surface and focal hemorrhage.

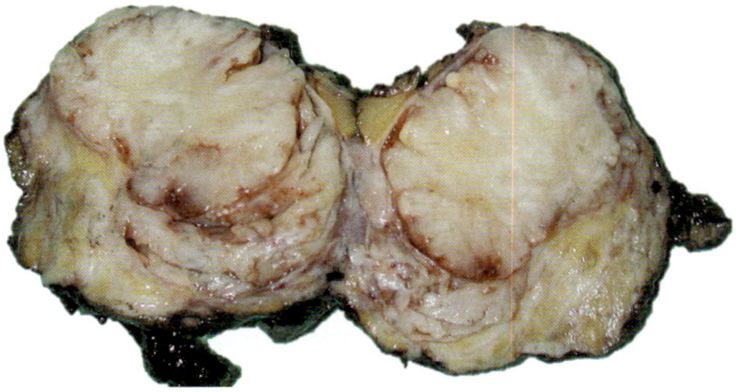

FIGURE 5.74. This lumpectomy specimen shows a tumor with irregular borders and a friable, fleshy cut surface.

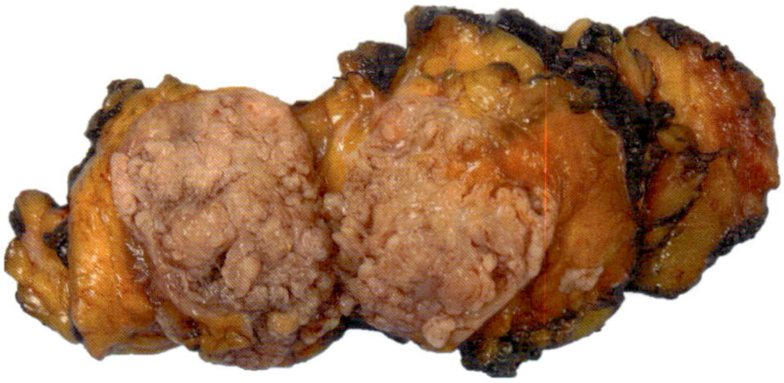

FIGURE 5.75. The cut surface of this large mass shows solid, papillary, cystic, myxoid, bony, necrotic, and hemorrhagic areas. Microscopy revealed stromal overgrowth with focal osteoid and cartilage formation.

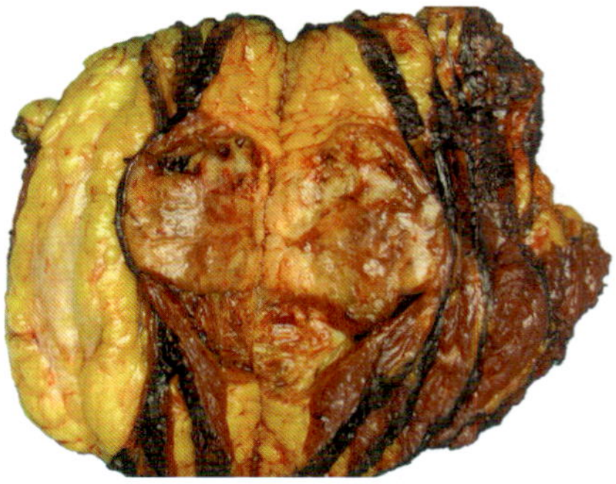

FIGURE 5.76. This resected specimen shows a large, irregular, lobulated tumor with extensive hemorrhage, necrosis, and cystic degeneration.

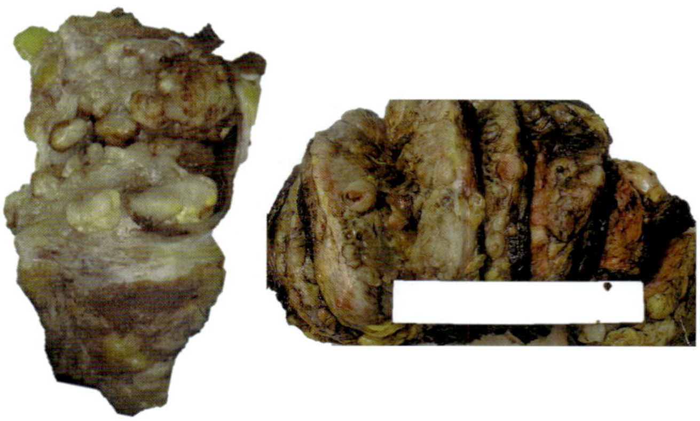

Nodular pseudoangiomatous stromal hyperplasia (PASH)

PASH is a breast mesenchymal lesion that is due to the proliferation of stromal myofibroblasts. Grossly, it can present as a palpable mass that can be either well circumscribed or ill defined. Histologically, the stromal fibroblasts can form prominent slit-like clefts that mimic vascular spaces.

FIGURE 5.77. This image shows a well-demarcated, firm, rubbery, white nodule.

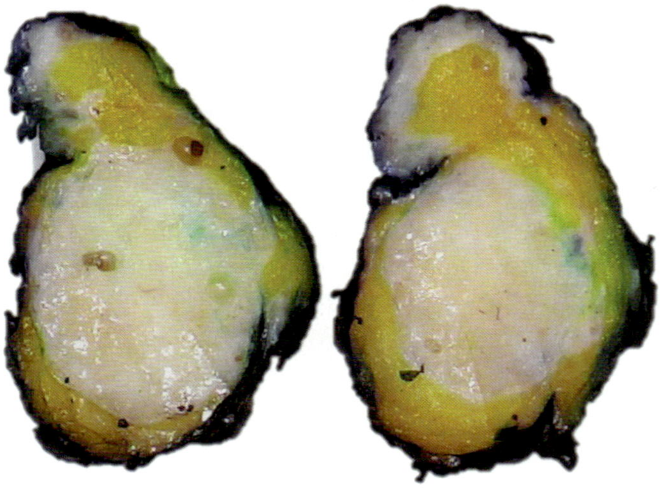

Granular cell tumor

A granular cell tumor is a mesenchymal soft tissue tumor thought to originate from Schwann cells. It occurs rarely in the breast, where it can present as a firm and hard mass that grossly resembles invasive carcinoma. The granular cells on histology contain fine eosinophilic granules. Immunohistochemistry for S100 is positive.

FIGURE 5.78. This specimen shows an ill-defined mass with a firm and tan cut surface.

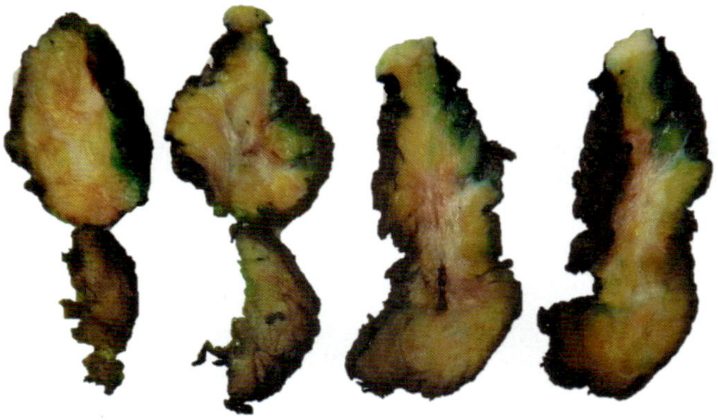

Angiosarcoma

PRIMARY ANGIOSARCOMA

Angiosarcomas are malignant mesenchymal tumors with endothelial differentiation. Primary lesions represent less than 0.1% of breast cancers.

FIGURE 5.79. This mastectomy specimen shows multiple irregular, red-purple, bruise-like skin lesions.

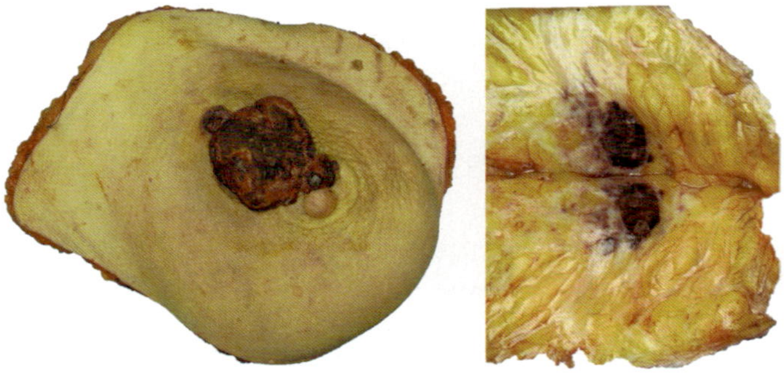

POSTRADIATION ANGIOSARCOMA

The occurrence of secondary angiosarcoma increases with radiation exposure. Postradiation angiosarcomas often present as patchy, irregular, blue-purple skin discolorations. The actual lesion is often more extensive than its skin appearance. In later stages, these lesions often became multiple nodules occurring deep in breast parenchyma or fungating out from the skin, often with ulceration. Most postradiation angiosarcomas are high grade and have poor prognosis.

FIGURE 5.80. This mastectomy specimen shows hemorrhagic lesions that have developed in an area of previous radiation therapy. Microscopic examinations demonstrate high-grade angiosarcoma with infiltration into the breast tissue.

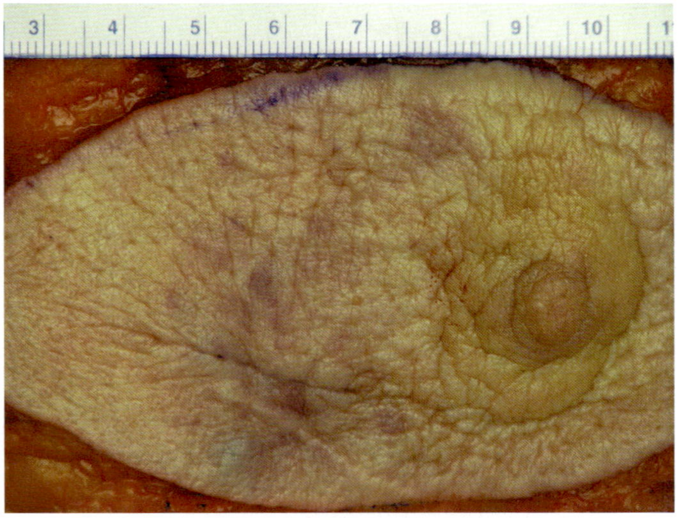

FIGURE 5.81. This lesion developed 7 years postradiation therapy for breast ductal carcinoma. In addition to multiple blue-purple nodular skin lesions, a large fungating lesion with surface ulceration and necrosis is present. On the cut surface, the lesion infiltrates deep into the breast parenchyma.

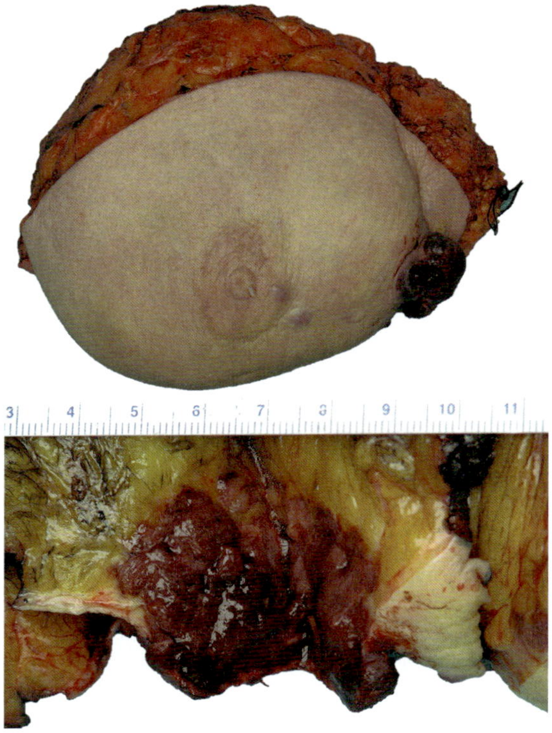

FIGURE 5.82. These are resection specimens of 2 postradiation angiosarcomas. This type of tumor is typically larger than it appears on gross examination, which makes radical surgical resection difficult.

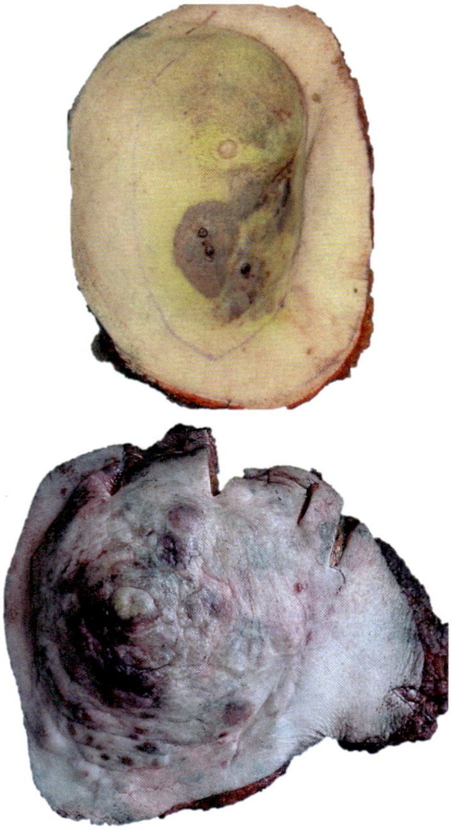

FIGURE 5.83. This patient developed multifocal cutaneous high-grade angiosarcoma 9 years postradiation therapy for breast carcinoma. Multiple hemorrhagic lesions involving the skin are present, and the skin surface appears bruised.

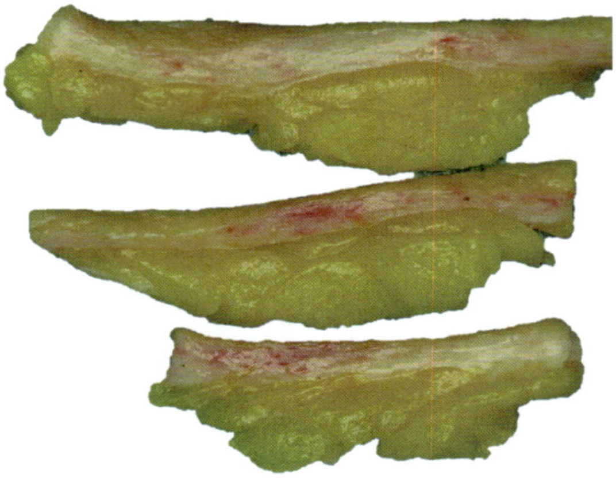

FIGURE 5.84. This lesion developed 10 years postradiation therapy for breast carcinoma. The cut surfaces show multiple ill-defined, hemorrhagic areas involving the full thickness of skin.

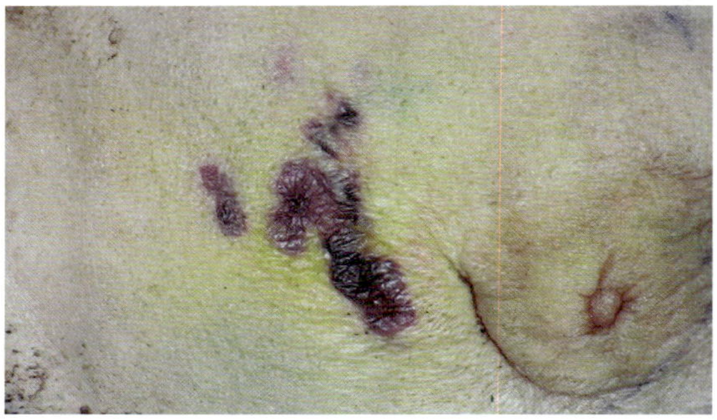

Nodular lymphocyte-predominant Hodgkin lymphoma

Both B-cell and T-cell lymphomas can involve the breast, but this is rare, comprising less than 0.5% of breast tumors. Nodular lymphocyte-predominant Hodgkin lymphoma occurs across a wide age range. Patients generally present after noticing a breast mass.

FIGURE 5.85. In this breast resection specimen, the cut surface demonstrates a solid, lobulated, and tan mass covered by a thin, smooth capsule.

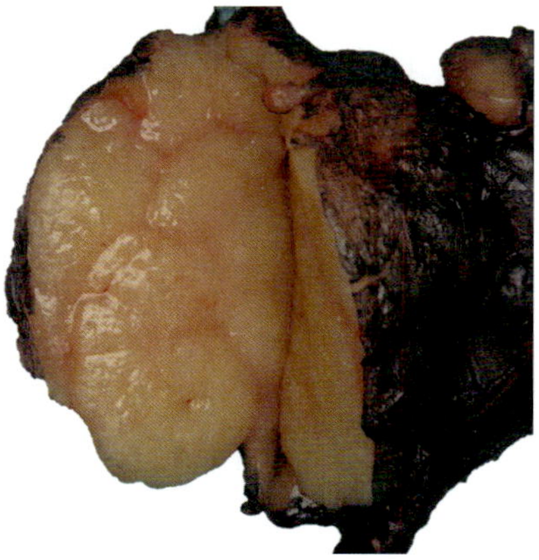

Sarcoma

Primary breast sarcomas are very rare, and a wide variety of types can occur. Many sarcomas that occur most commonly elsewhere in the body can rarely occur in the breast. Therefore this is a heterogeneous category of tumors, but size is an important prognostic factor for breast sarcomas in general.

FIGURE 5.86. In this mastectomy specimen, the low-grade spindle cell sarcoma appears well circumscribed with a firm, fleshy, and rubbery cut surface.

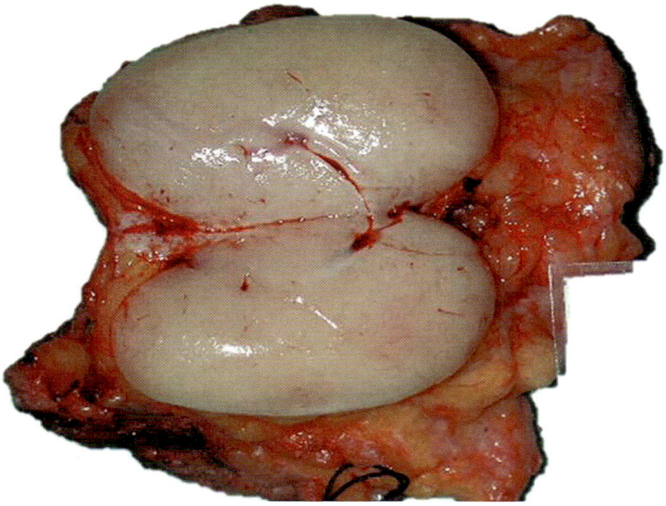

Malignant histiocytic sarcoma

Histiocytic sarcoma is a rare hematologic malignant neoplasia derived from histiocytic or dendritic cell clones. Diagnostic features include cellular positivity for the immunohistochemical markers CD163, CD68, CD4, and lysozyme.

FIGURE 5.87. This cut section demonstrates an ovoid mass with a tan, fleshy surface (arrow).

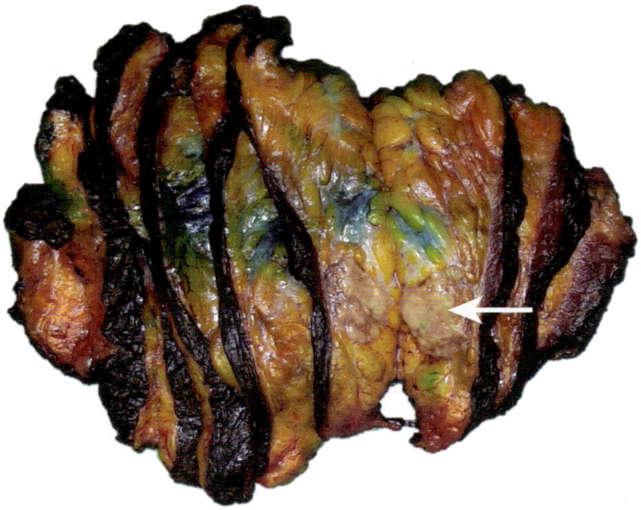

Metastasis to the breast

Metastatic tumors to breast tissue are rare. Melanoma, GI-tract tumors, and lung tumors are the usual suspects.

METASTATIC WELL-DIFFERENTIATED MUCINOUS ADENOCARCINOMA

FIGURE 5.88. This patient had a history of a mucinous appendiceal adenocarcinoma. The resected mass has a multilocular, mucinous, glistening appearance. Metastatic appendiceal carcinoma was confirmed histologically.

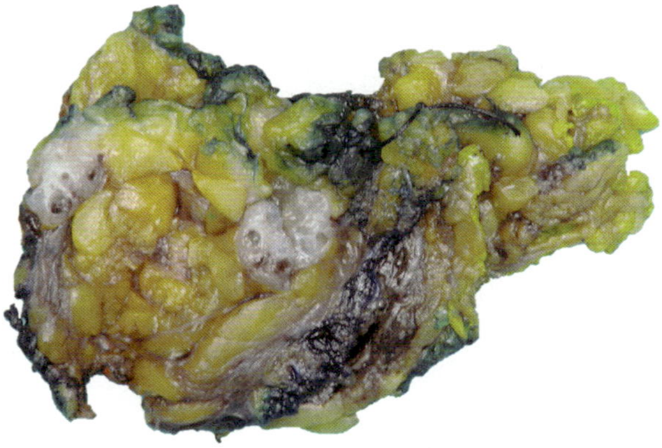

METASTATIC MELANOMA

The differential diagnosis for melanoma of the breast includes primary melanoma of the breast versus metastasis.

FIGURE 5.89. The cut surface of this mastectomy specimen shows a well-demarcated, soft, dark brown, and friable mass underlying the skin.

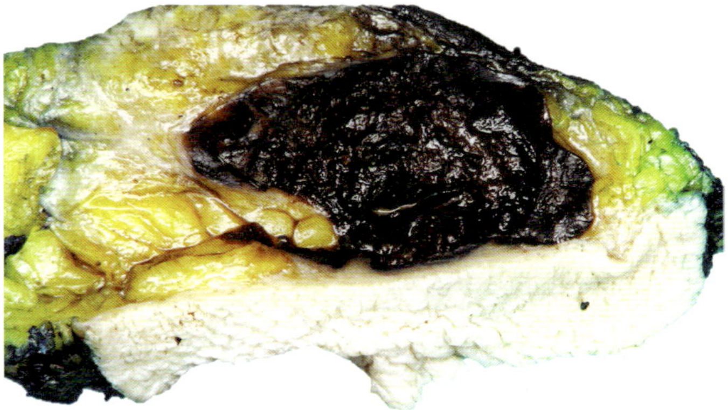

Metastasis from the breast to other sites

Breast cancer may metastasize to other sites, and the staging of tumors helps determine patient management and estimate prognosis. A distant metastasis is indicative of stage IV disease.

FIGURE 5.90. Image (A) shows the cut surface of a liver with multiple, small, and well-delineated metastases from the breast. In (B), a lytic lesion (arrow) is present between the vertebral bodies.

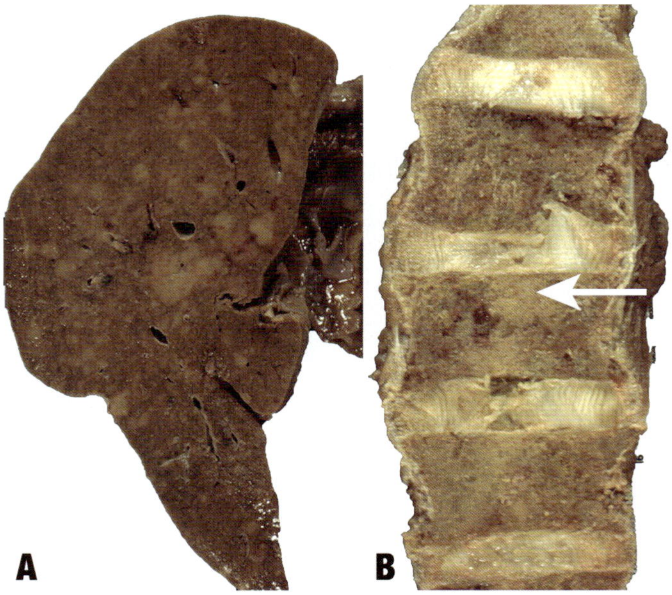

ACKNOWLEDGMENTS

We would like to thank the valuable contributions of Dr. Atilla Omeroglu, Dr. Gulbeyaz Altinel-Omeroglu, and Dr. Lili Fu, and the technical help of R. Gilot, E. Griss, A. Hossain, L. Korneichyuk Pasyuk, M. Mikhael, and E. Yaney.

Some of the images are from Calgary Laboratory Services' gross image file. The authors would like to thank all pathology technicians, residents, and staff pathologists from Calgary Laboratory Services for their contribution.

REFERENCES

Adem C, Reynolds C, Ingle JN, Nascimento AG. Primary breast sarcoma: clinicopathologic series from the Mayo Clinic and review of the literature. Br J Cancer. 2004;91(2):237–241. Medline:15187996

Foulkes WD. Inherited susceptibility to common cancers. N Engl J Med. 2008;359(20):2143–2153. https://doi.org/10.1056/NEJMra0802968. Medline:19005198

Kronowitz SJ, Kuerer HM. Advances and surgical decision-making for breast reconstruction. Cancer. 2006;107(5):893–907. https://doi.org/10.1002/cncr.22079. Medline:16862569

Kumar V, Abbas AK, Aster JC, Lester SC. The breast. In: *Robbins and Cotran pathologic basis of disease*. 9th ed. Philadelphia: Saunders/Elsevier; 2015. p. 1043–71.

Lakhani SR; International Agency for Research on Cancer, World Health Organization. *WHO classification of tumours of the breast*. Lyon, France: IARC Press; 2012.

Maxwell GP, Gabriel A. The evolution of breast implants. Clin Plast Surg. 2009;36(1):1–13, v. https://doi.org/10.1016/j.cps.2008.08.001. Medline:19055956

O'Malley FP, Pinder SE, Mulligan AM. *Breast pathology: a volume in the foundations in diagnostic pathology series*. 2nd ed. Philadelphia: Saunders/Elsevier; 2011. https://www.clinicalkey.com/dura/browse/bookChapter/3-s2.0-C20090418932

Page DL, Dixon JM, Anderson TJ, Lee D, Stewart HJ. Invasive cribriform carcinoma of the breast. Histopathology. 1983;7(4):525–536. https://doi.org/10.1111/j.1365-2559.1983.tb02265.x. Medline:6884999

Santen RJ, Mansel R. Benign breast disorders. N Engl J Med. 2005;353(3):275–285. https://doi.org/10.1056/NEJMra035692. Medline:16034013

Schnitt SJ, Collins LC. *Biopsy interpretation of the breast*. Philadelphia: Wolters Kluwer Health/Lippincott Williams & Wilkins; 2009.

Weidner N, Cote RJ, Suster S, Weiss LM. *Modern surgical pathology*. 2nd ed. Philadelphia: Saunders/Elsevier; 2009. https://www.clinicalkey.com/dura/browse/bookChapter/3-s2.0-B9781416039662X0001X

6

Diseases of the Lung, Pleura, and Mediastinum

PIERRE-OLIVIER FISET, LIVIA FLORIANOVA, GURDIP SINGH TAMBER, HANGJUN WANG, SOPHIE CAMILLERI-BROËT

Lung

Nonneoplastic lung diseases

Congenital pulmonary airway malformation (CPAM)

CPAM, also known as congenital cystic adenomatoid malformations (CCAM), are due to congenital abnormalities in lung morphogenesis.

FIGURE 6.1. This lobar resection from a young child shows thin-walled multilocular cysts with surrounding smaller cysts. The child was asymptomatic. This lesion was found in a prenatal ultrasound screen.

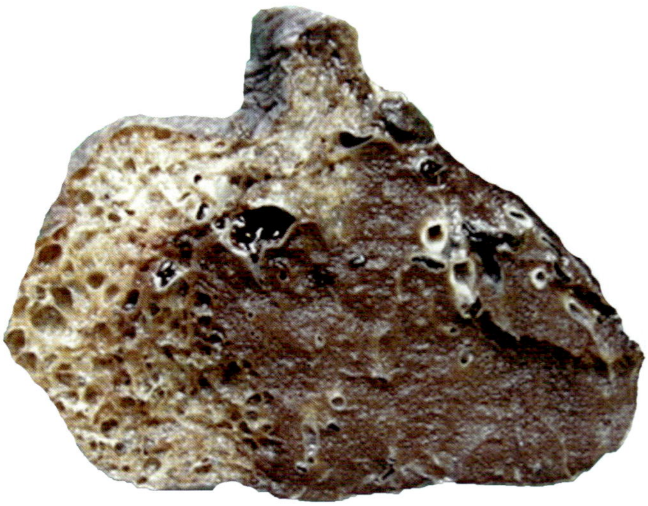

Bacterial pneumonia

BRONCHOPNEUMONIA

Bacterial pneumonia has 2 patterns of distribution: bronchopneumonia and lobar pneumonia.

FIGURE 6.2. In (A), an autopsy specimen of bronchopneumonia shows small, patchy, white-tan areas of consolidation involving both upper and lower lung lobes. Image (B) shows lobar pneumonia in another autopsy specimen. The entire lobe is consolidated, with delineation by the interlobar septa and fissure.

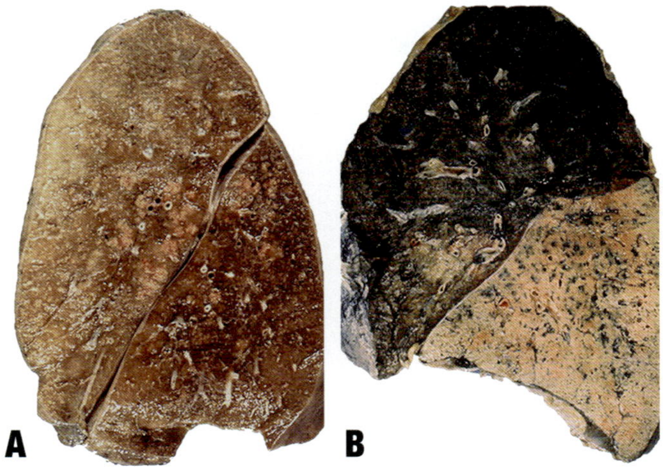

BACTERIAL PNEUMONIA WITH CHRONIC NECROSIS AND FIBROSIS

FIGURE 6.3. Serial sections of the lung demonstrate a consolidated lesion with central necrosis and small cavitations surrounded by a fibrotic rim, consistent with a chronic process. The surrounding lung parenchyma shows centrilobular emphysema.

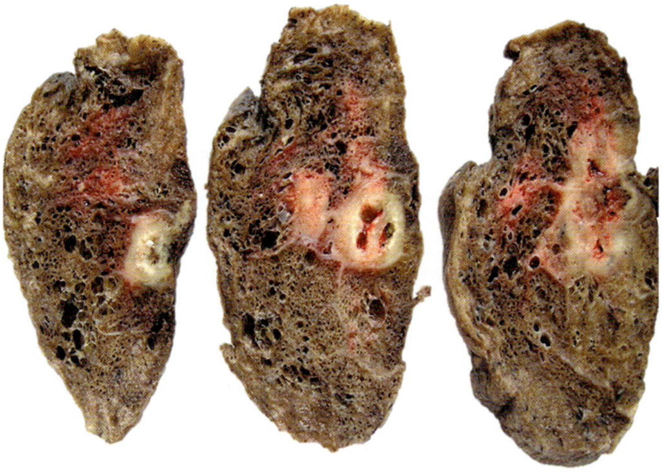

Lung abscess

FIGURE 6.4. This localized suppurative abscess may have several etiologies, including bacterial infection, aspiration, and septic embolism. This resection shows a solitary nodule with a sharply demarcated yellow-white abscess cavity containing pus.

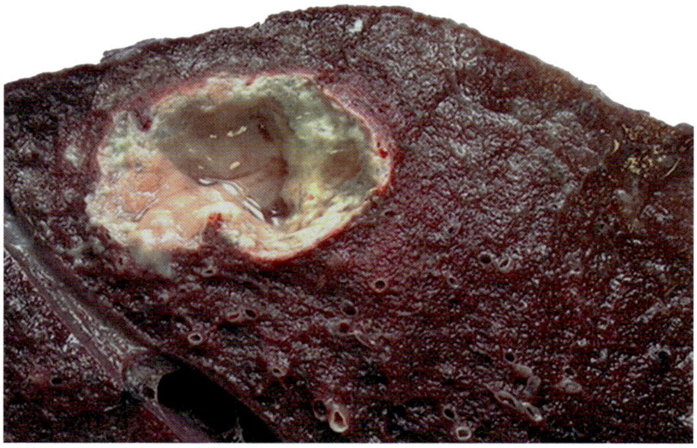

Mycobacterial infection

Mycobacterial infection may present as either solitary or multiple nodules that are often hypermetabolic on positron emission tomography (PET).

GRANULOMATOUS INFLAMMATION MIMICKING A TUMOR

FIGURE 6.5. This image shows a lung wedge resection performed because of a suspicious PET-avid lesion of the left upper lobe. Gross examination shows an ill-defined subpleural lesion with necrosis. Histology showed granulomatous inflammation with necrosis, suggestive of an infectious etiology (possibly tuberculosis). Although no organisms were detected with the use of special histological stains (which are difficult to identify on histological slide), an infectious process is still suspected.

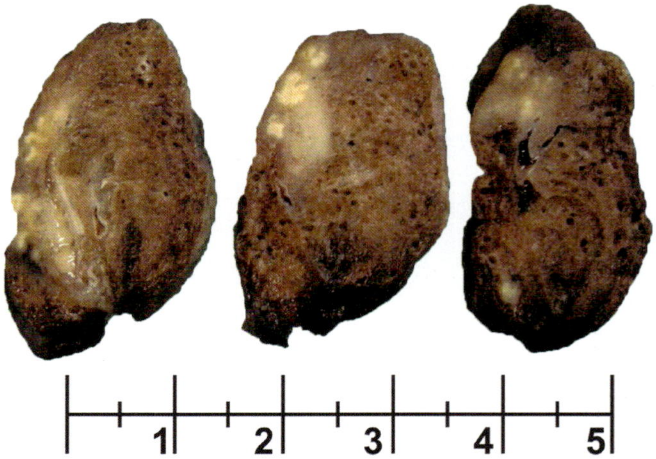

FIGURE 6.6. Image (A) shows a suspicious solitary lesion of the right upper lobe from a 45-year-old male smoker with severe chronic obstructive pulmonary disease (COPD). On gross examination, the lesion is central, solid, white, and ovoid. The background lung tissue shows severe emphysema. Histology revealed a granulomatous lesion with necrosis and fibrosis, suggestive of an infectious origin; however, special stains were negative. Image (B) shows another example of a lobectomy performed for a PET-positive lesion in a smoker. In this case, multiple lesions of granulomatous inflammation were present.

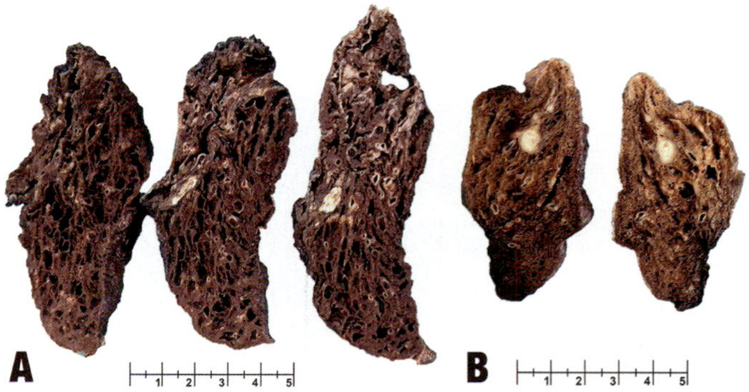

SPECIMEN WITH HILAR LYMPH NODE NECROTIZING GRANULOMA

FIGURE 6.7. This lung autopsy specimen shows a mycobacterial infection in an HIV-positive patient. Image (A) shows coalescent lymphadenopathy present at the hilum. In (B), an enlarged view of the hilar lymph nodes shows caseating necrosis and necrotic tissue drop-out. Numerous organisms were identified by special stains.

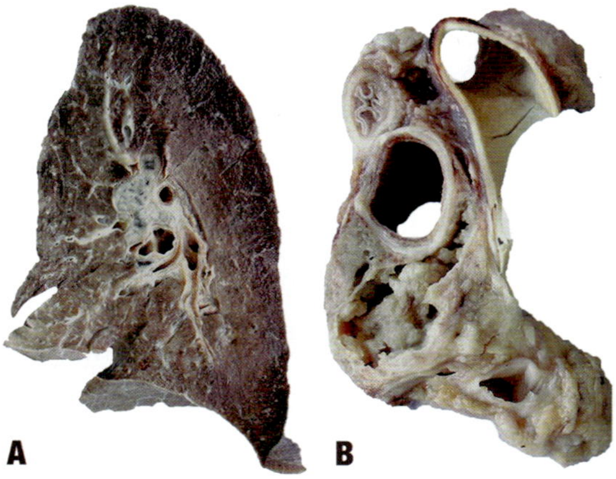

LUNG TUBERCULOMA

FIGURE 6.8. This autopsy specimen has a large, caseating apical lesion with a fibrotic rim in the right upper lobe. The rim was hard and had a laminar organization. Numerous organisms were seen by special stains.

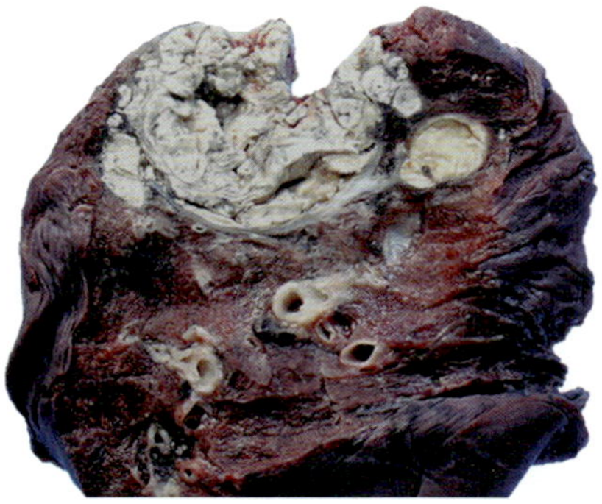

HEALED GRANULOMA

FIGURE 6.9. In this lobectomy for lung cancer, gross examination reveals multiple small (< 1 mm), diffuse, calcified subpleural nodules in the right, lower lobe. Histologically, these correspond to numerous healed granulomas from an infectious etiology (possibly previous tuberculosis or histoplasmosis infection).

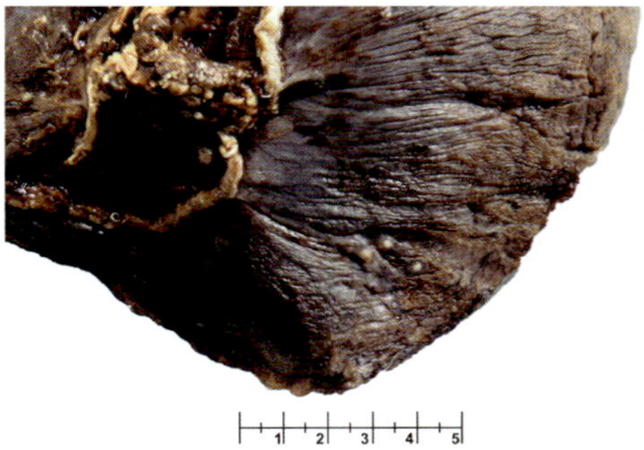

Fungal infection

BLASTOMYCOSIS

Inhalation of *Blastomyces dermatitidis* spores can lead to blastomycosis. Focal solitary nodules or diffuse miliary (disseminated) patterns may occur. In North America, the organism is predominantly found in the central and eastern United States and the Saint Lawrence basin.

FIGURE 6.10. Images (A) and (B) show miliary spread with numerous small, white nodules throughout the lung.

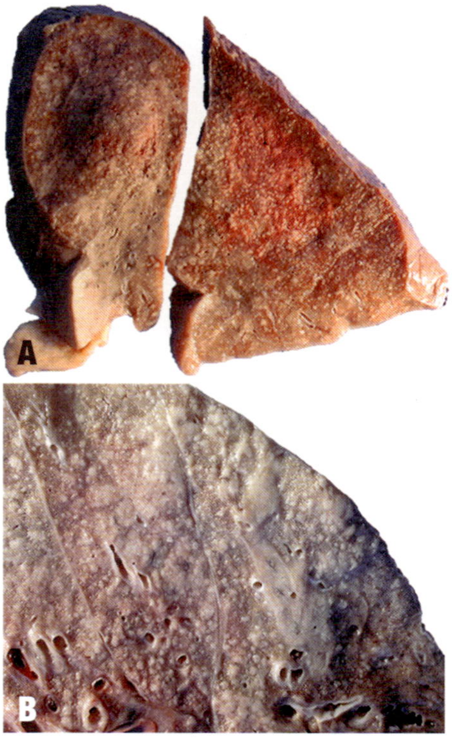

ASPERGILLOSIS

On gross examination, infection by *Aspergillus* species presents mainly as aspergillomas (fungus balls). These typically colonize preexisting cavities within the lung parenchyma.

FIGURE 6.11. The autopsy specimen in (A) shows an aspergilloma that formed via invasion in an immunocompromized patient. Image (B) shows another case of aspergillosis, with colonization of a complex cavity of the lung. Numerous *Aspergillus* organisms were observed in the friable, green, soft material present within the cavity.

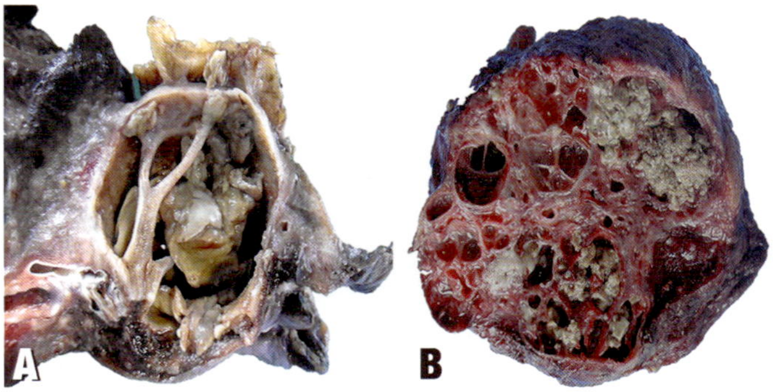

ZYGOMYCOSIS (MUCORMYCOSIS)

Zygomycosis is a life-threatening infection with a high mortality rate that is characterized by an angioinvasive pattern. This infection usually occurs in immunosuppressed patients (e.g., posttransplant patients, diabetics, or patients on corticosteroid therapy), burn victims, or patients suffering from renal failure.

FIGURE 6.12. This section of an autopsied lung shows lung mucormycosis infection causing vascular damage, hemorrhage, and vascular occlusion by thrombosis. Microscopy showed that the tissue consisted of large, irregular, ribbon-like fungi that were morphologically consistent with a diagnosis of mucormycosis.

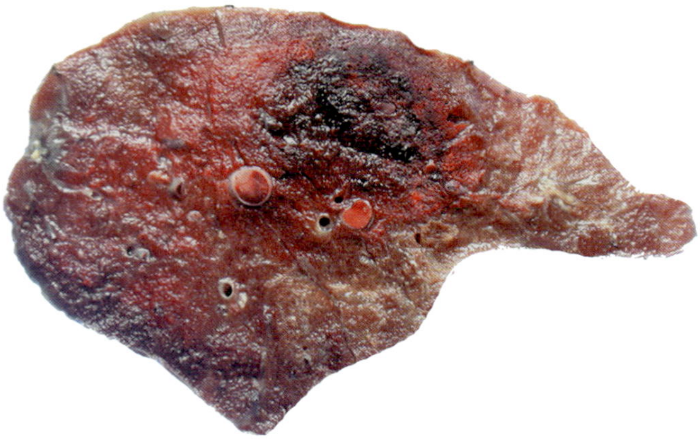

FIGURE 6.13. In this example, an autopsy was performed on an immunosuppressed patient who had acute respiratory decompensation. Radiological imaging showed possible thrombi formation and a suspicion of pulmonary embolism. Sections of the lung show that the lumens of both the pulmonary artery and veins are occluded by tan, irregular tissue that was confirmed to be mucormycosis (arrows).

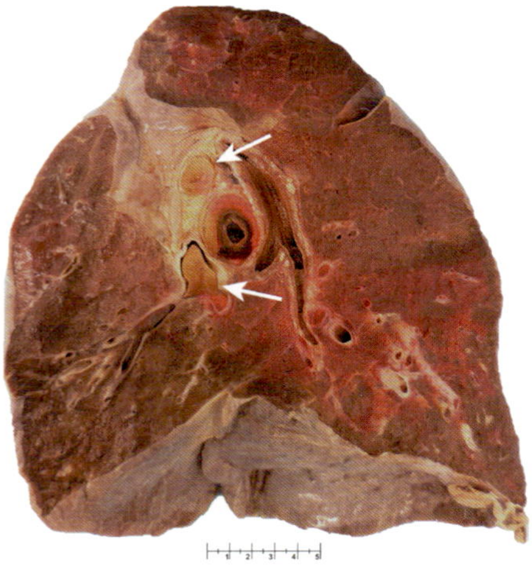

CRYPTOCOCCUS

Cryptococcus fungi are found in soil contaminated by bird droppings and decaying wood. Clinically important species include *C. neoformans* and *C. gatti*. In North America, infections are predominantly reported on the west coast.

FIGURE 6.14. This immunosuppressed patient had rapid postoperative decompensation with clinical suspicion of sepsis and acute respiratory distress syndrome. Grossly, the lungs are heavy and have a beefy-red color with a glistening aspect. Although diffuse alveolar damage was suspected, microscopy showed a diffuse *Cryptococcus* pneumonia.

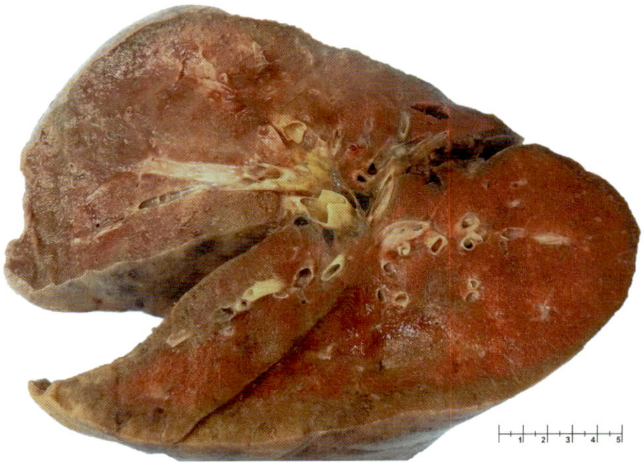

HISTOPLASMA CAPSULATUM

Histoplasma capsulatum can cause a deep fungal infection when dust or soil particles contaminated with bird or bat droppings are inhaled. In North America, infections are predominantly reported in the central and eastern United States and the Saint Lawrence basin in Canada.

FIGURE 6.15. This specimen shows a lesion with a pseudocapsule and central necrosis.

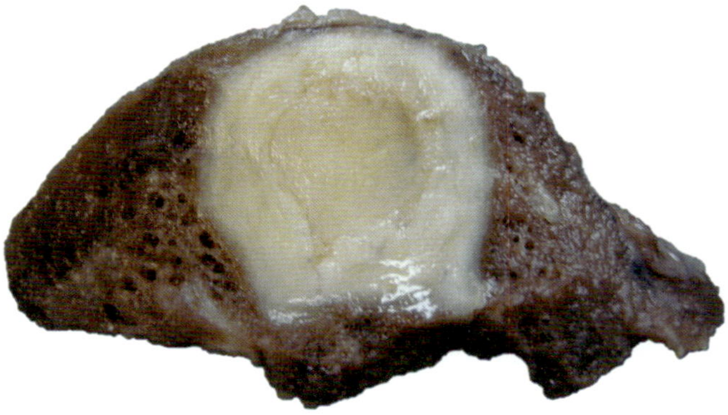

COCCIDIOIDOMYCOSIS

Coccidioides immitis mainly grows in hot and dry regions, and is endemic in the southwestern United States, Mexico, and Central and South America. Most primary pulmonary infections are asymptomatic. In cases of acute pneumonia, however, solitary nodules or a miliary pattern may develop.

FIGURE 6.16. This case of coccidioidomycosis shows a well-demarcated nodule with a fibrous wall and friable necrotic tissue.

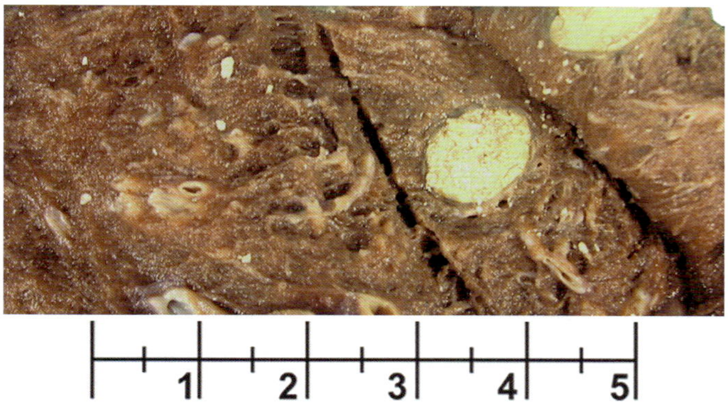

Parasitic infection

ECHINOCOCCOSIS (HYDATID CYST)

In adults, the lung is the second most common site of echinococcosis after the liver. Most patients are asymptomatic for many years, or present with nonspecific symptoms such as mild cough or chest pain. However, rupture of the cysts may cause severe complications such as anaphylactic shock, dissemination of the organism, or massive hemorrhage.

FIGURE 6.17. The lobectomy in (A) shows multiple well-demarcated, thick-walled cystic structures. The closer examination in (B) shows laminated membranes that corresponded to *Echinococcus* organisms.

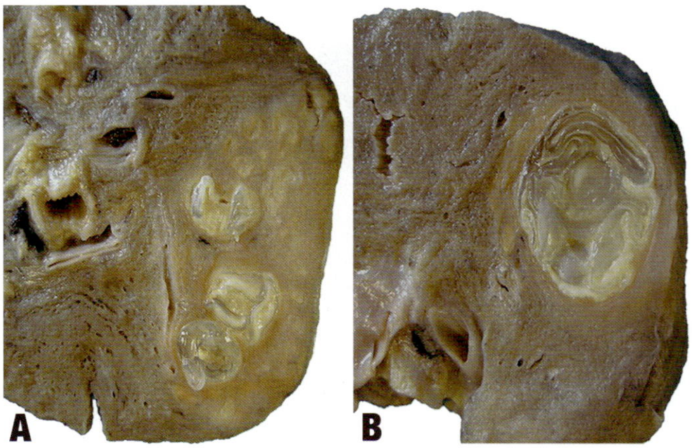

Viral infection

The lung is a frequent site of viral infections such as influenza. However, some infections can manifest as life-threatening disease and some as AIDS-defining diseases.

H1N1 INFLUENZA PNEUMONIA

FIGURE 6.18. This image shows the autopsied lungs of a patient who was found unresponsive and septic. A nasal swab was positive for H1N1 influenza A. The lungs show consolidation with a slippery texture. Microscopy confirmed the diagnosis as diffuse alveolar damage.

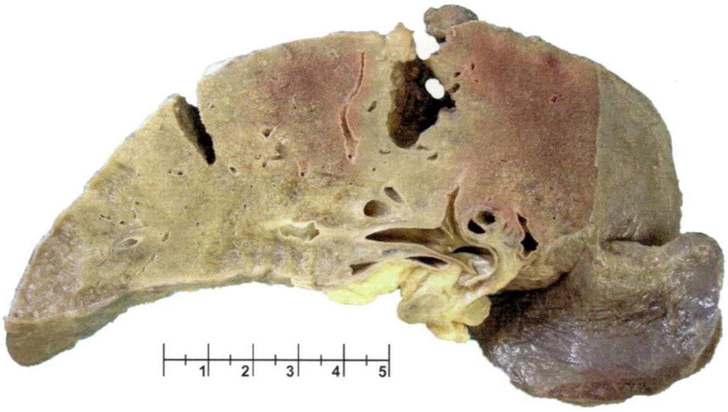

AIDS-RELATED KAPOSI SARCOMA

FIGURE 6.19. This specimen comes from a patient with human immunodeficiency virus (HIV). In (A), multiple irregular dark patches are visible in the mucosa of the trachea and within the subcarinal lymph node (arrow). Similarly, in (B), the visceral surface of the lung shows numerous dark patches. Multiple pleural adhesions are also present. Microscopically, the patches were confirmed to be Kaposi sarcoma.

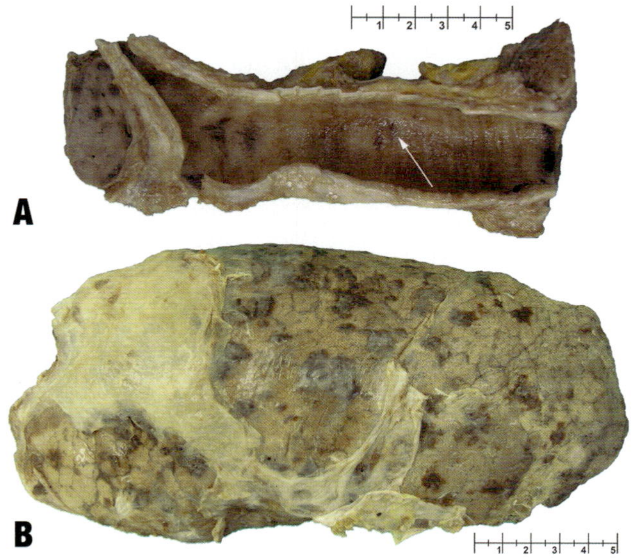

Centrilobular pulmonary emphysema

Permanent destruction of the lung parenchymal interstitium leads to formation of enlarged air spaces, termed emphysema. These do not usually show significant fibrosis.

FIGURE 6.20. In this lobectomy for lung cancer in a lifelong smoker, gross examination shows marked centrilobular emphysema.

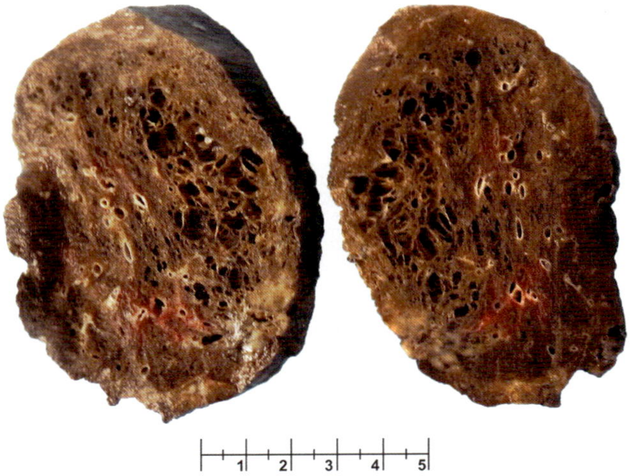

Subpleural bullae

Subpleural bullae are thin-walled, cyst-like spaces that bulge out of the lung. Pulmonary bullae can arise as a complication of emphysema. Rupture of these bullae leads to pneumothorax.

FIGURE 6.21. This image shows subpleural bullae in a patient with pneumothorax.

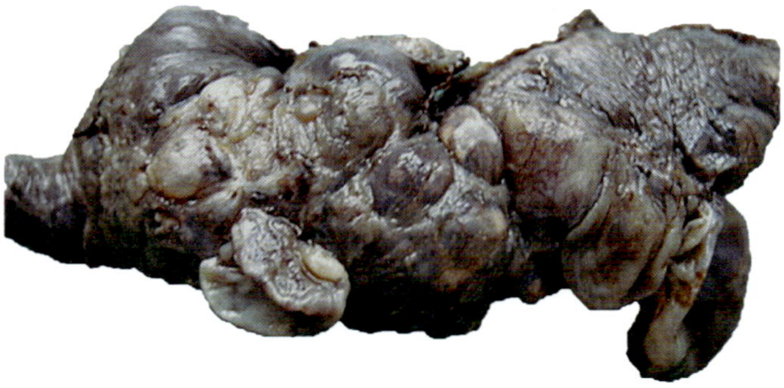

Bronchiectasis

Destruction of the larger airways with remodeling leads to tubular and saccular dilation of the bronchial tree, termed bronchiectasis. Most cases are related to cystic fibrosis or occur as a complication of pulmonary infection.

FIGURE 6.22. This autopsied lung demonstrates saccular bronchiectasis.

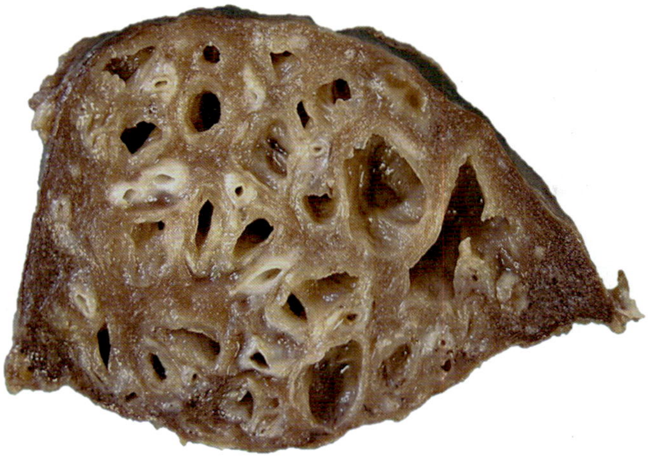

BRONCHIECTASIS WITH MUCINOUS PLUG FORMATION

Bronchiectatic airways can become completely occluded by thick mucinous plugs. The plugging can be so severe that a bronchial cast can form.

FIGURE 6.23. Image (A) shows complete occlusion of the bronchiectatic airways by thick mucinous plugs. Image (B) shows a bronchial cast expectorated by a patient suffering from bronchiectasis. It consists of mucus enmeshed with fibrin, red blood cells, and inflammatory cells.

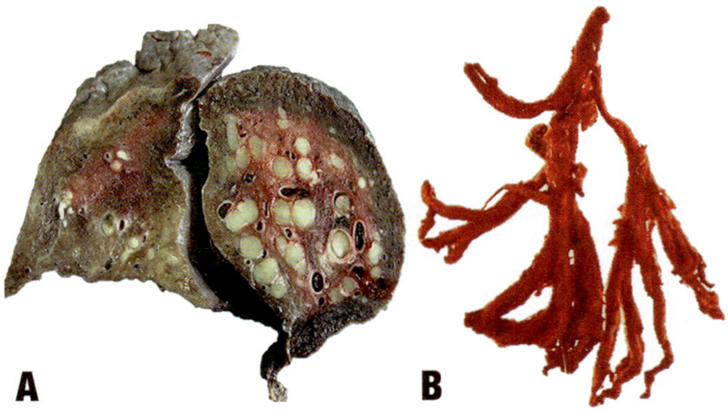

GRAFT VERSUS HOST DISEASE

FIGURE 6.24. This autopsy specimen was from a patient with acute myeloid leukemia who had undergone allogenic stem cell transplant. The specimen shows, grossly, cylindrical ulcerative bronchiectasis (arrow) with mucous plugging (removed). Microscopy showed necrotizing ulceration of the bronchiectatic segments. Additional findings on microscopy included extensive bronchiolitis obliterans of the lumens with fibrotic tissue: evidence of graft versus host disease.

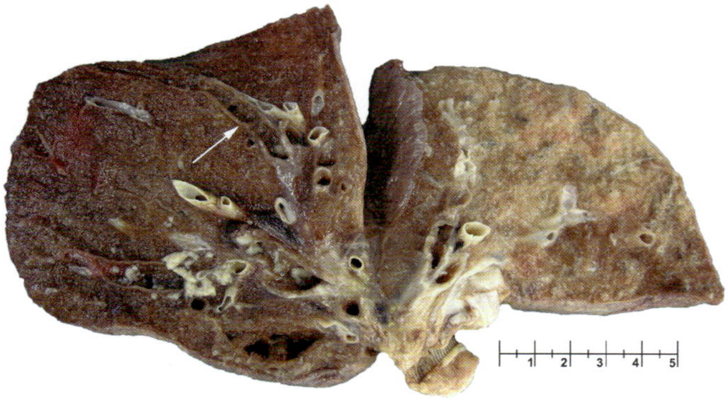

TRACTION BRONCHIECTASIS

This is another type of bronchiectasis, termed traction bronchiectasis. In this type, the segments are splayed open by mural fibrosis.

FIGURE 6.25. The autopsy specimen in (A) is from a patient with known end-stage pulmonary sarcoidosis. The lung tissue in (B) shows extensive cystic changes with traction-type bronchiectasis (arrow). Microscopic examination showed hyalinized nodules in the interstitium around the bronchioles, which were consistent with sclerosed sarcoid granulomas.

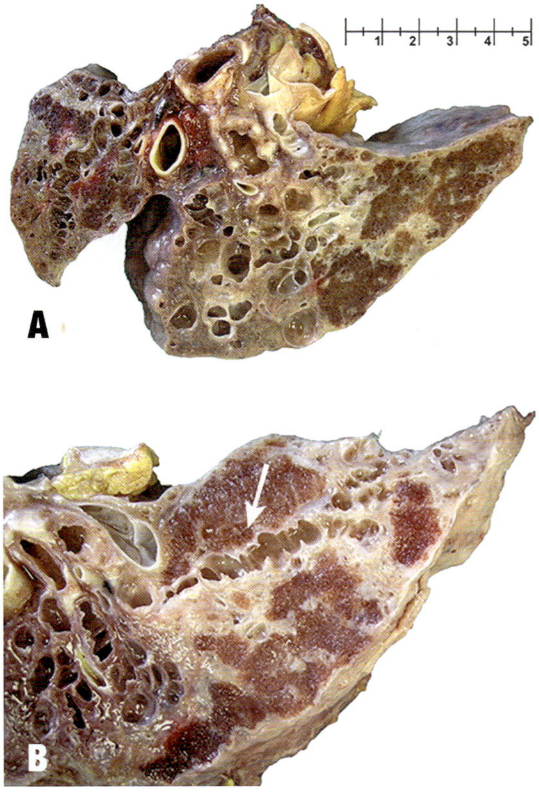

Diffuse alveolar damage

SEPSIS

FIGURE 6.26. This image shows specimens of autopsied lung from a patient who developed postoperative sepsis and acute hypoxia that was thought to be due to acute respiratory distress syndrome (ARDS). Grossly, the lungs were markedly heavy and enlarged. Sections show dark, beefy-red consolidation with areas of paler tan color and glistening appearance. The texture of the lung is slippery. Microscopic examination showed prominent hyaline membranes of the acute phases of diffuse alveolar damage.

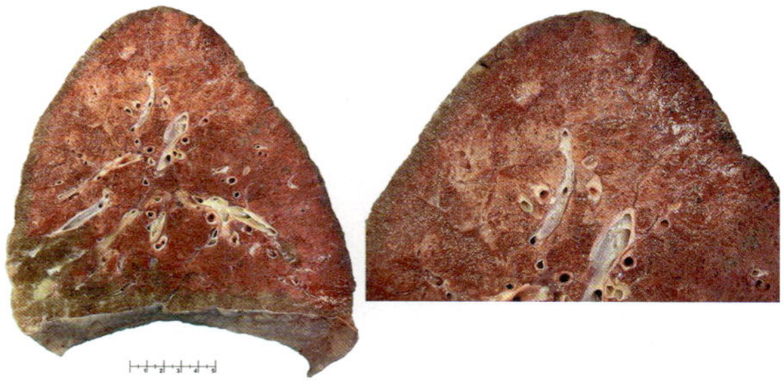

Usual interstitial pneumonia

FIGURE 6.27. This image shows lung sections from a patient who developed progressively worsening dyspnea. Computed tomography scans (CT scans) showed subpleural honeycombing fibrosis. The lung sections show a patchy disease process that is more pronounced in the lower lobes, and that consists of zones of subpleural fibrosis and cystic change. Between the areas of fibrosis are areas of relatively unaffected lung parenchyma. Histologically, the lung showed a temporal and spatial heterogeneity of fibrosis consistent with a usual interstitial pneumonia–type pattern. No underlying etiology could be discerned. The case was diagnosed as idiopathic pulmonary fibrosis.

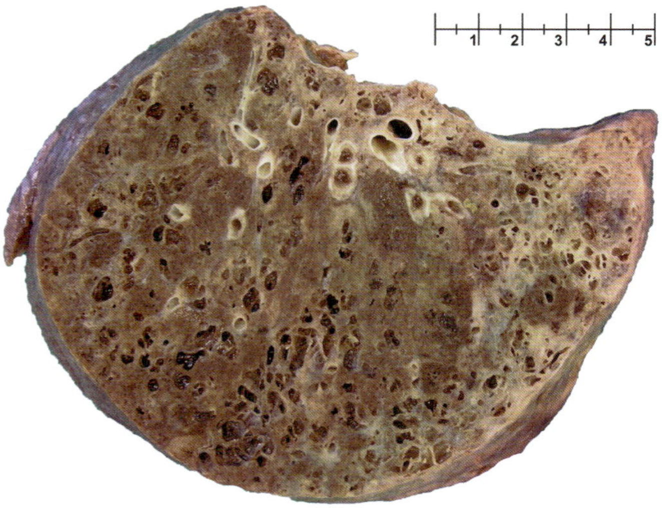

Coal worker's pneumonoconiosis

Coal worker's pneumoconiosis is a restrictive occupational lung disease that develops after prolonged exposure to coal dust particles and other types of dust. The spectrum of diseases includes anthracosis, simple-type pneumoconiosis, and complicated-type pneumoconiosis (progressive massive fibrosis).

FIGURE 6.28. In (A), the pleural surface of these autopsied lungs shows simple coal worker's pneumoconiosis with numerous coal dust macules and small black nodules. In (B), sections of the same lung show many parenchymal coal dust macules, which were shown microscopically to have developed adjacent to respiratory bronchioles.

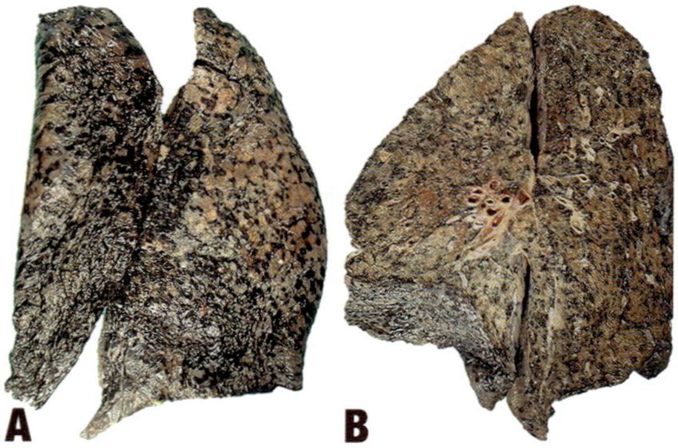

Bronchogenic cyst

Bronchogenic cysts are congenital cysts, mostly found in the hilum and anterior mediastinum. They are unilocular, do not communicate with the tracheobronchial tree, and have a fibrotic wall.

FIGURE 6.30. This image shows a typical bronchogenic cyst. Microscopy found respiratory epithelium in the cyst lining and cartilage within the cyst wall.

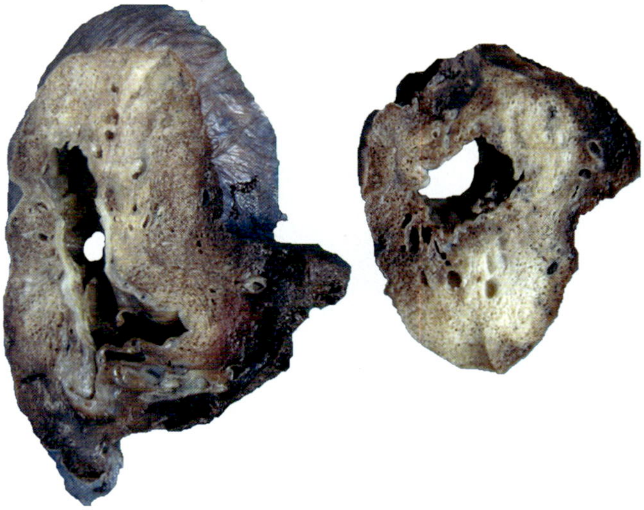

Bronchial mucocele (bronchocele)

Bronchocele results from a proximal obstruction, either congenital (e.g., bronchial atresia) or acquired (e.g., malignancy).

FIGURE 6.29. This lobectomy specimen was found to have a mucocele: a dilated bronchial segment completely filled with and expanded by mucus. In (A), the lobectomy shows a mucus-filled bronchocele. Image (B) shows the same lobectomy specimen with the mucus cleared. The dilated cyst-like architecture of the bronchocele is visible.

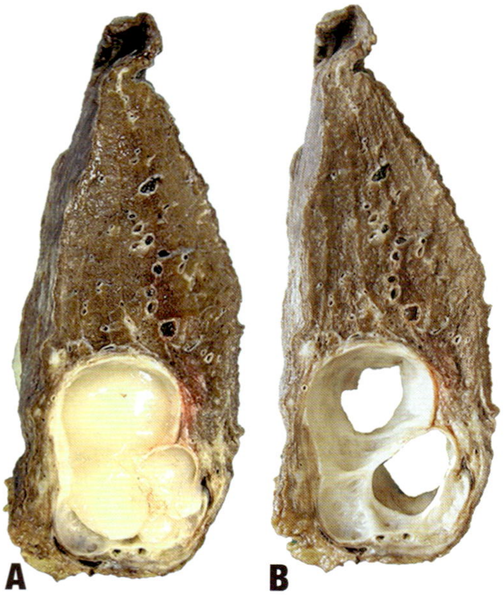

Light chain deposition disease

Light chain deposition disease is a nonamyloid immunoglobulin deposition disease, usually associated with a clonal plasma cell disorder (e.g., multiple myeloma). Deposits can range from a solitary lesion present in only 1 lobe to bilateral multiple diffuse nodules.

FIGURE 6.31. The wedge resection specimen in (A) shows a single, well-defined, tan-to-white, firm, and tumor-like lesion with nodular architecture and pseudoinvasion of the visceral pleura. Image (B) shows the cut section of the nodule. The diagnosis was confirmed on electron microscopy.

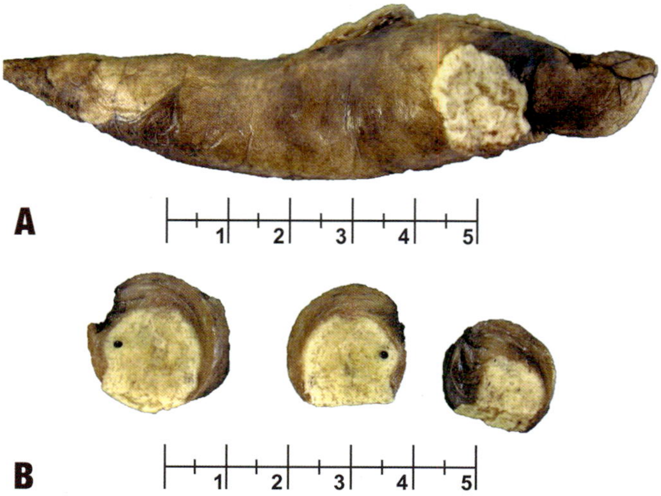

GRANULOMATOSIS WITH POLYANGIITIS

This vasculitis can present as a single focus, multiple discrete nodules (solid or cavitated), or hemorrhage (diffuse or localized).

FIGURE 6.32. In this example, the patient presented with bilateral lung cavitary nodules. A wedge biopsy was performed on the left lower lobe in which 2 separate nodules were present. This image shows that the smaller nodule is well circumscribed and contains a central cystic cavity. Microscopy revealed granulomatous inflammation with the vessels showing fibrinoid necrosis.

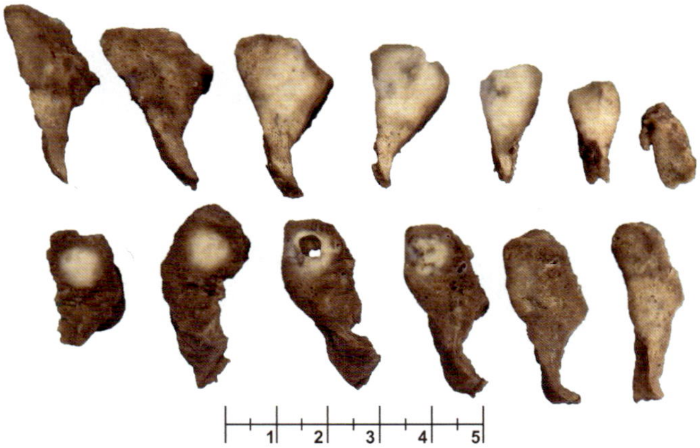

Pulmonary alveolar proteinosis

FIGURE 6.33. This image shows the autopsied lungs of a patient who developed respiratory distress and quickly succumbed to respiratory failure. The lungs show patchy and firm consolidations, thought to represent foci of bronchopneumonia. Histological examination showed PAS-positive, amorphous, granular, and eosinophilic material, which is consistent with pulmonary alveolar proteinosis.

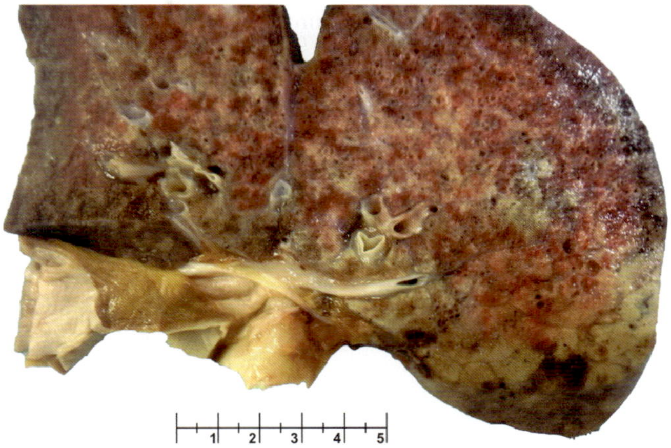

Neoplasms of the Lung

Adenocarcinoma

Adenocarcinoma of the lung is the most common subtype of lung cancer. Histologically, it shows the following architectures: glandular epithelial with noninvasive (lepidic), and invasive (e.g., acinar, papillary, micropapillary, and solid). Macroscopically, the distinction between these patterns can be difficult to predict. All cancers are staged according to the American Joint Committee on Cancer (AJCC) staging manual (8th edition).

PROCEDURE: SAMPLING ADENOCARCINOMA WITH PLEURAL PUCKERING

FIGURE 6.34. In this lobectomy, a pulmonary adenocarcinoma underlies the pleura surface where a desmoplastic reaction leads to retraction and distortion of the pleura. When sampling such a tumor, cut sections should be performed transverse to the long axis of the puckering to best demonstrate the relationship of the tumor with the pleura, including potential pleural invasion that may affect staging (double arrows).

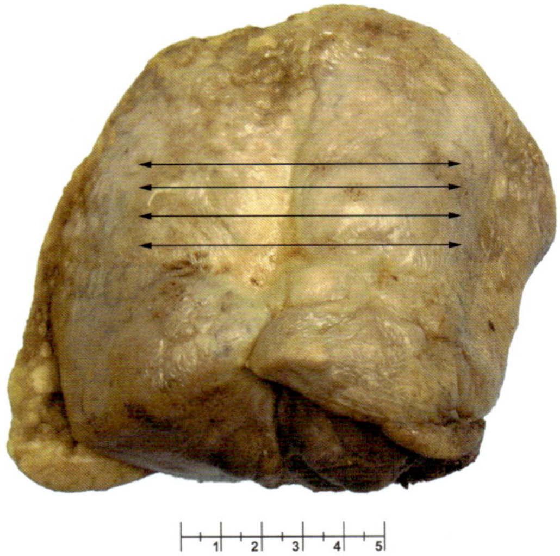

ADENOCARCINOMA IN SITU

In the 2015 World Health Organization (WHO) classification system, adenocarcinoma in situ is defined as a preinvasive lesion. It corresponds to growth of neoplastic cells (measuring < 3 cm) along alveolar structures (lepidic pattern) without any stromal, vascular, or pleural invasion. It occurs in the peripheral lung and usually corresponds to an incidental, small, "ground glass" lesion seen in radiological images. Wedge resection may be performed. Disease-free survival is achievable when the tumor is completely resected.

FIGURE 6.35. This tumor was staged pTis. Images (A) and (B) show a poorly defined, pleural-based, tan nodule measuring 1.1 cm and growing along the existing lung alveolar architecture. Gross examination must be performed carefully since small lesions are easily missed. The nodule must be entirely submitted for diagnosis to exclude any foci of invasion. Image (C) shows a microscopic examination of the adenocarcinoma in situ.

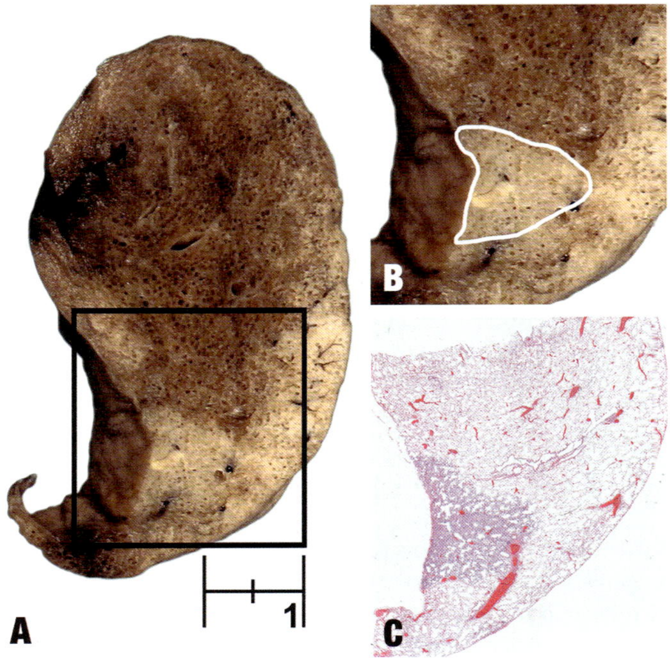

ACINAR-PREDOMINANT ADENOCARCINOMA, ASSOCIATED WITH ATYPICAL ADENOMATOUS HYPERPLASIA (AAH)

Differentiating AAH from adenocarcinoma in situ can be very difficult, even on histology, because these entities are on a continuous spectrum. Lesion size may help with diagnosis: lesions caused by AAH are usually < 0.5 cm; lesions caused by adenocarcinoma in situ are usually > 0.5 cm.

FIGURE 6.36. This left upper lobectomy was performed for a 3.6-cm adenocarcinoma. Gross examination shows a 0.5-cm, ill-defined nodule (arrows), corresponding histologically to AAH.

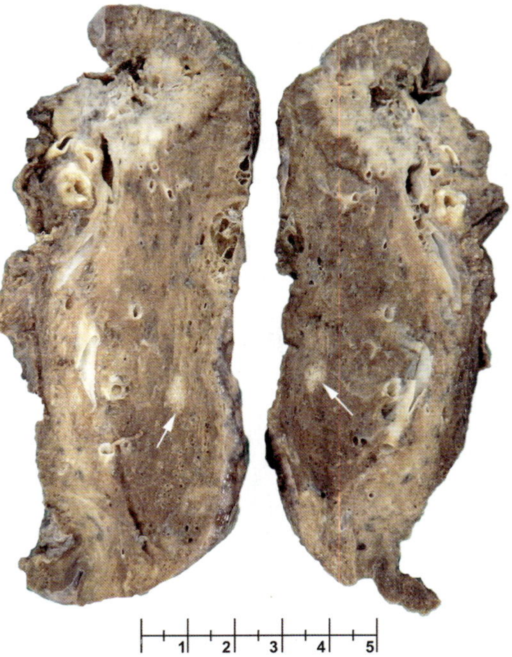

MINIMALLY INVASIVE ADENOCARCINOMA

This entity requires microscopic examination *in toto*, and shows predominantly a lepidic growth pattern combined with an invasive pattern where tumor cells infiltrate the myofibroblastic stroma. To make this diagnosis, the lesion must be solitary (i.e., absence of metastatic spread), ≤ 3 cm in size, and with the invasive component ≤ 0.5 cm. There must also be absence of lymphatic, blood vessel, or pleural invasion. In addition, there should be no spread that has occurred via air spaces or tumor necrosis.

FIGURE 6.37. Careful examination of this specimen reveals a 1.8-cm lesion (arrow), which corresponded histologically to a minimally invasive adenocarcinoma. This tumor was staged pT1mi.

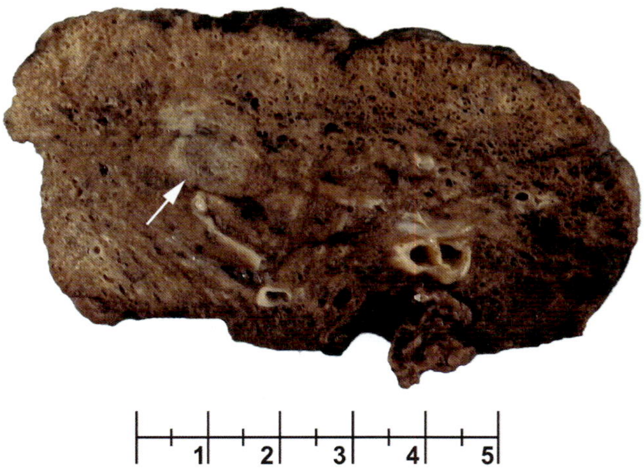

LEPIDIC-PREDOMINANT ADENOCARCINOMA

FIGURE 6.38. This right upper lobectomy shows a 1.5-cm, spiculated lesion (arrow) with central scarring fibrosis surrounded peripherally by a zone with partial preservation of the alveolar architecture. Histologically, the central portion of the adenocarcinoma consisted of an acinar component (evaluated at 30%, and 0.6 cm in diameter); the peripheral portion consisted of a lepidic pattern (evaluated at 70%). Pleural puckering was present, but no pleural invasion was detected. The tumor was staged pT1a.

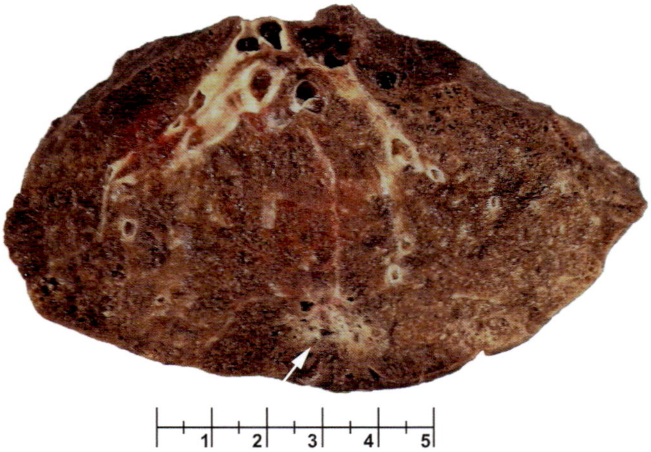

PAPILLARY-PREDOMINANT ADENOCARCINOMA

FIGURE 6.39. This right middle lobectomy shows a subpleural, heterogeneous, circumscribed tumor with anthracotic pigmentation. The puckered visceral pleura was not involved. Histologically, the adenocarcinoma showed papillary (50%), acinar (40%), and lepidic (10%) components. The tumor was staged pT1c.

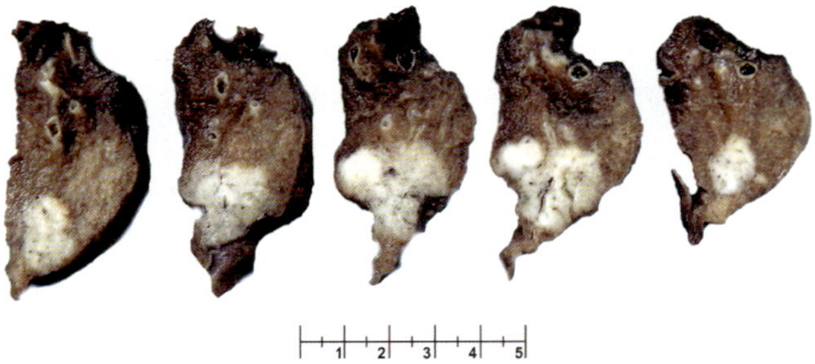

SOLID-PREDOMINANT ADENOCARCINOMA

FIGURE 6.40. This right upper lobectomy shows a 2.7-cm apical nodule with mixed histological subtypes (solid predominant). Severe centrilobular emphysema is also present. The tumor was staged pT1c.

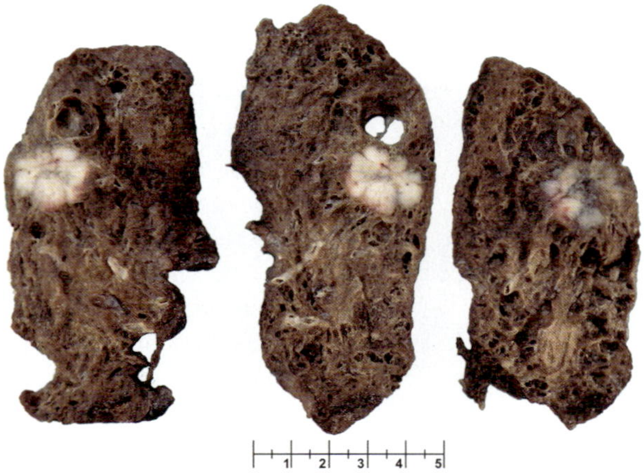

SOLID-PREDOMINANT ADENOCARCINOMA WITH NECROTIC AND CYSTIC CHANGES

FIGURE 6.41. This right lower lobectomy shows a 3.5-cm, well-circumscribed tumor at the pleural surface of the superior segment. Necrotic and cystic changes are present. Histologically, this specimen showed an adenocarcinoma with a solid predominant pattern and visceral pleura invasion. The tumor was staged pT2a.

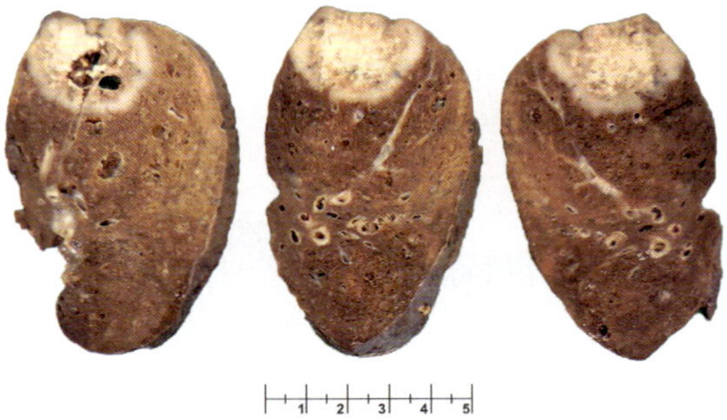

ACINAR-PREDOMINANT ADENOCARCINOMA

FIGURE 6.42. The left upper lobectomy in (A) shows prominent puckering of the visceral pleura. In (B), cut sections of the lung reveal a 5.5-cm lesion, which consisted of an acinar-predominant adenocarcinoma. Histologically, the visceral pleura was not involved by the tumor. Based on size criteria, the tumor was staged pT3.

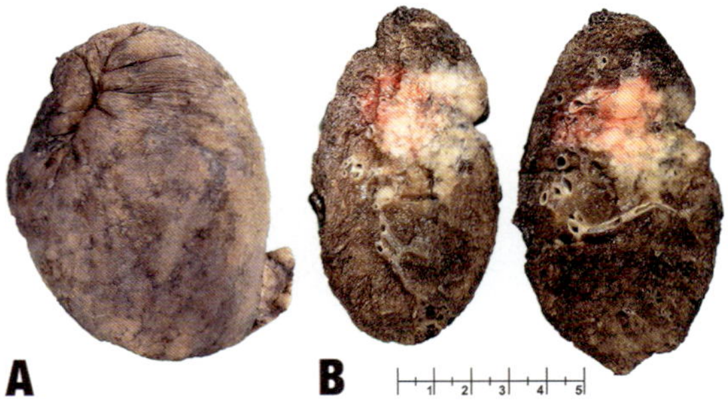

ACINAR-PREDOMINANT ADENOCARCINOMA WITH PARIETAL PLEURA INVASION

FIGURE 6.43. The black pigmentation seen in this specimen corresponds to anthracotic deposits within the visceral pleura (arrows). The tumor extends grossly into the parietal pleura, as can be seen by the white nodular area within yellow fat tissue (*). The tumor was staged pT3.

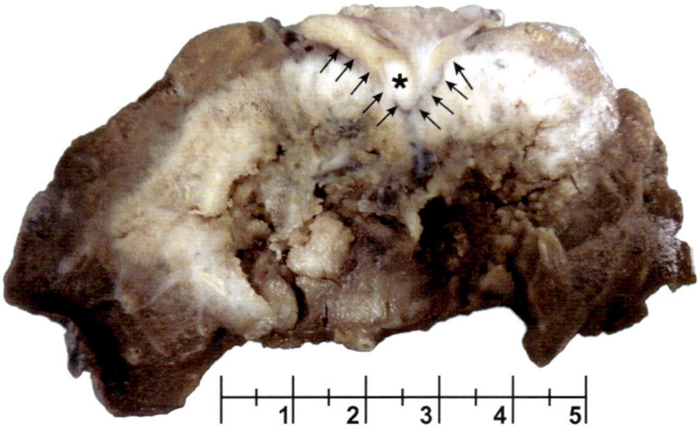

SOLID-PREDOMINANT ADENOCARCINOMA WITH INTERLOBAR LYMPH NODE INVOLVEMENT

FIGURE 6.44. This right pneumonectomy shows a peribronchial tumor with lymph node involvement by direct extension. Histologically, it consisted entirely of a solid pattern of poorly differentiated malignant cells. On immunohistochemistry, the cells stained positive for thyroid transcription factor 1 (TTF-1) and napsin A. Mucicarmine staining was also positive in the cells, consistent with mucosecretion. Overall, the findings were in keeping with a solid adenocarcinoma.

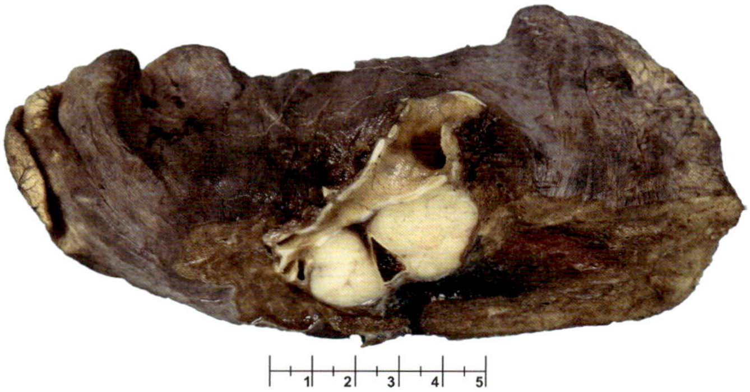

MULTIFOCAL LUNG ADENOCARCINOMA WITH LEPIDIC FEATURES

FIGURE 6.45. This image of a right upper lobectomy shows 5 separate nodules. The main tumor (1) is a 1.3-cm acinar adenocarcinoma with visceral pleura invasion. Two other, smaller nodules (2 and 3) are lepidic-predominant adenocarcinomas. The last 2 nodules (4 and 5) are adenocarcinoma in situ. In this entity, the lesions are considered synchronous primary tumors. The staging was pT2a (5) because of pleural invasion. Note the format of the stage designation, which follows the AJCC staging manual (8th edition): the highest-stage tumor (pT2a, in this case) followed by the total number of tumors in parentheses (5, in this case).

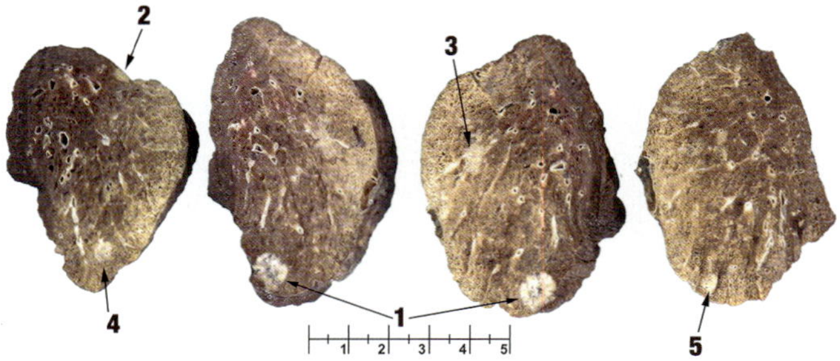

INVASIVE MUCINOUS ADENOCARCINOMA

In an invasive mucinous adenocarcinoma, the tumor cells have a columnar or goblet-cell morphology with abundant intracellular mucin. The tumors mostly exhibit a lepidic pattern, but also show other growth patterns including acinar, papillary, and micropapillary (but not solid). This tumor is thought to have aerogenous spread, and commonly grows in multiple foci within a single lobe, multiple lobes, or even in both lungs.

FIGURE 6.46. This lobectomy shows multiple small foci coalescing to involve the entire lobe. The cut surface has a glistening appearance.

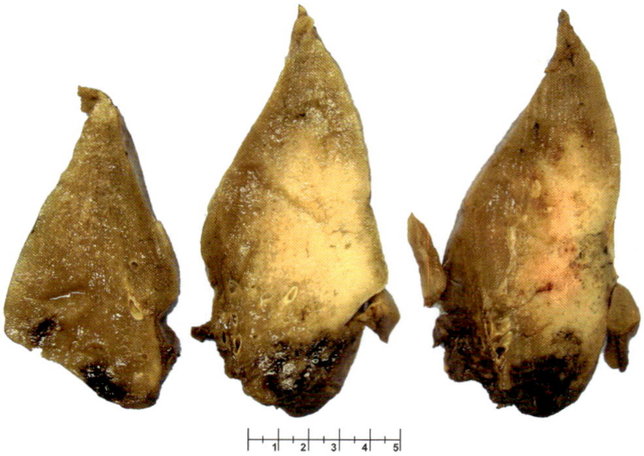

FETAL ADENOCARCINOMA

This variant of adenocarcinoma consists of glandular structures with glycogen-rich cells resembling the developing epithelium in the fetal lung. It often has morula formation.

FIGURE 6.47. This right upper lobectomy shows a solitary, well-demarcated, lobulated, tan tumor. Examination of the tumor did not show any necrotic or cystic changes. The tumor proved histologically to be fetal adenocarcinoma.

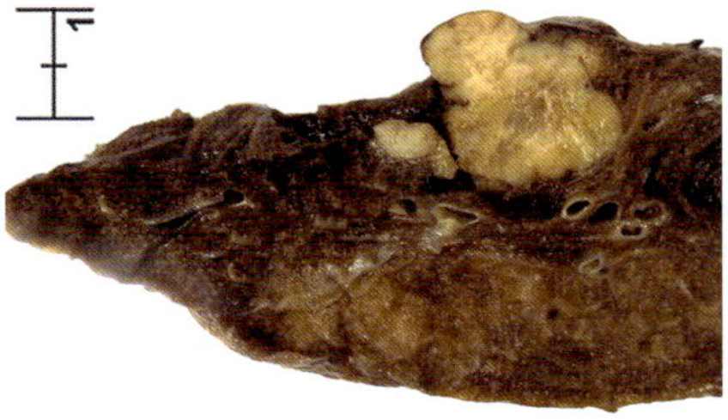

Squamous cell carcinoma (SCC)

Primary invasive lung SCC is often centrally located and corresponds histologically to a malignant epithelial tumor characterized by either keratinization and/or intercellular bridges. The classification of poorly differentiated carcinomas depends on the expression of squamous markers (i.e., p40, p63 or cytokeratin 5/6) by immunohistochemistry.

KERATINIZING SCC

FIGURE 6.48. Image (A) shows a lobectomy specimen with a centrally located, large, white, friable mass. Image (B) shows areas of necrosis and cavitation in the same specimen.

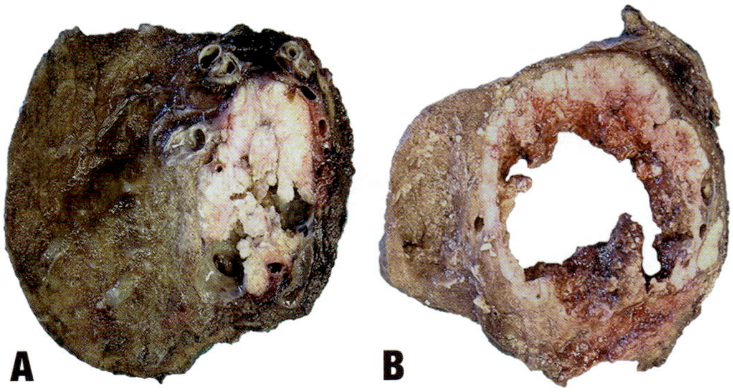

FIGURE 6.49. This lung lobectomy specimen shows a centrally located, well-defined, solid, white tumor with central cavitation (arrow). The lobar-associated lymph node shows metastatic carcinoma deposits and black anthracotic pigment (*). Histologically, the tumor was a keratinizing-type SCC with central necrosis.

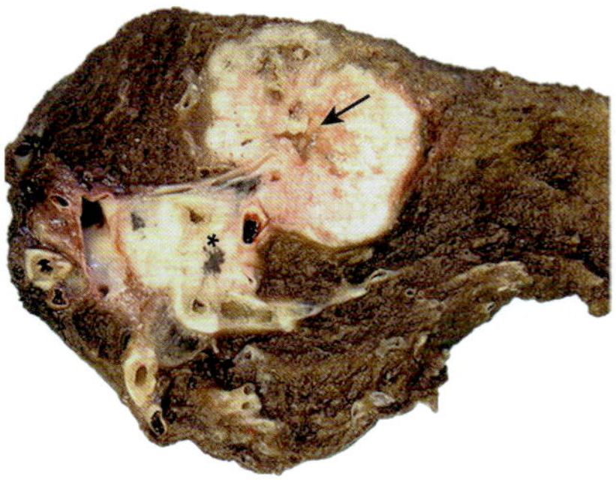

FIGURE 6.50. This bilobectomy of the right middle and lower lobes shows a 4.8-cm tumor obstructing the bronchus intermedius, which led to marked obstructive pneumonitis in the lung tissue peripheral to the tumor (*). Histologically, the tumor was a keratinizing-type SCC.

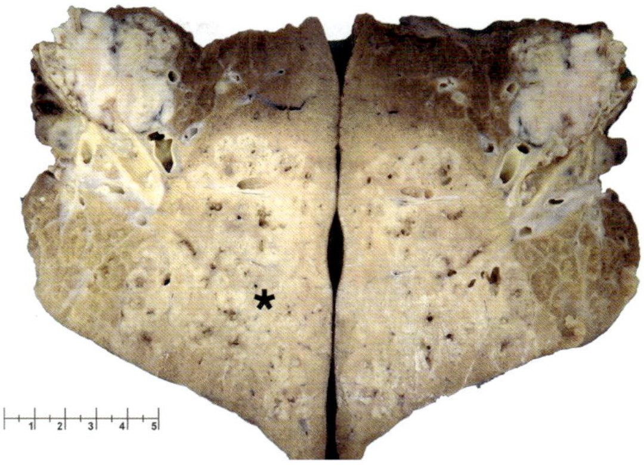

FIGURE 6.51. This image shows a centrally located carcinoma that led to airway obstruction, distal obstructive pneumonitis (*), and mucopurulent bronchiectasis. Histologically, the tumor was a keratinizing-type SCC.

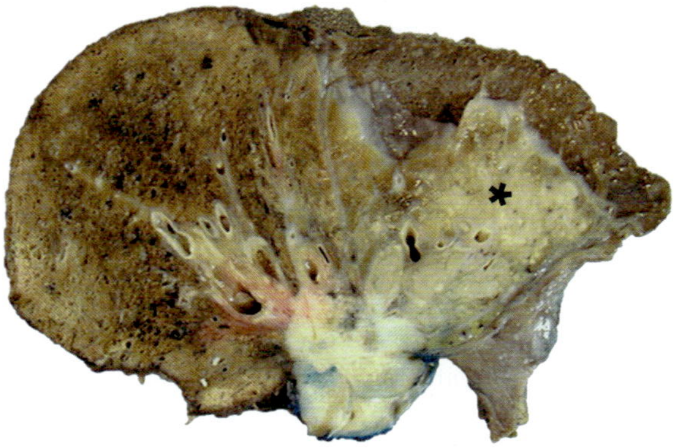

FIGURE 6.52. This right lower lobectomy was taken en bloc with posterior ribs 6 through 8 and their corresponding hemivertebrae. The patient had received neoadjuvant chemotherapy and radiation. The cut section of the specimen shows destruction of the bones with postneoadjuvant fibrosis and cystic degeneration. Histologically, the tumor proved to be a keratinizing-type SCC with extension of viable tumor into the vertebral body. It was classified as stage pT4.

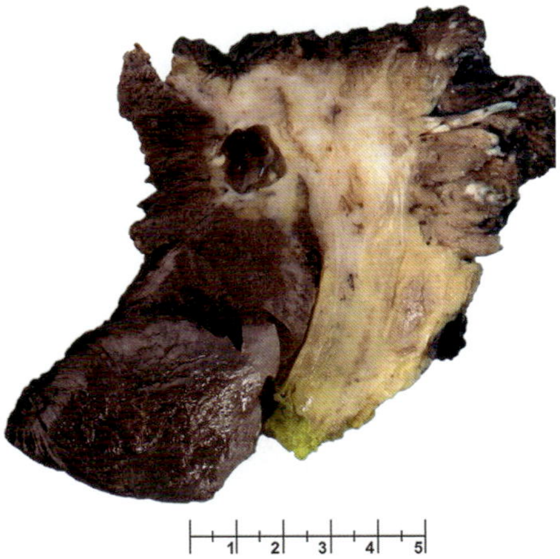

NONKERATINIZING SCC

FIGURE 6.53. The right upper lobectomy in (A) was resected en bloc with the first to fourth ribs of the lateral chest wall. The tumor, shown in (B), is 8.1 cm and invaded the chest wall. Histology showed this tumor to consist of a nonkeratinizing-type SCC. Due to its large size, this tumor is classified as stage pT4. If the tumor had been smaller, invasion into the chest wall would have led to a stage pT3 classification.

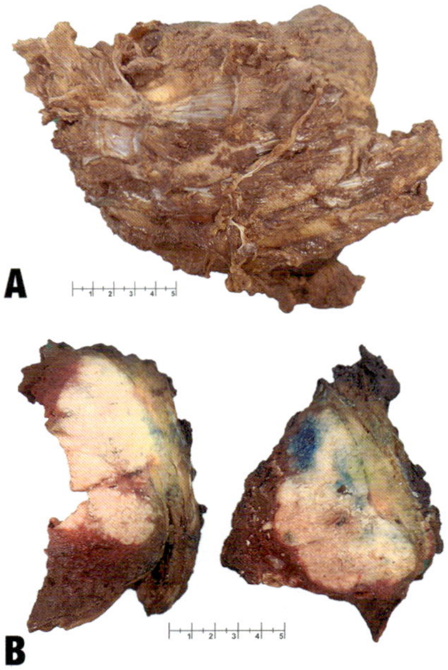

FIGURE 6.54. This is a right lower lobectomy combined with a right upper lobe wedge resection for a ruptured lung cancer. Outer examination in (A) shows empyema. The section in (B) shows a large, 7.2-cm tumor with necrotic and cystic changes crossing the fissure, as demonstrated by black, visceral pleura anthracotic deposits (arrow). Histologically, this tumor was a nonkeratinizing-type SCC and was classified as stage pT4.

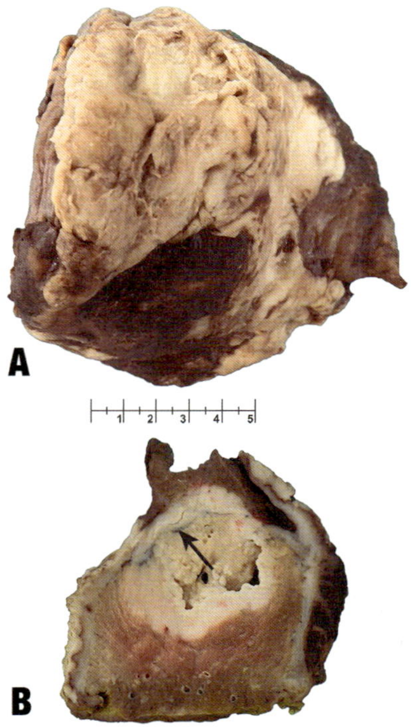

FIGURE 6.55. In this resection specimen, the tumor is invading the vasculature and extending via the lumen of the blood vessel to the left superior pulmonary vein as a tumoral thrombus. The tumor proved to be a nonkeratinizing-type SCC. Even though the tumor protruded out of the lumen in the postsurgical resection specimen, the true vascular margin of the pulmonary vein was histologically negative.

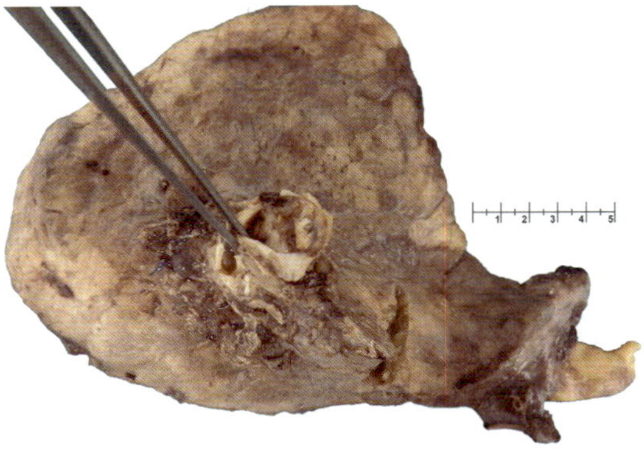

SCC OF THE PERIPHERAL LUNG

SCC often arises in the main or lobar bronchi; however, it can also occur at peripheral sites.

FIGURE 6.56. Image (A) shows a right upper bilobectomy that was performed for a right upper lobe SCC. Image (B) shows a peripherally located SCC that invaded the visceral pleura and caused pleural puckering.

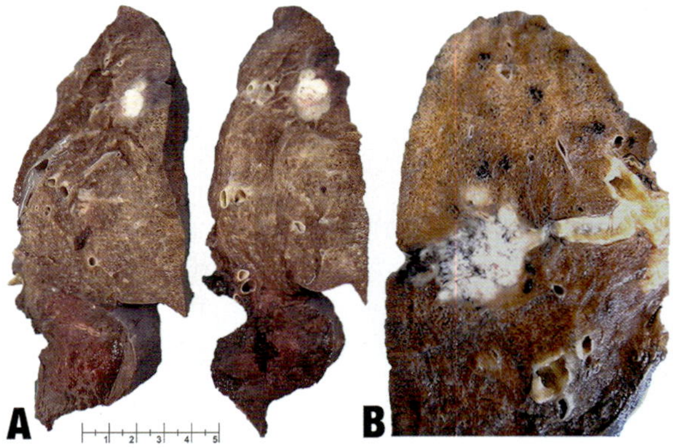

FIGURE 6.57. This image shows another example of peripheral SCC in a right lower lobectomy, where the tumor is in a subpleural location. Histology established the tumor as a keratinizing-type SCC, although the visceral pleura remained free of invasion.

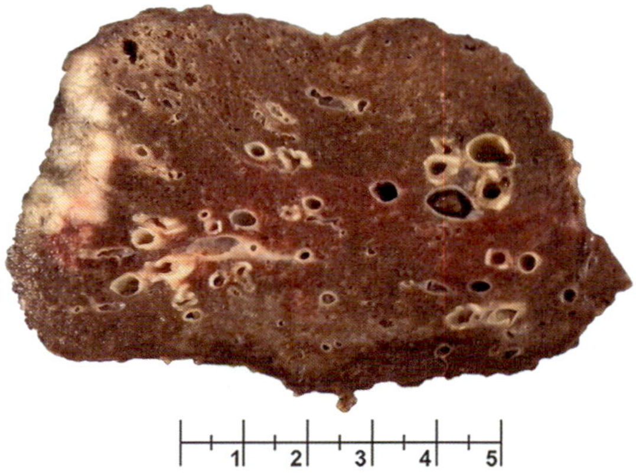

Large cell carcinoma

Large cell carcinomas are undifferentiated, non-small cell carcinomas, lacking either histological or immunohistochemical features of adenocarcinoma, SCC, or neuroendocrine carcinoma. Grossly, large cell carcinomas are usually large, high-stage tumors.

FIGURE 6.58. The pneumonectomy specimen in (A) shows a large, upper lobe tumor invading the main bronchus with associated mucopurulent bronchiectasis of the lower lobe (arrow). Image (B) shows another example of large cell carcinoma that is invading the bronchus and is associated with peribronchial lymph node invasion by contiguous spread (*).

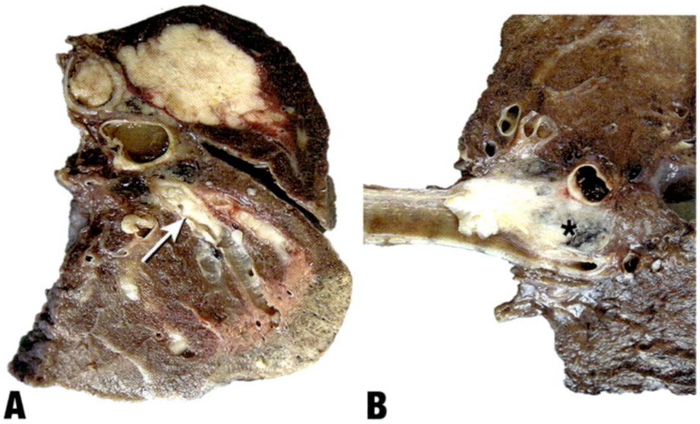

FIGURE 6.59. Gross examination of this lobectomy shows a 2.5-cm tumor with irregular borders. Bronchial and vascular margins are grossly free. Histological examination showed a large cell carcinoma without specific differentiation. Overall, the case was classified as stage pT1c.

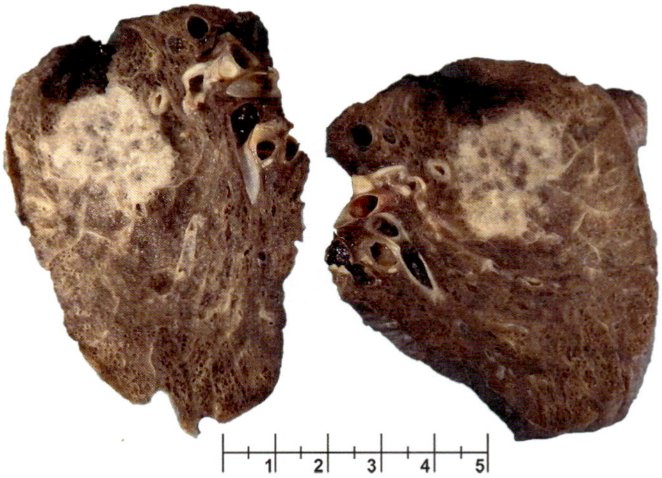

LARGE CELL CARCINOMA WITH INTRALOBAR LYMPH NODE METASTASES

The lung possesses a vast and complex network of lymphatic vessels with numerous lymph nodes. Metastases in ipsilateral hilar, interlobar, and peripheral lung lymph nodes are classified as stage pN1 according to the staging criteria of the AJCC staging manual (8th edition).

FIGURE 6.60. In this resection specimen, a large cell carcinoma had metastasized to lobar lymph nodes (pN1). This type of case must be distinguished from cases in which a separate tumor nodule is present in the same lobe, which would be classified as stage pT3.

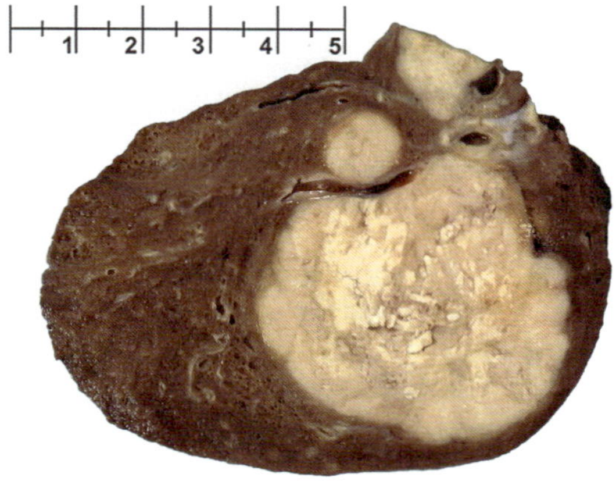

Typical carcinoid tumor

Carcinoids are tumors with neuroendocrine differentiation. Most proximal carcinoids occur in the main stem or lobar bronchi, growing as an endobronchial mass. Typical carcinoids can occur in the peripheral portions of the lung.

FIGURE 6.61. This lobectomy specimen shows a well-circumscribed, homogeneous, round tumor that is partially endobronchial. Histologically, the tumor proved to be a typical carcinoid.

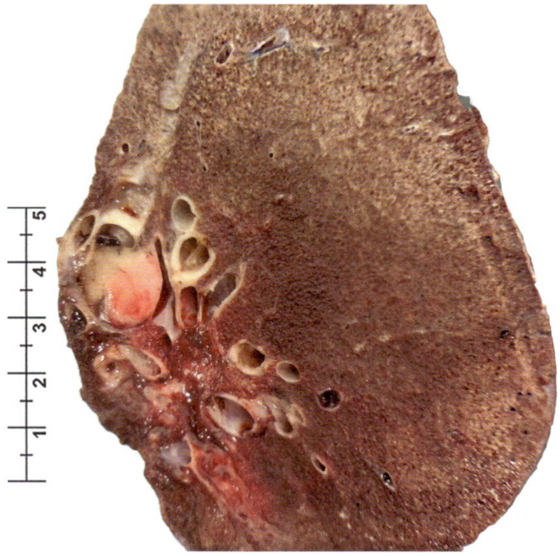

FIGURE 6.62. Gross examination of the lobectomy specimen in (A) demonstrates a polypoid endobronchial mass found mainly in the bronchus. Image (B) shows another example, where a carcinoid tumor has caused complete obstruction of the bronchial lumen.

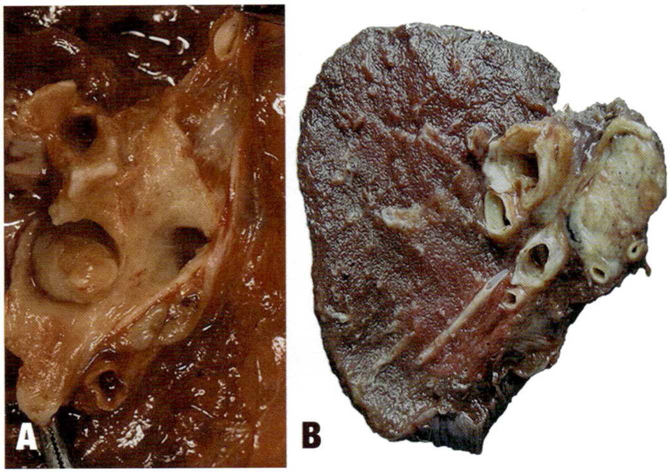

FIGURE 6.63. In (A), obstruction of the bronchial lumen by a centrally located carcinoid has led to distal obstructive pneumonitis. Image (B) shows the carcinoid exhibiting a well-delineated border with a homogenous cut surface.

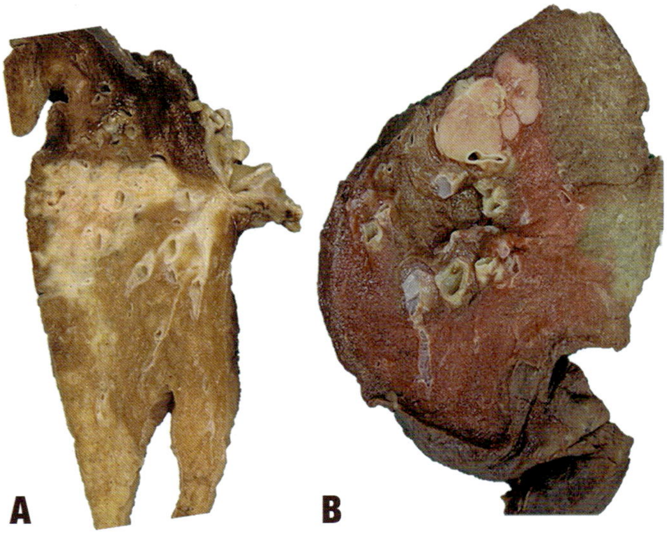

PEPTIDE-SECRETING CARCINOID TUMOR

Rarely, carcinoid tumors of the lung can secrete peptide hormones that can cause clinical symptoms such as carcinoid syndrome or Cushing syndrome.

FIGURE 6.64. In this example, a large, well-circumscribed carcinoid tumor with focal hemorrhage was resected from a patient with Cushing syndrome.

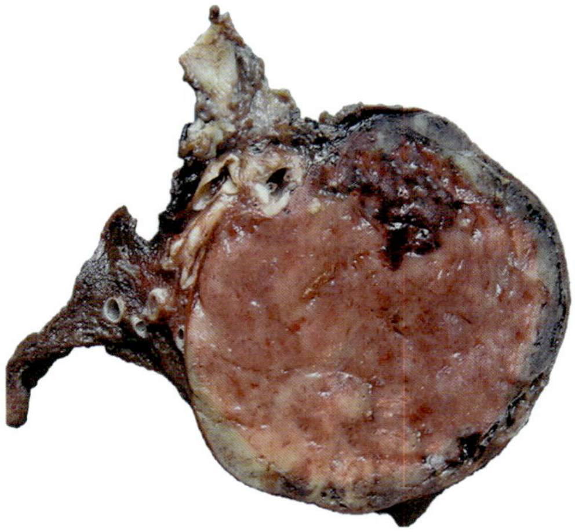

Atypical carcinoid tumor

Atypical carcinoids have an increased chance of metastasis, and confer a decreased survival rate, compared to typical carcinoids. They are larger and occur more often in the periphery of the lung. However, the distinction between typical carcinoids and atypical carcinoids requires microscopic examination for features of necrosis (usually punctate) and an increased mitotic count.

FIGURE 6.65. Images (A) and (B) show examples of atypical carcinoid tumors. The carcinoid tumor shows yellowish cut surface after formalin fixation (B).

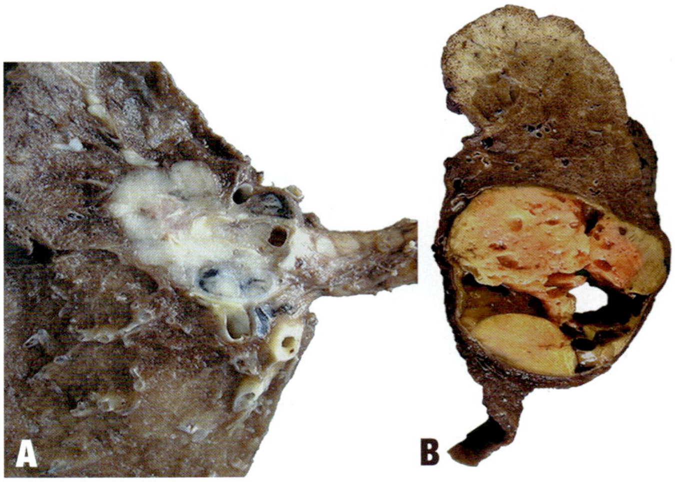

Small cell lung carcinoma (SCLC)

SCLC usually presents as a perihilar, mediastinal mass with lymphadenopathy. Resection is rarely performed; the diagnosis is most often made on biopsy.

FIGURE 6.66. This SCLC resection specimen shows a white, fleshy, and homogeneous peribronchial mass.

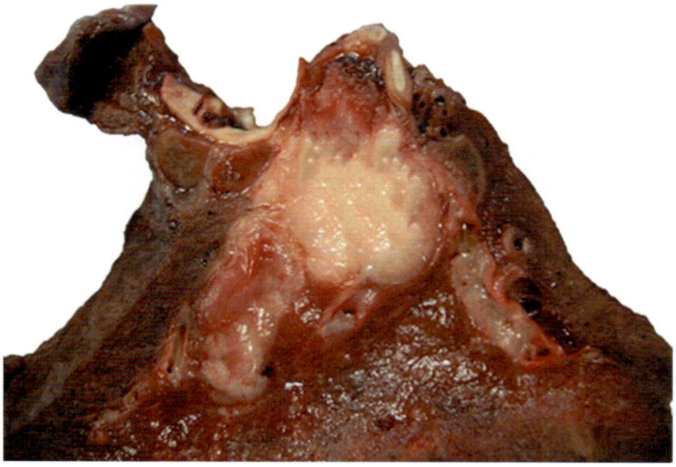

Large cell neuroendocrine carcinoma (LCNEC)

LCNEC is another type of high-grade neuroendocrine carcinoma. In contrast to SCLC, it occurs more often in the periphery of the lung (80% of cases). In many cases, the tumor is large and invades the pleura, chest wall, or adjacent structures, leading to a high stage classification. However, it cannot be distinguished from other carcinomas by macroscopic examination; definitive diagnosis requires histological examination and immunohistochemical staining (CD56, chromogranin, and synaptophysin).

FIGURE 6.67. In (A), a lobectomy of an LCNEC shows a peripherally located, well-circumscribed, white tumor with focal necrosis (arrow). Image (B) shows another LCNEC specimen in which most of the tumor mass has undergone necrosis, resulting in a cavitation.

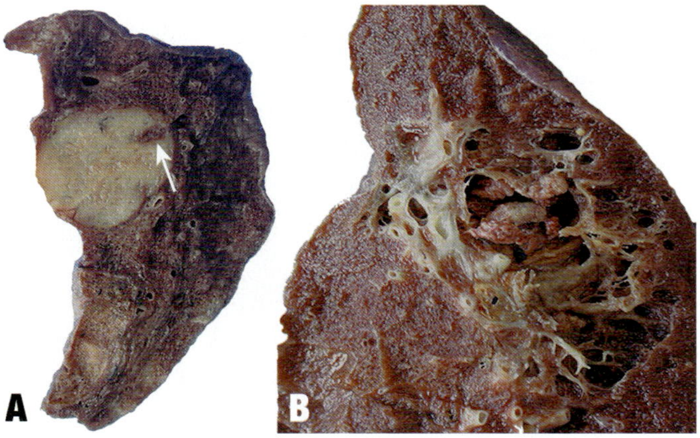

COMBINED NEUROENDOCRINE-NONNEUROENDOCRINE CARCINOMA

In rare cases, neuroendocrine carcinomas (SCLC and LCNEC) can combine with other carcinoma subtypes (e.g., adenocarcinoma, SCC, or pleomorphic carcinomas) to form combined neuroendocrine-nonneuroendocrine carcinomas. Diagnosis of these entities requires adequate sampling for identification of the different components of the tumor, and histological and immunohistochemical analysis.

FIGURE 6.68. This image shows a lung resection with a large, subpleural mass. Histological examination of this specimen showed a large cell neuroendocrine carcinoma combined with an adenocarcinoma.

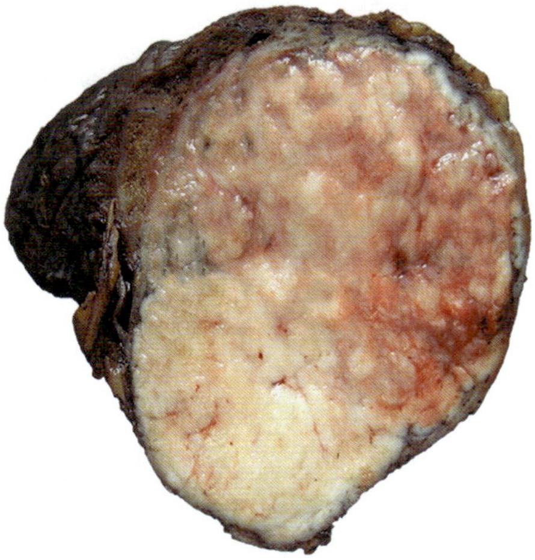

Pleomorphic carcinoma

Pleomorphic carcinoma is a poorly differentiated, non-small cell lung carcinoma. It consists of an SCC, adenocarcinoma, or undifferentiated non-small cell carcinoma with at least 10% spindle and/or giant cells, or a carcinoma with only spindle and giant cells. It is an aggressive type of tumor that often presents with large masses with a high stage.

FIGURE 6.69. This resection specimen shows a large, multinodular, hemorrhagic, and largely necrotic tumor invading the pulmonary artery and extending into the vascular lumen.

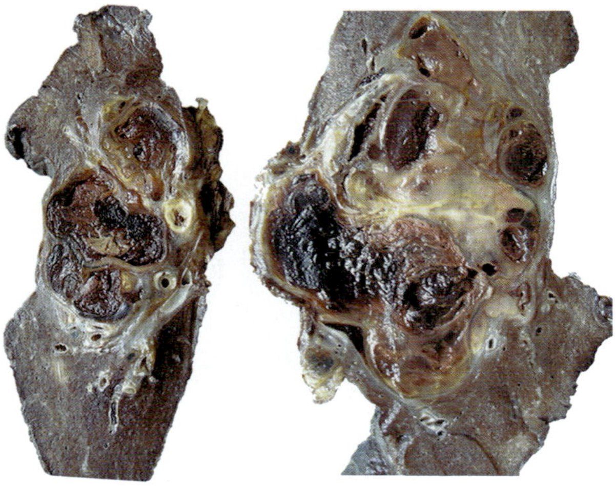

FIGURE 6.70. Image (A) shows a resection specimen with a large tumor extending into the bronchial tree. Image (B) shows a large tumor with necrosis and a peripheral white nodule. Histology established it as pleomorphic carcinoma.

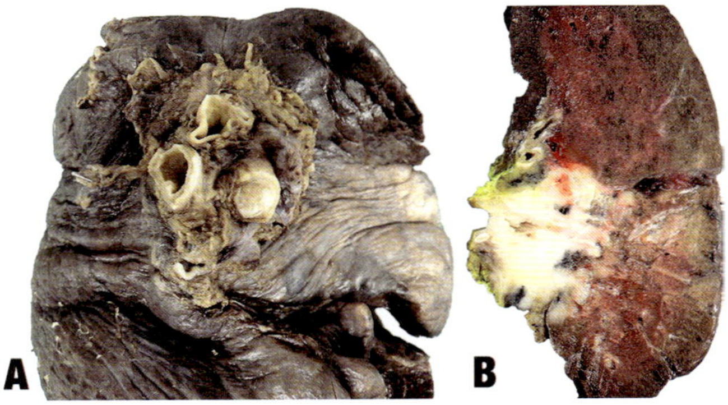

FIGURE 6.71. Image (A) shows a pleomorphic carcinoma found in an extended pneumonectomy with partial resection of the pericardium and mediastinal fat. The tumor was centrally located and filled the bronchial lumen. Image (B) shows that the tumor invaded both the pericardium and the perihilar fat (inked yellow).

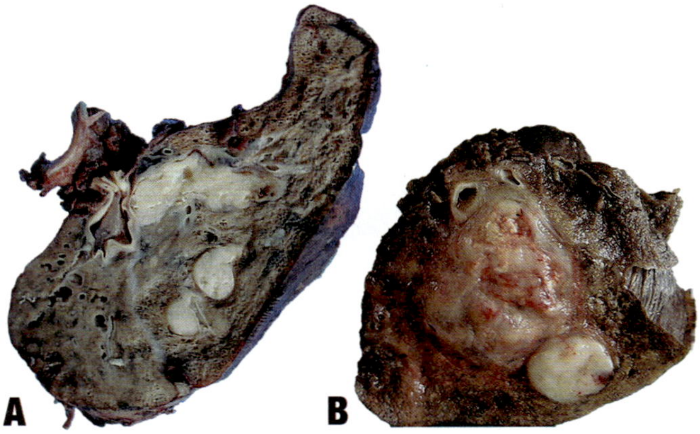

Salivary gland–type tumor

ADENOID CYSTIC CARCINOMA

FIGURE 6.72. Image (A) shows a distal tracheal resection specimen with an adenoid cystic carcinoma with polypoid morphology. In (B), the tumor has a white, homogeneous, vaguely nodular appearance on cut sections.

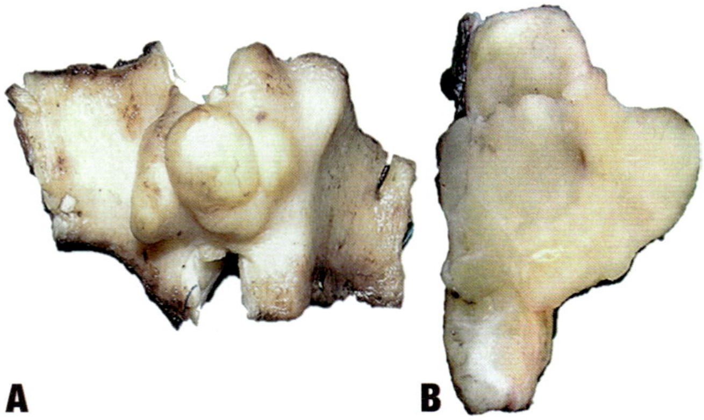

MUCOEPIDERMOID CARCINOMA

Mucoepidermoid carcinomas are rare intermingled collections of mucin-secreting glandular cells, intermediate-type cells, and squamoid cells. They are well-circumscribed tumors found in the proximal airways, and are usually endobronchial.

FIGURE 6.73. The pneumonectomy specimen shows a centrally located mucoepidermoid carcinoma within the bronchus.

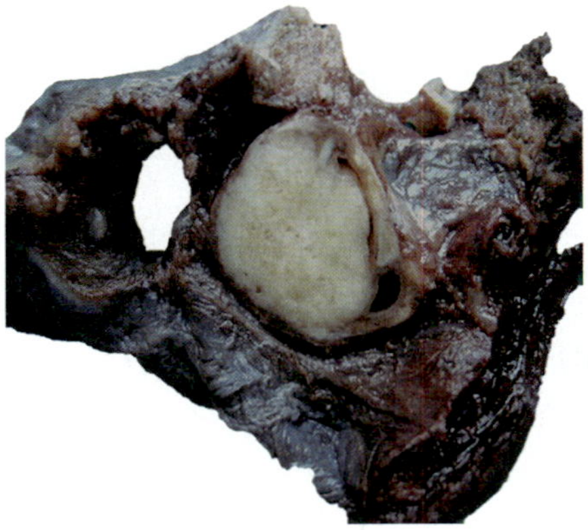

Mesenchymal tumors

PULMONARY HAMARTOMA

Pulmonary hamartomas are the most common benign lung tumors. They are sharply delineated and can have an irregular appearance. They have at least 2 mesenchymal components (cartilage is the most frequent component) with associated clefts of entrapped respiratory epithelium. Macroscopic examination shows pulmonary hamartomas to be firm with a multilobulated or round appearance and a grayish cut surface.

FIGURE 6.74. Image (A) shows a sharply delineated pulmonary hamartoma with an irregular appearance. In (B), a lobectomy specimen shows a pulmonary hamartoma with prominent internal clefts and cartilage.

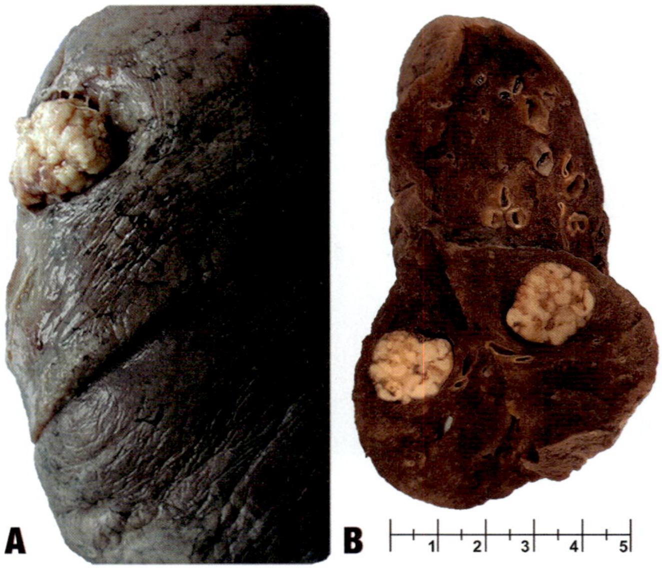

PERIVASCULAR EPITHELIOID CELL NEOPLASM (PEComa)

PEComatous tumors (also called clear cell tumors or sugar tumors of the lung) arise from perivascular epithelioid cells (PECs) and include lymphangioleiomyomatosis (LAM), PEComas, and mixed tumors with features of both.

FIGURE 6.75. This peripheral mass was found to be a PEComa on histology.

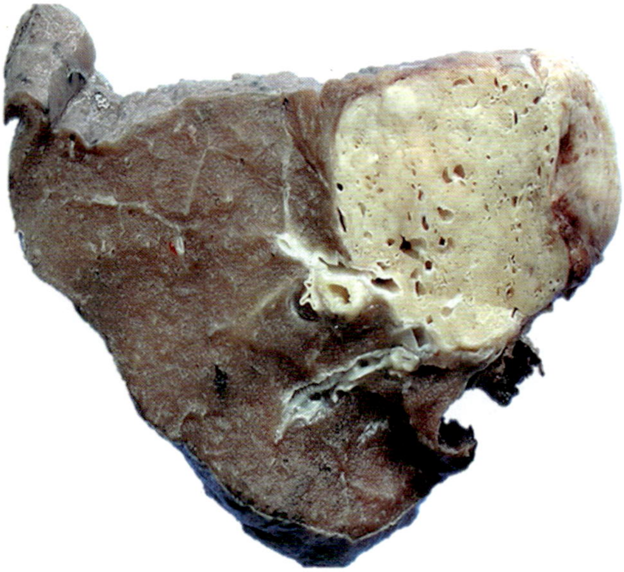

INFLAMMATORY MYOFIBROBLASTIC TUMOR (IMT)

IMT is a rare tumor composed of myofibroblastic spindle cells with rich inflammatory infiltrates.

FIGURE 6.76. The lobectomy specimen in (A) shows a large, well-delineated, firm mass with a white cut surface. Histology confirmed it as an IMT. Image (B) shows another example of an IMT.

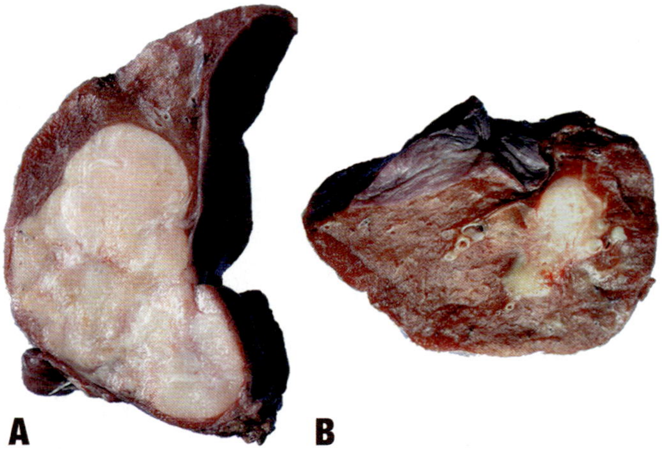

Lymphohistiocytic tumor

MUCOSAL-ASSOCIATED LYMPHOID TISSUE (MALT) LYMPHOMA

Small B-cell lymphomas affecting the lung include extranodal marginal zone lymphoma of mucosal-associated lymphoid tissue (MALT), follicular lymphoma, mantle cell lymphoma, and lymphoplasmacytic lymphoma. These all share similar macroscopic features, and can present as multiple ill-defined lesions or consolidations. MALT lymphoma is the most frequent lymphoma affecting the lung.

FIGURE 6.77. The autopsy specimen in (A) shows a MALT lymphoma with consolidated, yellow-tan areas delineated by interlobar septa. Image (B) gives another example of a MALT lymphoma.

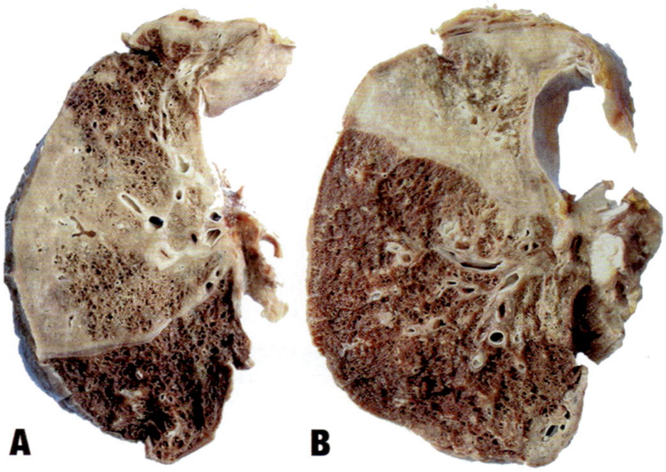

FIGURE 6.78. This wedge biopsy of the lingula shows multiple poorly defined areas of consolidation. Microscopic examination with immunohistochemical confirmation established this as an extranodal marginal zone MALT lymphoma.

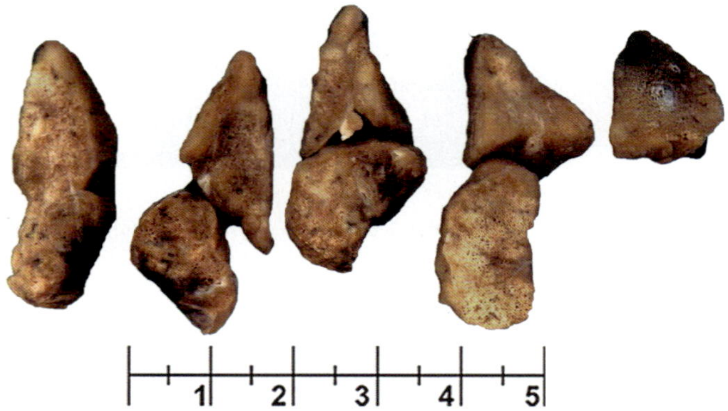

SMALL LYMPHOCYTIC LYMPHOMA

FIGURE 6.79. This lesion consists of a poorly defined area of consolidation. Histological examination with immunohistochemistry established this as a small lymphocytic lymphoma involving the lung parenchyma.

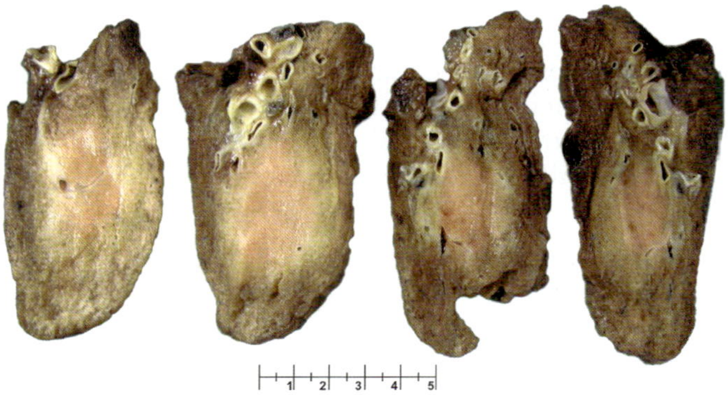

LYMPHOMATOID GRANULOMATOSIS

Lymphomatoid granulomatosis is a rare lymphoproliferative disorder associated with Epstein–Barr virus (EBV) that involves the lung in almost all cases. It usually manifests as multiple bilateral lung nodules; however, it can present as a single tumor.

FIGURE 6.80. In this lobectomy specimen, lymphomatoid granulomatosis presents as a solitary tumor.

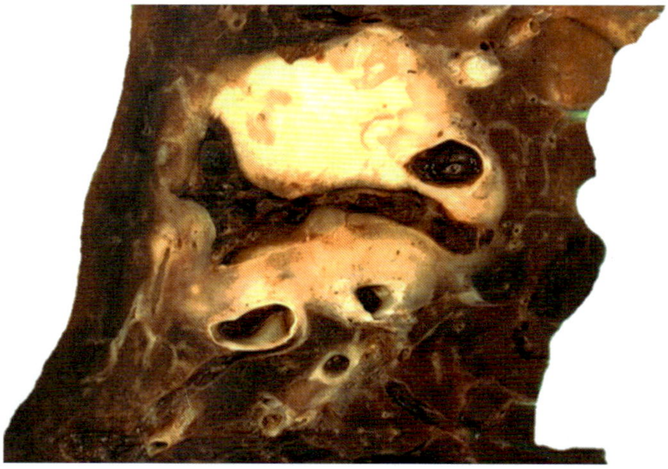

Metastasis to the lung

The lung, given its central role in gas exchange and its rich capillary bed network, is a frequent site of metastasis from other primary malignancies. Clinically, metastases present as multiple nodules or masses in 1 or both lobes and have well-circumscribed borders. In contrast, primary cancers of the lung present as solitary masses with infiltrative borders.

COLON CANCER METASTASIS

FIGURE 6.81. This left upper lobectomy shows a lobulated, irregular tumor with necrotic changes and an endobronchial component. This was a case of metastatic colon adenocarcinoma.

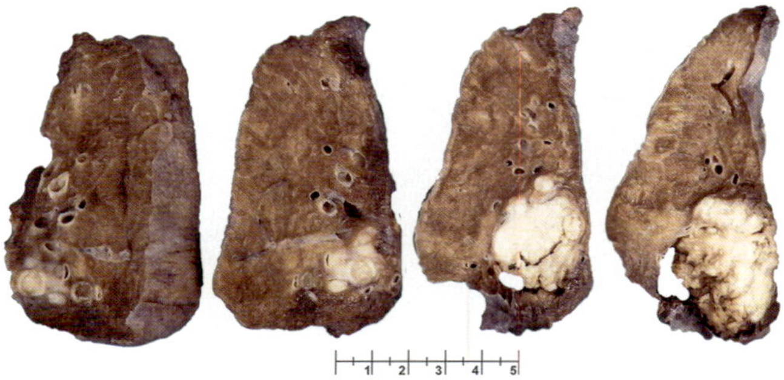

BREAST CANCER METASTASIS

FIGURE 6.82. This is a wedge resection of the right upper lobe for a small nodule incidentally detected on imaging. The patient had a remote history of breast carcinoma, but early stage lung carcinoma was the working diagnosis. Macroscopically, the nodule has irregular borders. Sections revealed that it was a metastasis from her former breast carcinoma. This case illustrates that not all metastatic lesions show well-circumscribed, expansile, growth-like characteristics. The irregular borders in this case were due to numerous sites of lymphatic invasion.

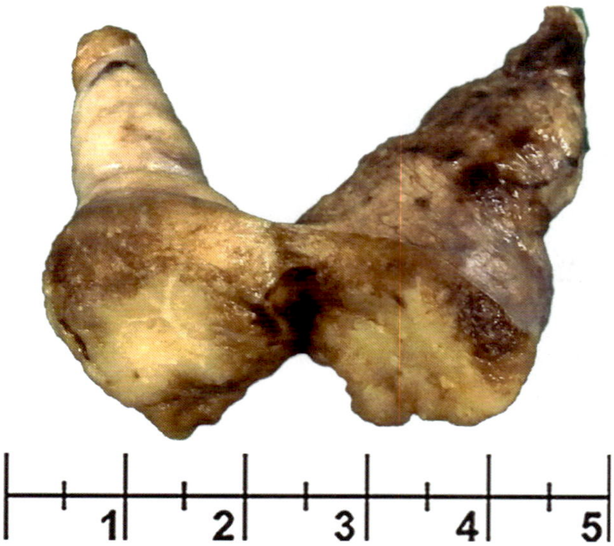

PLEOMORPHIC SARCOMA

FIGURE 6.83. In this case, the patient had a previous left upper limb amputation for a pleomorphic sarcoma. A large central metastasis was found in the left lower lobe and the patient received preoperative chemotherapy with 30% reduction in size. This left lower lobectomy shows a residual, circumscribed, hemorrhagic tumor. Less than 10% residual viable tumor was observed microscopically. Postneoadjuvant findings include hemorrhage, cystic degeneration, and fibrosis. Careful sampling and examination of sections is required in similar cases for evaluation of residual viable tumor.

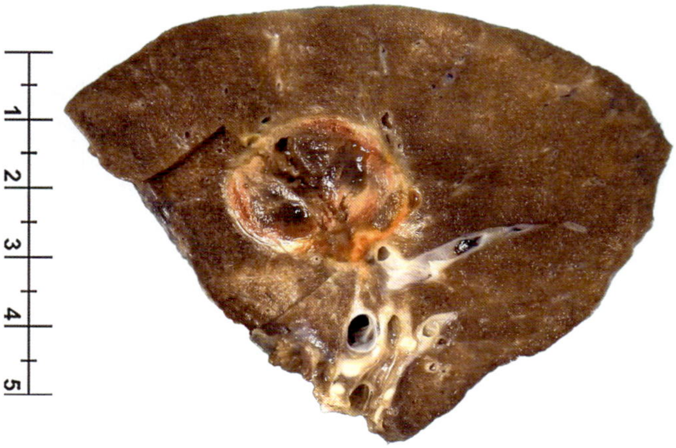

LEIOMYOSARCOMA METASTASIS

FIGURE 6.84. This tumor is metastasized from a uterine primary leiomyosarcoma. The cut sections show extensive necrosis and focal hemorrhage.

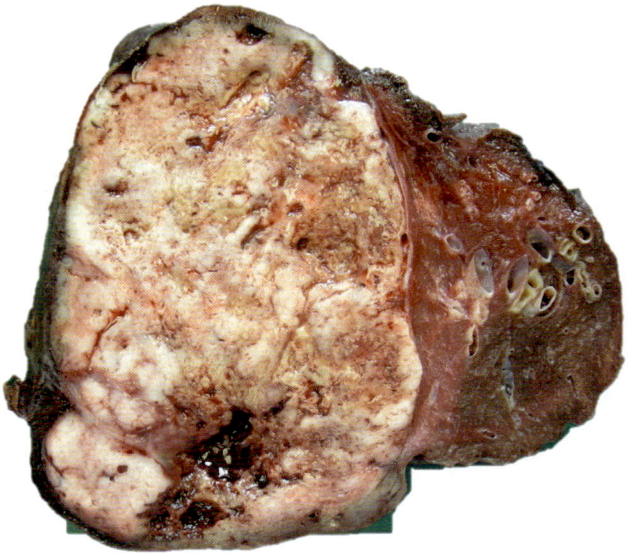

SYNOVIAL SARCOMA METASTASIS

FIGURE 6.85. This patient had a primary synovial sarcoma with a lung metastasis. Sections of the lung show a tumor that is firm and rubbery, with a hemorrhagic cut surface.

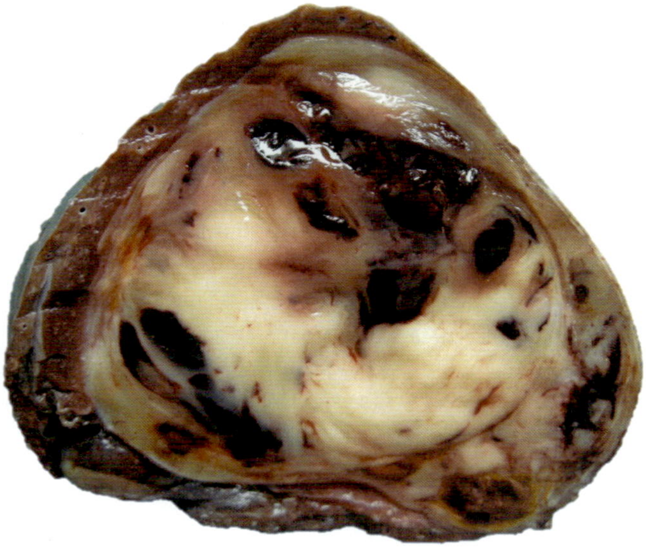

CHOLANGIOCARCINOMA METASTASIS

FIGURE 6.86. This autopsy specimen was obtained from a patient with cholangiocarcinoma. The carcinoma had widespread pulmonary metastasis that has led to a greenish color in the lung on gross inspection. This aspect is similar to diffuse pneumonic-type adenocarcinoma of the lung, which is most often invasive mucinous adenocarcinoma. Histologically, the metastatic cholangiocarcinoma was multifocal and had a lepidic growth pattern.

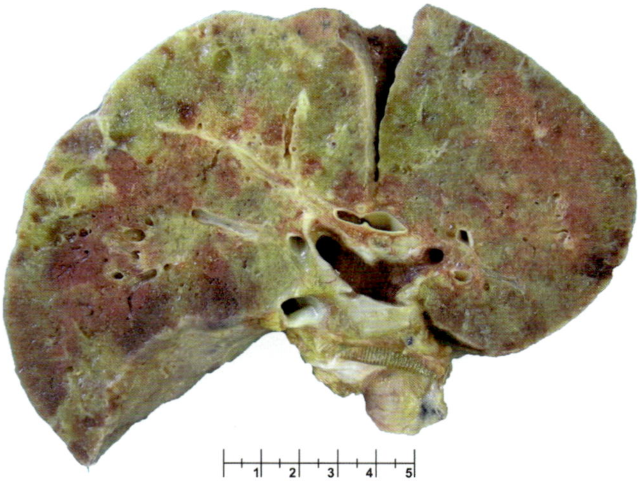

Pleura

Mesothelioma

Mesothelioma is a type of cancer caused by asbestos exposure. The most commonly affected area is the pleural lining of the lungs and chest wall and, less commonly, the peritoneal lining of the abdomen and, rarely, the pericardial lining of the heart. An extrapleural pneumonectomy may be performed in early stages of mesothelioma.

FIGURE 6.87. As seen in (A), the lung with all the surrounding structures lining the pleural cavity (parietal pleura, mediastinal pleura, pericardium, and diaphragm) are removed. In (B), a section from the pneumonectomy shows a pleural cavity diffusely filled with mesothelioma with extension into the fissures (arrows).

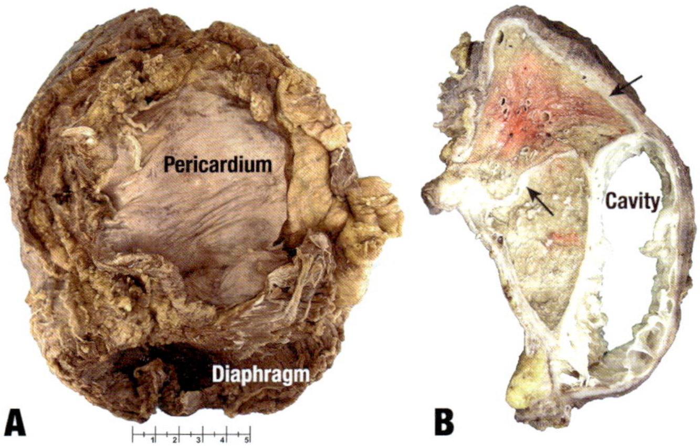

FIGURE 6.88. Image (A) shows a lateral view of the parietal pleura in an extrapleural pneumonectomy for a mesothelioma. The cut section in (B) shows the spread of the mesothelioma in the pleural space creating a rind-like appearance around the lung and in the fissures. The tumor can be seen grossly invading the lung.

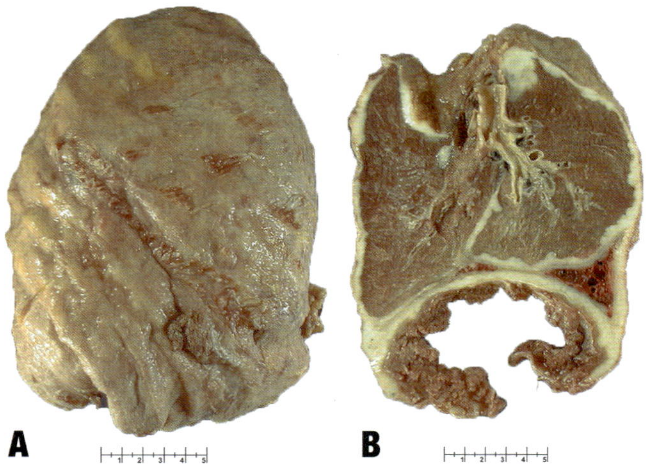

FIGURE 6.89. In (A), a mesothelioma has formed a very thick layer extending deep into the lung along a fissure. Image (B) shows a section of the lung with the mesothelioma forming parenchymal nodules that can mimic lung carcinomas both radiologically and by macroscopic examination.

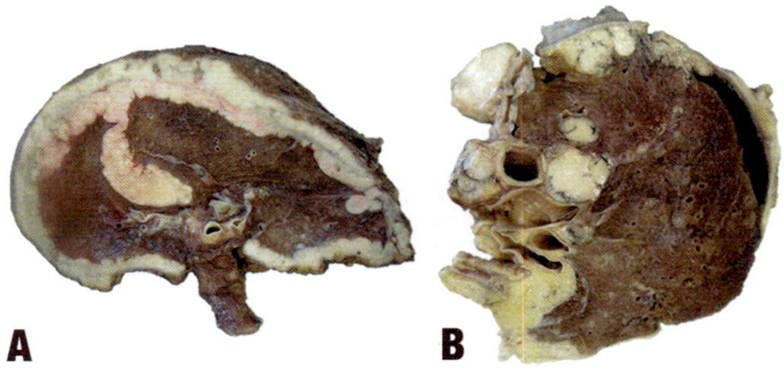

Pleura involvement by other malignancies

FIGURE 6.90. In this case, the patient had multiple myeloma that originated in the ribs of the chest wall and led to a pathological fracture. The myeloma seeded the pleural space and invaded the visceral pleura of the lung in a ring-like pattern, similar to mesothelioma. Although mesothelioma is the most frequent malignancy causing this pattern, other malignancies (usually metastatic carcinoma) are potential causes.

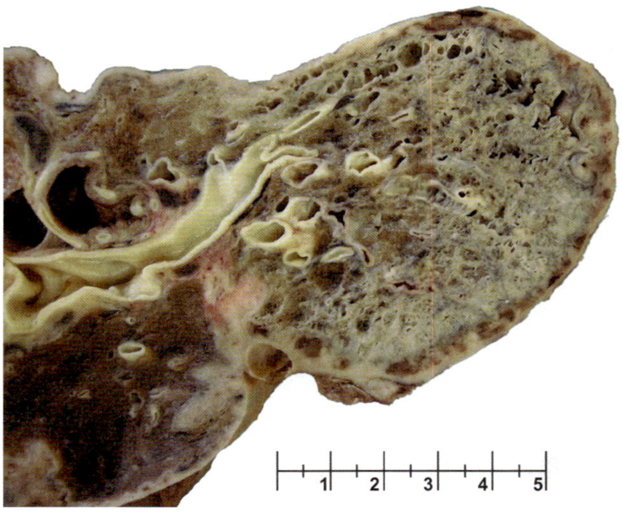

Solitary fibrous tumor (SFT) of the pleura

SFT is a pleural-based, slow-growing, fibroblastic mesenchymal tumor. It is often pedunculated via a stem attached to the lung's visceral pleura from which it arises. Most SFTs are benign, but 10% are malignant and have a more aggressive clinical course with risk of recurrence. Resectability is the most important indicator for clinical outcome.

FIGURE 6.91. Grossly, as in (A), SFTs are well-circumscribed, lobulated, and white-tan masses. This specimen shows an SFT with an attached wedge resection of the lung. In (B), a view of the same tumor shows the site of attachment of the pleural-based stalk.

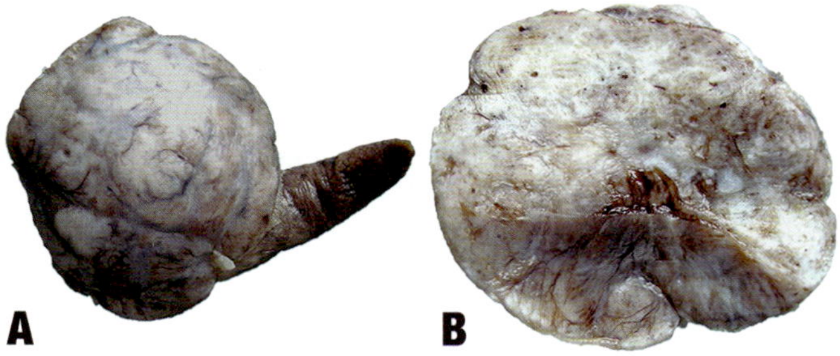

FIGURE 6.92. Image (A) shows a resected, large, 18-cm, pleural-based mass. In (B), the mass shows cystic and necrotic changes. Histologically, the mass was consistent with SFT; however, the large size (> 10 cm), the mitotic rate, and the necrosis are suspicious for aggressive behavior.

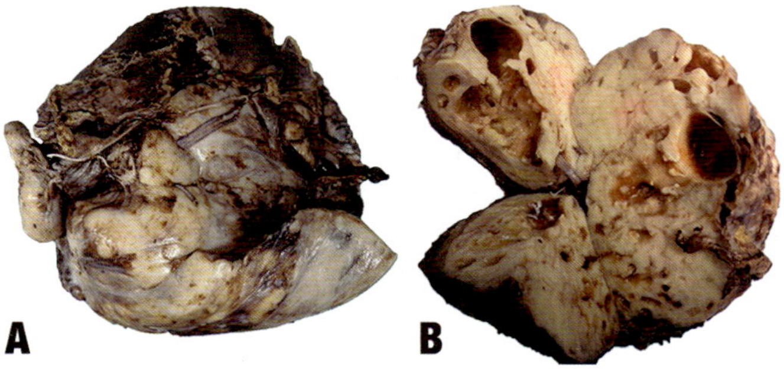

MALIGNANT SFT

FIGURE 6.93. The malignant SFT in (A) shows a large area of central necrosis and cavitation. Image (B) shows a malignant SFT that displays a variegated cut surface with necrosis (*) and hemorrhage.

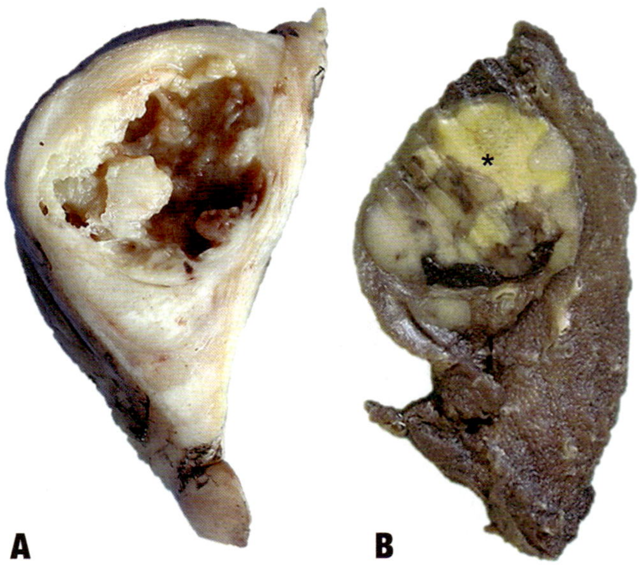

Desmoid-type fibromatosis

Desmoid-type fibromatosis (also called desmoid tumor) most commonly presents as deep-seated intraabdominal tumors. On very rare occasions, these can arise in the pleura.

FIGURE 6.94. The resection in (A) shows a large 18 cm × 10 cm × 10 cm thoracic mass arising from the chest wall and growing into the thoracic cavity. In (B), sections of the same tumor show a solid, white, and trabecular cut surface. Histologically, the tumor was consistent with desmoid-type fibromatosis.

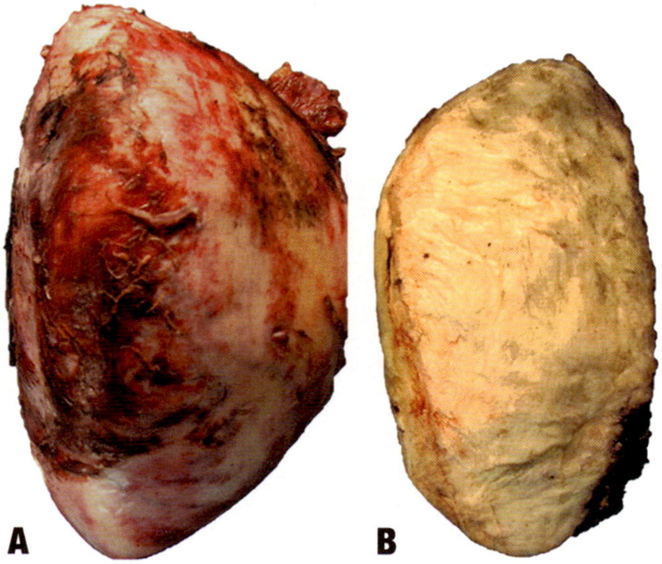

Courtesy of Dr. Zhaolin-Xu

Primary malignant peripheral nerve sheath tumor (MPNST)

MPNST is a rare type of sarcoma arising from the sheath cells surrounding nerves. It is highly aggressive and associated with patients with neurofibromatosis type 1 (NF1).

FIGURE 6.95. The specimen in (A) originated from the chest wall. In (B), a cut section of the mass shows a multilobate tumor with extensive hemorrhage and necrosis. Histology established the tumor as a primary MPNST of the chest wall.

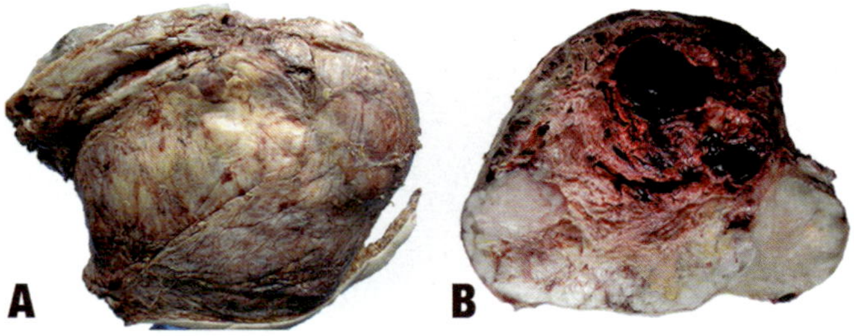

Mediastinum

REFERENCE: NORMAL THYMUS

The thymus is a bilobed organ found in the anterior and superior mediastinum. It functions as a lymphoid organ, important for development of T-cell responses of the adaptive immune system. Although variable, the mean organ weight at birth is 10 g to 20 g. The weight increases to 25 g to 35 g in early adulthood and decreases to about 15 g after age 30. With age, the thymus involutes with atrophy of the parenchyma and replacement by, largely, adipose tissue.

FIGURE 6.96. Image (A) shows a thymus from a term baby. Image (B) shows a rear view of the same specimen.

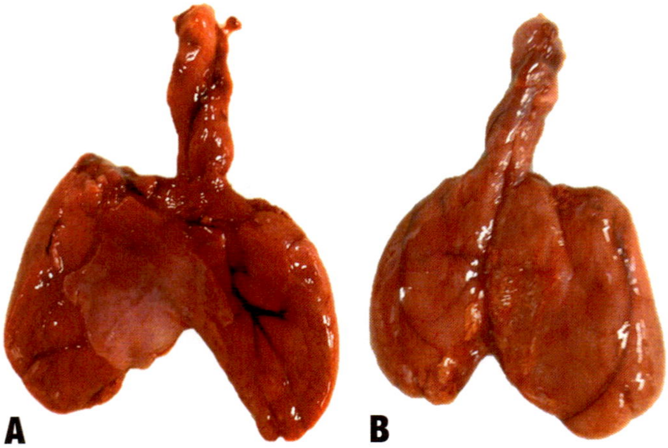

Thymic cyst

Unilocular thymic cysts are typically congenital and found in children; multilocular cysts are acquired or reactive. Causes of acquired cysts include trauma, systemic autoimmune diseases, Sjögren syndrome, systemic lupus erythematosus, and mediastinal neoplasms such as Hodgkin lymphoma.

FIGURE 6.97. This image shows a unilocular thymic cyst found in a patient with an anterior mediastinal mass.

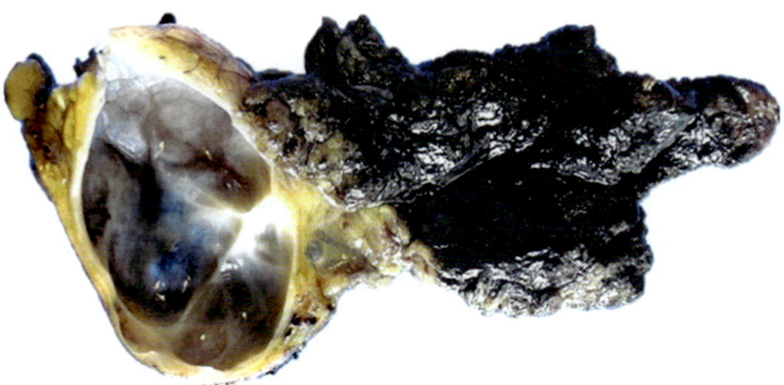

Retroperitoneal bronchogenic cyst

Bronchogenic cyst is the most common cystic lesion of the mediastinum. It results from a congenital malformation and forms without communication with the tracheobronchial tree.

FIGURE 6.98. Grossly, this mass demonstrates a unilocular cyst filled with mucinous secretions. Histologically, it was lined by pseudostratified epithelium with seromucinous glands.

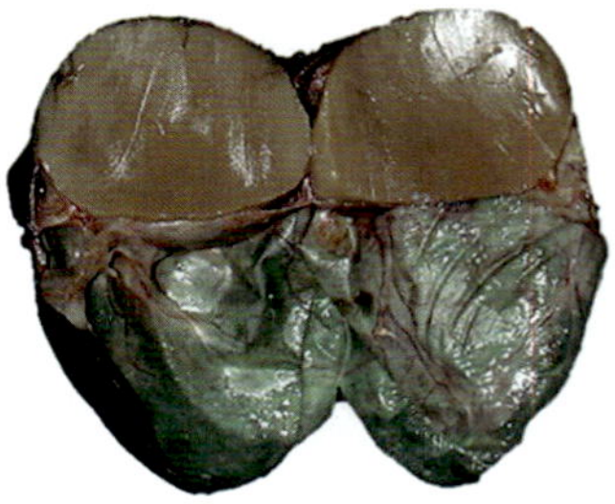

Thymoma

Thymomas are thymic epithelial tumors with variable histology; however, gross features are not specific for any histological type. Currently the AJCC staging manual (8th edition) is used to stage these tumors. Gross examination allows assessment of invasion of a thymoma into the mediastinal pleura, pericardium, and adjacent organs. It also serves to evaluate surgical margins and allows for adequate sampling for microscopic evaluation. Patients with thymomas often present with myasthenia gravis.

FIGURE 6.99. These images show an external view (A) and cut section (B) of a large thymoma. A well-formed capsule is visible and, although the thymoma capsule was adherent to the lung pleura, no invasion was found. The lung wedge resection is visible anteriorly (arrow).

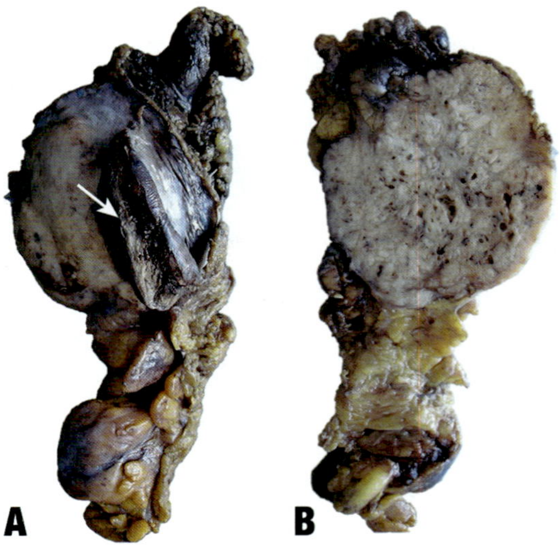

FIGURE 6.100. Most thymomas are encapsulated, unlike the thymoma in this image. The thymoma in (A), though well circumscribed, does not display a capsule. Grossly, the tumor is extending into the surrounding fat. In (B), the cut surface of the tumor shows a multinodular mass with fibrous bands. The tumor was staged pT1a.

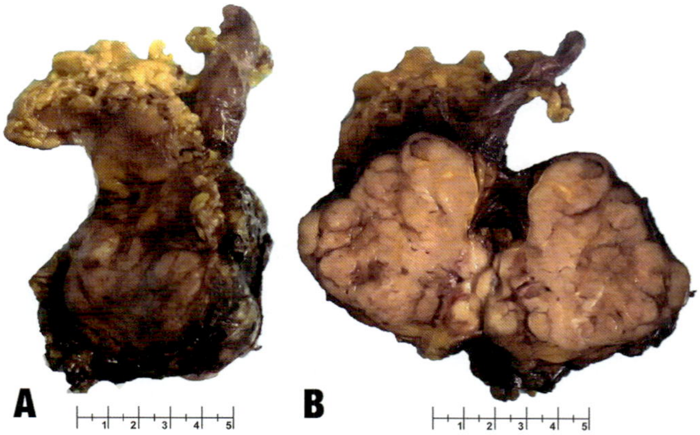

THYMOMA WITH CYSTIC CHANGES

Occasionally, thymomas can develop extensive cystic changes. Adequate sampling of the solid areas is necessary to correctly classify the tumor.

FIGURE 6.101. This resection specimen shows a large cyst (opened) with white solid tumor nodules in the cyst wall. The tumor was grossly and microscopically encapsulated, and staged pT1a.

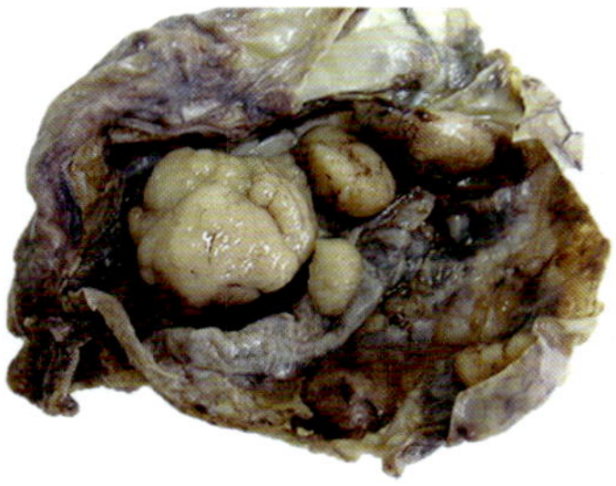

THYMOMA WITH MICROSCOPIC TRANSCAPSULAR INVASION

FIGURE 6.102. This thymoma has a lobulated, white-tan cut surface with some dissecting fibrous bands. Microscopically, transcapsular extension was identified that cannot be seen grossly. The tumor was staged pT1a.

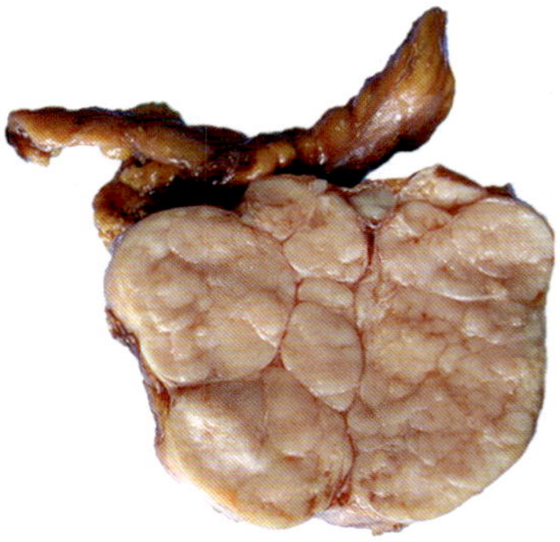

THYMOMA WITH MACROSCOPIC TRANSCAPSULAR INVASION

FIGURE 6.103. On gross examination, this tumor showed extension into the surrounding mediastinal fat. The tumor was staged pT1a.

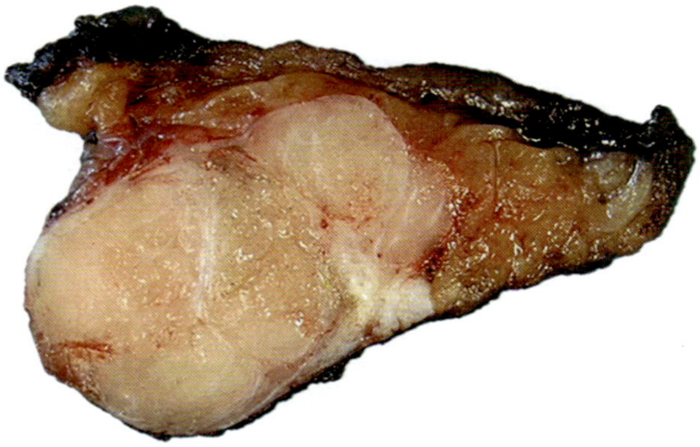

FIGURE 6.104. The mediastinal resection in the images below shows an irregular, poorly circumscribed tumor with invasion through the capsule into the surrounding fat. The gross differential diagnosis could include a thymic carcinoma. The tumor was staged pT1a.

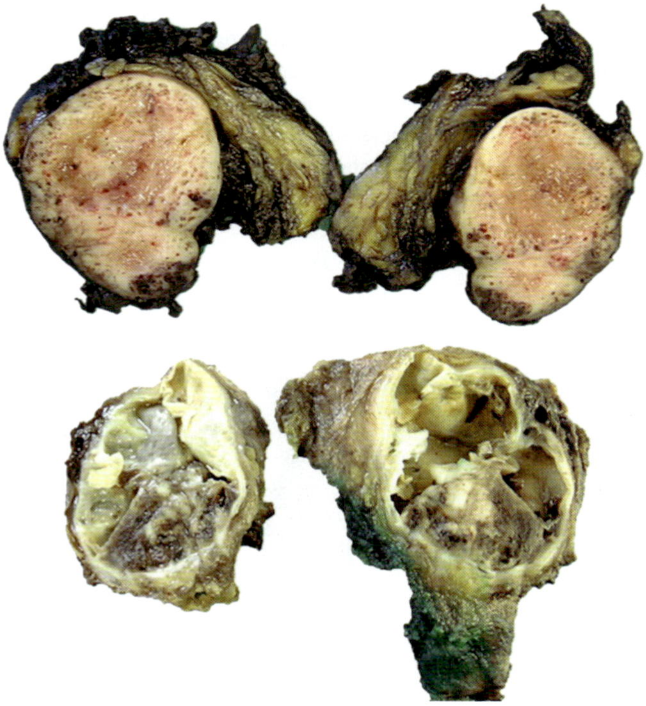

THYMOMA WITH INVASION INTO LUNG PARENCHYMA

To evaluate for invasion, a careful sampling of the tumor periphery, and the tissue or organs adjacent to the tumor, is necessary.

FIGURE 6.105. The specimen in this image shows a thymoma invading beyond its capsule and into the pleura and lung parenchyma. The tumor was staged pT3.

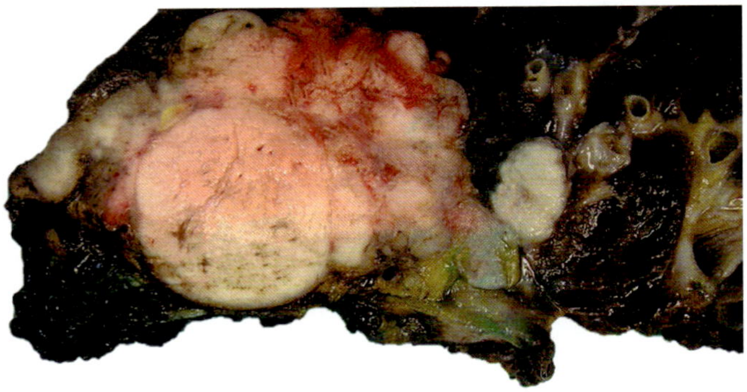

THYMOMA — TYPE A

Histologically, type A thymomas consist of epithelial cells with an oval or bland spindle cell morphology. Careful sampling establishes whether the tumor consists of a pure type A thymoma or a mixed thymoma.

FIGURE 6.106. Image (A) shows a mediastinal resection specimen with a portion of the mediastinal pleural surface (arrow). Image (B) shows cut sections from the same specimen: the thymoma is tan-white with a vague, lobulated architecture and a variegated appearance. Histology established this tumor as type A thymoma.

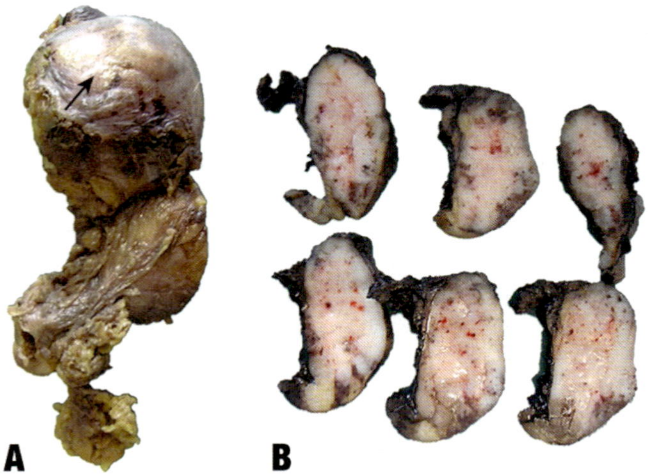

THYMOMA — TYPE B

Type B is the most common morphologic type of thymoma. Types B1, B2, and B3 reflect a progressive increase in the ratio of neoplastic epithelial cells versus lymphocyte numbers, and an increasingly aggressive clinical course.

FIGURE 6.107. Type B1 thymoma resembles normal thymus cortex, consisting of scattered neoplastic epithelial cells in the background of dense lymphocytic infiltrates. In this case, the patient also presented with myasthenia gravis. The surgical resection showed a large, bosselated thymoma. Histology established it as thymoma type B1.

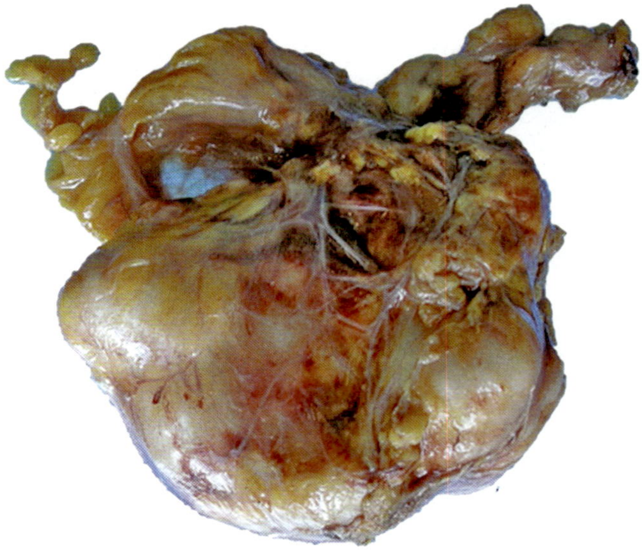

FIGURE 6.108. This mediastinal resection shows an irregular, poorly circumscribed tumor with necrotic changes and invasion through the capsule into the surrounding fat. The gross differential diagnosis could include a thymic carcinoma. Microscopic examination showed the tumor was composed mainly of polygonal thymoma epithelial cells, consistent with type B3. The tumor was staged IIb (by the modified Masaoka staging system).

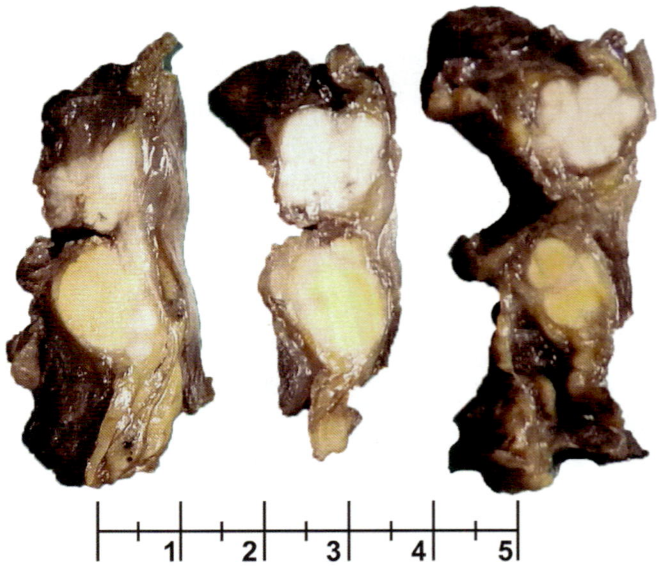

FIGURE 6.109. This large thymoma showed a lobulated architecture with both hemorrhagic and cystic degeneration. Histologically, it consisted of mostly large, atypical, polygonal cells in a solid growth pattern and with very few lymphocytes. This is consistent with thymoma type B3.

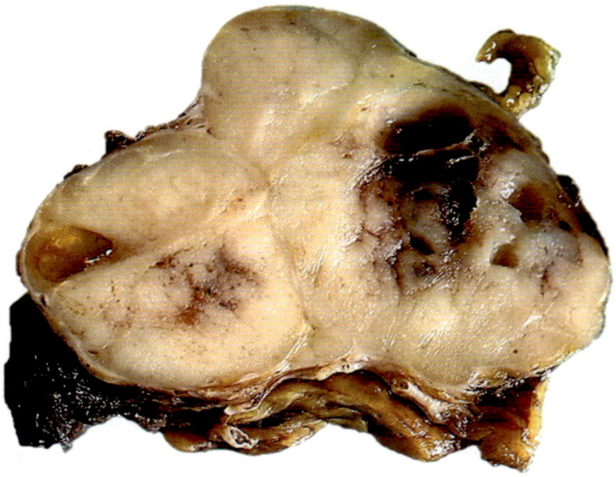

THYMOMA — TYPE AB

FIGURE 6.110. The specimen seen in (A) consists of a mediastinal resection with a wedge resection of the lung (arrow). In (B), the tumor found in the specimen is multilobulated and shows partial encapsulation with gross invasion of fat tissue (lower portion). Histologically, some lobules showed lymphocyte-poor areas with spindled cells (consistent with thymoma type A), as well as some lymphocyte-rich areas and a few epithelial cells (consistent with thymoma type B1). Overall, this is type AB morphology. Invasion of lung parenchyma by the thymoma was not observed. The tumor was staged pT1a.

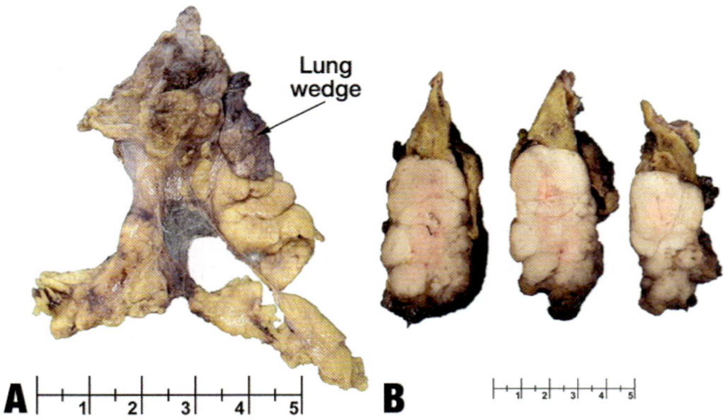

Thymic carcinoma

SCC is the most frequent subtype of thymic carcinoma. Unlike thymomas, thymic carcinomas are not associated with myasthenia gravis. Because thymic carcinomas tumors are very rare, it is important to first exclude mediastinal and thymic metastasis from an occult SCC in the lung or the head-and-neck area. On immunohistochemistry, primary thymic SCCs are usually positive for P40/P63, CD5, and C-kit (CD117).

FIGURE 6.111. The resection in (A) involves the mediastinum and part of the lung, and was thought to be a thymoma. Histology showed the tumor had SCC morphology, consistent with a thymic carcinoma. In (B), cut sections of the resection show a tan-white, firm tumor without a capsule, and broad-based invasion into the surrounding adipose tissue.

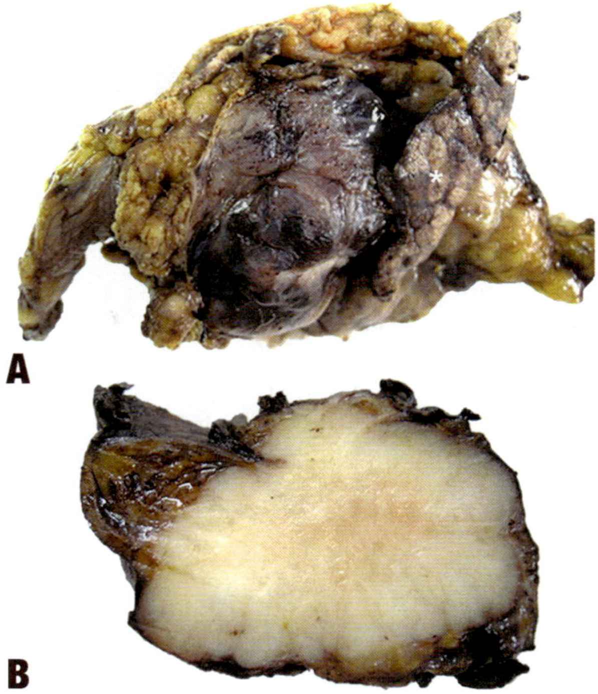

ATYPICAL CARCINOID OF THE THYMUS

Thymic neuroendocrine tumors are rare. Their classification follows nomenclature similar to lung tumors. However, thymic carcinoids are more frequently atypical and often show aggressive behavior.

FIGURE 6.112. This mediastinal mass consists of a large, poorly defined, heterogenous multinodular tumor with necrotic changes. It demonstrated perithymic fat invasion, pericardial invasion, lung invasion, and numerous lymph node metastases. The findings were suspicious for a thymic carcinoma, but histology established this tumor as an atypical carcinoid.

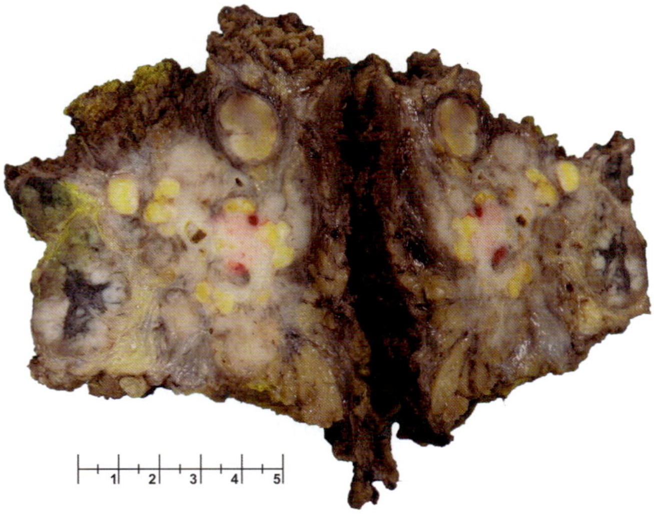

Ectopic mediastinal thyroid tumor

During the development of the thyroid gland, thyroid tissue can migrate to the mediastinum. This ectopic thyroid tissue can lead to benign and malignant mediastinal thyroid tumors, exactly like those that can occur in neck and thyroid gland itself.

FIGURE 6.113. This mediastinal mass was found to be a thyroid goiter.

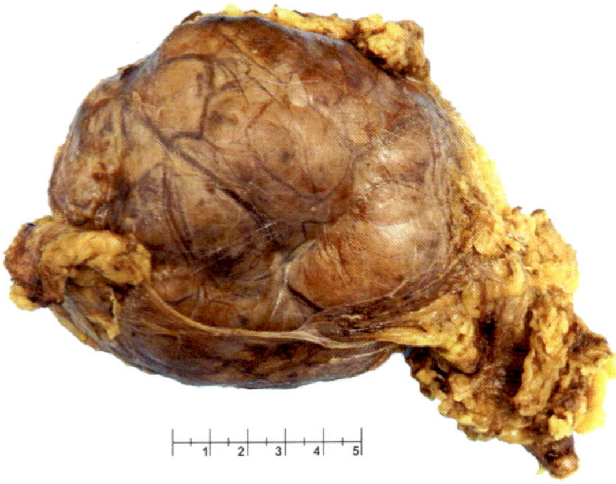

Multilocular thymic cyst with Hodgkin lymphoma

FIGURE 6.114. Image (A) shows an external surface of a mediastinal mass. In (B), cut sections of the mass show a multilocular thymic cyst. Growing within the walls of the cyst was a large, "fish flesh" lobular lesion with a lymphoid proliferation with Reed-Sternberg cells and a background of mixed inflammatory cells. Also present were some thymic epithelial cells. The findings were consistent with a nodular sclerosis–type of Hodgkin lymphoma. The diagnosis of mediastinal lymphoma rarely occurs with surgical resection: most are diagnosed via needle biopsy.

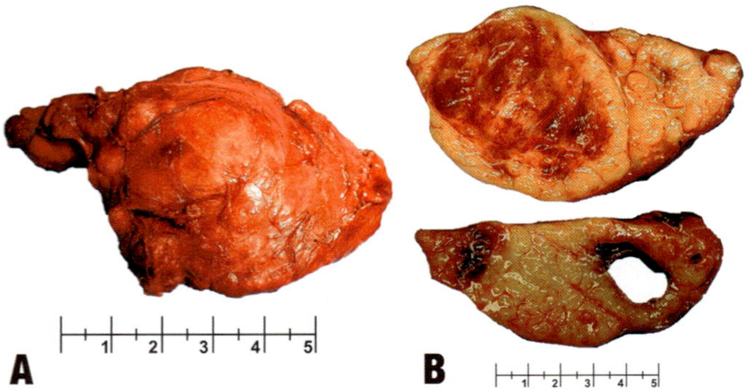

Mature teratoma

Teratomas of the mediastinum are rare and similar to those found in more common locations such as the ovary.

FIGURE 6.115. This specimen shows a large, sharply delineated tumor, with multilocular cysts with fatty and sebaceous material. Cases of mediastinal mature teratomas have very a good prognosis after complete resection.

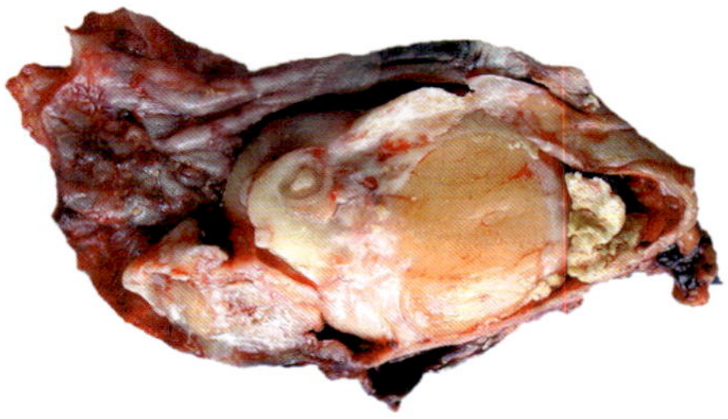

Schwannoma

Nerve sheath tumors are the most common soft tissue tumors of the mediastinum, arising in the posterior mediastinum.

FIGURE 6.116. This resection (A) shows a well-circumscribed lesion, which on cut surface (B) shows a capsule and punctate hemorrhages. Histologically, the tumor was consistent with a schwannoma.

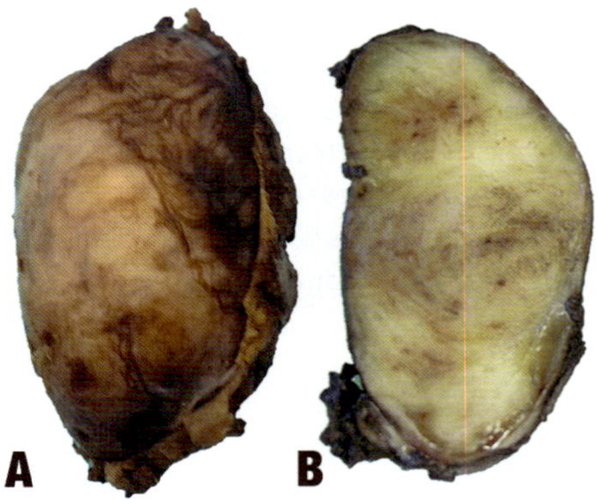

ACKNOWLEDGMENTS

We would like to thank the valuable input and contributions of Dr. B. Chergui and Dr. R. Fraser, and the technical help of R. Gilot, E. Griss, A. Hossain, L. Korneichyuk Pasyuk, M. Mikhael, and E. Yaney.

REFERENCES

Amin MB, Edge SB, editors. *AJCC cancer staging manual*. 8th ed. Chicago: Springer; 2018.

Hasleton P, Flieder DB, editors. *Spencer's Pathology of the lung*. 6th ed. United Kingdom: Cambridge University Press; 2013. https://doi.org/10.1017/CBO9781139018760.

Kumar V, Abbas AK, Aster JC, editors. *Robbins and Cotran pathologic basis of disease*. 9th ed. Philadelphia: Elsevier Saunders; 2015.

Travis WD, Brambilla E, Burke AP, Marx A, Nicoholson AG, editors. WHO classification of tumours of the lung. *Pleura, Thymus and Heart*. 4th ed. Lyon: International Agency for Research on Cancer; 2015.

Travis WD, Colby TV, Koss MN, Rosado-de-Christenson MI, Muller NL, King Jr TE, editors. *Non-neoplastic disorders of the lower respiratory tract (atlas of nontumor pathology)*. Washington: American Registry of Pathology; 2002.

7

Cardiac and Vascular Diseases

JOHN P. VEINOT

Heart

REFERENCE: NORMAL HEART

The heart is a muscular organ, the main function of which is to pump blood through the body. It has 3 layers: the epicardium (outer), the myocardium (middle), and the endocardium (inner). The myocardium is the thickest layer. A female adult heart weighs between 250 g and 300 g; a male adult heart weighs between 300 g and 350 g. The heart has 4 chambers, connected by valves. Valves are made of thin leaflets or cusps. Their main function is to prevent backflow of blood during heart contraction. An interatrial septum and an interventricular septum separate the right atrium and ventricle from the left atrium and ventricle. The normal thickness of the right ventricular wall is approximately 0.3 cm to 0.5 cm; this wall pumps blood to the pulmonary circulation. The normal thickness of the left ventricular wall is 1.3 cm to 1.5 cm; this wall pumps blood in the systemic circulation.

FIGURE 7.1. Image (A) shows an anterior view of the heart, with the left ventricle (LV) and right ventricle (RV) labeled. The cut surface in (B) shows the right and left ventricular cavities. Note that the right ventricular cavity (arrow) and wall thickness are smaller than their left-side counterparts.

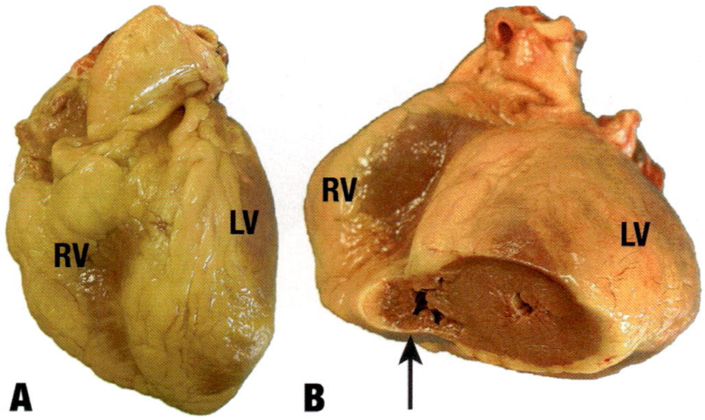

Normal right heart

FIGURE 7.2. Image (A) shows the right atrial cavity (top), which is separated from the right ventricular cavity (bottom) by the tricuspid valve. Image (B) shows the right ventricle (bottom), which is separated from the pulmonary artery (top) by the pulmonary artery valve. The tricuspid valve and the pulmonary valve are not connected: they are separated by the right ventricular infundibulum.

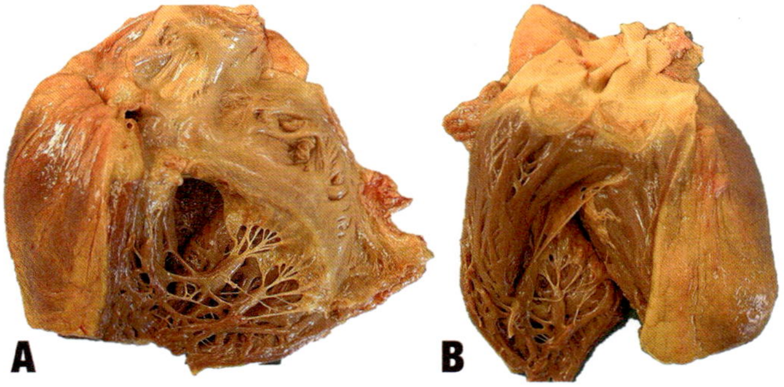

Normal left heart

FIGURE 7.3. These images show the left atrium and ventricle. Image (A) shows the separation of the left atrium (top) from the left ventricle (bottom) by the mitral valve. Image (B) shows the left ventricle (bottom) separated from the aortic root (top) by the aortic valve. Note the continuity between the mitral valve and the aortic valve (arrow).

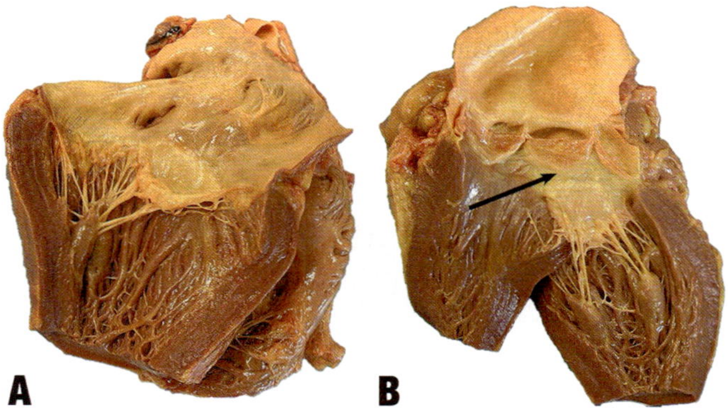

REFERENCE: CORONARY ARTERY CIRCULATION

Coronary arteries are the main vessels responsible for maintaining adequate blood flow. The left coronary artery (LCA) supplies the left side of the heart. The LCA divides into the left anterior descending artery and left circumflex artery. The right coronary artery (RCA) arises above the right cusp of the aortic valve in the aorta. It separates into the posterior descending artery and the right marginal artery.

FIGURE 7.4. In (A), an implant and cellophane technique is used to mold each vessel, revealing the complexity of the heart's circulation. Image (B) gives a rear view of the same specimen.

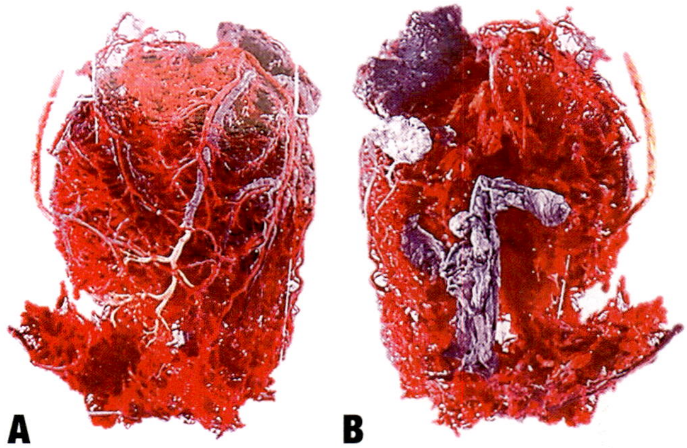

Nonneoplastic Heart Diseases

Eisenmenger syndrome

Eisenmenger syndrome (ES) is a pathologic process in which a long-standing left-to-right shunt, caused by a congenital heart anomaly, leads to severe pulmonary hypertension and reversal of the shunt to a right-to-left shunt. ES usually happens in young children with ventricular septal defect (VSD) or atrial septal defect (ASD).

FIGURE 7.5. This image shows a large ventricular septal defect (V). Dilation of the pulmonary trunk, a consequence of pulmonary hypertension, is present.

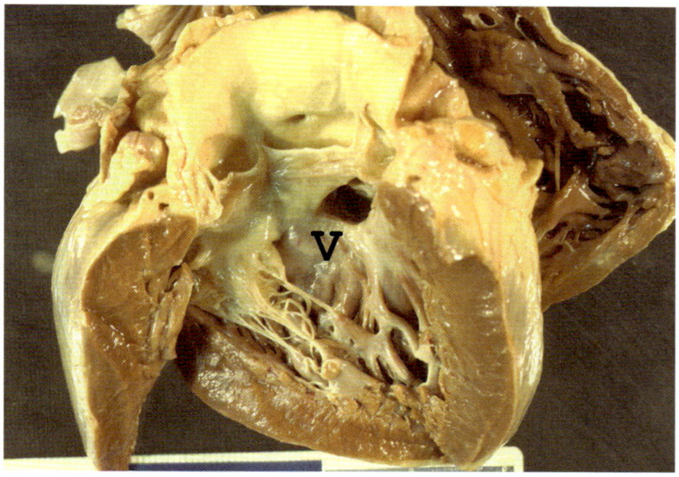

Secundum atrial septal defect

FIGURE 7.6. This specimen shows a persistent small opening that connects both atrial cavities (arrow).

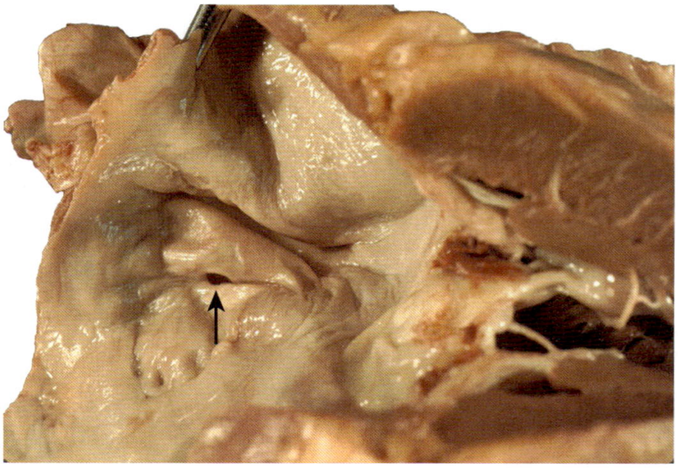

Patent ductus arteriosus

FIGURE 7.7. An anterior view of this heart reveals a large and widely patent ductus arteriosus (arrow), connecting the pulmonary artery (lower vessel) to the aorta (upper vessel).

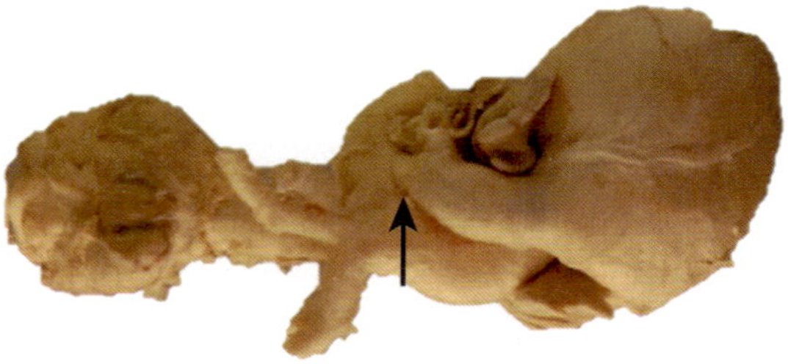

Coarctation of the aorta

Coarctation of the aorta is an abnormal narrowing of the aorta that commonly occurs near the area of the ductus arteriosus remnant. It is a congenital defect usually diagnosed in young children, but it can be diagnosed in adulthood. It may have severe complications including hypertension, stroke, aortic dissection, and heart failure.

FIGURE 7.8. Images (A) and (B) show near complete obliteration of the descending arch at the intersection of the ductus arteriosus (arrow). A bicuspid aortic valve (AV) is also visible.

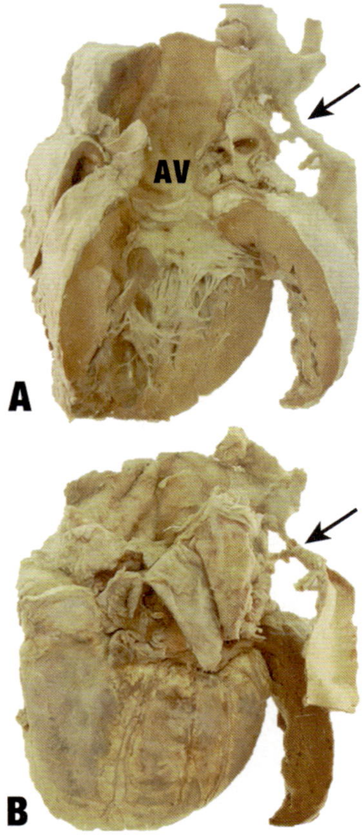

Tetralogy of Fallot

Tetralogy of Fallot is a congenital heart defect that consists of 4 characteristic heart abnormalities: overriding aorta, pulmonary stenosis, VSD, and right ventricular hypertrophy. Tetralogy of Fallot produces a right-to-left shunt, which can cause cyanosis. Tetralogy of Fallot accounts for approximately 10% of congenital heart diseases.

FIGURE 7.9. Images (A) and (B) show stenosis of the pulmonary artery infundibulum (arrow). Image (C) shows a ventricular septal defect. Image (D) shows a right ventricular hypertrophy.

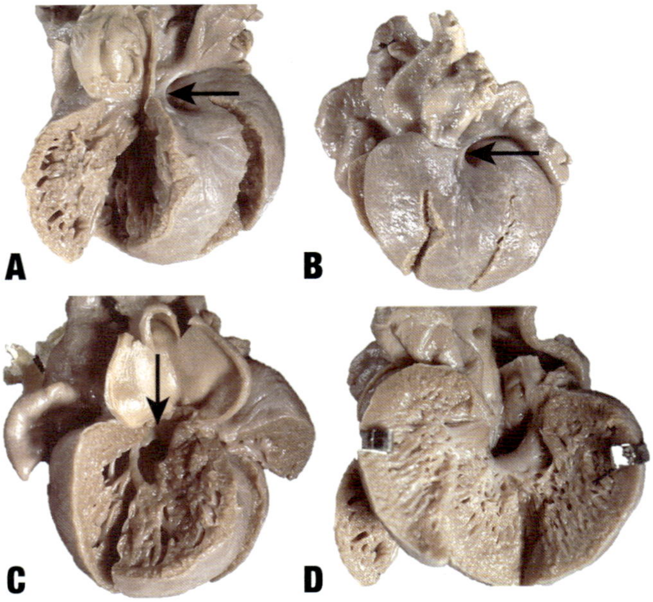

Congenital atresia of the aortic valve

Atresia of the aortic valve is a congenital narrowing of the aortic valve. It is often associated with other abnormalities, including hypoplasia of the ascending aorta, left ventricle, and mitral valve.

FIGURE 7.10. This image shows a front view of the heart in relation to surrounding thoracic structures. The aortic valve is absent (arrow). Hypoplasia of the ascending aorta and a rudimentary left ventricle are present.

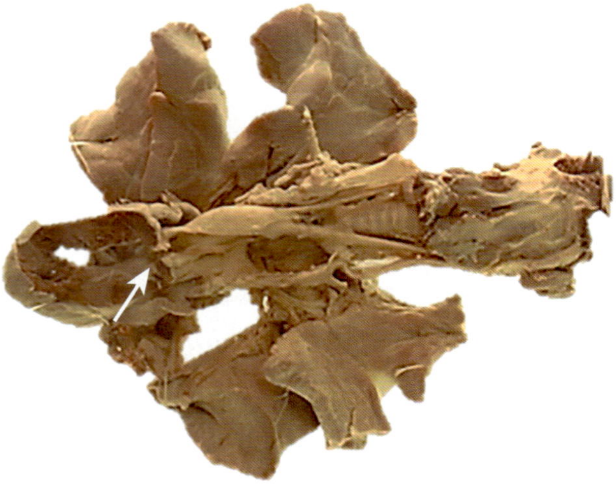

Interventricular diverticulum

Interventricular diverticulum is a rare cardiac malformation characterized by an outpouching of the ventricular myocardium. This cardiac defect is usually asymptomatic. It is often diagnosed incidentally when a patient undergoes imaging studies. The main differential diagnosis for this entity is ventricular aneurysm, which commonly follows myocardial infarction.

FIGURE 7.11. In this image, the heart chamber is opened and reveals a small opening (arrow) just below the aortic valve.

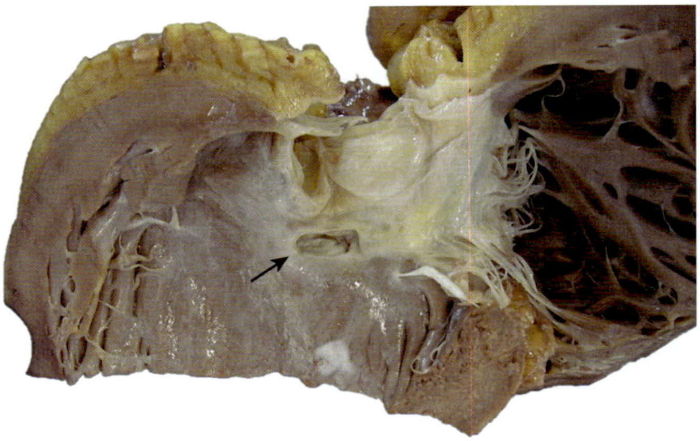

Left ventricular false tendon

Left ventricular false tendons are aberrant fibromuscular structures that cross the left ventricular chamber. Normal chordae tendineae run between the papillary muscles and the valve. False chords or tendons run from 1 ventricle wall to another wall. These are usually considered benign entities.

FIGURE 7.12. In this specimen, the left ventricle cavity is opened, exposing an aberrant fibrous tendon (arrow) that extends from the ventricular wall to another part of the ventricular wall.

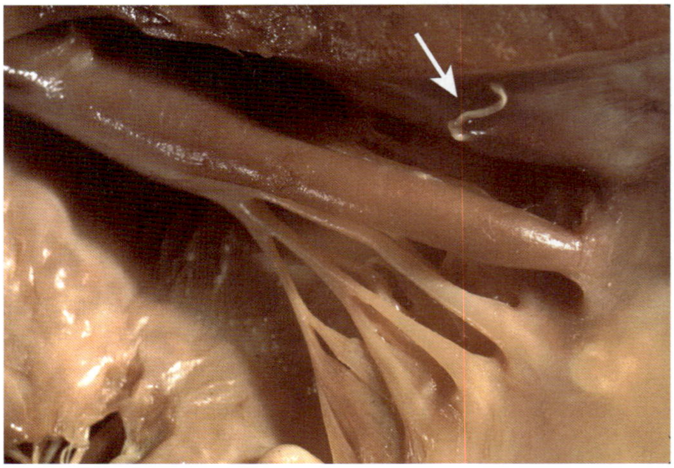

Ventricular hypertrophy

Ventricular hypertrophy is a thickening of the ventricular wall and an increase in muscle mass. It usually develops as an adaptive response to an increased demand on the heart's pumping ability. Both left and right ventricular hypertrophy can occur, but left-sided hypertrophy is more common. Ventricular hypertrophy can arise from a physiologic or pathologic process. An example of a physiologic process is hypertrophy from athletic training, called "athlete's heart." Pathological hypertrophy is associated with chronic hypertension, myocardial infarction, and valvular heart disease. A common cause of left ventricular hypertrophy is calcific aortic stenosis.

FIGURE 7.13. The left ventricular cavity in (A) is opened to reveal a marked diffuse thickening of the left ventricular wall. The cross-section in (B) shows significant and diffuse thickening of the ventricular myocardium in both the right and left ventricles.

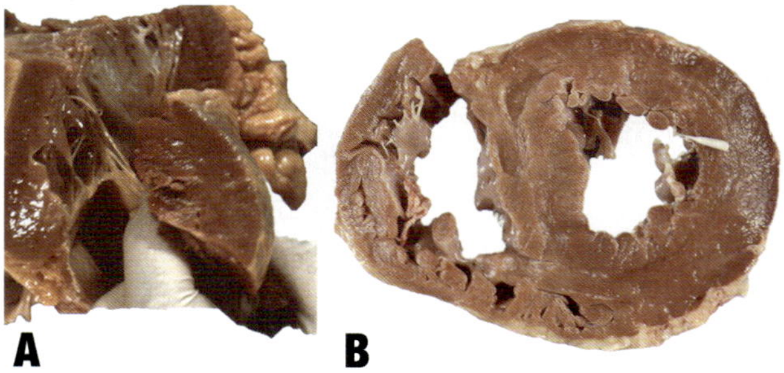

A B

LEFT VENTRICULAR HYPERTROPHY (LVH)

LVH can occur in cases of increased cardiac afterload in situations such as chronic hypertension, aortic stenosis, and aortic insufficiency.

FIGURE 7.14. Images (A) and (B) show diffuse thickening of the left ventricular myocardial wall and ventricular enlargement.

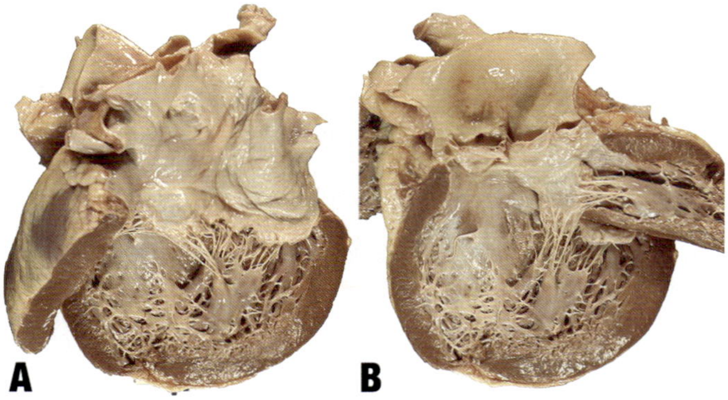

A B

Cardiomegaly

Cardiomegaly is defined as an enlargement of the heart. Cardiomegaly occurs in dilated and hypertrophic cardiomyopathy. Dilated cardiomyopathy (DCM) is the most common cardiomyopathy type, and is associated with gradual dilatation of the 4 heart cavities resulting in progressive congestive heart failure. Risk factors include myocarditis, and drug and alcohol toxicity. Some cases are familial or associated with extracardiac abnormalities such as myopathy or storage disease. Hypertrophic cardiomyopathy (HCM) is characterized by thickening or hypertrophy of the myocardium. HCM most frequently arises as part of an inherited condition. Other diseases, such as thyroid disease and diabetes, can cause hypertrophy.

FIGURE 7.15. Image (A) shows an anterior view of heart cardiomegaly (recorded weight 560 g) with biventricular hypertrophy. Image (B) shows the coronal cut surface of a specimen with biventricular hypertrophy.

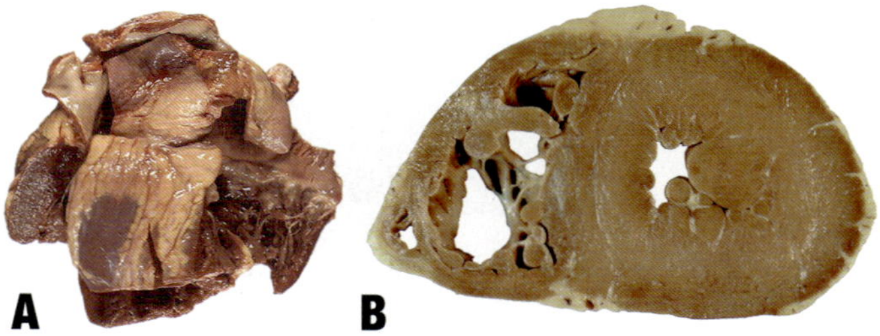

A B

CARDIOMEGALY AND CONGESTIVE HEPATOPATHY

Cardiomegaly can be associated with clinical congestive heart failure. In the setting of right-sided heart failure, a spectrum of hepatic disorders can arise, named cardiac congestive hepatopathy. In early stages, passive congestion occurs in the centrolobular regions (zone 3) followed by centrolobular necrosis due to ischemia. With chronicity, fibrosis develops and may lead to cirrhosis.

FIGURE 7.16. In this image, the heart is enlarged. The left ventricular cavity is opened to reveal left ventricular hypertrophy and dilatation.

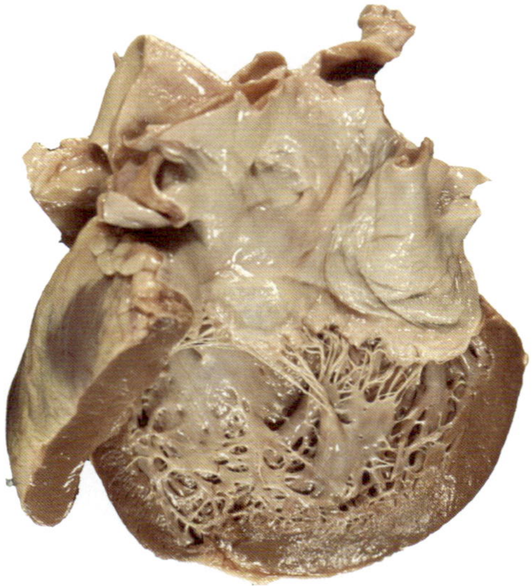

Dilated cardiomyopathy (DCM)

DCM has progressive 4-chamber dilation and contractile dysfunction. It may appear at any age, but manifests most commonly in the third and fourth decades. The possible causes are multiple: infectious entities (most commonly viral), familial entities (genetic abnormalities such as mutations in the gene that encodes for actin), toxic entities (e.g., antineoplastic drugs such as doxorubicin), collagen vascular diseases, granulomatous disease, carnitine deficiency, and storage diseases.

FIGURE 7.17. This specimen shows dilation of both ventricles and an enlarged heart size due to ventricular dilatation.

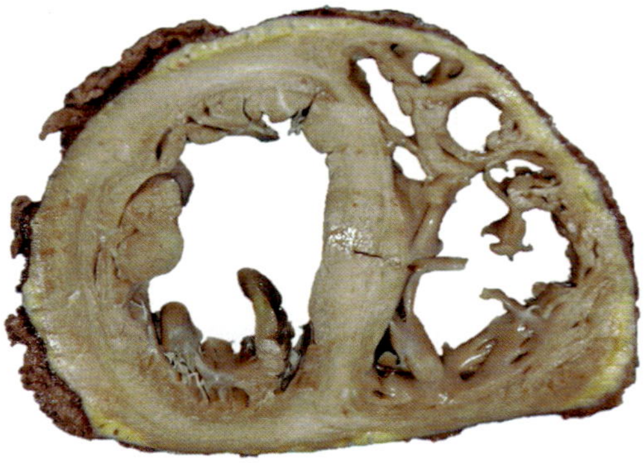

FIGURE 7.18. In (A), a specimen with dilated cardiomyopathy shows dilation of both ventricles, but dilation is accentuated on the right side, giving a rounded appearance to the heart. This specimen weighed 750 g. Image (B) shows a cross-section: note that the right ventricle (arrow) is dilated, and the wall is thickened and hypertrophied.

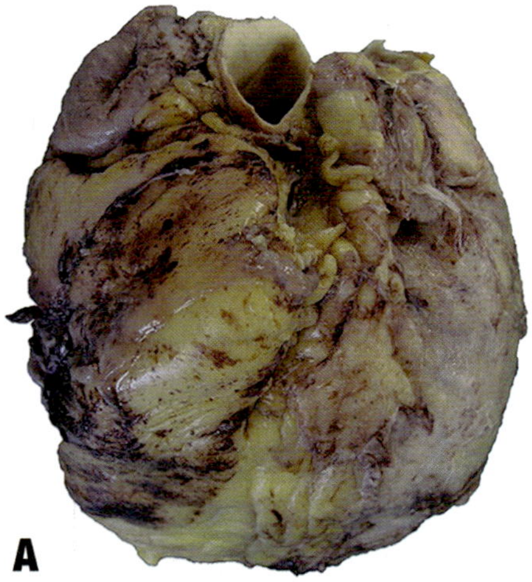

A

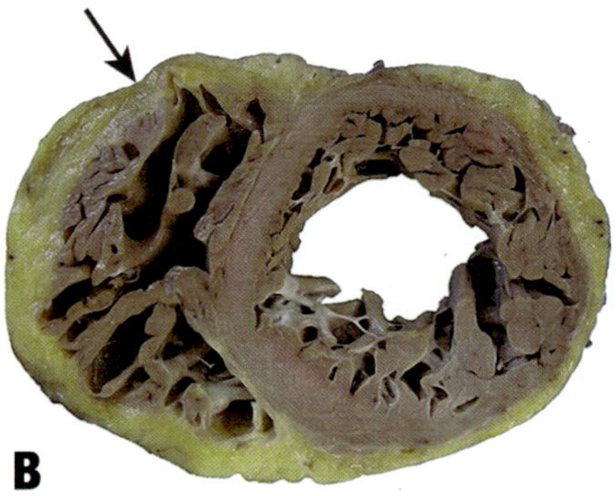

B

Dystrophinopathies

Dystrophinopathies are a spectrum of X-linked muscular diseases caused by mutation in the *DMD* gene (located at Xp21), which encodes for dystrophin (a protein that plays an important role in the support and function of muscle fibers). Dystrophinopathies fall on a spectrum: an asymptomatic form with elevated creatine kinase (CK) defines one end of the spectrum, and a severe form of muscle dystrophy with DCM defines the other.

FIGURE 7.19. This specimen shows a cross-section of the heart of a patient with *DMD*-associated dilated cardiomyopathy. Note the dilation of the left ventricle (arrow) without much increase in ventricular wall thickness.

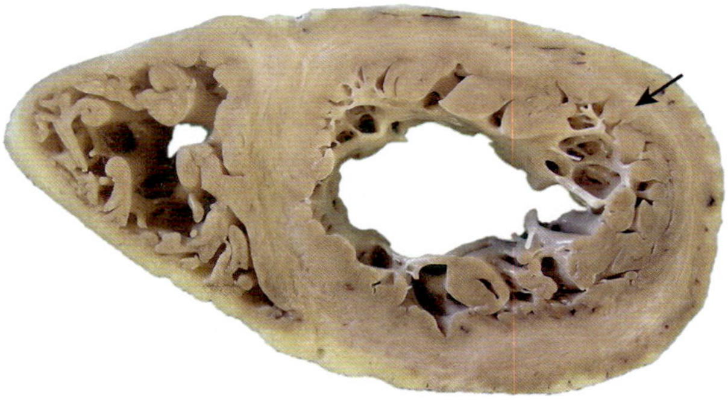

Arrhythmogenic cardiomyopathy

Arrhythmogenic cardiomyopathy is a disorder of the heart muscle characterized by fibrofatty replacement of the right ventricle and, often, the left ventricular subepicardial region. Its cause is related to genetic abnormalities associated with desmosomal mutations. It may result in ventricular tachyarrhythmias, sudden death, or heart failure.

FIGURE 7.20. This specimen shows thinning of the right ventricular wall with fatty replacement of the myocardial wall (arrow).

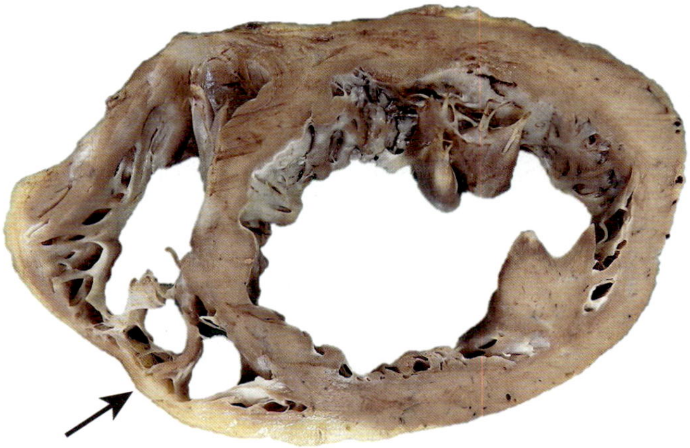

Myocarditis

Myocarditis is inflammation of the heart muscle. It may be idiopathic, infectious, or autoimmune mediated. Autoimmune myocarditis may be triggered by a viral response, or appear in the setting of connective tissue diseases such as rheumatoid arthritis or lupus. It may heal or may lead to heart failure, dilated cardiomyopathy, and even sudden death. Myocarditis and dilated cardiomyopathy are common causes of heart transplantation.

FIGURE 7.21. In (A), a right-side view of a heart shows autoimmune myocarditis. In (B), a left-side view of a heart with autoimmune myocarditis shows dilated ventricles and a discolored wall.

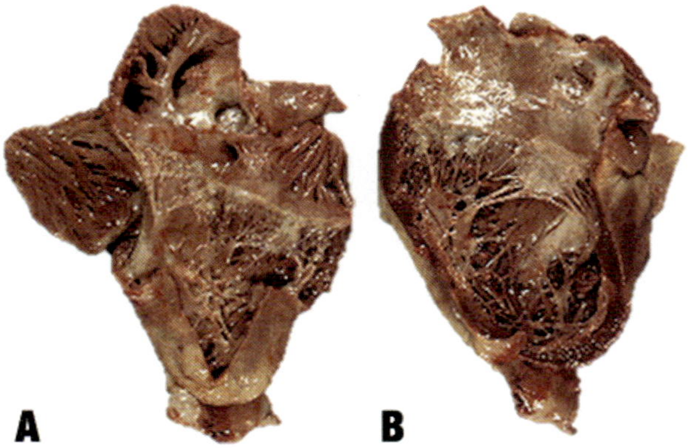

Pericarditis

Pericarditis is inflammation of the pericardium (the sac that contains the heart). It may be due to viral infection, tuberculosis, renal failure, trauma, cancer, or radiation therapy, or may occur post–myocardial infarction (including autoimmune Dressler syndrome). Depending on the type of fluid in the pericardial space, pericarditis may be classified as serous, fibrinous, hemorrhagic, purulent, or caseous.

FIBRINOUS PERICARDITIS

FIGURE 7.22. The heart specimen in (A) shows fibrinous, uremic (i.e., caused by renal failure) pericarditis. Image (B) shows the deposition of fibrin strands in the pericardium that are characteristic of this type of pericarditis. The fibrin gives the pericardium a roughened "bread and butter" appearance.

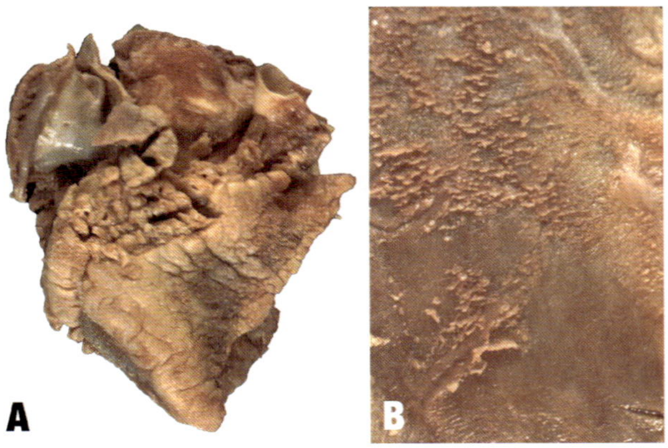

FIGURE 7.23. Note the tan-yellow, fibrinous exudate covering the whole surface of the heart, giving a roughened "bread and butter" appearance to the visceral pericardium.

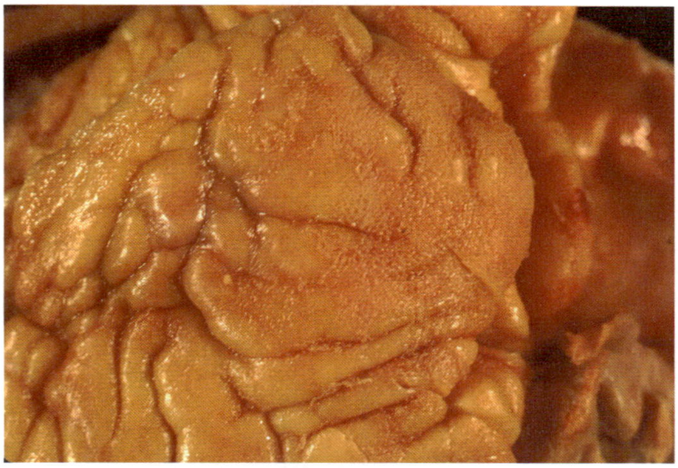

Tuberculosis

Tuberculosis (TB) is caused by *Mycobacterium tuberculosis,* which usually affects the lungs but may involve other organs including the heart. Tuberculous pericarditis, the most common way that TB affects the heart, may appear with inflammation of the pericardium and a fibrinous, bloody pericardial effusion. The infection is more frequent in developing countries and immunocompromised populations.

FIGURE 7.24. This specimen shows enlarged hilar lymph nodes (black arrows) with fibrocaseous tuberculosis. Both surfaces of the pericardium show white exudative caseous tuberculosis involvement (white arrow).

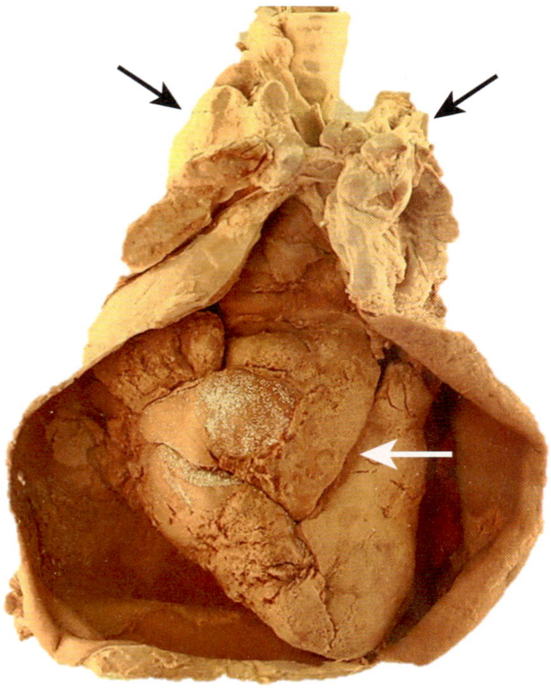

Specimen from Maude Abbott Medical Museum, McGill University

Myocardial infarction (MI)

MI is defined as the death of myocardial cells secondary to ischemia. The risk of MI increases with age.

SUBENDOCARDIAL INFARCTION

The subendocardial zone of the heart is anatomically quite susceptible to ischemia, because it is last to receive the coronary arterial supply. Infarction of this zone may be caused by atherosclerosis, thrombosis, sepsis, or shock.

FIGURE 7.25. This image shows subendocardial hemorrhage of the left ventricle.

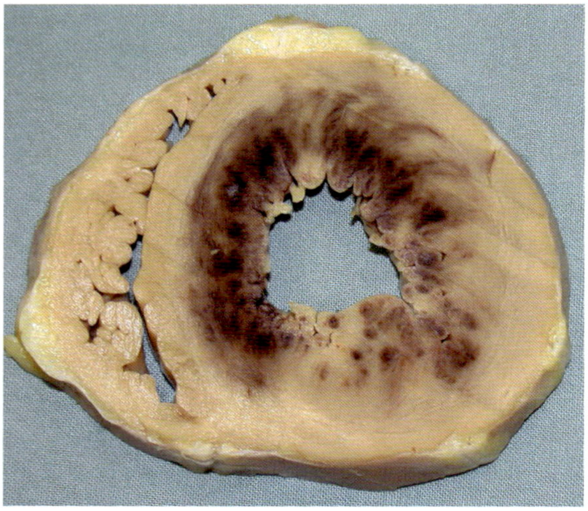

NONREPERFUSED AND REPERFUSED INFARCTION

Postinfarction, blood supply can be restored with reperfusion therapy, in which fibrinolytic agents or percutaneous interventional techniques are used to remove coronary artery stenosis or obstruction. Reperfusion may injure the myocardium after blood flow return, causing arrhythmias and a severe inflammatory response.

FIGURE 7.26. Image (A) shows a nonreperfused acute infarction with yellowish myocardial discoloration necrosis. Image (B) shows the reperfused infarction specimen: the cut surface of the myocardium reveals transmural dark myocardial hemorrhagic discoloration. Image (C) shows a specimen in which an old MI appears as a white, thin, transmural, fibrotic scar.

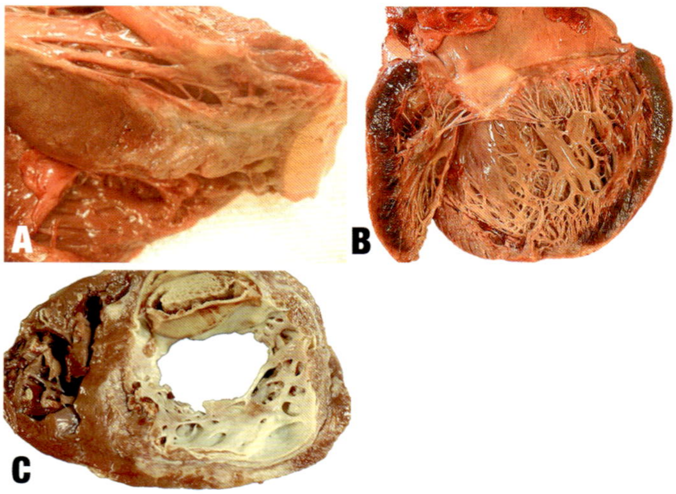

CORONARY ARTERY DISEASE WITH MI

Coronary artery disease is defined as stenosis or blockage of 1 or more coronary arteries secondary to the development of atheroma. The likelihood of developing atherosclerosis depends on modifiable and nonmodifiable risk factors. Modifiable risks factors include hypertension, tobacco use, smoking, diabetes mellitus, and hyperlipidemia. Nonmodifiable risk factors include family history, age, and male sex.

FIGURE 7.27. Image (A) shows a pale yellow plaque stenosing the lumen of the left anterior descending (LAD) artery (arrow). In (B), a heart cross-section shows a thin white subendocardial infarction scar (arrows) located along the septal and anterior region of the left ventricle.

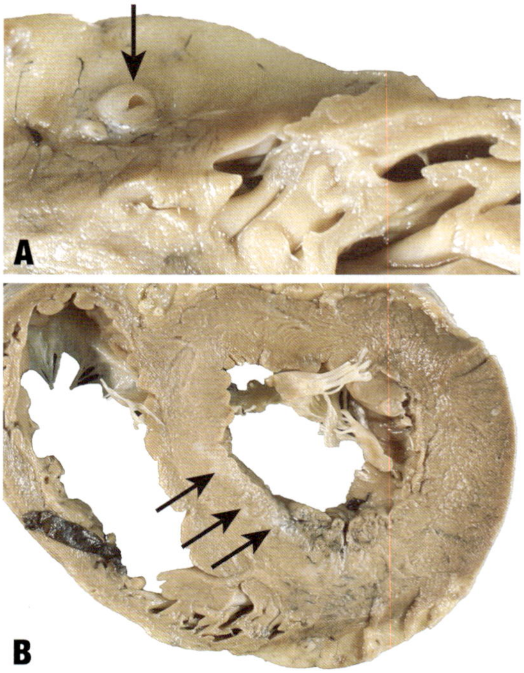

FIGURE 7.28. Images (A) and (B) show coronary arteries completely occluded by calcified atheroma (arrows). Image (C) shows additional cut sections of the grossly occluded arteries. In (D), a heart cross-section shows linear fibrosis (arrows) located in the lateral wall of the left ventricle, indicating an old MI.

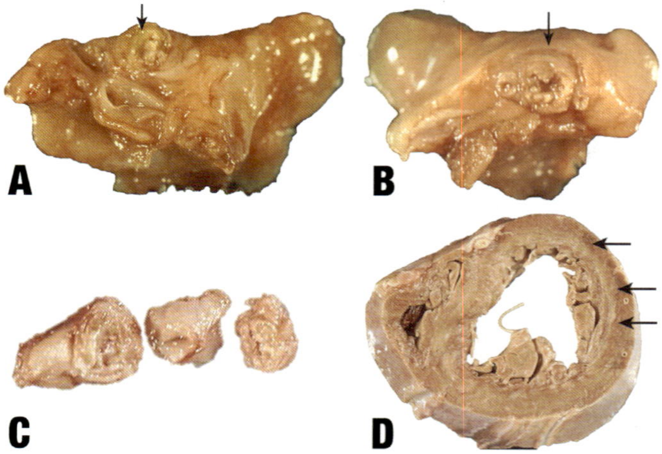

OLD MI

Gross features of MIs evolve over time. In the first 4 hours following an MI, gross and morphological examination may not reveal any changes. In the weeks following an MI, a series of changes become apparent, beginning with inflammation and ending in repair.

FIGURE 7.29. Image (A) shows an old subendocardial white scar indicating an old MI. Image (B) shows a small, old microinfarction, indicated by focal fibrosis (arrow) with calcification of the myocardium.

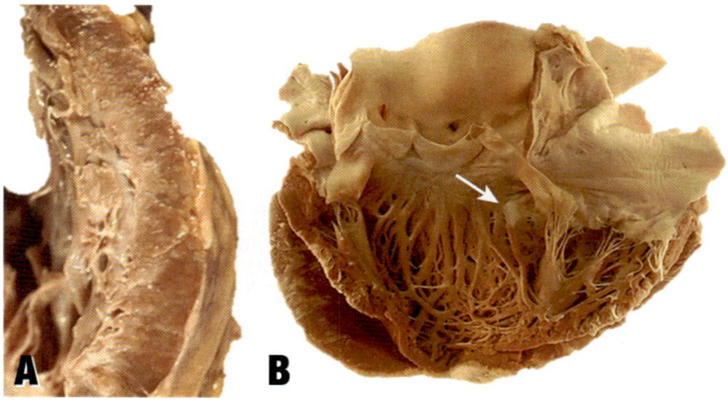

FIGURE 7.30. In (A), the patchy circumferential subendocardial pallor of the left ventricle suggests chronic severe ischemia with myocardial fibrosis and myocyte degeneration. Image (B) shows an old transmural inferior wall infarction (arrow).

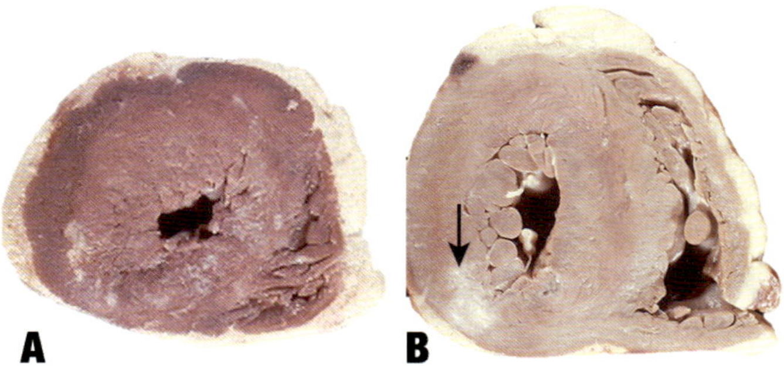

FIGURE 7.31. The cross-section in (A) shows an old septal discoloration suggestive of prior infarction. In (B), succinic dehydrogenase stain reveals a pale subendocardial infarction.

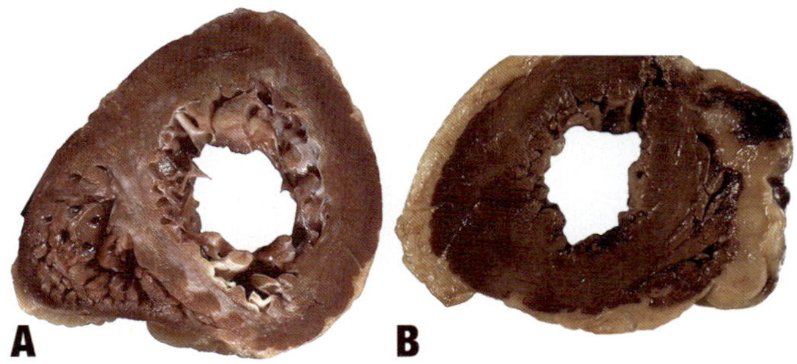

VENTRICULAR RUPTURE FOLLOWING MI

Following an MI, the myocardium may lose integrity: the wall may rupture, and cause hemopericardium and clinical tamponade. Risk factors for myocardial rupture include a recent transmural infarction without revascularization, older age, and female sex. An infarction may also cause a ventricular aneurysm, arrhythmias, valvular dysfunctions, heart failure, pericarditis, and cardiogenic shock. Ventricular wall rupture may occur in a wall weakened by an infarction. Common areas where ruptures occur include the free walls of the ventricle, the ventricular septum, and the papillary muscles.

FIGURE 7.32. This image shows a free wall transmural rupture of the ventricular wall. Blood clots adhere to the heart surface, which indicates hemopericardium.

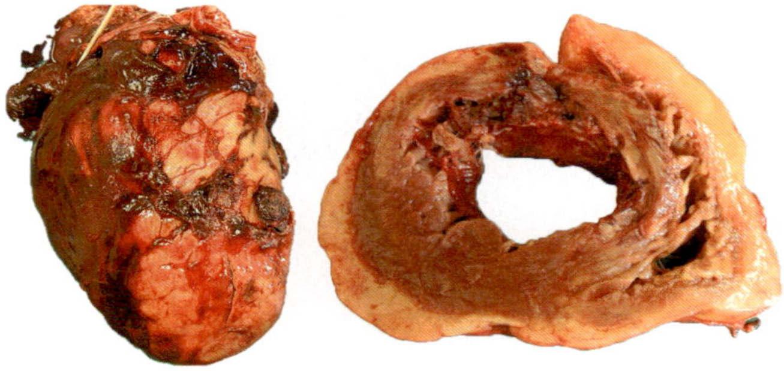

FIGURE 7.33. In (A), an injection of black ink in the left circumflex branch colors the vessel trajectory and allows easy recognition of coronary lesions. The black ink extravasation reveals the infarction location in the left ventricular wall. Images (B) and (C) show cut surfaces of an anterior transmural infarction (arrows); in (C), a small fissure connects to the surface.

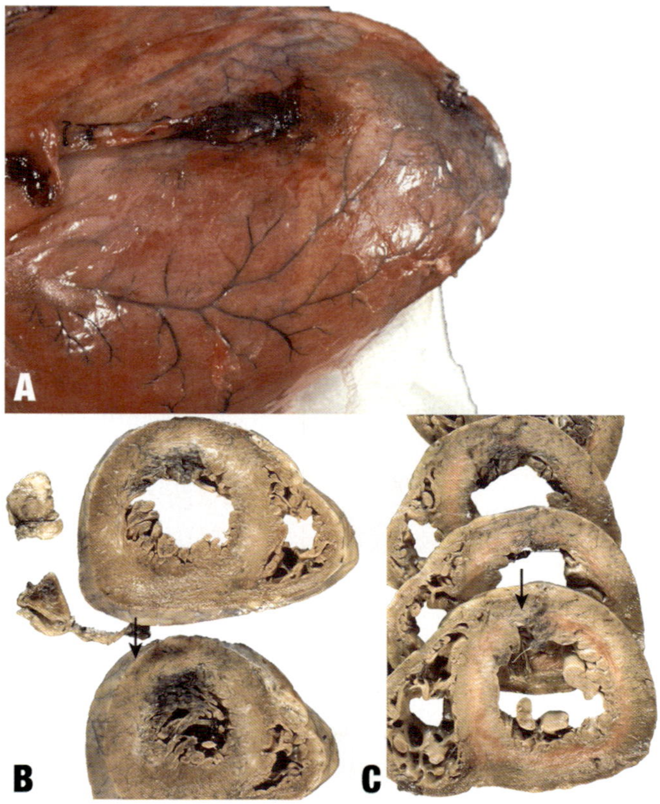

FIGURE 7.34. Image (A) shows stenosis of the left anterior descending coronary artery, secondary to a calcified atheroma (arrow). In (B), succinic dehydrogenase stain highlights the infarcted zone and rupture site (arrow).

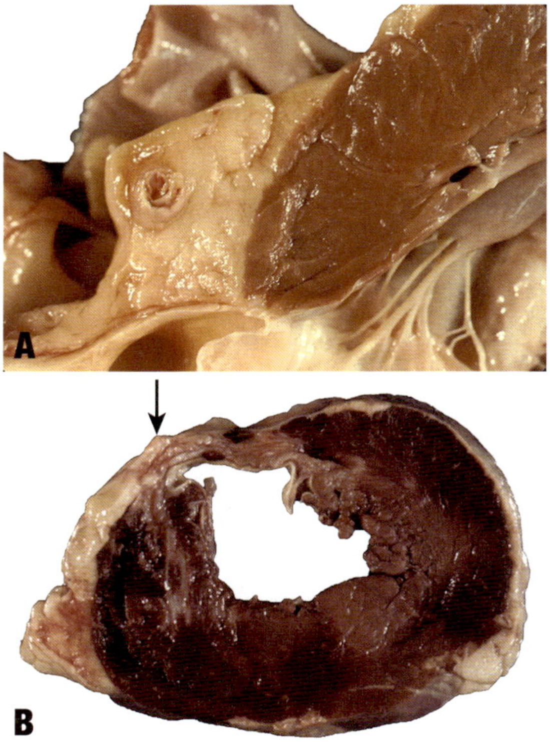

FIGURE 7.35. This image shows epicardial hemorrhage secondary to myocardial rupture. In this case, an incomplete myocardial rupture close to the heart apex led to an accumulation of blood within the epicardium. The patient had an occlusion of a distal branch of the left coronary artery.

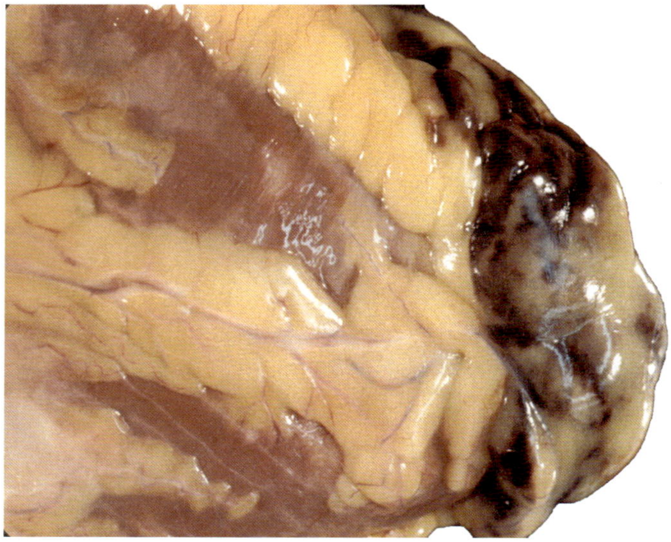

OBSTRUCTED CORONARY ARTERY BYPASS GRAFT (CABG)

CABG surgery grafts sections of the leg saphenous vein to a coronary artery to restore blood flow. The grafted vein may become obstructed.

FIGURE 7.36. In this image, a left saphenous graft is completely occluded by thrombus and is cut in cross-section (arrows) 10 days after CABG.

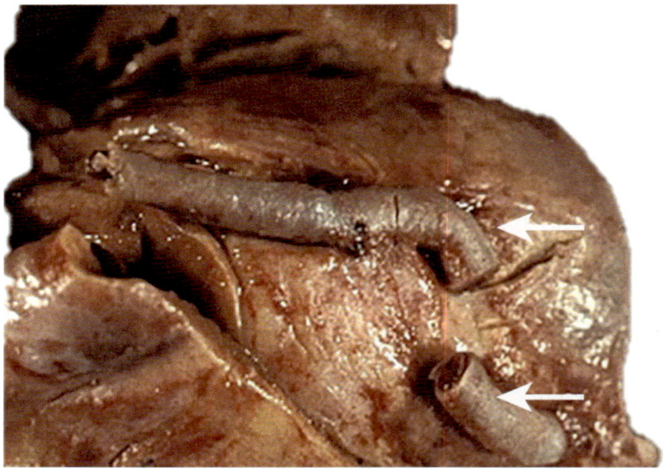

APICAL ANEURYSM FROM OLD MI

Myocardial aneurysms usually arise from an infarcted myocardium with fibrosis. Fibrosis and scarring from old infarctions alter the wall dynamics and may predispose the heart to aneurysm formation.

FIGURE 7.37. An incision into the apex of the ventricle of this specimen reveals an aneurysm of the myocardium.

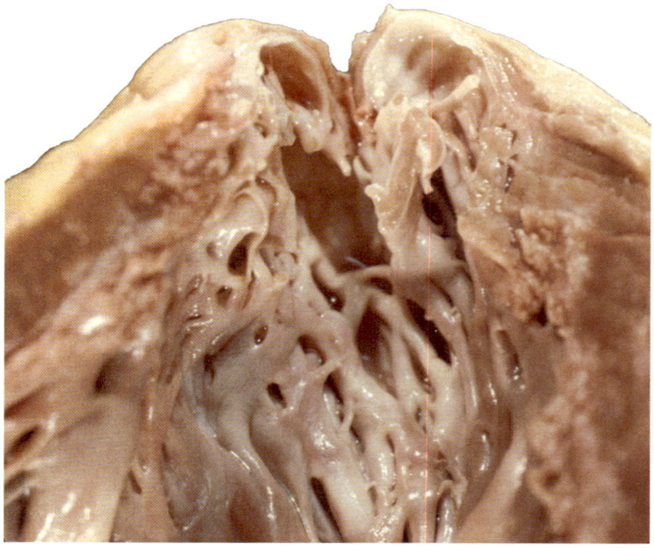

MI WITH ANEURYSM AND MURAL THROMBUS

Following an MI, the affected portion of the wall may become akinetic or dyskinetic. This decrease of motion may lead to blood stagnation, which can predispose the heart to thrombus formation.

FIGURE 7.38. This cut surface illustrates an old MI with wall thinning and an organized lamellated thrombus (arrow).

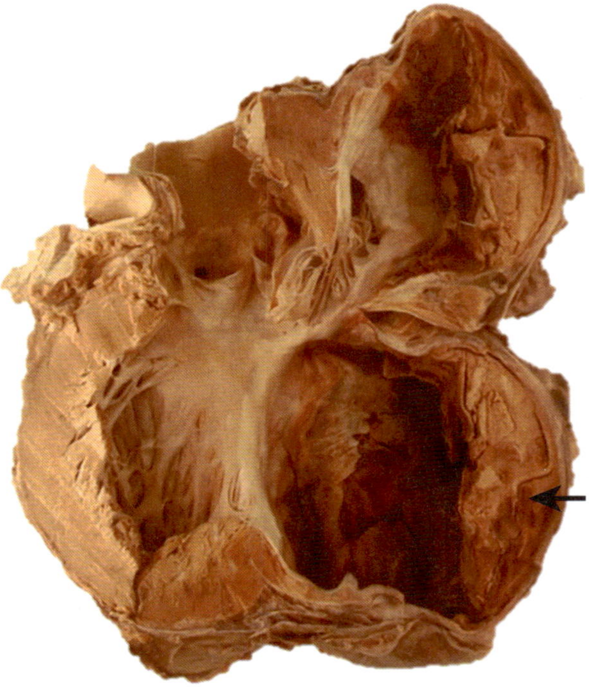

VENTRICULAR ANEURYSM FROM OLD MI

FIGURE 7.39. This image shows left ventricular aneurysmal dilatation, especially in the apical region, with a thin fibrotic wall due to an old healed infarction. A large, organized thrombus is observed in the aneurysm.

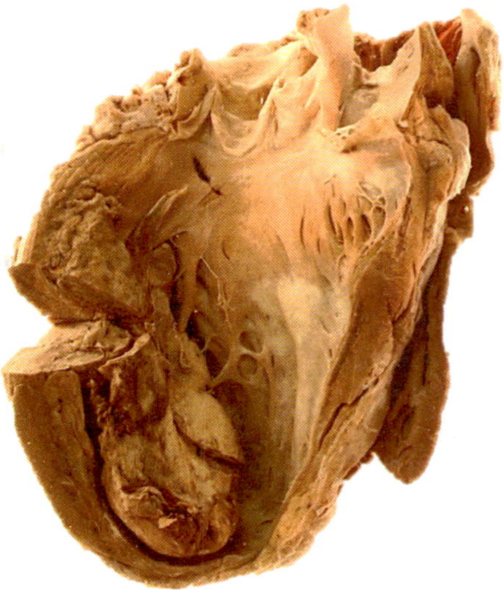

Specimen from Maude Abbott Medical Museum, McGill University

Aortic stenosis (AS)

AS is the most common valvular heart disease in the developed world. AS involves narrowing of the outflow region of the left ventricle into the aorta. The aortic valve normally has 3 cusps, and lies between the left ventricle and the aorta. The most common valvular abnormality is calcific aortic stenosis, which appears due to degeneration in a 3-cusp valve or in a congenitally bicuspid valve. AS can occur above, below, or at the aortic valve level. It is a progressive condition that leads to left-sided heart failure, angina, ischemia, and syncope.

FIGURE 7.40. Image (A) shows a 3-cusp aortic valve with calcific, degenerative deposits. Image (B) shows a congenitally bicuspid aortic valve with degenerative changes and stenosis. The valve is thickened and shows a dull, irregular surface and multiple small foci of calcification. The right cusp has a raised raphe (arrow); this is the region of failed cusp division.

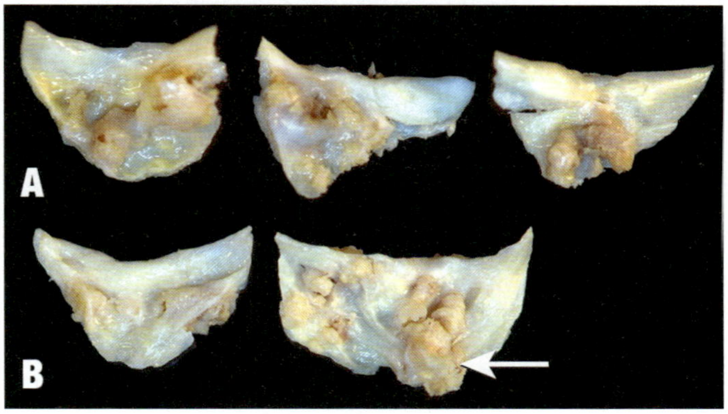

FIGURE 7.41. Images (A) and (B) show calcific aortic stenosis of the aortic valve.

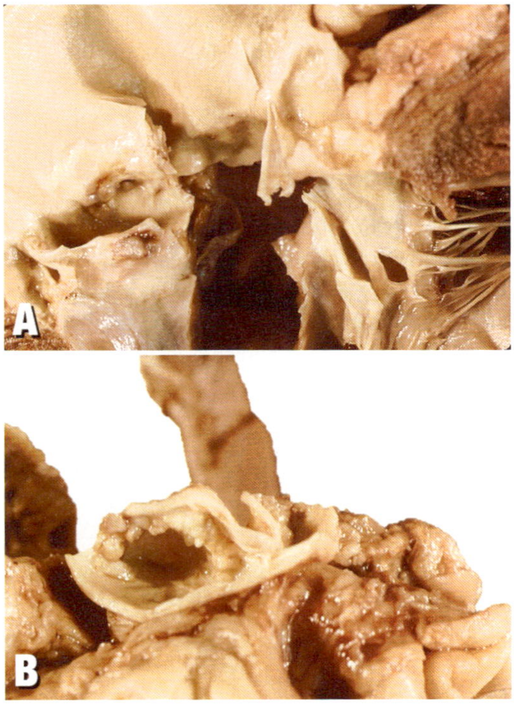

CONGENITALLY BICUSPID AORTIC VALVE

The aortic valve normally has 3 cusps. In 1% to 2% of the population, the aortic valve has only 2 cusps (congenitally bicuspid aortic valve). This condition is an important risk factor for developing aortic stenosis, which tends to appear in these patients 10 years earlier than in the general population.

FIGURE 7.42. Images (A) and (B) show 2 specimens of congenitally bicuspid aortic valve with degenerative changes: fibrous thickening and calcification.

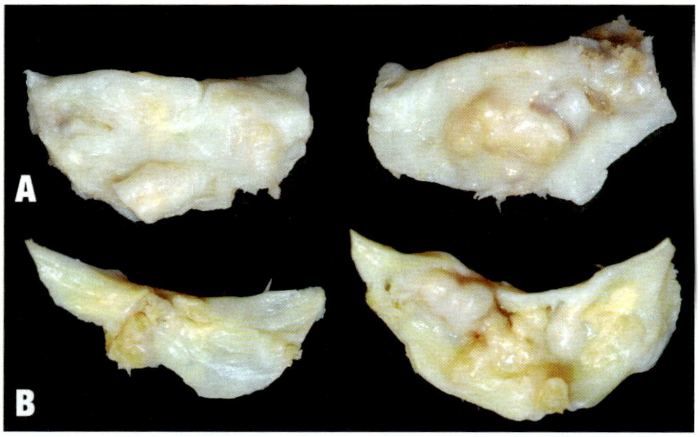

Myxomatous degeneration

Myxomatous degeneration of the mitral valve is a common cause of mitral valve insufficiency. There is thickening of the spongiosa layer of the valve due to myxoid material deposition. It affects 2% to 3% of adults, occurring more frequently in females than males (7:1 ratio), and can be associated with inherited disorders of connective tissue such as Marfan syndrome, Ehlers–Danlos syndrome, and osteogenesis imperfecta. Myxoid degeneration in the valves may be complicated by mitral valve insufficiency, infective endocarditis, systemic embolism of leaflet thrombi, and ventricular and atrial arrhythmias.

FIGURE 7.43. Image (A) shows a specimen with a myxoid mitral valve in a patient with regurgitation; the leaflet appears white, thickened, and rubbery, and shows upward hooding (ballooning) toward the left atrium. Image (B) shows a myxoid mitral valve leaflet with fibrosis, thickening, and chordal elongation.

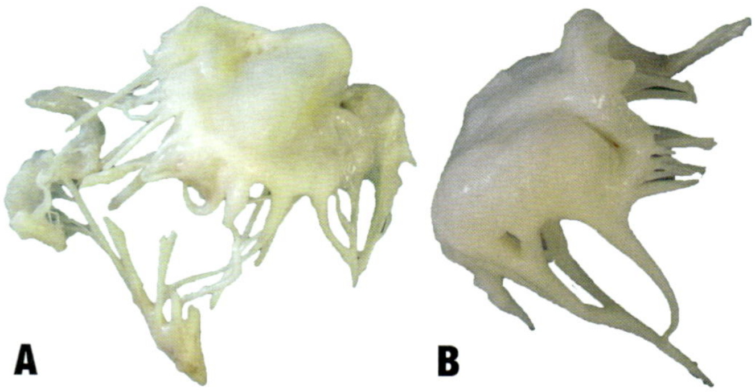

FIGURE 7.44. In (A), myxoid changes in a mitral valve show valve enlargement, thickening, and ballooning due to accumulation of myxoid ground substance. The specimen in (B) shows excised myxoid mitral valve leaflets with fibrosis and myxoid degeneration.

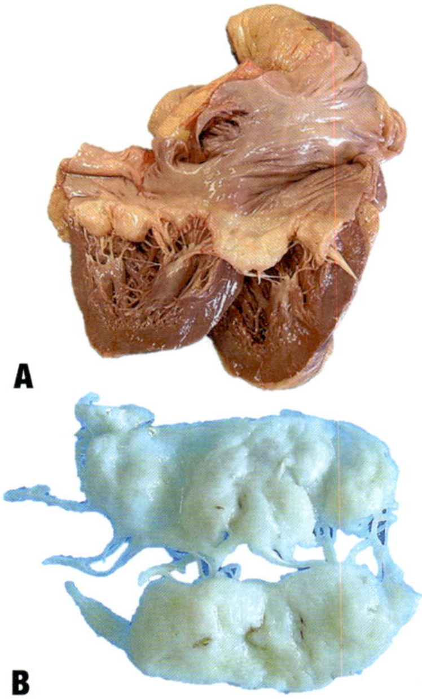

Valvular amyloidosis

Valvular amyloidosis consists of extracellular deposition of amyloid in the cardiac valves. It may cause valve regurgitation or stenosis, or even lead to the rupture of chordae. It may also have no functional effect. Valvular amyloidosis happens most frequently in the aortic and mitral valves, and is usually due to amyloid light chain (AL) amyloidosis (90% of cases).

FIGURE 7.45. This image shows valvular amyloid. Note the translucent, waxy, beaded surface.

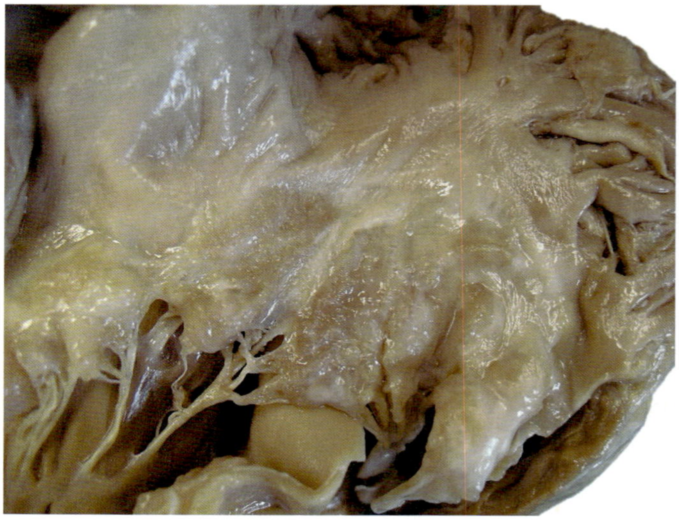

Calcification of the mitral annulus

Calcification of the mitral annulus results from aging, and involves progressive calcium deposition on and under the valve leaflet. It affects the posterior leaflet, occurs in a "C" shape, and spares the anterior leaflet.

FIGURE 7.46. This image shows mitral valve annular calcification as a calcified irregular mass of gritty material along the posterior leaflet (black arrow), sparing the base of the anterior leaflet (*). There is an uninfected, red-brown thrombotic vegetation along the posterior leaflet annulus ring (white arrow). This heart came from an elderly woman with chronic renal failure and secondary hyperparathyroidism.

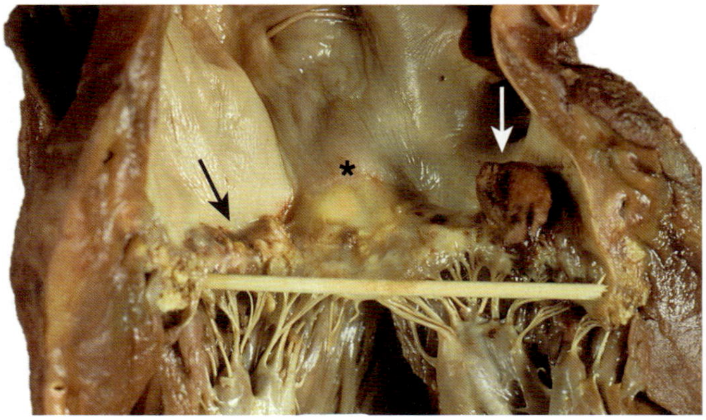

Valve vegetation

There are 3 types of valve vegetations (endocardial or valvular thrombi): 1) vegetations of infective endocarditis; 2) vegetations of nonbacterial thrombotic endocarditis (NBTE, also called marantic endocarditis because associated with debilitating diseases such as cancer and sepsis); and 3) Libman–Sacks endocarditis, which is often related to systemic lupus erythematosus.

VEGETATIONS OF INFECTIVE ENDOCARDITIS

FIGURE 7.47. Image (A) shows mitral valve infective vegetations; they appear as soft, friable, nodular-irregular lesions in the line of closure that can extend to the chordae tendineae (black arrow). There is also an annular abscess (white arrow) and intramyocardial abscess (*). Image (B) shows a resected infected mitral valve with vegetations.

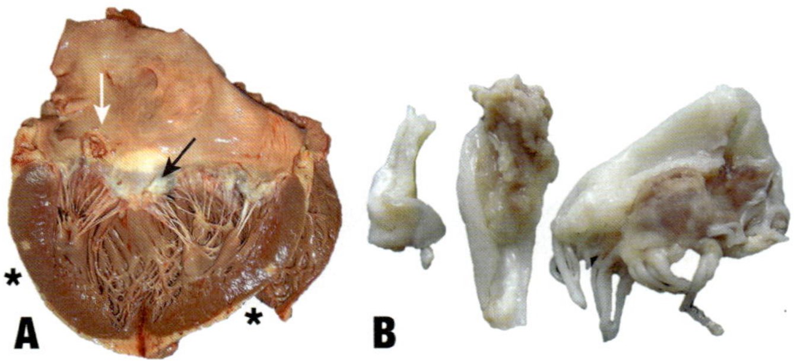

VEGETATIONS OF NBTE

Noninfectious vegetations with thrombus attached to the underlying valve occur in cases of NBTE, and in conditions that induce a hypercoagulable state such as immune thrombocytopenic purpura and malignancy-induced coagulopathy (especially mucinous adenocarcinoma). Their strong association with mucinous adenocarcinoma is due to the procoagulant effects of mucin or tissue factors derived from the tumor, which can also cause migratory thrombophlebitis (a condition called Trousseau syndrome).

FIGURE 7.48. This image shows a mitral valve with thrombotic vegetations along the line of closure (arrow). Note the absence of destruction of the underlying valve.

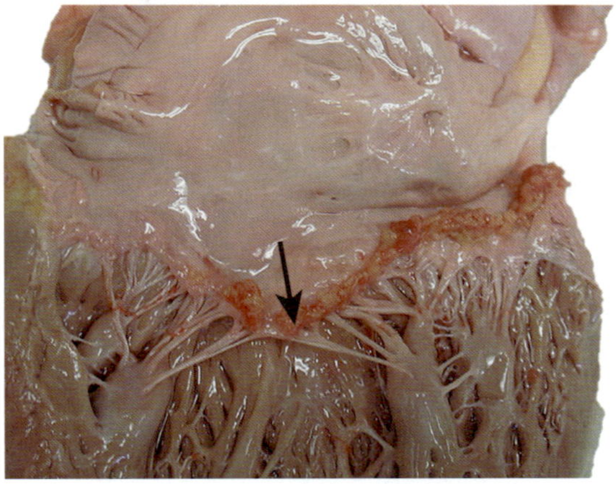

FIGURE 7.49. This image shows a mitral valve with nonbacterial vegetations appearing as red, firm, irregular vegetations at the line of closure (arrows).

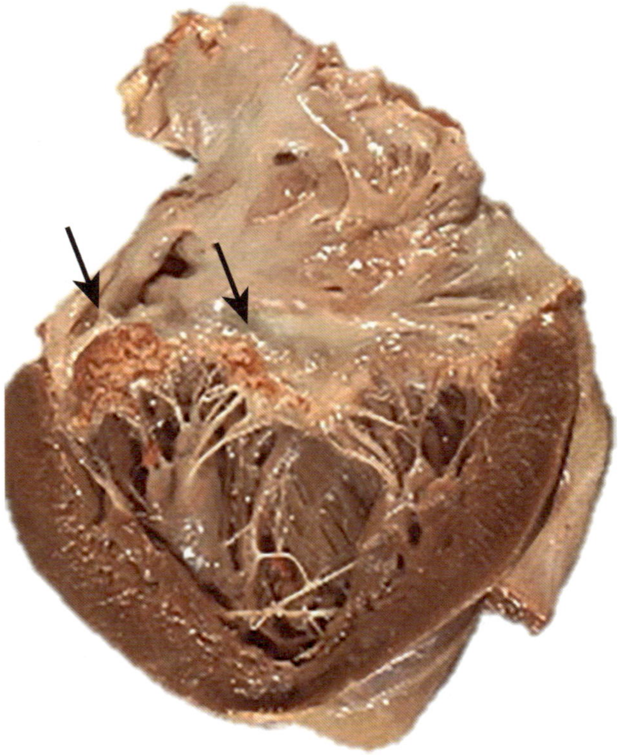

FIGURE 7.50. In this image of mitral valve marantic endocarditis (A), note the pink, granular, bland vegetations superficially deposited along the line of closure (arrows). No inflammation or destruction of the valve is caused by this kind of vegetation, but there is thickening of the valve and the chordae tendineae. Image (B) shows a closer view of the mitral valve marantic endocarditis.

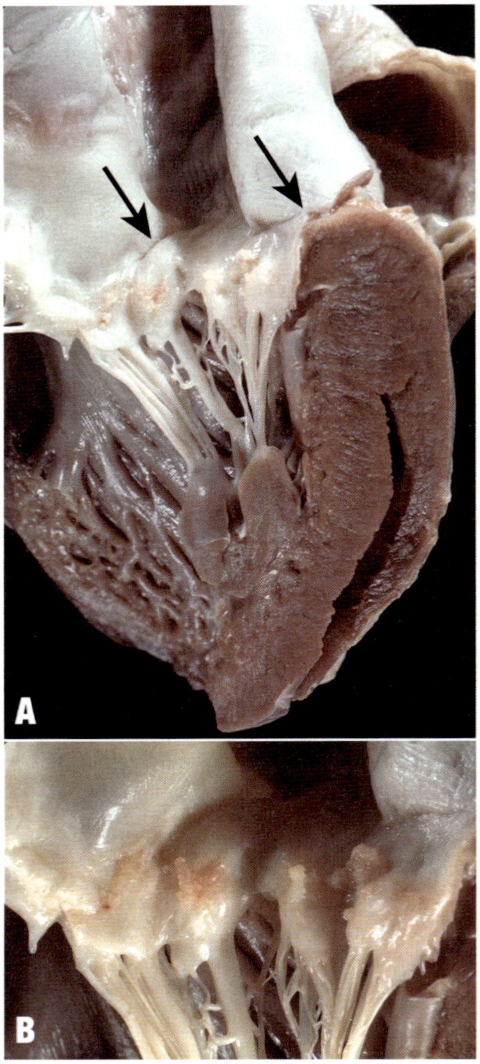

Infective endocarditis (IE)

IE is an infection of the internal surface of the heart (the endocardium). It may affect the heart valves or mural endocardium, or involve septal defects. The valves most commonly affected by IE, in descending order, are the mitral valve, the aortic valve, the tricuspid valve, and (rarely) the pulmonic valve. IE vegetation may be anywhere on the valve and may cause destruction of the valve. IE develops from a triad of factors: 1) bacteremia or fungemia; 2) adherence of the organisms to the endocardium; and 3) invasion of the valve. (Staphylococci and streptococci are common bacterial organisms that cause IE. They cause vegetations: masses composed of fibrin, platelets, and infecting organisms, and are held together by agglutinating antibodies produced by the bacteria.) Patients may show signs of systemic infection. Although IE can appear in a normal heart, 60% of patients have a predisposing cardiac condition. The most frequent risk factors are mitral valve prolapse, mitral and aortic regurgitation, rheumatic disease, hypertrophic cardiomyopathy, ventricular septal defect, bicuspid aortic valve, and coarctation of the aorta.

FIGURE 7.51. This image shows an aortic valve vegetation (arrow) on the noncoronary cusp due to IE. Note the small red nodular lesion (measuring 0.2 cm) sitting on an otherwise normal-looking aortic valve.

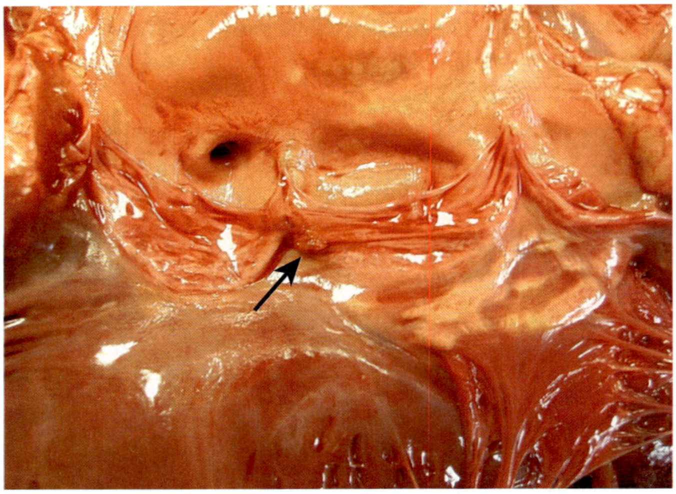

FIGURE 7.52. Images (A) and (B) show bacterial endocarditis. Note the polypoid white-pink vegetations attached to the mitral valve. Image (C) shows a left ventricle intramural abscess (arrow). Image (D) shows a spleen septic infarction. Note the wedge-shaped, tan-white lesion with a necrotic dark center.

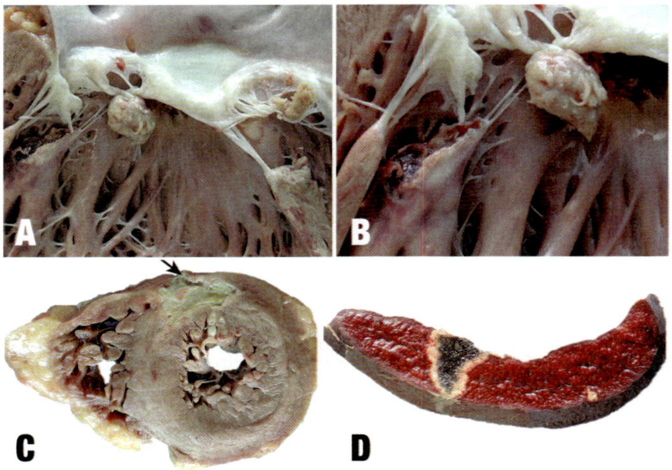

FIGURE 7.53. This image shows bacterial endocarditis on a rheumatic mitral valve.

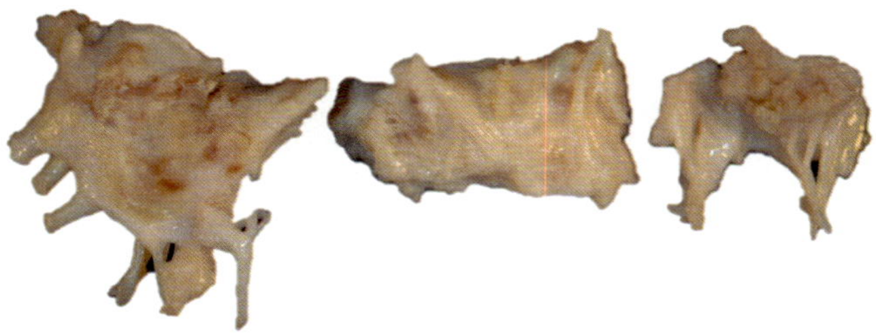

FIGURE 7.54. This image shows a resected aortic valve with organizing IE. Note the white-tan polypoid vegetations with tissue destruction in this congenitally bicuspid valve.

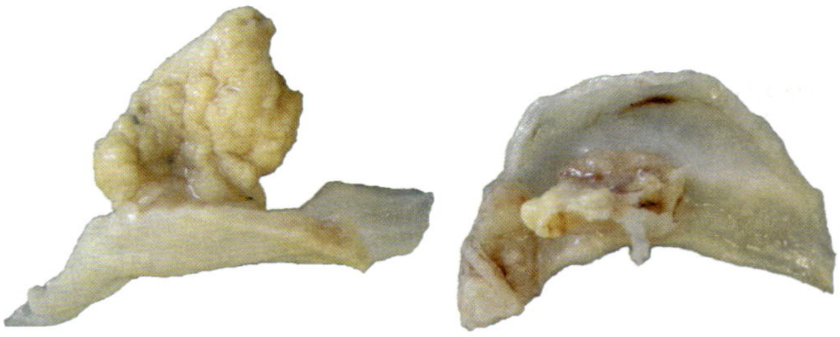

FIGURE 7.55. Image (A) shows a case of pneumococcal IE with polypoid vegetations of the mitral valve and left atrium. Note the large, red, polypoid excrescences (arrows). Image (B) shows IE in the heart of a 56-year-old male. *Staphylococcus pyogenes* was cultured; subsequently, bacteremia led to endocarditis of the mitral valve. Note the beige vegetation in the mitral leaflet (arrow).

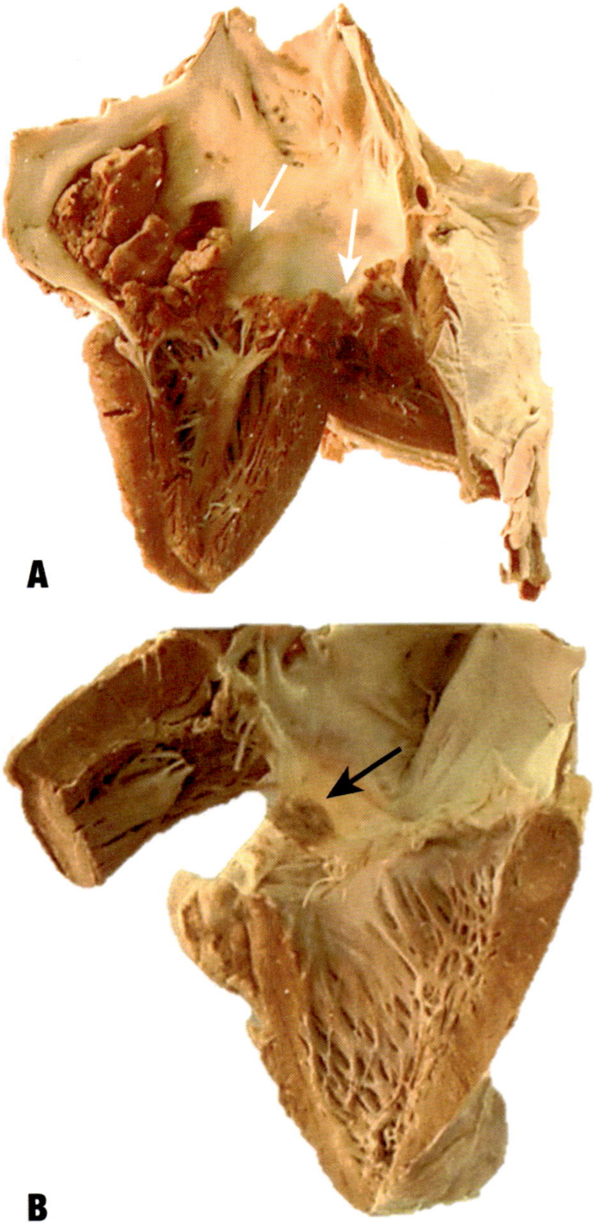

IE AND VALVE DESTRUCTION

As inflammation continues, IE may lead to ulceration with erosion or perforation of the valve cusps.

FIGURE 7.56. This image shows large vegetations on the aortic cusps with reddish excrescences growing onto the ventricular surface (arrows).

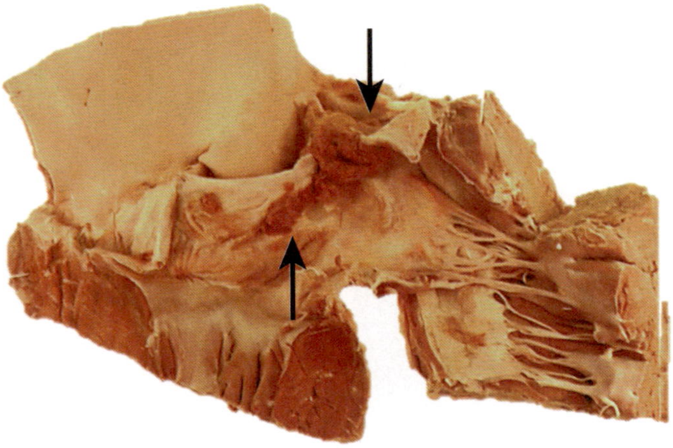

BACTERIAL IE OF THE MITRAL VALVE AND ENDOCARDIUM

FIGURE 7.57. Image (A) shows heart bacterial endocarditis involving the mitral valve and atrial endocardium. Note the red excrescences on the mitral valve (white arrow) and the white, thickened, and wrinkled left atrial endocardium (black arrow). Image (B) shows a kidney with an IE-related infarction. There is a light, wedge-shaped, depressed lesion (arrow). In (C), a cut section of the same kidney infarction gives a closer view of the wedge-shaped infarction, the base of which is near the renal cortex (arrow).

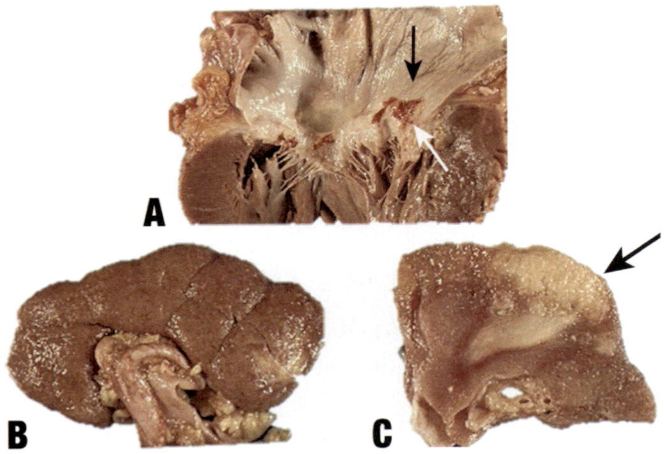

EFFECTS OF IE ON OTHER ORGAN SYSTEMS

FIGURE 7.58. Image (A) shows lung bronchopneumonia of a patient with acute bacterial endocarditis. Note the patchy, lighter areas of pulmonary consolidation. Image (B) shows the brain of a patient with acute bacterial endocarditis, which has a right parietal cerebral-cortical septic infarction.

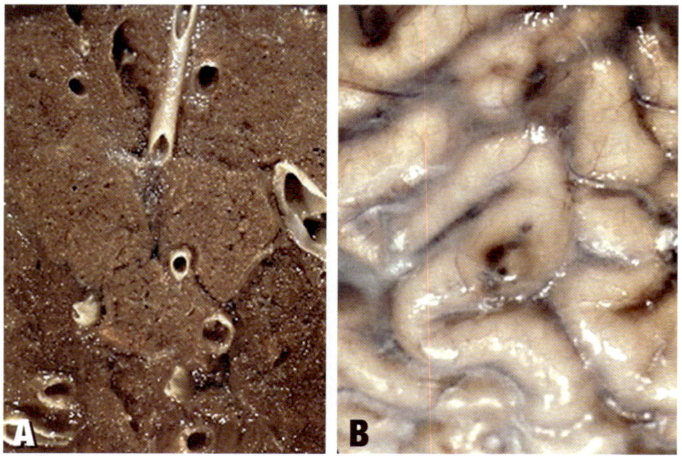

IE OF THE AORTIC VALVE

FIGURE 7.59. This image shows red, friable vegetations located on the aortic cusp (white arrow) and a hypertrophied left ventricle with ventricular wall thickening (black arrow). This patient had a history of rheumatic fever and a recent *Streptococcus viridans* septicemia.

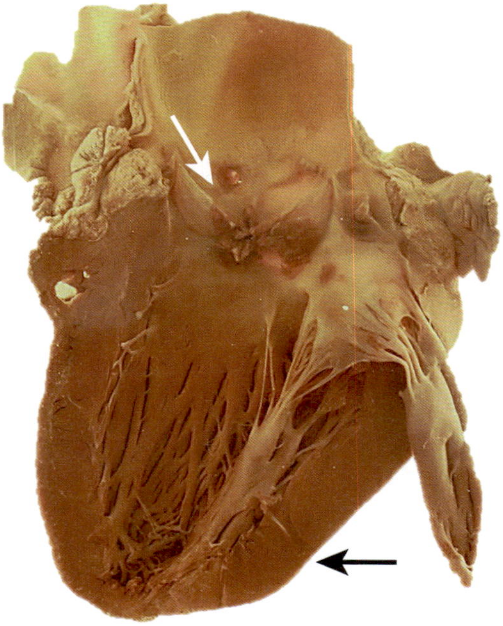

Rheumatic heart disease

Rheumatic fever occurs in 0.3% of cases of group A ß-hemolytic streptococcal pharyngitis in children (aged 5 to 17 years). Its most serious complication is rheumatic heart disease. Rheumatic heart disease is caused by an autoimmune reaction to group A streptococci. Rheumatic heart disease was the main cause of cardiac valve replacement in the past; since 1960, it has become fairly rare due to widespread use of antibiotics to treat streptococcal infections. In the acute stage, rheumatic heart disease leads to pancarditis. In the chronic stage, it leads to valve fibrosis resulting in stenosis and/or insufficiency of the affected valve (most commonly the mitral valve, followed by the aortic).

FIGURE 7.60. In (A), a surgical specimen shows the pathognomonic changes seen in rheumatic valves: thickened leaflets and a "fish mouth" appearance with fused commissures. Image (B) shows rheumatic mitral valve calcifications, commissural fusion, and erosion of calcium with ulceration (arrow). Images (C) and (D) demonstrate chordae tendineae that have thickened and fused (arrows).

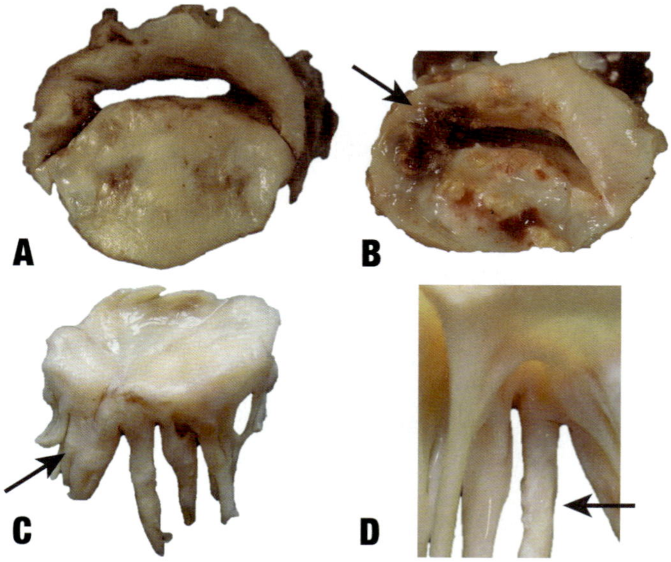

FIGURE 7.61. Images (A) through (D) are examples of rheumatic mitral valves, showing thickening of the valves with fused chordae tendineae. Image (D) also demonstrates erosion of the leaflet calcium.

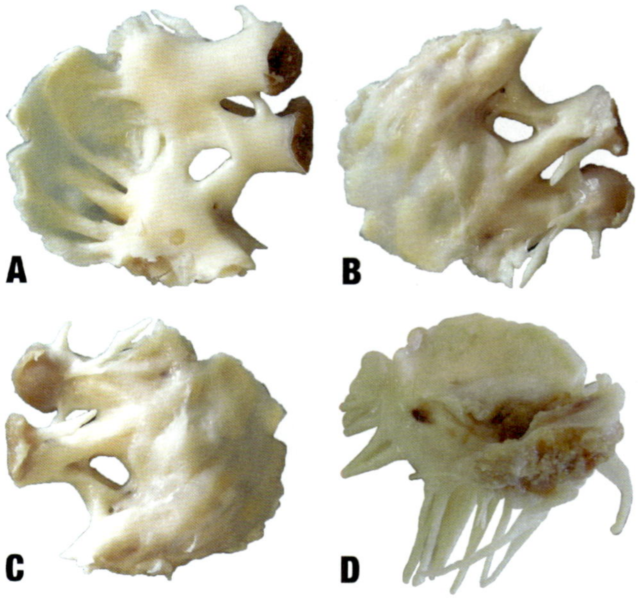

MITRAL VALVE RHEUMATIC STENOSIS

Most mitral stenosis is due to rheumatic heart disease. However, mitral stenosis may also be congenital, or a result of calcific degeneration, systemic lupus erythematosus, or rheumatoid arthritis.

FIGURE 7.62. In this example, mitral valve rheumatic stenosis leads to obstruction of the blood flow from the atrium to the ventricle.

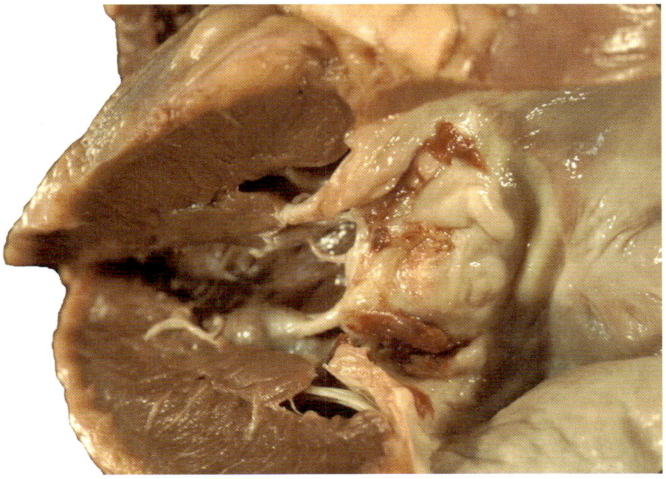

FIGURE 7.63. This excised mitral valve demonstrates mitral valve rheumatic stenosis, showing severe chordal fibrosis and fusion that practically obliterates the subvalvular apparatus.

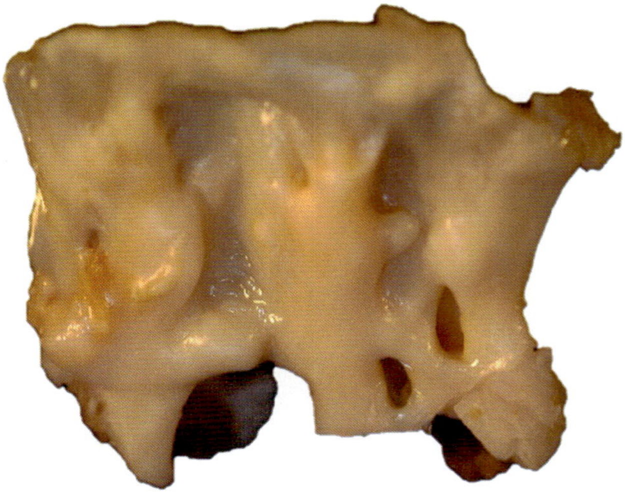

AORTIC RHEUMATIC STENOSIS

Aortic stenosis is narrowing of the orifice of the aortic valve that leads to obstruction of blood flow from the ventricle to the aorta and the systemic circulation. Calcific degeneration is the main cause in the developed countries, but rheumatic heart disease is still the most common cause worldwide.

FIGURE 7.64. Image (A) shows an example of rheumatic aortic stenosis due to fusion of cusp commissures with fibrous thickening and focal calcification. Image (B) shows degenerative aortic stenosis with calcific degeneration without cusp commissural fusion. White, hard, calcifications are present in all 3 aortic cusps (arrows).

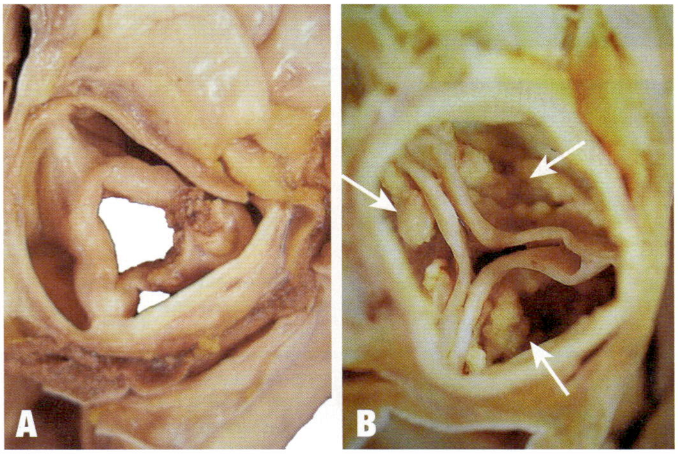

Cardiovascular syphilis

Cardiovascular syphilis is infection of the heart and related blood vessels by *Treponema pallidum*. Cardiac manifestations are part of tertiary syphilis. This may appear 10 to 30 years after the initial primary infection. The most common manifestation of tertiary cardiovascular syphilis is syphilitic aortitis with aneurysm formation.

FIGURE 7.65. Image (A) shows an MI of the left ventricular wall in a patient with syphilitic aortic valve disease. Note the pale discoloration of the myocardium (arrow). Image (B) shows a mural thrombus in the right atrium due to heart failure. Image (C) shows an example of syphilitic aortic valve with fibrosis.

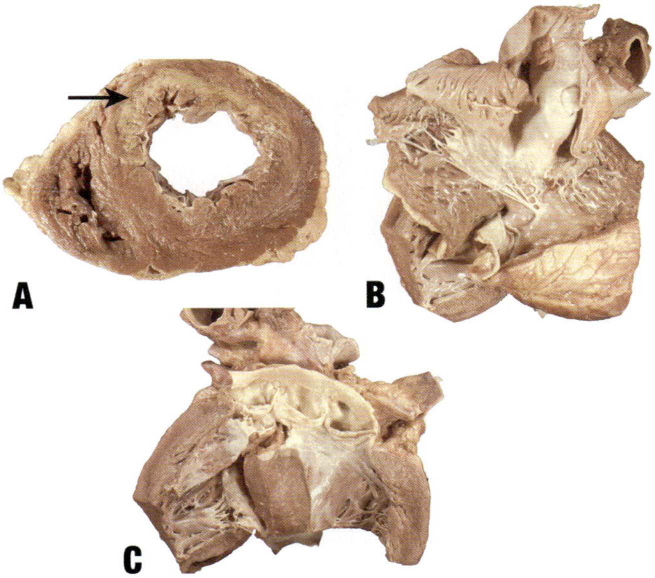

TERTIARY SYPHILIS

Tertiary syphilis is a late stage of syphilis that manifests 3 to 15 years after the initial infection. It affects many organs and systems, including the cardiovascular system, with gumma formations, and causes aortitis in the heart.

FIGURE 7.66. This image shows the heart of a 36-year-old male with chronic aortic insufficiency and aortic aneurysm. The inner intimal surface of the aorta shows distortion from plaques and fibrosis related to underlying aortitis.

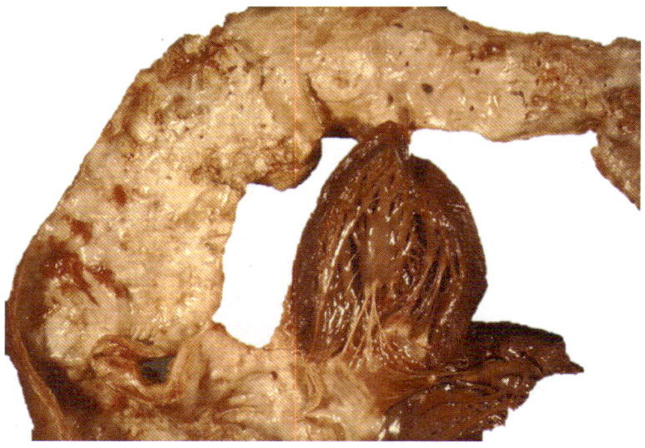

Heart Surgery and Prosthetics

Glenn shunt, or anastomosis of the superior vena cava (SVC) to the pulmonary artery

Anastomosis of the SVC to the pulmonary artery, also called a Glenn shunt, is a palliative cardiac surgery for infants with right-sided congenital heart anomaly, such as tricuspid atresia. This surgery aims to increase systemic oxygen saturation without placing additional strain on the left ventricle.

FIGURE 7.67. These images show: (A) anastomosis of the SVC to the pulmonary artery; (B) a calcific aortic valve; and (C) increased pleural vasculature.

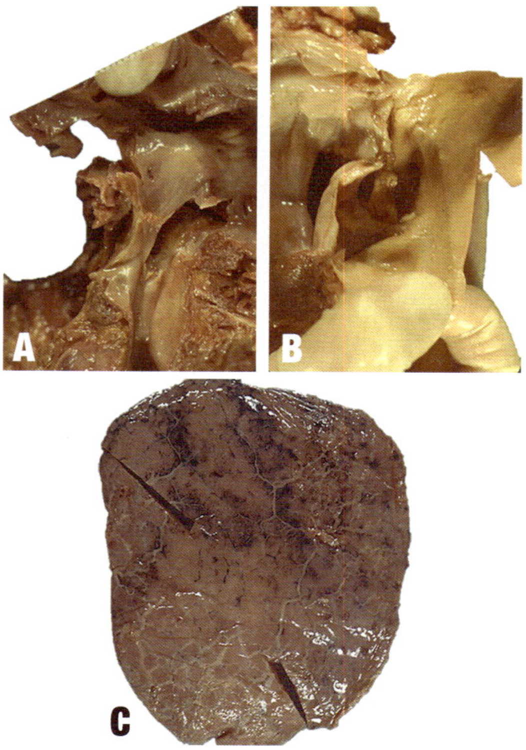

Pacemaker lead

Pacemaker leads may incorporate into the adjacent valve leaflets or chords causing distortion and fibrosis. They may give rise to thrombosis or become infected.

FIGURE 7.68. In this specimen, a pacemaker lead (arrow) crosses the tricuspid valve (TV).

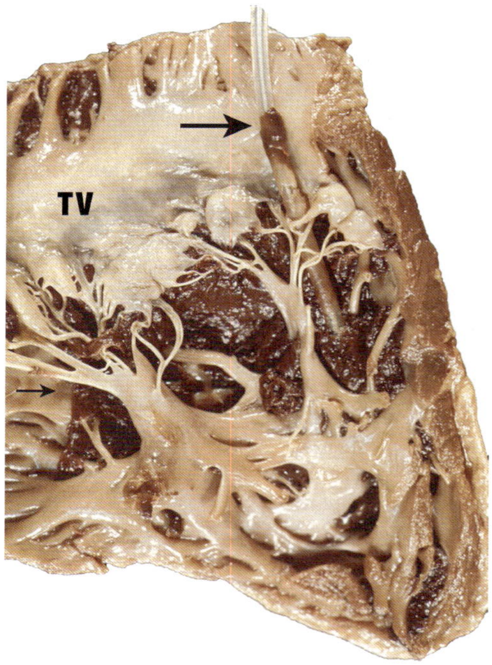

Valve replacement

The aortic and mitral valves are the most commonly replaced valves. Replacement valves may be mechanical heart valves or tissue bioprosthetic (human or animal) heart valves. Either option has advantages and disadvantages. Mechanical heart valves last longer, but patients need lifelong anticoagulation. Tissue heart valves do not require anticoagulation therapy, but have a shorter lifespan.

FIGURE 7.69. Image (A) shows an aortic valve mechanical prosthesis. Image (B) shows a rheumatic mitral valve with mitral commissurotomy.

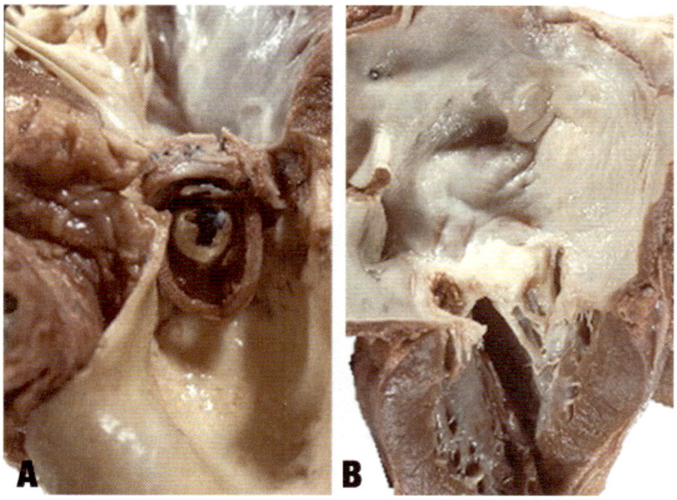

MECHANICAL HEART VALVE

Mechanical heart valves may last 20 to 30 years and are considered very reliable.

FIGURE 7.70. Image (A) shows a mitral valve mechanical bileaflet prosthesis, with 2 semicircular leaflets, which move, attached to the valve housing. Image (B) shows a "caged ball" aortic valve, called a Starr–Edwards valve. It consists of a metal cage that houses a silicone ball; when blood pressure in the ventricle exceeds that of the aorta, the ball is pushed against the cage and allows blood to flow. This valve is no longer used for valve replacements, but there are still patients who are living with these older valves.

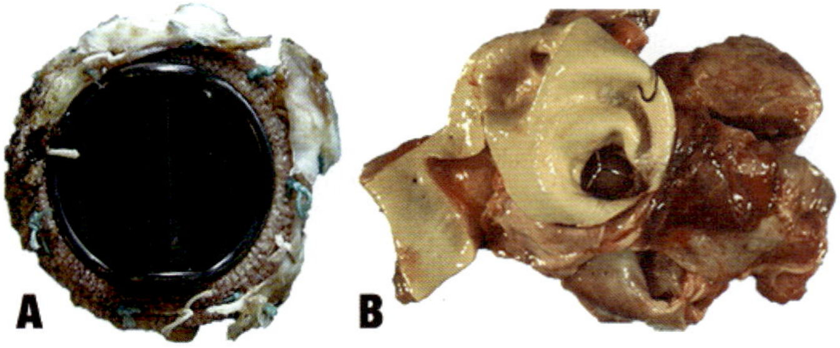

FIGURE 7.71. Image (A) shows a mechanical prosthetic valve. Note the suture on the valve strut (arrow). Image (B) shows a mitral valve prosthesis complicated by subendocardial necrosis. Note the gray-tan discoloration in the myocardial wall (arrow). Image (C) shows a heart valve replacement with a suture around the valve strut (arrow). Image (D) shows a heart mitral valve prosthesis with subendocardial necrosis.

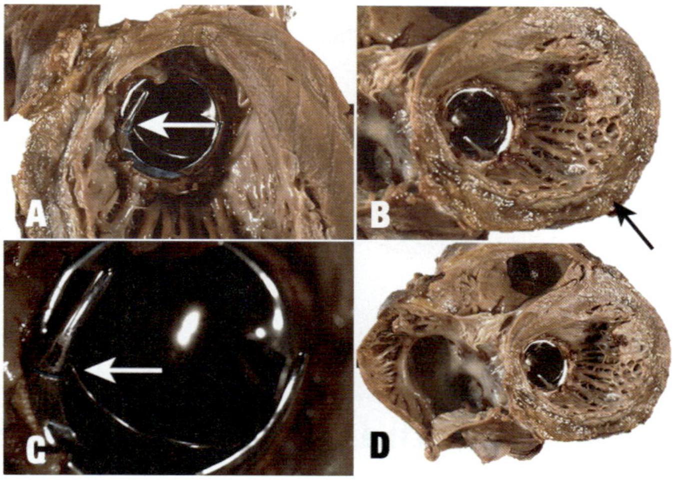

FIGURE 7.72. Image (A) shows the lung of a patient with rheumatic valve disease and mitral stenosis. Pulmonary edema occurred post–valve replacement. In (B), a mitral valve mechanical prosthesis is complicated by multiple thrombi. Image (C) is a close-up view of a mitral valve prosthesis.

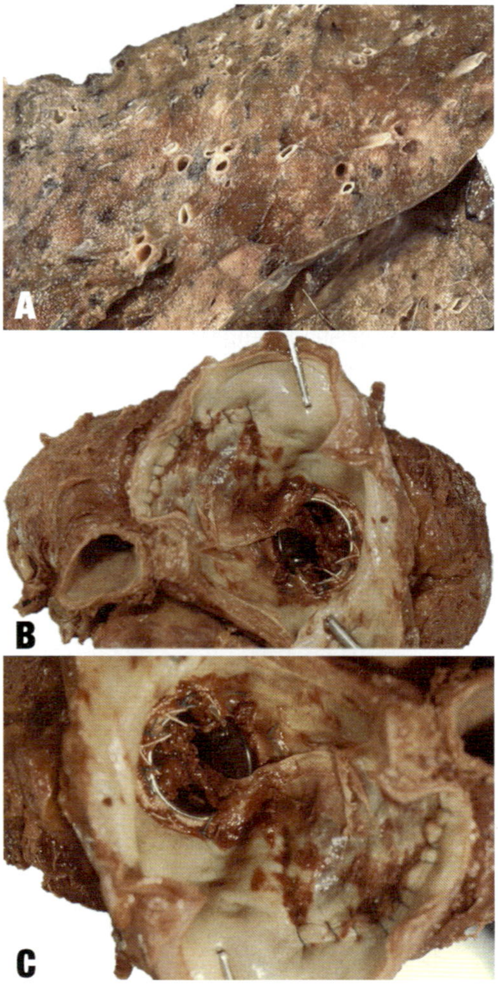

BIOPROSTHETIC HEART VALVE

Bioprosthetic valves may result in different complications than mechanical valves. They may lead to primary valve leaflet degenerative failure, prosthetic valve endocarditis, cr thrombosis.

FIGURE 7.73. In this image, a bioprosthetic valve shows complications of leaflet degeneration and insufficiency. The right valve leaflets, taken from a prosthesis, have thrombi formation.

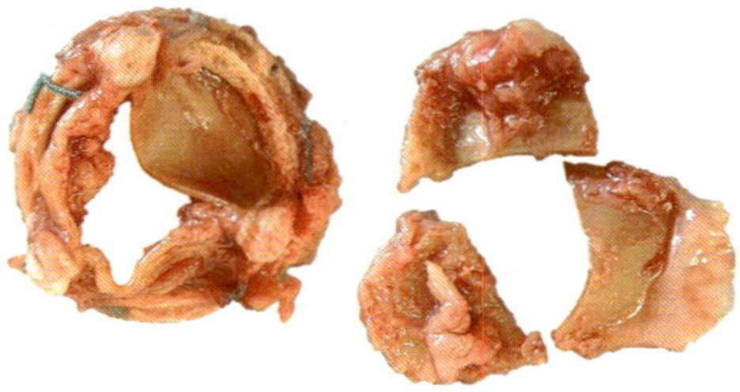

PROSTHETIC VALVE COMPLICATIONS

A serious complication of any prosthetic valve is infective endocarditis.

FIGURE 7.74. Images show a bioprosthetic valve with infectious endocarditis. Leaflet thickening, vegetations, and leaflet destruction are present.

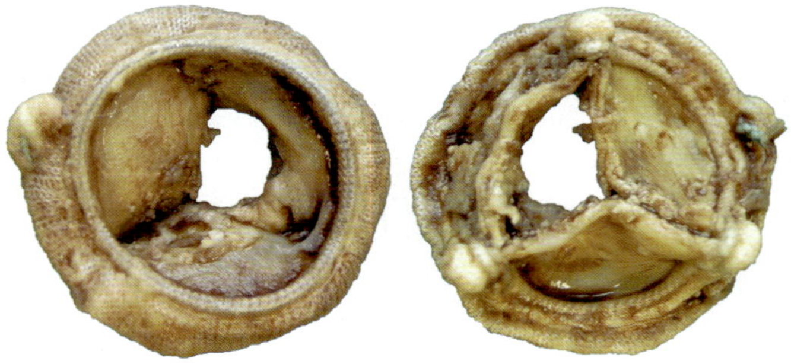

Neoplasms and Masses of the Heart

Cardiac myxoma

Cardiac myxoma, also called atrial myxoma, is the most common primary heart tumor, and most commonly occurs in the left atrium on the septum. It is benign, but it may cause sudden death due to tumor embolization, and it may recur if incompletely resected. Myxomas are polypoid tumors with a smooth or lobulated surface of gelatinous consistency, and are usually white, yellow, or brown. The most common complications of myxomas include heart failure, sudden death, arrhythmias, infection, and embolization.

FIGURE 7.75. The left atrial myxoma in (A) has an irregular surface, tan color, and small focal areas of hemorrhage. The cut surface in (B) has the gelatinous appearance and focal areas of hemorrhage characteristic of cardiac myxoma.

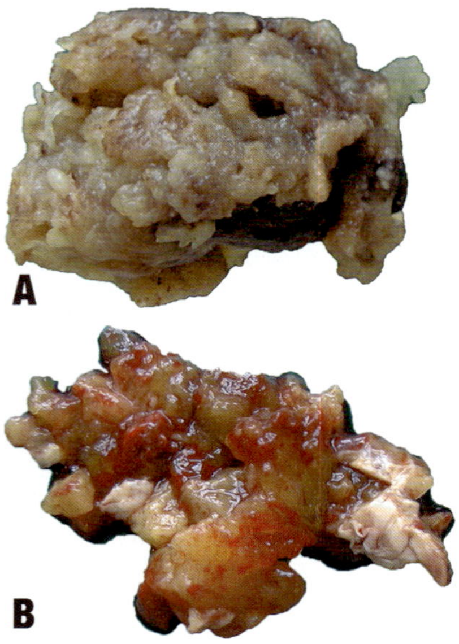

FIGURE 7.76. These images show 2 cardiac myxomas and their cut surfaces. Image (A) shows a polypoid tumor with a white-to-tan and slightly lobulated surface, focal hemorrhage, and a short stalk; image (B) shows the yellow, gelatinous cut surface of this tumor. Image (C) shows a polypoid tumor with white fibrous areas intermingled with red, hemorrhagic areas; image (D) shows the cut surface of this tumor.

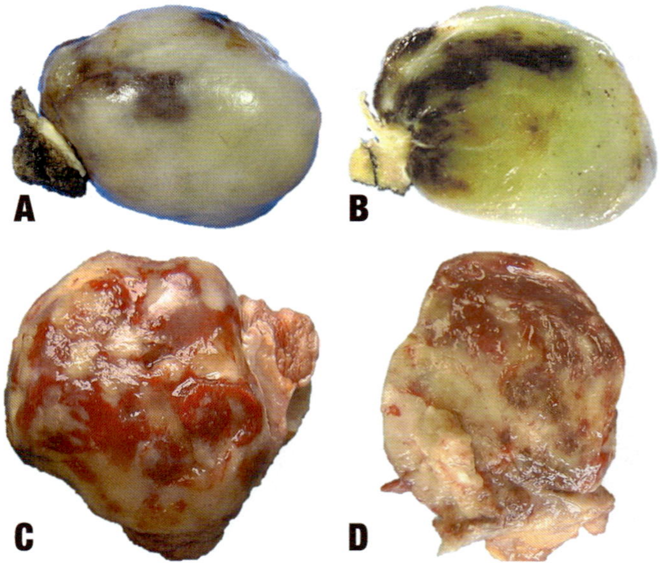

FIGURE 7.77. Image (A) shows an atrial view of a left atrial myxoma with a large, brown tumor (arrow). Image (B) shows an abdominal aorta containing an embolic myxoma tumor; image (C) shows the embolic myxoma material removed from the aorta. Image (D) shows a cardiac myocardial infarction due to myxoma emboli in the coronary artery, showing pale myocardial discoloration. In (E), a myxoma embolus completely occludes a hepatic vessel (arrow).

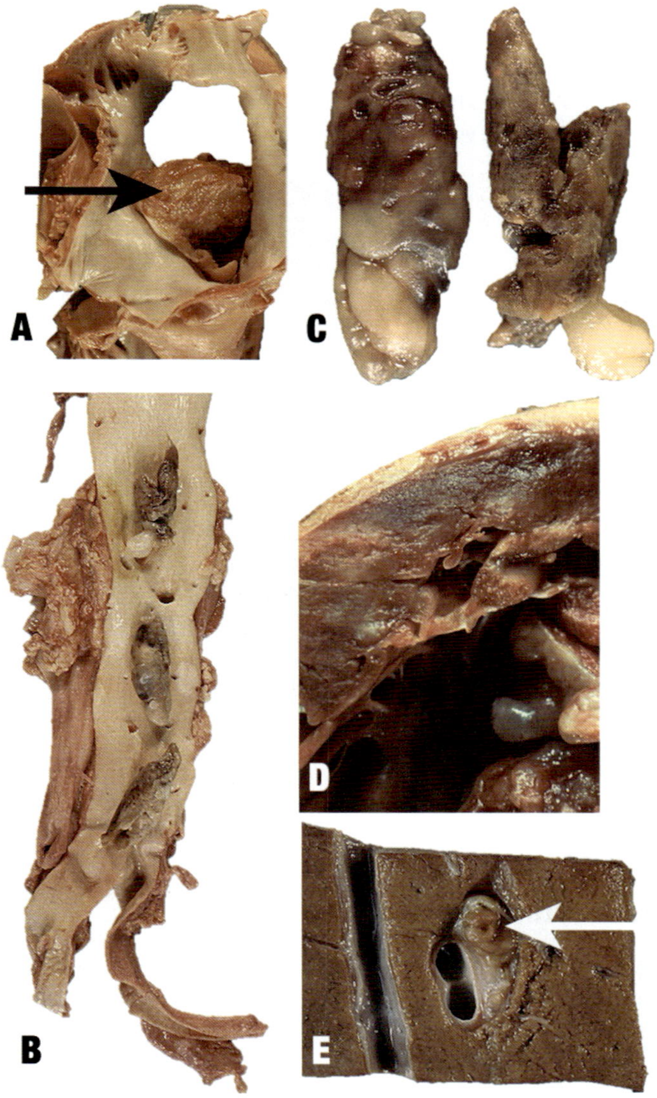

ATRIAL MYXOMA

Atrial myxoma is the most common primary heart tumor. The tumors are benign and most commonly occur in the left atrium on the septum. About 10% are familial, occurring as an autosomal dominant condition, and the rest are sporadic. The mean age of occurrence is 50 years in sporadic cases and 24 years in familial cases.

FIGURE 7.78. The atrial myxoma in (A) is round and brown with a smooth surface. Image (B) shows a gelatinous cut surface with some cysts and solid areas.

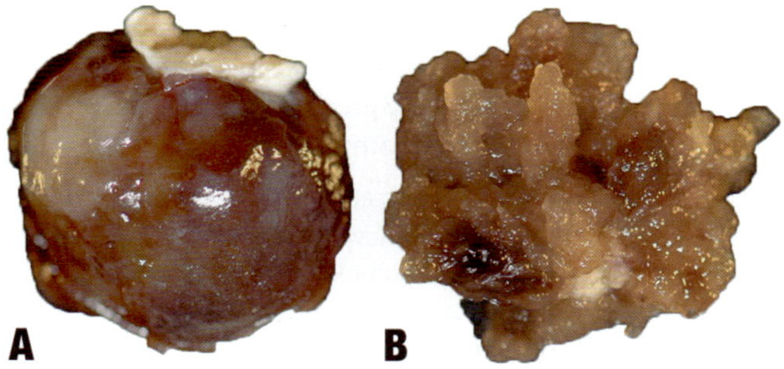

FIGURE 7.79. This image shows left atrial myxoma with *Streptococcus viridans* endocarditis in a 42-year-old male with a history of rheumatic fever. The patient presented with 1 year of malaise, weakness, and weight loss; clubbed fingers; an enlarged spleen; and a positive *S. viridans* blood culture. A large pedunculated tumor (arrow) is attached to the atrium and obstructs the mitral opening. The tumor is ragged and has friable material on the surface.

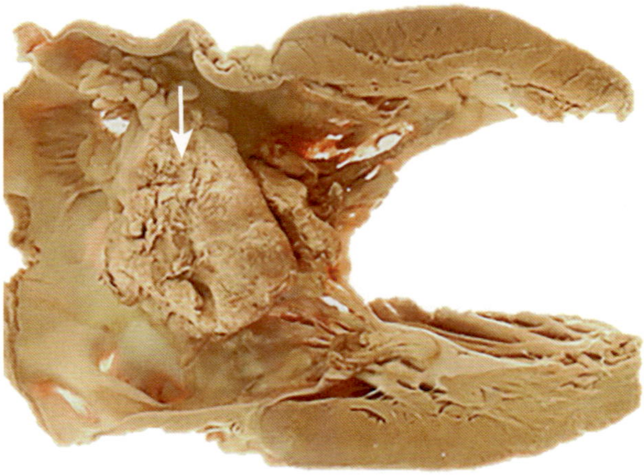

CARNEY SYNDROME

About 7% of atrial myxomas are part of Carney syndrome, recently found to have mutations in *PRKAR1A*. The syndrome consists of cardiac myxoma, breast neoplasms, spotty skin pigmentation, endocrine overactivity, schwannomas, and epithelioid blue nevus.

FIGURE 7.80. The cardiac myxoma shown in (A) is white with a gelatinous, transparent surface. There are focal areas of hemorrhage, and the image shows the site of endocardial attachment (arrow). Image (B) shows the gelatinous appearance of the cut surface.

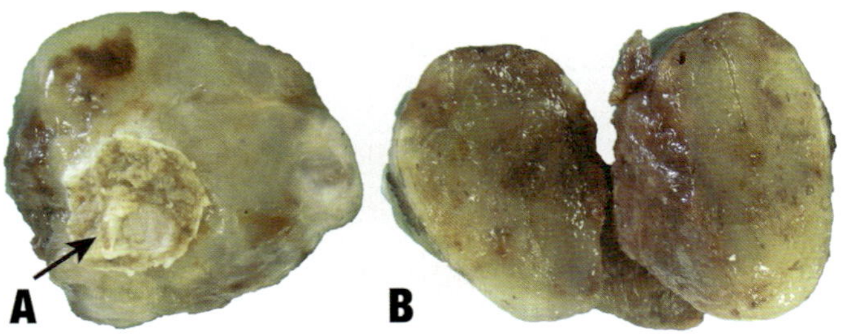

Papillary fibroelastoma

Papillary fibroelastoma is a benign valvular endocardial tumor. It may be related to thrombus or occur postinjury, but often the etiology is unclear. Papillary fibroelastomas arise on valve cusps or leaflets, most often on the aortic valve, as yellow-white papillary projections. They may be associated with neurological complications.

FIGURE 7.81. Image (A) shows an aortic valve with papillary fibroelastoma (arrow). Image (B) shows another example of papillary fibroelastoma with multiple fibroelastic fronds and papillae. Image (C) shows papillary fibroelastoma with characteristic white projections and a short pedicle.

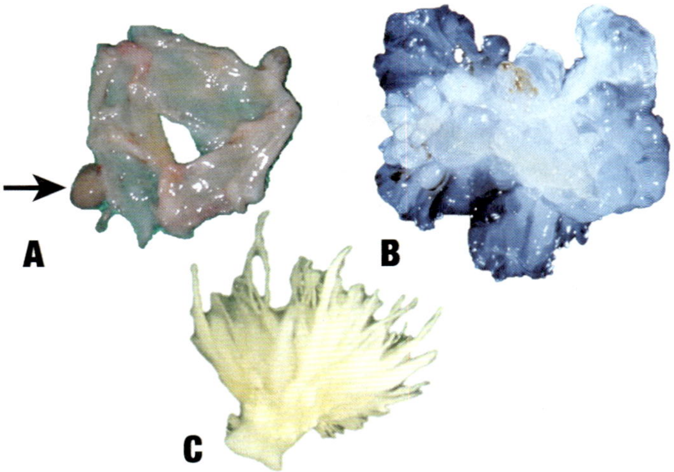

Pericardial hemangioma

Pericardial hemangioma is a rare, benign cardiac tumor characterized by endothelial cells that line interconnecting vascular channels. It can be capillary, cavernous, or arteriovenous. It is often asymptomatic, but may cause pericardial effusion, arrhythmia, cardiac tamponade, and even sudden death.

FIGURE 7.82. Image (A) shows a heart with a left-sided pericardial mass with multiple red-brown nodules, which is a pericardial hemangioma. Image (B) shows a cross-section of the same heart demonstrating the multiple blood-filled, thin-walled channels that form this tumor.

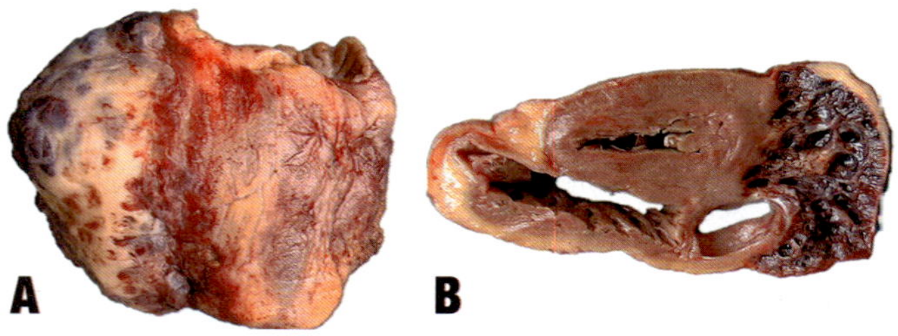

Rhabdomyoma

Rhabdomyoma is considered a hamartoma. It is the most common pediatric cardiac tumor. It is usually detected either in utero or within the first year. When located in the left ventricle or septal areas, tumors may lead to arrhythmias or chamber obstruction. Rhabdomyoma may be associated with tuberous sclerosis (TS), which is either inherited as an autosomal dominant condition or appears sporadically. TS patients show multiple organ hamartomas, including in the brain, kidneys, heart, and skin.

FIGURE 7.83. This heart shows multiple white, well-circumscribed nodules in the left ventricle and septum.

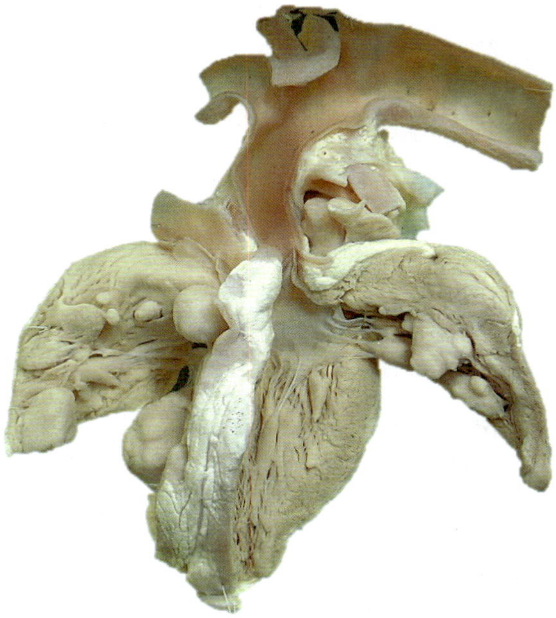

Pericardial cyst

Pericardial cyst is a benign lesion. It can, however, become a mass lesion that displaces local structures, and it may be associated with effusion, pericarditis, and constrictive pericarditis.

FIGURE 7.84. This heart has a bisected pericardial cyst.

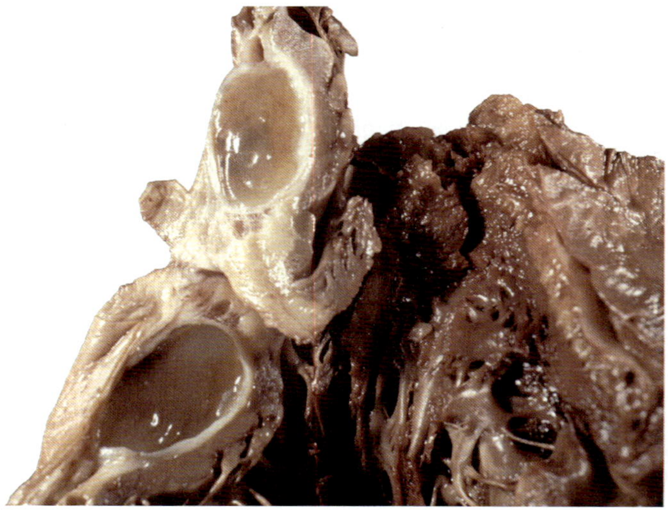

FIGURE 7.85. This is an epicardial view of a heart with a large, protuberant pericardial cyst.

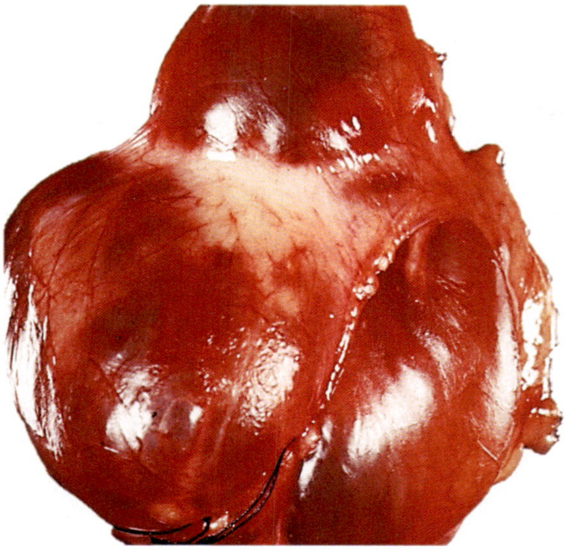

PERICARDIAL PSEUDOCYST

FIGURE 7.86. This image shows a thin capsule and a white, granular, cheese-like, cholesterol-material content.

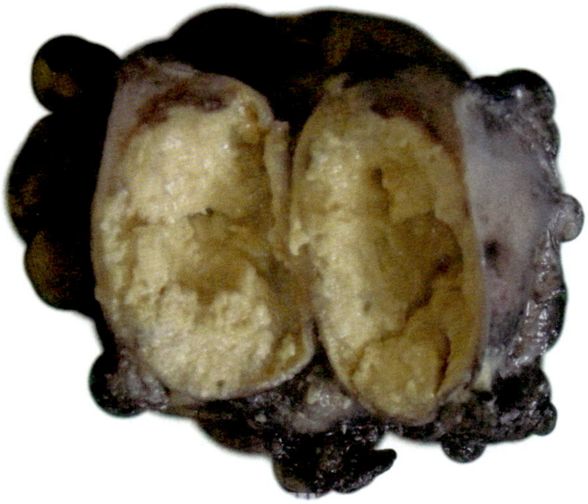

Primary cardiac malignancies

Primary cardiac malignancies are rare. Sarcoma is the most common primary malignancy of the heart and pericardium. Several subtypes exist, including angiosarcoma (the most frequent subtype), rhabdomyosarcoma, fibrosarcoma, leiomyosarcoma, myxosarcoma, and schwannoma.

CARDIAC SARCOMA

Cardiac angiosarcoma has shown p53 mutations. Sarcomas may occur in any chamber. They may present as obstructive lesions that mimic valvular stenotic lesions.

FIGURE 7.87. This image shows a left atrial sarcoma that is high grade and pleomorphic with a white-gray, irregularly lobulated surface.

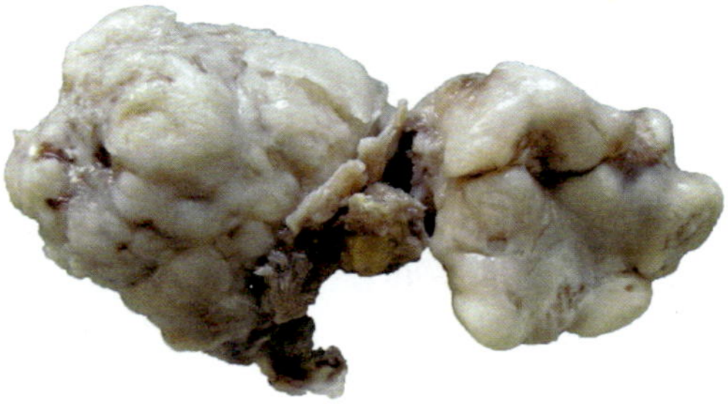

FIGURE 7.88. This heart has a large polypoid right atrial cardiac sarcoma (arrow).

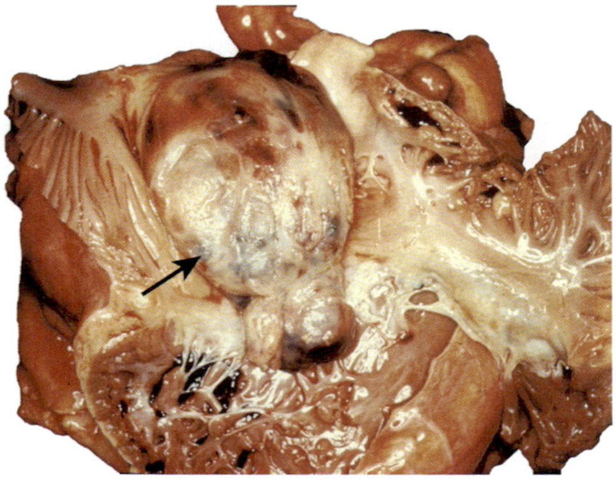

CARDIAC RHABDOMYOSARCOMA

Cardiac rhabdomyosarcoma is a malignant tumor that arises anywhere in the myocardium and often invades the pericardium. It is the most common sarcoma in infants and children. Cardiac rhabdomyosarcoma may metastasize to the lungs, adjacent soft tissues, and liver.

FIGURE 7.89. This heart has a large tumor (arrow) in the right ventricle myocardium extending from the apex to the tricuspid valve.

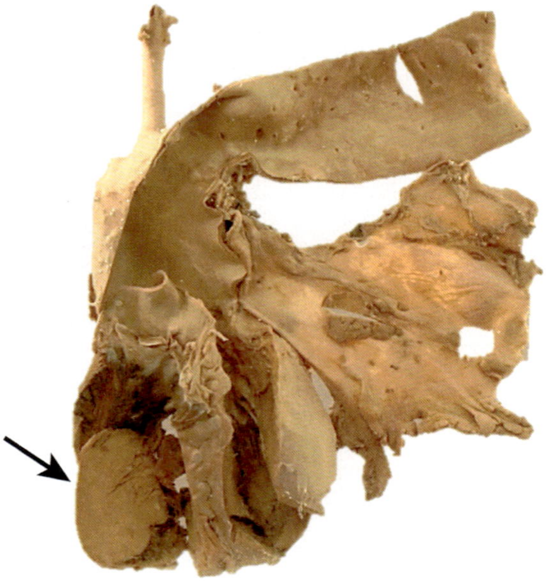

CARDIAC OSTEOSARCOMA

Cardiac osteosarcoma is very rare. It may be mixed with other types of sarcoma differentiation.

FIGURE 7.90. Image (A) shows a left ventricle high-grade osteosarcoma, chondroblastic type, with an irregular lobulated surface. The cross-section in (B) shows a central, firm, bony area with focal cystic change and hemorrhage.

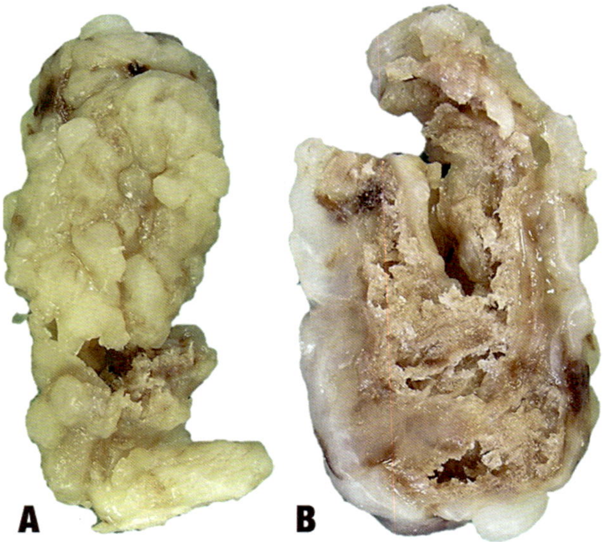

Metastasis to the heart

Secondary neoplastic metastases to the heart and pericardium are more frequent than primary cardiac malignancies. Carcinomas and sarcomas can spread to the heart. Metastases may occur to the epicardium, myocardium, or endocardium. Pericardial and epicardial deposits are quite common and may be accompanied by effusion.

FIGURE 7.91. This image shows a heart with epicardial nodules (arrows), which are more pronounced at the base.

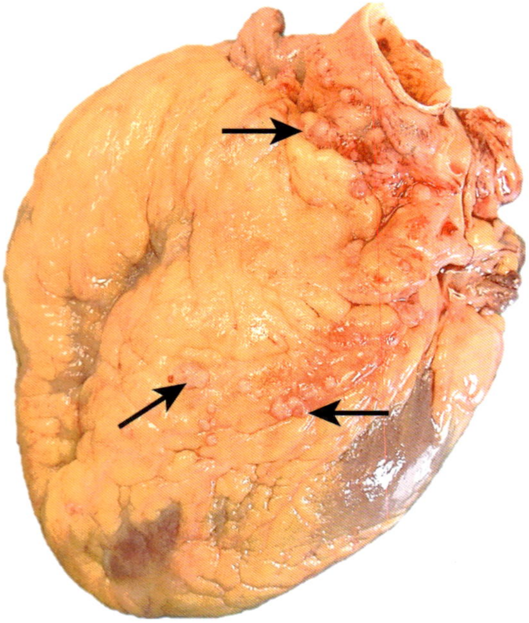

METASTATIC CARCINOMA

FIGURE 7.92. This heart shows an epicardial mass of metastatic carcinoma (arrow).

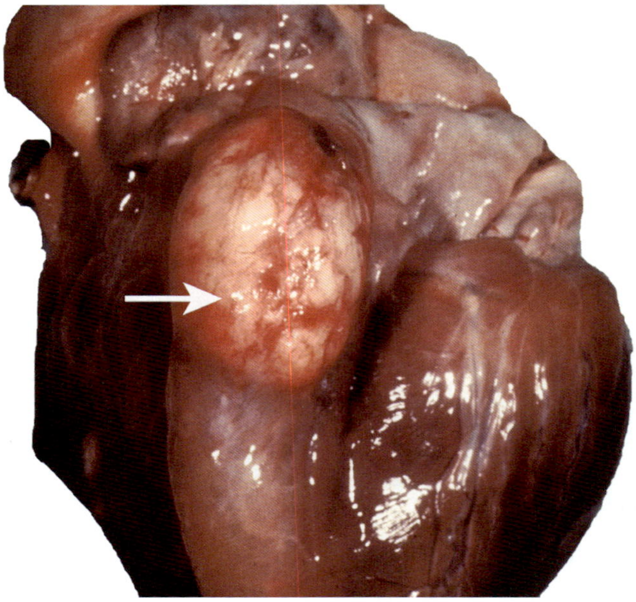

Other lesions

PATENT DUCTUS ARTERIOSUS

The ductus arteriosus is a fetal vessel that connects the pulmonary artery to the heart prior to birth. After birth, the ductus closes, as mature pulmonary circulation takes over. Patency of the ductus may require interventional cardiology or surgical closure.

FIGURE 7.93. This image shows a patent ductus arteriosus with probe.

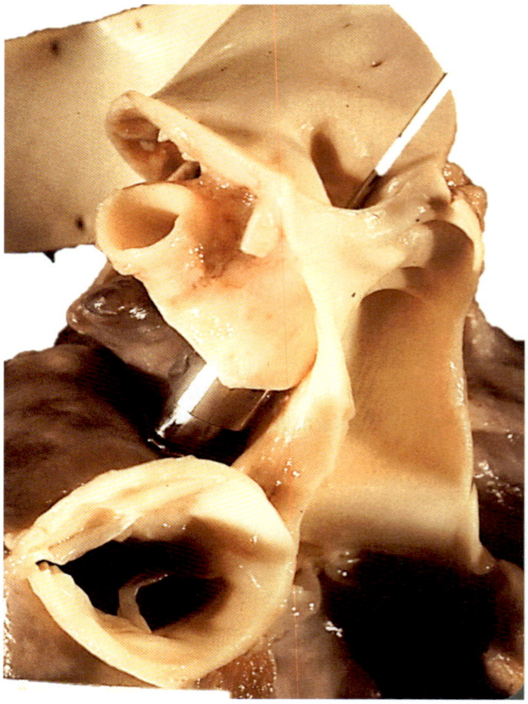

PATENT FORAMEN OVALE

The foramen ovale connects the 2 atria during fetal life. Normally, after birth, left-atrial pressure increases and the defect closes. It is not, however, uncommon for the foramen ovale to remain patent for a short time after birth. A patent foramen ovale may become important if right-atrial pressure increases and the defect opens, causing shunting.

FIGURE 7.94. This image shows a patent foramen ovale, which is open (arrow).

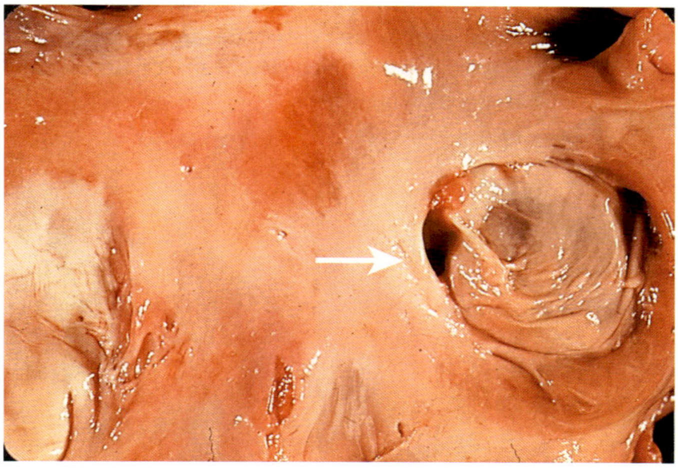

Vessels

Atherosclerosis

Atherosclerosis is a process causing plaque formation in large and medium-sized arteries. It commonly involves the lower abdominal aorta, coronary arteries, popliteal arteries, internal carotid arteries, and vessels of the circle of Willis. The abdominal aorta is usually more affected than the thoracic aorta.

FIGURE 7.95. The specimen in (A) shows atherosclerosis of the abdominal aorta (arrow) mainly below the renal arteries. Image (B) shows a closer view of irregular plaque deposition in the lumen of the aorta.

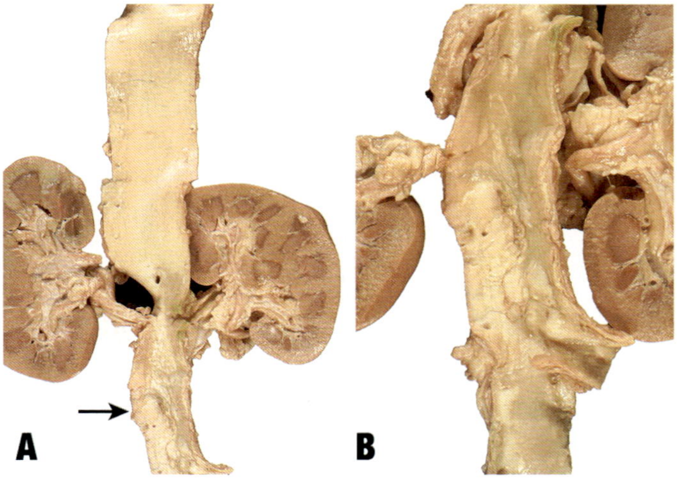

ULCERATION OF ATHEROSCLEROTIC PLAQUES

Atherosclerotic plaques may rupture or ulcerate; the exposure of the plaque may lead to thrombosis, which may compromise the vessel lumen partially or completely. Thrombosis often happens in arteries of the heart (leading to MI, or heart attack), the brain (leading to cerebral infarction, or stroke), and inferior limbs (leading to peripheral vascular disease and, eventually, gangrene of the legs). Atherosclerotic plaques may also be complicated by hemorrhage, embolism, and/or aneurysm formation.

FIGURE 7.96. Image (A) shows severe aortic atherosclerosis obstructing the renal arteries. Image (B) shows a low abdominal aortic thrombus occluding the vessel lumen (arrow indicates vessel cross-section).

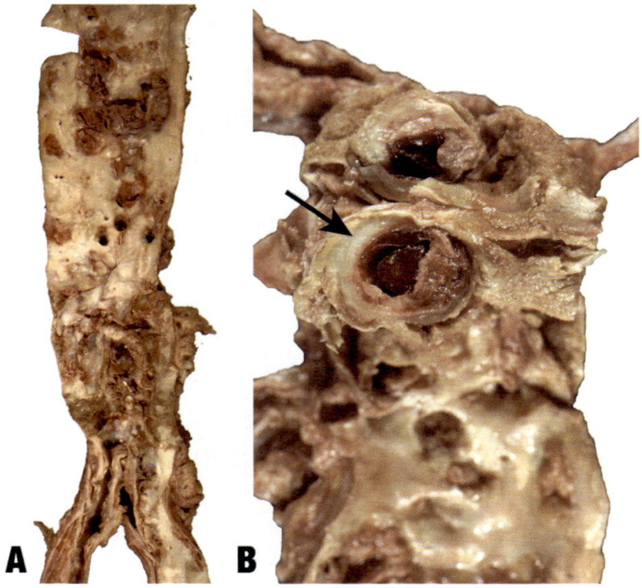

FIGURE 7.97. The specimen in (A) shows a severely complicated aorta atherosclerosis with multiple ulcerated thrombosed plaques. Image (B) shows an abdominal aorta atherosclerotic aneurysm (arrow); (C) gives a closer view of this abdominal aorta aneurysm. Image (D) shows a close-up view of an ulcerated aorta atheromatous plaque with thrombosis.

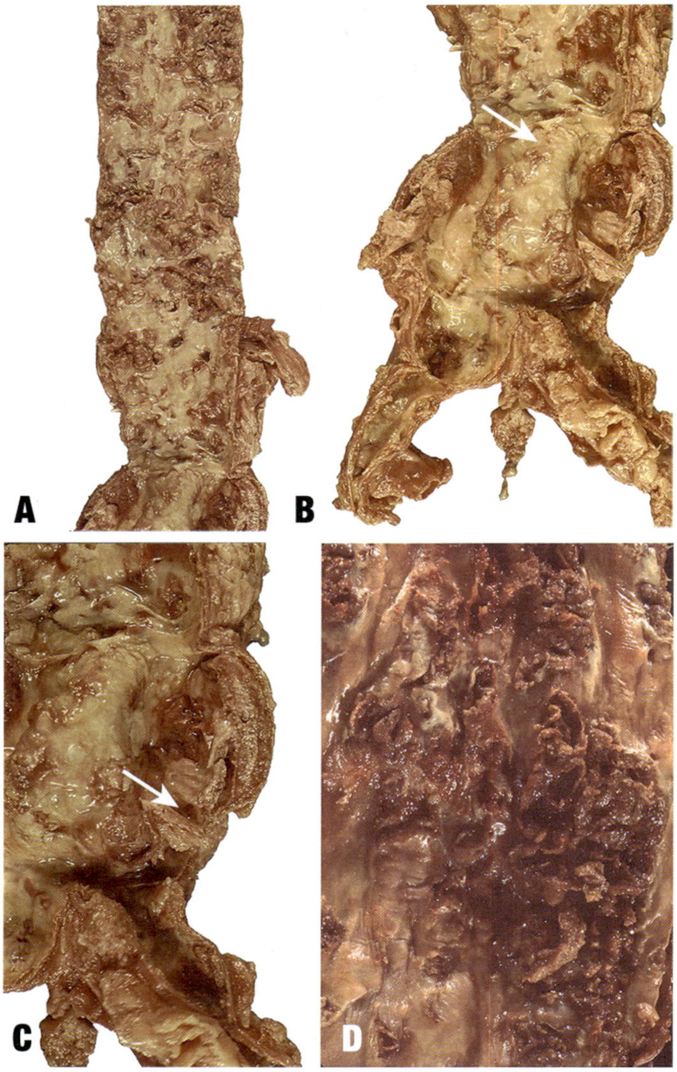

Aneurysm

Morphologically, aneurysms are classified as saccular and fusiform. Saccular aneurysms are round protruding regions affecting only a portion of a vessel wall. They vary in size from 5 cm to 20 cm, and often contain thrombus. Fusiform aneurysms are circumferential dilatations of long segments of an artery; they vary in size.

SACCULAR ANEURYSM

FIGURE 7.98. The specimen in (A) shows multiple saccular aortic aneurysms (arrows). Note the thin, saccular, protrusions of the aortic wall above the renal arteries. Image (B) shows a posterior view of these aneurysms.

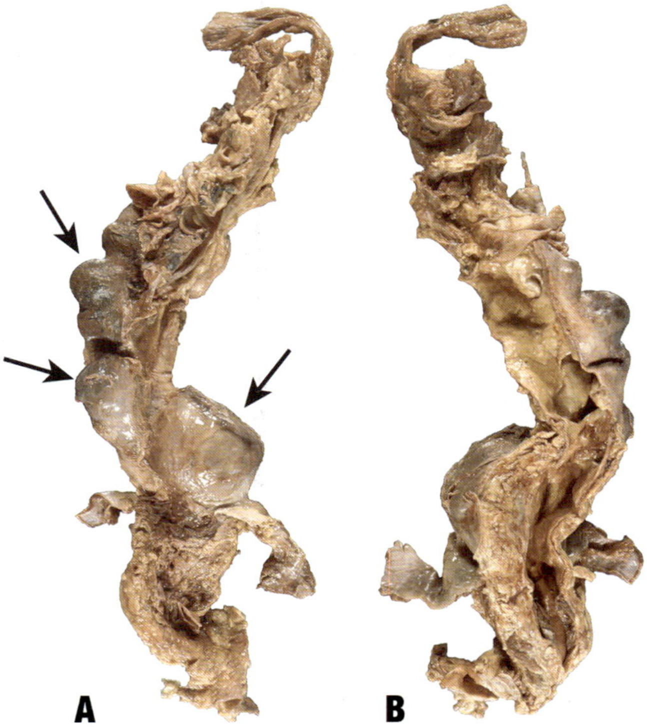

ABDOMINAL AORTIC ANEURYSM (AAA)

AAA is a focal dilation of the aorta that enlarges the diameter of the aorta by 50% or more. It results from degeneration of the medial layer of the arterial wall, which is mainly due to atherosclerosis. The incidence of AAA increases after age 50 and peaks in the eighth decade of life; the male-to-female ratio is 2:1 before age 80, and 1:1 after.

FIGURE 7.99. Image (A) shows AAA (arrow) with fusiform dilatation of the arterial wall; the aneurysm contains organizing thrombus. Image (B) shows another example of an atherosclerotic AAA. Image (C) shows an infrarenal aneurysm that has stenosed the ostia of the renal arteries resulting in bilateral renal atrophy.

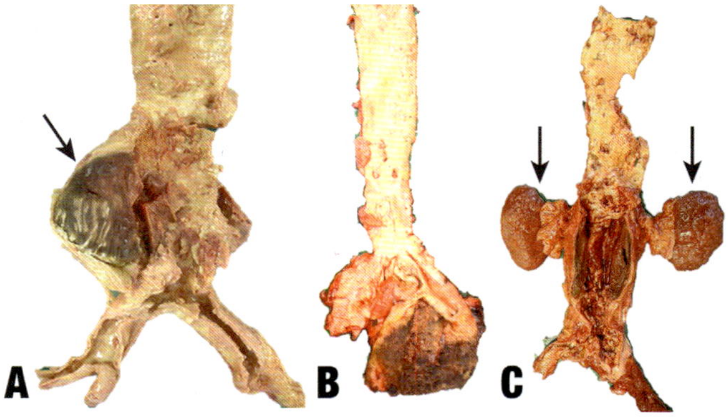

POPLITEAL ARTERY ANEURYSM

Leg claudication or ischemia occurs with popliteal artery aneurysm, which may also involve embolization of the aneurysm thrombus contents.

FIGURE 7.100. Image (A) shows a large, excised popliteal artery aneurysm with an adjacent normal artery. Image (B) shows the opened aneurysm containing thrombus material.

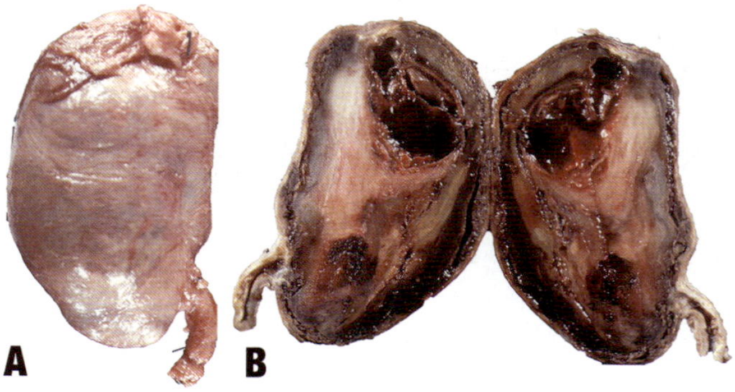

ANEURYSM REPAIR

There are 2 methods for aneurysm surgical repair: 1) open surgical repair (through the abdomen or retroperitoneal approach), and; 2) endovascular aneurysm repair (EVAR). In both procedures, a graft is placed in the arterial lumen. EVAR involves stent grafts.

FIGURE 7.101. Image (A) shows an ascending aorta prosthetic graft replacing an excised atherosclerotic aneurysm. Image (B) shows AAA thrombus content with stent graft.

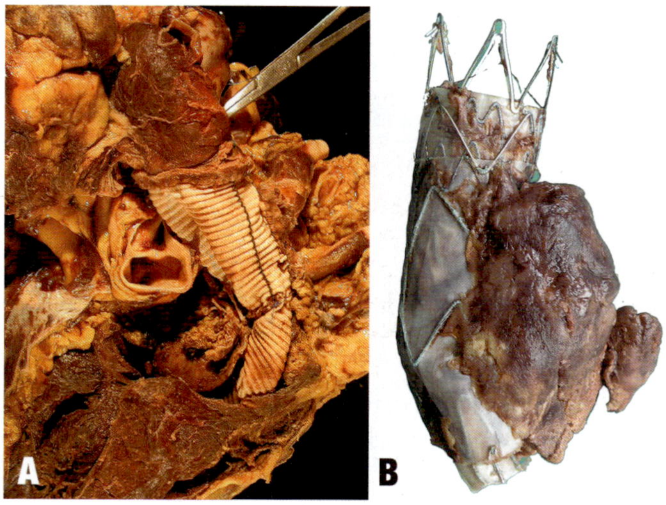

Aortic dissection

An aortic dissection occurs when blood separates the layers of the media and forms a blood-filled channel within the aortic wall. Incidence of aortic dissection is highest in patients with hypertension, congenitally bicuspid aortic valve, and connective tissue disorders such as Marfan and Ehlers–Danlos syndromes. Aortic dissections are also more frequent between the ages of 40 and 70, with a peak at age 65; Marfan patients may present in the third and fourth decades of life.

FIGURE 7.102. Image (A) shows an old aortic dissection with separation of the media layer (arrow). Image (B) shows a posterior view of the same aortic dissection. The false lumen contains thrombus.

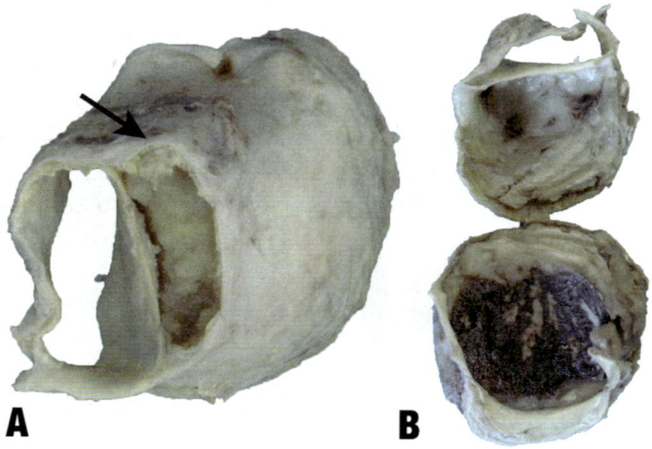

Aortic rupture and Ehlers–Danlos syndrome

Ehlers–Danlos syndrome is associated with arterial rupture and visceral perforation.

Ehlers–Danlos syndrome is a group of more than 10 inherited connective tissue disorders. Clinical manifestations are joint hypermobility, skin hyperelasticity, and weakness of tissues including blood vessels. Type IV Ehlers–Danlos involves a decrease of type III collagen, which is linked to *COL3A1* gene mutation. It is due to an autosomal dominant disorder.

FIGURE 7.103. This specimen shows aortic rupture in a patient with Ehlers–Danlos syndrome.

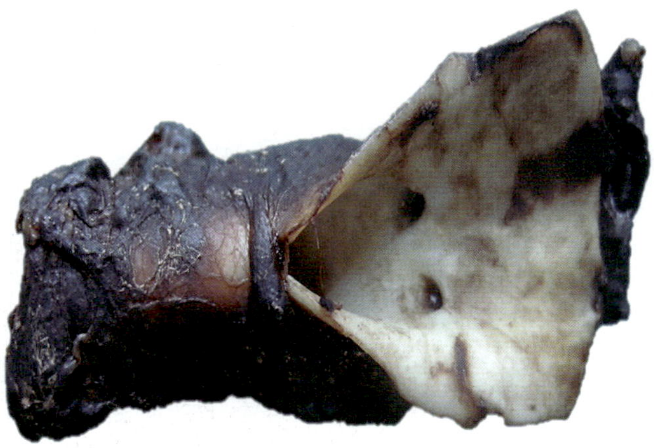

Aortic graft

Aortic grafts may thrombose or become chronically occluded. Distal vessel disease may progress and the grafts can fail.

FIGURE 7.104. In (A), aortic and distal branch prosthetic grafts are occluded by thrombus (arrows). Image (B) shows severe aortic atherosclerosis, and peripheral vascular-surgery grafts that are occluded by thrombus. Image (C) shows aortic bifurcation with occlusion of aortic iliac grafts.

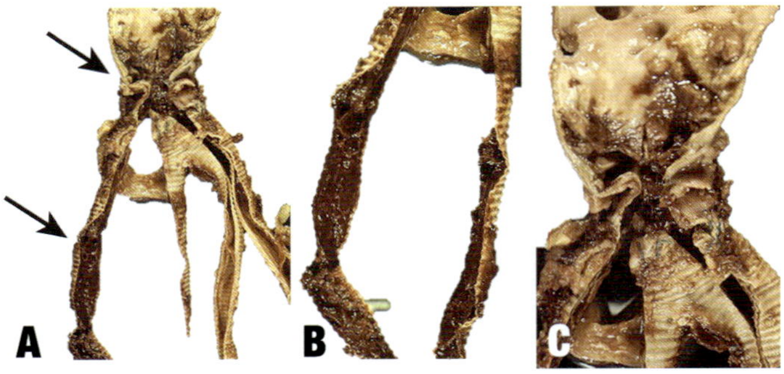

FIGURE 7.105. Image (A) shows severe aortic atherosclerosis with an aortofemoral prosthetic bypass graft (arrow). Image (B) gives another example of an aortofemoral prosthetic bypass graft (arrow).

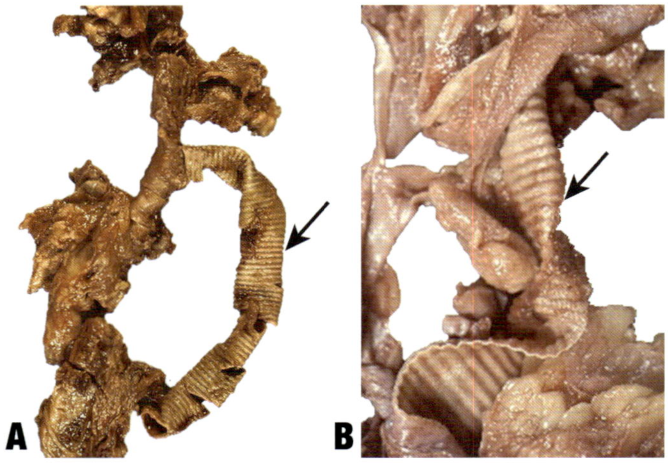

Peripheral arterial disease

Peripheral arterial disease is a manifestation of insufficient tissue perfusion. It is usually secondary to atherosclerosis. The most common manifestations are claudication (reproducible lower-limb pain triggered by exercise and relieved by rest), and ulcers of the toes and/or pressure points.

FIGURE 7.106. Image (A) shows a below-the-knee amputation that was performed due to ischemia with ulcers of the medial aspects of the heel and foot. Image (B) shows toe ulceration due to ischemia. Image (C) shows a digit amputation due to ischemia.

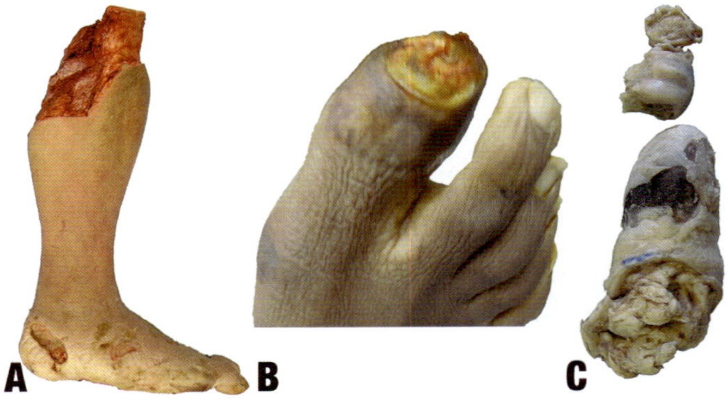

Aortic tumor infiltration

Lymphomas, sarcomas, and carcinomas may lead to aortic infiltration by local extension and invasion of the vessel.

FIGURE 7.107. Images (A) and (B) show adventitial infiltration of the aorta by tumors (arrow). Image (C) shows infiltration of the aorta by a tumor (arrow).

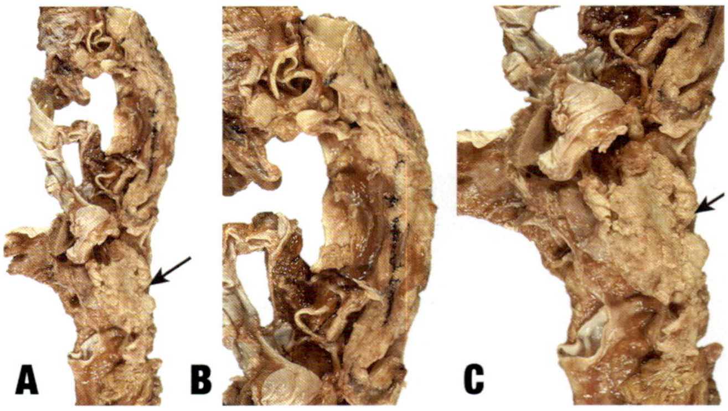

REFERENCES

Cunningham KS, Veinot JP, Butany J. An approach to endomyocardial biopsy interpretation. J Clin Pathol. 2006;59(2):121–129. https://doi.org/10.1136/jcp.2005.026443. Medline:16443725

DiPatre PL, Carter D. *Sternberg's diagnostic surgical pathology review*. Philadelphia: Lippincott Williams & Wilkins; 2004.

Haber MH, Paolo Gattuso P, David O, Spitz DF, Betlej T. *Differential diagnosis in surgical pathology*. 1st ed. Philadelphia: Saunders; 2002.

Kumar V, Abbas AK, Fausto N, Aster J. *Robbins and Cotran pathologic basis of disease*. 8th ed. Philadelphia: Saunders/Elsevier; 2010.

Lester SC. *Manual of surgical pathology*. 2nd ed. Philadelphia: Elsevier Churchill Livingstone; 2006.

Silver MD, Gottlieb AL, Schoen FJ. *Cardiovascular pathology*. 3rd ed. Philadelphia: Churchill Livingstone; 2001.

8

Skin Diseases

SUNGMI JUNG, MARGARET REDPATH, KATHERINE LACH, ELIZABETH O'BRIEN, AIMILIOS LALLAS

Psoriasis

Psoriasis is an autoimmune disease that can be localized or it can cover the entire body surface. It has 5 main types: plaque, guttate, inverse, pustular, and erythrodermic. The plaque form is the most common, also known as psoriasis vulgaris.

FIGURE 8.1. This image shows the characteristic white scales of psorasis vulgaris.

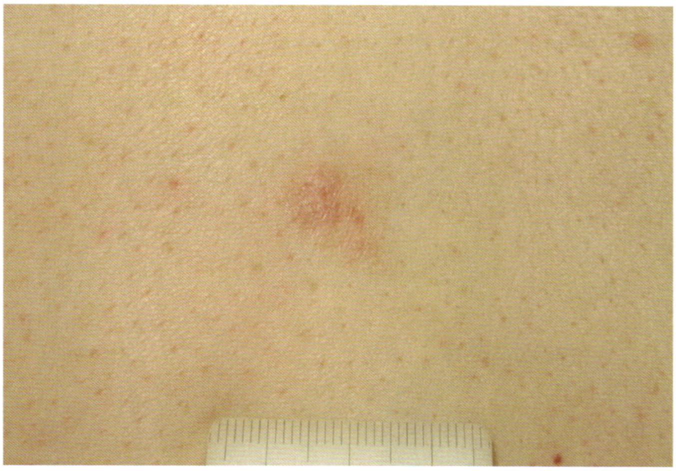

Mycosis fungoides

Mycosis fungoides is a common form of cutaneus T-cell lymphoma with unknown etiology. It is more commonly seen in men than women and can progress from patches to plaques or tumor-like lesions and can involve the entire body.

FIGURE 8.2. This image shows a red patch with the characteristic linear vessels of mycosis fungoides.

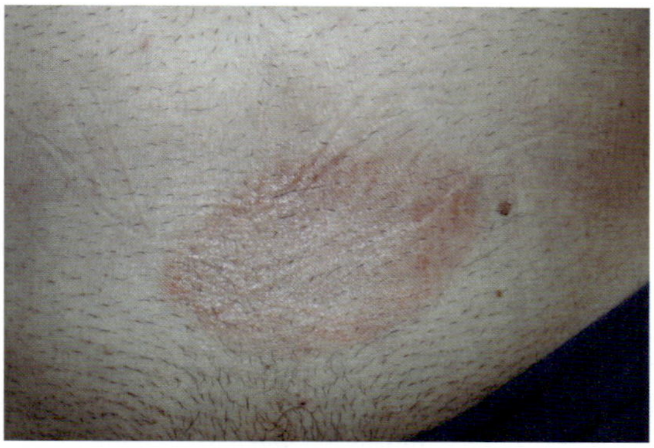

Discoid lupus erythematosus (DLE)

DLE is the skin manifestation of an autoimmune disease named systemic lupus erythematosus (SLE) that can also affect the joints, kidneys, brain, and other organs. It typically presents with coin-shaped inflamed skin patches with a scaling crust on the surface. DLE can lead to severe scarring, and without treatment, it can last for years.

FIGURE 8.3. This image shows an early stage of DLE with characteristic folicular keratin plugs.

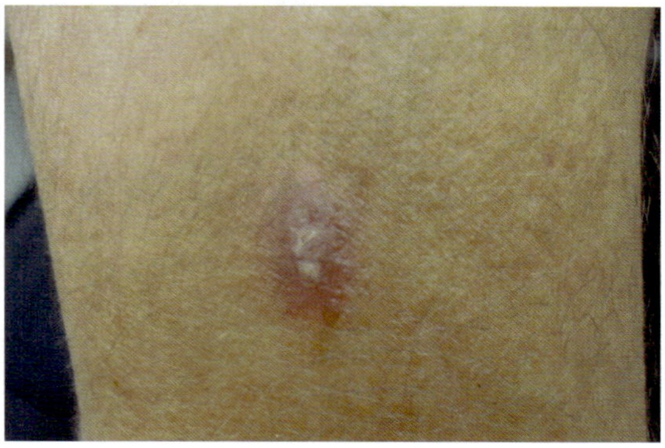

Lichen sclerosus (LS)

LS is a chronic skin disorder that is most common in postmenopausal women, affecting the vulva or the area around the anus. In men, it typically affects the tip of the penis.

FIGURE 8.4. This image of LS shows characteristic white-yellowish keratotic follicular plugs over a white background.

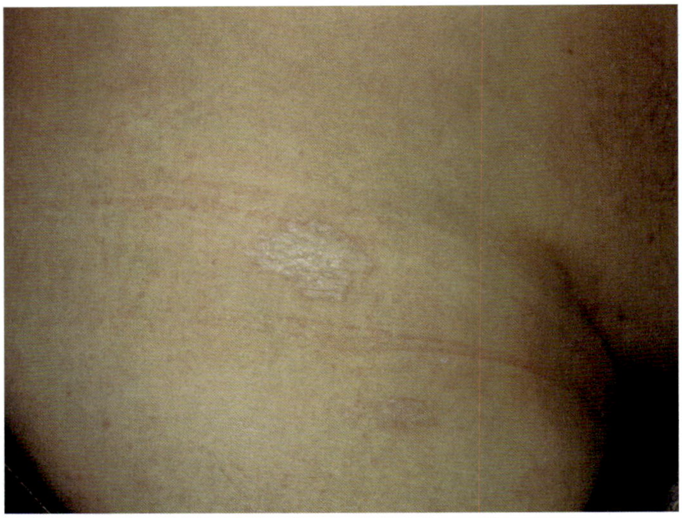

Rosacea

Rosacea is a chronic inflammatory skin disease involving the face, commonly seen in 30- to 50-year-old Caucasians. It is characterized by redness, pimples, swelling, and small, superficial dilated blood vessels.

FIGURE 8.5. This image of rosacea shows facial redness with fine linear vessels arranged in horizontal and vertical lines.

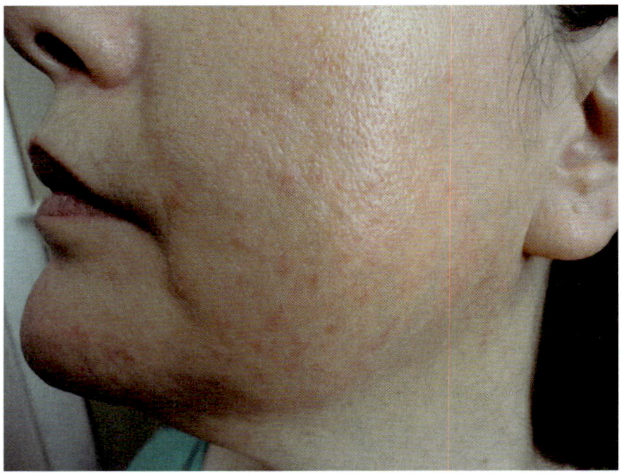

Porokeratosis

Porokeratosis is a rare skin disorder that typically presents as small, round skin patches with a thin, raised border. Although it is usually benign, a small number of people may develop skin cancer within the lesion.

FIGURE 8.6. This image shows a characteristic well-defined, thin, white-yellow peripheral annular rim.

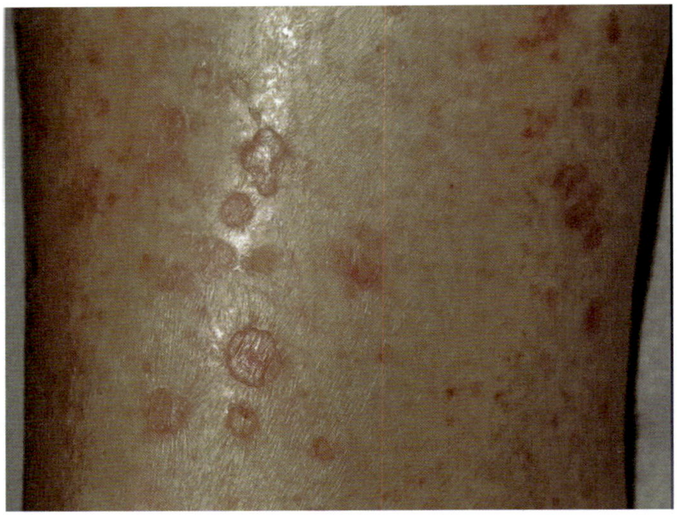

Neonatal lupus

Neonatal lupus is a rare syndrome associated with antinuclear and anti-SSA/Ro antibodies. A rash develops in utero, or soon after birth, that tends to resolve after several weeks or months. The infant is at risk of developing heart block and bradycardia. The rash commonly involves the extremities, scalp, and periorbital region.

FIGURE 8.7. These images show examples of how neonatal lupus may present: (A) erythematous annular papulosquamous rash; (B) periorbital erythema and edema resulting in neonatal lupus "owl eye" or "eye mask"; and (C) crusted erythematous plaques.

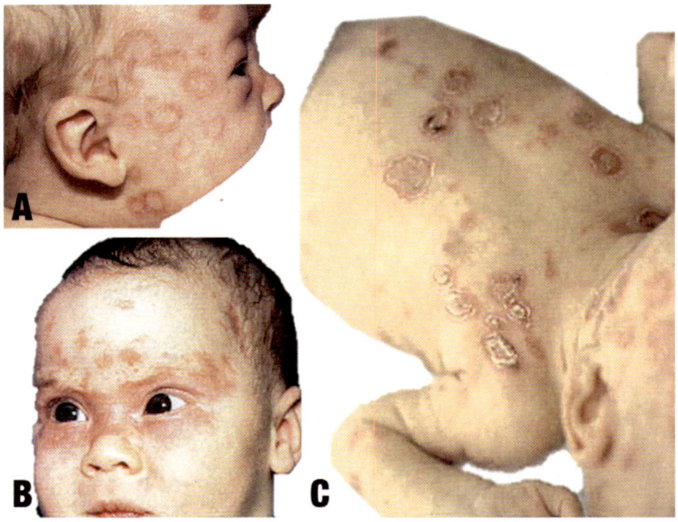

Diabetes-induced ulceration

Diabetic patients develop macrovascular and microvascular angiopathy, making them prone to ulcer formation. Macrovascular disease includes endothelial dysfunction and atherosclerosis that can impair perfusion; this can lead to ischemia of tissue, or inadequate delivery of inflammatory cells or proteins required for tissue repair. Microvascular disease involves increased permeability and thickening of the capillary basement membrane, leading to distal symmetric peripheral neuropathy of the extremities. This makes patients less sensitive to injuries in the "glove and stocking" distribution. Toe ulceration is a common complication of poorly controlled diabetes.

FIGURE 8.8. The image shows an amputated ulcerated toe from a diabetic patient.

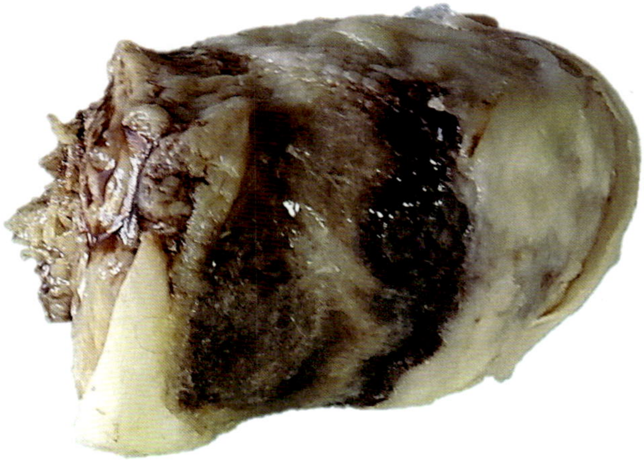

Cutaneous horns

Cutaneous horns are clinically diagnosed keratinized protrusions of skin that may result from a wide variety of underlying benign and malignant conditions. The horn is typically conical in shape with a hardened texture. As the horn becomes longer, it is common for it to curve. A cutaneous horn is at least half as tall as its widest diameter; the height of this type of lesion distinguishes it from similar, flatter lesions such as warts. A height less than the diameter of the base, particularly in an erythematous horn, may indicate the presence of squamous cell carcinoma.

FIGURE 8.9. This image shows well-developed horny processes removed from the skin of a scalp. The processes are hard and bony in consistency, and consist of keratinized material.

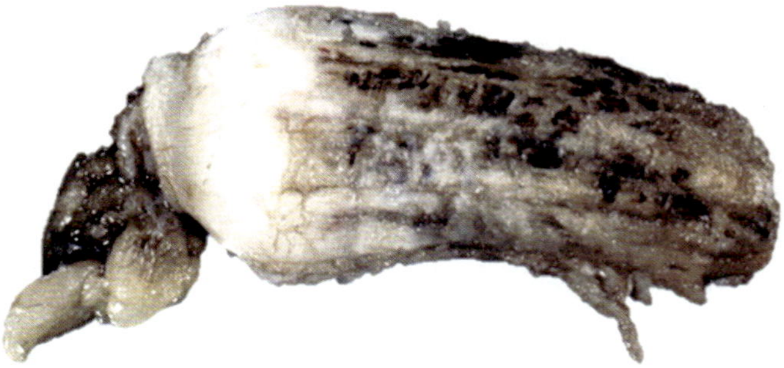

Verruca vulgaris

Verruca vulgaris is caused by human papilloma virus (HPV) — most commonly HPV-2, although types 1, 4, and 7 may also be implicated. It most frequently occurs in children and adolescents. Typically, it is a self-resolving lesion that produces only cosmetic problems for the patient.

FIGURE 8.10. This image shows an ellipse of skin featuring an excised growth composed of heaped-up smooth, skin-colored, coalescing projections with finger-like morphology.

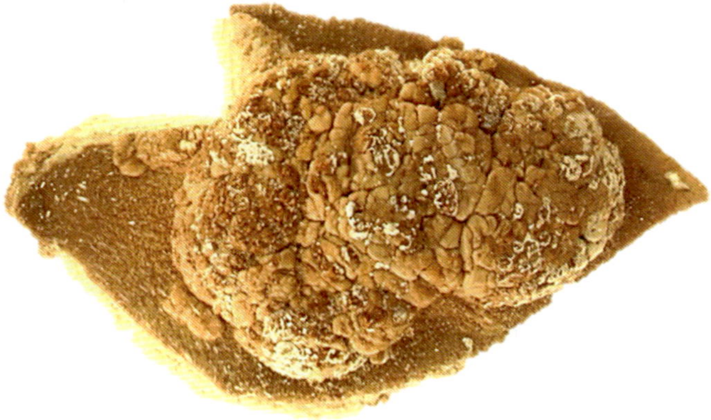

Seborrheic keratosis

Seborrheic keratoses are very common benign lesions that present as sharply delineated, brown-black, warty plaques on the face, chest and/or back of middle-aged and elderly people. Their dark pigmentation can be clinically mistaken for melanoma. Sudden onset of numerous seborrheic keratoses (known as the Leser–Trélat sign) may occur in association with internal malignancy; gastric adenocarcinoma is the most commonly related malignancy.

FIGURE 8.11. This case of seborrheic keratosis was related to gastric adenocarcinoma.

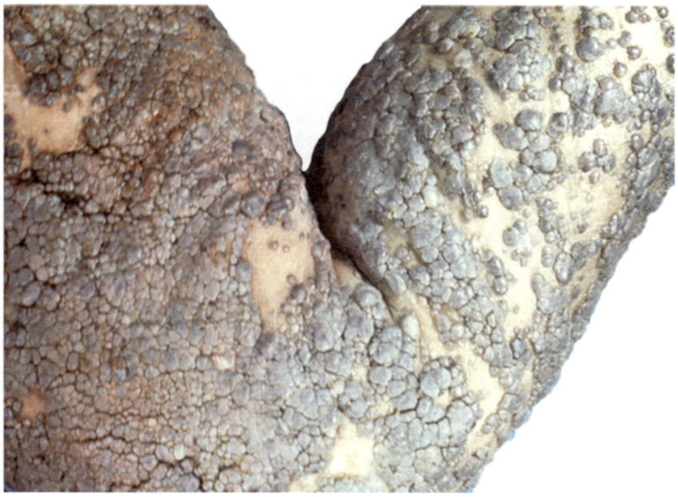

Bowenoid actinic keratosis

Bowenoid actinic keratosis is a premalignant lesion secondary to excessive sun exposure, particularly ultraviolet B radiation. It presents as multiple erythematous-to-pigmented, scaly lesions on frequently sun-exposed areas of the body in middle-aged or elderly people. The word *bowenoid* refers to histologic findings displaying a full-thickness, keratinocytic dysplasia.

FIGURE 8.12. This image shows a bowenoid actinic keratosis of the scalp. Multiple macules and papules that are hyperpigmented and scaly appear on a background of Caucasian, hairless skin.

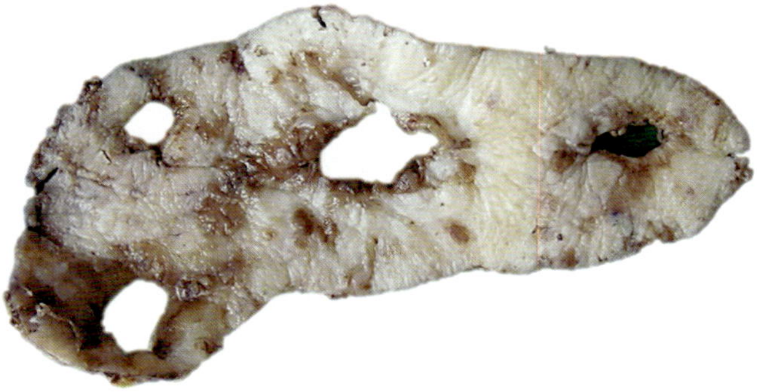

Squamous cell carcinoma (SCC)

The pathogenesis of SCC can include direct sun exposure, immunosuppression, chronic irritation, inflammation, and HPV infection. SCC begins in the superficial epidermis and invades downward into the dermis. Occasionally, infiltration may extend along blood vessels and nerves, and aggressive tumors may invade the subcutaneous tissues. Perineural invasion, deep spread, poor differentiation, and acantholysis, along with narrow surgical margins, increase the risk of metastasis. SCC has a spectrum of clinical presentations: on one end, it may present as sharply defined scaly plaques (in situ); on the other, as invasive, protuberant, nodular lesions with ulceration and keratin production.

FIGURE 8.13. Image (A) shows an ulcerated endophytic tumor with rolled, thickened borders. Image (B) shows a wide excision of a nodular exophytic tumor with a smooth, lobulated surface and without ulceration.

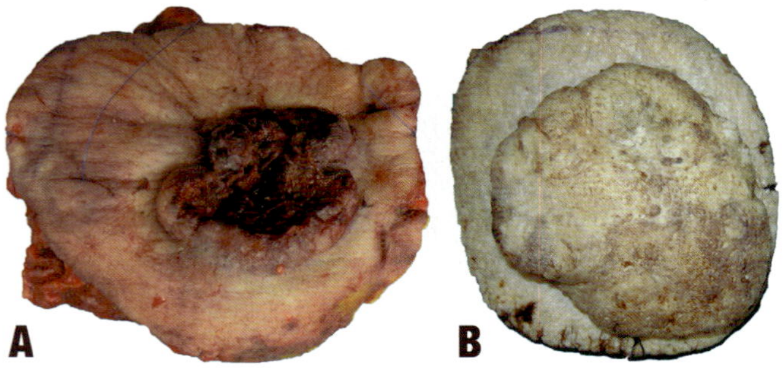

FIGURE 8.14. This image shows a wide excision of a tumor with surrounding normal tissue. The tumor has rolled, thickened, keratinized borders surrounding a deep ulcer crater.

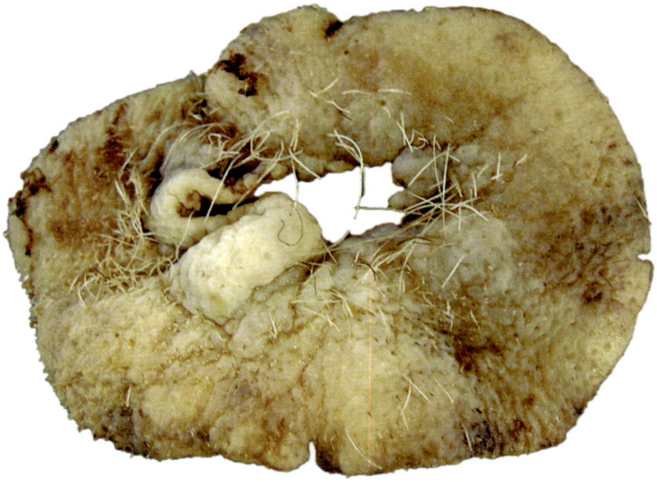

FIGURE 8.15. Image (A) shows a wide excision of a nodule of exophytic tumor with surrounding plaque and scale on hair-bearing skin. Image (B) shows SCC from a lip that has twin nodules of exophytic, skin-colored tumors. The left nodule has apical ulceration and overlying hyperkeratotic ulceration.

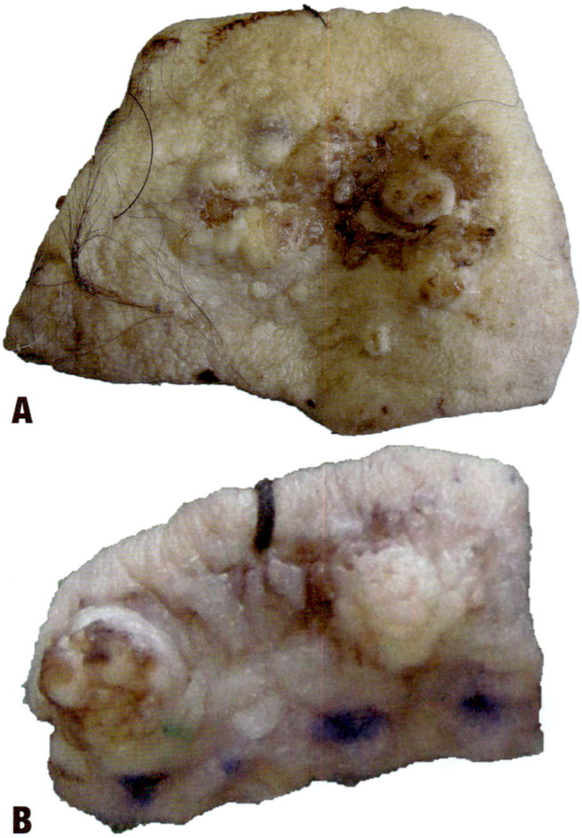

HIGH-RISK SCC

High-risk factors of SCC include anatomic site, degree of differentiation, anatomic thickness, anatomic level, and perineural and lymphovascular invasion. High-risk anatomic sites include the maxilla, mandible, orbit, and temporal bone. Invasion of the skeleton or perineural invasion of the skull base is staged T4. Tumor thickness, or Breslow depth, is measured at a right angle from the granular layer to the point of deepest tumor invasion. When a tumor is ulcerated, the base of the ulcer constitutes the upper point of reference. SCC with invasion > 4 mm and diameter > 2 cm is considered high risk.

FIGURE 8.16. Images (A) and (B) show elliptical excisions of hair-bearing skin with ulcerated craters. Note the keratin-like gray debris filling the crater in (A).

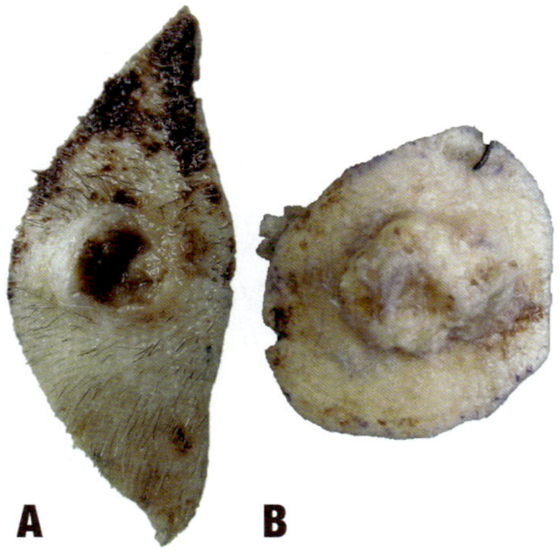

FIGURE 8.17. Image (A) shows an SCC of the right lateral canthus. Congested, nodular, rolled borders overhang a central ulcer with an indurated and hemorrhagic base. In (B), the destructive lesion has invaded deep into the dermis and subcutaneous tissue.

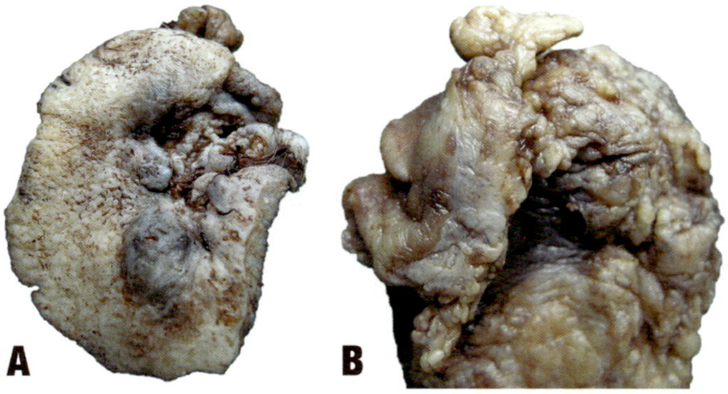

METASTATIC SCC

SCC causes local tissue destruction and has the potential to metastasize, primarily to regional lymph nodes; in-transit metastases also occur. The overall metastatic rate is in the range of 3% to 4%, but in transplant patients on immunosuppressive therapies, metastases have often already occurred by the time of primary tumor detection. Higher rates of metastatic spread are also found in SCCs arising from radiation dermatitis, chronic osteomyelitis sinus tracts, and burn scars.

FIGURE 8.18. This image shows a deeply invasive SCC of the manubrium. The tumor itself is not visible, but excised deep tissue and bone involved with SCC are visible.

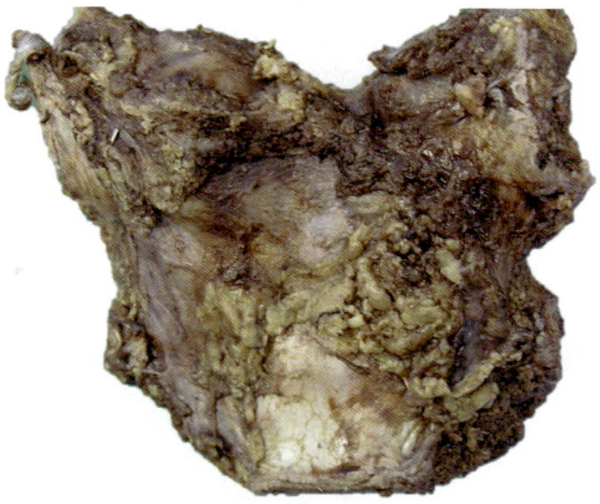

PROCEDURE: ELLIPTICAL SURGICAL EXCISION OF SCC

Elliptical surgical excisions allow for stepwise histopathologic examination for depth of invasion and permit easy therapeutic reexcision, if necessary. They can be sutured closed without undue tension on the skin.

FIGURE 8.19. This image shows an elliptical excision of a nodular, exophytic growth.

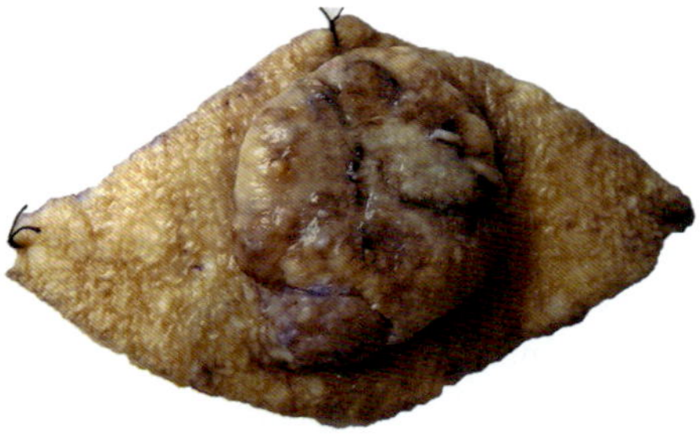

MARJOLIN ULCER

Marjolin ulcer is an aggressive, ulcerating SCC that arises from chronically inflamed and scarred skin from prior trauma, burn, vascular stasis, varicose vein, osteomyelitis, or radiation. Marjolin ulcer may be difficult to distinguish clinically from other etiologies of ulceration. Any chronic, nonhealing ulcerated lesion merits a biopsy to rule out SCC.

FIGURE 8.20. This image shows an irregular, ulcerative lesion with dirty exudate at its central base and raised edge, in an inflamed and scarred skin. This lesion was diagnosed as Marjolin ulcer.

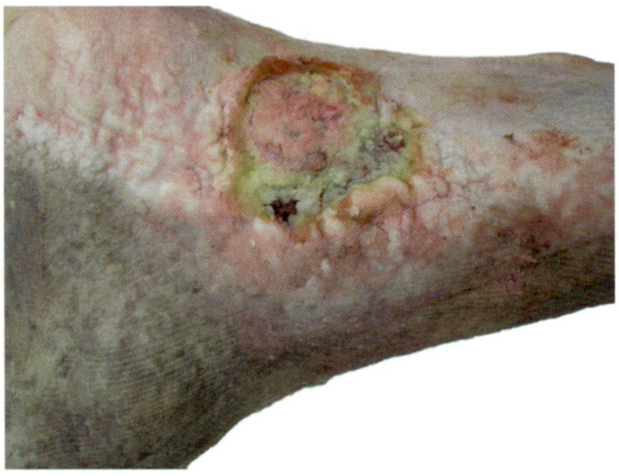

VERRUCOUS CARCINOMA OF THE BUCCAL MUCOSA

Verrucous carcinoma is a slow-growing variant of SCC that commonly affects the oral cavity secondary to chronic irritation or inflammation from ill-fitting dentures, poor oral hygiene, or the use of chewing tobacco or betel nut. Prognosis is excellent with complete excision.

FIGURE 8.21. The lesion in this image is a white-tan, cauliflower-like, fungating mass of the interior oral mucosa. Local spread is evident in adjacent heaped-up lobules of tan tissue.

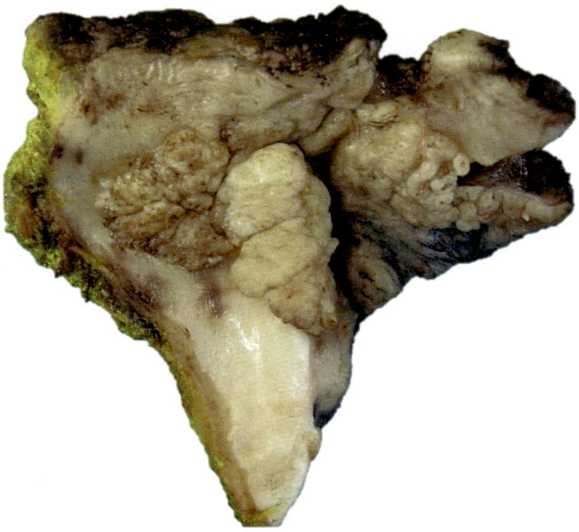

KERATOACANTHOMA

Keratoacanthoma is appropriately considered a low-grade SCC. It is clinically characterized by a rapidly growing, but self-regressing, tumor on sun-damaged skin. It rarely recurs and has essentially no metastasis.

FIGURE 8.22. Images (A) and (B) show flesh-colored, umbilicated nodules with keratin-filled central craters. Image (C) shows the typical development of a keratoacanthoma on a background of sun-damaged skin.

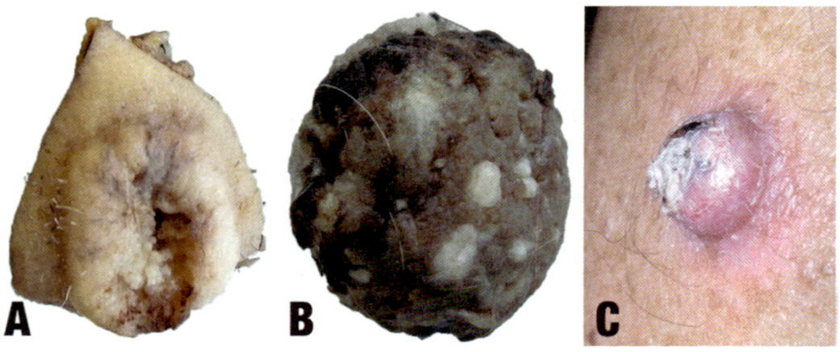

Basal cell carcinoma (BCC)

BCC is the most common tumor in humans. It may invade locally, but metastasis is very rare. The typical appearances of BCC include nodular, ulcerating, sclerosing, superficial multicentric, and pigmented types. Risk factors for BCC include ultraviolet-radiation exposure, arsenic exposure, radiation therapy, immunosuppression, and Gorlin syndrome. BCC occurs most frequently on the face: the nasolabial folds, the medial and lateral canthi, and the posterior ear are the most high-risk areas. BCC on the extremities is not as common; however, any skin surface with trichoblasts is susceptible. Clinically, BCC can present as pearly white, dome-shaped nodules or papules with prominent telangiectatic surface vessels. Later, surface ulceration can occur. Histologically, BCC is characterized by lobules, columns, bands, or cords of basaloid cells.

FIGURE 8.23. Image (A) shows a wide excision of an exophytic, skin-colored tumor with a rolled, elevated, translucent, and well-delineated border. The lesion in (B) has irregular borders and variegated coloration with hues from chalky white to hemorrhagic brown. When BCCs are pigmented, as in (B), they mimic melanoma.

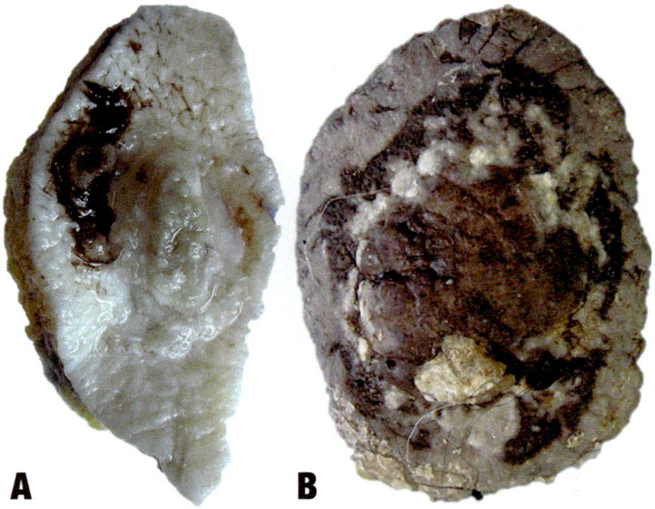

FIGURE 8.24. Images (A) and (B) show wide excisions of exophytic, skin-colored tumors with surrounding normal tissue and underlying dermis.

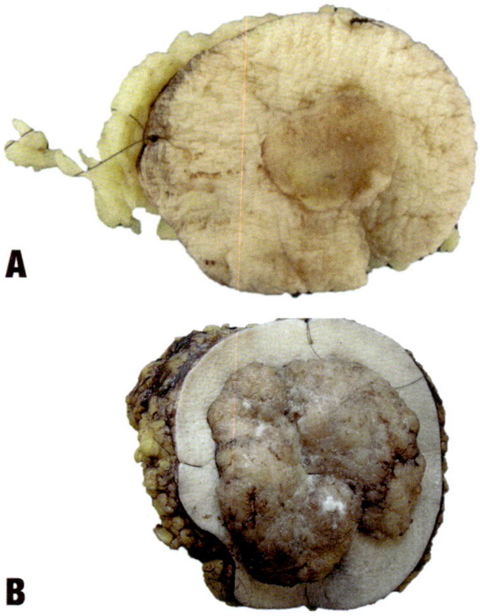

FIGURE 8.25. Images (A) and (B) show BCC presenting as a pearly white, dome-shaped nodule (A) or papule (B) with prominent telangiectatic surface vessels. Image (C) shows surface ulceration.

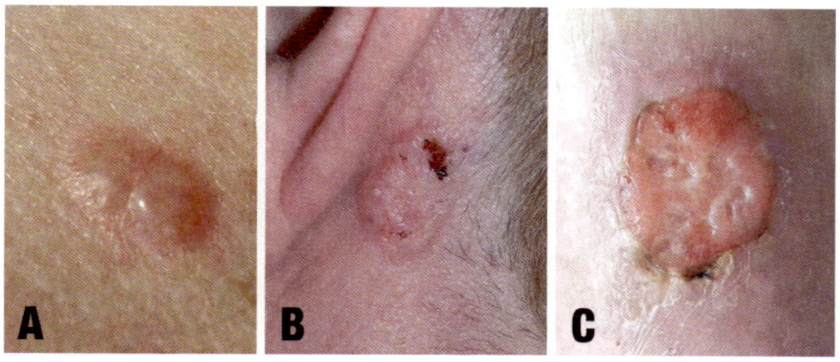

FIGURE 8.26. This image shows a wide excision of a pearly nodule with inked margins of normal tissue, demonstrating the locally aggressive nature of this slow-growing but invasive tumor with nodular effacement of the normal architecture.

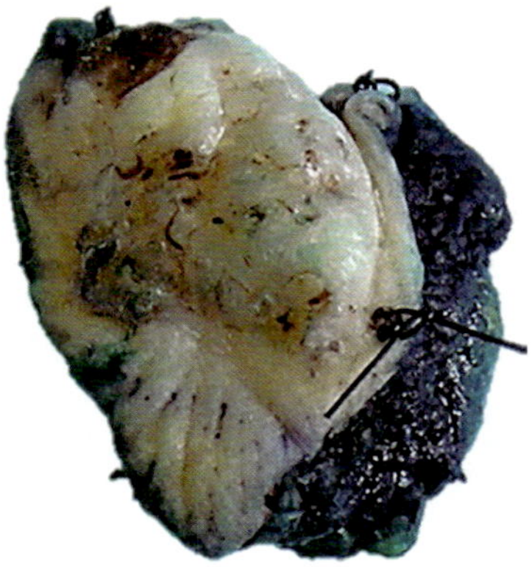

ATYPICAL BCC

Clinically atypical lesions may be difficult to distinguish from SCC or melanoma without biopsy. Rolled, elevated, translucent, and well-delineated borders are typical of ulcerating BCC.

FIGURE 8.27. Image (A) shows an elliptical excision of a multinodular, skin-colored to red-black, erosive lesion of the epidermis. Image (B) shows BCC on a posterior auricle, which is a common site for cancers induced by sun exposure.

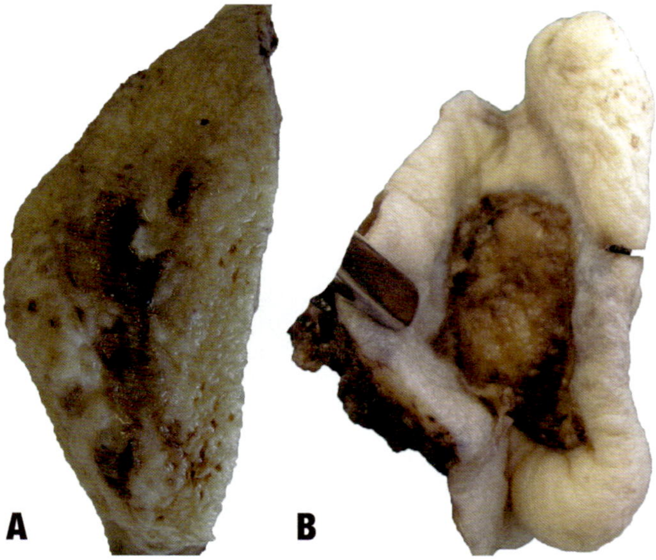

NEVOID BCC (GORLIN) SYNDROME

Also called Gorlin–Goltz syndrome, nevoid BCC (Gorlin) syndrome is a rare syndrome characterized by the early onset of multiple nevoid BCCs, as well as odontogenic keratocysts, palmoplantar pits, calcification of the falx cerebri, and skeletal deformities. It is also associated with medulloblastoma, which occurs in about 5% of cases. The syndrome is transmitted in an autosomal dominant fashion, caused by a loss-of-function mutation in the *PTCH1* gene localized to 9q22.3.

FIGURE 8.28. This image shows multiple BCCs with a fleshy-to-brown color clustered about the nape of the neck in a young adult. This presentation is typical of this disorder.

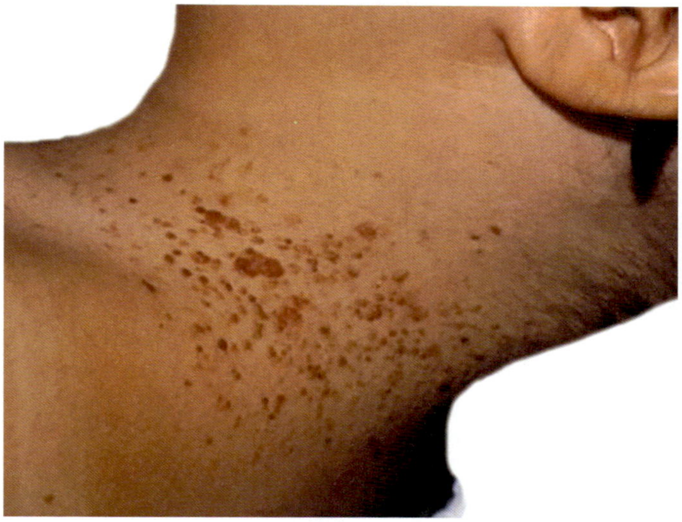

Scar

Exuberant scar formation leads to hypertrophic scars and keloids. Keloids are much more common in those of African descent and present as disfiguring, raised, indurated lesions, usually on the head and neck, upper chest, and arms. Local recurrence is very common.

FIGURE 8.29. This scar tissue appears atrophic and shiny.

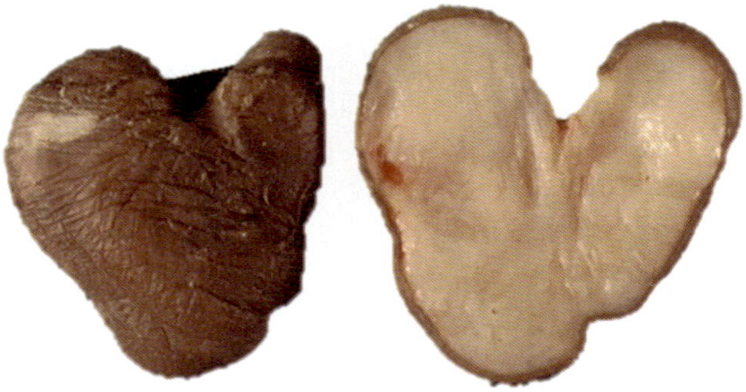

Tattoo complications

Tattoo complications include infections, allergic reactions to tattoo pigments, and photosensitivity reactions. In some cases, these complications are so important that the tattoo is resected to ameliorate the side effects.

FIGURE 8.30. These tattoos were resected due to complications.

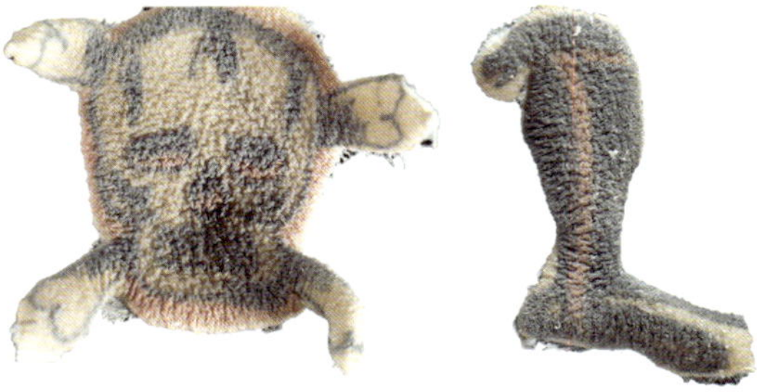

Cutaneous leiomyoma

Cutaneous leiomyoma commonly presents as multiple, small, slow-growing, painful papules.

FIGURE 8.31. This surgical resection specimen shows cutaneous leiomyoma arising from arrector pili muscles. It displays involvement of both epidermis and subcutis by a firm, multilobulated, well-circumscribed mass of smooth muscle nodules and bundles with associated subcutaneous fat.

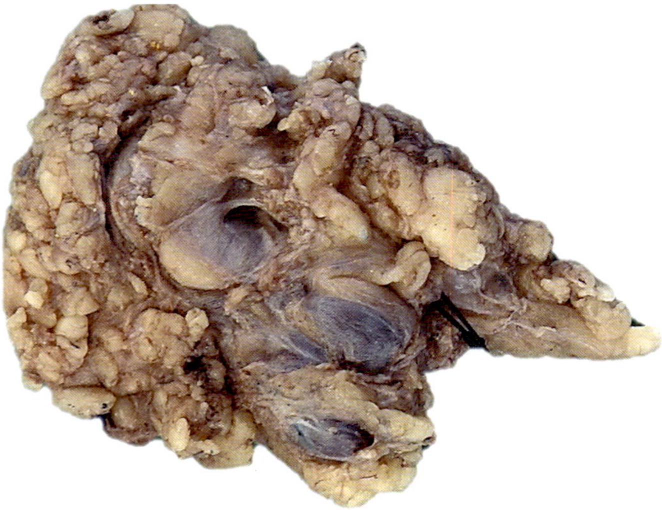

Hyaline fibromatosis

JUVENILE HYALINE FIBROMATOSIS

Juvenile hyaline fibromatosis is an exceedingly rare autosomal recessive connective tissue disease. The syndrome also presents with gingival hyperplasia, joint contractures, and osteolytic bone involvement. It has been mapped to chromosome 4q21 and is hypothesized to stem from aberrant synthesis of glycosaminoglycans.

FIGURE 8.32. Image (A) shows a characteristic skin finding in this disease: skin-colored, boggy, nontender, waxy nodules and papules. The cut surface in (B) shows a grayish-white, solid tumor.

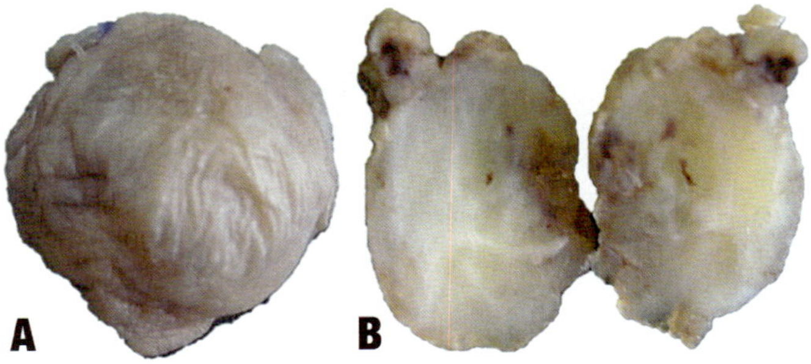

SKIN HYALINE FIBROMATOSIS

The cutaneous tumors of hyaline fibromatosis can measure centimeters in size. They occur in young patients. The life expectancy of most patients is into the fourth decade.

FIGURE 8.33. These cut surfaces of cutaneous nodules of hyaline fibromatosis demonstrate the solid, granular, white, and yellow-and-gray inner surface of the tumor involving the dermis and subcutis. The brown-red punctate spots on the interior are transected vessels.

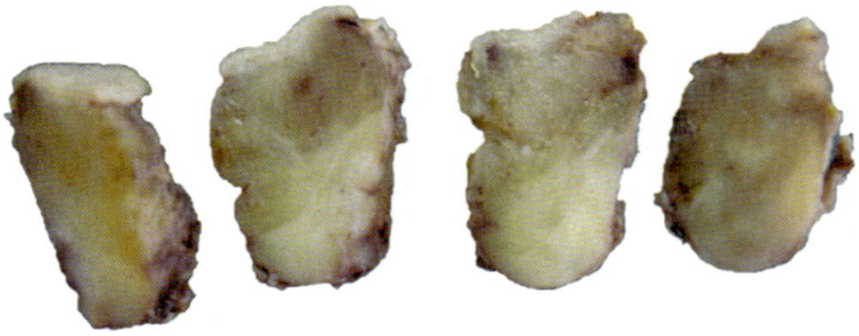

Atypical fibroxanthoma

Atypical fibroxanthoma usually occurs on sun-damaged skin of the head and neck of elderly patients. Rarely, it occurs in young patients and children with xeroderma pigmentosum. It is histologically indistinguishable from sarcoma, but is restricted to the dermis with minimal subcutaneous extension. It has an excellent prognosis with rare recurrences (less than 5%) and no metastasis. Excision is curative.

FIGURE 8.34. This image shows an excision of skin with underlying subcutaneous fat. The surface shows thinned epidermis with a hypopigmented macule or patch.

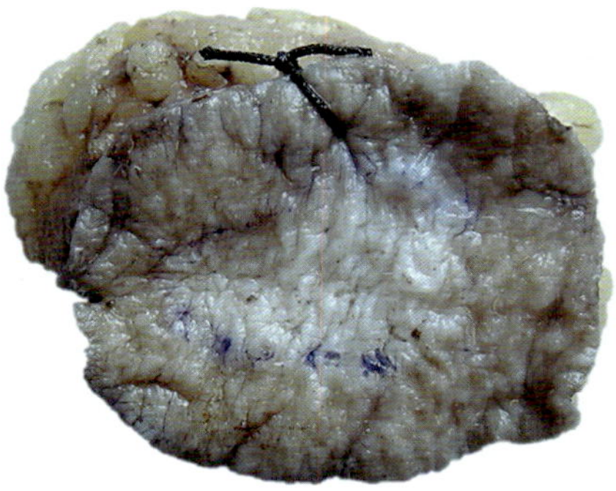

High-grade myxofibrosarcoma

High-grade myxofibrosarcoma is a common superficial sarcoma in the elderly. Approximately 50% of cases occur in the dermal and subcutaneous tissue. The name refers to a spectrum of tumors with variably prominent myxoid stroma and cellular pleomorphism; all of these tumors share a characteristic curvilinear vascular pattern.

FIGURE 8.35. This mass shows a multilobulated architecture and gelatinous myxoid exudate.

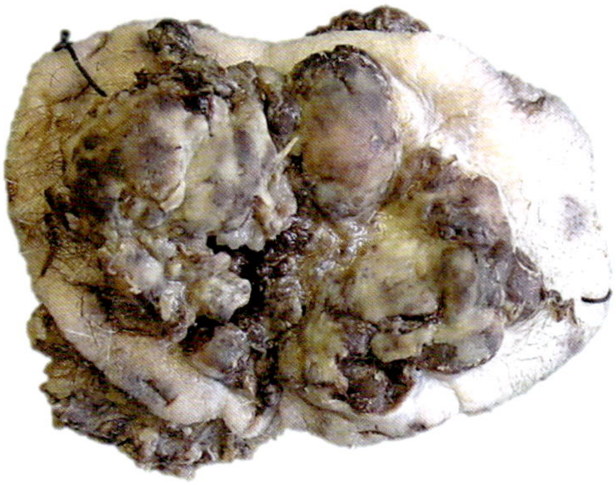

Pyogenic granuloma (lobular capillary hemangioma)

Pyogenic granuloma, also called lobular capillary hemangioma, is a proliferation of vessels that clinically presents as rapidly growing lesions that bleed easily and favor the fingers, face, gingiva, lips, and mucosa of the nose. They are benign growths that resolve spontaneously over the course of months, but can also be easily removed with electrodessication. Deep lesions with dermal involvement may recur.

FIGURE 8.36. These examples show well-delineated, exophytic vascular red nodules.

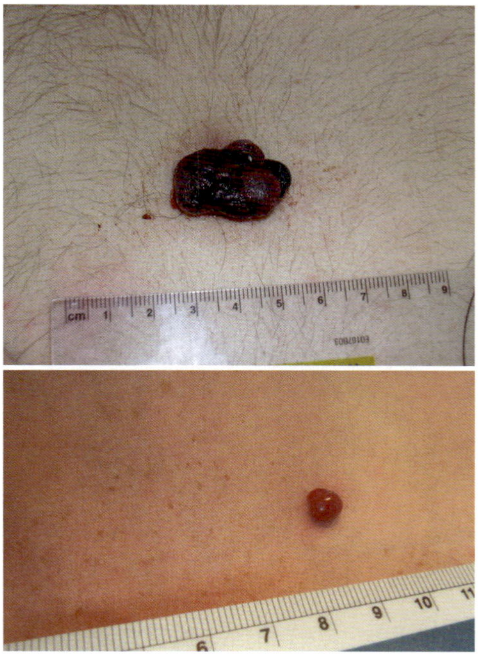

Lymphangioma circumscriptum

Lymphangioma circumscriptum is a lymphatic vessel malformation of the superficial dermis that may occur anywhere in the body. Lymphangioma circumscriptum has a predilection for the neck and can occur on the genitals. Other common areas include the axillary folds, shoulders, proximal extremities, and tongue. These are benign lesions that do not require excision, although they may be cosmetically troublesome. Clinically, the lesion appears as grouped vesicles forming a plaque with verrucous areas. The lesion is usually congenital, but may occur in early childhood.

FIGURE 8.37. This tumor was located on the thigh. The violaceous component is due to vascular thrombus and hemorrhage.

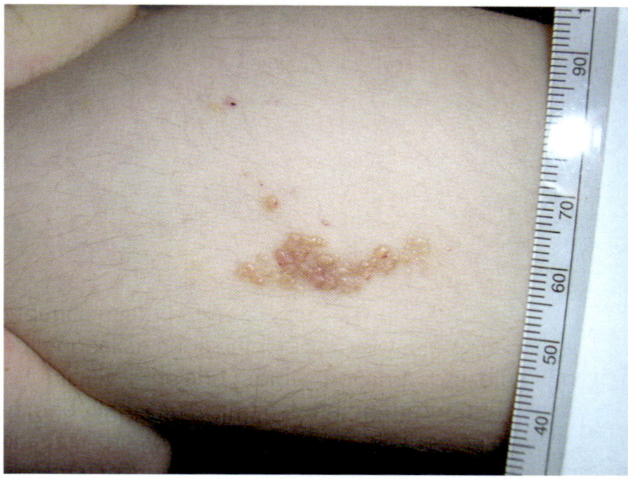

Cutaneous angiosarcoma

Cutaneous angiosarcoma is a malignant tumor of the endothelial cells lining blood vessels, and predominantly involves the scalp and central face in late adulthood. The lesions initially present as bruise-like plaques. They may extend several centimeters beyond what is visible, and the development of nodules is variable. Metastasis is hematogenous and prognosis is poor.

FIGURE 8.38. Image (A) shows a wide excision of multinodular subcutaneous nodules with apical ulceration and visible vasculature. Image (B) shows the opposite side, which demonstrates the highly vascular, blood-filled nature of the tumor.

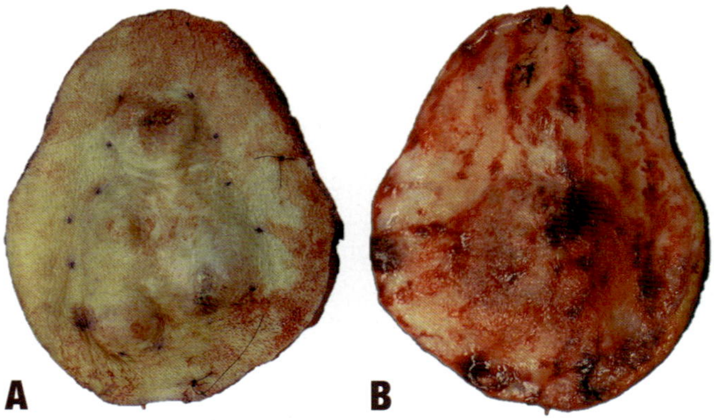

Eccrine poroma

Eccrine poroma most commonly occurs as a tan-to-red nodule on the foot in middle-aged adults. Grossly, it appears as a well-delineated, dome-shaped papule with a shiny, micronodular, exophytic surface.

FIGURE 8.39. This distal amputation of the toe displays a periungual, skin-colored, multilobular firm nodule.

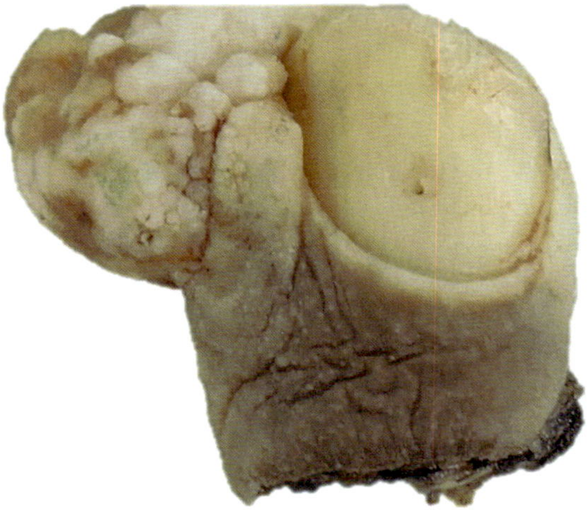

Hidradenoma

Hidradenoma is a benign adnexal tumor that may arise from both eccrine and apocrine ducts. It presents as a slow-growing, solid-to-cystic nodule on the head and neck or extremities.

FIGURE 8.40. This image shows an elliptical excision of a skin-colored, multinodular tumor of the trunk.

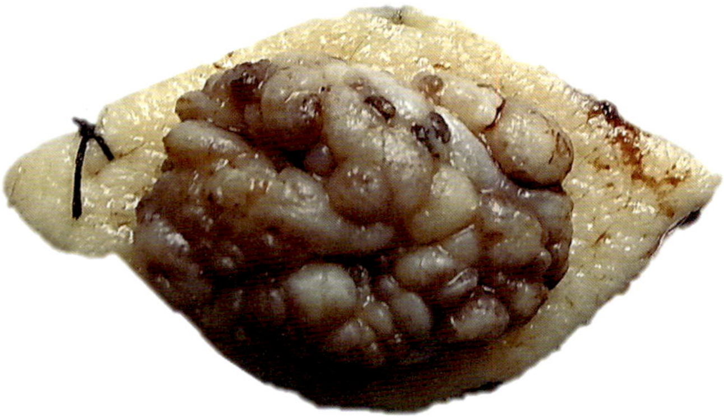

Syringoma

Syringomas are benign adnexal neoplasms that are almost always multiple, with a predilection for the lower eyelid area. Histologically, syringomas may be differentiated from microcystic adnexal carcinomas by their small size, symmetry, and restriction to the upper two-thirds of the reticular dermis.

FIGURE 8.41. This image shows multiple skin-colored irregular papules at the neck.

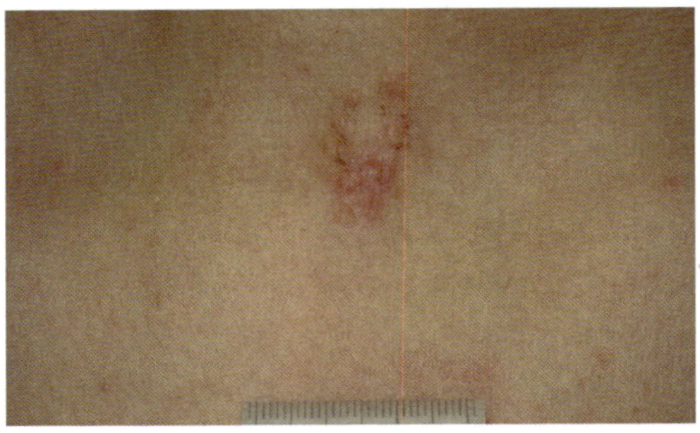

Hidrocystoma

Hidrocystomas are typically periorbital, benign cystic proliferations originating either from retention of an eccrine cyst duct or from an apocrine secretory coil. They may also afflict other areas of the head and neck. The exact cause for these fluid-filled cysts is unknown. Excision or drainage is curative.

FIGURE 8.42. This image shows a skin-colored fluid-filled cystic lesion.

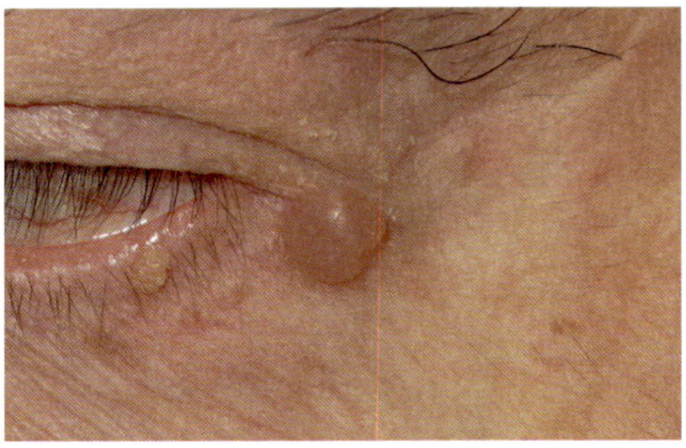

Pilomatricoma

Pilomatricomas are benign neoplasms derived from hair follicles and sheaths that display positive staining for LEF-1, a marker of hair matrix cells. Rare cases of multiple pilomatricoma are associated with myotonic dystrophy, Rubinstein–Taybi syndrome, Goldenhar syndrome, sternal cleft defects, coagulative defects, and sarcoidosis.

FIGURE 8.43. This image shows a shiny, solitary, tan, well-circumscribed nodule. When cut open, this type of lesion reveals various quantities of chalky, white-to-yellow keratinous material.

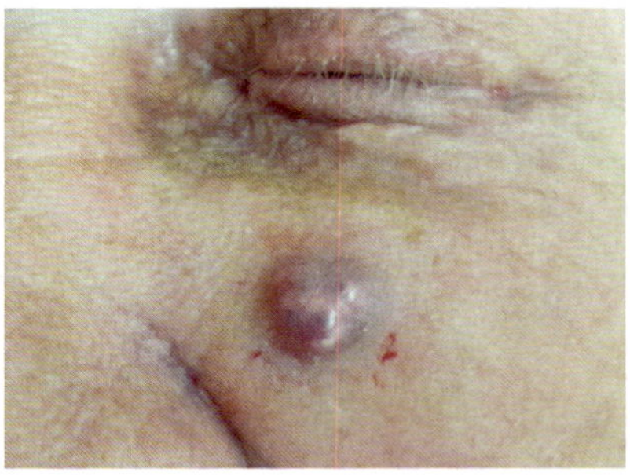

Photo courtesy of Dr. Kevin Pehr.

Epidermoid cyst

Epidermoid cysts are common, solitary, benign lesions in adults. They affect the face, upper trunk, neck, and scrotum. Histologically, they are characterized by a stratified squamous epithelium enclosing keratin- and lipid-rich debris within the dermis, often with a central punctum. The natural history is to spontaneously rupture, leading to inflammation and pain. Excision is curative.

FIGURE 8.44. Image (A) shows an excision of a cyst with underlying dermis and subcutaneous tissue. The cut section in (B) shows the thickly encapsulated cyst filled with crumbly, white-yellow keratin.

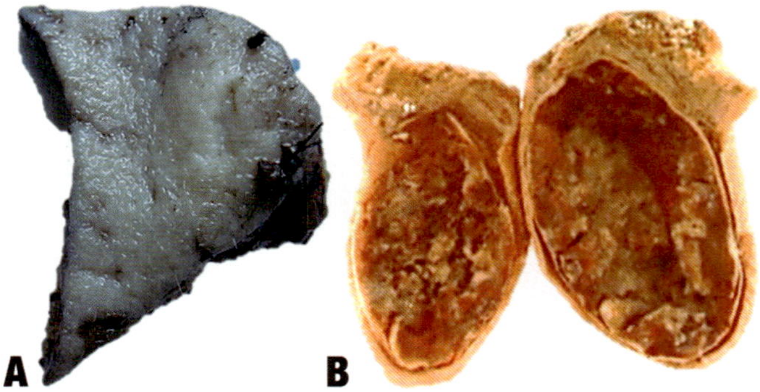

Trichilemmal cyst (Pilar cyst)

Trichilemmal cyst, also called Pilar cyst, is a common cyst arising from a hair follicle and most often found on the scalp.

FIGURE 8.45. Grossly, the encapsulated cyst is smooth, mobile, and filled with keratinous contents.

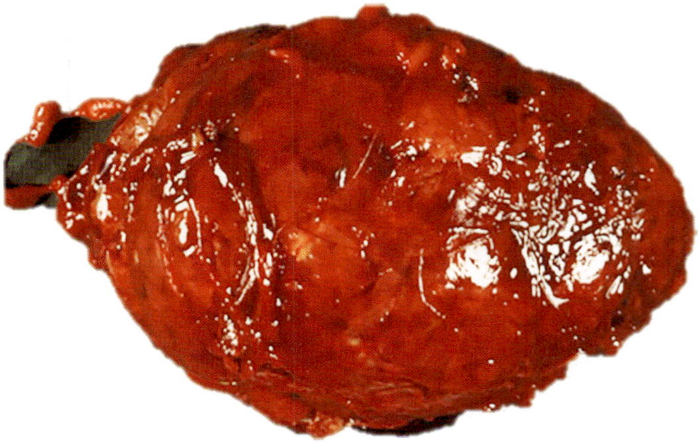

Pilonidal sinus

Pilonidal sinus typically occurs in the intergluteal cleft after chronic or acute trauma of a hair follicle, resulting in formation of a pore. Negative pressure and mechanical forces contribute to the collection of debris and entrapment of bacteria, leading to abscess formation and the creation of a sinus tract. Acute management involves incision and drainage; chronic recurrent pilonidal disease requires surgical excision of the entire sinus tract.

FIGURE 8.46. Image (A) shows a surgically excised sinus tract. Image (B) shows a readily visible sinus tract cavity.

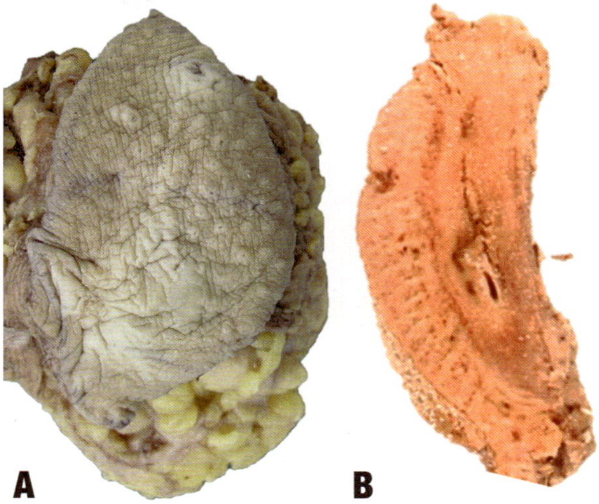

Paget disease

EXTRAMAMMARY PAGET DISEASE

Extramammary Paget disease is either a primary adenocarcinoma in situ of the apocrine gland-bearing skin or an underlying internal malignancy. The 2 types are histologically indistinguishable; on diagnosis, patients must be investigated to rule out malignancy. Primary disease can invade the dermis and potentially metastasize. Extramammary Paget disease commonly occurs in areas rich in apocrine sweat glands, including the vulva and perianal region.

FIGURE 8.47. This image shows a wide excision of involved tissue of the perianal area and surrounding normal skin with inked margins.

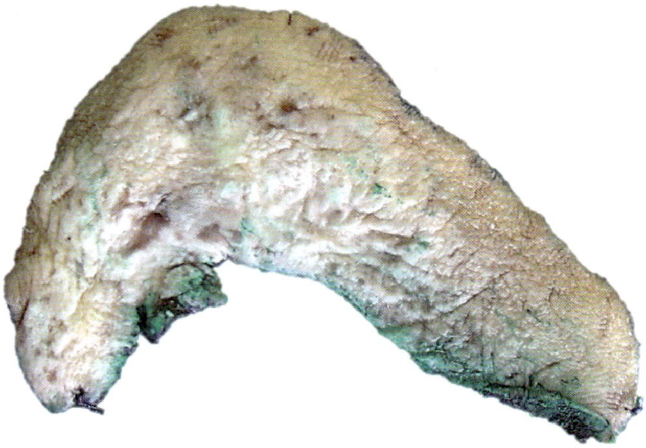

FIGURE 8.48. Grossly, the skin in this image is extensively involved with multicentric and erosive, eczematous lesions with scale crusts.

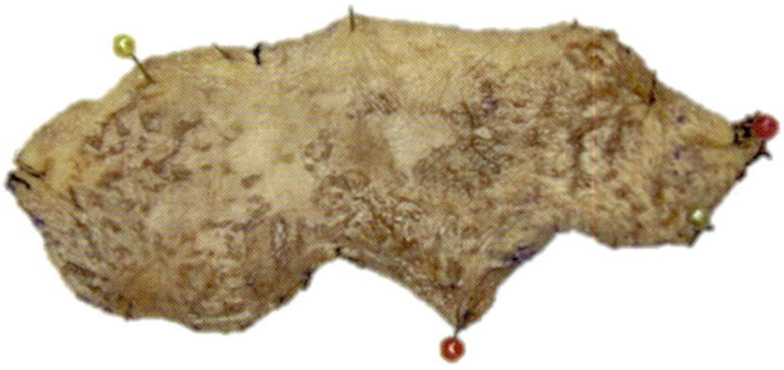

Blue nevi

Blue nevi — also called mongolian spots, nevi of Ota, and nevi of Ito — are dendritic melanocytic lesions with a bluish hue that are located primarily in the reticular dermis. Blue nevi typically develop in childhood and commonly occur on the distal extremities. They may present as macules or well-circumscribed dome-shaped papules.

FIGURE 8.49. This blue nevus presents as a well-circumscribed, dome-shaped papule.

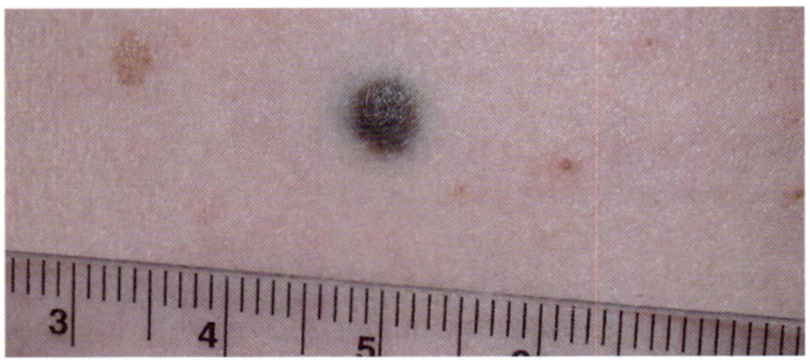

Melanoma

Melanoma is a malignant proliferation of melanocytes with an extremely poor prognosis. Thin melanomas, < 1 mm in thickness, can be cured by wide local excision alone, so early recognition and removal is important. Clinically suspicious lesions are characterized by the ABCDE mnemonic: **a**symmetry, **b**order irregularity, **c**olor variation, **d**iameter (large), and **e**volution (or change).

FIGURE 8.50. These excised lesions show asymmetry.

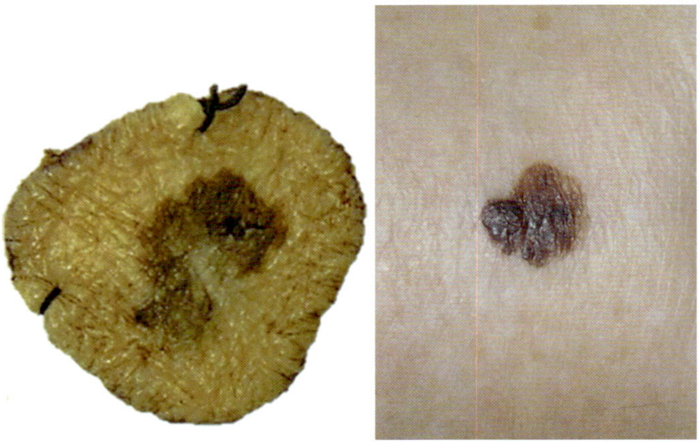

FIGURE 8.51. These melanoma lesions clearly demonstrate border irregularity.

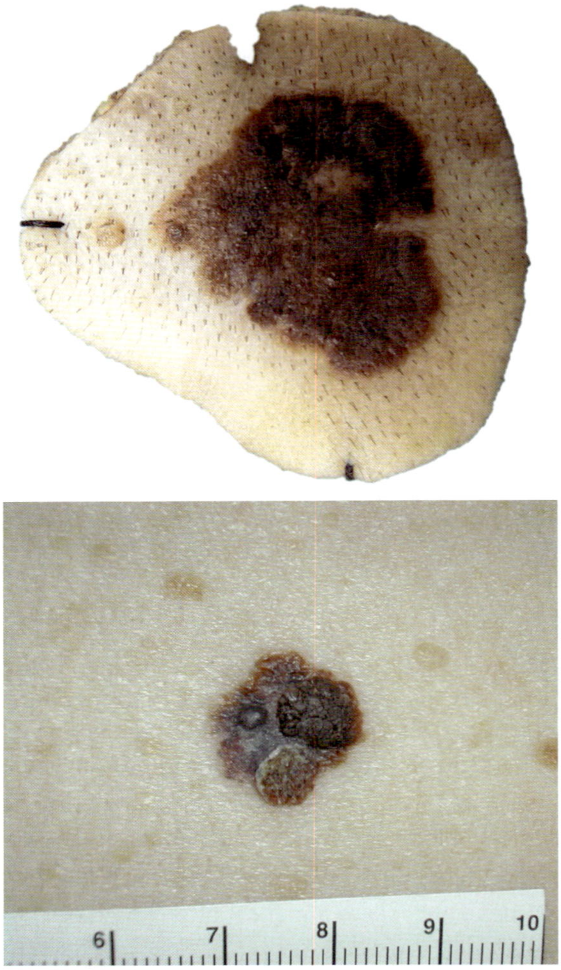

FIGURE 8.52. These lesions demonstrate color variation: the presence of more than 1 color.

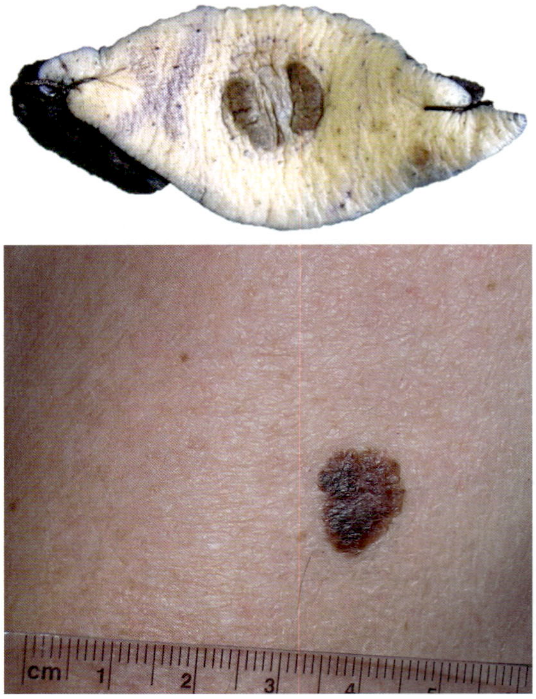

FIGURE 8.53. This image shows a melanoma with a large diameter. This melanoma does not demonstrate the final letter in the mnemonic, "E", which stands for rapid evolution or change in lesion color or size.

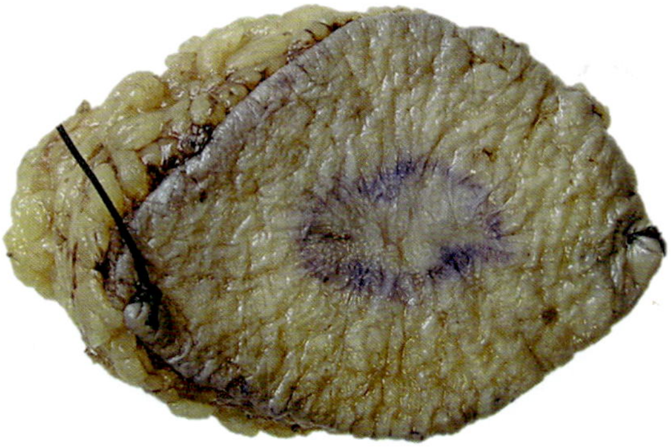

LENTIGO MALIGNA (HUTCHINSON MELANOTIC FRECKLE)

Lentigo maligna, also called Hutchinson melanotic freckle, is an in situ melanoma presenting as irregularly pigmented and enlarging macules on sun-damaged skin in elderly patients. After a long period (10 to 15 years), it progresses to invasive melanoma (lentigo maligna melanoma). The development of lentigo maligna melanoma is directly proportional to sun exposure. It is therefore sometimes called "solar melanoma." This subtype is characterized by a lentiginous proliferation of atypical melanocytes that has a propensity to extend down hair follicles and sweat ducts. These lesions are associated with epidermal atrophy and prominent solar elastosis.

FIGURE 8.54. Image (A) shows a large, irregularly pigmented, flat lesion on the face (a Hutchinson melanotic freckle). Image (B) shows an excision of a pigmented irregular flat lesion.

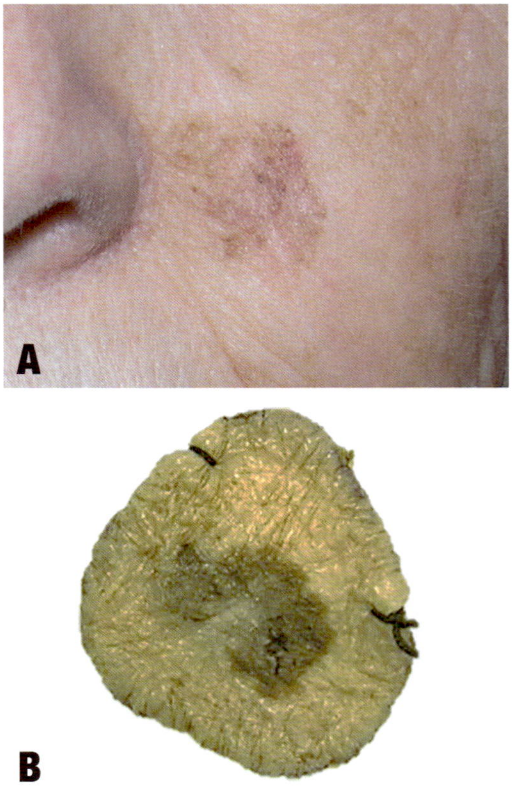

FIGURE 8.55. Images (A) and (B) show excisions of lentigo maligna melanomas: (A) a flat and pigmented lesion; and (B) a pigmented irregular lesion located on the anterior lower groin.

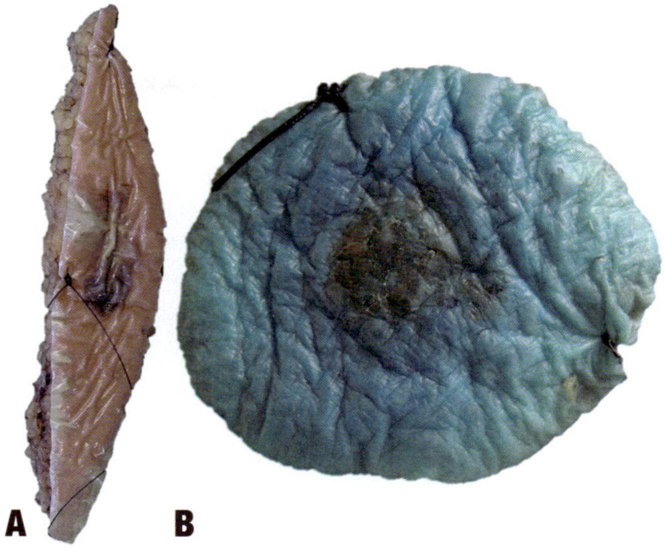

FIGURE 8.56. In (A), a flat melanoma of the mid-back shows hypopigmented areas of regression. Image (B) shows an asymmetric pigmented growth on the lower back.

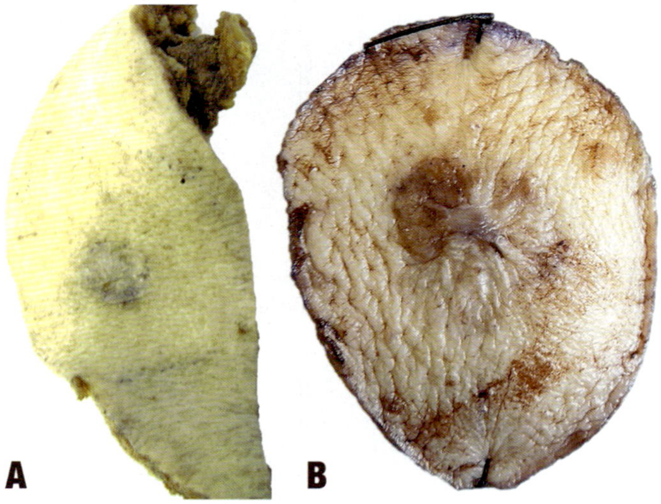

SUPERFICIAL SPREADING MELANOMA

Superficial spreading melanoma is the most common subtype of melanoma. It typically arises on sun-exposed skin and is characterized by a variably pigmented nodule with asymmetry, irregular borders, and satellite nodules. Satellitosis is defined by the location of tumor nodules within a 2-cm radius of the primary lesion, differentiating it from in-transit metastases (nodules more than 2 cm from the primary lesion). Histologically, superficial spreading melanoma is characterized by pagetoid melanocytosis and the intraepidermal extension of melanocytes more than 3 rete ridges beyond the dermal component.

FIGURE 8.57. This is a wide excision of a darkly pigmented lesion with multiple satellite nodules.

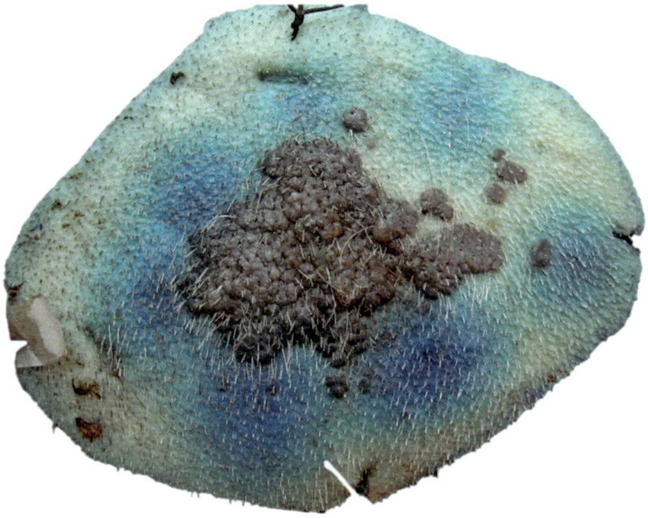

FIGURE 8.58. These images show wide local excisions of superficial spreading melanoma of the left cheek (A) and back (B).

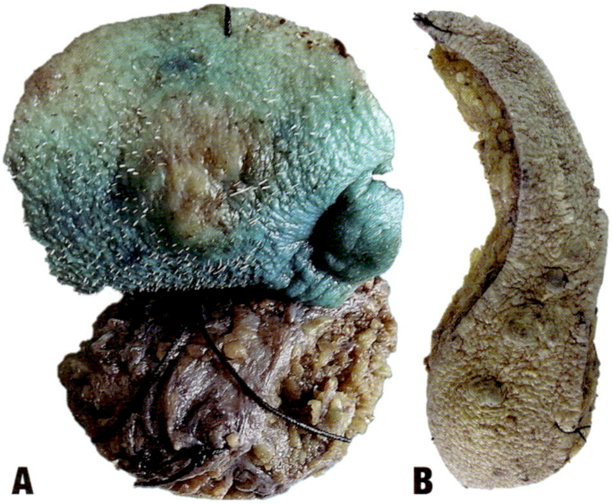

NODULAR MELANOMA

Nodular melanoma is the second most common subtype of melanoma. Clinically, it presents as a raised lesion of nodules of atypical dermal melanocytes that have an expansile growth pattern and cause thinning, effacement, and/or ulceration of the epidermis. Histologically, atypical melanocytes may be present in the epidermis, but should not extend significantly (i.e., more than 3 rete ridges) beyond the dermal component. The nodular appearance represents a shift from the radial to the vertical growth phase with extension deep into the dermis.

FIGURE 8.59. Images (A) and (B) show black, dome-shaped nodules with ulceration on the back.

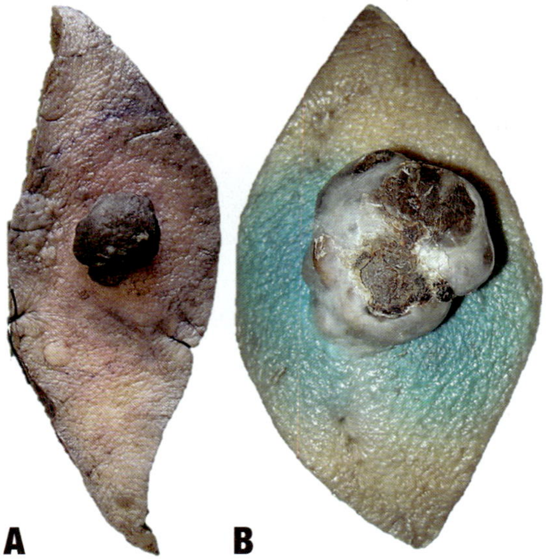

FIGURE 8.60. These images show nodular melanomas on the shoulder (A), right thigh (B), and neck (C).

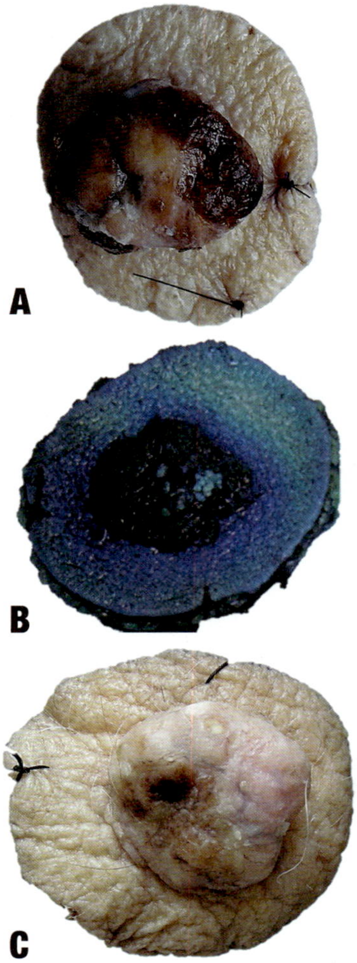

FIGURE 8.61. This image shows an excision of a nodular melanoma with extensive hemorrhagic ulceration.

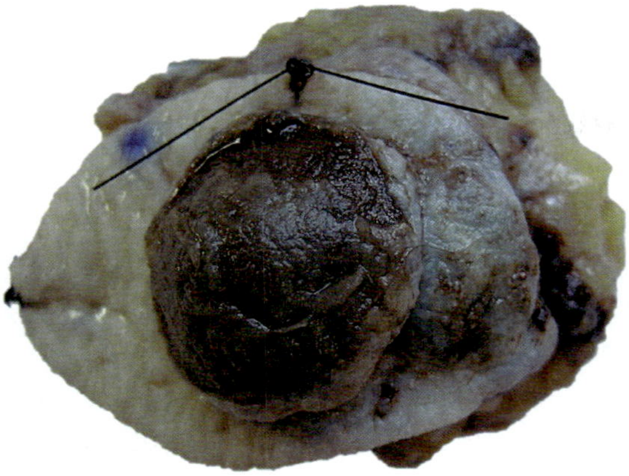

ACRAL LENTIGINOUS MELANOMA

Acral lentiginous melanoma is typically unrelated to sun exposure or *BRAF* mutation. It involves skin on the palms, soles, digits, and/or nail beds, with 90% of cases occurring on the feet.

FIGURE 8.62. Images (A) and (B) show 2 views of an irregularly pigmented nodule on the toe.

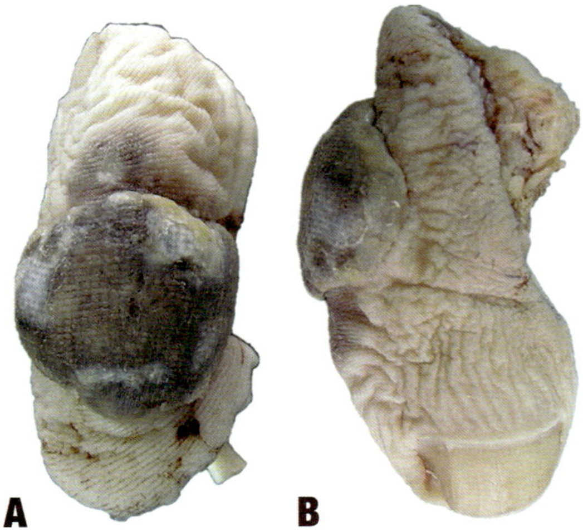

FIGURE 8.63. This image shows acral lentiginous melanoma on the right heel.

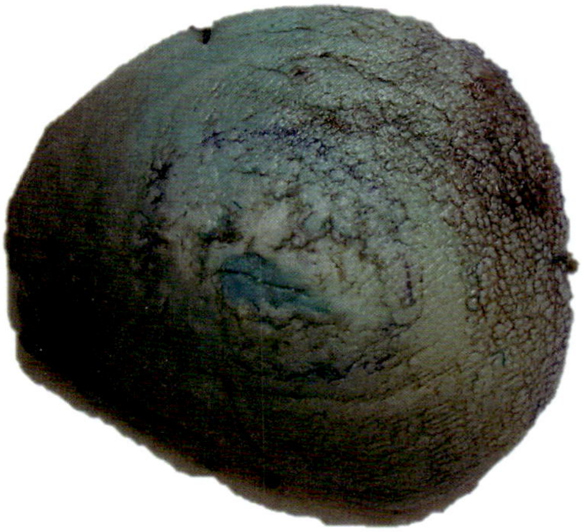

FIGURE 8.64. These images of acral lentiginous melanoma show (A) an intact toe amputation specimen; and (B) the cut surface of a small, pigmented lesion arising in the junction between toes.

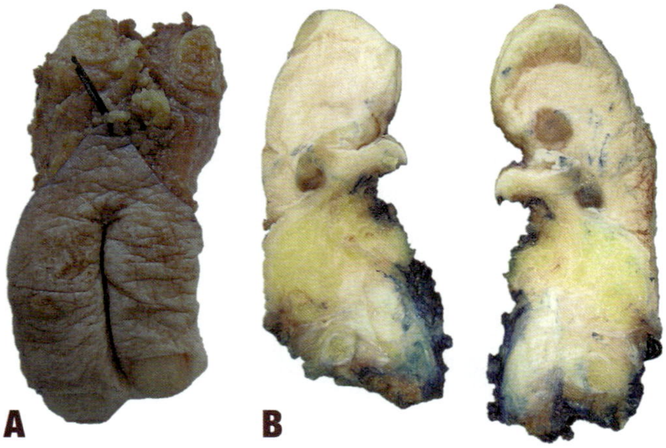

DESMOPLASTIC MELANOMA

Desmoplastic melanoma is a variant of spindle cell melanoma with a predilection for sun-exposed skin. It most commonly arises on a background of lentigo maligna and often presents as firm, amelanotic, indurated plaques or nodules that mimic scarring. Desmoplastic melanoma is notorious for deep infiltration; at diagnosis, it has often already extended widely.

FIGURE 8.65. This image shows a firm, indurated plaque located on the back.

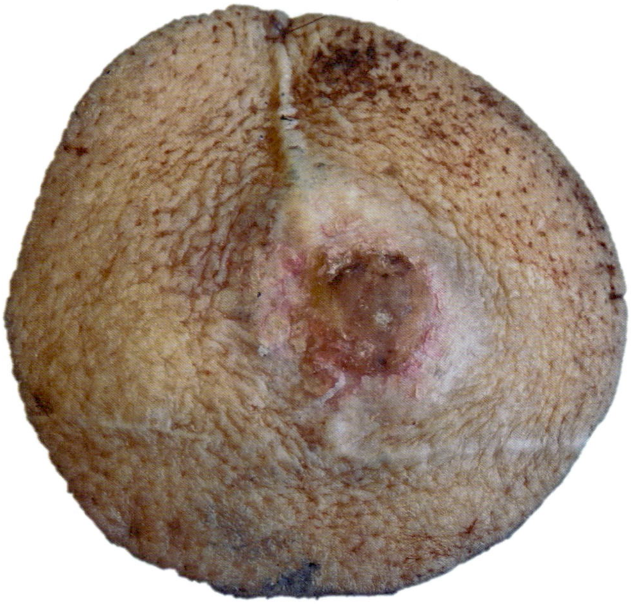

POSTRESECTION RESIDUAL MELANOMA

Residual melanoma postresection requires reexcision with an optimal margin of uninvolved tissue. The optimal margin depends on the depth of invasion of the primary tumor: melanoma in situ should have 5 mm of tumor-free tissue circumferentially; a tumor with a depth of 4 mm should have margins of at least 2 cm.

FIGURE 8.66. Images (A), (B), and (C) show examples of irregularly pigmented lesions with associated scarring from previous surgeries.

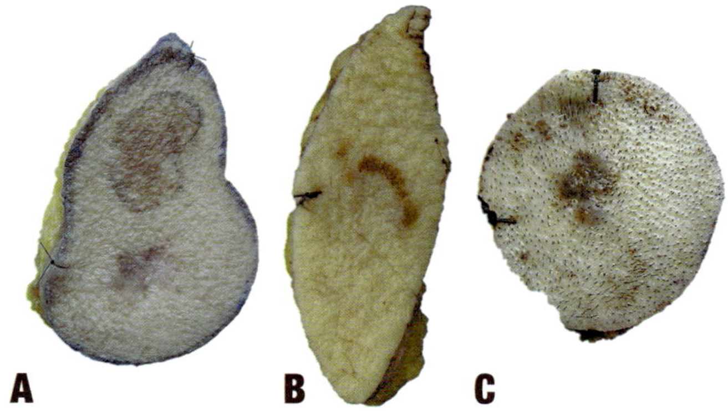

FIGURE 8.68. This nodular lesion protrudes into the skin surface with surface necrosis and dark pigmentation. Because of the dark color of this lesion, melanoma should be included in the differential diagnosis.

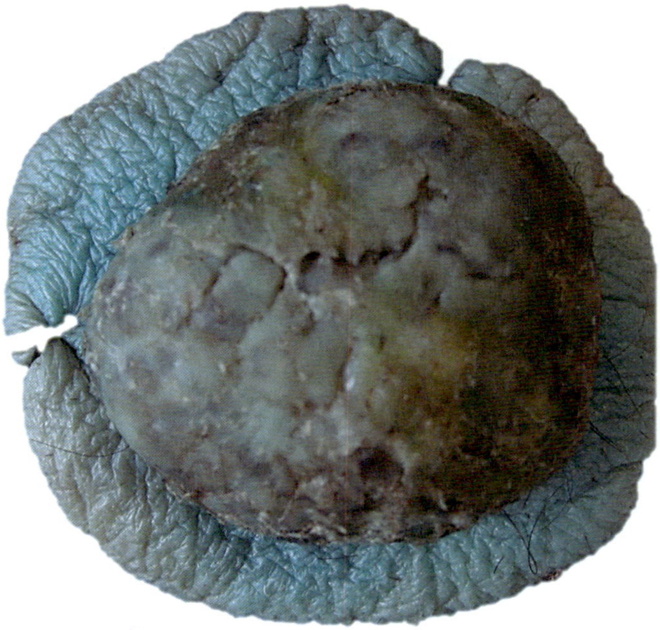

Merkel cell carcinoma

Merkel cell carcinoma is a highly aggressive cutaneous neuroendocrine carcinoma with a high mortality rate. It clinically presents as a firm, painless, solitary nodule on sun-damaged skin, most often on the head and neck of elderly patients. Surgical excision is the primary mode of management; however, the aggressive nature of this lesion necessitates adjuvant radiotherapy and chemotherapy.

FIGURE 8.67. Grossly, this elliptical excision shows an irregular, multinodular lesion of the left cheek with focal ulceration.

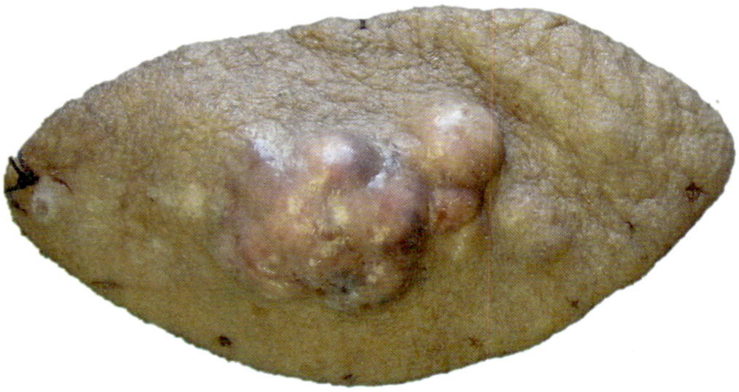

ACKNOWLEDGMENTS

We would like to acknowledge the valuable contributions of Dr. Kevin Watters and the technical help of R. Gilot, E. Griss, A. Hossain, L. Korneichyuk Pasyuk, M. Mikhael, and E. Yaney.

REFERENCES

Bai XL, Zhang Q, Masood W, et al. Sister Mary Joseph's nodule as a first sign of pancreatic cancer. World J Gastroenterol. 2012;18(45):6686–6689. https://doi.org/10.3748/wjg.v18.i45.6686. Medline:23236247

Fletcher CDM, Bridge JA, Hogendoorn PCW, Mertens F. *WHO classification of tumours of soft tissue and bone*. 4th ed. Lyon, France: IARC Press; 2013.

Krishnamurthy J, Dalal BS, Sunila, Gubanna MV. Juvenile hyaline fibromatosis. Indian J Dermatol. 2011;56(6):731–733. https://doi.org/10.4103/0019-5154.91840. Medline:22345782

Kumar V, Abbas AK, Aster JC. *Robbins and Cotran pathologic basis of disease*. 9th ed. Philadelphia: Saunders/Elsevier; 2015.

Lawrence PE. *Essentials of general surgery*. 4th ed. Philadephia: Lippincott Williams & Wilkins; 2006.

LeBoit PE, Burg G, Weedon D, Sarasin A, editors. *World Health Organization classification of tumours: pathology and genetics of skin tumours*. Lyon, France: IARC Press; 2006.

Soriano LF, Piansay-Soriano ME. A rapidly growing giant cutaneous horn on the chest. J Dermatol Case Rep. 2015;9(4):113–115. https://doi.org/10.3315/jdcr.2015.1217. Medline:26848321

Wolff K, Johnson RA, Saavedra AP. *Fitzpatrick's color atlas and synopsis of clinical dermatology*. 7th ed. New York: McGraw-Hill Companies; 2013.

Yu RC, Pryce DW, Macfarlane AW, Stewart TW. A histopathological study of 643 cutaneous horns. Br J Dermatol. 1991;124(5):449–452. https://doi.org/10.1111/j.1365-2133.1991.tb00624.x. Medline:2039721

9

Soft Tissue Diseases

SUNGMI JUNG, MARTIN CHEVRIER, LISA M. DIFRANCESCO

Lipoma

Lipoma is a common benign tumor of adipose tissue. It occurs in various locations but is usually superficial (i.e., above the fascia). While deep lipomas do exist, retroperitoneal lipomas are rare; bland, fatty tumors in this location therefore may require molecular tests to rule out well-differentiated liposarcoma. Lipomas typically appear as well-circumscribed, soft, yellow, greasy tumors reminiscent of benign adipose tissue.

FIGURE 9.1. A typical, well-circumscribed lipoma appears soft, yellow, and greasy, reminiscent of benign adipose tissue.

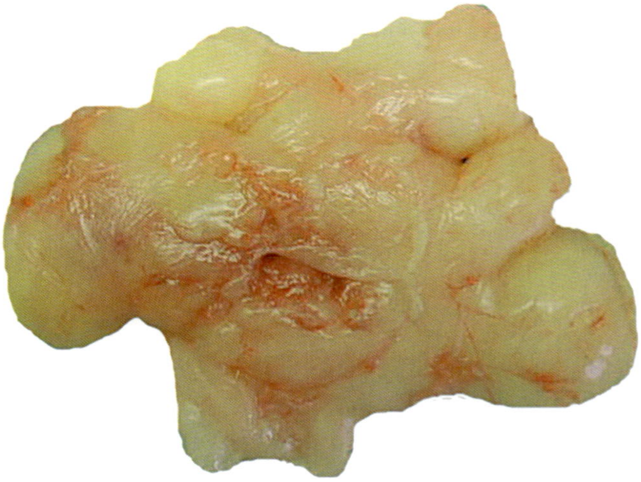

SPINDLE CELL LIPOMA (PLEOMORPHIC LIPOMA)

Spindle cell, or pleomorphic, lipoma is a variant of lipoma with a particular predilection for the shoulder, back, and posterior neck regions of older males. In contrast to the usual lipoma, spindle cell lipoma shows interspersed white-gray, fibrous bands, and is slightly firmer in consistency.

FIGURE 9.2. In (A), the outer surface of a specimen shows a well-circumscribed, pseudoencapsulated tumor. In (B), white-gray, fibrous bands are visible on the cut surface.

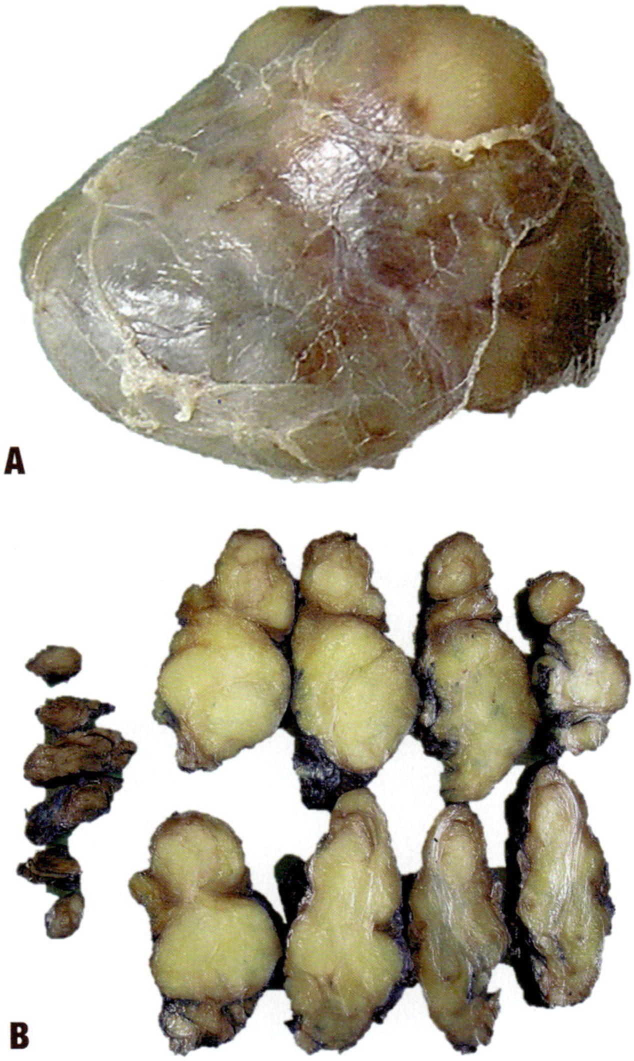

MYELOLIPOMA

Myelolipoma is a benign tumor containing hematopoietic and adipocytic elements. It mostly occurs in the adrenal gland, and occasionally in other locations such as the liver and retroperitoneum. Most myelolipomas are incidental radiologic findings. They are well-demarcated tumors with a variegated, yellow-to-brown cut surface, depending on the relative proportions of fat (yellow) and myeloid (brown) tissue within.

FIGURE 9.3. This image shows a myelolipoma from the retroperitoneum.

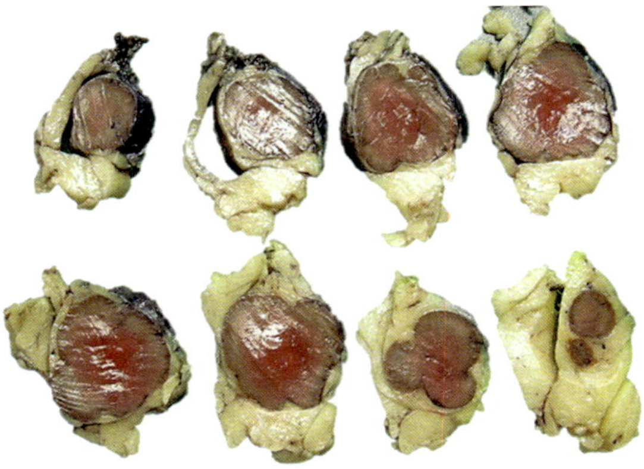

Liposarcoma

Liposarcoma is a malignant neoplasm that mostly occurs in the retroperitoneum and the thigh.

ATYPICAL LIPOMATOUS TUMOR (ALT)

ALT is a low-grade malignant, fatty tumor characterized by an *MDM2* amplification involving chromosome 12. ALT and well-differentiated liposarcoma are nearly synonymous; the difference lies in the location and resectability of the tumors. The name *ALT* is reserved for tumors in surgically amenable locations such as the limbs or trunk. The macroscopic features of ALT are relatively nonspecific. Cytogenetic findings in ALT include supernumerary ring and giant marker chromosomes, which contain amplified or overexpressed sequences (typically *MDM2*) from chromosome 12.

FIGURE 9.4. This image shows an ALT from the thigh. Macroscopic features of ALT are nonspecific, as this large, pseudoencapsulated, well-delineated lipomatous tumor shows.

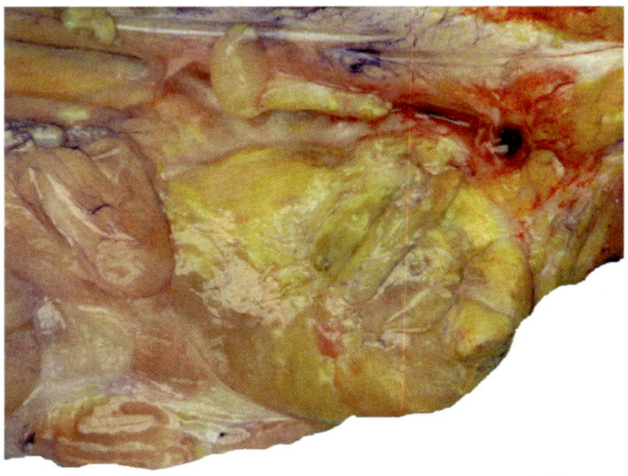

WELL-DIFFERENTIATED LIPOSARCOMA

Well-differentiated liposarcoma is cytologically identical to ALT, but is less amenable to resection because of its location (the most common location is the retroperitoneum). This means it has higher rates of recurrence and dedifferentiation.

FIGURE 9.5. This well-differentiated liposarcoma comes from the retroperitoneum. The image shows a large, perinephric, lobulated, yellow-tan, adipocytic neoplasm with no evidence of direct invasion of the kidney.

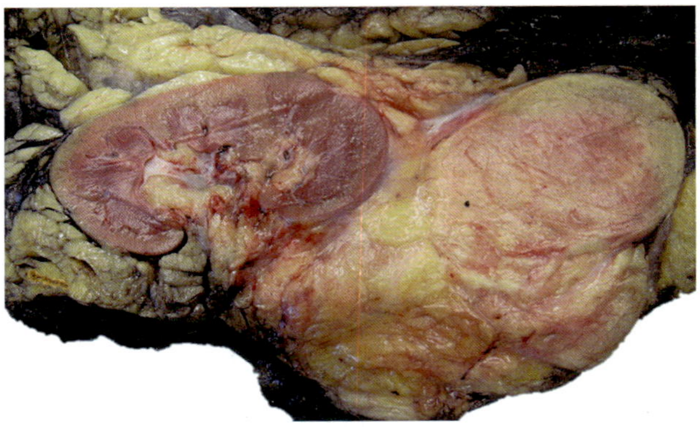

DEDIFFERENTIATED LIPOSARCOMA

Dedifferentiated liposarcoma arises in a background of low-grade liposarcoma, and may occur years later, after multiple recurrences. Transition from lipogenic to nonlipogenic areas may not be obvious grossly; thorough sampling to rule out higher-grade foci is, therefore, necessary. Cytogenetic findings in dedifferentiated liposarcoma are the same as in ALT and well-differentiated liposarcoma.

FIGURE 9.6. A nonlipogenic area (upper half of image) transitions to a lipogenic area (lower half of image).

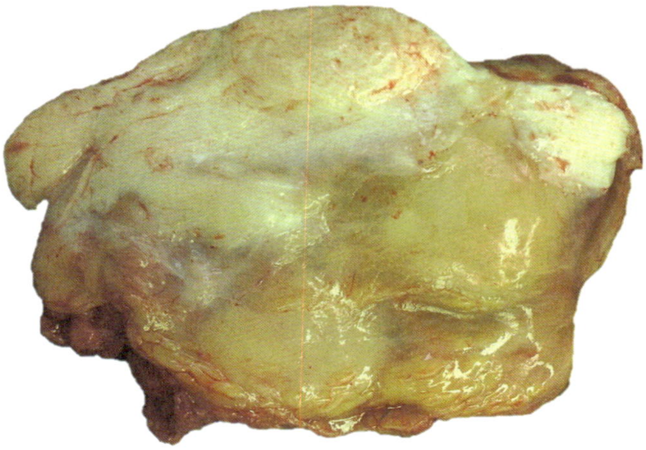

MYXOID LIPOSARCOMA

Myxoid liposarcoma is a distinct subtype of liposarcoma characterized by a prominent myxoid stroma; small, round, univacuolar lipoblasts; a delicate vasculature; and a specific chromosomal rearrangement in t(12;16). It tends to affect younger individuals, usually aged 30 to 50 years, and occurs most commonly in the large muscles of the proximal extremities.

FIGURE 9.7. The cut section here shows a homogenous, well-circumscribed tumor with a glistening, tan, gelatinous appearance. This tumor arose in the thigh.

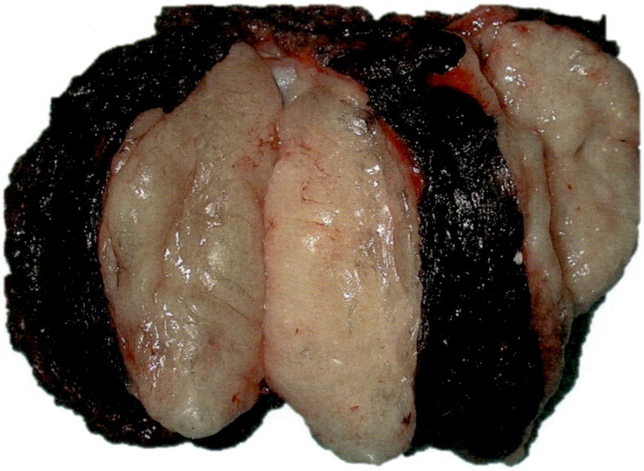

MYXOID / ROUND CELL LIPOSARCOMA

The presence of a more cellular and primitive round cell component signifies a higher-grade tumor and a worse prognosis. In myxoid / round cell liposarcoma, cytogenic findings show a recurrent t(12;16) that most commonly results in a *FUS-DDIT3 (CHOP)* fusion.

FIGURE 9.8. This specimen from the thigh shows a deep, intramuscular mass with glistening, gelatinous low-grade (myxoid) areas and a tan, fleshy, high-grade (round cell) component.

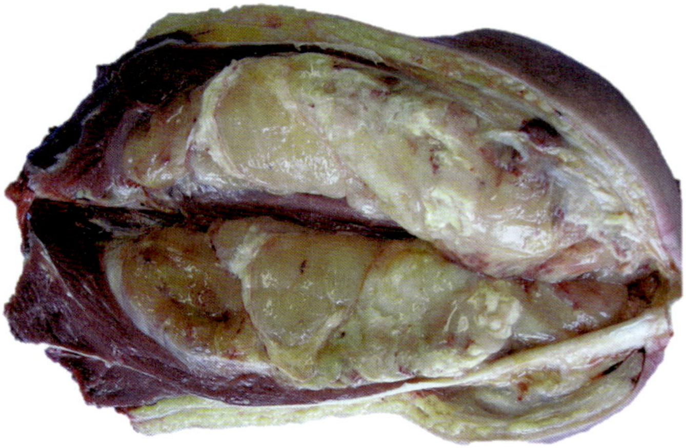

PLEOMORPHIC LIPOSARCOMA

Pleomorphic liposarcoma is a rare variant of liposarcoma involving the deep soft tissue of the extremities in elderly patients. It does not have a specific cytogenetic signature.

FIGURE 9.9. This specimen from the thigh shows an intramuscular, multinodular tumor with a variegated hemorrhagic and necrotic cut surface.

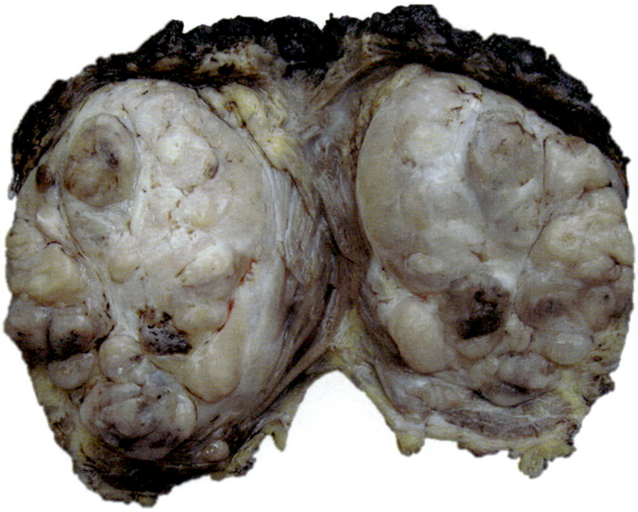

Desmoid-type (deep) fibromatosis

Desmoid-type, or deep, fibromatosis is a locally aggressive, but nonmetastasizing, myofibroblastic tumor. It develops in locations such as the deep soft tissue of the extremities, abdominal wall, and mesentery. Some desmoid tumors, especially those in the mesentery, are associated with Gardner-type familial adenomatous polyposis (FAP). Microscopic examination of these tumors reveals infiltrative borders, accounting for frequent local recurrences.

FIGURE 9.10. Grossly, this tumor, located on the thigh, is deceptively well circumscribed. It is tan-white with a trabeculated, firm cut surface.

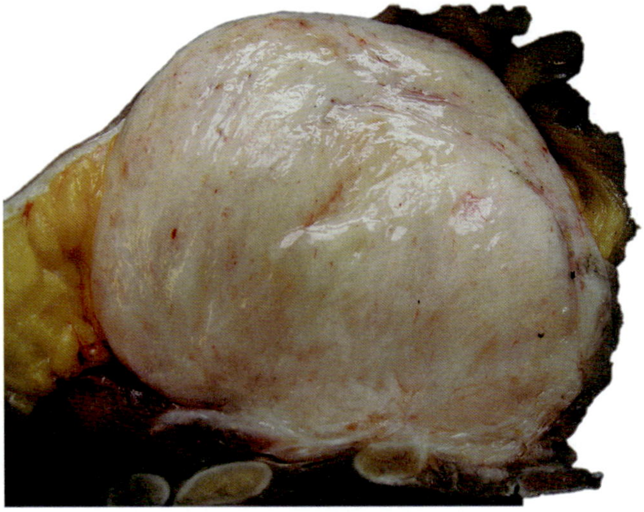

Dermatofibrosarcoma protuberans (DFSP)

DFSP is a superficial, low-grade, fibroblastic neoplasm associated with *COL1A1-PDGFB* gene fusion. The trunk and proximal extremities are the most common sites. DFSP is a locally aggressive neoplasm, but almost never metastasizes. A slightly increased metastatic potential (13%) is reported in cases with fibrosarcomatous transformation; these cases are called fibrosarcomatous DFSP.

FIGURE 9.11. This specimen, located on the shoulder, shows a multinodular tumor centered in the dermis with a firm, tan-white, homogenous cut surface.

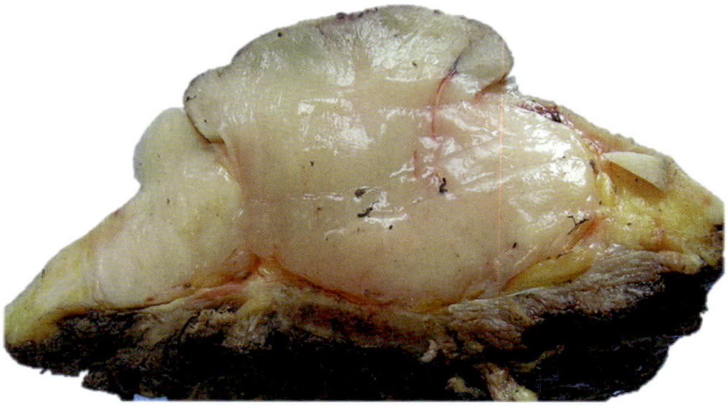

Solitary fibrous tumor (SFT)

SFT is an intermediate, rarely metastasizing, fibroblastic tumor containing prominent, hemangiopericytoma-like, branching blood vessels. SFT is most commonly pleural based. Extrapleural SFT occurs in subcutaneous tissue, and the deep soft tissues of the head and neck and/or extremities.

FIGURE 9.12. This well circumscribed extrapleural SFT shows a firm, white-tan, gritty cut surface.

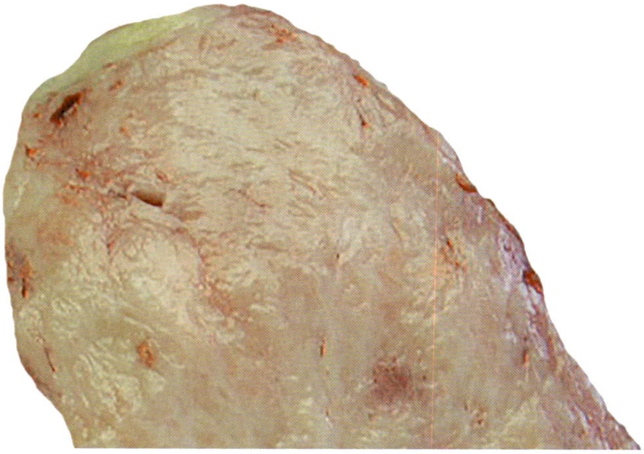

Myxoinflammatory fibroblastic sarcoma (MIFS)

MIFS is a rarely metastasizing, locally aggressive sarcoma occurring primarily in the distal extremities of middle-aged adults. Although the local recurrence rate is high (up to 70%), metastatic disease is exceedingly rare.

FIGURE 9.13. This specimen displays a subcutaneous, multinodular myxoid tumor involving the tenosynovial structures of the finger.

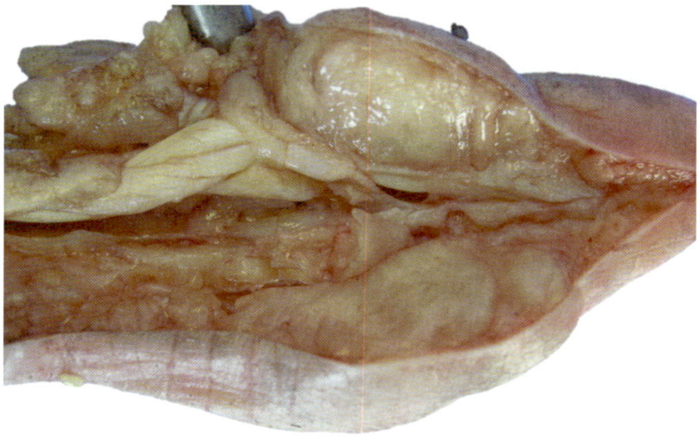

Myxofibrosarcoma

Myxofibrosarcoma is a relatively common sarcoma in elderly patients. Most myxofibrosarcomas arise in the limbs and limb girdles, and at least 50% of cases occur above the fascia (unusual for sarcomas in general). Myxofibrosarcomas tend to extend along fibrous septa, making them difficult to resect and accounting for multiple local recurrences. As with most sarcomas, these tumors can metastasize to the lungs; in addition, myxofibrosarcomas may spread to bones or even lymph nodes. Prognosis is closely tied to tumor grade.

FIGURE 9.14. This specimen, adjacent to the tibia, shows an infiltrative, multinodular myxoid tumor extending to the periosteum.

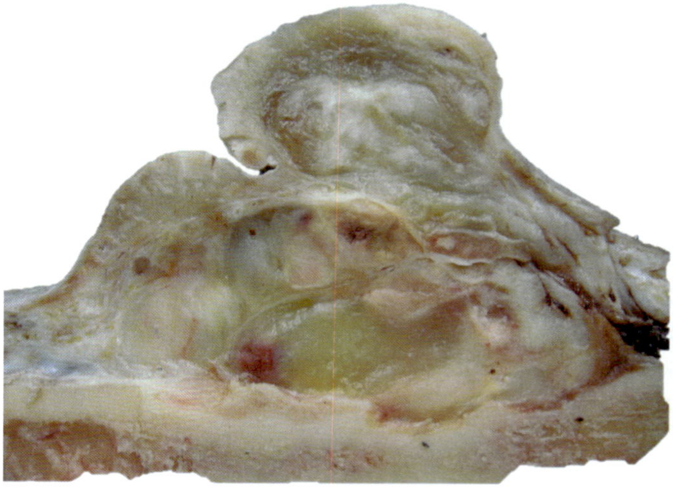

FIGURE 9.15. This deep myxofibrosarcoma of the arm has necessitated an amputation.

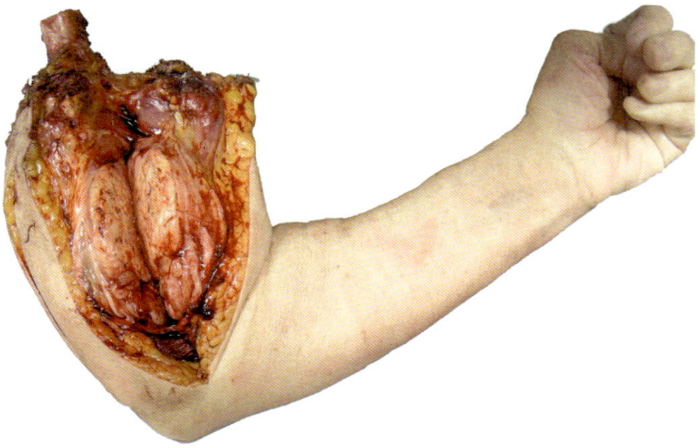

Low-grade fibromyxoid sarcoma

Low-grade fibromyxoid sarcoma is an unusual, deceptively bland, low-grade sarcoma with frequent t(7;16) (*FUS-CREB3L2*) rearrangement. Most patients are young adults. The thigh, shoulder, and chest wall are preferential locations for this type of sarcoma, and recurrence and metastasis can occur late after the primary excision.

FIGURE 9.16. This image shows a homogenous, tan, fibromyxoid tumor with a trabeculated cut surface.

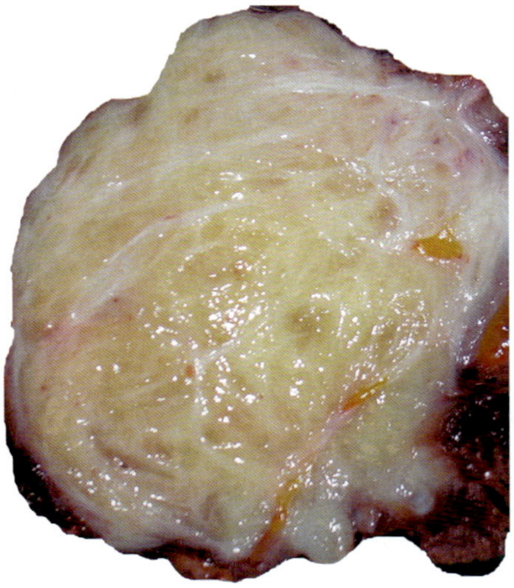

Tenosynovial giant cell tumor — diffuse type

Diffuse-type tenosynovial giant cell tumor is a locally aggressive, destructive neoplasm involving joints and periarticular soft tissue. It is commonly called pigmented villonodular synovitis when it occurs within a joint.

FIGURE 9.17. Image (A) shows gross findings of a large multinodular proliferation with a variegated yellow and tan-to-brown cut surface, and a villous appearance. In (B), a T2-weighted MRI shows a circumscribed bright mass arising posterior to the joint.

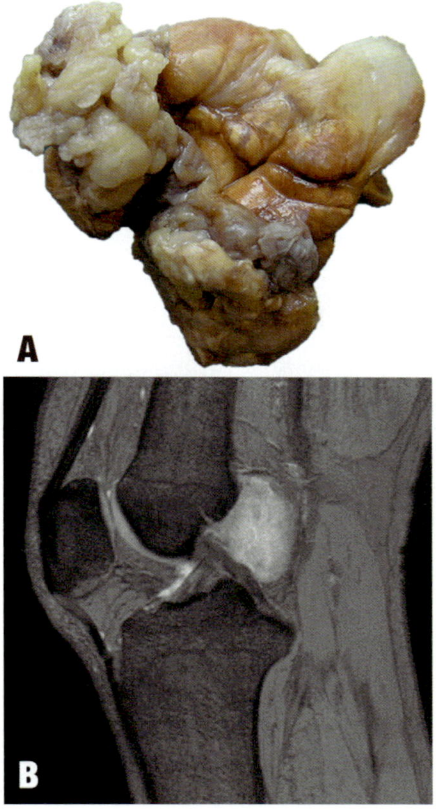

Deep benign fibrous histiocytoma

Deep benign fibrous histiocytoma is a deep-seated variant of benign fibrous histiocytoma that extends beyond the dermis. Although benign, the deep form can recur in up to 20% of cases, but very rarely metastasizes.

FIGURE 9.18. This specimen shows a well-defined subcutaneous tumor with focal hemorrhage and necrosis.

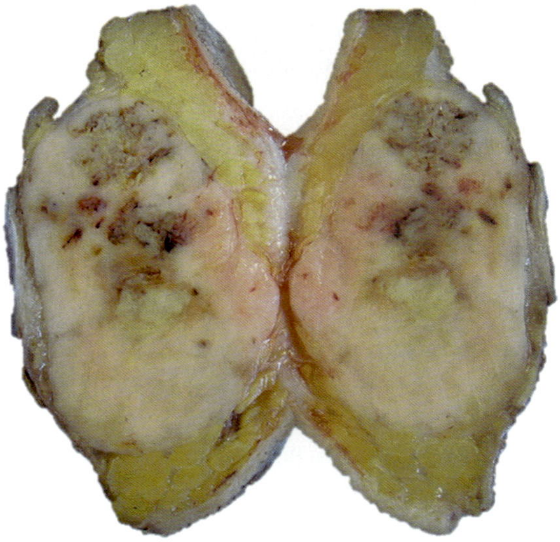

Leiomyosarcoma

Leiomyosarcoma commonly occurs in the retroperitoneum and pelvis. It is predominantly diagnosed in females.

FIGURE 9.19. Grossly, this tumor, located in the retroperitoneum, appears as a well-defined, homogeneous mass with a whorled or trabeculated cut surface reminiscent of a leiomyoma.

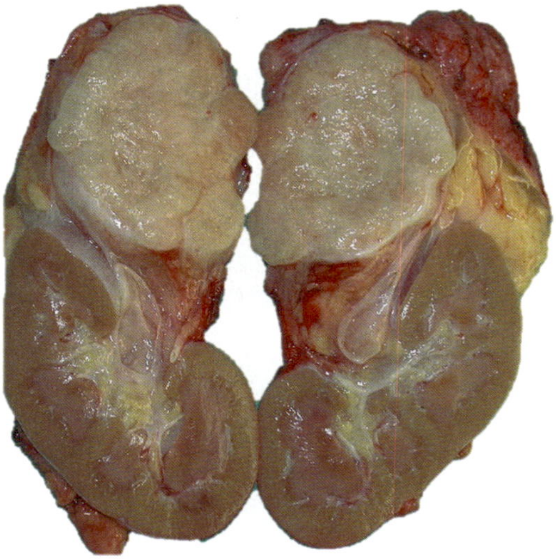

SUPERFICIAL LEIOMYOSARCOMA

Superficial leiomyosarcoma occurs above the fascia and generally has a better prognosis than its deep counterpart.

FIGURE 9.20. This image shows a well-circumscribed, fleshy, gray-tan tumor, centered in the dermis and subcutis.

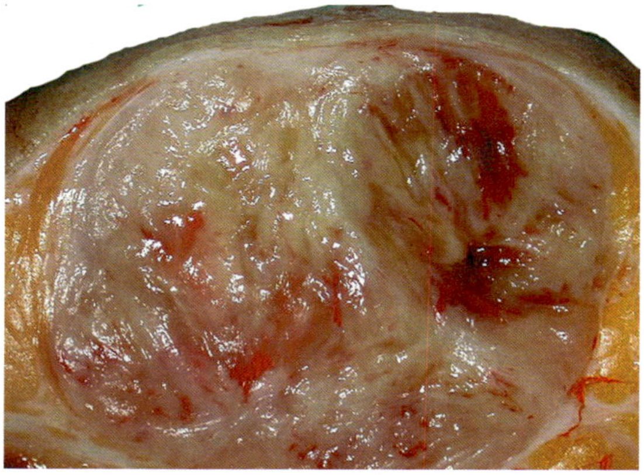

Embryonal rhabdomyosarcoma

Embryonal rhabdomyosarcoma is a malignant proliferation of primitive skeletal muscle cells. Most are diagnosed in children aged 5 to 15 years. Common sites are the head, neck, pelvis, and genital area. No consistent cytogenetic abnormality has been described; the alveolar subtype, however, has been associated with *FOXO1* rearrangement on chromosome 13. Grossly, embryonal rhabdomyosarcoma appears as a large, fleshy, tan mass with occasional cystic and hemorrhagic changes.

FIGURE 9.21. This image of an embryonal rhabdomyosarcoma from the genital area shows a large, fleshy, tan mass with some cystic and hemorrhagic changes.

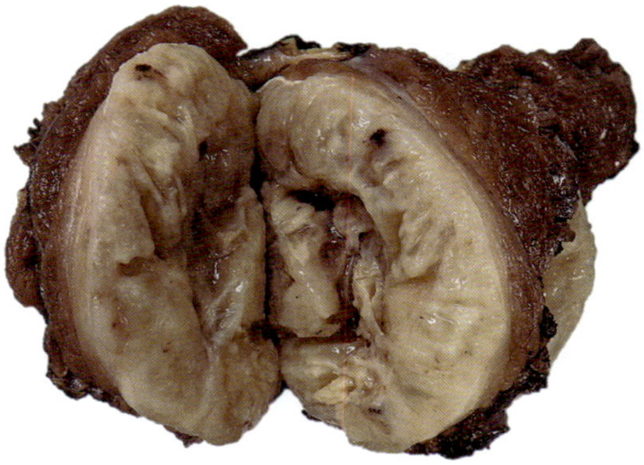

Cutaneous angiosarcoma

Cutaneous angiosarcoma is a malignant vascular neoplasm that typically occurs in sun-damaged skin of the head and neck of elderly patients. It is usually multifocal and poorly delineated, making macroscopic evaluation of margins and complete excision very difficult.

FIGURE 9.22. The cut surface of this scalp specimen reveals extensive horizontal and deep infiltration by a diffuse hemorrhagic lesion.

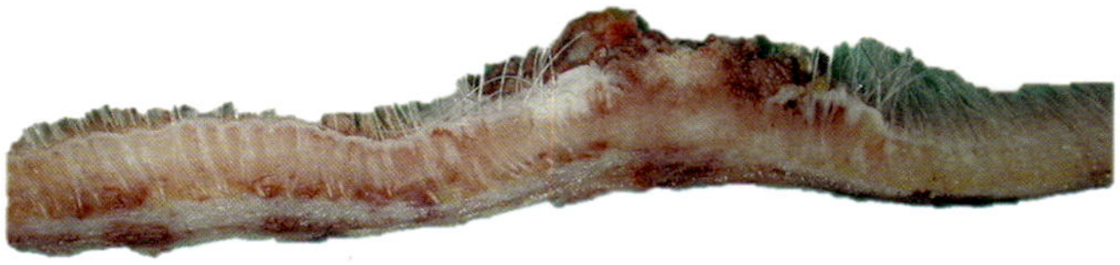

ANGIOSARCOMA OF DEEP SOFT TISSUE

Angiosarcomas of deep soft tissue are commonly found in the lower extremities, where no specific causative factor is identified. Risk factors for angiosarcoma in other specific contexts include Thorotrast exposure (liver), vascular implants, radiation (breast, skin), and lymphedema (breast, skin).

FIGURE 9.23. Grossly, this tumor from the buttock appears as a large ill-defined, hemorrhagic mass reminiscent of a hematoma.

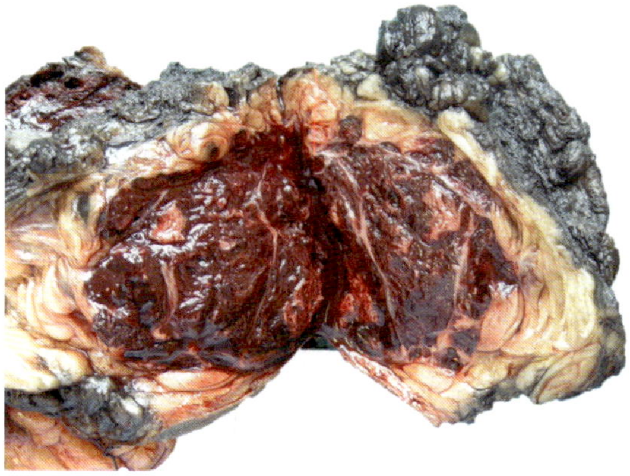

Soft tissue chondroma

Soft tissue chondromas are benign, extraskeletal and extrasynovial proliferations of chondrocytes and chondroid matrix. They most commonly occur in the fingers, and also in the hands, feet, and toes.

FIGURE 9.24. This example shows a well-demarcated and lobulated firm, gray-white nodule with central myxoid change in the hand.

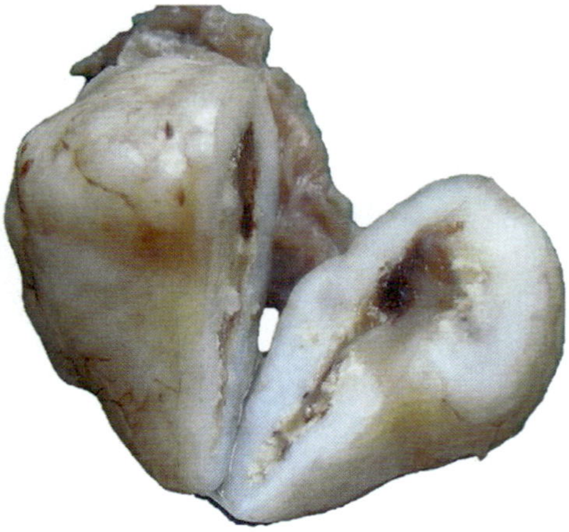

Ganglioneuroma

Ganglioneuroma is a benign tumor of the sympathetic nervous system characterized by an admixture of mature ganglion cells (neurons) and abundant Schwann cells. It usually occurs in the adrenal gland, retroperitoneum, and posterior mediastinum. Most ganglioneuromas are thought to develop de novo rather than from maturing neuroblastomas.

FIGURE 9.25. This tumor from the retroperitoneum is encapsulated and has a homogenous, gray-tan cut surface.

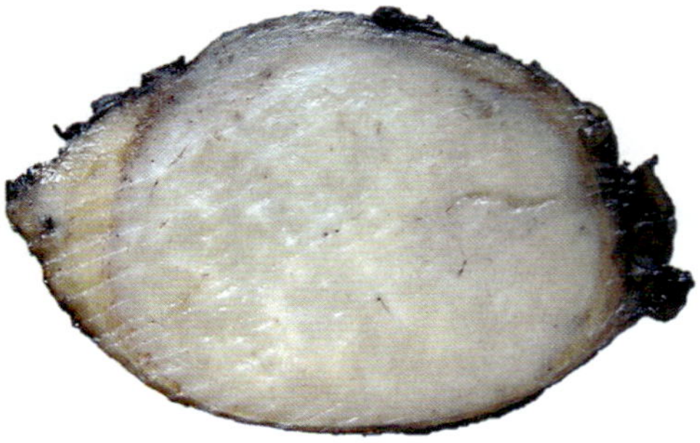

Schwannoma

Schwannoma is a common, benign, mesenchymal tumor that arises from the nerve sheath in middle-aged adults. Most tumors are solitary and found close to peripheral nerves, nerve plexuses, or spinal roots. Multiple schwannomas occur as part of neurofibromatosis type 2 (NF2).

FIGURE 9.26. In this solitary tumor, a globoid, eccentric nodule (left) distorts the associated nerve (right).

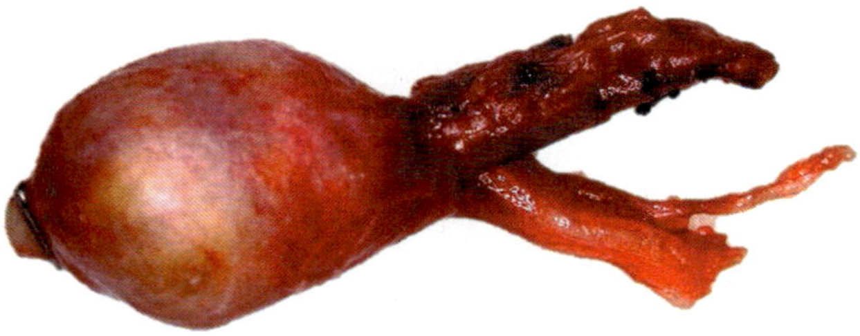

Neurofibroma

Neurofibroma is a benign tumor of the peripheral nerve sheath that expands native nerve fibers. Most are solitary and occur sporadically, but they also present as multiple tumors in patients with neurofibromatosis type 1 (NF1).

FIGURE 9.27. Grossly, this localized, cutaneous tumor of the thigh shows a tan, semitranslucent, and glistening cut surface.

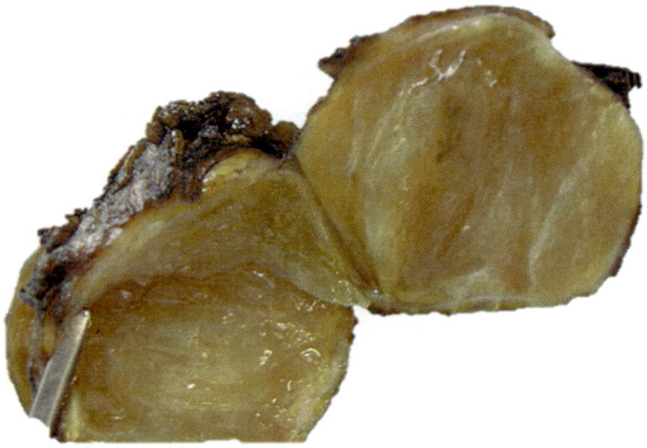

Dermal nerve sheath myxoma

Dermal nerve sheath myxoma is a rare, benign nerve sheath tumor, commonly found in superficial locations of the distal extremities, such as the fingers. It affects patients across a wide age range. Grossly, these tumors are small and multinodular.

FIGURE 9.28. This specimen, located on the shoulder, shows a well-circumscribed, yellow-tan myxoid tumor with surrounding subcutaneous adipose tissue.

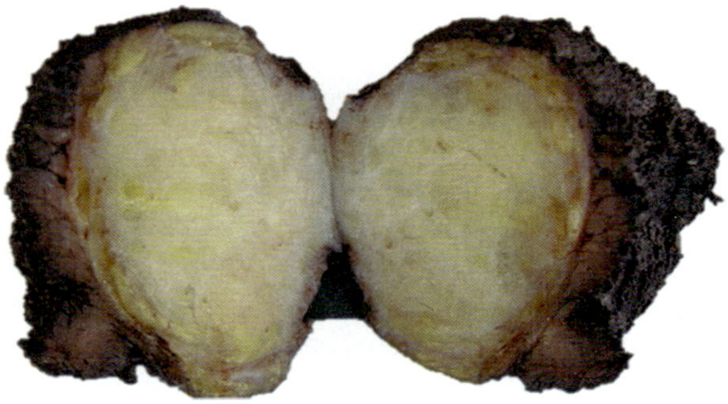

Malignant peripheral nerve sheath tumor (MPNST)

MPNST can arise in the setting of radiation, or result from transformation (either sporadic or in the setting of NF1) of a neurofibroma. Most are diagnosed in middle-aged adults and located in the extremities, trunk, and/or neck. Grossly, MPNSTs are large and heterogeneous tumors with hemorrhage and necrosis.

FIGURE 9.29. This MPNST has arisen in a large nerve; native nerve is visible at both ends of the specimen, with the tumor expanding the specimen's central portion.

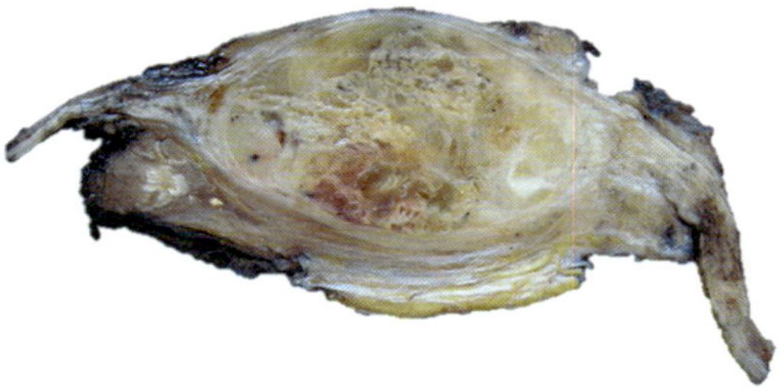

Retrorectal cystic hamartoma (tailgut cyst)

Retrorectal cystic hamartoma, or tailgut cyst, is a rare, benign, congenital lesion typically identified in the retrorectal space in young women. Absence of neural and dermal elements distinguish it from teratoma in a similar location.

FIGURE 9.30. This tailgut cyst occurred in the sacrum. The cut surface shows a multinodular, solid, and cystic lesion with mucoid content.

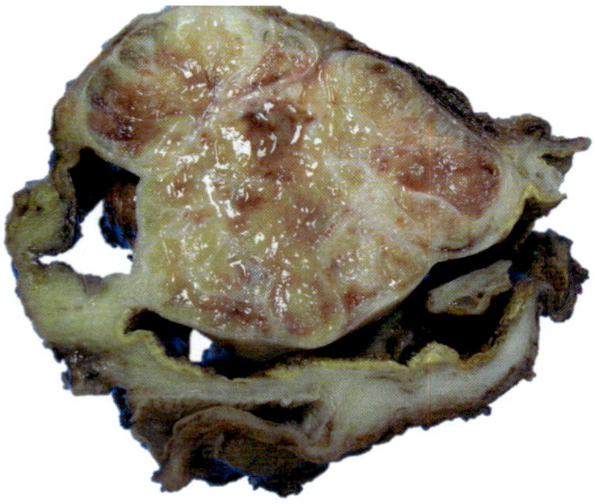

Intramuscular myxoma

Intramuscular myxoma is a benign, paucicellular, myxoid neoplasm that tends to involve large muscles of the shoulder and hip girdles. Point mutations in the *GNAS* gene are commonly identified. When these lesions occur along with fibrous dysplasia, they are characteristic of Mazabraud syndrome. Although myxomas appear well defined, microscopic examination often reveals infiltration into the adjacent skeletal muscle.

FIGURE 9.31. This cut surface shows a well-circumscribed intramuscular gelatinous mass with fine internal septations.

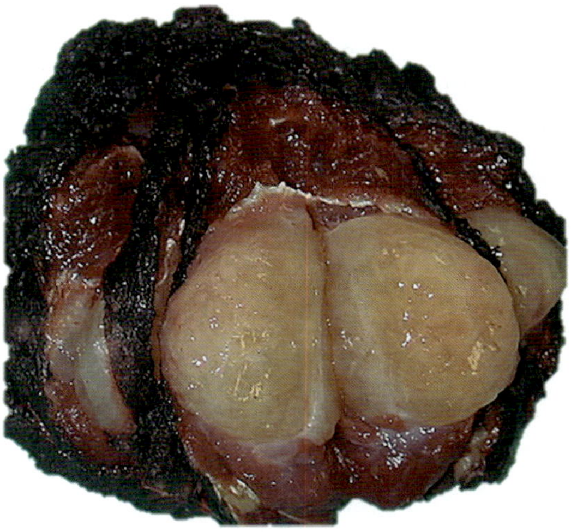

Angiomatoid fibrous histiocytoma (AFH)

AFH is a fibrohistiocytic tumor of intermediate malignancy with a low potential for metastasis. It typically affects young patients, and presents as a subcutaneous lesion adjacent to lymph nodes (antecubital fossa, popliteal fossa, inguinal, or neck) where it may mimic a hematoma. More than 90% of cases harbor a specific t(2;22), resulting in *EWSR1-CREB1* fusion.

FIGURE 9.32. This specimen, found in the arm, shows a nodular, rubbery, tan, subcutaneous tumor in which the typical blood-filled spaces are not apparent.

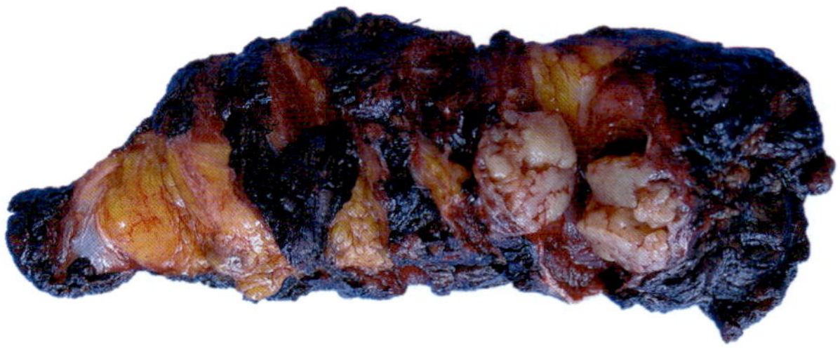

Myoepithelioma (mixed tumor, parachordoma)

The majority of myoepitheliomas behave in a benign fashion, but tumors with prominent cytological atypia may be more aggressive. *EWSR1* gene rearrangement is found in many tumors. Malignant myoepithelioma is an uncommon soft tissue tumor sharing many histologic features with its salivary gland counterpart. Most patients are young adults presenting with palpable soft tissue masses in the hip and thigh.

FIGURE 9.33. This image shows a benign myoepithelioma: a well-circumscribed, fleshy, hemorrhagic tumor with a peripheral rim of gelatinous-to-solid tissue. The gelatinous tumor is more typical for a benign myoepithelioma.

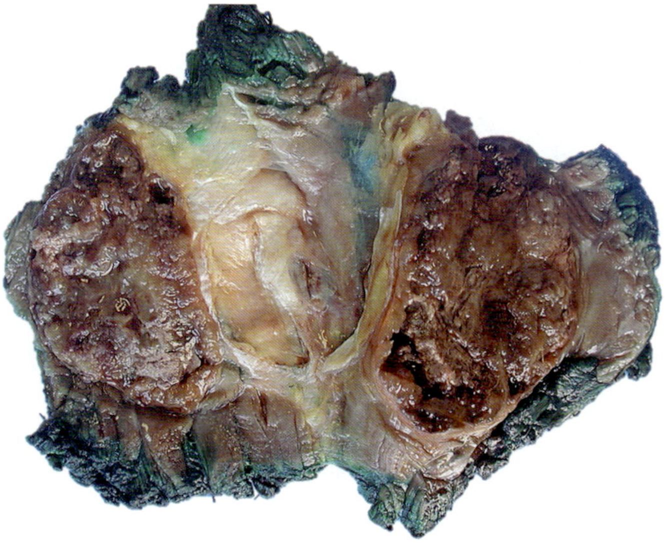

Synovial sarcoma (SS)

SS is a malignant biphasic tumor showing both epithelial (not synovial) and mesenchymal differentiation. It commonly arises adjacent to large joints, and primarily affects teenagers and young adults. SS harbors a defining (X;18) translocation.

FIGURE 9.34. Image (A) shows SS arising near the ankle. In (B), the cut surface shows a tan-pink, nodular mass intimately associated with tendons and soft tissue.

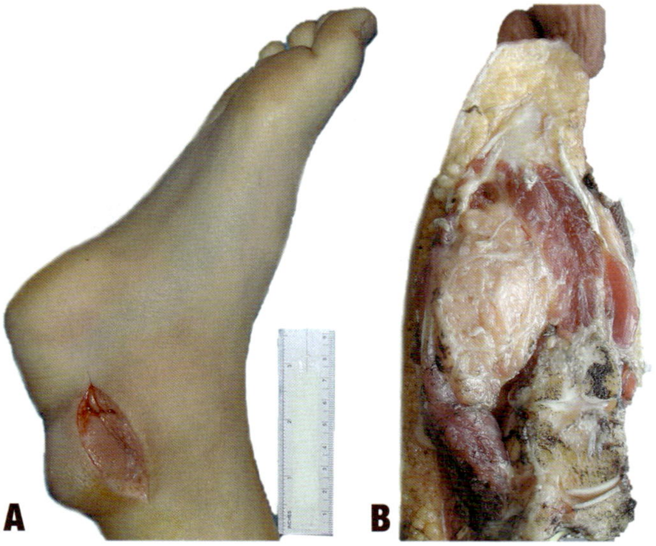

Epithelioid sarcoma

Epithelioid sarcoma is a malignant mesenchymal tumor with epithelial features associated with loss of the tumor suppressor gene *SMARCB1* on chromosome 22. The proximal type occurs in the pelvic and genital regions, in contrast to the more common distal type, which presents as small ulcerating lesions in the fingers and hands.

FIGURE 9.35. The cut section of this proximal-type epithelioid sarcoma shows a gray-tan, solid tumor with areas of hemorrhage and necrosis encasing a large femoral vessel.

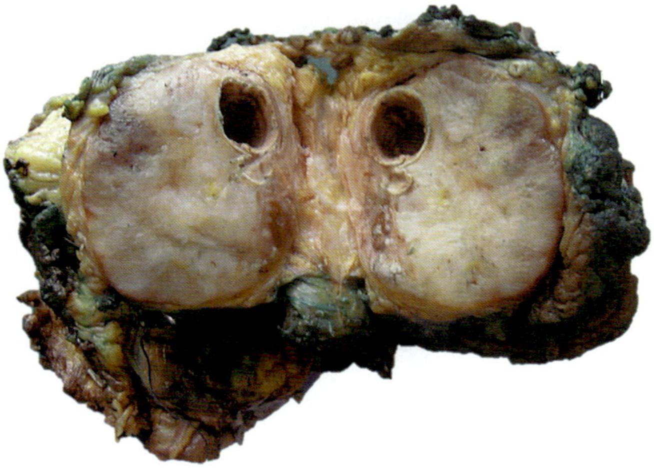

Clear cell sarcoma (CCS) (malignant melanoma of soft parts)

CCS, also called malignant melanoma of soft parts, is a rare sarcoma of young people and has a poor prognosis. Histologically, it mimics malignant melanoma, but is distinguished by the demonstration of t(12;22)(*EWSR1-ATF1*). Lymph node metastasis develops in half of patients.

FIGURE 9.36. As this image from a lower limb demonstrates, CCS is nonpigmented, and often arises and spreads along tendon sheaths.

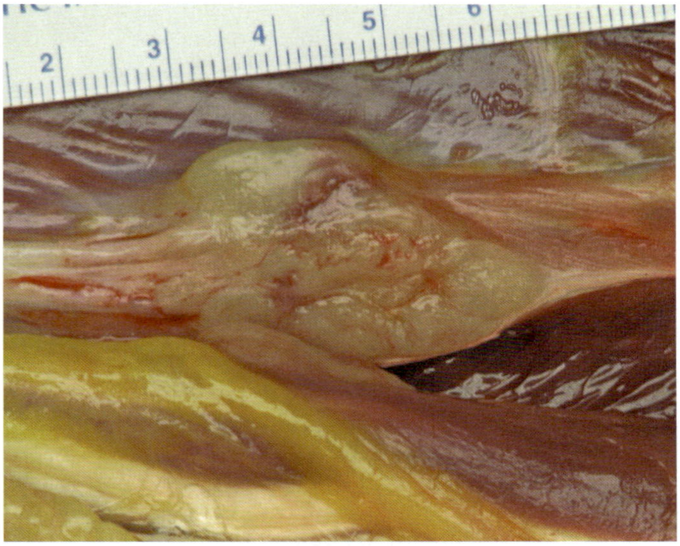

Extraskeletal myxoid chondrosarcoma (ESMC)

ESMCs are rare, malignant tumors. They do not, despite their name, demonstrate cartilaginous differentiation. Grossly, they appear as gray-tan, multinodular masses with a glistening, myxoid texture. Hemorrhage is common, and therefore these tumors can be mistaken for hematomas.

FIGURE 9.37. This image shows a gray-tan, multinodular mass with a glistening, myxoid texture.

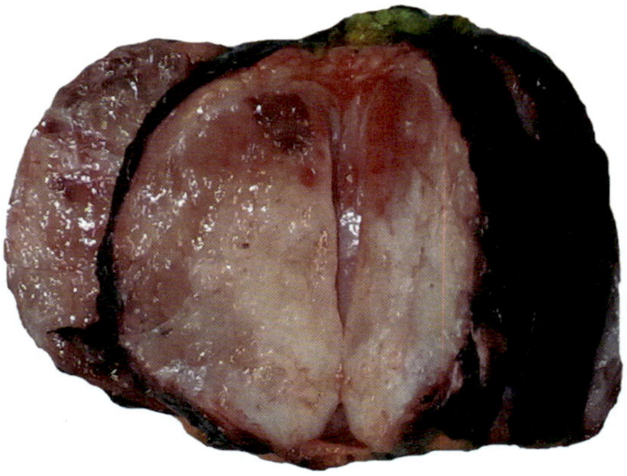

Undifferentiated pleomorphic sarcoma (UPS)

UPS refers to a group of high-grade sarcomas without signs of specific differentiation. UPS is a diagnosis of exclusion, when histology, immunohistochemistry, and molecular analysis fail to reveal specific differentiation. In the most common clinical scenario, older patients present with a deep lower limb mass.

FIGURE 9.38. This UPS demonstrates a large, solid, heterogeneous tumor with hemorrhage and necrosis.

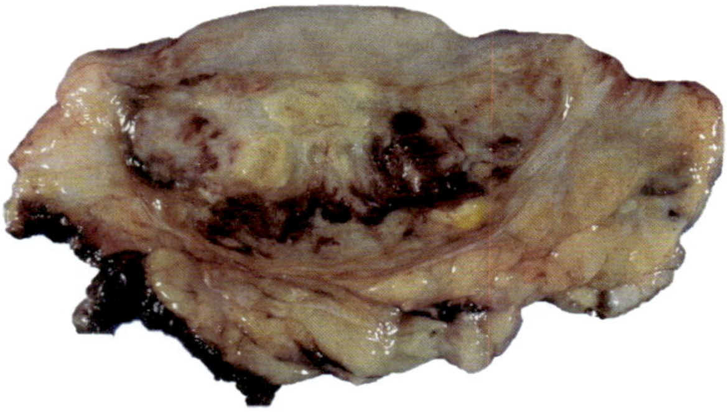

Metastasis

TESTICULAR TERATOMA METASTATIC TO RETROPERITONEUM

Teratoma and other germ cell tumors identified outside the gonads can be either primary or metastatic. Extragonadal teratoma may be found anywhere along the body's midline, especially in the mediastinum and sacrococcygeal area.

FIGURE 9.39. This cut surface reveals a multinodular mass filled with mucinous and yellow keratinous material. Thick septations and calcifications are also visible.

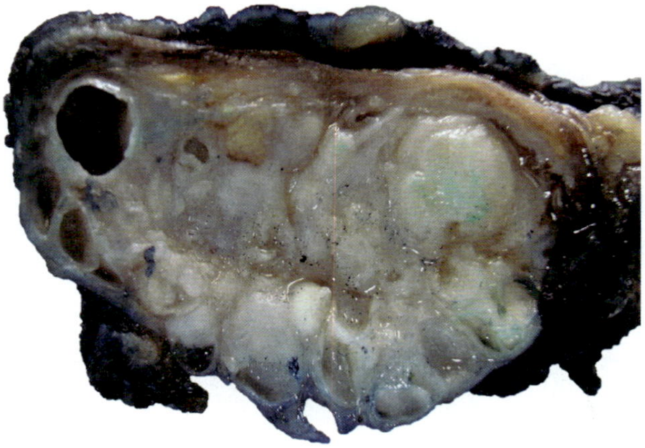

RENAL CELL CARCINOMA METASTATIC TO DERMIS

Melanoma and carcinomas of the kidney, lung, and breast are the most common malignancies that metastasize to skin.

FIGURE 9.40. This image shows a subcutaneous brown nodule with foci of hemorrhage.

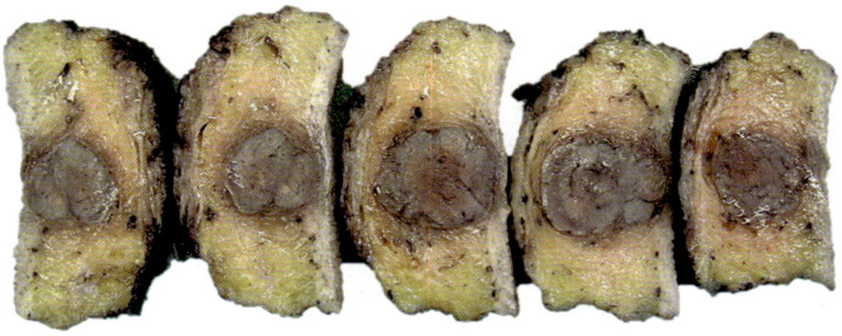

ACKNOWLEDGMENTS

We would like to thank the valuable contributions of Dr. A. Nahal and Dr. O. Ajise, and the technical help of R. Gilot, E. Griss, A. Hossain, L. Korneichyuk Pasyuk, M. Mikhael, and E. Yaney.

REFERENCES

Bullough PG. *Orthopaedic pathology*. Maryland Heights, MO: Mosby/Elsevier; 2010.

Fletcher CDM. *Diagnostic histopathology of tumors*. Philadelphia: Saunders/Elsevier; 2013.

Fletcher CDM, Bridge JA, Hogendoorn PCW, Mertens F. *WHO classification of tumours of soft tissue and bone*. 4th ed. Lyon, France: IARC Press; 2013.

Folpe AL, Inwards CY. *Bone and soft tissue pathology*. Philadelphia: Saunders/Elsevier; 2010.

Goldblum JR, Weiss SW, Folpe AL. *Enzinger and Weiss's soft tissue tumors*. 6th ed. Philadelphia: Saunders/Elsevier; 2014.

Rosai J. *Rosai and Ackerman's surgical pathology*. 10th ed. Philadelphia: Mosby/Elsevier; 2011.

10

Bone Diseases

SUNGMI JUNG, MARTIN CHEVRIER, LISA M. DIFRANCESCO

Fractures

Nonunited femoral neck fracture

Fracture nonunion can have many causes, including infection, inadequate immobilization, and disrupted blood flow. Bones such as the proximal femur and scaphoid (wrist) are especially vulnerable to disrupted blood flow and subsequent malunion or necrosis.

FIGURE 10.1. Images (A) and (B) show the cut surfaces of 2 specimens. After approximately 2 months, abundant internal and external callus is evident. Portions of the neck and head have been resorbed and the ends of the fractures are not joined.

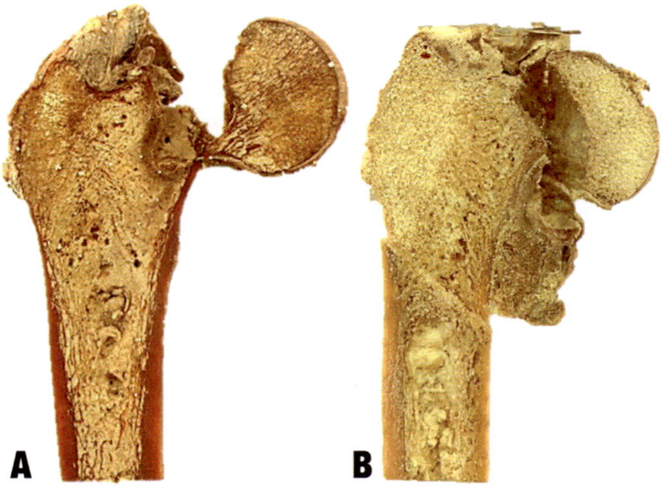

Transverse sternal fracture

This fracture is most often seen in the context of high-velocity trauma, especially motor vehicle accidents. Vigorous resuscitation maneuvers can cause rib and sternal fractures.

FIGURE 10.2. Image (A) shows a transverse sternum fracture; image (B) gives a close-up view. Contusion around edges is consistent with an antemortem fracture.

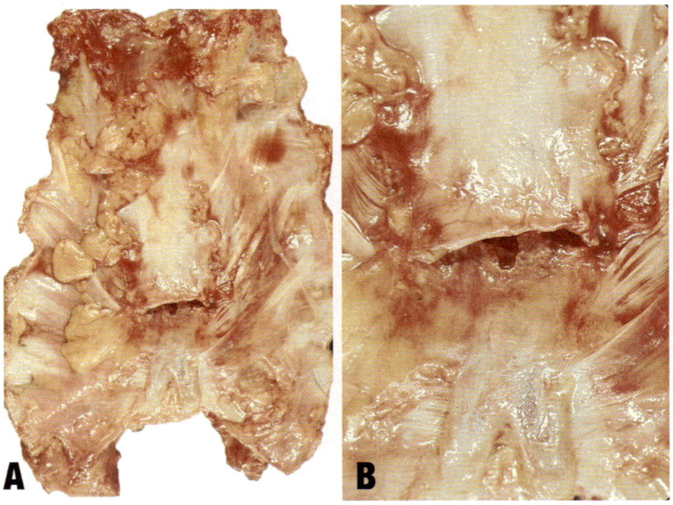

Nonneoplastic Bone Diseases

Rickets

Rickets is a disease of the immature (i.e., child) skeleton characterized by the abnormal mineralization of bone (hyperosteoidosis). Causes include nutritional or metabolic abnormalities that affect uptake of vitamin D, phosphorus, or calcium, which can disrupt normal mineralization. This leads to growth abnormalities, deformation, and pathological fractures.

FIGURE 10.3. These images show cases of rickets involving the femur (A), humerus (B), and ribs (C). Image (A) shows shortening of the femoral neck and prominent widening or flaring of the distal growth plate / metaphysis. Image (B) shows bowing of the shaft of the humerus. Image (C) shows marked thickening of the costochondral junctions (rachitic rosary) with irregular lines of ossification.

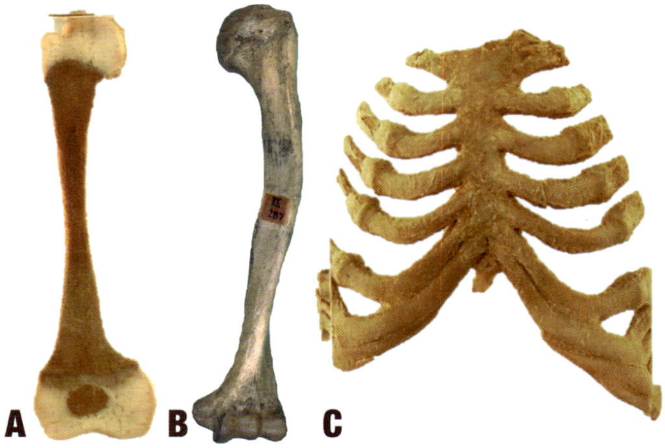

Osteoporosis

Osteoporosis is defined as a decrease in density of bone that is otherwise properly mineralized microscopically. Unbalanced osteoclastic to osteoblastic activity is central to loss of bone density in the mature skeleton. Postmenopausal women are at highest risk of osteoporosis, and can suffer fractures and spinal deformities secondary to vertebral collapse.

FIGURE 10.4. Image (A) shows vertebral osteoporosis; image (B) gives a close-up view. Grossly, spongy bone is the first to be lost, and bony trabeculae appear very thin and sparse.

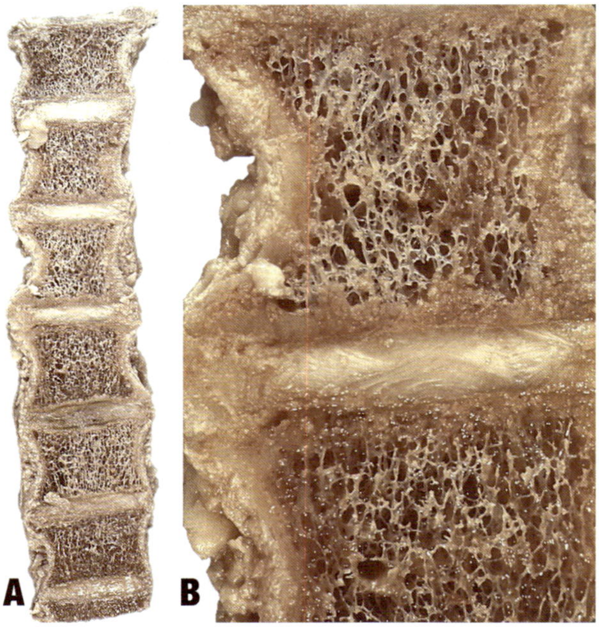

Gouty tophus

Gout is defined by hyperuricemia and deposition of monosodium urate crystals in joint spaces, soft tissues, and the kidneys. Clinically, gout may be asymptomatic, but can present with acute arthritis, renal disease, and chronic tophaceous gout. The small joints of the extremities are preferentially affected, particularly the metatarsophalangeal joint of the big toe.

FIGURE 10.5. This image shows gouty tophus near an elbow joint. Chalky, amorphous, yellow-white deposits of urate crystals (tophi) are visible in the soft tissue.

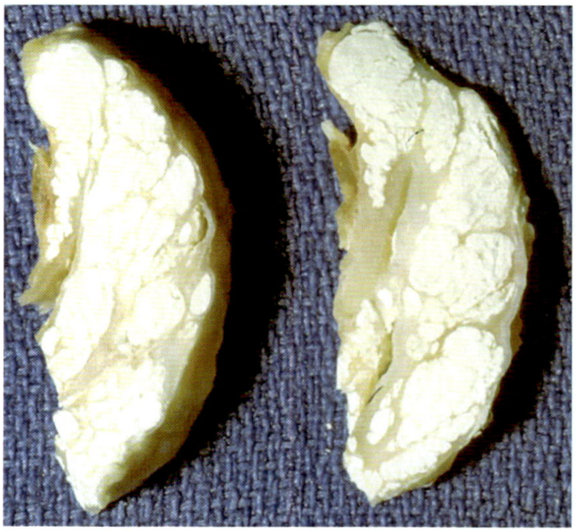

Osteonecrosis

Osteonecrosis is most commonly caused by fracture or corticosteroid administration. Vascular insufficiency due to mechanical injury, infection, or thromboembolism can all be predisposing factors.

FIGURE 10.6. This image shows a soft, yellow, necrotic focus in the small bones of the foot in a diabetic patient.

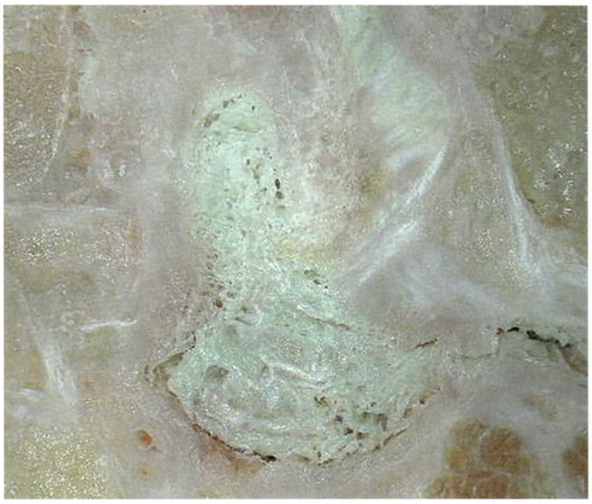

Osteoarthritis (OA)

OA is a degenerative joint disease characterized by progressive destruction and loss of articular cartilage resulting in structural and functional failure of synovial joints.

FIGURE 10.7. Image (A) shows complete cartilage loss in the medial plateau of the tibia, with eburnation (ivory-like "polishing"), scoring, and pitting of the underlying bone. Image (B) shows a cross-section of a femoral head in which advanced OA changes are seen, including cartilage thinning and loss, deformation, pseudocyst formation, and osteophyte development.

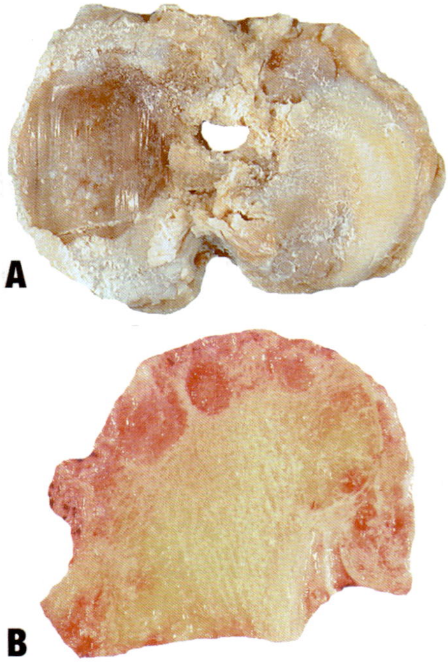

Ankylosing spondylitis

Ankylosing spondylitis is a chronic inflammatory joint disease of the spine, sacroiliac, and large proximal joints. It typically affects young males of Caucasian descent who have the major histocompatibility complex associated with human leukocyte antigen B27 (HLA-B27).

FIGURE 10.8. The spine is typically involved in an ascending fashion, and shows thinning of intervertebral discs, thickening of surrounding ligaments, and fusion of adjacent vertebral bodies.

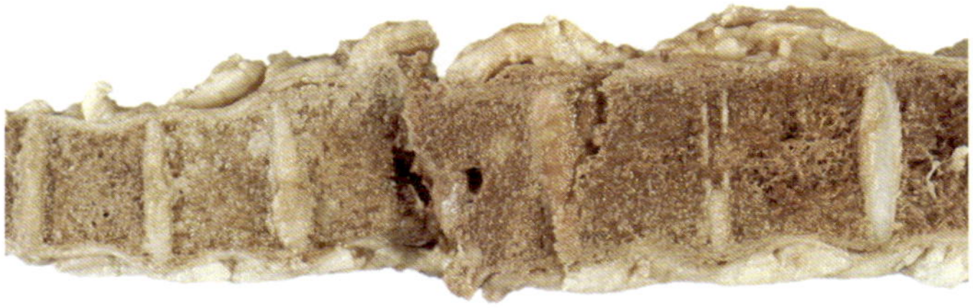

Paget disease (osteitis deformans)

Paget disease, or osteitis deformans, is a multiphasic and usually polyostotic skeletal disease affecting older individuals of Caucasian descent. It especially affects the bones of the skull, spine, and pelvis. The disease is characterized by abnormal remodeling of the bone; mutations involving p62 / sequestosome 1 are present in some cases.

FIGURE 10.9. These images show the inner (A) and outer (B) surfaces of a skull with Paget disease. There is marked irregular thickening of the inner surfaces of both frontal bones.

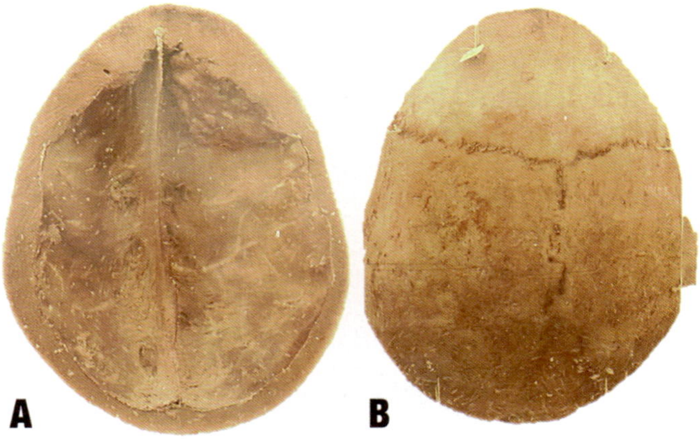

Specimen from Maude Abbott Medical Museum, McGill University

Bone Neoplasms

Osteochondroma

Osteochondroma is a common, benign bone tumor of young individuals. It is characterized by a bony outgrowth from the medullary cavity covered by a thin layer of cartilage.

FIGURE 10.10. The x-ray in (A) shows a mushroom-shaped projection arising at an acute angle to the surface of the fibula. Grossly, in (B), these lesions may be sessile or pedunculated, and are covered by a cartilaginous cap.

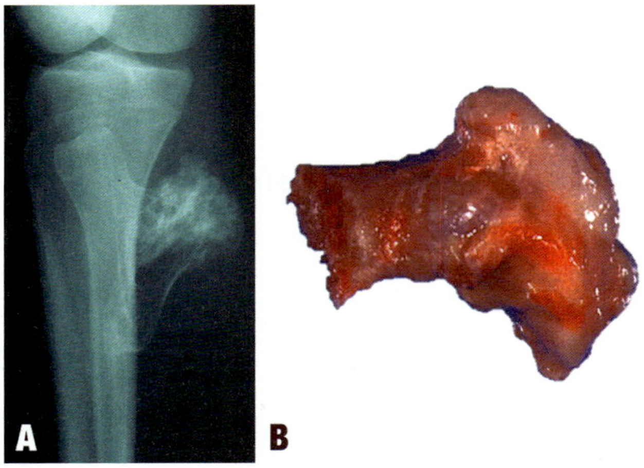

PERIPHERAL CHONDROSARCOMA ARISING FROM PREEXISTING OSTEOCHONDROMA

While solitary osteochondromas have a low risk of transformation to chondrosarcoma, patients with hereditary osteochondromatosis have an increased risk of up to 5%. A thickened cartilaginous cap (> 1.5 cm), increased pain, and rapid growth are worrisome signs that may indicate malignant transformation.

FIGURE 10.11. This cut surface of a large, gray, translucent chondrosarcoma shows a markedly thickened cartilaginous cap and periosteal lifting.

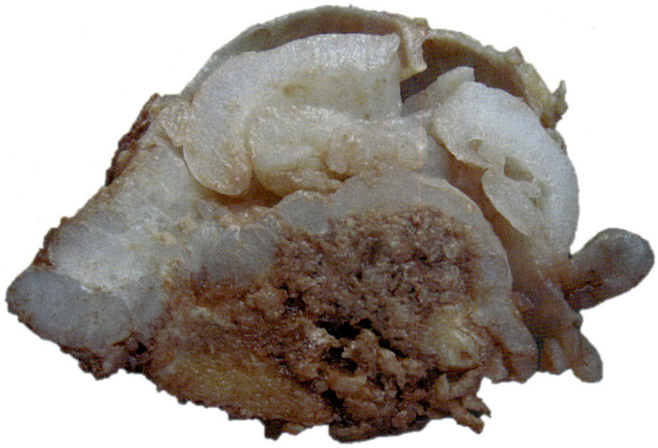

Enchondroma

Enchondromas are benign, cartilaginous tumors that classically develop within the medullary cavity of small bones of the hands and feet, although occasionally they occur in the long bones. Most are single, small (< 5 cm) lesions. The presence of multiple enchondromas is characteristic of Ollier disease and Maffucci syndrome (which is characterized by multiple enchondromas and soft tissue hemangiomas).

FIGURE 10.12. This image of a finger lesion shows a circumscribed, white-gray, rubbery mass without cortical disruption.

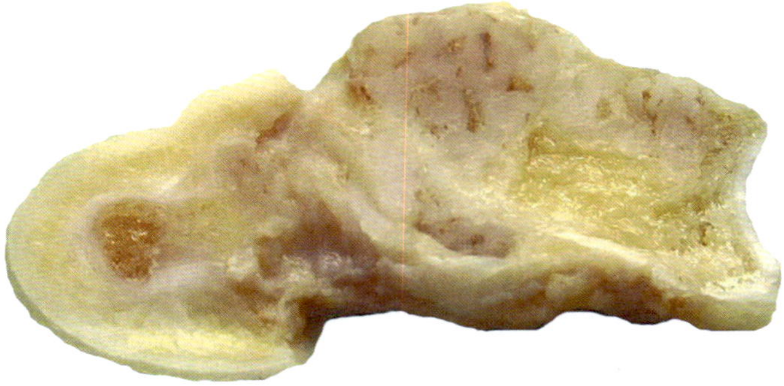

SECONDARY CHONDROSARCOMA (CS) AND ENCHONDROMA

Secondary CS arising within a solitary enchondroma is rare.

FIGURE 10.13. Image (A) shows a solitary enchondroma with adjacent secondary CS on the tibia. The CS — an infiltrative, gray, gelatinous mass — is invading the cortex alongside a well-defined white nodule: the enchondroma. In (B), an x-ray depicts a case of Ollier disease (i.e., multiple enchondromas) confined to 1 limb. No malignancy is present here, but the rate of transformation to secondary chondrosarcoma in Ollier disease is high: approximately 40%.

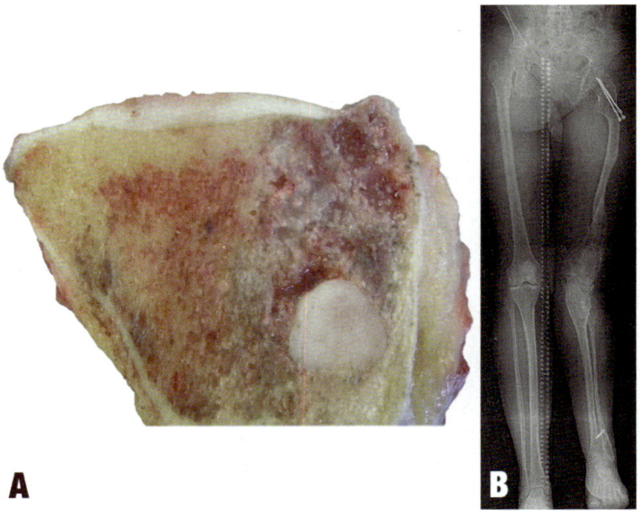

Bizarre parosteal osteochondromatous proliferation (Nora lesion)

Bizarre parosteal osteochondromatous proliferation, also called Nora lesion, is a rare, benign, osteochondromatous proliferation found mainly on the outer surface of small bones of the hands and feet in middle-aged adults (usually aged 30 to 40 years).

FIGURE 10.14. This specimen in the distal fibula shows a lobulated cartilaginous cap stuck on the surface of the bone. Unlike osteochondroma, there is no connection with the underlying medullary cavity.

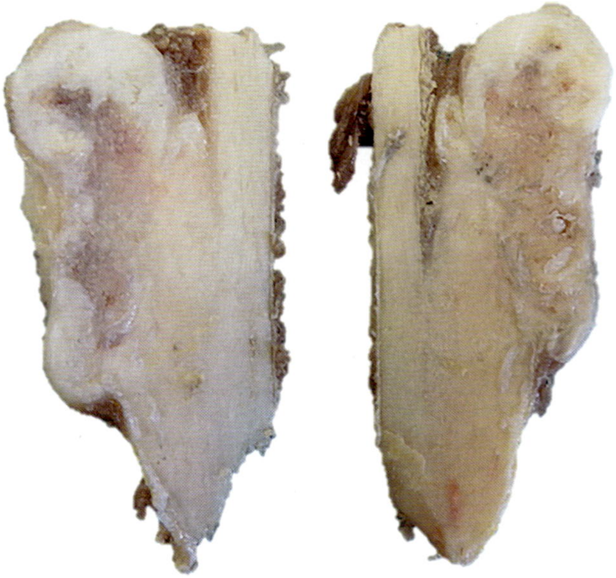

Fibrous dysplasia

Fibrous dysplasia is a benign, fibroosseous lesion with a predilection for the craniofacial and femoral bones. The disease is most commonly monostotic and found in young patients aged 10 to 30 years. The less frequent polyostotic form affects younger patients, and may be associated with endocrine abnormalities and skin pigmentation (McCune-Albright syndrome), or with intramuscular myxomas (Mazabraud syndrome). A specific recurrent mutation in the *GNAS1* gene has recently been identified, which indicates a neoplastic process.

FIGURE 10.16. In (A), an x-ray of the femur shows a benign, lytic lesion with sclerotic borders. In (B), long-standing fibrous dysplasia has markedly expanded this rib; typical white-yellow fibrous areas and secondary cyst formation are visible.

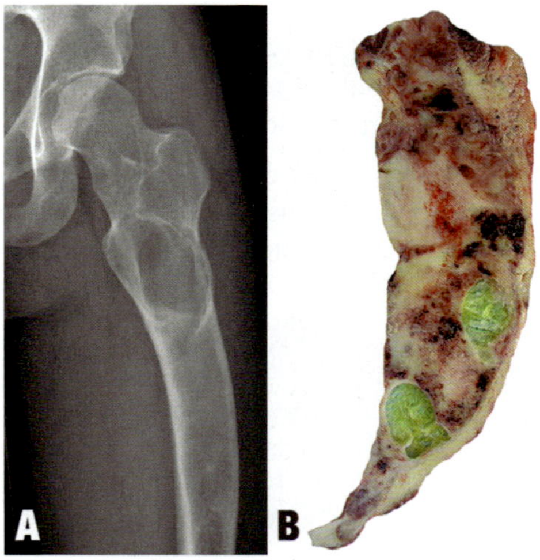

Synovial chondromatosis

Synovial chondromatosis is a subsynovial, multinodular proliferation of benign hyaline cartilage that typically affects the knee joint. It generally occurs in the third to fifth decade, and is twice as common in males. Local recurrences are seen in 20% of cases.

FIGURE 10.15. In this specimen from a knee joint, numerous cobblestone-like, white, cartilaginous nodules partially covered by synovial membrane are present.

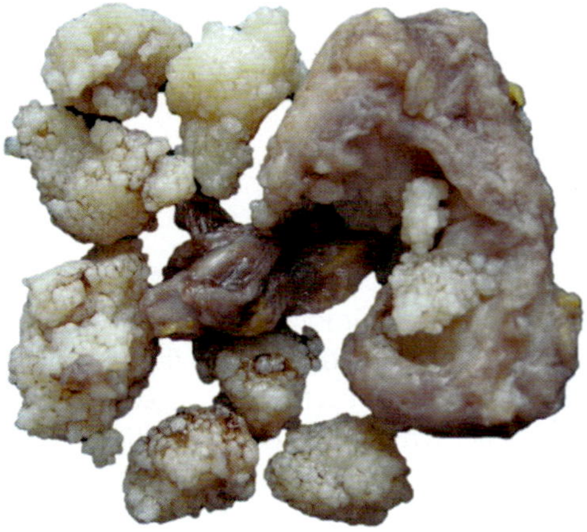

Chondroblastoma

Chondroblastoma is a benign neoplasm of immature chondrocytes (chondroblasts) that typically arises in the epiphysis or apophysis of the immature skeleton. Recently, a mutation in the histone family *K36M H3F3* gene has been found in this condition.

FIGURE 10.17. These images show x-rays of chondroblastoma of the proximal femur (A) and distal humerus (B). The x-rays demonstrate well-circumscribed, radiolucent lesions with sclerotic rims.

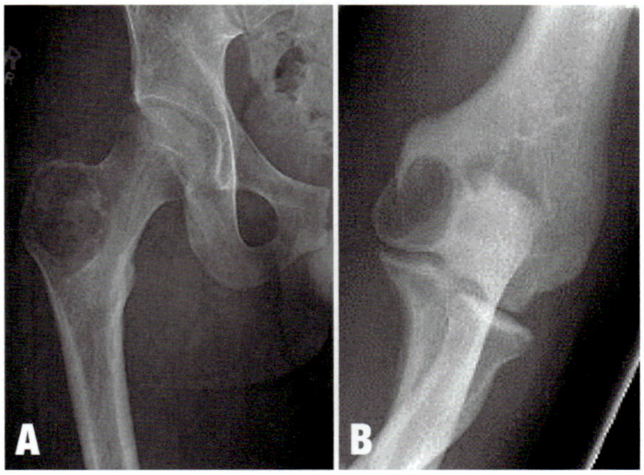

Chondrosarcoma (CS)

Primary CS is typically identified in the femur, humerus, ribs, and pelvic bones, where it accounts for approximately 20% of primary malignant tumors of the bone. It clinically presents with a long history of pain and swelling. Conventional CS does not harbor recurrent cytogenetic change, but many have *IDH1* or *IDH2* mutation.

PROCEDURE: GRADING CS

CS is graded on a 3-grade scale. Low-grade CS is a locally aggressive cartilaginous neoplasm with minimal metastatic potential. The diagnosis requires close clinical, radiological, and pathological correlation. Features that suggest malignancy include older age (older than 45 years), proximal location, pain, and cortical scalloping or breakthrough. CS needs to be sampled thoroughly for grading: grading is important in determining prognosis. Curettage or limited resection is the treatment plan for grade 1 CS. Higher-grade tumors require radical resection.

FIGURE 10.18. This gross image of grade 1 CS of the proxima humerus shows an ill-defined, blue-gray, translucent tumor invading through cortical bone into surrounding soft tissue.

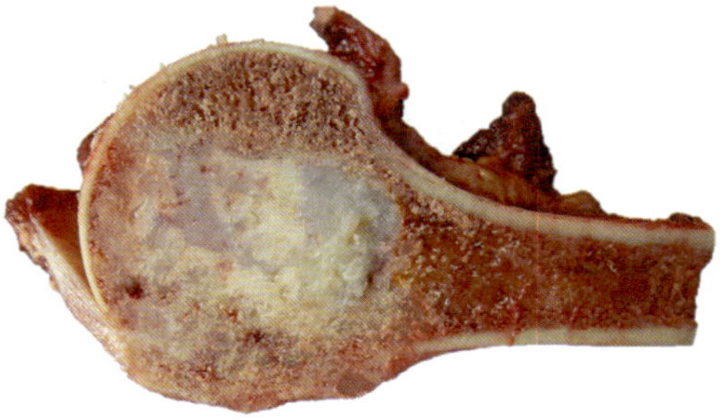

FIGURE 10.19. Grossly, this image of grade 2 CS of the manubrium sternum shows a gray-white, translucent, destructive tumor invading cortical bone and adjacent soft tissue.

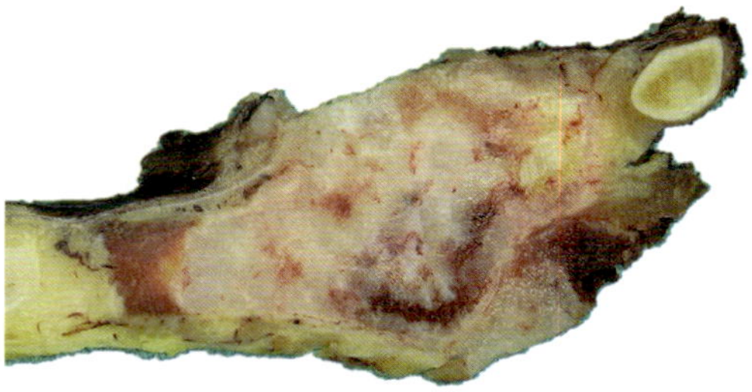

FIGURE 10.20. As seen in this specimen, higher-grade tumors tend to show prominent soft tissue extension, necrosis, and hemorrhage.

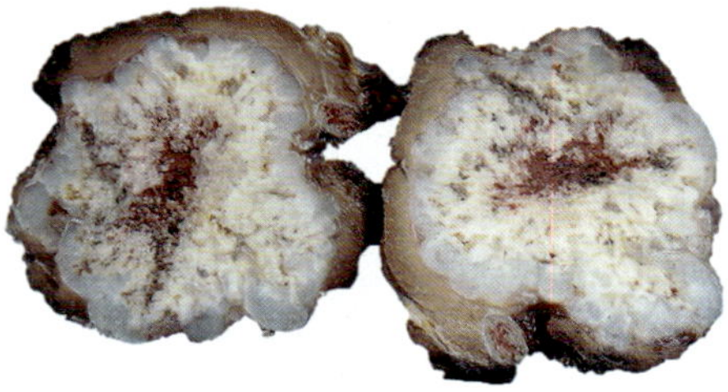

MESENCHYMAL CHONDROSARCOMA

Mesenchymal chondrosarcoma is a rare variant of chondrosarcoma that occurs in younger individuals in their second to third decade. It is characterized by a biphasic pattern of well-differentiated hyaline cartilage juxtaposed with a small-round-blue-cell component. Up to 20% of cases occur in the soft tissues.

FIGURE 10.21. This image shows a lobulated, glistening, gray tumor arising in the soft tissue adjacent to the fibula.

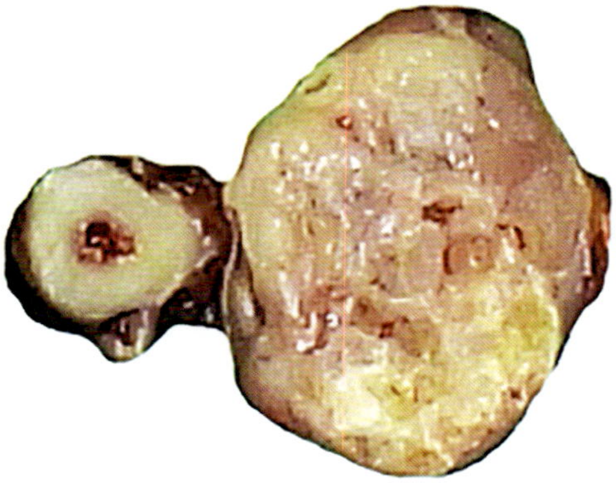

CLEAR CELL CHONDROSARCOMA

This rare but distinctive variant of chondrosarcoma arises most commonly in the epiphysis of the proximal humerus or femur in young males. Given the location and the age group affected, these tumors can be confused with chondroblastoma.

FIGURE 10.22. This large tumor, located in the glenoid fossa, has an infiltrative, myxoid, and hemorrhagic quality.

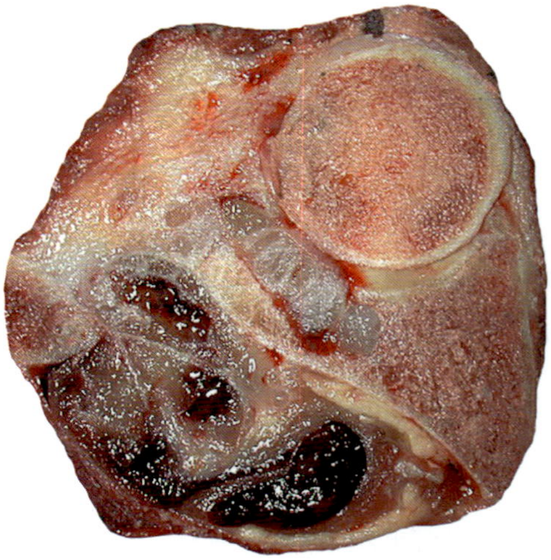

Enostosis and osteoma

Enostoses occur in the epimetaphysis of long bones. Despite their benign course, they may grow or light up on bone scan, causing concern for metastatic disease. Osteomas are benign, generally asymptomatic proliferations of compact bone found almost exclusively in the skull, facial bones, and sinuses. They can cause mass effect or obstructive symptoms. Familial adenomatous polyposis can occur in association with Gardner syndrome, which is characterized by multiple osteomas.

FIGURE 10.23. In (A), enostoses appear as small, spiculated foci of dense bone, seen here in the femoral head. Image (B) shows a bosselated osteoma of the sinus that has caused obstruction. It is made of dense, white, marble-like bone.

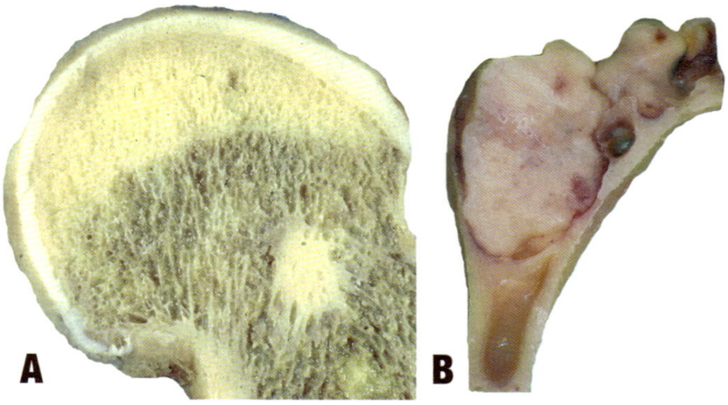

OSTEOID OSTEOMA

Osteoid osteoma is a benign, bone-forming tumor identified most commonly in young males (aged 10 to 30 years). It is characterized by intense nocturnal pain that is typically relieved by acetylsalicylic acid (ASA) or nonsteroidal antiinflammatory drugs (NSAIDs). Long bones and vertebrae are preferential sites, where the lesions often occur in a cortical and metaphyseal location.

FIGURE 10.24. This x-ray shows a typical osteoid osteoma: a small, circumscribed lesion with a central lytic nidus and an outer sclerotic rim. This osteoid osteoma measures approximately 1 cm.

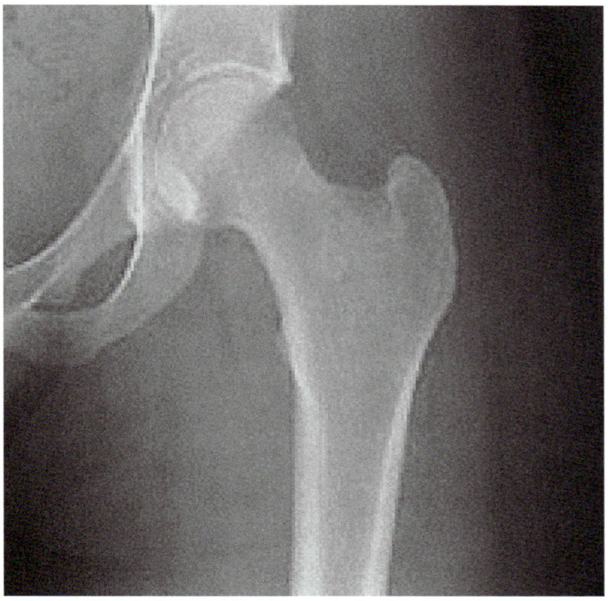

Osteoblastoma

Histologically identical to osteoid osteoma, osteoblastoma differs in location and size (osteoblastoma is typically larger). It is classically found in the intramedullary, posterior vertebral arch, and sacrum, and may be > 2 cm. Osteoblastoma also lacks the classic clinical symptomatology of osteoid osteoma, and has no nidus on imaging.

FIGURE 10.25. The external surface of this skull displays an ovoid, expansile, dark brown, and richly vascularized lesion.

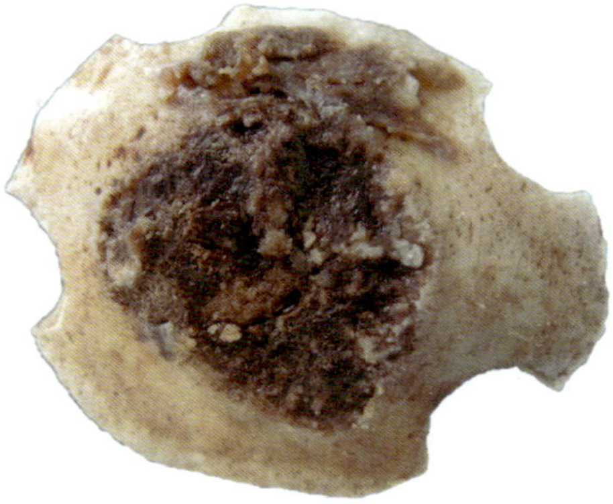

Osteosarcoma (OS)

OS is the most common primary sarcoma of bone. The incidence peaks between age 10 and 14 years, with a second smaller peak in adults older than 40 years. Osteosarcomas are typically large and rapidly growing, spreading within the medullary cavity and extending through the cortical bone into the adjacent soft tissue, eliciting an exuberant periosteal reaction. Skip or satellite lesions can occur within the same bone, leading to a worse prognosis.

CONVENTIONAL OS

FIGURE 10.26. In (A), a sagittal section of a distal femoral metaphysis shows a classic OS with hemorrhage, necrosis, and a prominent periosteal reaction. In (B), the corresponding x-ray highlights the periosteal reaction. Spicules of reactive bone are oriented perpendicular to the long axis of the bone in a characteristic "sunburst" fashion.

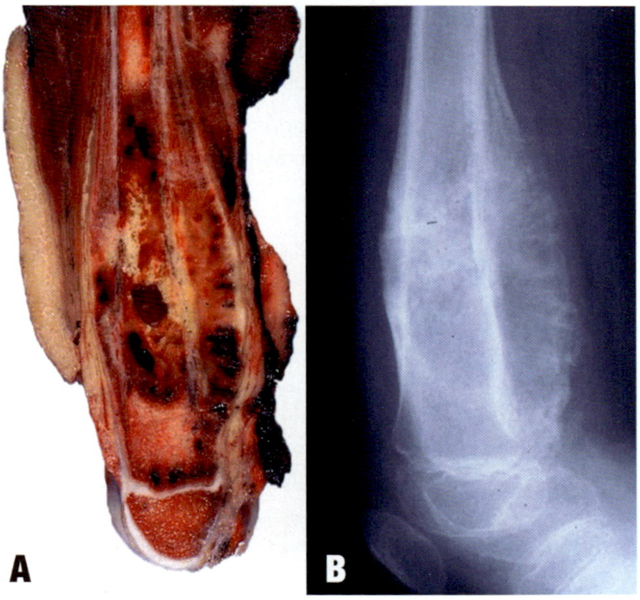

FIGURE 10.27. This tumor of the distal femur is centered in the metadiaphysis, and presents a heterogeneous, fleshy, myxoid, and hemorrhagic cut surface.

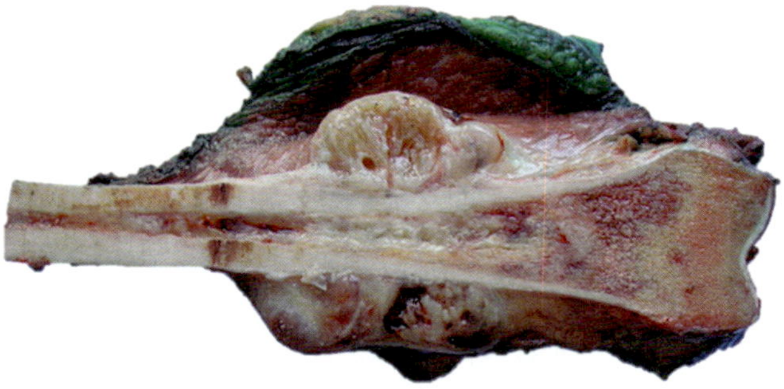

CONVENTIONAL OS POSTTREATMENT

Modern therapy revolves around preoperative chemotherapy and wide surgical resection. Posttreatment tumor regression has become a key factor in determining prognosis. Systematic mapping and extensive sampling are necessary for precise assessment.

FIGURE 10.28. This coronal cut section of a distal tibia shows a relatively homogeneous, firm, gritty, tan metaphyseal tumor — a common appearance after chemotherapy.

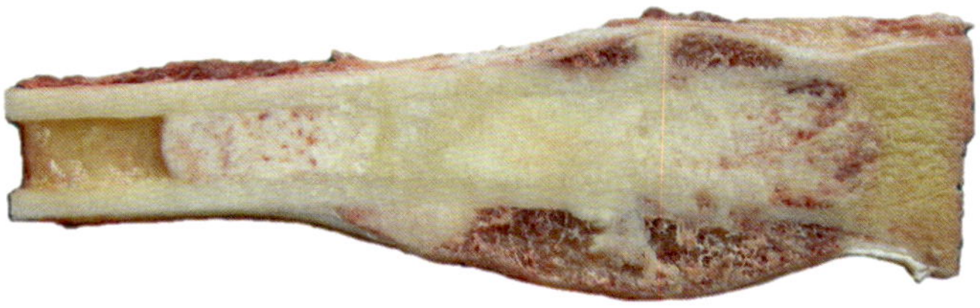

SECONDARY OS

In young patients, OS usually develops without an identifiable predisposing factor, although patients with a history of retinoblastoma or Li–Fraumeni syndrome are at an increased risk. In older patients, secondary OS is more common. Tumors may arise in a setting of radiation or previously abnormal bone due to, for example, Paget disease, a foreign body, or fibrous dysplasia.

FIGURE 10.29. In this image, an aggressive tumor arises in a background of long-standing Paget disease with a characteristic "saber shin" deformity of the tibia.

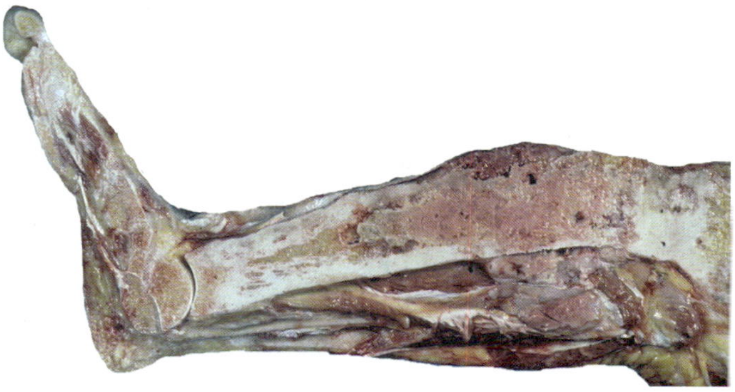

CHONDROBLASTIC OS

Chondroblastic osteosarcoma is an OS variant that contains malignant cartilage. This subtype is often seen in surface osteosarcomas (parosteal, periosteal). Despite the presence of cartilage, the histological finding of malignant osteoid leads to a diagnosis of osteosarcoma.

FIGURE 10.30. This image shows lobules of an infiltrative, white-gray, translucent tumor.

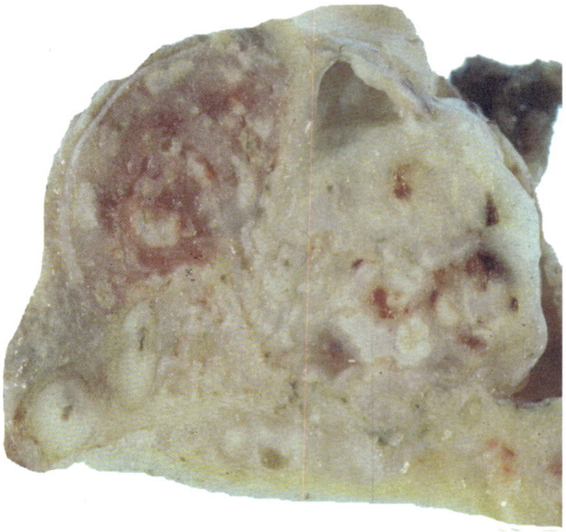

TELANGIECTATIC OS

Telangiectatic osteosarcoma is an OS variant with prominent hemorrhage and blood-filled cystic spaces. On radiological imaging, it appears as an ill-defined, invasive, and lytic neoplasm, and can mimic an aneurysmal bone cyst.

FIGURE 10.31. This coronal section of a distal femur shows a widely invasive sarcoma with numerous hemorrhagic loculations.

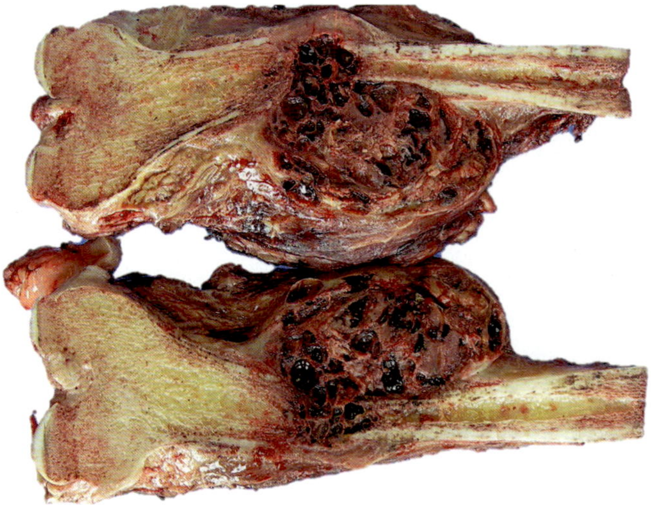

PAROSTEAL OS

Parosteal osteosarcoma is a distinct subtype of low-grade OS generally identified on the posterior surface of the distal femur. Parosteal and periosteal osteosarcoma subtypes have a better prognosis than conventional OS, given their limited involvement of the medullary cavity.

FIGURE 10.32. This sagittal cut section demonstrates a broad-based surface OS with focal medullary cavity extension. It is tan, firm, and calcified with elements of gray, translucent cartilage.

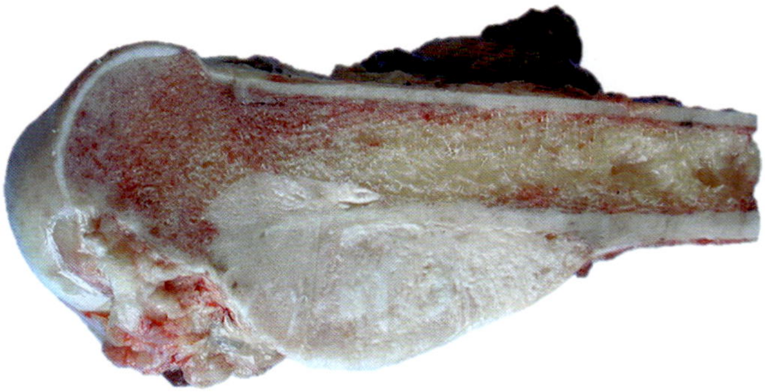

HIGH-GRADE SURFACE OS

High-grade surface OS is rare. The epidemiology of this lesion is similar to conventional OS, and the femur, tibia, and humerus are preferential sites. Although the histological appearance is not unique, this variant does not involve the medullary cavity.

FIGURE 10.33. Grossly, a large variegated and necrotic tumor surrounds the proximal tibia with minimal erosion of cortical bone, and no extension into the underlying bone.

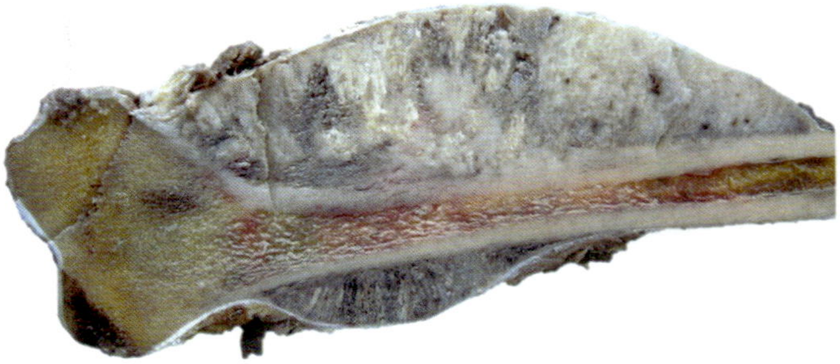

Ewing sarcoma (ES) / primitive neuroectodermal tumor (PNET)

ES, also called PNET, is a high-grade, small-round-blue-cell tumor that peaks in the teenage years. ES tends to involve the diaphysis of the long bones, pelvis, and ribs. Fever, pain, swelling, and leukocytosis are frequent clinical features, and can simulate osteomyelitis. ES is associated with a classic translocation: t(11;22).

FIGURE 10.34. This image shows an extensive, permeative tumor in the proximal humerus with cortical thickening and a large soft tissue component.

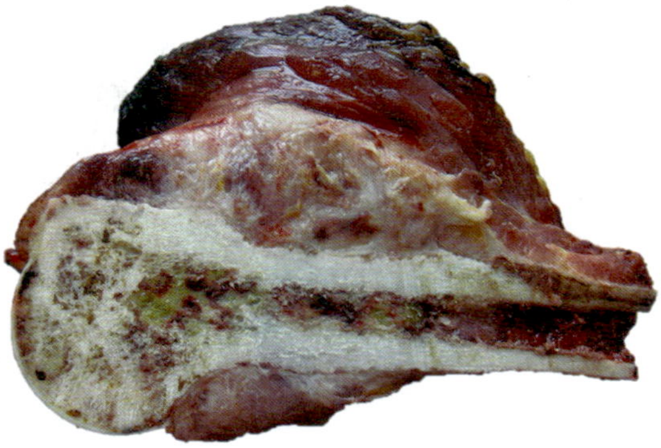

POSTTREATMENT ES/PNET

Modern treatment protocols with high-dose radiation and multidrug chemotherapy have dramatically improved survival in patients with ES. Measuring posttreatment tumor regression and necrosis is important in determining prognosis; unfavorable prognostic factors include metastatic disease, older age, and large tumors.

FIGURE 10.35. Grossly, after partial regression, this diaphyseal tumor of the fibula demonstrates diffuse cortical bone permeation and periosteal reaction.

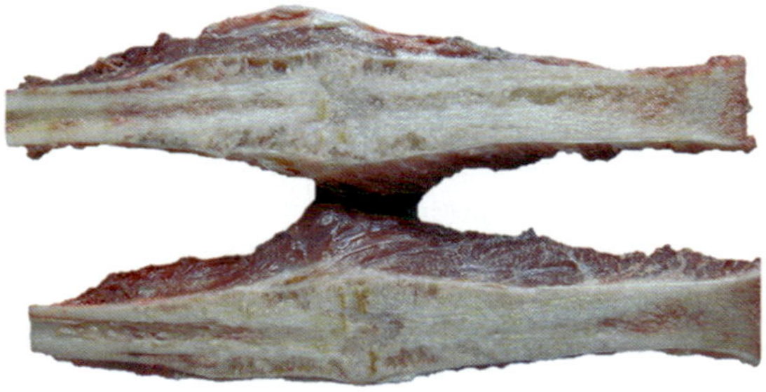

Angiosarcoma

Angiosarcoma involving bone is a rare, aggressive malignancy that most often presents as a painful lesion. It occurs throughout adulthood. One-third of cases may have multiple lesions.

FIGURE 10.36. This scapular tumor shows multiple punched-out, vascular lesions with surrounding sclerosis.

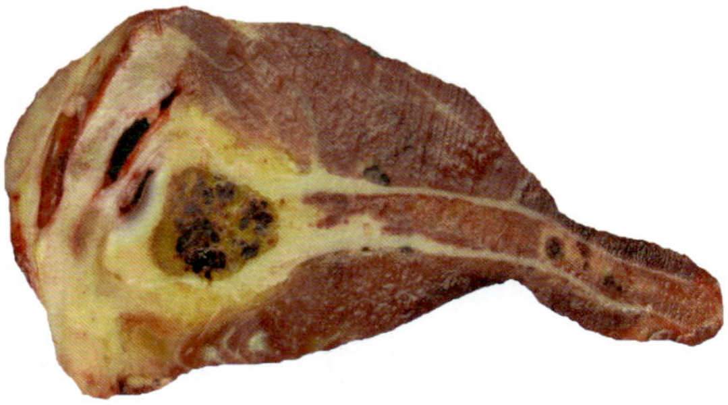

Leiomyosarcoma

Leiomyosarcoma is a rare bone malignancy showing smooth muscle differentiation. It occurs across a spectrum of ages, and may be associated with Epstein–Barr virus (EBV) infection (in the immunosuppressed) or previous radiation therapy. Given the much higher incidence of soft tissue leiomyosarcoma, a metastatic focus to the bone should always be considered first.

FIGURE 10.37. This example shows a nonspecific, firm, white-gray, infiltrative tumor of the distal radius with cortical breakthrough. Note that the yellow material in the lower aspect is bone cement placed following an open biopsy.

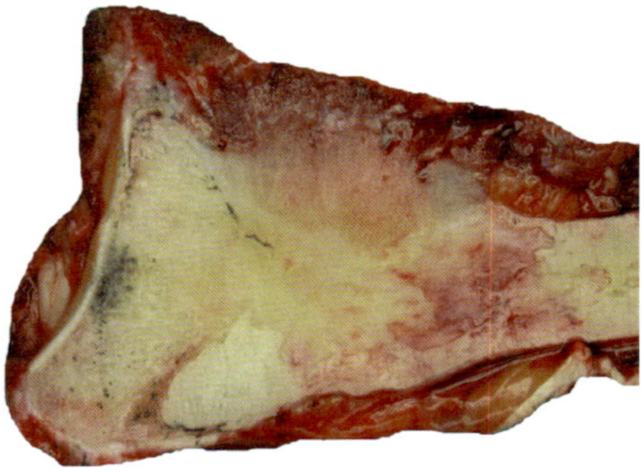

Undifferentiated pleomorphic sarcoma of bone

Undifferentiated pleomorphic sarcoma is a high-grade bone sarcoma devoid of specific signs of differentiation. The long bones of the lower extremities are preferential sites of involvement, and older adults are typically affected. Some of these tumors represent malignant transformation in the context of Paget disease, bone infarction, or radiation therapy. Undifferentiated pleomorphic sarcoma of bone is a diagnosis of exclusion. Extensive sampling is necessary, because the gross appearance of these lesions is nonspecific.

FIGURE 10.38. This specimen in the humeral diaphysis shows a tan-gray, heterogeneous, and necrotic tumor with cortical bone destruction and soft tissue invasion.

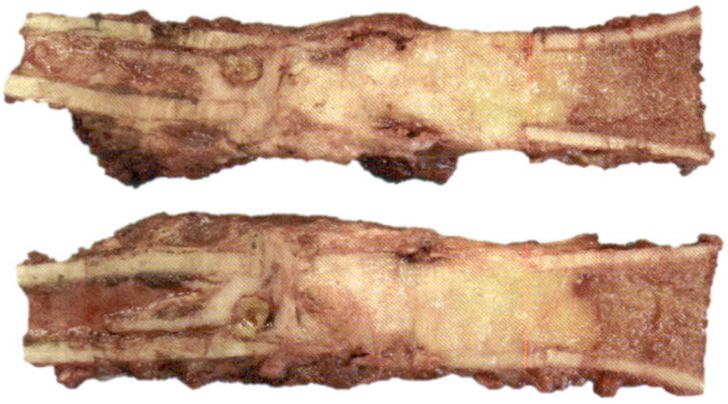

Desmoplastic fibroma (DF) of bone

DF of bone is a benign but locally aggressive fibroblastic neoplasm, arising most commonly in the pelvis and jaw bones of young people. It is microscopically identical to its soft tissue counterpart. It is an intermediate-type tumor with common local recurrences.

FIGURE 10.39. This image shows a deceptively circumscribed, white-yellow, fibrous lesion.

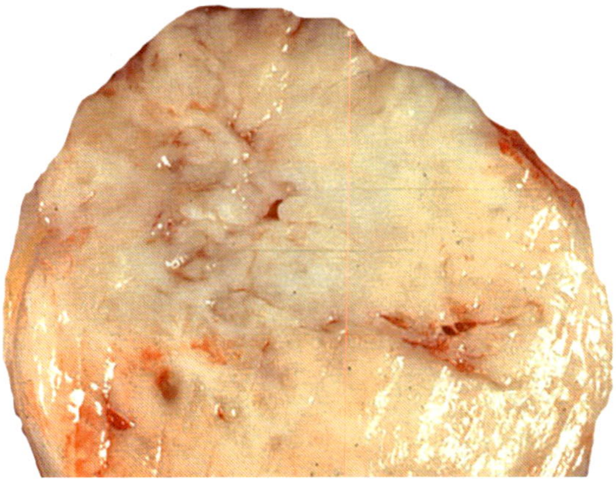

Nonossifying fibroma

Nonossifying fibroma is a common lesion in children. It is often found incidentally, and can generally be diagnosed based on radiology alone. Resection is reserved for cases involving clinical concerns or a pathological fracture.

FIGURE 10.40. Nonossifying fibroma, as presented in this image, classically appears on x-ray as an eccentric, cortically based, lytic lesion with benign, sclerotic borders. This lesion occurred in the tibia.

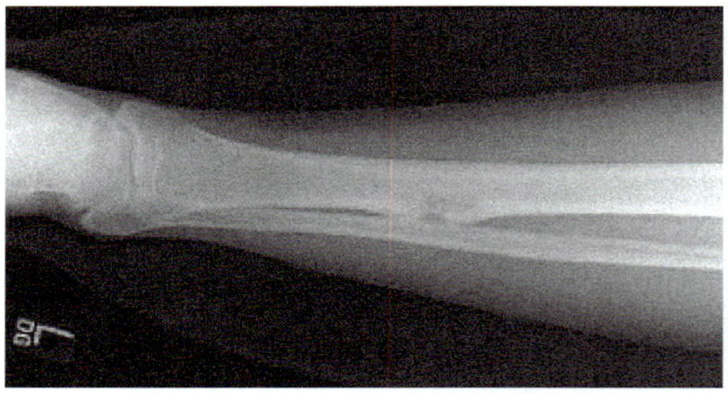

Plasma cell neoplasm

FIGURE 10.41. This lesion occurred in the proximal femur.

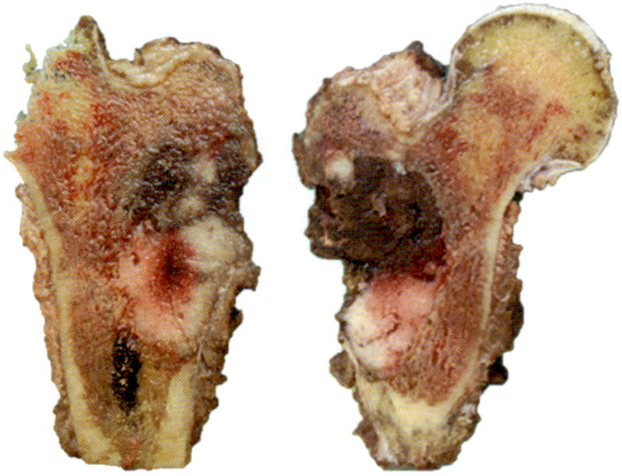

Giant cell tumor (GCT) of bone

GCT of bone is a benign, but locally aggressive, tumor that typically involves the epiphysis of long bones or the sacrum in a mature skeleton. Pulmonary metastasis (also benign) can develop in up to 2% of patients.

FIGURE 10.42. In (A), imaging shows a lytic, expansile tumor in the epiphysis of the proximal tibia. Image (B) shows a GCT involving the fibula. The tumor is soft, but gritty and hemorrhagic, which is typical of GCT.

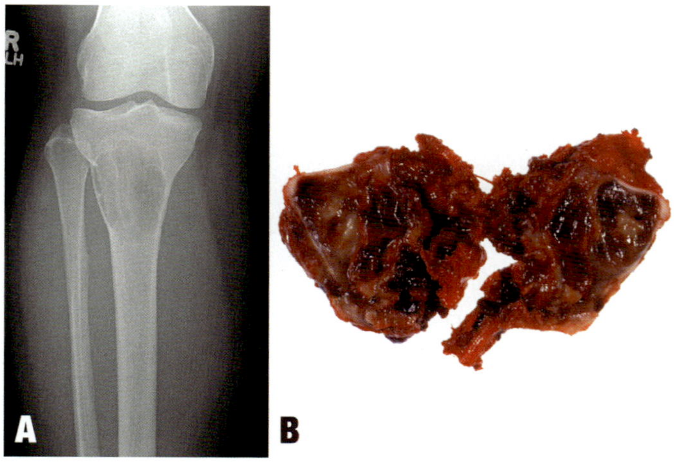

Chordoma

Chordoma is a malignant tumor showing notochordal differentiation. It arises predominantly in the bones of the skull base, vertebral bodies, and the sacrococcygeal area. While metastases are not common, the location of these tumors makes them difficult to excise with adequate margins, leading to frequent local recurrences.

FIGURE 10.43. The sacral chordomas in (A) and (B) appear as large, hemorrhagic, lobulated masses with focal gelatinous and myxoid areas.

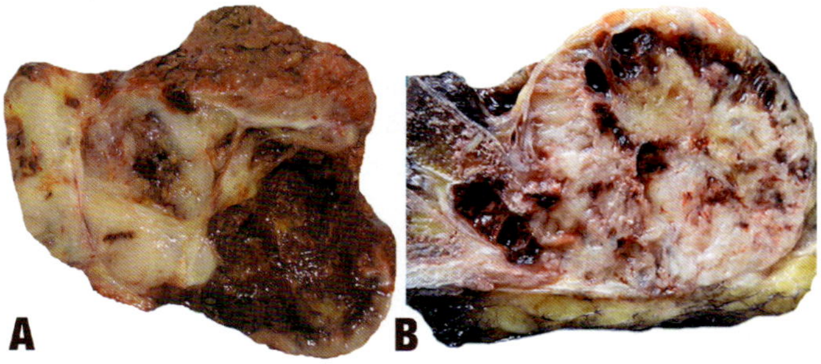

Hemangioma

Hemangiomas of bone, like their soft tissue counterparts, represent benign proliferations of small- or large-caliber blood vessels. They are common lesions, and most often occur in the vertebral bodies, followed by the craniofacial and long bones. Multiple lesions are frequent.

FIGURE 10.44. This example in the skull shows a well-circumscribed, hemorrhagic mass with a vague, honeycomb appearance.

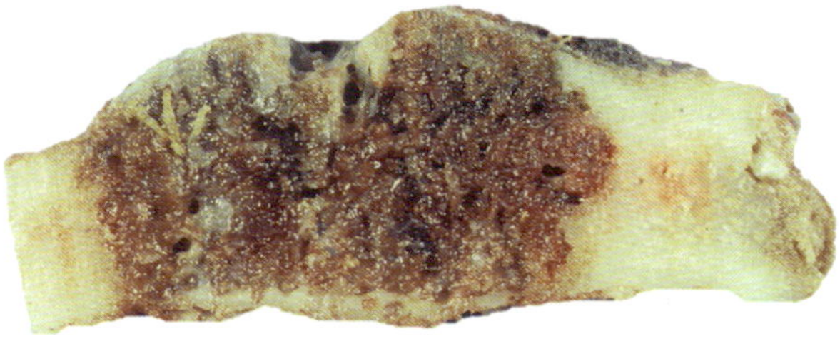

Epithelioid hemangioendothelioma (EHE)

EHE is a low-grade, malignant, vascular neoplasm commonly found in the liver, lungs, lymph nodes, and soft tissue, and, rarely, in bone. EHE harbors a unique chromosomal rearrangement: t(1;3).

FIGURE 10.45. This example involves the sternum. The cut surface shows an ill-defined, white-gray lesion with prominent soft tissue extension, but few hints of its vascular nature.

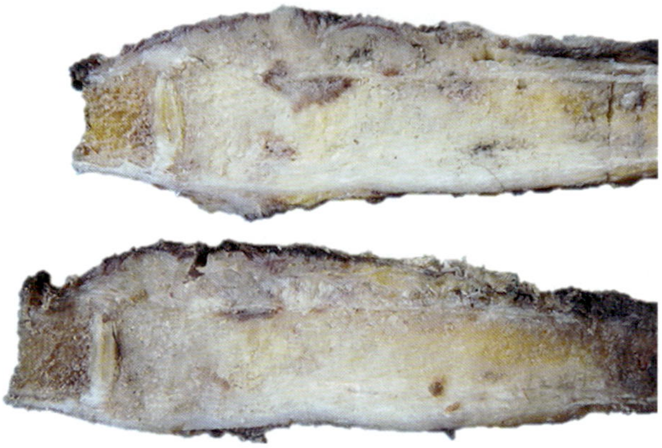

Adamantinoma

Adamantinoma is a peculiar malignant bone tumor that occurs almost exclusively in the anterior tibia. It presents with swelling and/or pain, and may be present for many years before diagnosis. Adamantinoma is associated with a classic, biphasic, histological pattern combining spindle cells with an epithelial component.

FIGURE 10.46. While smaller lesions may be limited to cortical involvement, this adamantinoma of the anterior tibia shows medullary extension by a tan-red, gritty tumor.

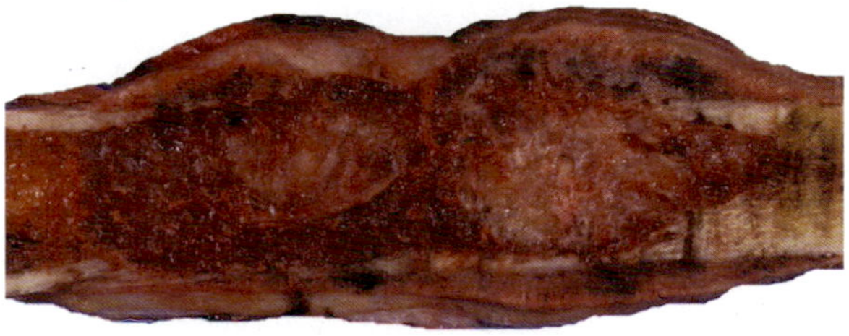

Aneurysmal bone cyst (ABC)

ABC is a blood-filled, multilocular lesion with numerous septations containing giant cells, reactive bone, and chronic inflammation. A recurrent *USP6* gene rearrangement on chromosome 17 supports its neoplastic nature. It is commonly diagnosed in the first 2 decades of life.

FIGURE 10.47. In (A), an x-ray of the humerus shows a multiloculated, cystic lesion with a "blow out" appearance. Grossly, the ABC of the fibula in (B) is expanded by a hemorrhagic, cystic lesion with sclerotic borders.

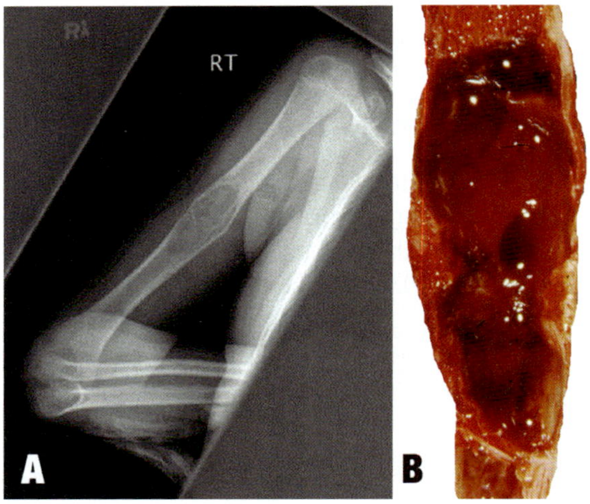

Metastasis to bone

Unremitting pain, swelling, and pathologic fractures are the main clinical features of bone metastasis. Metastases usually seed the medullary cavity and then grow centrifugally, with cortical destruction and soft tissue invasion.

FIGURE 10.48. These images are examples of carcinomas that have metastasized to bone: (A) vertebrae with metastatic breast carcinoma; (B) metastatic prostate carcinoma involving the spine; (C) sternum with metastatic squamous cell carcinoma. The normal, spongy bone is replaced by solid, fleshy or firm tumor, which destroys normal bone structure.

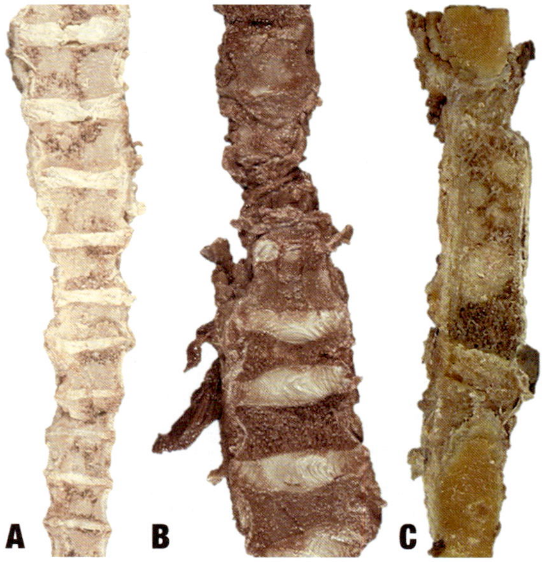

FIGURE 10.49. This image shows renal cell carcinoma metastatic to the humerus. Grossly, this osteolytic-type metastasis is destructive, soft, and hemorrhagic.

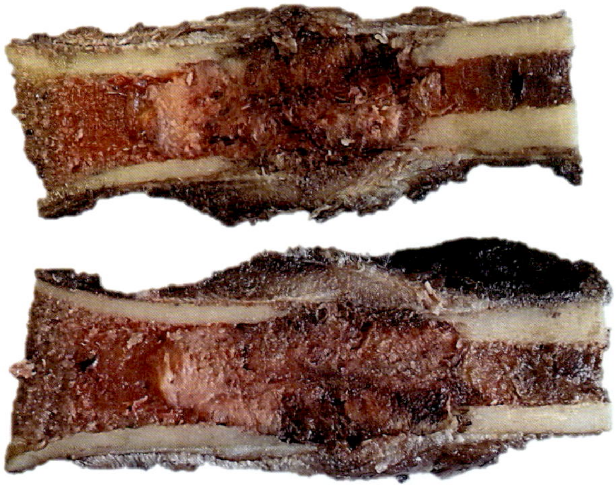

FIGURE 10.50. This image shows colon adenocarcinoma metastatic to femoral diaphysis. A large, soft, and hemorrhagic lesion has grown outward, destroying the cortical bone and invading the surrounding soft tissue. A superimposed pathologic fracture is present as well.

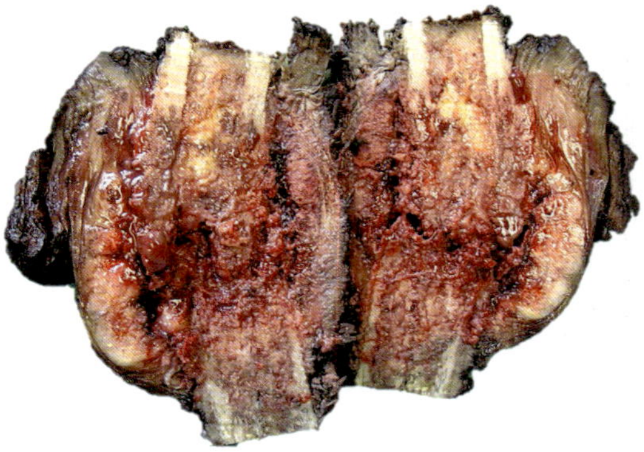

ACKNOWLEDGMENTS

We would like to thank the valuable contributions of Dr. A. Nahal and Dr. O. Ajise, and the technical help of R. Gilot, E. Griss, A. Hossain, L. Korneichyuk Pasyuk, M. Mikhael, and E. Yaney.

REFERENCES

Bullough PG. *Orthopaedic pathology*. Maryland Heights, MO: Mosby/Elsevier; 2010.

Fletcher CDM. *Diagnostic histopathology of tumors*. Philadelphia: Saunders/Elsevier; 2013.

Fletcher CDM, Bridge JA, Hogendoorn PCW, Mertens F. *WHO classification of tumours of soft tissue and bone*. 4th ed. Lyon, France: IARC Press; 2013.

Folpe AL, Inwards CY. *Bone and soft tissue pathology*. Philadelphia: Saunders/Elsevier; 2010.

Goldblum JR, Weiss SW, Folpe AL. *Enzinger and Weiss's soft tissue tumors*. 6th ed. Philadelphia: Saunders/Elsevier; 2014.

Rosai J. *Rosai and Ackerman's surgical pathology*. 10th ed. Philadelphia, PA: Mosby/Elsevier; 2011.

11

Diseases of the Esophagus, Stomach, and Intestine

VICTORIA MARCUS, YU SHI, ZU-HUA GAO

Esophagus

REFERENCE: NORMAL ESOPHAGUS

The esophagus is a muscular tubular structure that is, on average, 25 cm long in adults, as measured from the cricopharyngeus muscle of the pharynx to the gastroesophageal junction in the upper abdomen.

FIGURE 11.1. Image (A) shows the esophageal mucosa, which is whitish and contrasts with the salmon-pink gastric mucosa below the gastroesophageal junction. Image (B) gives a closer view of the esophageal mucosa.

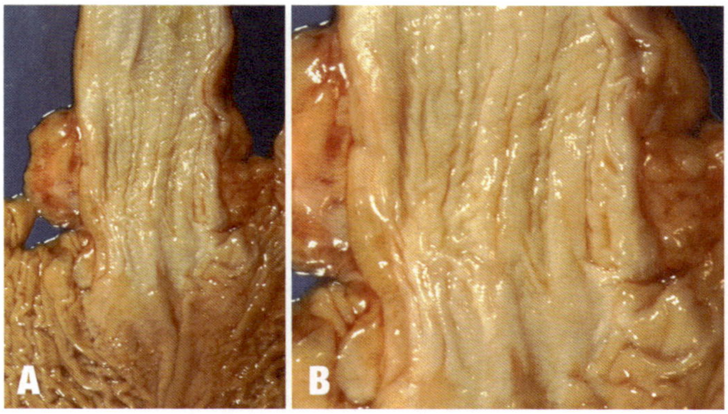

Nonneoplastic Diseases of the Esophagus

Zenker diverticulum

Zenker diverticula are more common in the elderly and account for about 70% of esophageal diverticula. They are usually located on the posterior wall at the junction between the pharynx and esophagus (known as the Killian triangle), an area of wall weakness. Zenker diverticula are acquired "false" diverticula: they do not contain all the layers of the wall.

FIGURE 11.2. This image shows a Zenker diverticulum with a red pill obstructing the lumen.

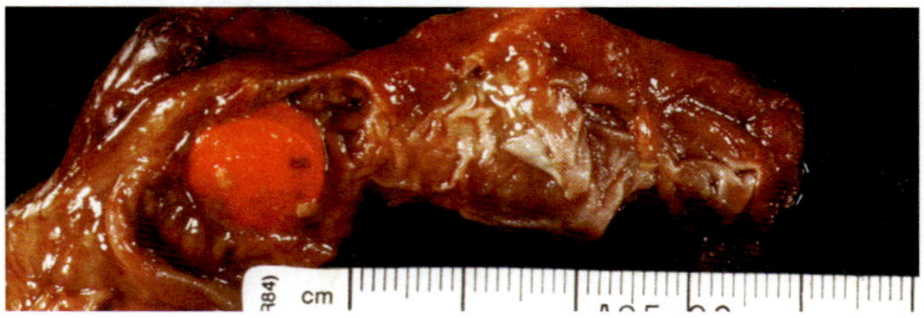

Esophageal perforation

Perforation of the esophagus is usually due to foreign body ingestion (most commonly a fish bone) or to malignancy. The adjacent thoracic aorta can be involved to form an aortoesophageal fistula, which is often lethal.

FIGURE 11.3. A probe is placed through a perforated tract above the gastroesophageal junction.

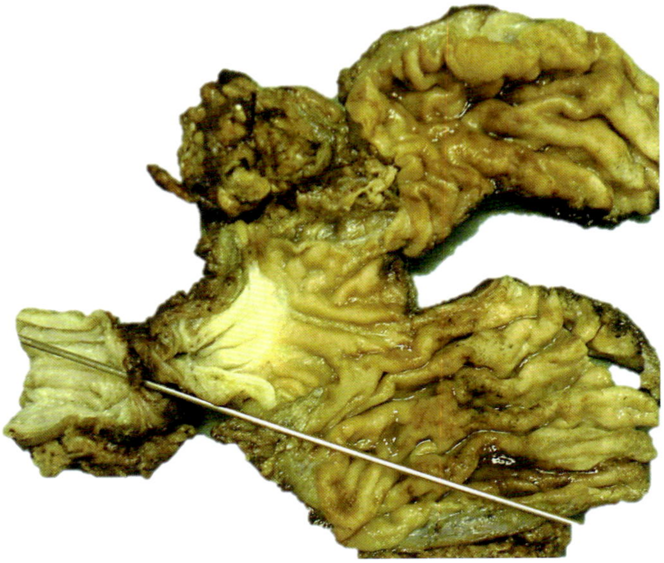

Achalasia

Achalasia is an esophageal motor disorder due to loss of ganglion cells in the myenteric plexus, and is characterized by lack of progressive peristalsis and impaired relaxation of the lower esophageal sphincter (LES) muscle.

FIGURE 11.4. These images show fresh (A) and formalin-fixed (B) achalasia specimens. Both specimens show marked dilatation with stenosis and LES muscular hypertrophy.

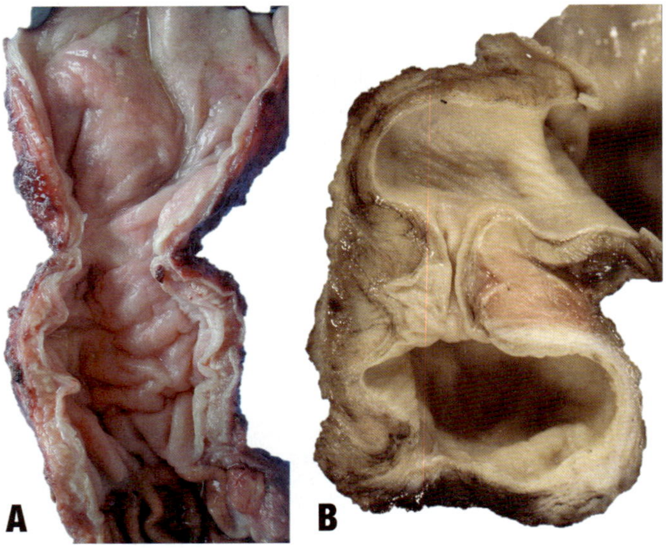

Esophageal varices

Portal hypertension due to liver cirrhosis leads to shunting of blood from the portal system to the systemic venous system. Esophageal varices are examples of portosystemic shunts. They may bleed, and result in massive hematemesis and death.

FIGURE 11.5. Images (A) and (B) show dilated veins bulging the esophageal mucosa.

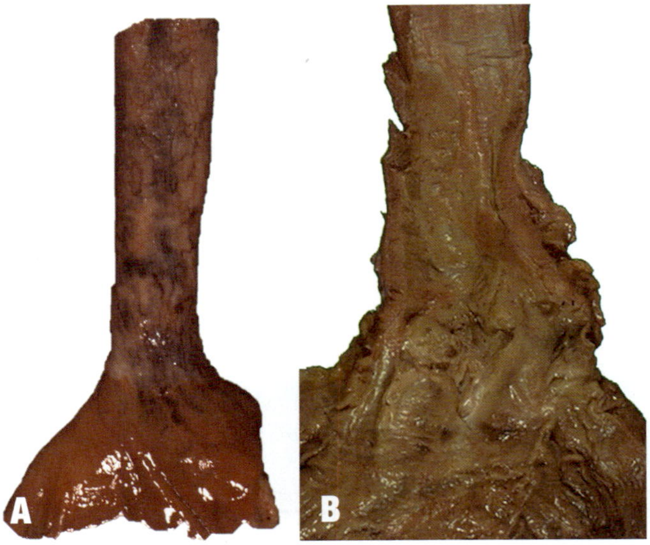

FIGURE 11.6. The cross-sections of this distal esophagus show dilated submucosal veins with thrombosis.

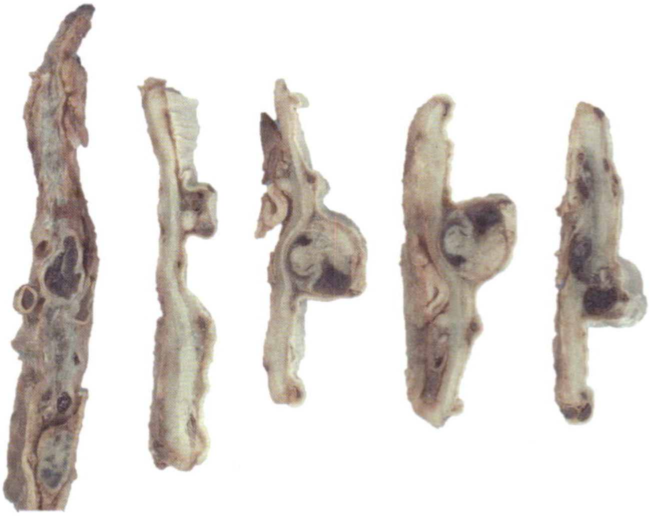

Mucosal erosions and ulceration of the esophagus

Erosion is a defect that involves only the superficial portion of the mucosa. Ulceration is a full thickness mucosal defect. The causes of esophageal erosions and ulcerations include gastroesophageal reflux disease (GERD), infectious esophagitis, chemical injury, mechanical trauma, and underlying cancer.

FIGURE 11.7. Image (A) shows mucosal erosions with residual white, pale, squamous mucosal islands. Image (B) shows a close-up of an ulcer caused by a nasogastric tube.

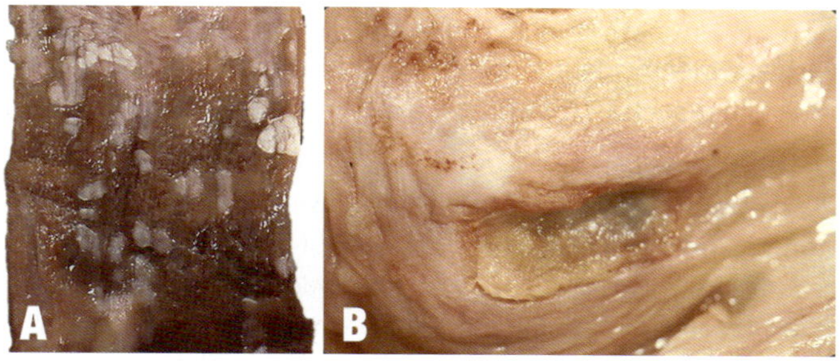

Esophagitis

CANDIDAL ESOPHAGITIS

Candida albicans is the most common cause of infectious esophagitis.

FIGURE 11.8. Note the white membrane-like exudate at the distal esophagus (toward the right of the image) within eroded and ulcerated hemorrhagic mucosa.

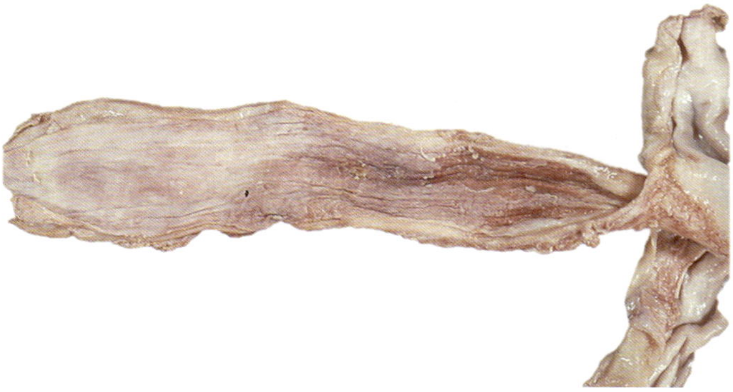

HERPES ESOPHAGITIS

Common manifestations of herpes simplex virus type 1 (HSV-1) include painful sores, blisters, and ulcers in the mouth and lips. HSV-1 may also affect the esophagus.

FIGURE 11.9. This image shows characteristic punctate ulcerations with areas of normal intervening mucosa.

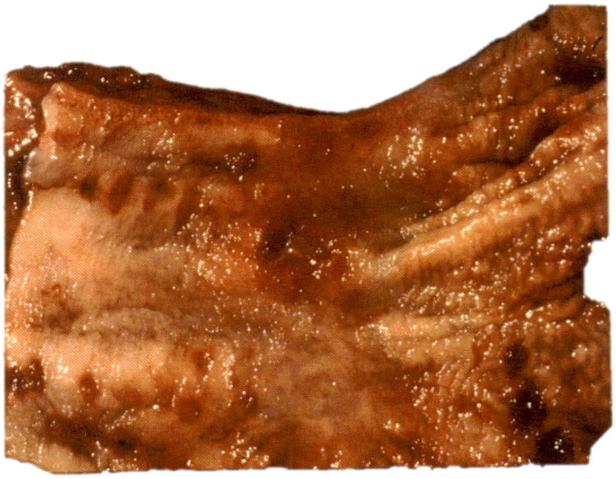

PILL-INDUCED ESOPHAGITIS

Certain medications may damage the esophagus, including antibiotics (particularly doxycycline), nonsteroidal antiinflammatory drugs (NSAIDs), alendronate, and iron pills. Pills stuck on the esophageal surface may cause isolated ulcers; repeated injury causes fibrosis and, rarely, stricture formation.

FIGURE 11.10. Image (A) shows an endoscopic view of isolated round ulcers caused by pills on the esophageal surface. Image (B) shows fibrosis and stricture caused by repeated injury.

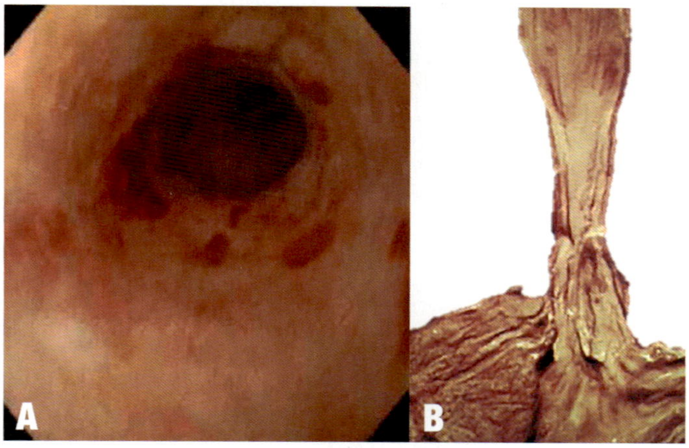

EOSINOPHILIC ESOPHAGITIS (EoE)

EoE is an atopic inflammatory condition characterized by increased numbers of eosinophils in the esophageal epithelium. EoE patients have enhanced production of cytokines against both food and environmental allergens. Clinically, they usually present with dysphagia.

FIGURE 11.11. This endoscopic image of EoE shows the classic concentric esophageal rings (trachealization or felinization) with vertical linear ridges (furrows).

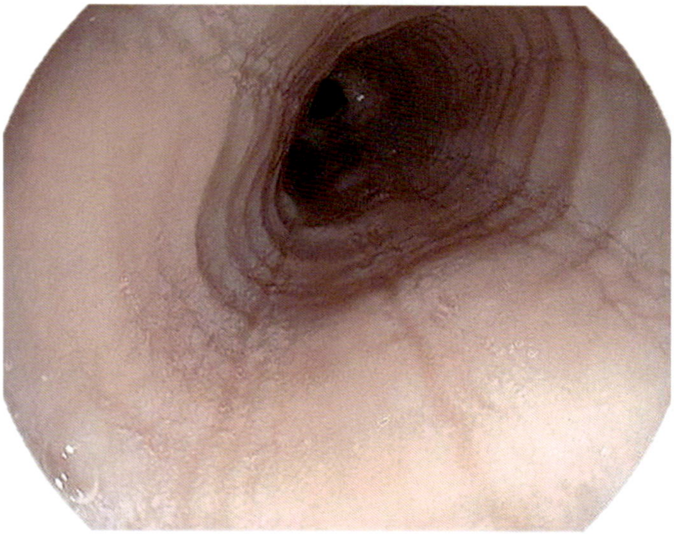

GASTROESOPHAGEAL REFLUX DISEASE (GERD)

GERD is the most clinically encountered esophagitis. It is caused by chronic exposure to gastric acid. Endoscopically, GERD may show a spectrum of changes from normal endoscopy to ulcerations with stenosis.

FIGURE 11.12. This example of GERD shows patchy mucosal erosions (dark red) interspaced by relatively healthy (white) squamous mucosa.

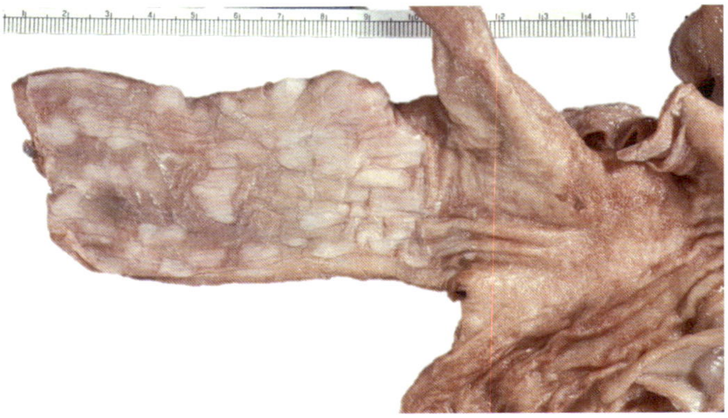

Barrett esophagus (BE)

Defined by the presence of intestinal metaplasia (specifically goblet cells) in the esophagus, BE is a complication of chronic GERD. It is considered a precancerous condition that requires regular endoscopic screening to identify glandular dysplasia, a premalignant lesion for adenocarcinoma. In addition to sampling BE at regular intervals, any nodularity within BE should be biopsied, and its size and location documented.

FIGURE 11.13. The endoscopic image in (A) shows an irregular Z-line (squamocolumnar junction), with tongue-shaped intrusions of salmon-colored mucosa into the distal esophagus. In (B), a resected esophagus shows pale squamous mucosa surrounded, more distally, by salmon-pink BE mucosa.

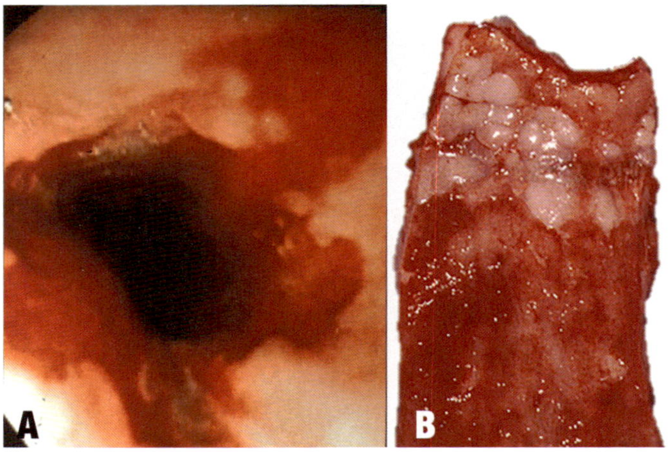

BE WITH DYSPLASIA

Low- and high-grade dysplasia in the setting of BE are diagnosed microscopically and usually require confirmation by a second pathologist. High-grade dysplasia is treated with various modalities including local ablation, endoscopic mucosal resection (EMR), and even esophagogastrectomy.

FIGURE 11.14. In (A), a formalin-fixed specimen of the distal esophagus (white, pale mucosa, above) and proximal stomach (below) shows short-segment BE (< 3 cm above the gastroesophageal junction) with high-grade dysplasia. Image (B) illustrates an EMR specimen: a glistening, slightly elevated mucosa. On histology, it contained intestinal metaplasia with focal high-grade dysplasia. No invasive cancer was seen.

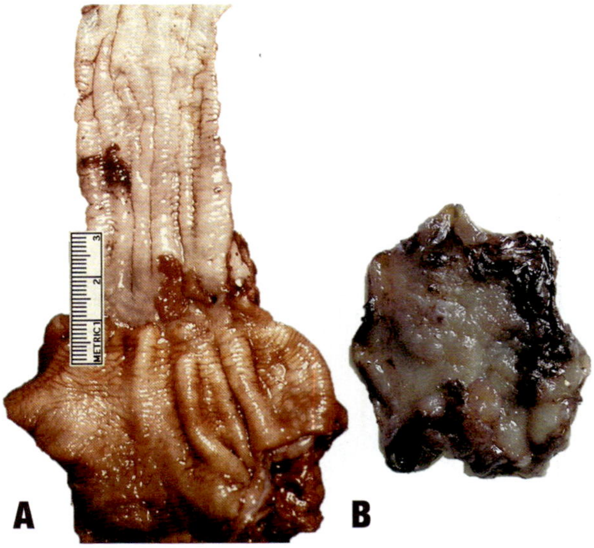

Scleroderma

Esophageal dysfunction develops in approximately 90% of patients with scleroderma (progressive systemic sclerosis). Abnormal esophageal motility is usually the earliest manifestation, due to involvement of the smooth muscle wall and the lower esophageal sphincter by the disease process.

FIGURE 11.15. These images show mucosa ulceration at the lower end of the esophagus.

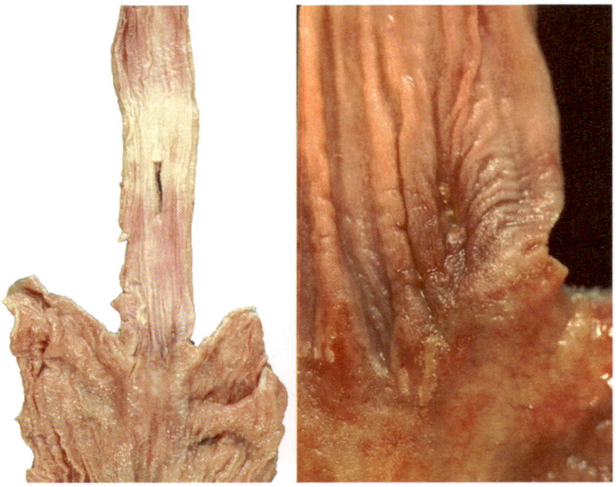

Esophageal Cancer

Adenocarcinoma

Esophageal adenocarcinoma is presently the most common type of esophageal cancer in the developed world. It is a tumor with glandular differentiation, often occurring in a background of BE and GERD. BE–associated adenocarcinoma usually occurs in the distal esophagus, the region most severely affected by GERD.

FIGURE 11.16. This gross image shows BE with an ill-defined thickening of the distal esophagus that was histologically confirmed to be adenocarcinoma. Adenocarcinomas arising in BE may be difficult to identify endoscopically.

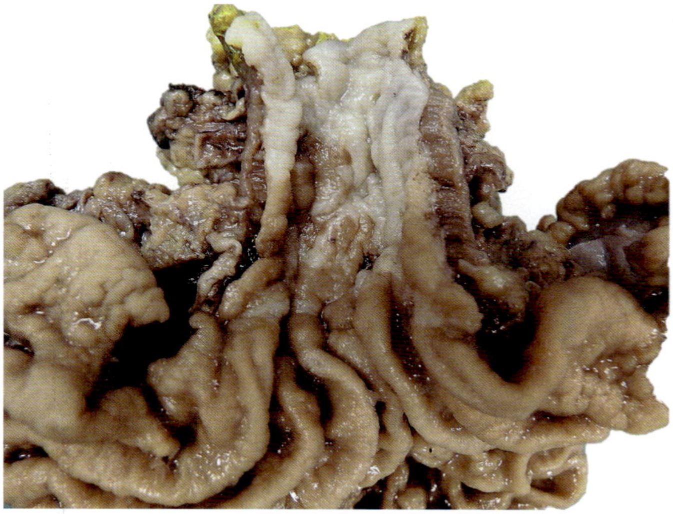

FIGURE 11.17. This adenocarcinoma, arising in long-segment BE (> 3 cm in length), shows as subtle granularity just above the gastroesophageal junction. Such poorly visualized tumors can be detected by adequate surveillance biopsies.

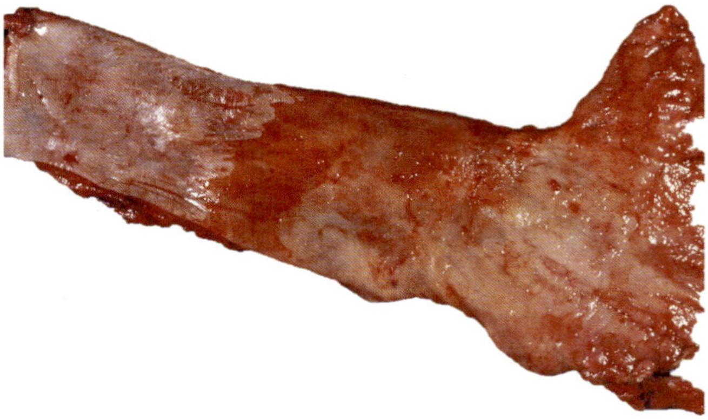

FIGURE 11.18. This ulcerated BE–associated tumor, just proximal to the gastroesophageal junction, caused stenosis of the distal esophagus. Marked narrowing of the esophageal lumen may lead to dysphagia (difficulty swallowing).

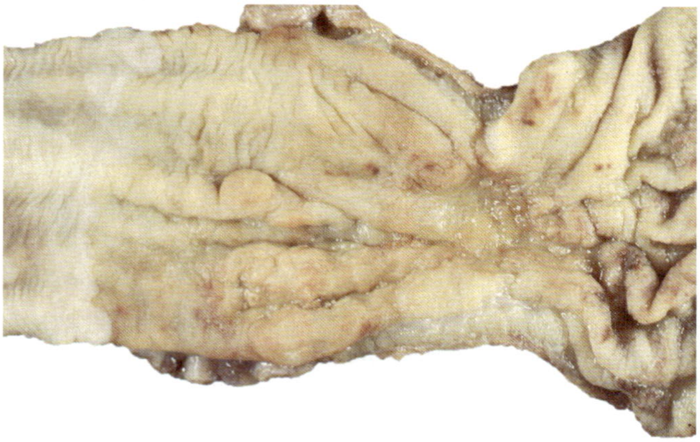

FIGURE 11.19. These examples of esophageal adenocarcinoma are more well developed, with raised borders and central ulceration. Image (A) shows a resection specimen photographed fresh during an intraoperative consultation to ensure adequate margins of resection. Image (B) shows a formalin-fixed resection specimen.

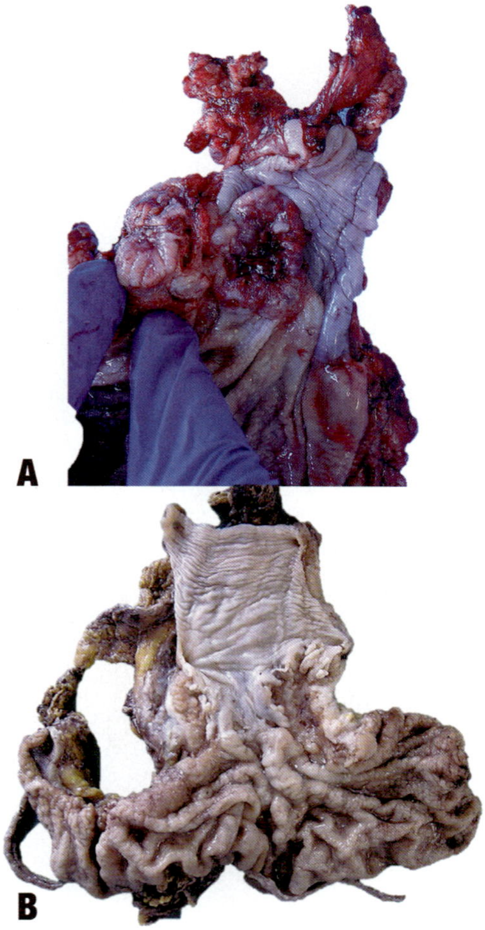

A

B

Squamous cell carcinoma (SCC)

SCC is the most common carcinoma of the esophagus worldwide. Esophageal SCCs are commonly seen in the middle and proximal esophagus and are usually associated with consumption of alcohol or tobacco, rather than with GERD or Barrett esophagus.

FIGURE 11.20. Image (A) shows esophageal SCC surrounded by unremarkable squamous mucosa. Image (B) shows a formalin-fixed tumor located at the middle segment of the esophagus. No associated Barrett esophagus is present.

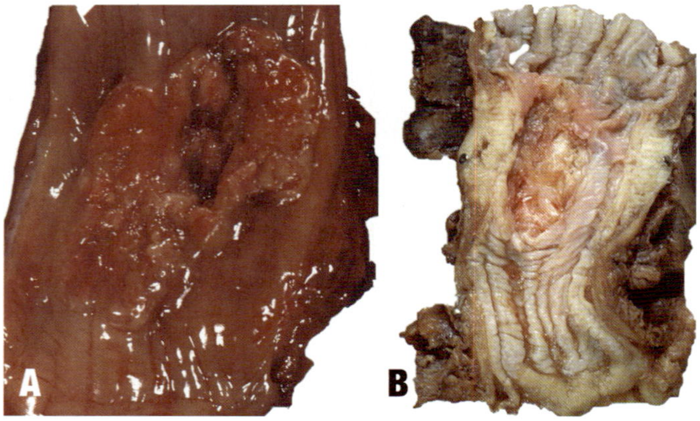

FIGURE 11.21. This example of SCC is hemorrhagic. The tumor had perforated through the esophageal wall.

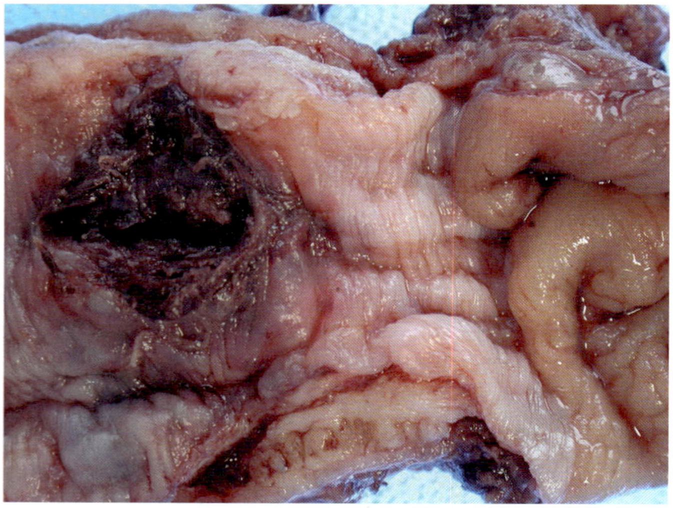

FIGURE 11.22. This example of esophageal SCC was located in the midesophagus. The tumor shows central ulceration with raised borders.

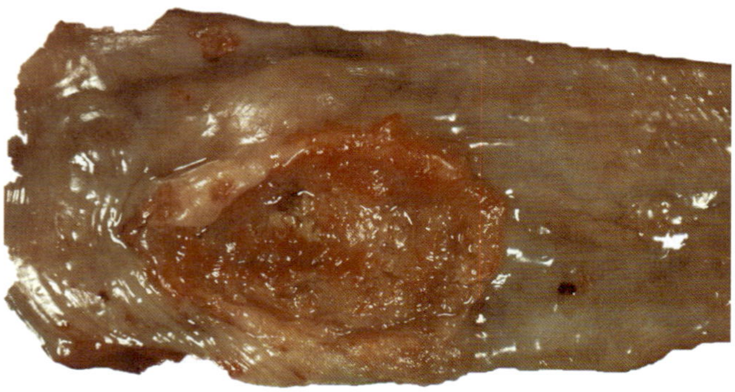

PROCEDURE: STAGING OF ESOPHAGEAL CARCINOMA

Appropriate sampling must be performed after formalin fixation to properly assess and stage a tumor by the TNM staging system. The depth of invasion through the different layers of the esophageal wall determines the tumor stage (T stage) in the TNM system. For example, an esophageal carcinoma that invades into, but not beyond, the muscle wall is staged T2; a tumor invading into adjacent organs is staged T4 (the highest T stage). N-stage malignancy has metastasis to regional lymph nodes; M-stage malignancy has distant metastasis.

FIGURE 11.23. Cross-sections of an esophageal adenocarcinoma show a dense, white invasive tumor in the center of the specimen with surface ulceration. The tumor invades throughout the wall of the esophagus to the radial (circumferential) margin.

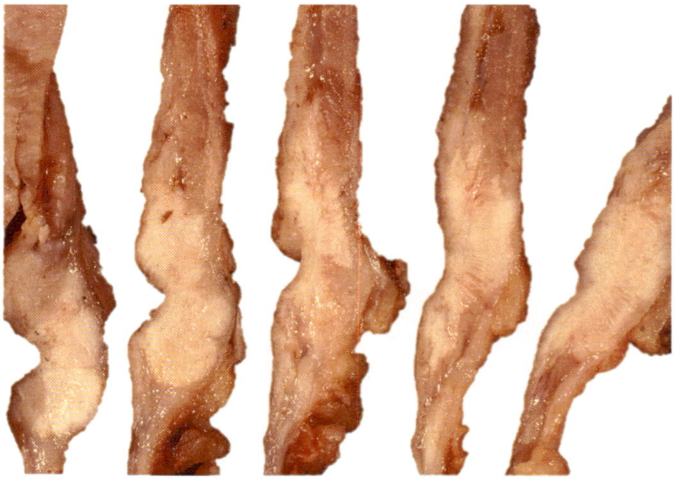

FIGURE 11.24. These serial cross-sections of an esophagogastrectomy specimen after fixation show dense, white tumor occluding the lumen and invading through the full thickness of the esophageal wall. Clinically, the patient had dysphagia. Histologically, this tumor was an invasive SCC.

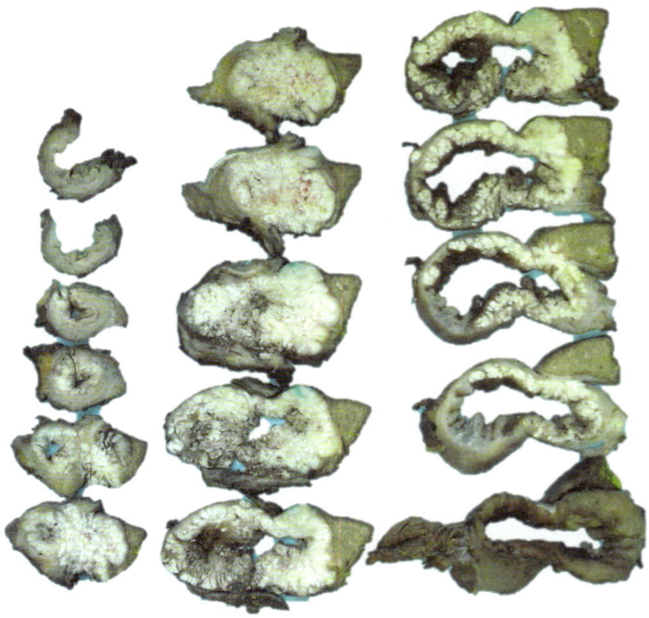

Stomach

REFERENCE: NORMAL STOMACH

The stomach is situated between the esophagus and the duodenum. The stomach is divided into cardia, fundus, body, antrum, and pylorus.

FIGURE 11.25. This image shows a stomach opened along the greater curvature. Note that the mucosal folds (rugae) are more prominent in the fundus and body area.

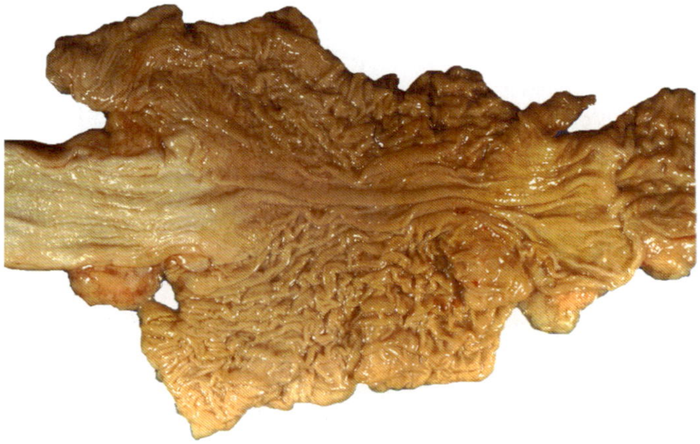

Nonneoplastic Diseases of the Stomach

Surgically reduced stomach (laparoscopic sleeve gastrectomy)

Laparoscopic sleeve gastrectomy removes a sizable portion of the stomach along the greater curvature and permanently reduces the stomach to about 20% of its original size. It is a form of bariatric surgery performed in obese patients attempting to lose weight.

FIGURE 11.26. The majority of the stomach is resected in this type of surgery and a narrow tube ("sleeve") is created from the remaining stomach. This partial gastric resection shows normal mucosa folds.

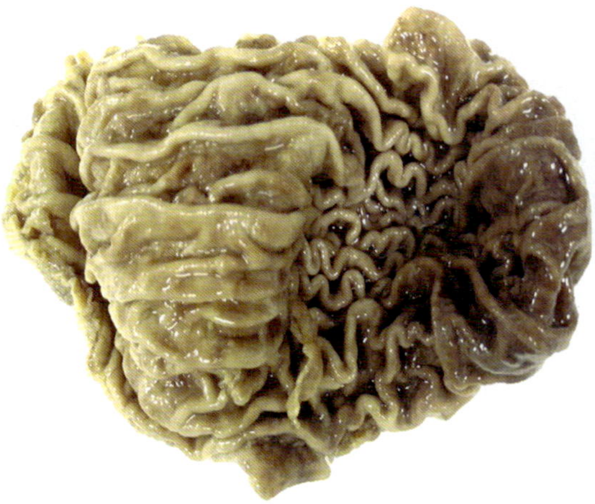

Erosions and erosive gastritis

Erosions represent acute mucosal injury with damage to the superficial epithelial lining. Hemorrhage often occurs and may lead to upper gastrointestinal bleeding. Risk factors include smoking, alcohol, NSAIDs, shock, and severe stress (e.g., extensive burns or trauma), among others.

FIGURE 11.27. Image (A) shows multiple erosions in the gastric antrum. Image (B) shows erosive (acute hemorrhagic) gastritis. This specimen was everted to demonstrate the mucosal side that has a diffusely hemorrhagic surface with loss of the mucosal folds.

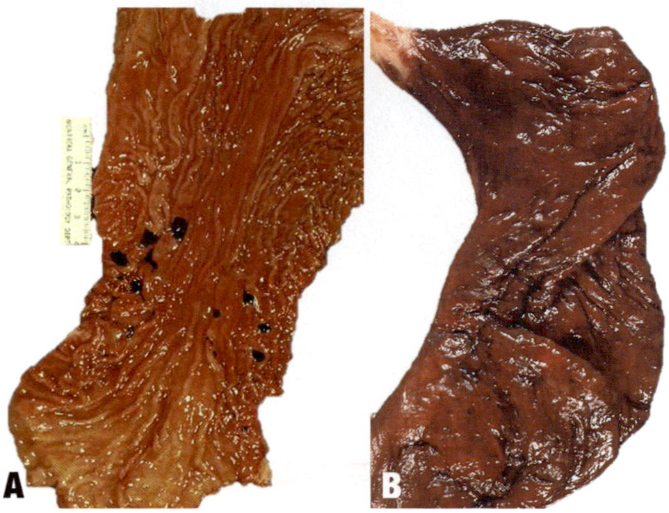

Peptic ulcer

Gastric ulcers are associated with *Helicobacter pylori*, alcohol, NSAIDs, and smoking, among other factors. A chronic peptic ulcer is due to excessive acid and/or compromised mucosal protection.

FIGURE 11.28. This image shows a small, deep, oval-shaped, sharply demarcated ulcer; the surrounding mucosal folds radiate from the ulcer's center. Biopsy confirmation is required to completely exclude malignancy.

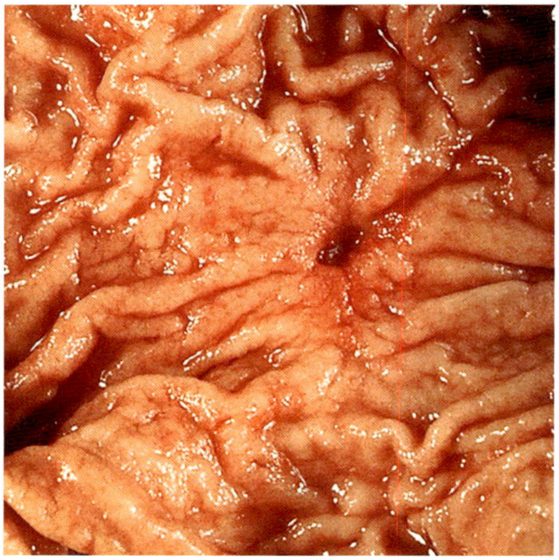

PERFORATED GASTRIC ULCER

Sometimes peptic ulcer is so severe that it penetrates through all the layers of the stomach wall. Gastric perforation allows food and gastric juices to spill into the abdominal cavity, which leads to acute peritonitis. It is a medical emergency that requires immediate surgery.

FIGURE 11.29. This image shows a large perforated ulcer.

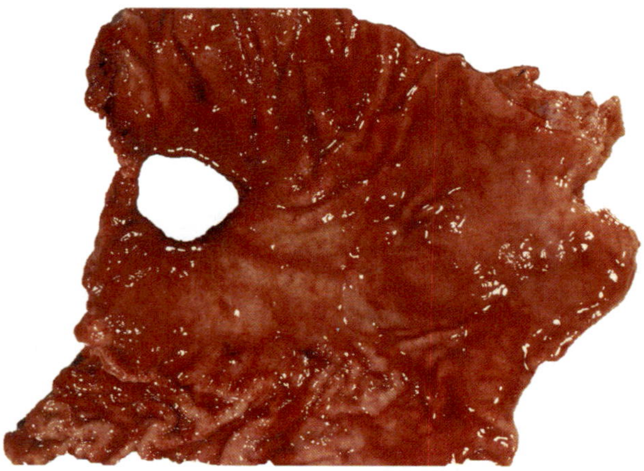

IATROGENIC GASTRIC ULCER FROM NASOGASTRIC (NG) TUBE

NG tubes provide access to the stomach for diagnostic and therapeutic purposes. However, long-term contact with NG tubes can damage mucosal tissue.

FIGURE 11.30. This image shows loss of the mucosal folds with focal ulceration corresponding to the contact area with an NG tube.

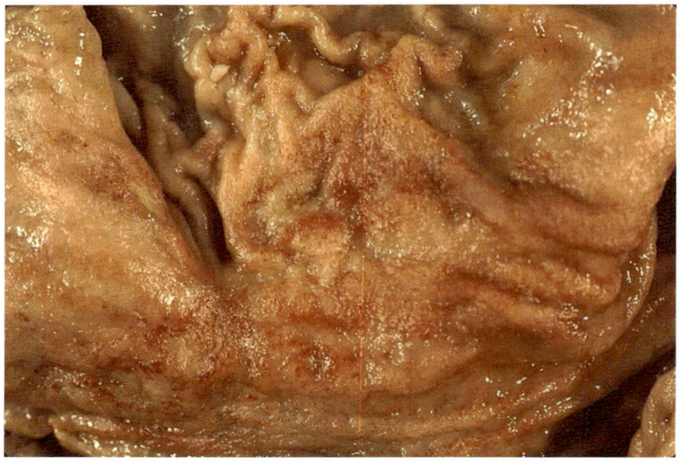

Gastric antral vascular ectasia (GAVE)

GAVE is an uncommon cause of blood loss and iron-deficiency anemia. It mainly occurs in elderly women. Also known as "watermelon stomach," GAVE endoscopically shows red stripes on the mucosa due to congested ectatic mucosal vessels. It has no association with esophageal varices or with gastric neoplasia.

FIGURE 11.31. Note the red tortuous ectatic vessels along prominent longitudinal folds of the antrum, resembling watermelon stripes.

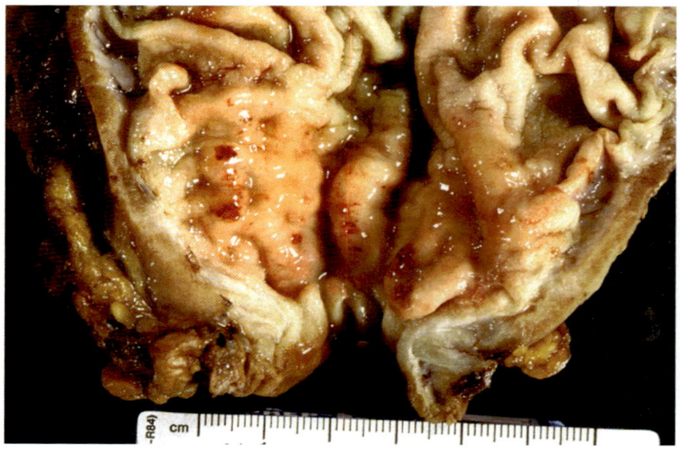

Pancreatic heterotopia in the stomach

Nonneoplastic pancreatic tissue may occur outside the pancreas, including in the stomach. Usually discovered incidentally as a nodule, pancreatic heterotopia may present with bleeding or obstruction, particularly if the nodule is large.

FIGURE 11.32. This image shows ectopic pancreas tissue presenting as yellowish tissue under the mucosa.

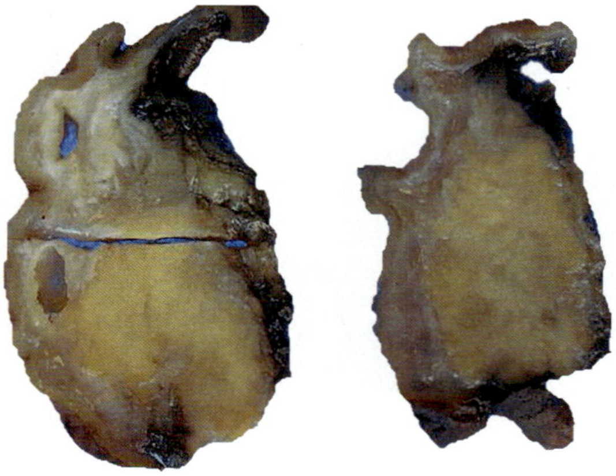

Trichobezoar

A bezoar is a mass of material trapped in the gastrointestinal tract. A trichobezoar (more commonly known as a hair ball) is a bezoar composed of indigestible hair and/or animal fur. Trichobezoars most commonly occur in psychiatric patients.

FIGURE 11.33. This is an example of a trichobezoar that took on the shape of the stomach.

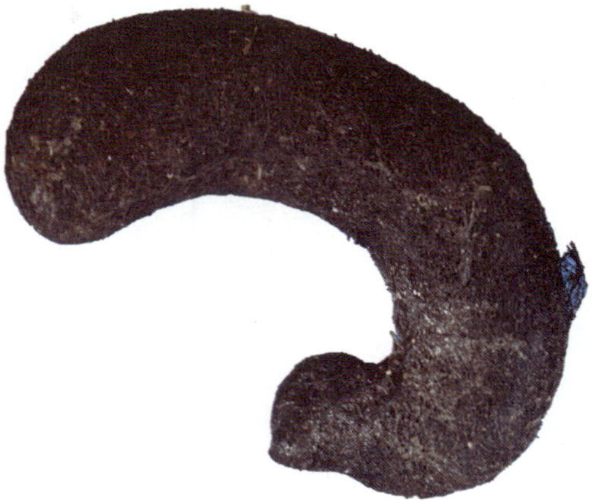

Gastric Nodules and Neoplasms

Hyperplastic polyp of the stomach

Gastric hyperplastic polyps are thought to be inflammatory or regenerative lesions of foveolar cells. Hyperplastic polyps are smooth, dome shaped, or stalked with an average size range of 0.5 cm to 1.5 cm. They may develop anywhere in the stomach, are commonly associated with chronic gastritis, and are characterized by proliferation of foveolar epithelium.

FIGURE 11.34. This image shows multiple mucosal nodules (upper portion of image). Histology confirmed the nodules as hyperplastic polyps.

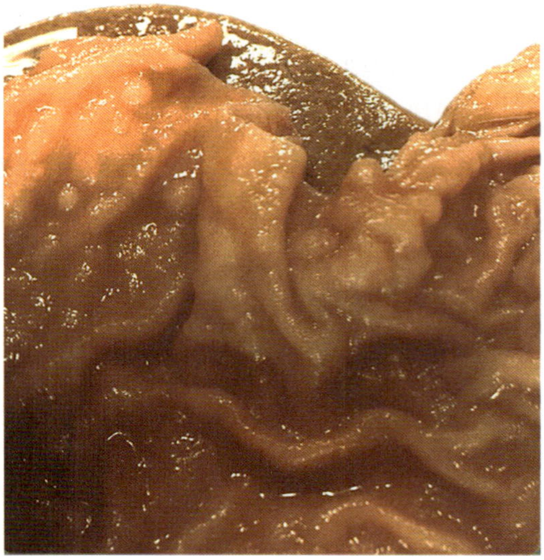

FIGURE 11.35. This image shows several large edematous hyperplastic polyps on the gastric mucosa, some with a distinct stalk.

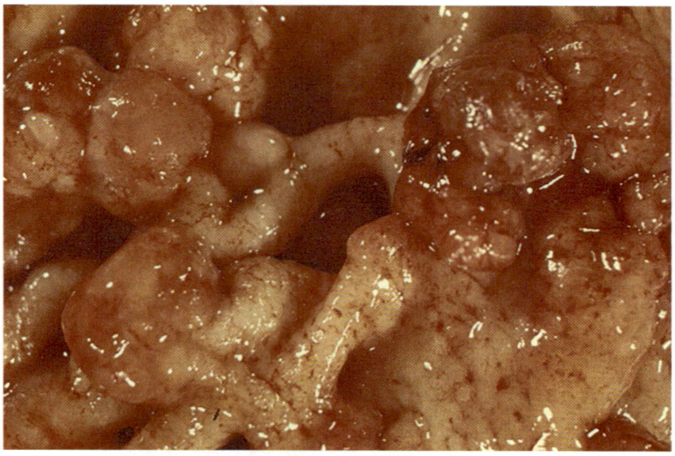

Fundic gland polyp

Fundic gland polyps are commonly associated with proton pump inhibitor treatment, and are characterized by proliferation of parietal and chief cells with microcyst formation. Fundic gland polyps could also be associated with familial adenomatous polyposis (FAP) syndrome.

FIGURE 11.36. This image shows fundic gland polyps.

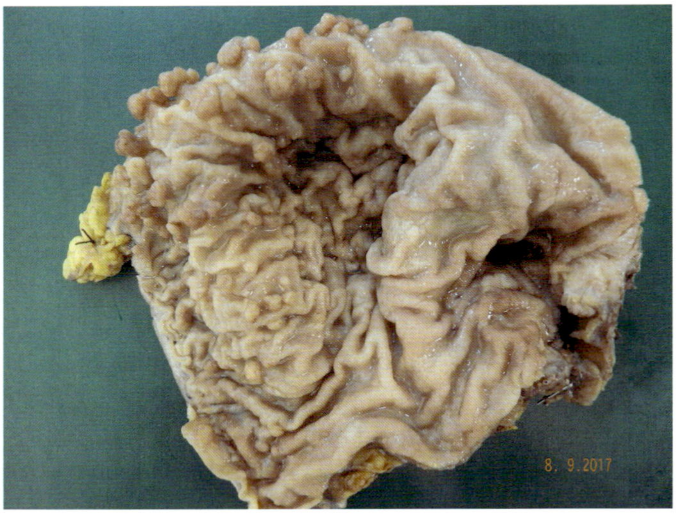

Gastric polyposis

Gastric polyposis may be associated with hamartomatous polyposis syndromes such as juvenile polyposis syndrome (*SMAD4* mutation), Peutz–Jeghers syndrome (*STK11* mutation), and Cowden disease (*PTEN* hamartoma tumor syndrome). Dysplasia and adenocarcinoma may arise in a background of gastric polyposis.

FIGURE 11.37. This image shows numerous mucosal polyps. Focally, dysplasia was found on histology; however, this cannot be identified grossly.

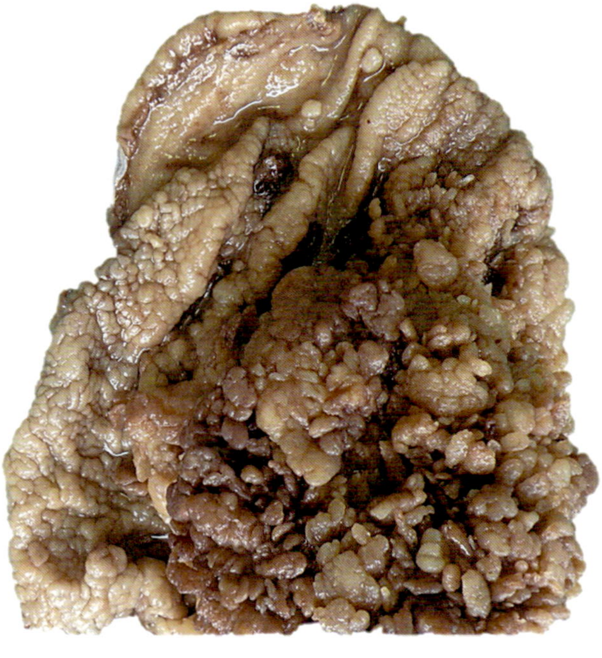

FIGURE 11.38. This total gastrectomy specimen is blanketed with innumerable nodules and finger-like villous projections with an edematous appearance. Extensive sampling was required to identify the invasive adenocarcinoma.

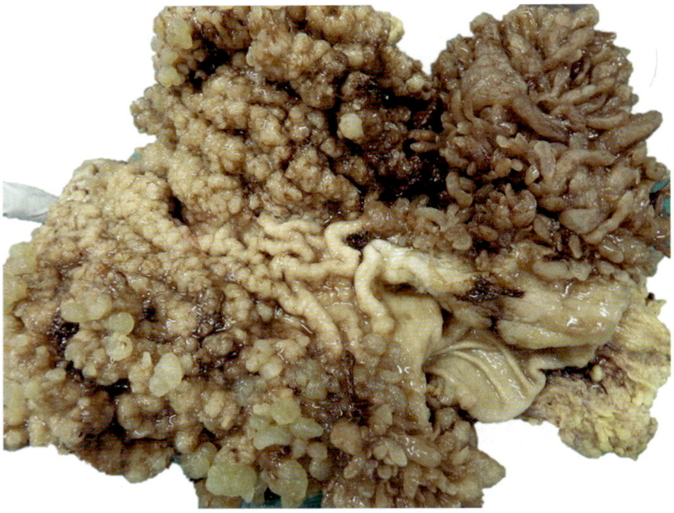

Gastric adenoma

Gastric adenoma represents about 10% of gastric polyps in Western countries. Four main types of adenomas have been reported: intestinal, foveolar, pyloric, and oxyntic gland types. The intestinal type is the most common and resembles a colonic tubular adenoma.

FIGURE 11.39. In this specimen, note the rigid polyp without edema or inflammatory appearance.

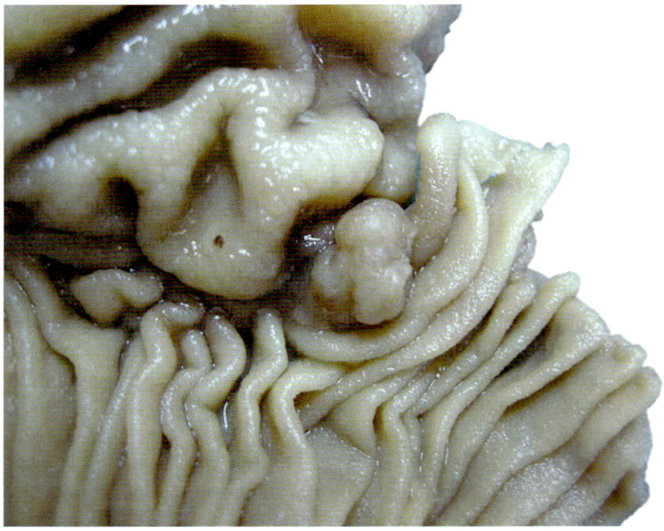

Gastric adenocarcinoma

More than 90% of gastric cancer is gastric adenocarcinoma. The strongest risk factor for developing gastric adenocarcinoma is *H. pylori* infection. The macroscopic appearance of gastric adenocarcinoma varies from a subtle ulcer to an exophytic lesion, and even to diffuse thickening of the stomach.

ULCERATED GASTRIC CANCER

FIGURE 11.40. Endoscopy does not reliably differentiate a benign ulcer from a malignant ulcer: accurate diagnosis requires histological assessment. This irregular-shaped mucosal ulcer was histologically confirmed to be invasive adenocarcinoma.

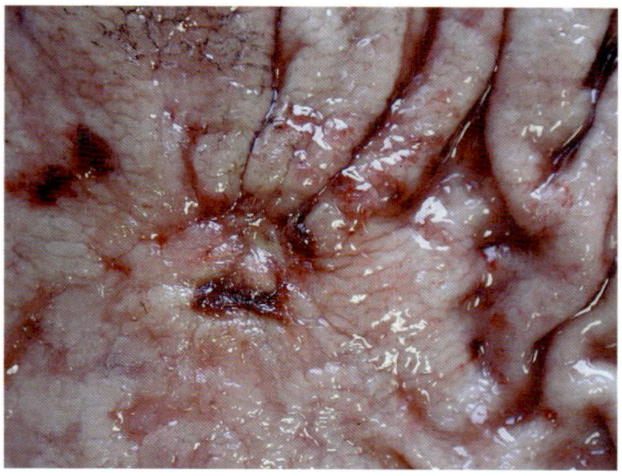

FIGURE 11.41. Images (A) and (B) show gastrectomy specimens which have large, irregular ulcers with heaped-up edges and uneven bases. The ulcer beds are necrotic and fibrotic. These lesions were histologically confirmed as adenocarcinomas.

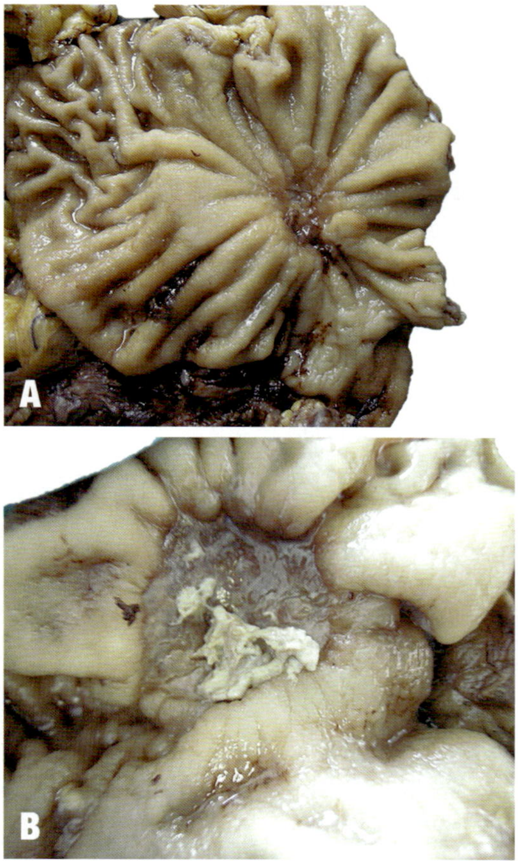

INTESTINAL-TYPE GASTRIC ADENOCARCINOMA

The Lauren classification divides gastric adenocarcinomas into 3 types based on histology: intestinal, diffuse, and mixed. The intestinal type makes up the majority of gastric adenocarcinoma.

FIGURE 11.42. This example of intestinal-type gastric adenocarcinoma is exophytic and more easily recognized as a tumor. The location of this tumor is the proximal stomach, just below the gastroesophageal junction.

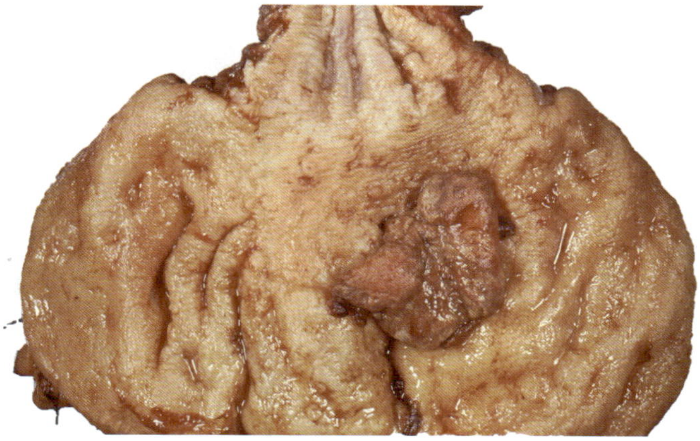

DIFFUSE-TYPE GASTRIC ADENOCARCINOMA

The World Health Organization calls diffuse-type adenocarcinoma "poorly cohesive carcinoma." Previously termed signet-ring cell adenocarcinoma, diffuse-type gastric adenocarcinomas include (but are not limited to) signet-ring cell carcinomas in which signet ring cells account for more than half the tumor. They are poorly differentiated and often show an infiltrative growth pattern. Diffuse-type gastric adenocarcinomas may lead to a "linitis plastica" appearance grossly (a "leather bottle" appearance), with firm, thickened gastric walls sometimes involving the entire stomach. A hereditary form of this type of gastric adenocarcinoma exists, called hereditary diffuse gastric cancer (HDGC), often involving the E-cadherin gene *CDH1*. Prophylactic gastrectomy is recommended in HDGC patients.

FIGURE 11.43. Images (A) and (B) show an infiltrative tumor resulting in gastric wall thickening and loss of mucosal folds.

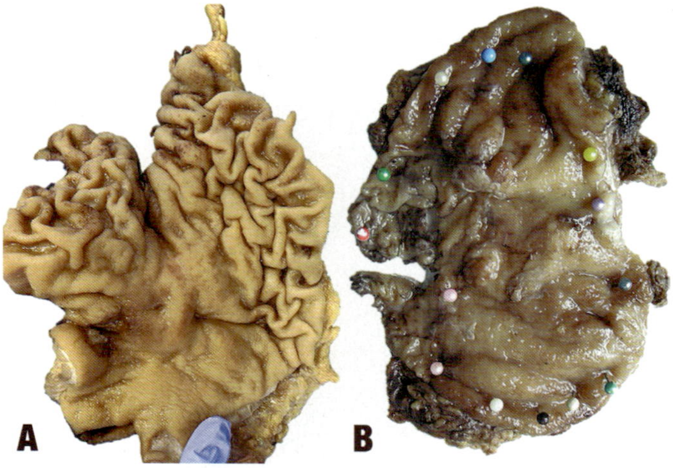

FIGURE 11.44. These images illustrate the thickening of the gastric wall and the "leather bottle" appearance of diffuse-type gastric adenocarcinoma.

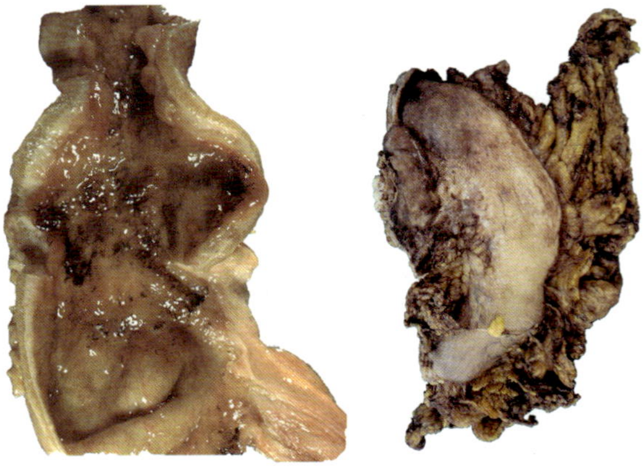

FIGURE 11.45. This specimen was opened along the greater curvature and was pinned for better fixation. This is an example of diffuse-type gastric adenocarcinoma postchemotherapy. The specimen has an ill-defined pale granular area lacking folds, particularly along the lesser curvature (middle of the specimen). Extensive sampling is required to identify residual adenocarcinoma postneoadjuvant therapy.

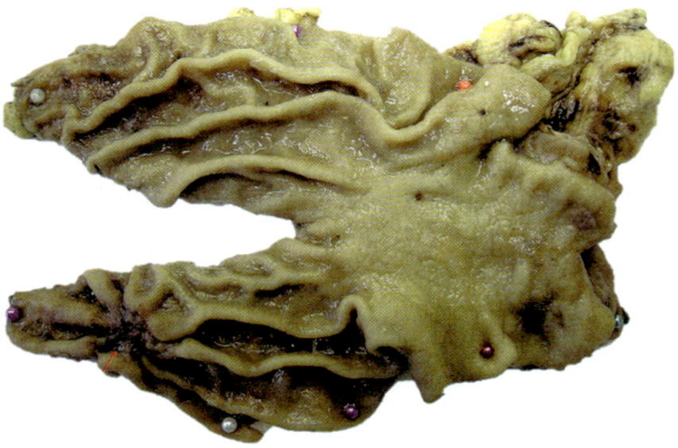

RECURRENT GASTRIC ADENOCARCINOMA

Tumor recurrence after surgical resection portends a poor prognosis and often occurs at the surgical anastomosis.

FIGURE 11.46. This specimen is a resection of a gastrojejunostomy. Note the tumor recurrence at the gastrojejunal anastomotic line, as well as more proximally in the stomach.

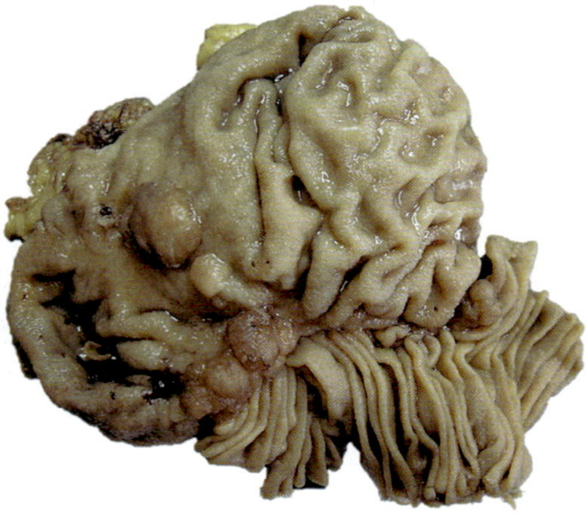

Gastric lymphoma

The stomach is the most common site for gastrointestinal lymphoma.

FIGURE 11.47. These cut sections show the characteristic "fish flesh" appearance of lymphomas. Image (A) shows a specimen in fresh state and (B) shows the specimen after formalin fixation.

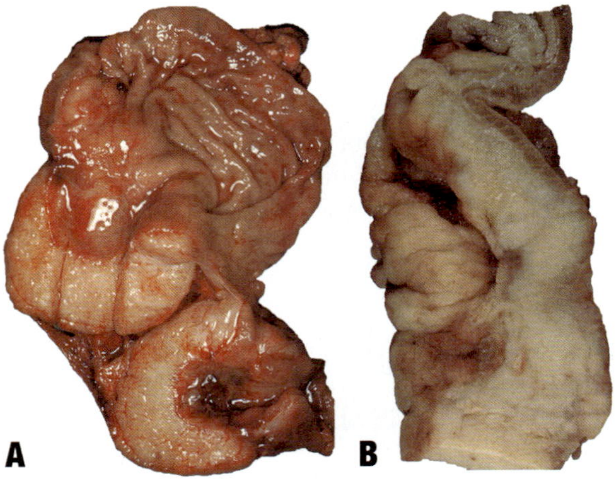

DIFFUSE LARGE B-CELL LYMPHOMA (DLBCL) OF THE STOMACH

DLBCL is the most common type of gastric lymphoma. It is an aggressive malignancy.

FIGURE 11.48. Image (A) shows a total gastrectomy specimen with multiple umbilicated nodules of lymphoma. Image (B) shows that the nodules are well circumscribed with a central ulcerating depression (umbilication) to the otherwise intact overlying mucosa.

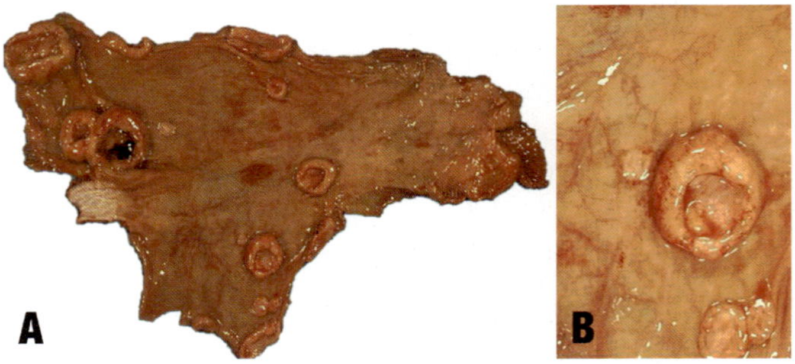

FIGURE 11.49. This image shows an irregular ulcer with an elevated edge and uneven ulcer base.

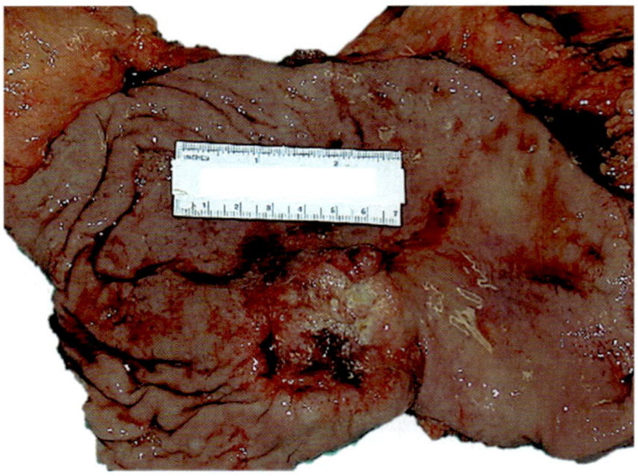

MUCOSA-ASSOCIATED LYMPHOID TISSUE (MALT) LYMPHOMA OF STOMACH

This extranodal marginal zone B-cell lymphoma involving mucosa-associated lymphoid tissue (MALT) is usually slow growing and indolent. MALT lymphoma is the second most common gastric lymphoma. Gastric MALT lymphoma is associated with *H. pylori* infection and is treated with antibiotics. However, gastric MALT lymphomas with t(11;18) are resistant to antibiotics, and may require chemotherapy, radiotherapy, and, rarely, surgery.

FIGURE 11.50. Image (A) shows an enucleated nodule from the gastric wall. The cut surface in (B) is yellow-white and homogeneous, characteristic of lymphoma.

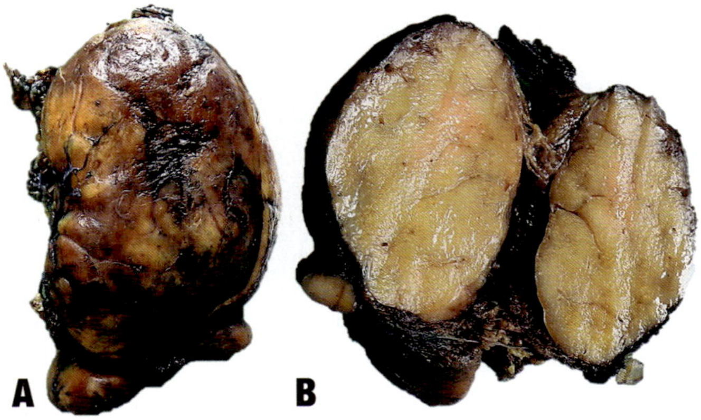

Gastrointestinal stromal tumor (GIST) of the stomach

GIST arises from interstitial cells of Cajal, the pacemaker cells of the GI tract. It mostly occurs in the stomach, but it can occur anywhere in the GI tract. Most GISTs are sporadic: only a minority (< 5%) have a hereditary predisposition. GIST is subtyped into spindle cell type, epithelioid type, and mixed type. Most gastric GISTs have an underlying *c-Kit* gene mutation, but a minority has a *PDGFRA* mutation; these 2 gene mutations are mutually exclusive. Less than 5% of GISTs have a succinate dehydrogenase mutation. GISTs need to be differentiated from leiomyoma and schwannoma. Immunohistochemistry for *c-Kit* (*CD117*), *DOG1*, and *CD34* aid diagnosis.

FIGURE 11.51. Image (A) shows a polypoid nodule with a smooth surface and normal mucosal covering. The cut surface (B) is homogeneous white.

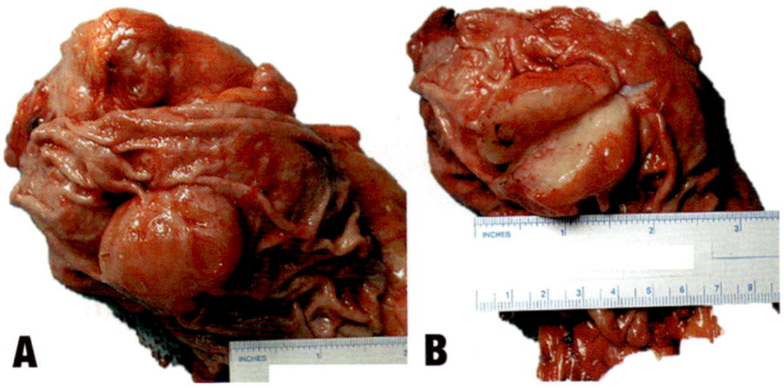

FIGURE 11.52. This GIST is characterized by a submucosal nodule with central umbilication (depression) and ulceration. The main differential diagnosis of an umbilicated gastric nodule includes pancreatic heterotopia, GIST, lymphoma, neuroendocrine tumor, and metastatic tumor.

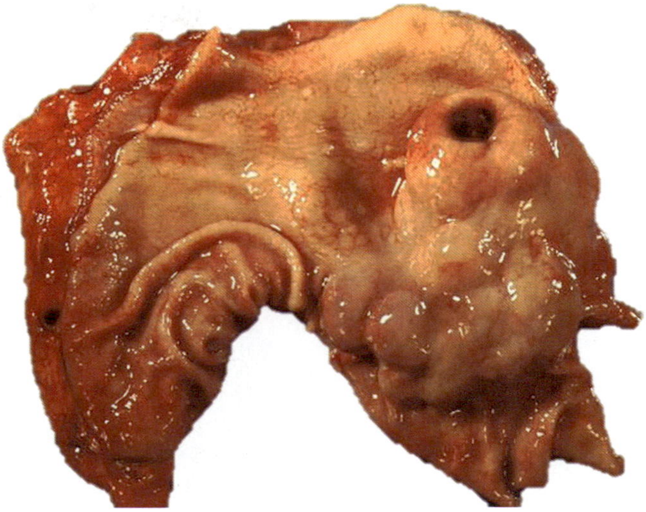

FIGURE 11.53. Image (A) shows a well-circumscribed, solid nodule. In (B), the cut surface is white and homogeneous with focal hemorrhage.

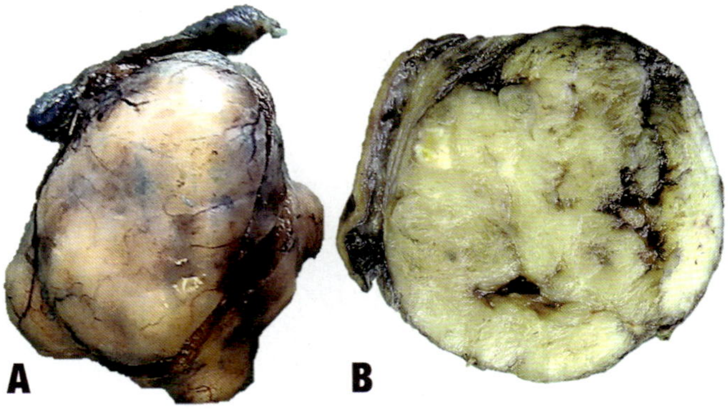

FIGURE 11.54. Image (A) shows a well-circumscribed GIST. Image (B) shows the cut surface with focal hemorrhage.

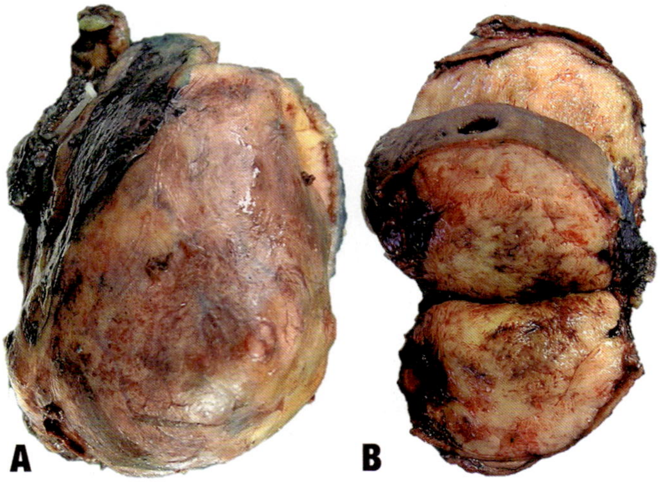

GIST WITH HIGH MALIGNANT POTENTIAL

Assessment of the malignant potential of GIST depends on tumor size, location, and mitotic count. GIST at high risk of progressive disease has a mitotic rate greater than 5 per 5 mm^2 and/or a size of 5 cm to 10 cm or more, depending on the location in the GI tract. Macroscopically, GIST with high malignant potential generally has more extensive necrosis and hemorrhage.

FIGURE 11.55. Image (A) shows a well-circumscribed nodule. In (B), the cut surface shows extensive hemorrhage and necrosis.

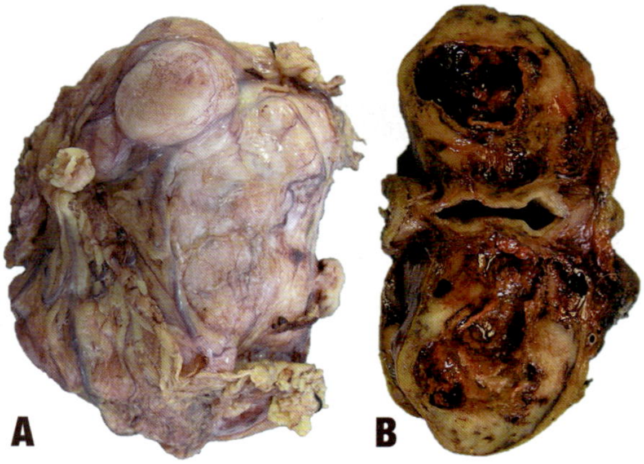

FIGURE 11.56. Image (A) shows a large GIST (24 cm). In (B), its cut surface shows hemorrhage and necrosis. Given the size and the high mitotic count, this gastric GIST was considered to have a high risk of aggressive, malignant behavior.

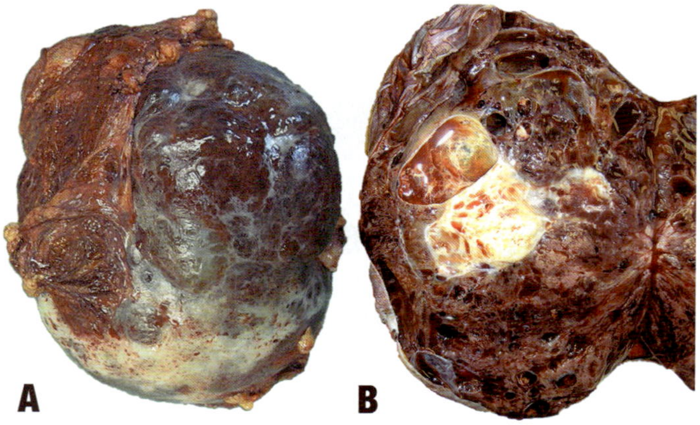

Submucosal lipoma of the stomach

Submucosal lipoma is a benign polypoid mesenchymal lesion that consists of mature adipose tissue. These lesions must be differentiated from other submucosal lesions such as GIST, pancreatic heterotopia, and lymphoma.

FIGURE 11.57. This image shows erythematous, but intact, mucosa overlying the submucosal lesion.

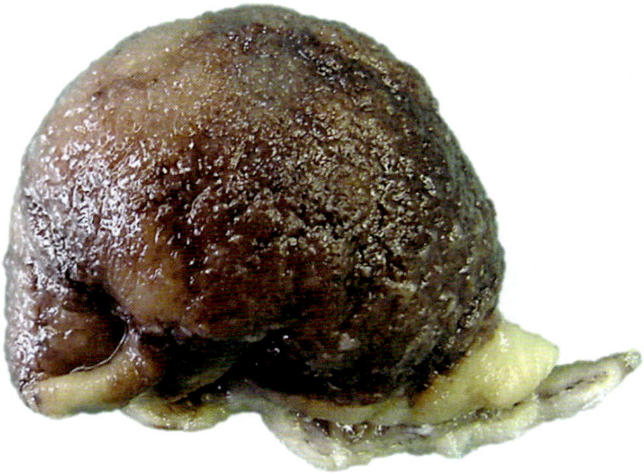

Kaposi sarcoma of the stomach

Kaposi sarcoma is a low-grade vascular neoplasm due to human herpesvirus type 8 (HHV-8) infection and may occur anywhere in the gastrointestinal tract. Kaposi sarcoma is categorized into subtypes according to clinical setting, including immunocompromised and AIDS patients.

FIGURE 11.58. These examples show hemorrhagic masses. Immunohistochemistry for HHV-8 would confirm the diagnosis.

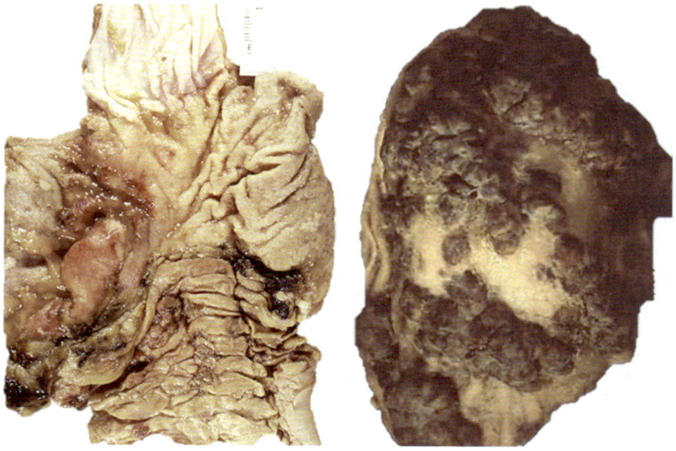

Ménétrier disease

Ménétrier disease is a rare disorder characterized by diffuse hyperplasia of gastric foveolar epithelium of gastric body and fundus associated with hypoproteinemia due to protein-losing enteropathy.

FIGURE 11.59. This image shows marked hypertrophy of rugal folds.

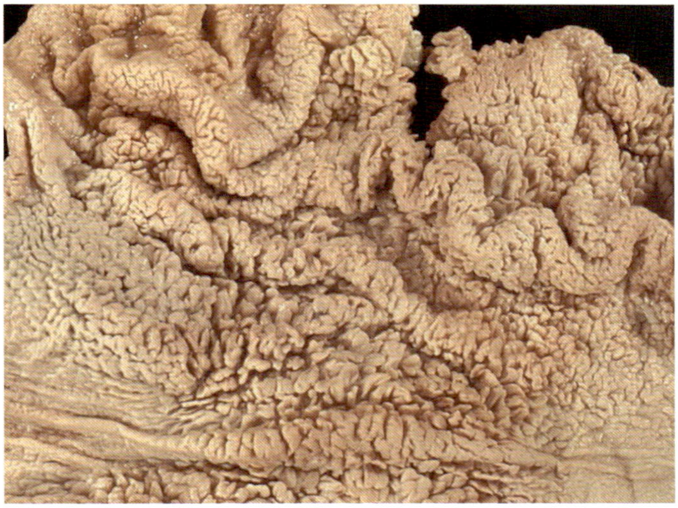

Mallory–Weiss syndrome

Mallory–Weiss syndrome is also called gastroesophageal laceration syndrome. It refers to bleeding from a laceration in the mucosa at the junction of the stomach and esophagus, usually caused by severe vomiting due to alcoholism or bulimia.

FIGURE 11.61. This image shows multiple mucosa lacerations and a perforation.

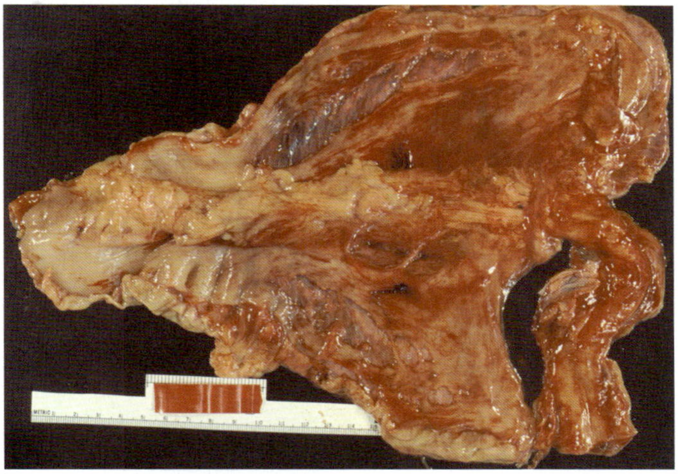

Gastromalacia

Gastromalacia is a softening of the mucosa coats of the stomach. This is usually seen postmortem and could be caused by digestion of mucosa tissue.

FIGURE 11.60. This specimen shows softening and flattening of the gastric mucosa folds.

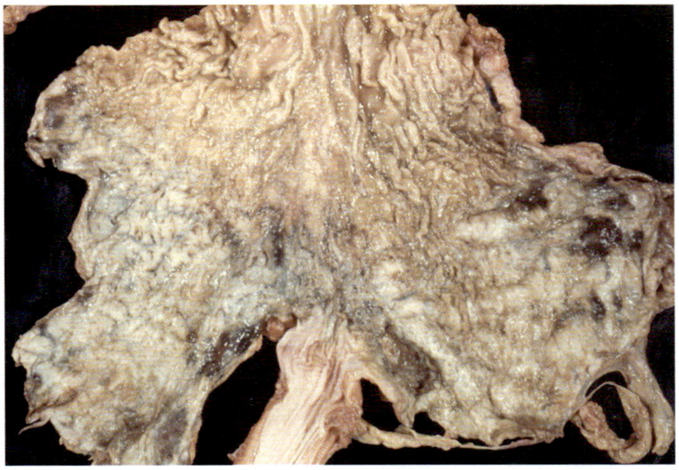

Pyloric stenosis

Pyloric stenosis is an uncommon condition that occurs in infants, in which the stomach pylorus opening is too narrow and blocks food from moving from the stomach to the small intestine. Symptoms become obvious in the first 2 weeks of life and include projectile vomiting without the presence of bile after feeding.

FIGURE 11.62. This image shows the thick smooth muscle wall and narrowed lumen of the pylorus.

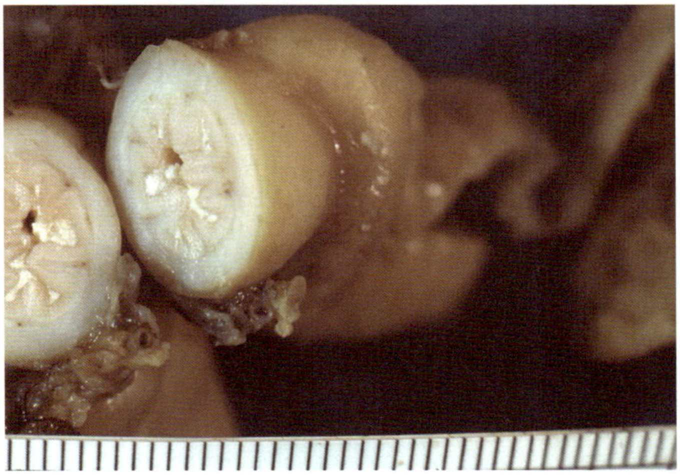

Small Bowel

REFERENCE: NORMAL SMALL BOWEL (SMALL INTESTINE)

The small bowel lies between the stomach and the colon (large bowel), and consists of the duodenum, jejunum, and ileum.

FIGURE 11.63. Image (A) shows a normal external aspect of the small bowel with a smooth peritoneal surface and attached mesenteric fat. Image (B) shows a normal small bowel luminal surface with dense folds called the plicae circulares, which increase the mucosal surface area and help with the absorption of nutrients.

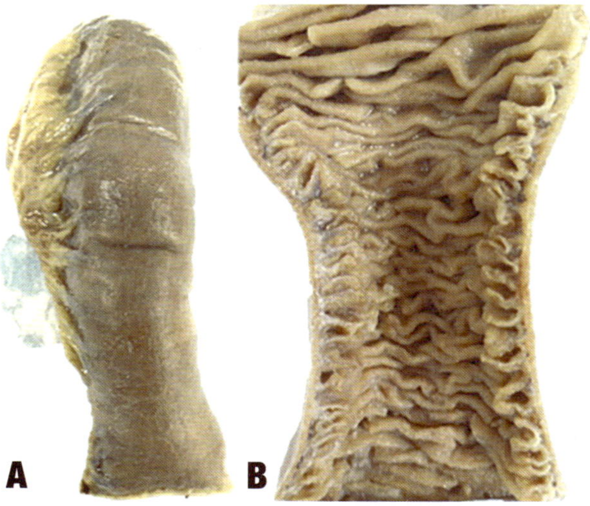

REFERENCE: NORMAL AMPULLA OF VATER

The ampulla of Vater is located at the confluence of the distal common bile duct and the main pancreatic duct. The ampulla protrudes into the second part of the duodenum at the major duodenal papilla, and its opening is controlled by muscles called the sphincter of Oddi.

FIGURE 11.64. This image shows the ampulla of Vater (arrow). The distal stomach is to the left of the image.

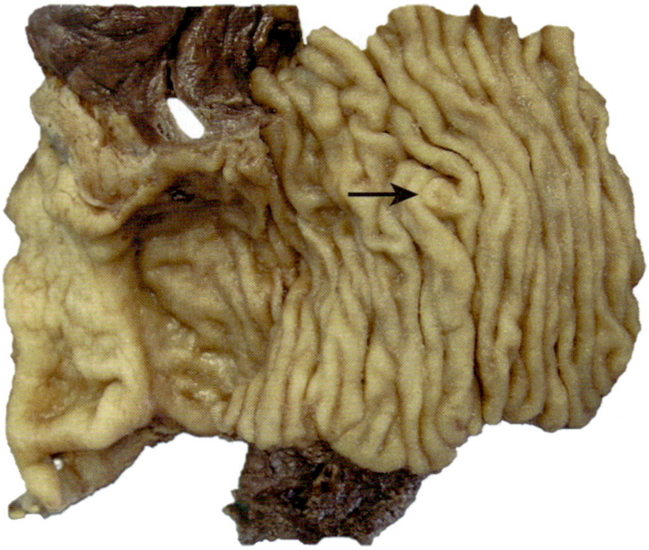

Nonneoplastic Diseases of the Small Bowel

Meckel diverticulum

This congenital lesion is a narrow outpouching of the small bowel wall, on its antimesenteric side. It involves all the layers of the bowel wall including the muscularis propria — that is, it is a "true" diverticulum. The "rule of 2s" applies in the context of Meckel diverticulum: it affects 2% of the population, is 2 inches long, is located within 2 feet of the ileocecal valve, often presents at 2 years of age, and occurs 2 times as often in males. Additionally, there are 2 common types of ectopic tissue in Meckel diverticula: gastric and pancreatic heterotopia. Meckel diverticula may become inflamed and, rarely, neuroendocrine tumors may arise from the ectopic epithelium.

FIGURE 11.65. In (A), a 2-inch, tube-like diverticulum protrudes from the small bowel wall. Image (B) shows the cut opening of a diverticulum, revealing the mucosal lining and the muscular wall.

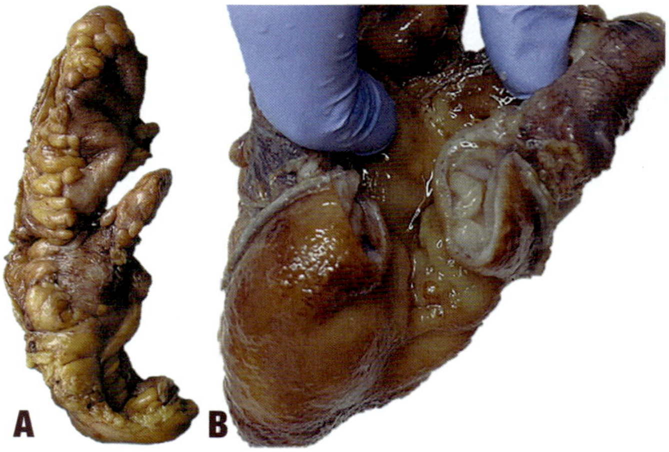

FIGURE 11.66. This image shows a Meckel diverticulum with pancreatic heterotopia (bottom right-hand side).

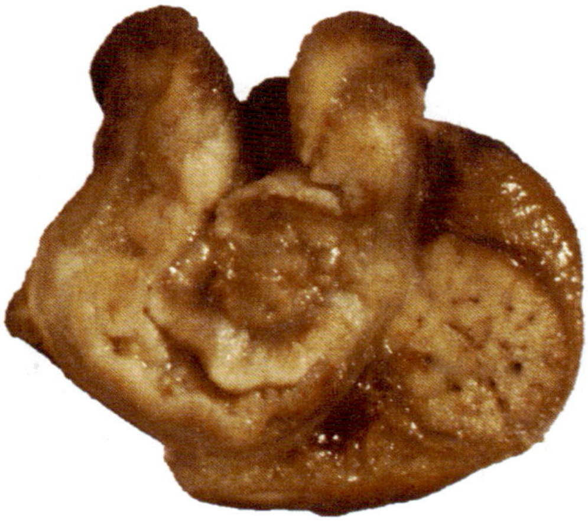

Diverticular disease

Small intestinal diverticula are usually not congenital. They are acquired "false" diverticula: they do not involve all the layers of the bowel wall. Instead, only the mucosa and submucosa form the outpouching that protrudes through the muscular wall. Complications include inflammation, hemorrhage, and perforation. Small intestinal diverticular disease is much less common than its colonic counterpart.

FIGURE 11.67. This image shows the serosal aspect of 3 diverticula in the jejunum. The largest occupies the center.

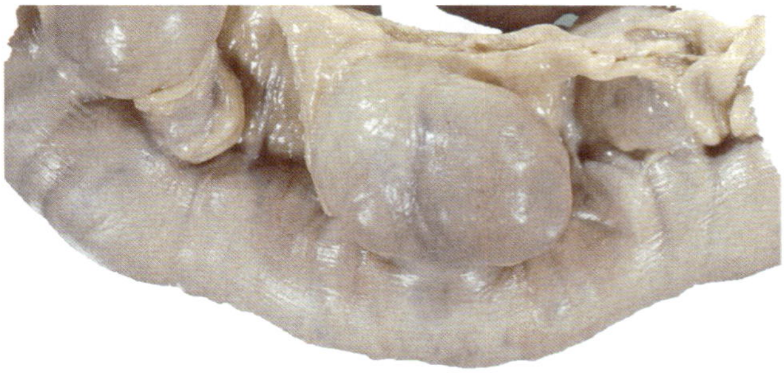

FIGURE 11.68. This resected small bowel segment was opened to reveal a tumor-like lesion, which is actually an inflamed and perforated diverticulum with a surrounding fibro-inflammatory reaction.

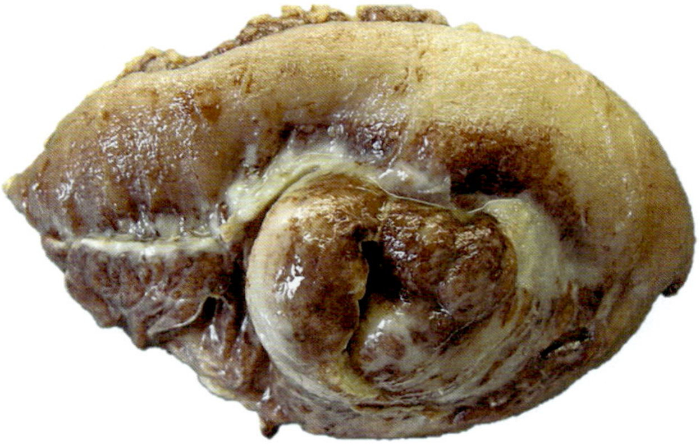

Duplication of the small intestine

Gastrointestinal duplication is an uncommon congenital malformation. The small bowel is the most frequent site of alimentary duplication. Patients may present with abdominal distension or a painless abdominal mass, and they may have other associated congenital anomalies.

FIGURE 11.69. The tweezers in this image illustrate a separate lumen parallel to the main intestinal lumen, indicating a duplicated segment of small intestine.

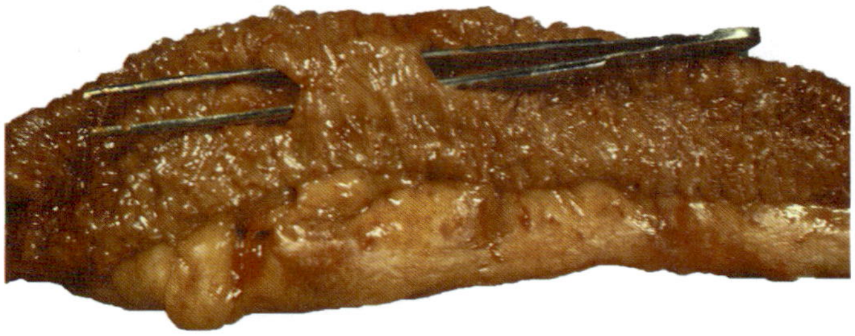

Phytobezoar

Undigested vegetable matter may, uncommonly, form a solid intraluminal mass, called a phytobezoar. Phytobezoars may obstruct the small bowel lumen, especially at the relatively narrowed terminal ileum.

FIGURE 11.70. The image shows vegetable matter in the lumen that obstructed the small bowel.

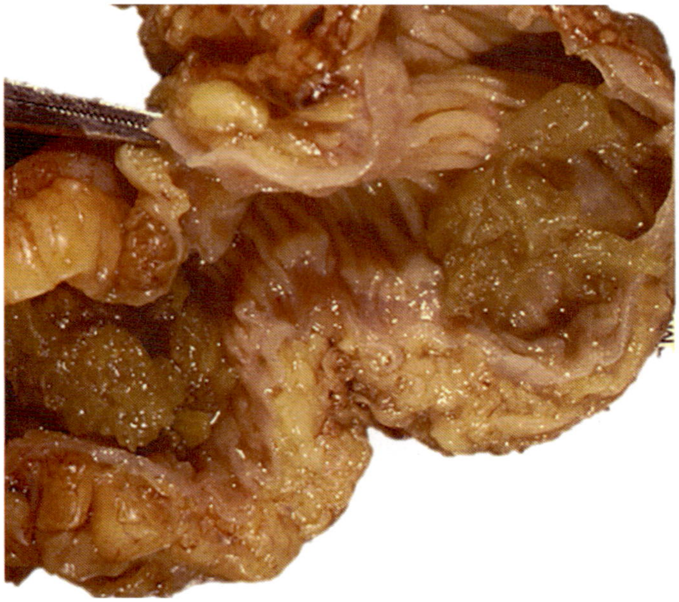

Richter hernia of the small bowel

Richter hernia is the protrusion and/or strangulation of only part of the circumference of the intestine's antimesenteric border through a rigid, small defect of the abdominal wall. It is a form of partial enterocele.

FIGURE 11.71. A portion of the small bowel wall is protruding into a defect in the abdominal wall, where it is incarcerated. The small bowel lumen is partially obstructed.

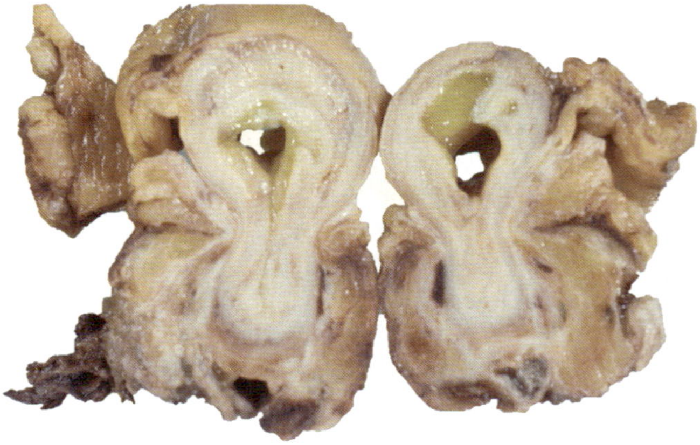

Intussusception of the small bowel

Intussusception is the telescoping of a proximal bowel segment into the adjacent bowel lumen (which is often retroperitoneal or fixed from adhesions). The telescoping can obstruct the lumen and compress blood vessels, thus causing ischemia and infarction. Small bowel intussusception occurs more frequently in infants and young children. Patients may present with abdominal pain, bloody diarrhea, and a palpable tender mass. In adults, intussusception is more commonly associated with a neoplasm.

FIGURE 11.72. This image shows typical telescoping of a small bowel segment into the adjoining lumen.

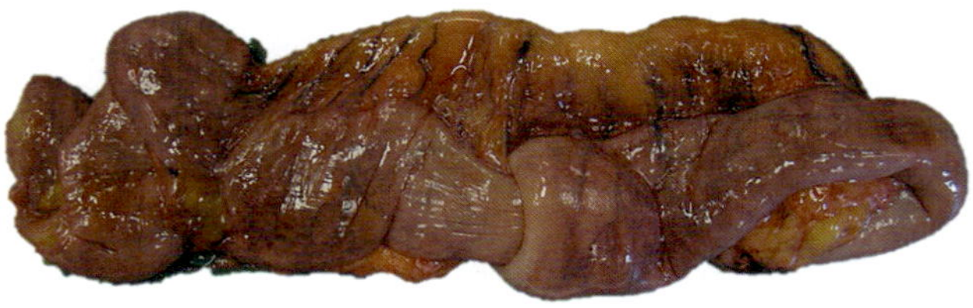

Small bowel adhesions

Small bowel adhesions are areas of fibrous connective tissue on the external surface of the small bowel that adhere to adjacent sites, including other segments of small bowel. Adhesions are usually scar tissue from prior surgery. They are the most common cause of small bowel obstruction. Adhesions may also lead to volvulus, ischemia, and subsequent small bowel perforation.

FIGURE 11.73. This image shows a segment of small bowel with fibrous adhesions. The serosa appears rough, due to the presence of fibrous tissue, in contrast to the normal smooth, shiny surface.

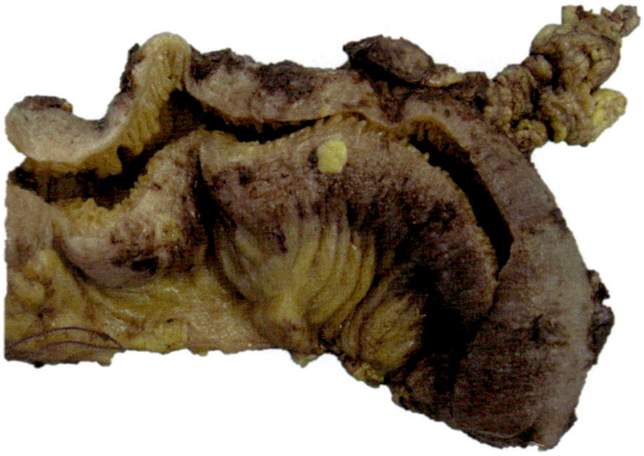

Ischemic small bowel

Small bowel ischemia has many possible causes, including adhesions, hernia, thromboemboli, atherosclerosis, and hypotension. Perforation may result when ischemia leads to transmural necrosis.

FIGURE 11.74. This small bowel segment shows dark serosa and dusky mucosal tissue, consistent with transmural ischemic injury.

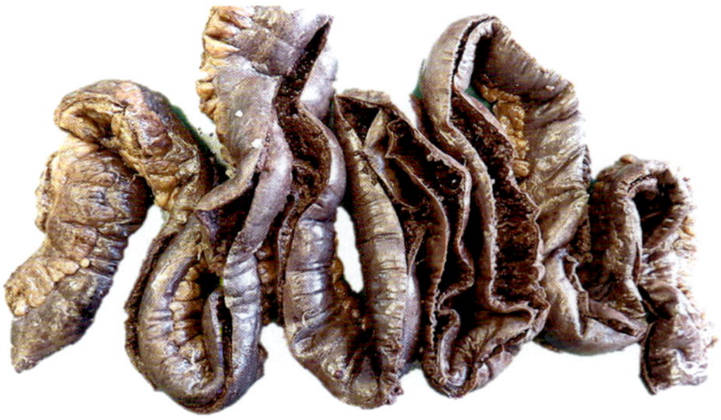

FIGURE 11.75. Image (A) shows dark, dusky discoloration of the small bowel serosa and mesenteric fat. In (B), an opened lumen shows mucosal and mural necrosis (dark discoloration).

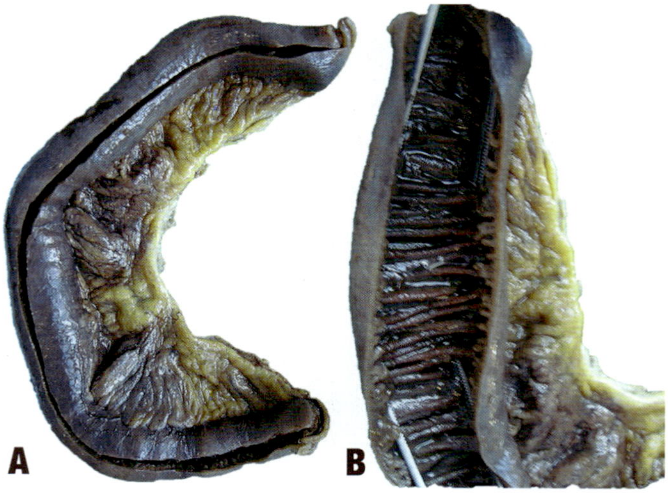

Volvulus

Volvulus occurs when a portion of intestine twists around itself and the mesentery. It may cause obstruction, and severe bowel ischemia and necrosis, all of which are surgical emergencies. Small bowel volvulus occurs more commonly in children. In adults, volvulus more frequently affects the sigmoid colon followed by the cecum. Risk factors for small bowel volvulus include congenital intestinal malrotation and adhesions.

FIGURE 11.76. In this image, the twisted bowel segment (left) appears dark and necrotic, and is clearly distinguished from the paler viable bowel.

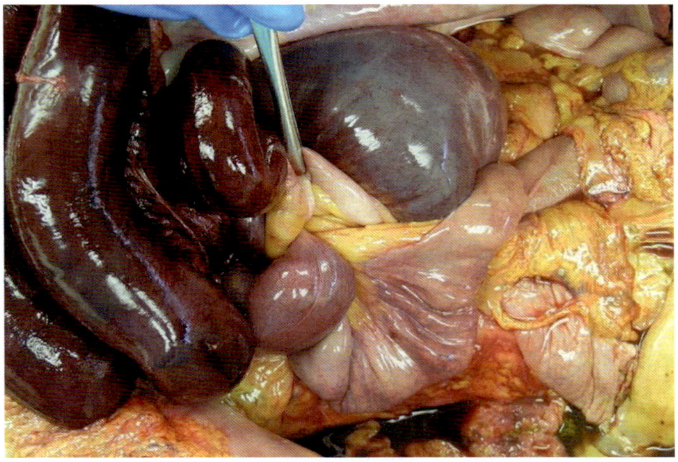

Courtesy of Dr. Evan Matshes

Small bowel trauma

Laparotomy is needed to survey the location of traumatic bowel injury; repair or resect the wound; and stabilize hemostasis.

FIGURE 11.77. This image shows penetrating trauma involving the bowel wall and mesentery caused by a bullet.

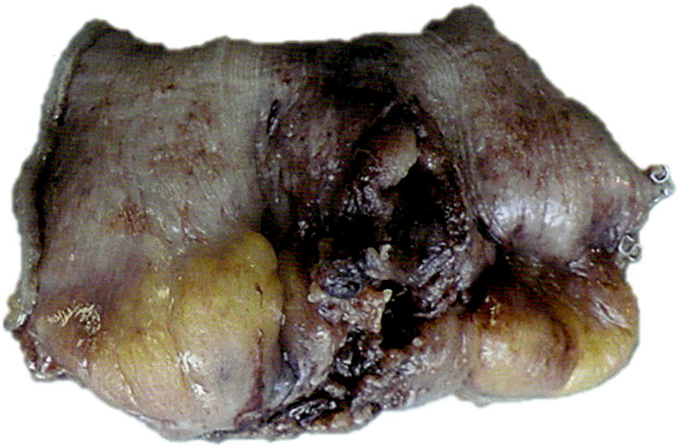

Duodenal ulcer

Duodenal ulcers are rarely neoplastic and usually caused by underlying *H. pylori* infection of the stomach. A biopsy of the stomach is usually indicated.

FIGURE 11.78. Image (A) shows multiple sharply demarcated ulcerative lesions. Image (B) shows transmural perforation of an ulcer against a background of white gauze.

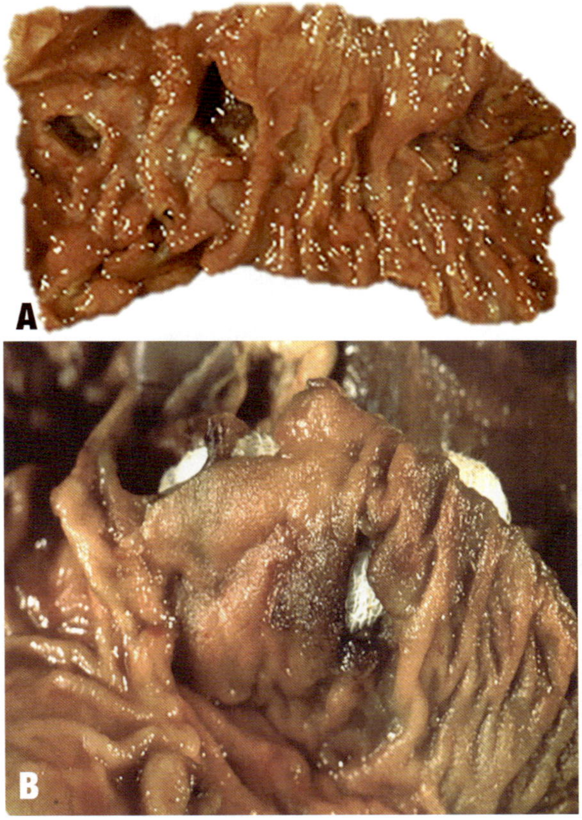

Angiodysplasia of the small bowel

Angiodysplasia is characterized by vascular distortion and dilatation in thin-walled blood vessels. It is more common in the proximal colon. In the elderly, angiodysplasia is thought to be a relatively common cause of obscure gastrointestinal bleeding. Its pathogenesis is poorly understood.

FIGURE 11.79. Grossly, this resected small bowel segment shows erythematous mucosal changes (redness) corresponding to ectatic blood vessels.

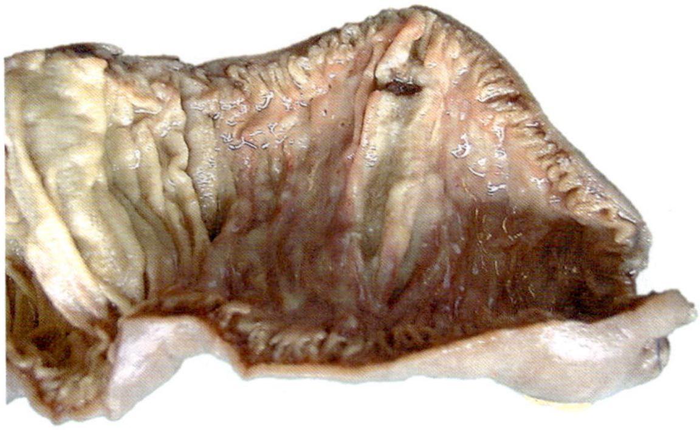

Crohn disease

Crohn disease is a type of chronic idiopathic inflammatory bowel disease (IBD). It frequently involves the terminal ileum, ileocecal valve, and cecum, but may occur anywhere in the GI tract, from mouth to anus. It is characterized by transmural lymphoid inflammation, granulomas, skip lesions, stricture formation, and ulceration. Other possible complications include perforation, abscesses, and fistula formation. "Creeping fat" — fat wrapping around more than 50% of the bowel circumference — is a characteristic finding of Crohn disease involving the small bowel.

FIGURE 11.80. The external surface of this terminal ileum demonstrates creeping fat. The fat is enveloping the entire circumference of the small bowel, including the antimesenteric surface.

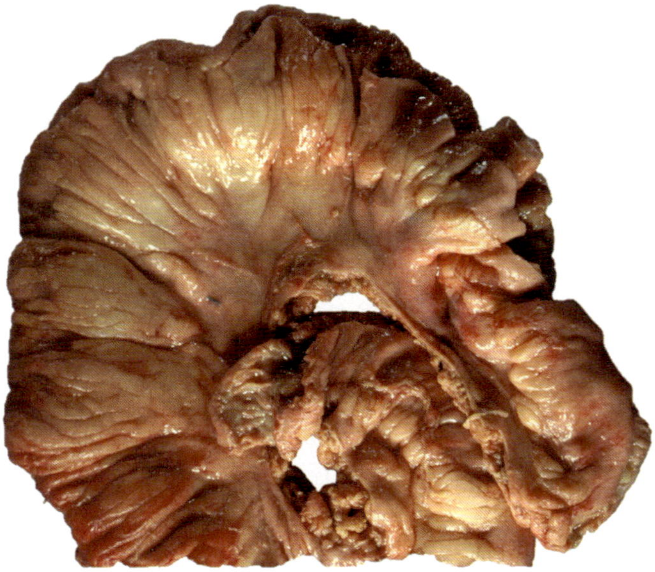

FIGURE 11.81. Creeping fat is present in this terminal ileum specimen from a patient with Crohn disease. In addition, the small bowel wall is thick and its mucosa (lower right) has a cobblestone appearance.

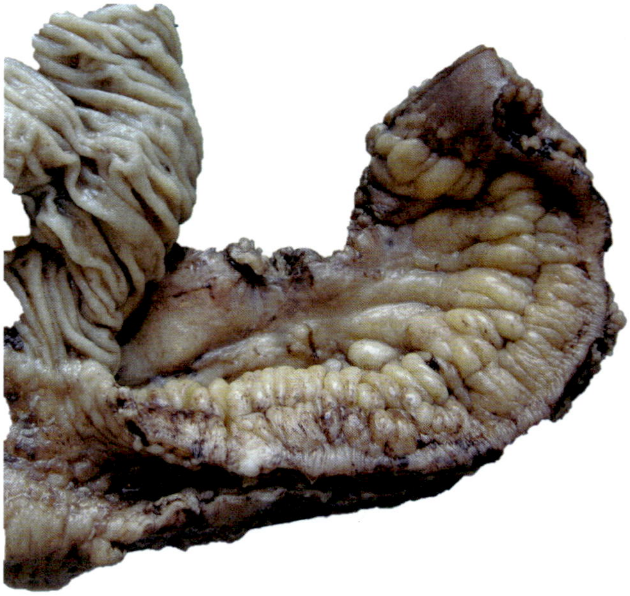

FIGURE 11.82. Circumferential and longitudinal ulcers divide the mucosa in this specimen, resulting in a cobblestone appearance.

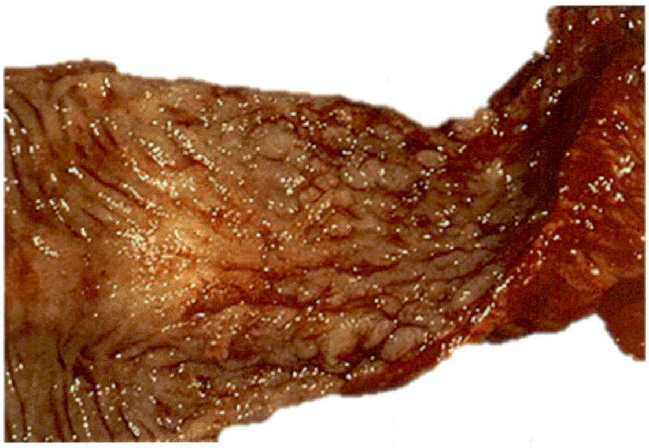

FIGURE 11.83. The small bowel mucosa in this specimen is erythematous, inflamed, and ulcerated. The small bowel wall is thickened and the lumen is stenosed, leading to obstruction.

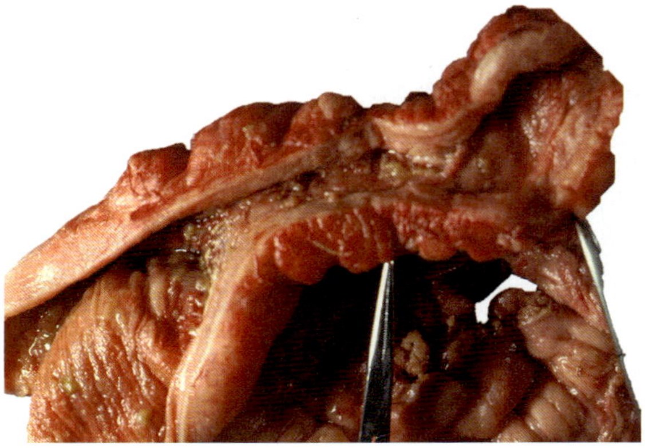

Granulomatosis with polyangiitis (GPA) of small bowel

Previously termed Wegener granulomatosis, GPA is a form of pauci-immune vasculitis. Cytoplasmic antineutrophil cytoplasmic antibody (c-ANCA) is thought to be responsible for the inflammation and is the specific serological test for diagnosis. The small- and medium-sized arteries are involved by necrotizing granulomatous inflammation.

FIGURE 11.84. This image shows partial effacement of mucosa folds and mucosal ulceration as a result of vascular compromise.

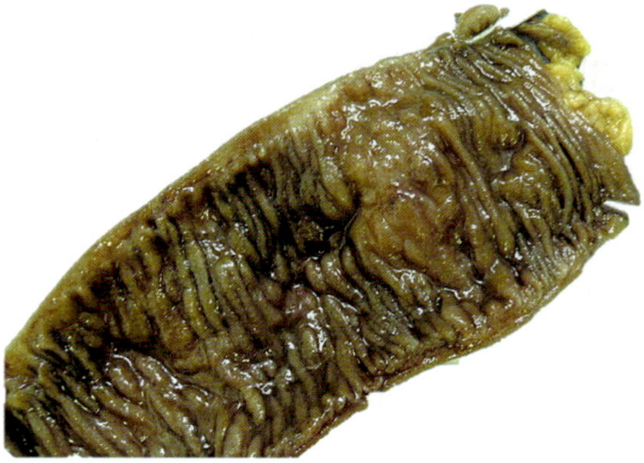

Yersinia enteritis

Yersinia is present in contaminated water, milk, and meat. The ileum, right colon, and appendix are common sites for infection. *Y. enterocolitica* infection causes elongated ulcerations and small aphthous ulcers overlying lymphoid hyperplasia, thus resembling Crohn disease. *Y. pseudotuberculosis* typically produces necrotizing granulomas in the bowel wall and mesenteric nodes mimicking tuberculosis. The bacteria are gram-negative rods and negative on acid-fast stain.

FIGURE 11.85. This example of *Yersinia* enteritis shows multiple ulcers and enlarged mesenteric lymph nodes with white, cheese-like necrosis (caseation) mimicking tuberculosis.

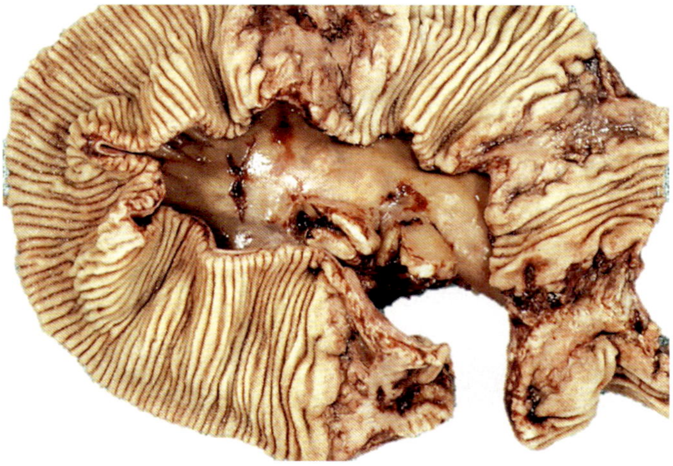

Tuberculosis

Mycobacterium tuberculosis (TB) of the GI tract is much less common than pulmonary TB. The terminal ileum and mesenteric lymph nodes are the most frequently affected locations in the GI tract, due to the rich lymphoid tissue of these locations and the lymphotropic nature of the organism. Ulcerations and luminal narrowing are the predominant lesions found in this region.

FIGURE 11.86. This image shows enlarged mesenteric lymph nodes with caseation.

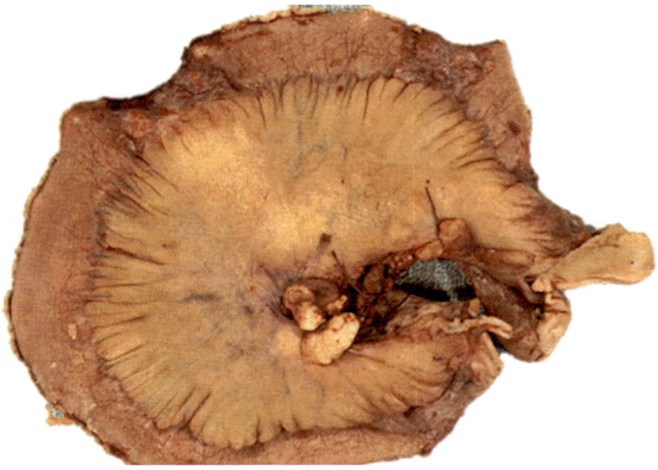

Typhoid perforation

Typhoid fever is an acute illness caused by *Salmonella typhi*. The prevalence of typhoid fever is decreasing worldwide, but still remains endemic in the Indian subcontinent. Intestinal hemorrhage is the most common complication of typhoid fever. Intestinal perforation is a serious complication that requires urgent surgery.

FIGURE 11.87. Image (A) shows the mucosal side of perforated ulcers. Image (B) shows the serosal aspect of the perforated ulcers.

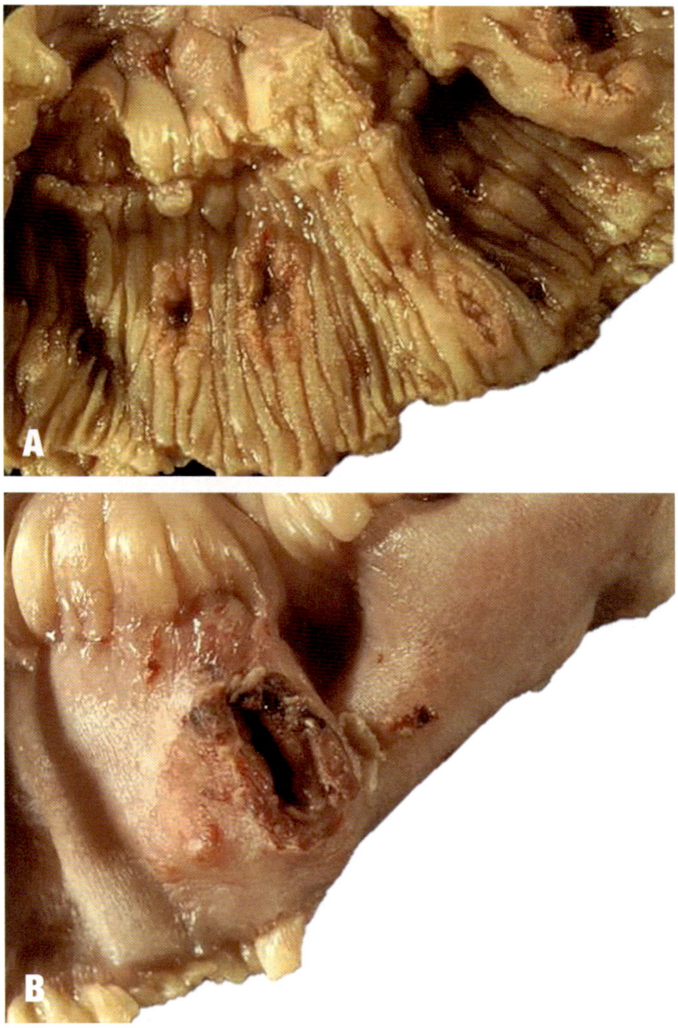

Neoplasms of the Small Bowel

Adenoma of the small bowel

Adenomas are precursor lesions of small bowel adenocarcinomas. Most small bowel adenomas occur in the region of the ampulla of Vater. Ampullary and periampullary adenomas may lead to obstruction of the biliary and pancreatic ducts.

FIGURE 11.88. This image of a periampullary adenoma shows a multinodular mass in the middle of the second part of the duodenum. It has grown so large that the ampulla of Vater is unrecognizable. The adenoma contained high-grade dysplasia, but there was no underlying invasive adenocarcinoma.

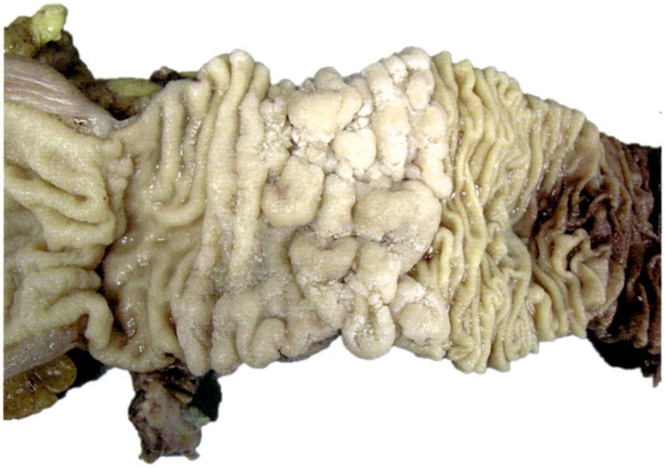

FIGURE 11.89. This image shows a 9-cm villous adenoma in the first part of the duodenum. On histology, the adenoma contained high-grade dysplasia and focal invasive adenocarcinoma.

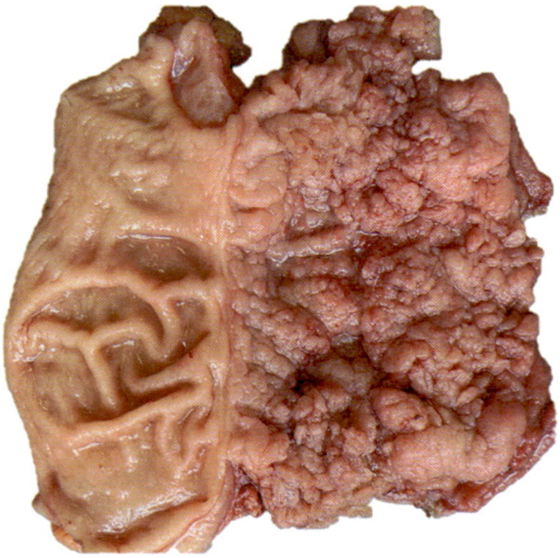

Adenocarcinoma of the small bowel

The incidence of adenocarcinoma in the small bowel is much lower than in the colon. Small bowel adenocarcinomas may be associated with Lynch syndrome (hereditary nonpolyposis colorectal cancer), familial adenomatous polyposis (FAP), and hamartomatous polyposis syndromes, such as Peutz–Jeghers syndrome and juvenile polyposis. Adenocarcinomas of the small bowel most commonly arise at the ampulla of Vater in the second part of the duodenum; these are called ampullary carcinomas.

FIGURE 11.90. This segmental resection specimen of the small bowel shows a stricture caused by adenocarcinoma invading through full thickness of bowel wall to the serosa.

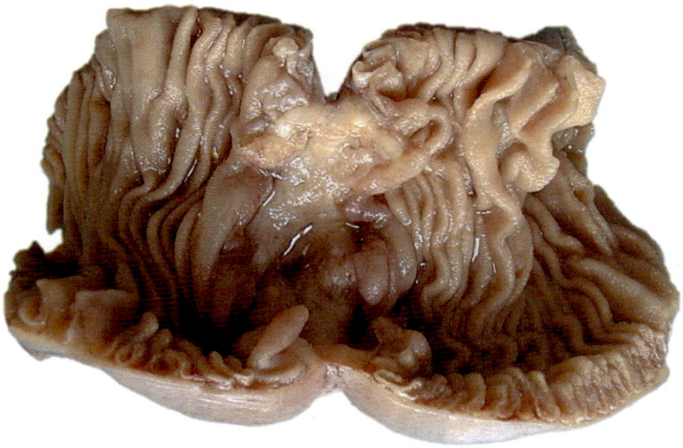

FIGURE 11.91. An opened small bowel segment shows an irregular, ulcerated tumor with overlying green necroinflammatory material. This tumor was a poorly differentiated adenocarcinoma on histology: only a minority of the tumor cells formed glands.

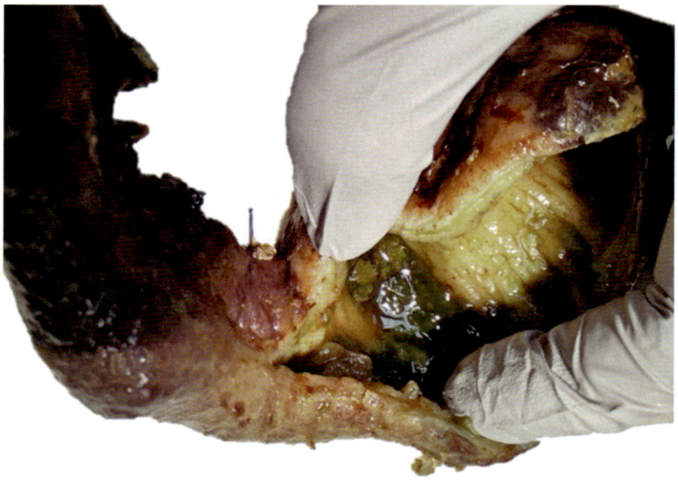

SIGNET-RING CELL ADENOCARCINOMA OF THE DUODENUM

By definition, more than 50% of cells in this tumor are signet ring cells. This type of adenocarcinoma is also known as poorly cohesive carcinoma. It is a rare form of small bowel cancer with poor prognosis.

FIGURE 11.92. This diffusely infiltrating adenocarcinoma of the duodenum caused thick mucosal folds and a rigid bowel wall. On histology, this was a signet-ring cell adenocarcinoma.

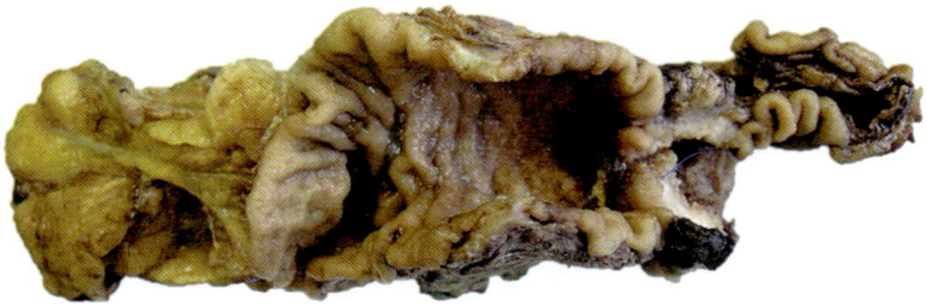

Ampullary carcinoma

The College of American Pathologists recognizes 3 categories of ampullary tumors based on location: periampullary (on the duodenal surface of the ampullary papilla), intraampullary, and mixed types. Ampullary carcinomas may obstruct the distal common bile duct and the pancreatic duct, leading to jaundice, pancreatitis, and other complications.

FIGURE 11.93. In this Whipple resection specimen, there is a nodular mass at the ampulla of Vater where a probe was inserted.

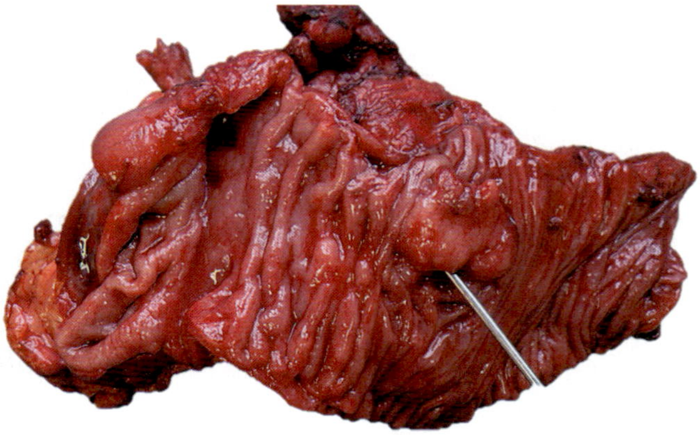

FIGURE 11.94. This Whipple resection specimen was sectioned to demonstrate the relationship of the tumor with adjacent structures. This solid white ampullary carcinoma invaded into the pancreatic head, the duodenum, and the distal common bile duct. It caused obstruction and dilatation of the common bile duct (seen with an inserted probe).

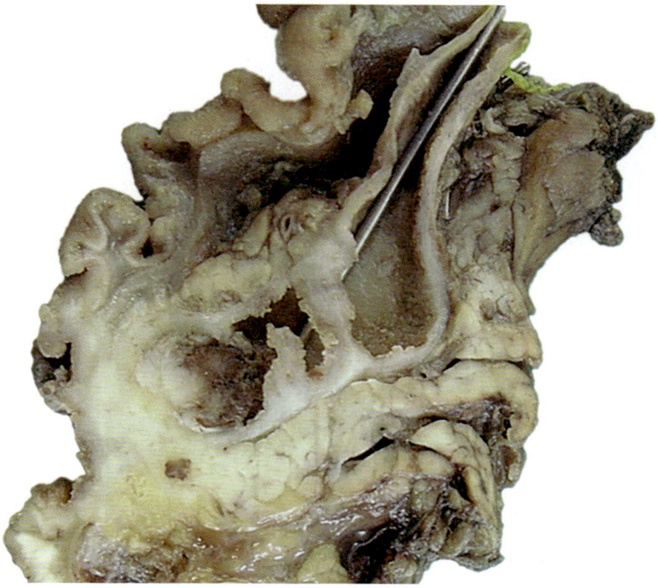

FIGURE 11.95. These images are cross-sections that demonstrate tumor location and extent of invasion. The intraampullary carcinoma in (A) involves the ampulla and sphincter of Oddi. The intraampullary carcinoma in (B) invades the duodenal wall.

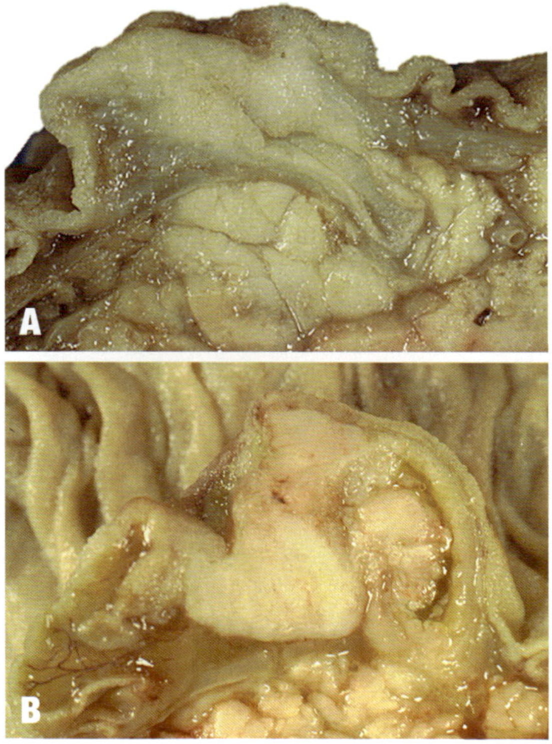

FIGURE 11.96. The image of a Whipple resection specimen shows a periampullary carcinoma. This type of ampullary tumor demonstrates a prominent exophytic growth pattern on the surface of the ampullary papilla, which may obstruct the orifice. There is a probe in the lumen of the stenosed ampulla.

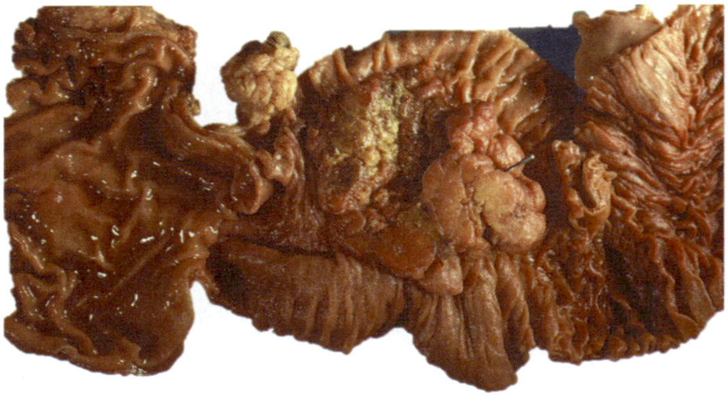

Neuroendocrine tumor (NET) of the small bowel

Neuroendocrine neoplasms have variably aggressive behaviors. Well-differentiated NETs generally have better prognosis than low-grade adenocarcinomas of the small bowel. NETs are graded by their mitotic count and proliferation rate (Ki-67 index), and are staged by their size, depth of invasion, and metastases. Neuroendocrine neoplasms express neuroendocrine markers such as synaptophysin and chromogranin by immunohistochemistry. Not uncommonly, lymph nodal metastases of small bowel NETs are larger than the primary tumor. Sometimes, NETs may be the lead point for intussusception.

FIGURE 11.97. This image shows a segmental resection of small bowel with a polypoid NET covered by normal mucosa.

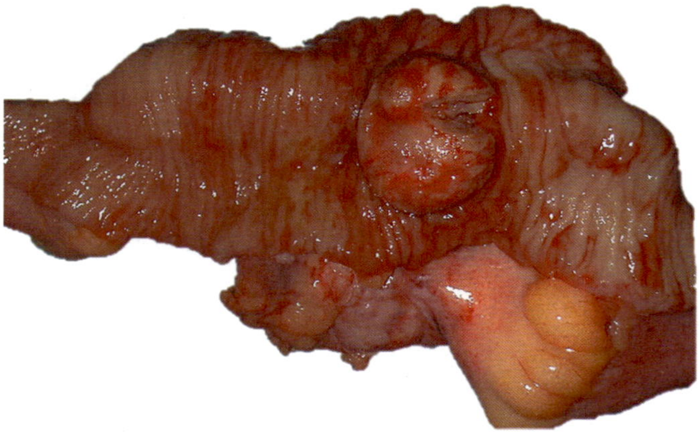

FIGURE 11.98. This segmental resection shows a small polypoid nodule covered by nonneoplastic mucosa with a central ulcerated depression, histologically confirmed as NET.

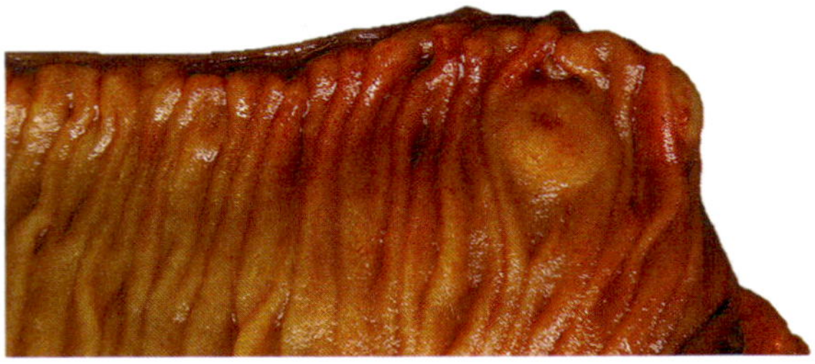

FIGURE 11.99. This 1.2-cm NET of the small intestine had a metastasis in 1 lymph node resulting in a 5-cm mesenteric mass.

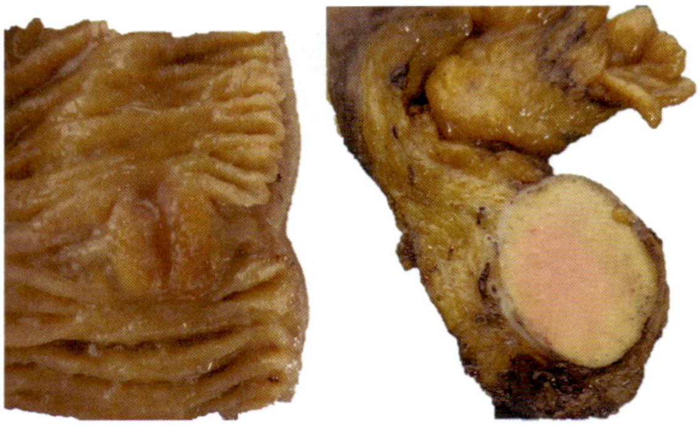

FIGURE 11.100. The NET in (A) bulges into the cecum (in fresh state). Image (B) shows the NET in cross-section (after formalin fixation). These are examples of NETs in the ileum with early intussusception into the cecum.

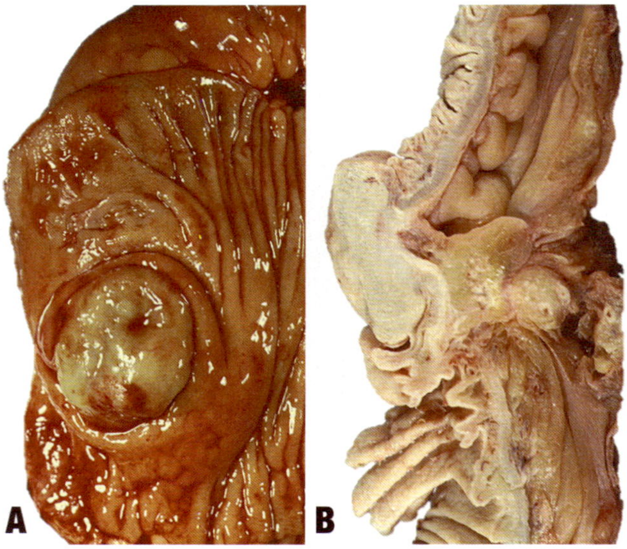

Non-Hodgkin lymphoma (NHL) of the small bowel

The small bowel may be the site for primary extranodal lymphoma or may be secondarily involved by NHL. Primary B-cell lineage NHLs vastly outnumber T-cell lymphomas in the GI tract. Diffuse large B-cell lymphoma (DLBCL) is the most common type of gastrointestinal lymphoma.

It is a high-grade aggressive lymphoma. Other types of NHL seen in the small bowel include marginal zone MALT lymphoma, mantle cell lymphoma, follicular lymphoma, and Burkitt lymphoma. Immunohistochemistry is necessary to accurately classify lymphomas and to help determine their prognosis.

FIGURE 11.101. This image shows a whitish solid tumor extending from the ulcerated mucosa to the serosa, including involvement of regional lymph nodes.

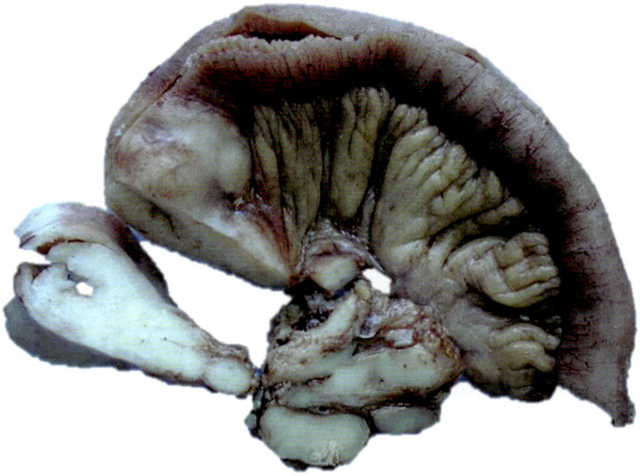

FIGURE 11.102. This example of NHL shows a circumferential ulcerating mass. The wall of the small bowel is thickened by tumor and has a "fish flesh" appearance.

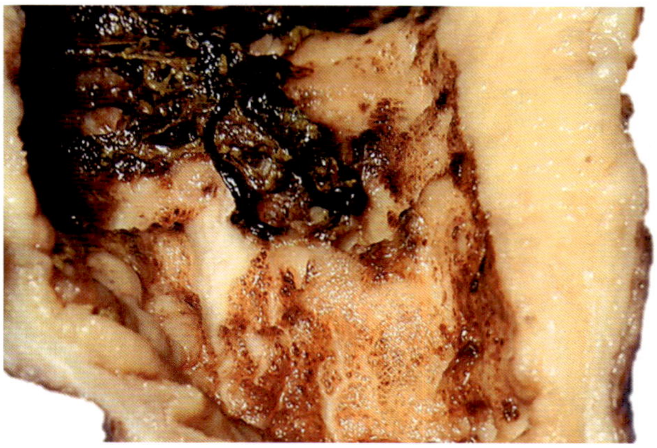

FIGURE 11.103. This small bowel segmental resection specimen shows a multifocal nodular mass extending into the lumen with a fleshy cut surface. This is an example of DLBCL.

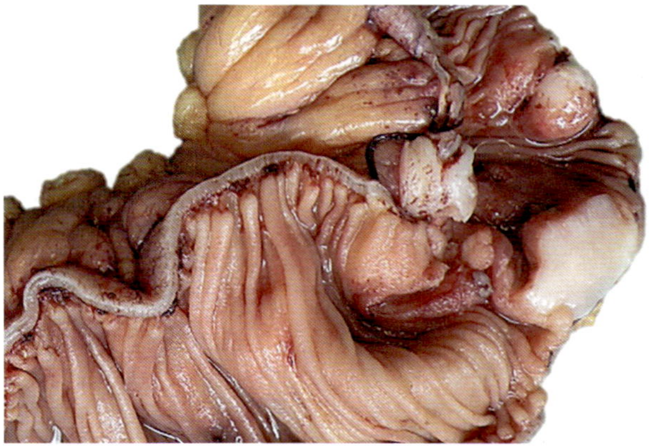

Gastrointestinal stromal tumor (GIST) of the small bowel

This mesenchymal tumor is derived from interstitial cells of Cajal, which are the pacemaker cells of the GI tract. On histology, GISTs may be spindle cell or epithelioid type. The spindle cell type may be confused with leiomyoma or schwannoma. Confirmatory immunohistochemical markers include *c-Kit* and *DOG-1*. Risk assessment of GISTs takes into consideration tumor size, mitotic count, and location. GISTs of the small bowel are considered at high risk for progressive disease if they are > 10 cm, or have a mitotic count > 5 per 5 mm^2.

FIGURE 11.104. This image shows a tumor nodule with a smooth surface bulging from the subserosa of the ileum.

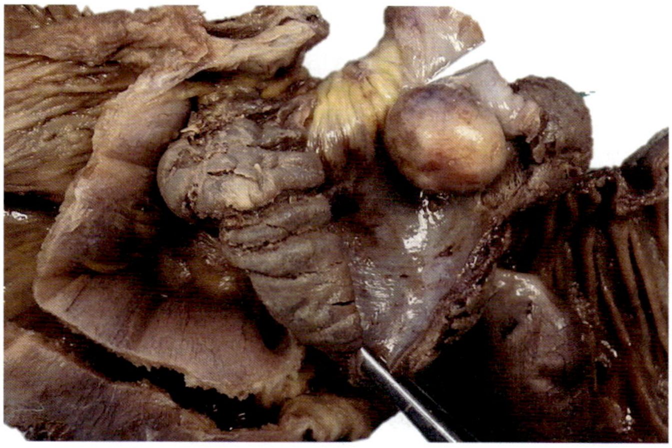

FIGURE 11.105. Image (A) shows a segmental resection of small bowel with a small subserosal nodule, histologically confirmed as GIST with a low risk of malignant behavior. Image (B) shows a large multinodular tumor attached to the small bowel; this large tumor has a high risk of progression.

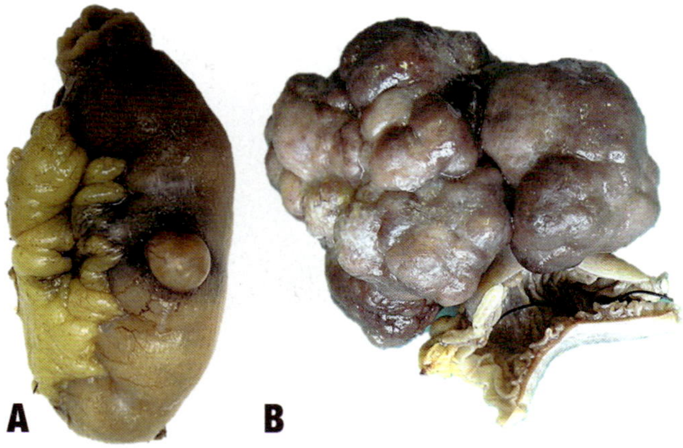

FIGURE 11.106. This is a cross-section of a small bowel GIST showing a typical firm, whitish, "fish flesh" appearance with focal hemorrhage.

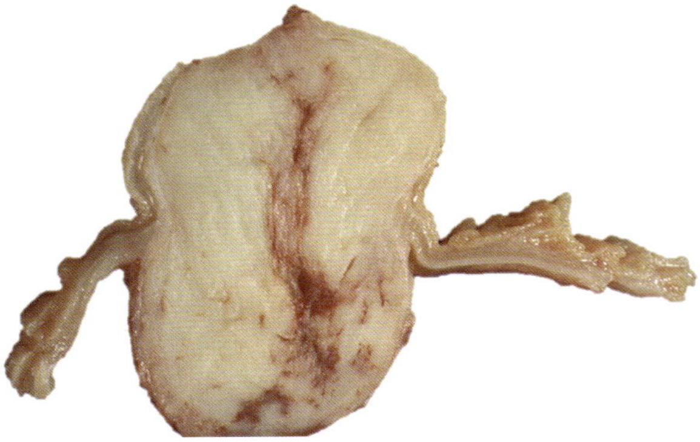

FIGURE 11.107. Image (A) shows a well-defined submucosal and mural nodule with normal overlying mucosa. In (B), the cut surface of this GIST has a whitish "fish flesh" appearance with focal hemorrhage and necrosis.

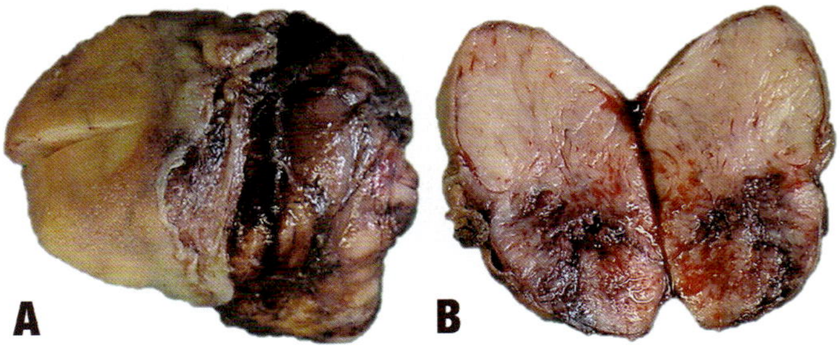

FIGURE 11.108. In (A), a small bowel segmental resection specimen shows a large dark multinodular GIST attached to the small bowel. In (B), the cut surface of the specimen shows a tumor with more extensive hemorrhage and necrosis, suggesting a more aggressive behavior.

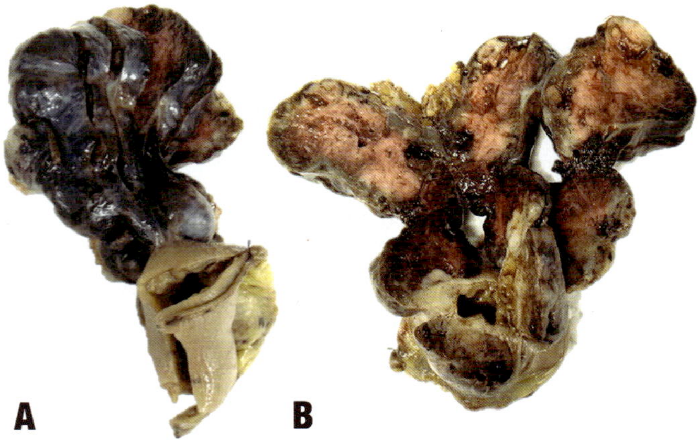

Gangliocytic paraganglioma of the duodenum

This rare tumor, nearly always located in the ampullary area, is characterized by a mixed proliferation of epithelioid, ganglion, and spindle cells on histology. It is usually benign, although local recurrence may follow incomplete excision.

FIGURE 11.109. This example of gangliocytic paraganglioma appears as a polypoid lesion protruding into the intestinal lumen. The lesion is overlain by stretched normal duodenal mucosa.

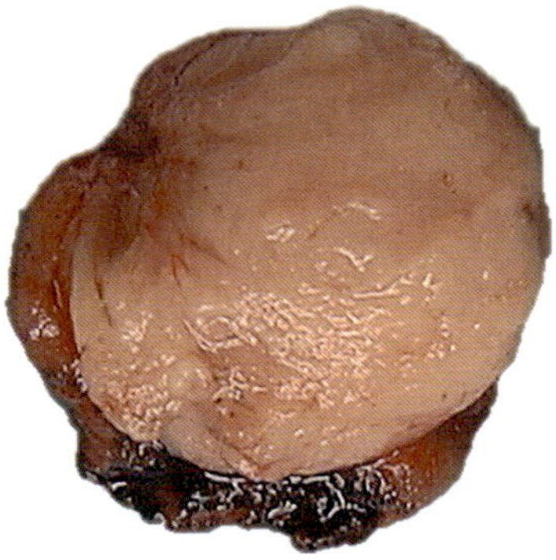

Lipohyperplasia of ileocecal valve

The ileocecal valve is situated at the most distal end of the terminal ileum, and indicates the end of the small intestine and the start of the colon. Lipohyperplasia of the ileocecal valve (lipomatous hyperplasia) is characterized by diffuse prominence of the ileocecal valve due to increased submucosal adipose tissue. It may rarely lead to recurrent intussusception and obstruction.

FIGURE 11.110. This image shows a prominent ileocecal valve containing fat (arrow).

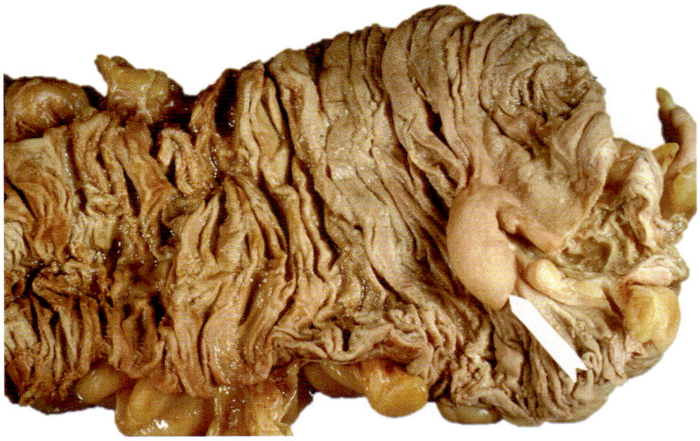

Lipoma of the small bowel

Lipomas are common benign neoplasms and are the most common mesenchymal tumors of the GI tract. Lipomas are less frequent in the small bowel compared with the colon. Unlike lipohyperplasia of the ileocecal valve, an ileocecal lipoma is a distinct polypoid neoplasm arising from an otherwise normal ileocecal valve.

FIGURE 11.111. This ileocecal resection specimen shows a solitary, spherical, and smooth nodule at the ileocecal valve. This is a lipoma.

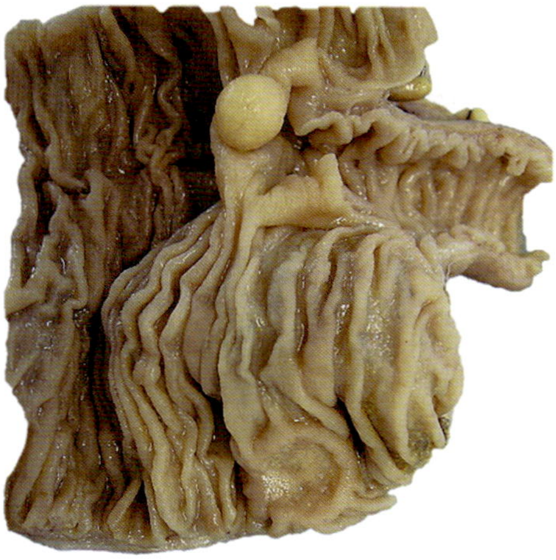

FIGURE 11.112. In (A), a small bowel segmental resection shows a tumor on the luminal surface with intussusception. Image (B) shows a yellow and lobulated cut surface with intact overlying mucosa. This example of lipoma occurred in the jejunum.

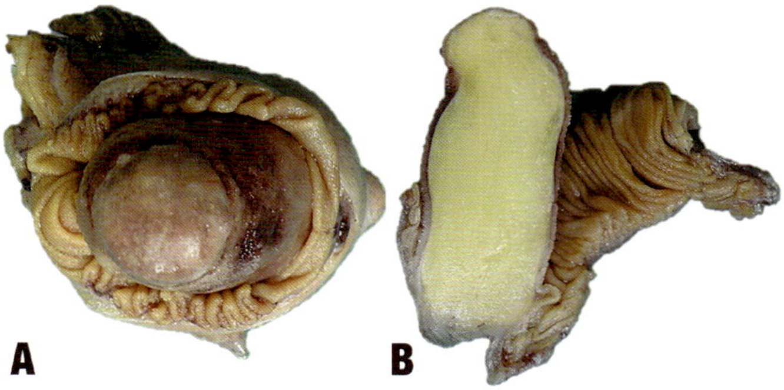

Inflammatory fibroid polyp of the small bowel

These benign tumors are polypoid and based in the submucosa. Histologically, they contain eosinophils, spindle cells, and prominent capillaries. They are not thought to be premalignant.

FIGURE 11.113. The image shows a polypoid neoplasm with a narrow stalk protruding into the lumen of the small bowel.

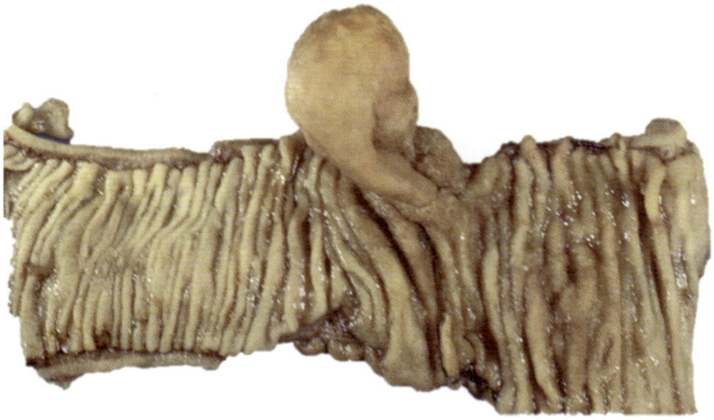

Inflammatory myofibroblastic tumor (IMT) of the small bowel

IMT is a rare soft tissue tumor that may arise in various organs. IMTs are characterized by spindle cell fibroblastic and myofibroblastic proliferations with an inflammatory infiltrate. These tumors often have an *ALK* gene rearrangement.

FIGURE 11.114. A small bowel segmental resection specimen shows an ill-defined lesion on the serosal surface, histologically diagnosed as IMT.

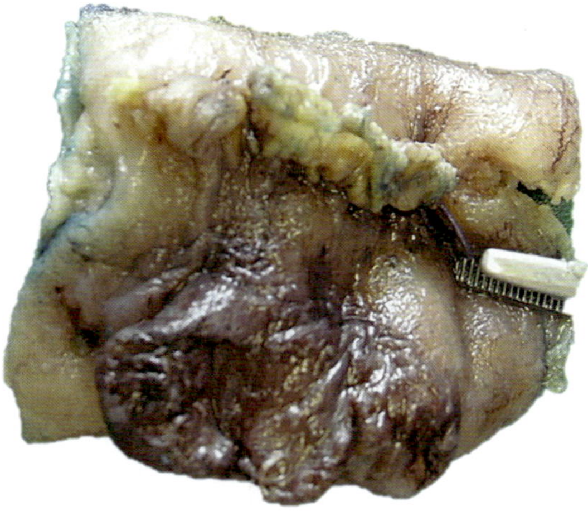

Mesenteric fibromatosis

Mesenteric fibromatosis is also known as intraabdominal desmoid. It is rare and locally aggressive. These tumors do not metastasize, but tend to recur locally. Mesenteric fibromatosis may be associated with Gardner syndrome and familial adenomatous polyposis.

FIGURE 11.115. This 7-cm mass in the mesentery surrounds a diverticulum in the jejunum.

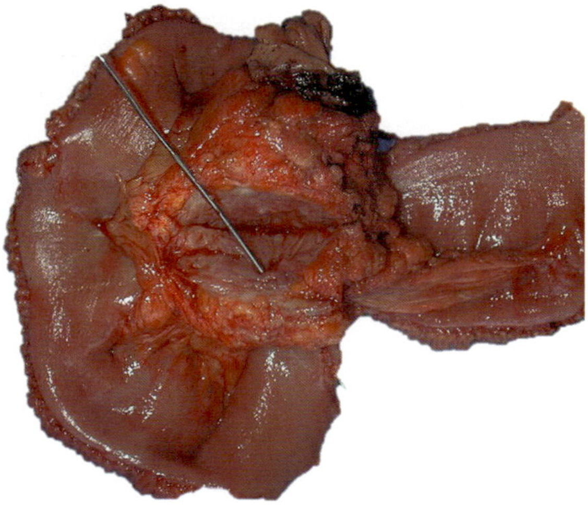

Lymphangioma

Lymphangiomas are uncommon, benign malformations of the lymphatic system that rarely occur in the small bowel. On histology, they demonstrate a proliferation of thin-walled lymphatic channels.

FIGURE 11.116. This small bowel segmental resection specimen of jejunum shows a yellowish lesion on the luminal aspect.

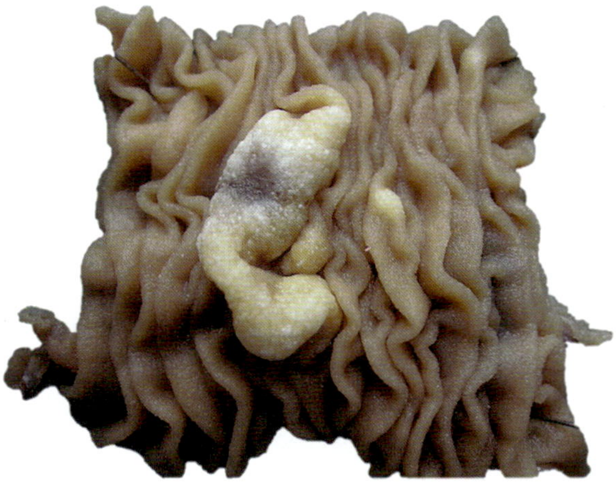

Kaposi sarcoma of the small intestine

This low-grade vascular neoplasm is caused by human herpesvirus type 8 (also called Kaposi sarcoma–associated herpesvirus, or KSHV). Kaposi sarcoma is categorized into subtypes according to clinical setting, including immunocompromised and AIDS patients.

FIGURE 11.117. Note the multiple erythematous small bowel mucosal lesions.

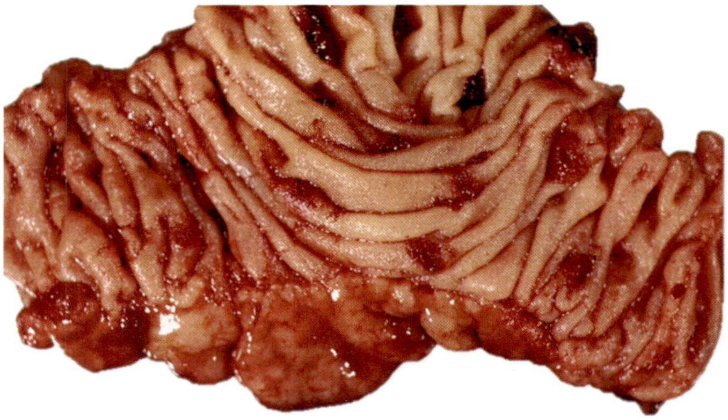

Gastrointestinal neuroectodermal tumor (GNET) of the small bowel

This rare malignant neoplasm (also called primary clear cell sarcoma–like tumor of the small bowel) is associated with *EWSR1* gene rearrangement. On immunohistochemistry, GNETs are S100 positive, but are negative for other melanoma markers.

FIGURE 11.118. In (A), a small bowel specimen shows a polypoid mass extending into the lumen. Image (B) shows the cut surface of the tumor.

A

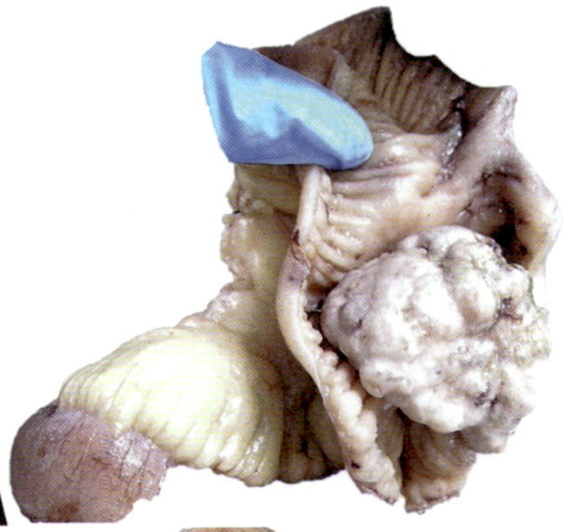

B

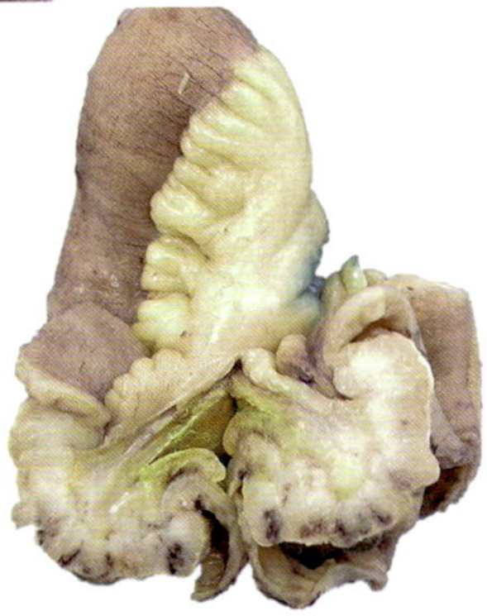

Metastasis to the small bowel

Tumors may metastasize to the small bowel from other sites, including the skin (melanoma), lung, breast, colon, and kidney. Such secondary tumors are as common as primary small bowel tumors. Metastatic tumors to the small bowel may appear as solitary tumors, or multiple luminal or subserosal tumors. Immunohistochemical markers help confirm the diagnosis.

FIGURE 11.119. Image (A) shows a breast lobular carcinoma that metastasized to the small bowel; multiple luminal masses are present. In (B), a sarcoma that metastasized to the small bowel shows multiple dark red masses with necrosis protruding into the lumen.

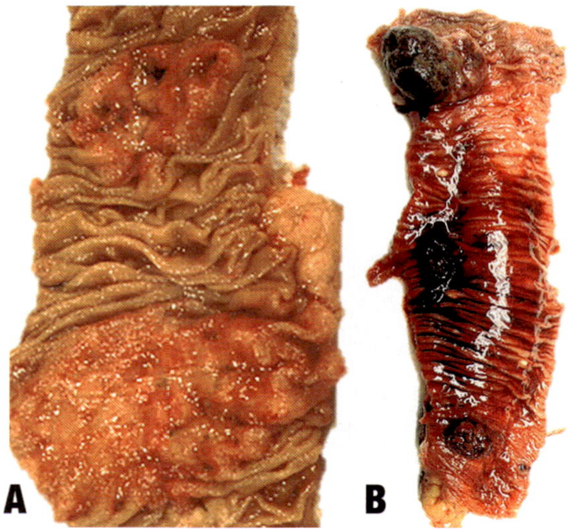

A B

FIGURE 11.120. Image (A) shows metastatic melanoma as a large luminal mass. In (B), metastatic melanoma presents as subserosal tumors.

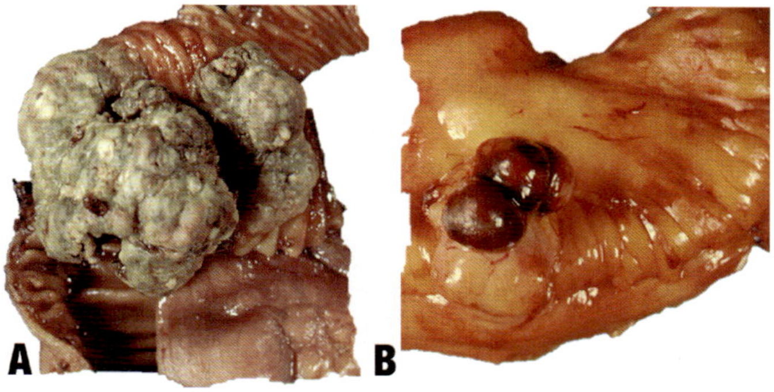

FIGURE 11.121. This cross-section of metastatic melanoma shows an ulcerated, variably pigmented tumor with transmural involvement from the mucosa (right), through the bowel wall, and into the mesentery (left).

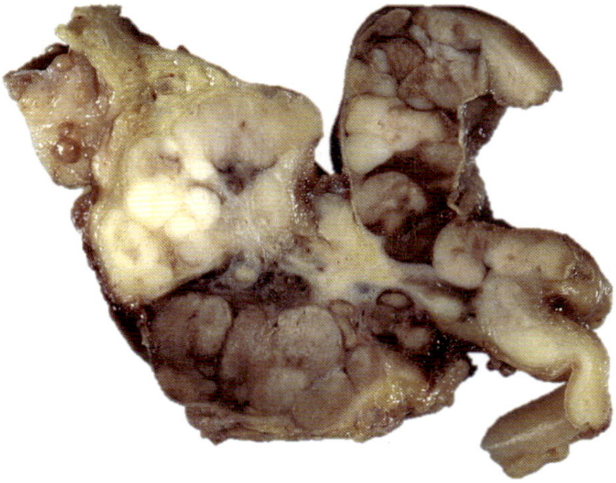

FIGURE 11.122. This small bowel segmental resection specimen shows a vascular polypoid lesion. Histological and immunohistochemical evaluations, and the patient's clinical history of renal cell carcinoma (RCC), confirmed the diagnosis of metastatic RCC.

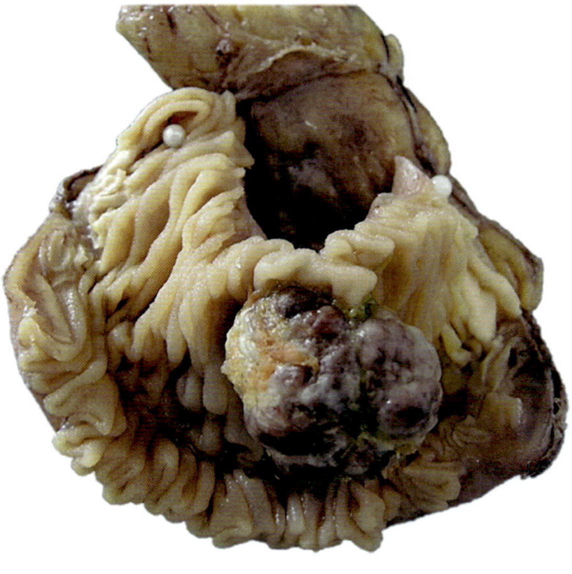

FIGURE 11.123. These images show autopsy-acquired specimens of metastatic undifferentiated carcinoma to the (A) small intestine and (B) para-aortic lymph nodes.

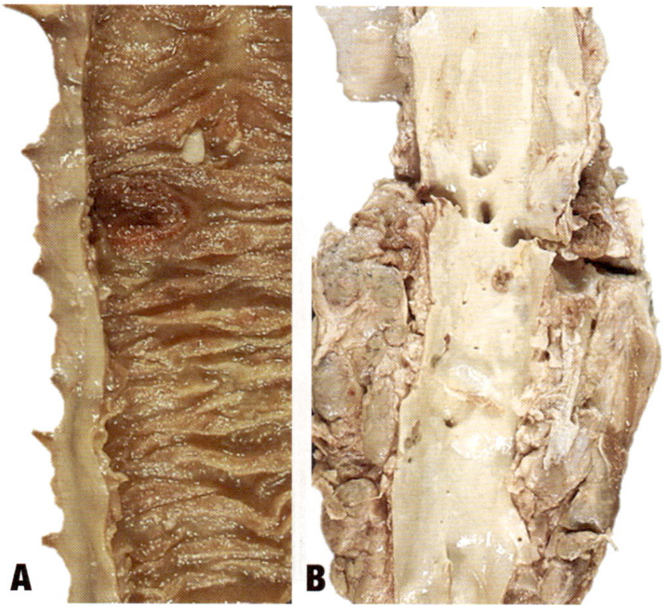

PRIMARY MULLERIAN-TYPE ADENOCARCINOMA OF THE PERITONEUM

This entity is also known as peritoneal papillary serous carcinoma, peritoneal mesothelioma, primary peritoneal carcinoma, and diffuse carcinomatosis. Carcinoma of the peritoneum resembling papillary serous carcinoma of the ovary is considered to originate from the Mullerian system, and is staged with the ovarian and tubal cancer guidelines.

FIGURE 11.124. An autopsy-acquired organ block shows peritoneal cancer with diffuse micronodular spread on the surface.

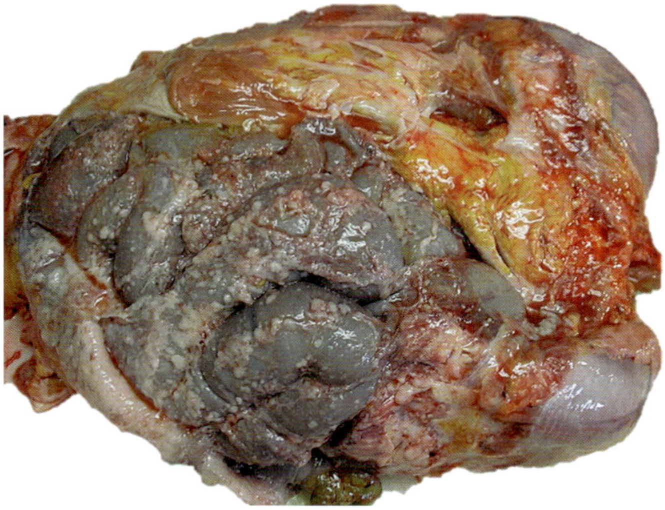

Colon, Rectum, and Anus

REFERENCE: NORMAL COLON (LARGE BOWEL)

Situated between the terminal ileum and rectum, the colon's main function is to extract water and salt from solid waste prior to elimination from the body. The normal adult colon measures approximately 1.5 meters and is divided into 4 anatomical parts: the ascending, transverse, descending, and sigmoid colon. The rectum stores the feces temporarily and the anus is the last part of the gastrointestinal tract.

FIGURE 11.125. The colon or large bowel has a larger diameter than the small bowel. In (A), the external surface of a large bowel shows abundant adipose tissue posteriorly. In (B), the luminal mucosal surface of a large bowel shows circular folds (plicae).

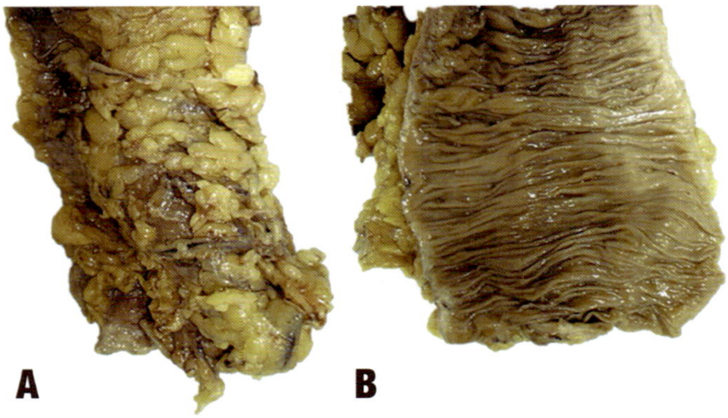

Nonneoplastic Diseases of the Colon and Rectum

Colonic duplication

This congenital anomaly is rare. Patients may remain asymptomatic or may present with obstruction, bleeding, or constipation.

FIGURE 11.126. The probe in this image identifies the lumen of the duplicated bowel.

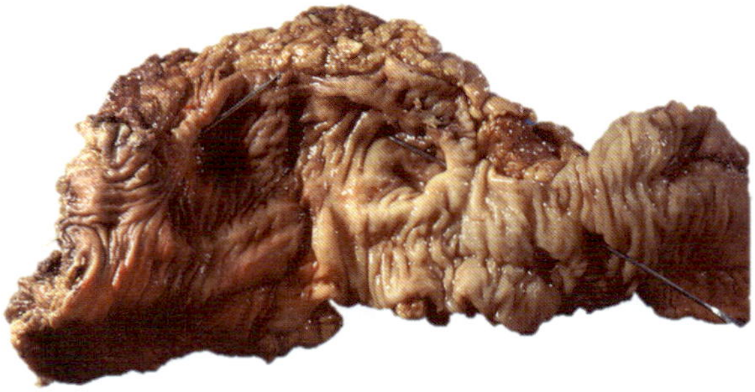

FIGURE 11.127. This brown discoloration of the colon contrasts with the pale mucosal polyps (adenomas), which are not affected by this process.

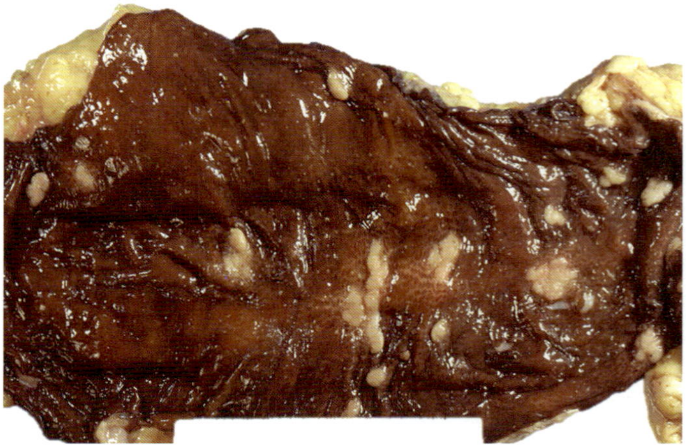

Melanosis coli (MC)

MC is characterized by brown discoloration of the colon secondary to long-standing ingestion of laxatives (usually containing senna). Histology shows an accumulation of pigment-laden macrophages in the colonic mucosa. Interestingly, polyps are more easily identified within MC, because they generally do not accumulate the lipofuscin pigment. MC has no known association with cancer and its clinical significance is unclear.

FIGURE 11.128. The dark brown discoloration of the colon may be confused with ischemic injury. Note that most of the mucosal polyps (adenomas) are not affected by the process.

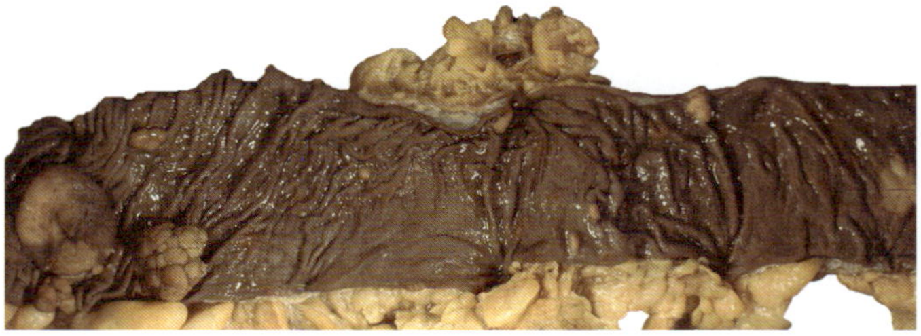

Ischemic colitis

Ischemia may lead to hemorrhage, duskiness, and dark brown discoloration of the colon. Ischemic colitis is potentially life-threatening and must be distinguished from MC. The splenic flexure, or "watershed" area, is at the junction of the superior and inferior mesenteric artery blood supplies, and is the area in the colon most commonly affected by ischemia. Colonic dilatation and purulent exudate (also known as pseudomembranes) may be present in ischemic colitis. Transmural ischemic necrosis may lead to thinning of the colonic wall and even perforation.

FIGURE 11.129. This image shows mucosal dark discoloration and erosions due to ischemia.

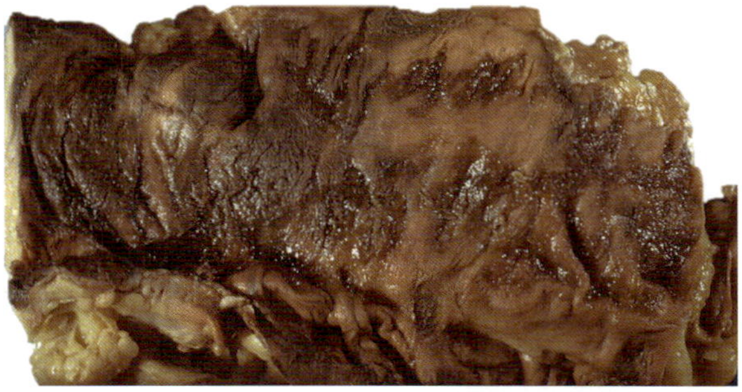

FIGURE 11.130. The overlying pseudomembranes in this example of ischemic colitis may be difficult to differentiate from those seen in *Clostridium difficile* pseudomembranous colitis on gross examination.

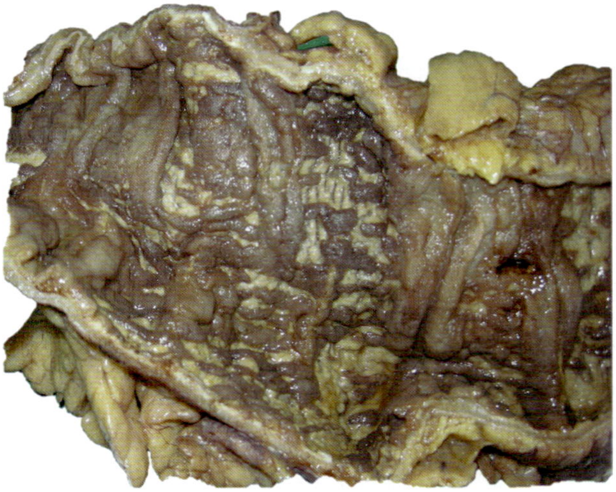

Clostridium difficile pseudomembranous colitis

Clostridium difficile pseudomembranous colitis typically occurs after antibiotic use. *C. difficile* overgrows other intestinal flora and produces toxins that cause acute colitis with adherent overlying necroinflammatory exudates (pseudomembranes). Severe cases may lead to toxic megacolon.

FIGURE 11.131. This example of *C. difficile* pseudomembranous colitis shows characteristic multiple spots of yellow-white material (pseudomembranes) attached to the mucosal surface.

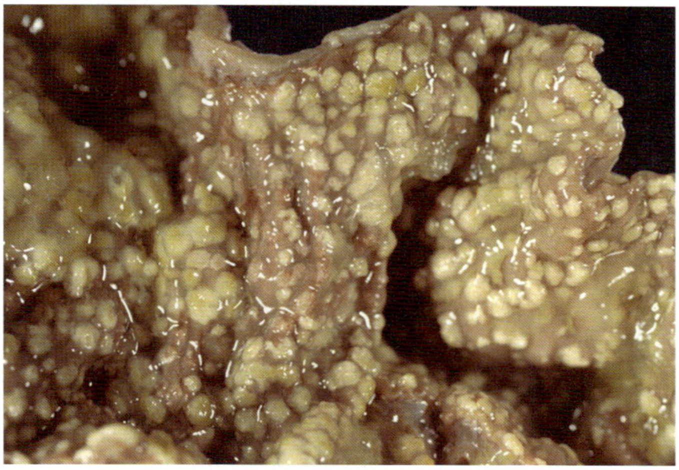

FIGURE 11.132. This is an example of a fulminant case that required resection. Note the involvement of the entire colon, even with extension into the distal terminal ileum.

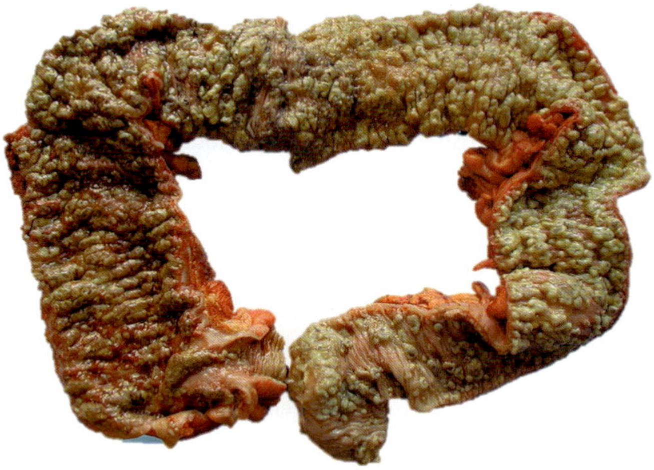

Tapeworm (Cestoda)

There are several types of tapeworm that can infect humans, including fish (broad) tapeworm (*Diphyllobothrium latum*), beef tapeworm (*Taenia saginata*), and pork tapeworm (*Taenia solium*). Infection occurs by eating undercooked, infected fish, beef, or pork. Tapeworms may cause chronic malnutrition, anemia, weight loss, restlessness, and sleep disturbance. Adult worms may be more than 20 meters long.

FIGURE 11.133. This is a tapeworm recovered from the stool of an infected patient.

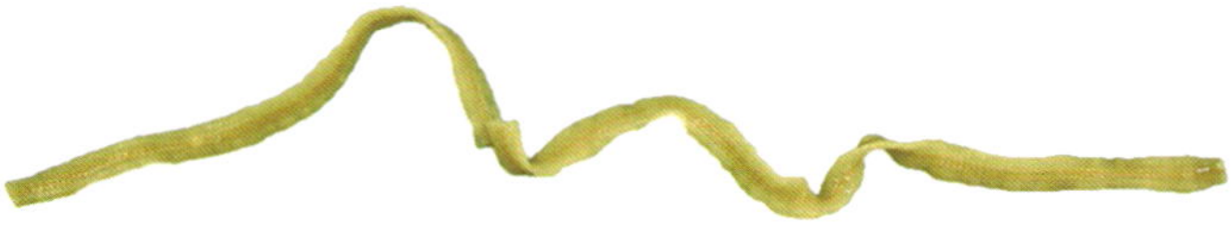

Graft versus host disease (GVHD)

GVHD occurs after hematopoietic stem cell (bone marrow) transplantation when the donor is genetically different from the recipient patient. The donor's immune cells recognize the recipient's cells as foreign and attack the new host, causing damage. GVHD may involve organs such as the skin, lung, liver, and gastrointestinal tract. Severe GVHD leads to mucosal necrosis.

FIGURE 11.134. This is a case of severe GVHD with mucosal necrosis.

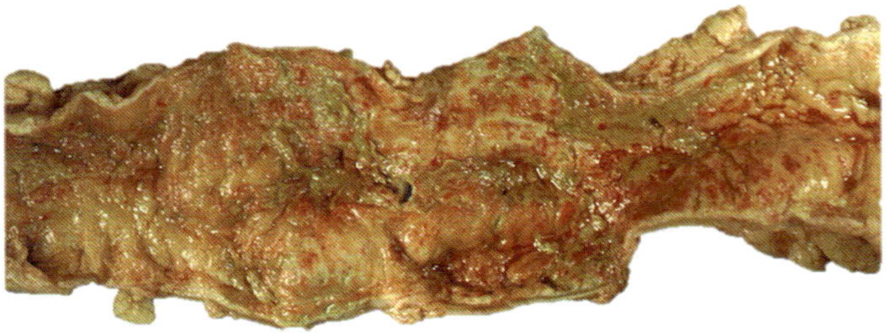

Angiodysplasia

This entity is characterized by tortuously dilated blood vessels in the colonic mucosa or submucosa, best diagnosed by angiography. The most commonly affected site is the cecum and proximal ascending colon. It is the second most common cause of lower GI bleeding, after diverticular disease.

FIGURE 11.135. Images (A) and (B) show cases of a right hemicolectomy with hemorrhage in the cecum and ascending colon. The bulging dilated blood vessels of angiodysplasia may not be easily identified in specimens, because the vessels may collapse after surgical resection. It requires careful examination to identify angiodysplasia.

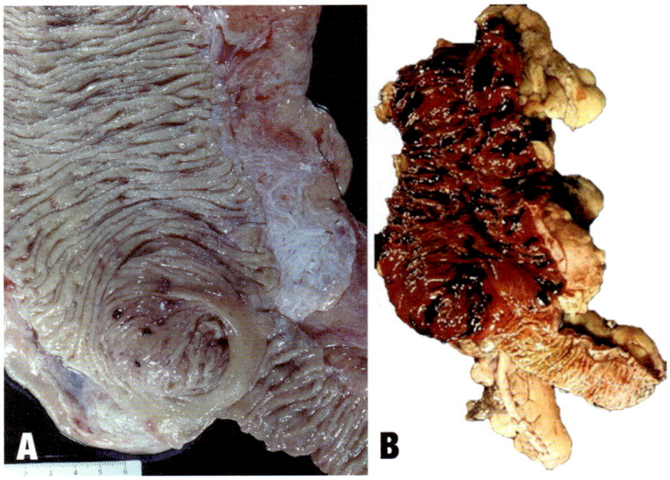

Amyloidosis of the colon

Amyloid protein is characterized by amorphous, waxy, pink material on hematoxylin and eosin stain (H&E stain). Systemic amyloidosis is usually of the following types: AL amyloidosis (light chains associated with myeloma); AA amyloidosis (acute phase proteins secondary to chronic inflammation or familial Mediterranean fever); or β_2-microglobulin amyloidosis (chronic dialysis). In the colon, amyloid deposition in vessel walls compromise vessel contraction and can cause bleeding.

FIGURE 11.136. This image shows patchy mucosal hemorrhage from extensive amyloidosis, which involves small- to medium-sized vessels throughout the bowel.

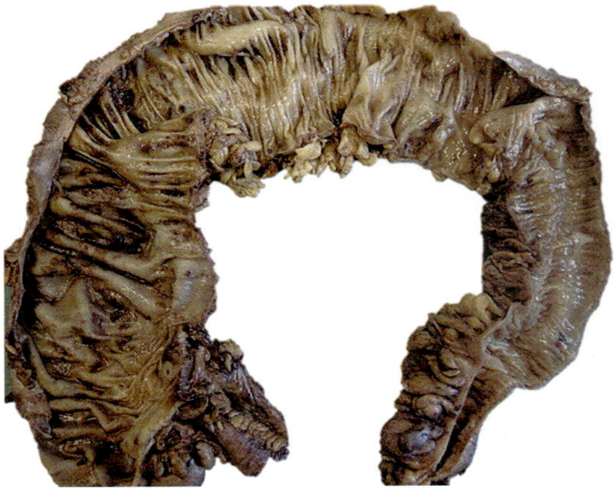

Pneumatosis coli

Pneumatosis coli is characterized by intramural gas that accumulates in the colon. It is thought to be due to mucosal necrosis and bacterial fermentation, or to dissection of pulmonary gas from a pulmonary bulla. It may be fulminant in children. In adults, it may be idiopathic or associated with ischemic colitis, obstruction, infection, chronic lung disease, and other entities.

FIGURE 11.137. This image shows round, smooth, empty air spaces in the bowel wall and submucosa.

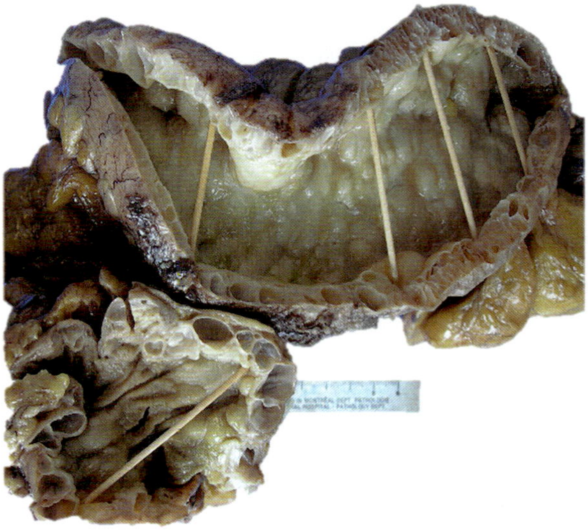

FIGURE 11.138. Image (A) shows air-filled cystic structures in the subserosa. Image (B) shows air-filled cystic structures in the submucosa.

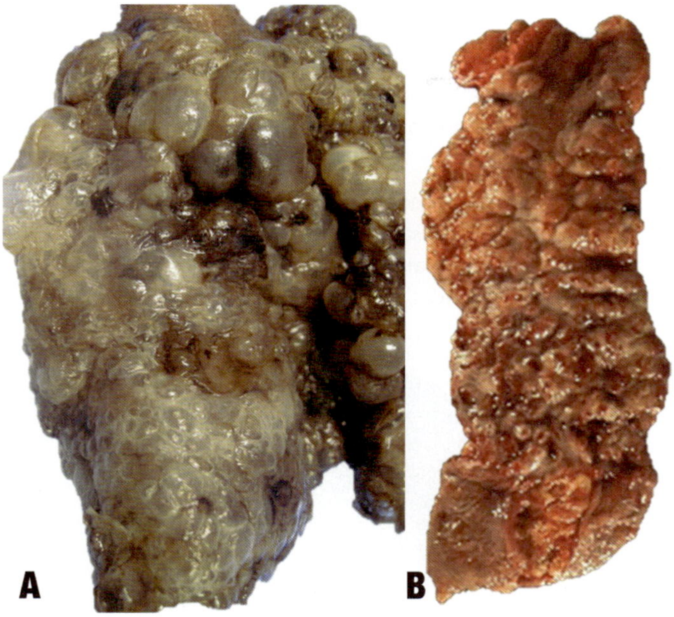

Megacolon

By definition, megacolon is the abnormal dilatation of the large intestine. It may be congenital or acquired.

FIGURE 11.139. This massively dilated colorectum is an autopsy specimen from a diabetic patient. No physical cause of obstruction was identified. The megacolon was determined to be secondary to autoimmune neuropathy due to underlying diabetes mellitus in this patient.

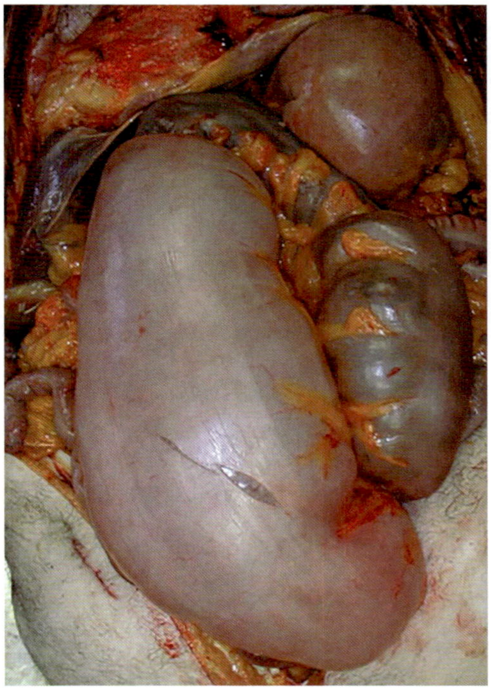

Inflammatory Bowel Disease (IBD)

IBD refers to a group of inflammatory diseases that affect the GI tract. Common symptoms in IBD include abdominal pain, diarrhea, weight loss, rectal bleeding, and anemia. IBD includes 2 main conditions: ulcerative colitis and Crohn disease. Ulcerative colitis mostly affects the colon and rectum. Crohn disease may affect any part of the GI tract, from mouth to anus.

Crohn disease

FIGURE 11.140. This case of Crohn colitis shows characteristic "bear claw" ulceration. These are deep longitudinal ulcers along the length of the colon.

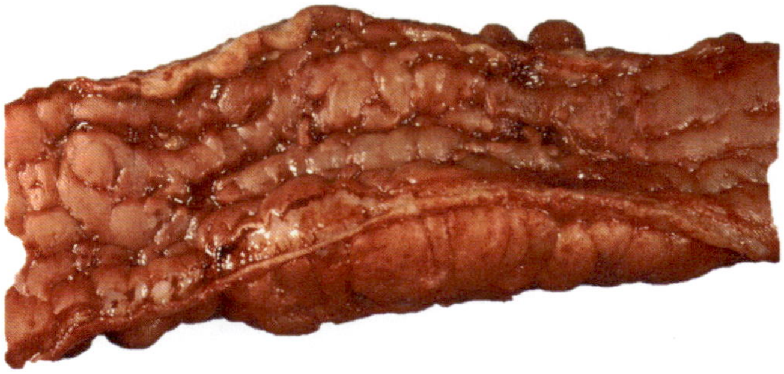

FIGURE 11.141. This resected large bowel shows a "cobblestone" mucosal surface. This appearance is due to intersecting circumferential and longitudinal mucosal ulcers.

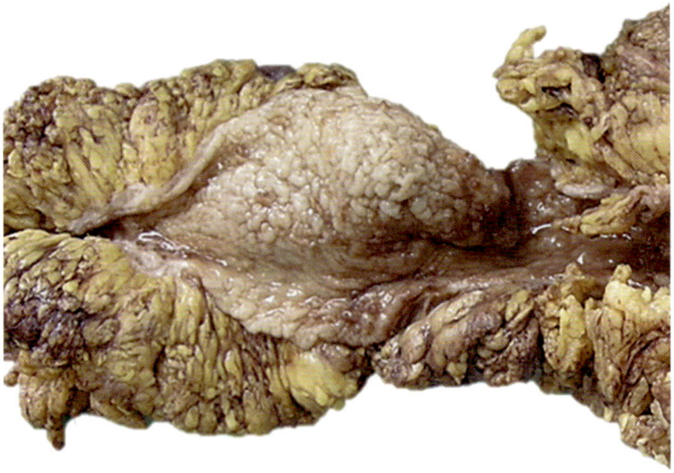

Ulcerative colitis (UC)

FIGURE 11.142. Image (A) shows typical disease distribution from distal to proximal. Image (B) shows the mucosal aspect of chronic active UC.

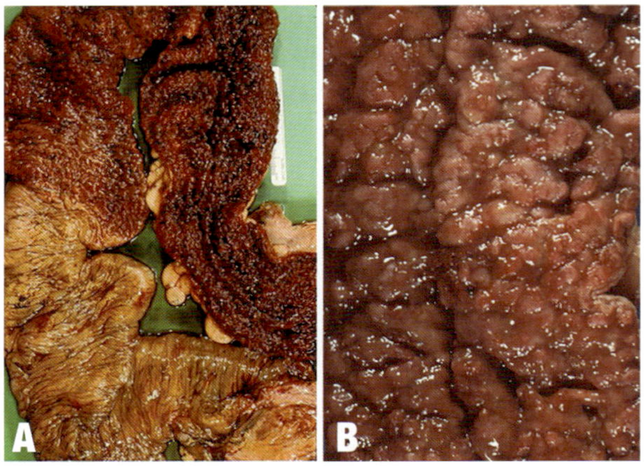

FIGURE 11.143. This resected large bowel segment shows inflamed mucosal islands mixed with flatter areas of mucosal loss corresponding to ulcerated mucosa.

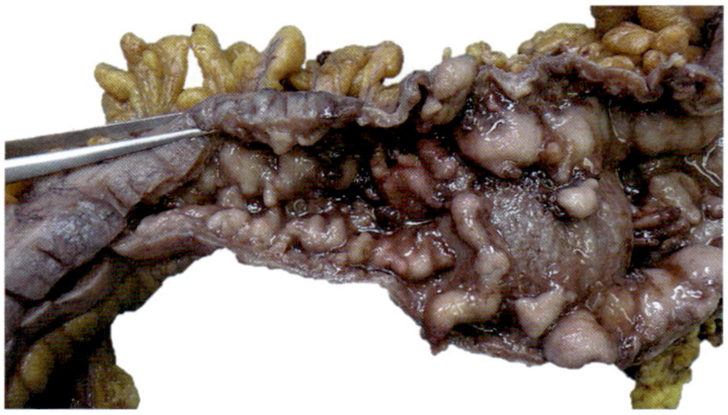

FULMINANT UC

Fulminant UC is a severe acute flare of the disease associated with specific clinical criteria: more than 10 stools per day, abdominal pain, distension, bleeding, and fever, among others. Patients may progress to toxic megacolon (massive colonic dilatation), perforation, and shock.

FIGURE 11.144. This image shows fulminant colitis with ulcers, friable granular mucosa, and extensive inflammatory pseudopolyp formation.

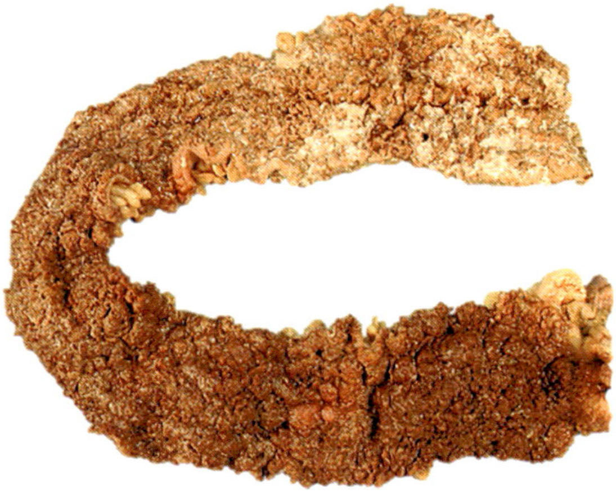

Inflammatory pseudopolyp in chronic IBD

Inflammatory pseudopolyps are formed by protrusion of regenerating mucosal epithelium and granulation tissue after repeated ulceration. Histology can help to distinguish inflammatory pseudopolyps from polyps that show dysplasia. Patients with UC or Crohn disease may develop mucosal dysplasia and cancer; regular surveillance biopsies are necessary.

FIGURE 11.145. This image shows the right colon, cecum, and ileocecal valve. The mucosa is erythematous and granular, with numerous small inflammatory pseudopolyps. The ileocecal valve is spared in this case of UC.

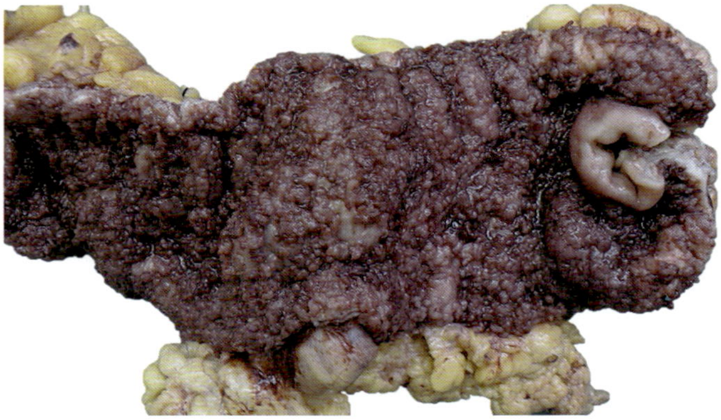

FIGURE 11.146. Numerous inflammatory pseudopolyps are seen in (A), a case of actively inflamed IBD. Image (B) shows a case of quiescent disease.

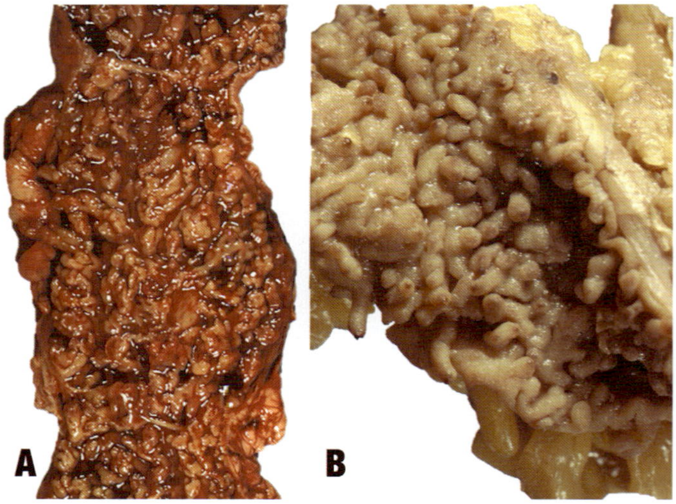

FIGURE 11.147. This resected large bowel segment shows numerous variably sized polyps and finger-like projections intermingled with areas of flat mucosa. It is difficult to distinguish inflammatory pseudopolyps from polyps that show dysplasia.

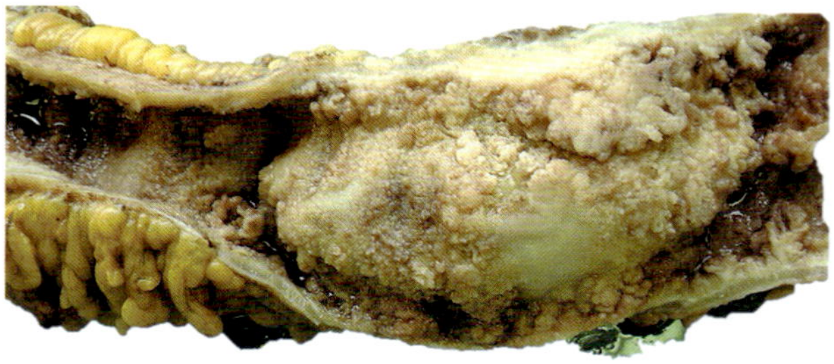

Polypoid dysplasia and cancer arising in chronic IBD

Patients with UC and Crohn disease may develop mucosal dysplasia and cancer. For this reason, regular surveillance biopsies are recommended for early detection. Dysplasia in IBD may be visible or invisible, polypoid or nonpolypoid; it may also be endoscopically resectable or unresectable. Histological evaluation is required to differentiate low-grade dysplasia, high-grade dysplasia, and adenocarcinoma. The diagnosis of dysplasia in IBD should be confirmed by a second pathologist with expertise in IBD.

FIGURE 11.148. This image shows an area of polypoid dysplasia. Note the background cobblestone-like edematous mucosa and the thick colonic wall.

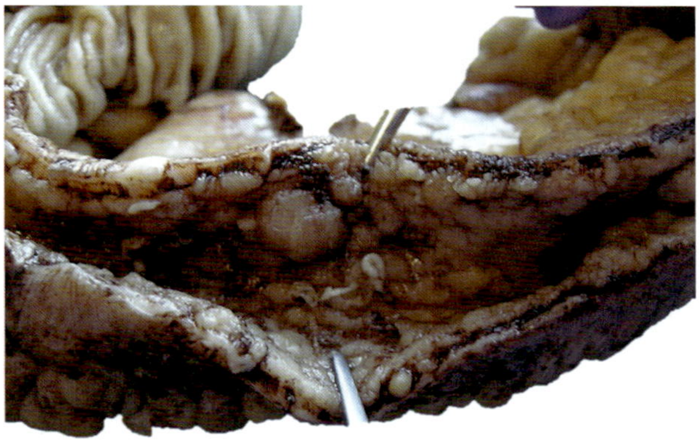

Diverticular Diseases of the Colon

Colonic diverticulosis

Unlike true congenital diverticula, acquired "false" colonic diverticula lack muscularis propria, or have only an attenuated muscle lining. Colonic diverticulosis is usually due to focal weakness in the bowel wall and increased intraluminal pressure.

FIGURE 11.149. This resected large bowel segment shows multiple sac-like diverticula, which are outpouchings from the gut lumen.

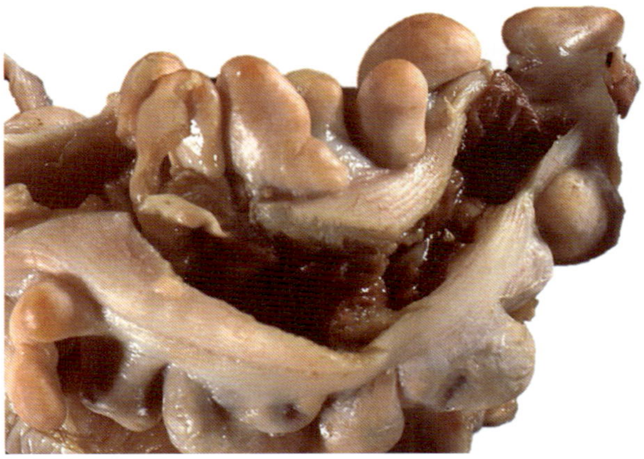

Colonic diverticulitis with perforation

Diverticula may become acutely inflamed (diverticulitis), and may perforate due to obstruction and high pressure. Acute diverticulitis with perforation may lead to abscesses, sepsis, fistulas, and suppurative peritonitis. Colonic perforation is a surgical emergency.

FIGURE 11.150. In (A), a resected large bowel segment shows the bowel lumen with a diverticulum indicated by a probe. The peritoneal aspect in (B) shows the perforation site.

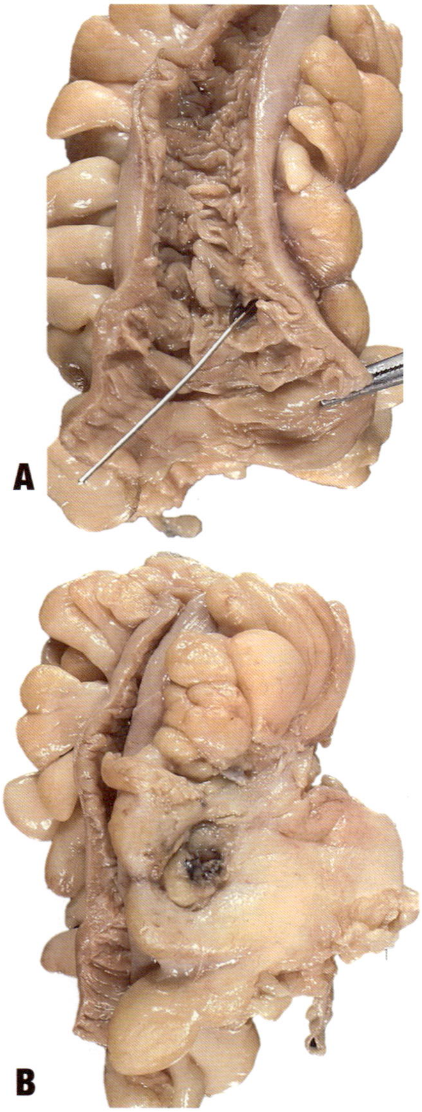

FIGURE 11.151. This resected large bowel segment shows sac-like diverticula with focal rupture and fibrinopurulent exudate.

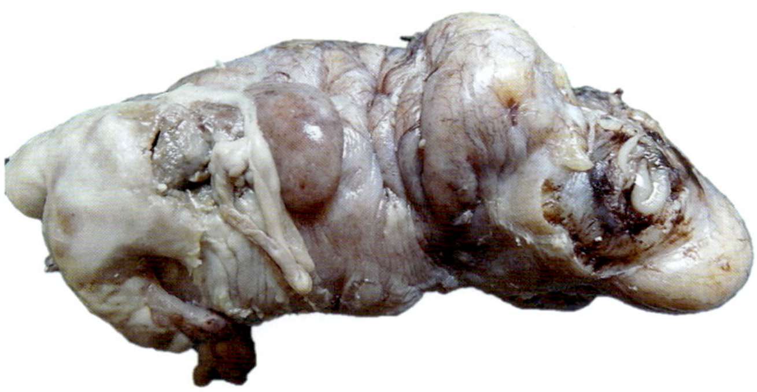

Prolapse, Intussusception, and Hernias

Mucosal prolapse of the rectum

This entity is associated with straining during defecation, and is defined as the protrusion of rectal mucosa (not the entire rectal wall) through the anus. The clinical presentation includes pain, and mucus or blood from the rectum on defecation.

FIGURE 11.152. In these images, note the erythematous polypoid distal end (bottom) of the specimens.

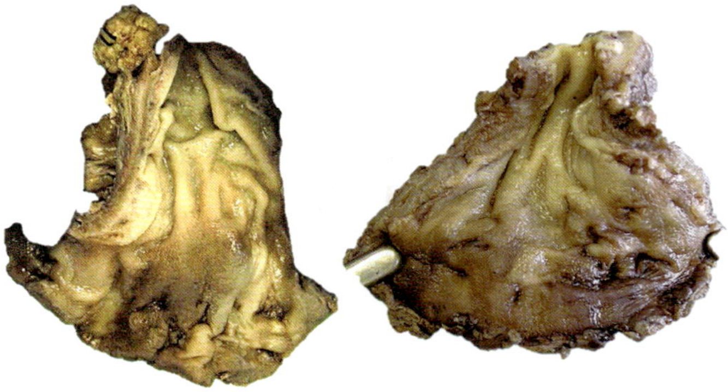

Intussusception of the rectum

Intussusception is the telescoping of a proximal bowel segment into the adjacent bowel lumen. It is a full-thickness prolapse.

FIGURE 11.153. This resected rectum shows bowel-in-bowel and inside-out mucosa with ulceration.

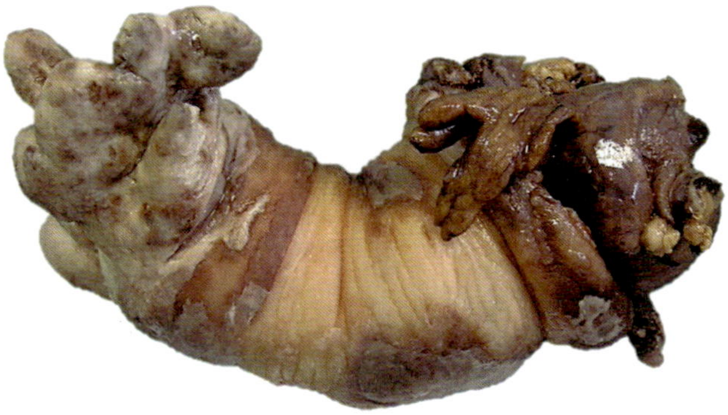

Prolapsed/intussuscepted colostomy

Colostomies are surgically created openings in the abdominal wall used to bypass a damaged part of the colon or rectum.

FIGURE 11.154. This colostomy stoma prolapsed out of the abdominal wall.

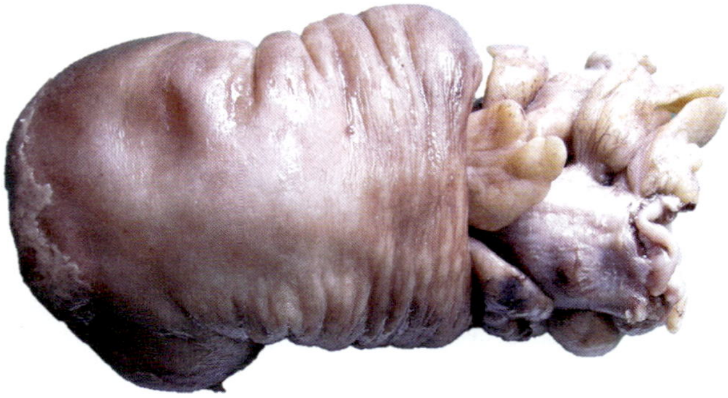

Intussusception of a lipoma

It is important to examine the lead point of any intussusception, especially in adults, because a neoplasm may have initiated the full-thickness prolapse.

FIGURE 11.155. This lipoma was the lead point of the intussusception that caused intestinal obstruction.

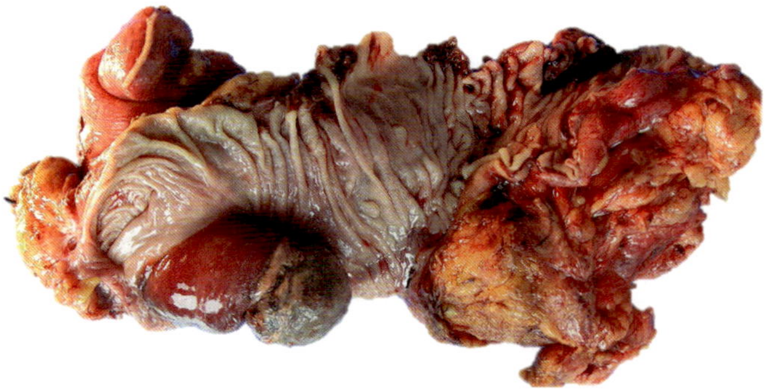

Umbilical hernia, incarcerated and strangulated

Hernias are a form of bowel protrusion. The bowel may become trapped (incarcerated), sometimes leading to bowel obstruction. It may lose blood supply, leading to ischemia (strangulation). Types of hernias include inguinal, femoral, umbilical, and incisional, among others.

FIGURE 11.156. This resected umbilical hernia shows hernia-sac contents (black necrotic tissue) protruding through the umbilicus surrounded by a rim of resected skin.

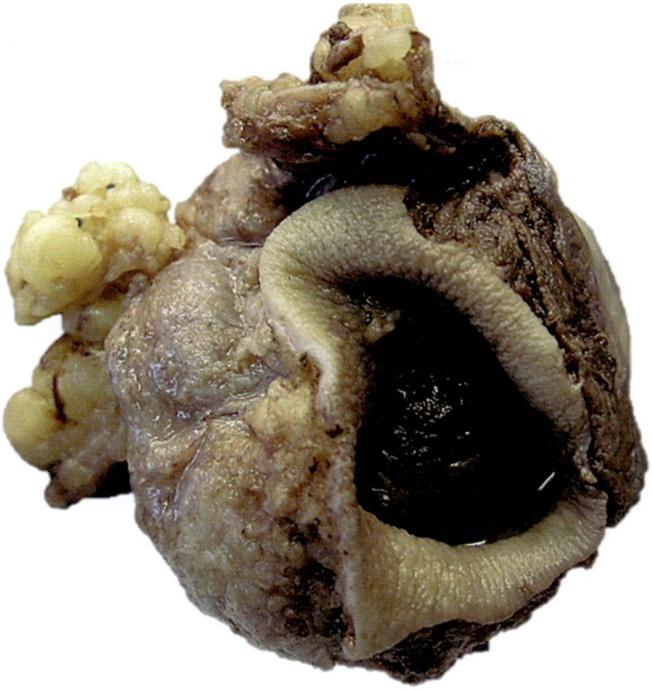

Richter hernia of sigmoid colon, incarcerated and strangulated

Richter hernia is the protrusion and/or strangulation of only part of the circumference of the intestine's antimesenteric border through a rigid small defect of the abdominal wall.

FIGURE 11.157. This resected large bowel segment shows a rough and focally necrotic surface on the side of the antimesenteric wall due to a Richter hernia that was incarcerated and strangulated.

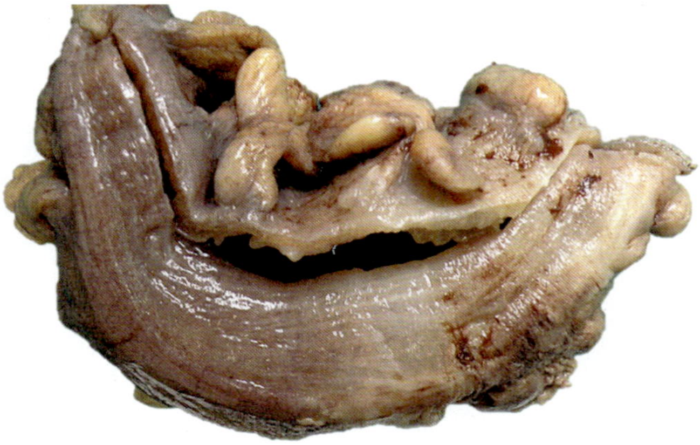

Colorectal Polyps

Peutz–Jeghers syndrome (PJS)

PJS is an autosomal dominant disorder associated with *STK11* gene mutation. Clinically, patients present with intestinal hamartomatous polyps and mucocutaneous pigmentation. On histology, Peutz–Jeghers polyps demonstrate normal-looking glandular epithelial cells interspaced by lamina propria and arborizing smooth muscle. Patients with PJS are at risk for gastrointestinal tract cancer, and cancers of the pancreas, bile duct, breast, ovaries, uterus, cervix, testicles, and lungs.

FIGURE 11.158. This image shows a lobulated polyp with a rigid contour and smooth surface.

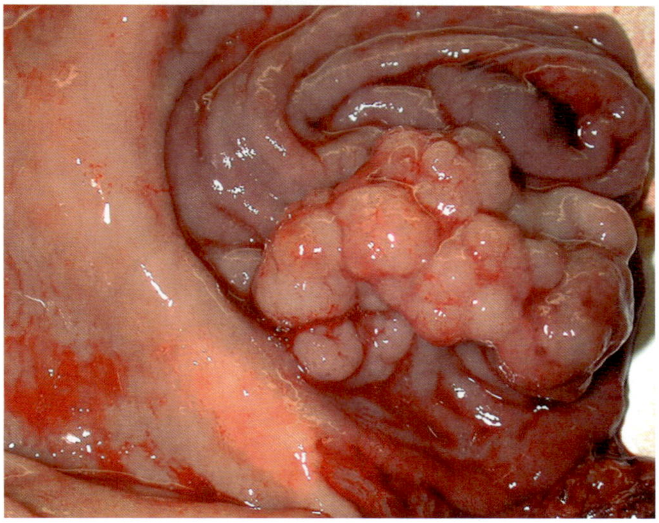

FIGURE 11.159. In this example of multiple Peutz–Jeghers polyps, note the well-circumscribed pedunculated polyps. Large Peutz–Jeghers polyps increase the risk of intussusception.

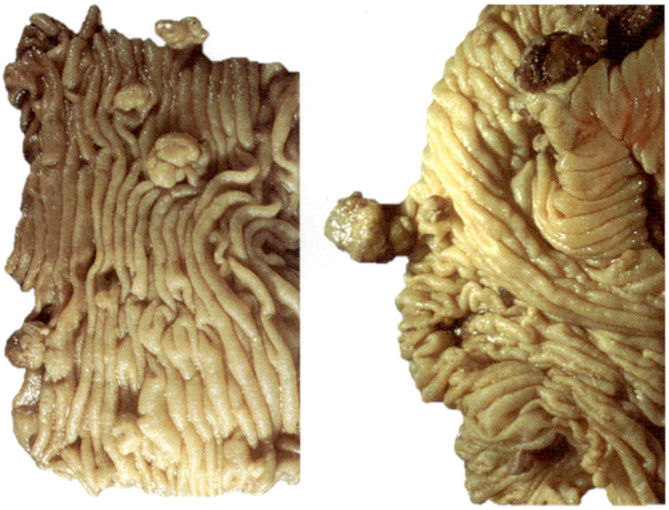

Juvenile polyp

Isolated juvenile polyp, also called retention polyp, is the most common pediatric intestinal polyp and is often found in the rectum. When multiple (more than 5) polyps are present, they are classified as juvenile polyposis, a rare autosomal dominant hamartomatous polyposis associated with germ-line mutations in *SMAD4* or *BMPR1A* genes. This condition confers increased risk of gastrointestinal cancers.

FIGURE 11.160. This image of a juvenile polyp shows a characteristic smooth, edematous, round contour, and the presence of mucin-containing cysts.

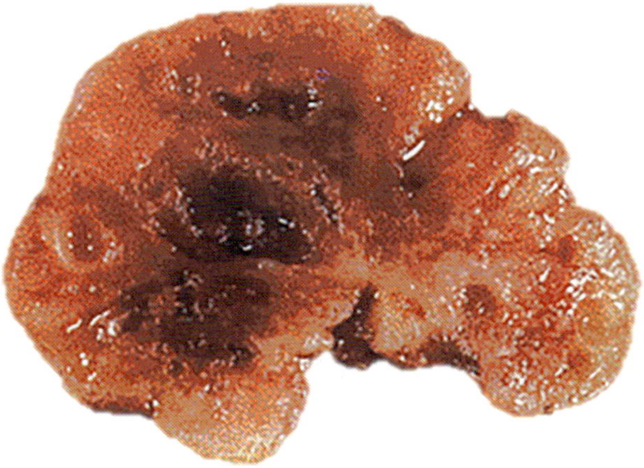

Hyperplastic polyp in the rectum

Hyperplastic polyps are the most common type of benign colorectal polyp in adults. They usually occur in the distal colon and rectum, are typically small (< 0.5 cm), and may be multiple. On histology, they demonstrate serration of gland epithelium, which in cross-section forms a star-shaped, glandular lumen.

FIGURE 11.162. This image shows multiple small sessile polyps with smooth surfaces. The color of the polyps is the same as the background mucosa.

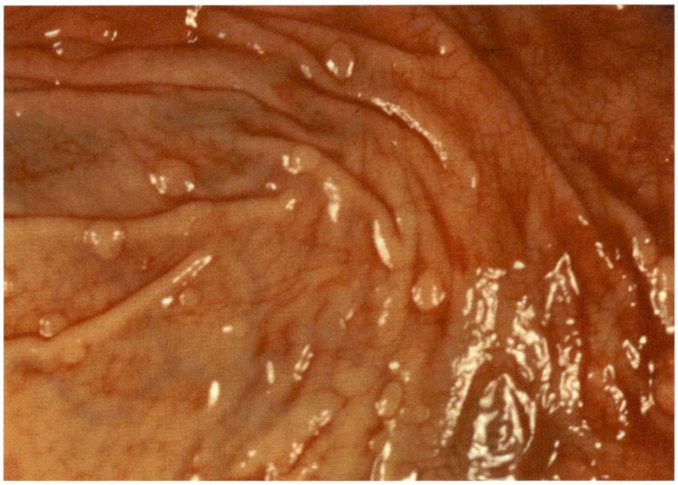

Cowden syndrome

Cowden syndrome is a rare autosomal dominant disorder associated with *PTEN* germ-line mutation. Clinically, patients typically present with oral mucosal fibromas, trichilemmomas, and acral keratosis. They have an increased risk for cancer (mainly breast, thyroid, and endometrial). Patients with Cowden syndrome can have inflammatory (juvenile) polyps (most common), expansive lymphoid follicle polyps, ganglioneuromatous polyps, and intramucosal lipomas.

FIGURE 11.161. This image shows multiple intramucosal lipomas in a patient with Cowden syndrome.

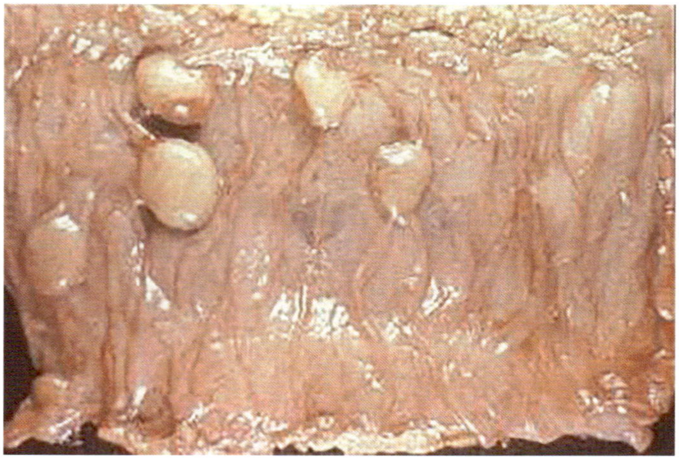

Sessile serrated lesion (SSL)

SSL, also known as sessile serrated adenoma/polyp, refers to a sessile lesion that most commonly occurs in the cecum and ascending colon. On histology, it demonstrates basal crypt dilation and serration, horizontal crypts, and crypt branching. It is a premalignant lesion that may lead to microsatellite unstable adenocarcinomas of the colon.

FIGURE 11.163. This image shows a sessile polyp with a characteristic flat glistening surface. Endoscopically, this area is frequently covered with mucin. This specimen is from a patient who also had a cecal adenocarcinoma.

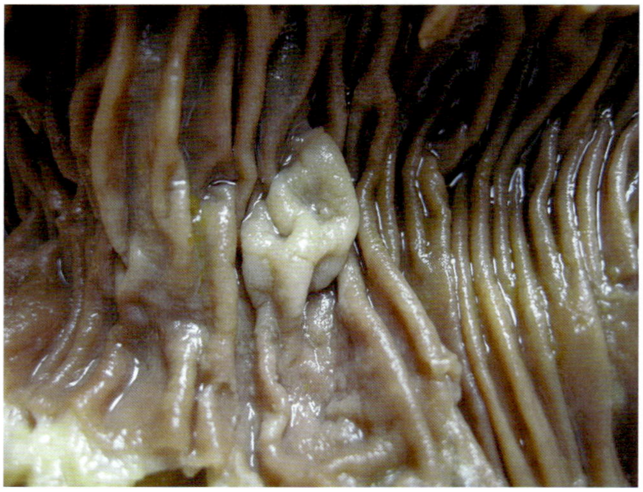

Adenomatous polyp

Adenomas are the second most common type of colorectal polyp after hyperplastic polyps. They are considered premalignant: they may progress to adenocarcinoma. *APC* is the most common gene mutated early in the colorectal adenoma–carcinoma sequence. Adenoma can gain further gene mutations such as K-*ras* and *TP53* to progress to adenocarcinoma. Grossly, these polyps can be pedunculated (with a stalk) or sessile (without a stalk). Histologically, they can be tubular, villous, or tubulovillous. Villous adenomas (more than 75% villous component) are usually sessile. Colorectal adenomas, by definition, have at least low-grade dysplasia. Cancer incidence increases in colorectal adenomas with the presence of high-grade dysplasia, increased number of adenomas (at least 3), size (≥ 1 cm), and villous architecture. Colonoscopy is a way to screen for colorectal cancer and its precursor lesions. Keep in mind, however, that accurate differentiation of a hyperplastic polyp from an SSL or a small tubular adenoma usually requires histology.

FIGURE 11.164. This image shows a large pedunculated tubular adenoma.

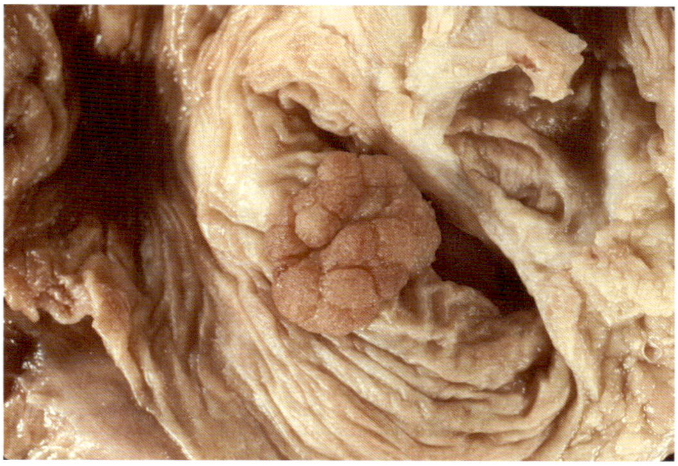

FIGURE 11.165. This image shows a large sessile villous adenoma. There is no invasion into the submucosa or deeper layers.

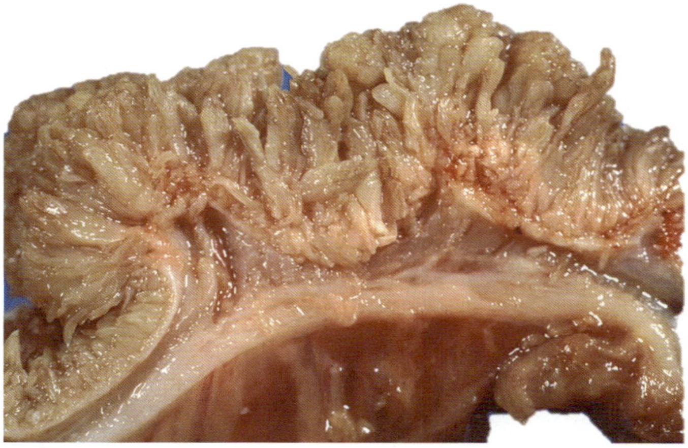

FIGURE 11.166. This right hemicolectomy specimen shows a massive villous adenoma with numerous finger-like villous projections. This endoscopically unresectable adenoma required surgical resection because of its increased risk of developing adenocarcinoma.

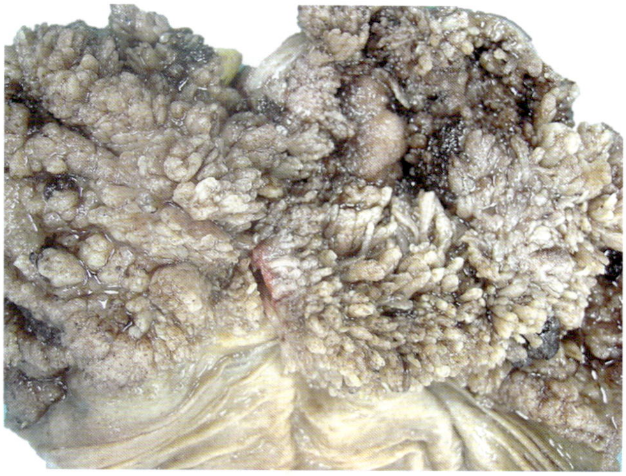

FIGURE 11.167. This right hemicolectomy specimen shows a large, irregularly shaped tubulovillous adenoma. Focal high-grade dysplasia was identified histologically. High-grade dysplasia is diagnosed histologically when there is architectural complexity, loss of cell polarity, and increased cytological atypia. No invasive adenocarcinoma was present.

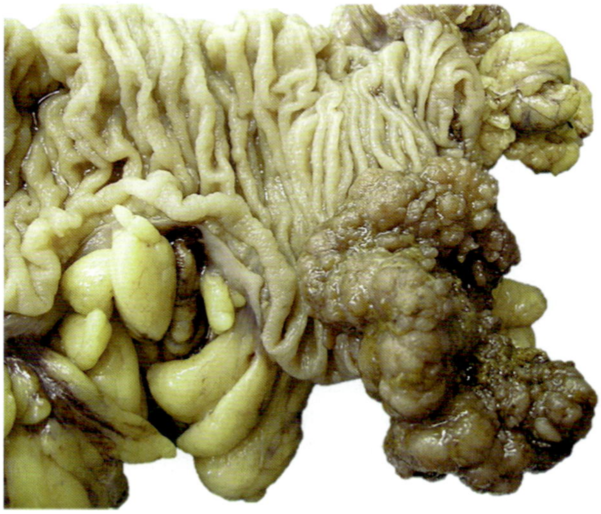

FIGURE 11.168. This resected large bowel segment shows many adenomas of different sizes and shapes. Macroscopically, the larger and more irregular adenomas are at a higher risk of progressing to invasive adenocarcinoma.

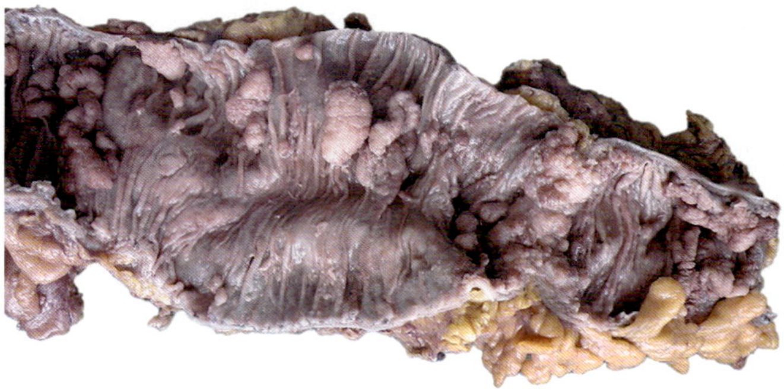

Familial adenomatous polyposis (FAP)

FAP is an autosomal dominant disease that is due to a germ-line mutation in the *APC* gene on chromosome 5q. FAP patients characteristically have numerous adenomas (more than 100) throughout the colorectum and a guaranteed lifetime risk of developing colorectal cancer (CRC); CRC usually occurs before age 40. The attenuated form of FAP has fewer than 100 adenomas, is mainly right-sided, and has an older age of CRC onset. Patients with FAP usually undergo prophylactic colorectal surgery at around age 20 to reduce the risk of CRC.

FIGURE 11.169. Images (A) and (B) are examples of colons of FAP patients with numerous adenomas.

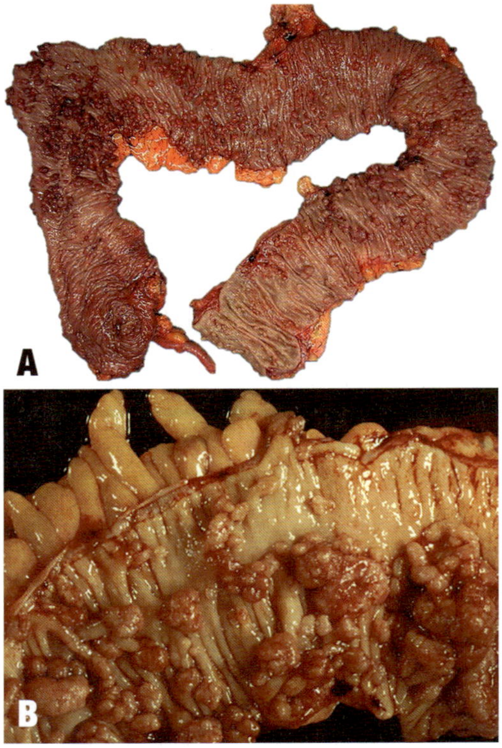

FIGURE 11.170. Invasive cancer may be difficult to identify when the colorectum is packed with polypoid lesions. The cancer in this case was first identified in a lymph node and further sampling revealed a rectal primary tumor.

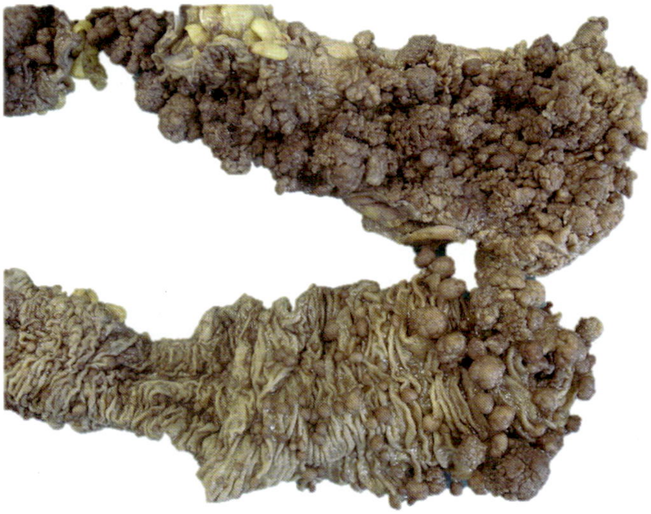

Cancers of the Colon and Rectum

Most cancers in the colon and rectum are adenocarcinomas. Colorectal cancer (CRC) is the third most common newly diagnosed cancer and the third most common cause of cancer death. CRC is associated with numerous risk factors, including dietary and lifestyle factors, adenomas, FAP, Lynch syndrome, and IBD. CRC may be asymptomatic. Symptomatic CRC varies in clinical presentation, depending on the site and growth pattern: right-sided polypoid CRC may present with iron deficiency anemia; left-sided stenosing CRC may present with bowel obstruction or bleeding.

PROCEDURE: COLORECTAL SCREENING VIA COLONOSCOPY

Colonoscopy is a way to screen for colorectal cancer and its precursor lesions. Accurate differentiation of a hyperplastic polyp from an SSL or a small tubular adenoma usually requires histology. Indications for increased surveillance of adenomas include large size (≥ 1 cm), multiple lesions (3 or more), or presence of high-grade dysplasia or a villous component.

FIGURE 11.171. Colonoscopy reveals adenomas warranting surveillance.

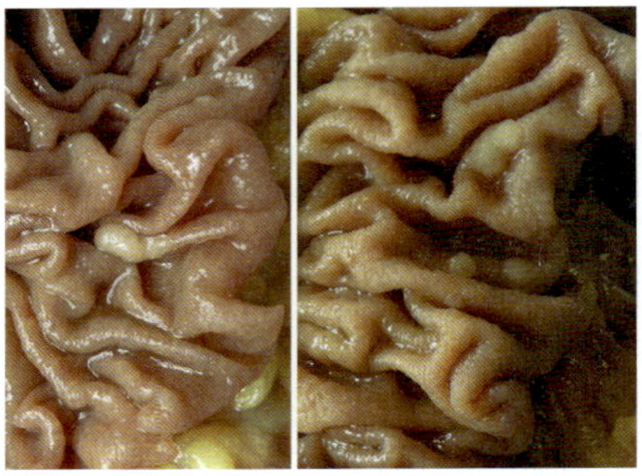

REFERENCE: COLORECTAL CANCER (CRC) GROWTH PATTERNS

CRC has 3 common growth patterns: polypoid luminal protrusions, ulcerated fungating tumors, and annular lesions with circumferential stricture.

FIGURE 11.172. These images illustrate the 3 common growth patterns of CRC: (A) polypoid luminal protrusion; (B) ulcerated fungating tumor with raised edges; and (C) annular, encircling lesions causing circumferential stricture.

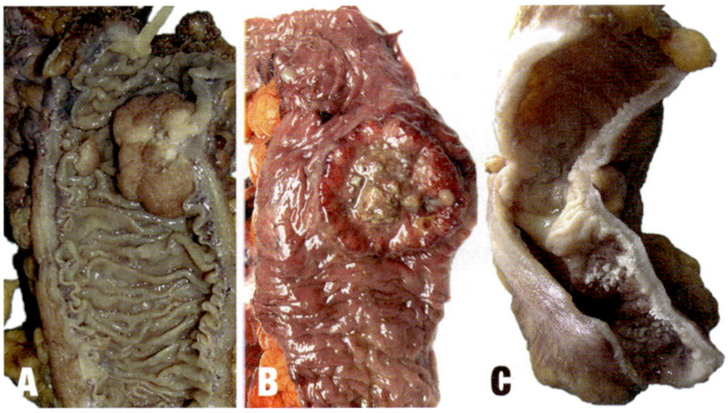

Colorectal adenocarcinoma

FIGURE 11.173. This tumor is centrally ulcerated and involves the entire circumference of the large bowel.

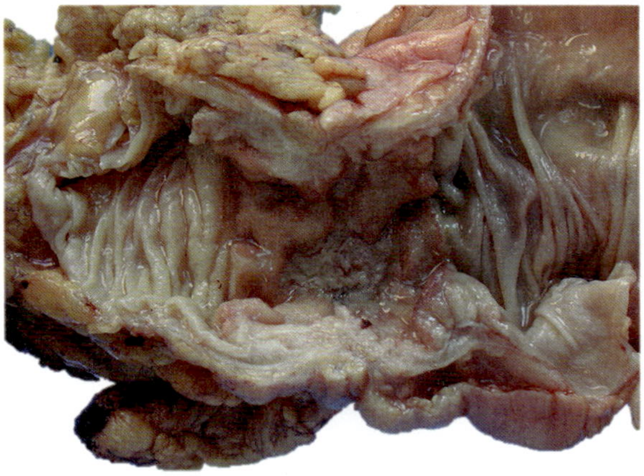

FIGURE 11.174. This sigmoid resection illustrates circumferential involvement of a nodular mass with central necrosis.

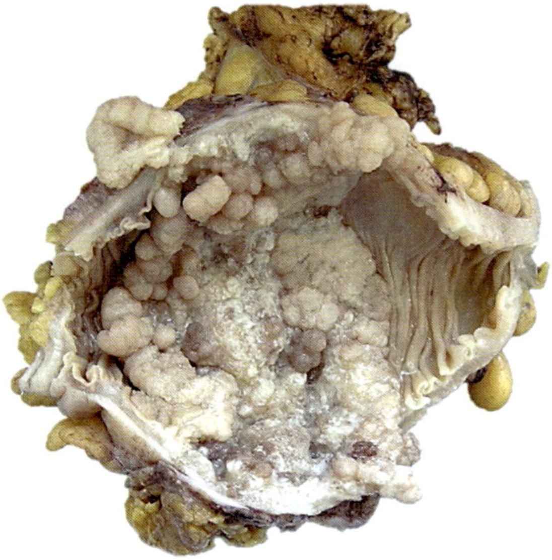

FIGURE 11.175. This resected large bowel segment shows an exophytic mass with irregular border. The tumor is located on the anterior aspect of the sigmoid colon and was cut when opening the lumen to inspect the tumor.

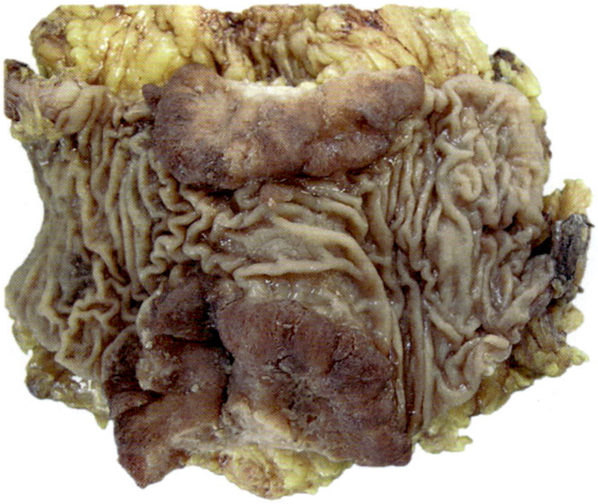

FIGURE 11.176. The cross-section of this CRC shows that the tumor invades through the muscle layer into the pericolic adipose tissue and focally comes very close to the serosal lining. Microscopy was required to determine the exact depth of invasion and its T stage.

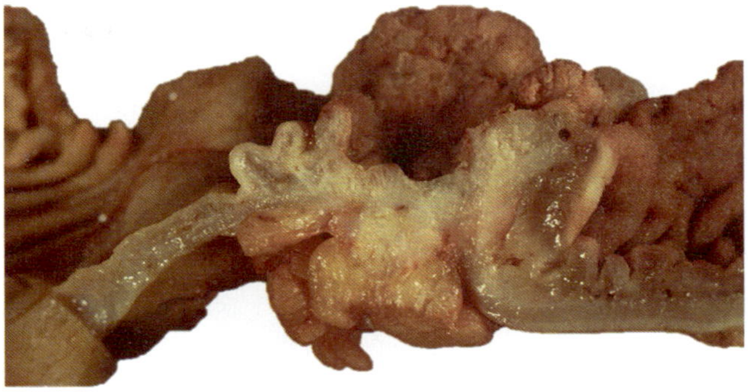

FIGURE 11.177. This right hemicolectomy specimen with the appendix (left background) and the cecum shows a large mass in the center. Some cecal tumors may obstruct the appendiceal orifice.

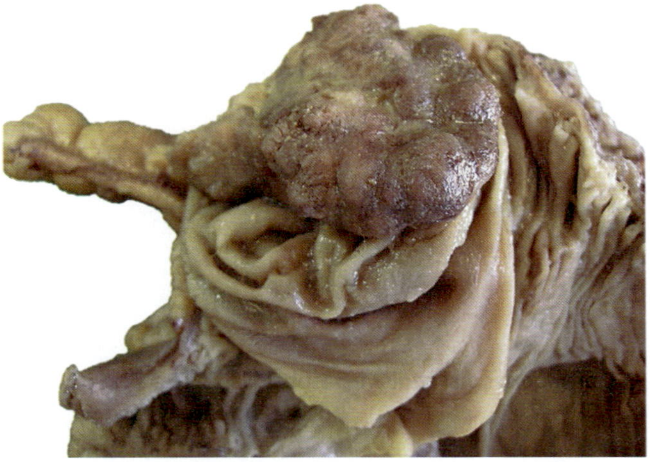

CRC, MUCINOUS TYPE

CRC with more than 50% extracellular mucin is called mucinous CRC.

FIGURE 11.178. This image shows a thick bowel wall diffusely infiltrated by a characteristic white homogenous translucent tumor, best illustrated on the left.

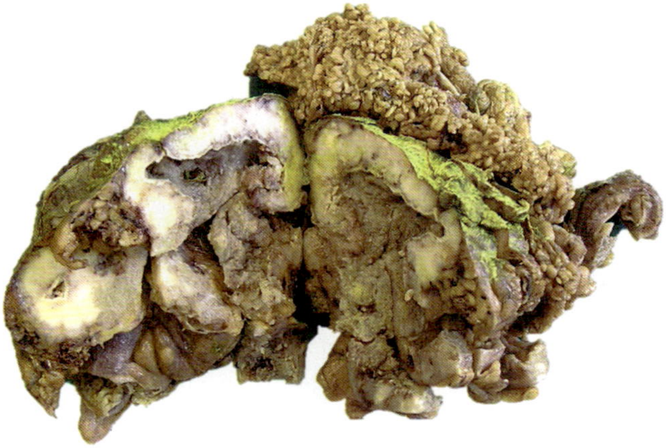

CRC WITH INTUSSUSCEPTION

FIGURE 11.179. The lead point of intussusception, where the intestine invaginates into the adjacent bowel, is sometimes a tumor. In this case, a cecal adenocarcinoma initiated the intussusception.

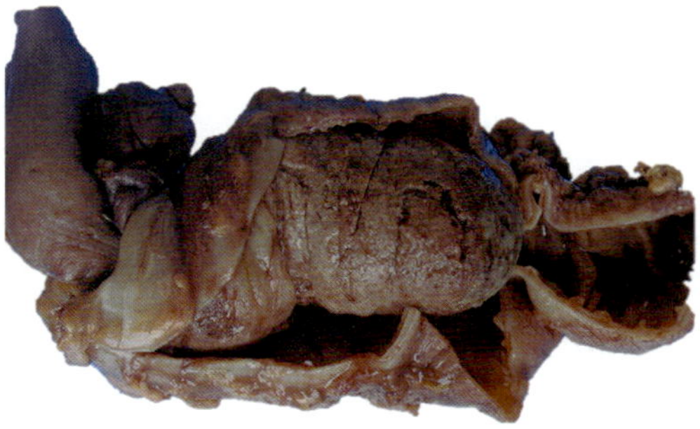

CRC WITH BACKGROUND MELANOSIS COLI

Melanosis coli does not increase the risk for colorectal adenocarcinoma, but it makes tumors and polyps easier to identify because their pallor contrasts with the background dark colon.

FIGURE 11.180. The dark pigmentation of the colon is due to laxative abuse in this case. Note the contrasting, pale color of the tumor.

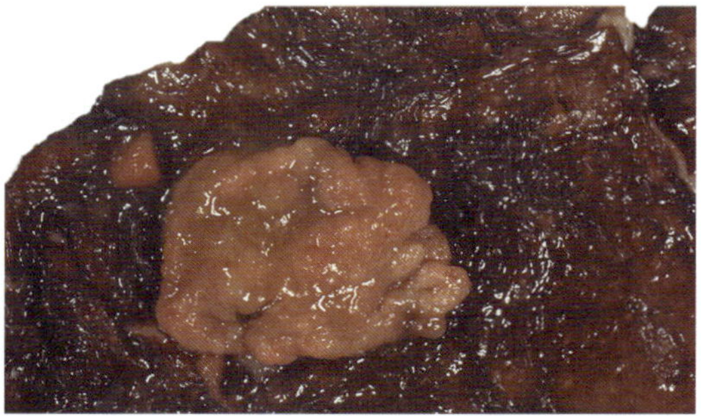

CRC WITH INFLAMMATORY BOWEL DISEASE

FIGURE 11.181. This resected colon shows multiple large polypoid lesions with dysplasia, and focal adenocarcinoma. Note the background cobblestone-like mucosa and thick colon wall indicating long-term IBD. Patients with IBD are at increased risk for adenocarcinoma. Patients with IBD undergo regular surveillance to detect dysplasia and early cancer.

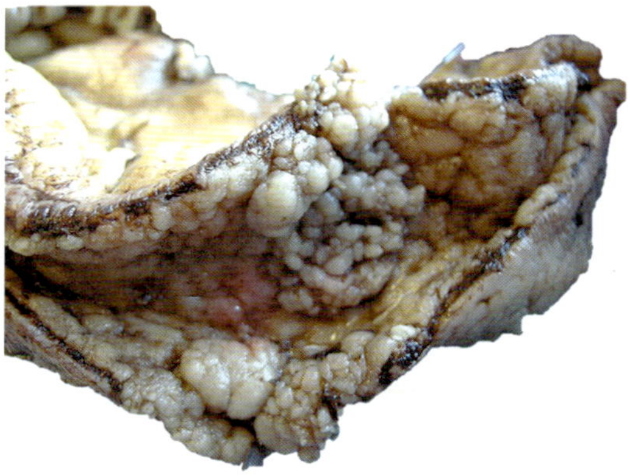

PROCEDURE: TREATMENT OPTIONS FOR RECTAL CANCER

Transanal excision

Since rectal surgery carries a high morbidity risk, a transanal excision through the anus may be indicated for endoscopically unresectable adenomas or early adenocarcinomas of the distal rectum, thereby leaving the sphincter and anus intact.

FIGURE 11.182. This transanal resection specimen shows a dark irregular lesion that histology confirmed as an early rectal adenocarcinoma.

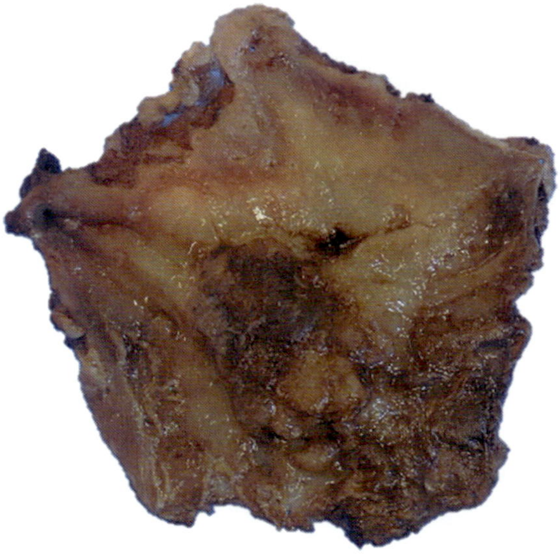

Neoadjuvant therapy

Prior to rectal surgery, patients may undergo neoadjuvant therapy, such as radiotherapy. If the tumor is responsive, it may shrink, ulcerate, and even disappear. Careful sampling of the ulcerated lesion is required to confirm the presence of residual viable cancer. The treatment effect (such as fibrosis) should be documented in the pathology report, along with tumor staging and other parameters.

FIGURE 11.183. This is an example of rectal cancer postradiotherapy. An ulcer is present (right), surrounded by a slightly raised edge.

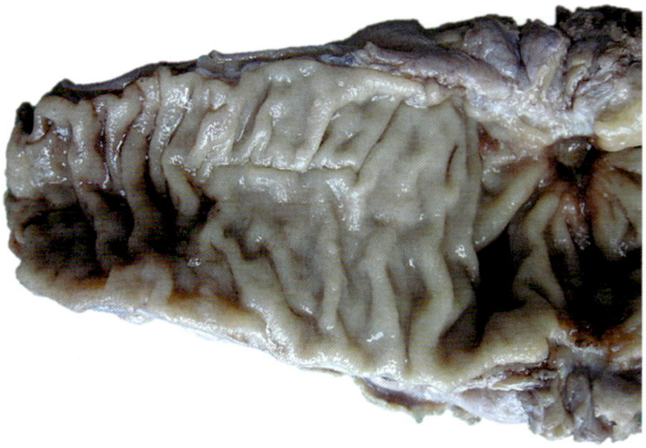

Lower anterior resection (LAR)

LAR is a type of surgical resection that includes the distal sigmoid colon and the rectum, but not the anus.

FIGURE 11.184. These images show LAR specimens of the rectum and distal sigmoid colon. Note the large fungating (A) and polypoid (B) tumors toward the distal resection margin.

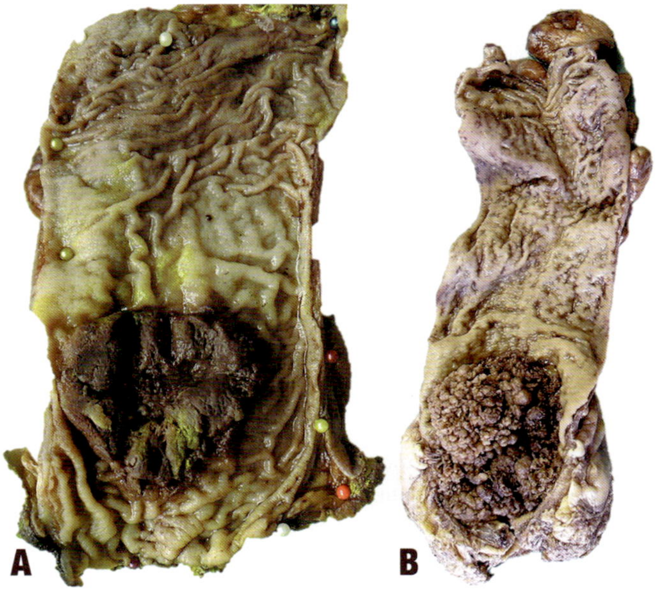

Abdominoperineal resection (APR)

APR is a procedure usually reserved for distal rectal and anal tumors.

FIGURE 11.185. This image shows a fungating, nearly circumferential, tumor in the rectum. This specimen is from an APR. Note the dentate line indicating the anal canal (toward the right).

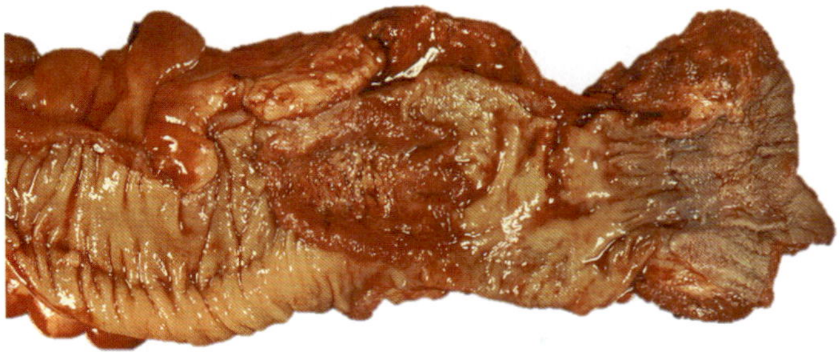

Resection of recurrent carcinoma

Follow-up colonoscopy after surgery is performed to identify local recurrence at an early stage and allow for resection.

FIGURE 11.186. This image of a resection shows an irregular ulcer at an anastomosis site, where mucosal folds are discontinuous. Histology confirmed this as adenocarcinoma.

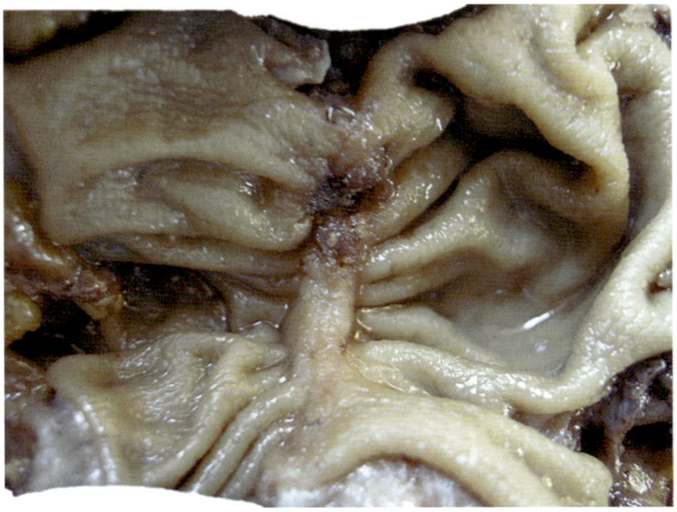

Total mesorectal excision (TME)

TME is a surgical technique in which the rectum and the entire mesorectum are dissected. The mesorectum of the TME includes all the regional nodes and all the perirectal adipose tissue, including the fascial envelope around the rectum. TME has been shown to reduce the rate of local recurrence and to prolong survival.

FIGURE 11.187. The cross-sections of this LAR with TME show a mucinous adenocarcinoma with 2 positive lymph nodes, 1 of which is at the radial resection margin. Note the translucent cut surface.

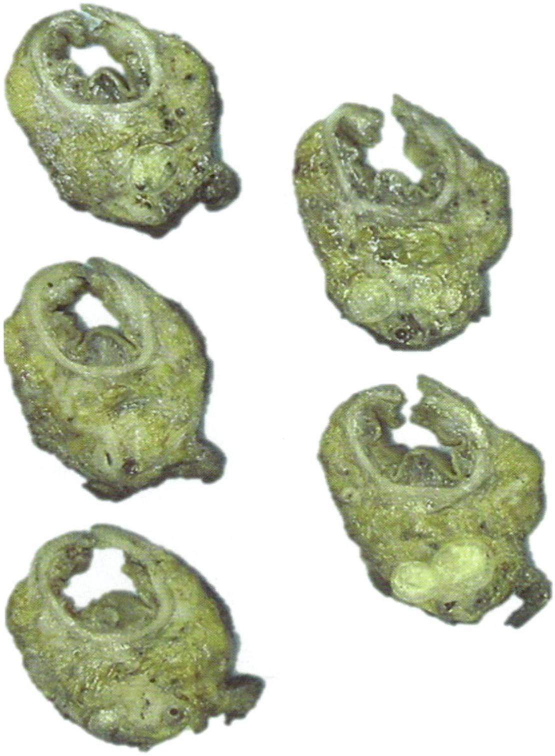

PROCEDURE: PATHOLOGY ASSESSMENT OF TME

The Quirke method of grossly assessing and sampling TME specimens includes an assessment of TME quality. The quality of a TME depends on the intactness of the mesorectum on macroscopy; the assessment focuses on the least-intact area, which is graded complete, nearly complete, or incomplete. Patients with incomplete TMEs have a higher rate of local recurrence and worse outcomes. After assessment of TME quality, the radial margin and the serosa underlying the tumor are inked different colors. The specimen is opened anteriorly, leaving the circumferential area closest to the tumor intact. After 72 hours of fixation, cross-sections are made in the TME. They are assessed for tumor size, location, depth of invasion, lymph nodes, and proximity to the radial margin by tumor, tumor deposits, or involved nodes.

FIGURE 11.188. The Quirke method of grossly assessing and sampling TME specimens includes the assessment of TME quality, ideally in both the fresh and intact state, and after formalin fixation on the cross-sections. Image (A) shows a fresh TME. Image (B) shows cross-sections of the fixed TME.

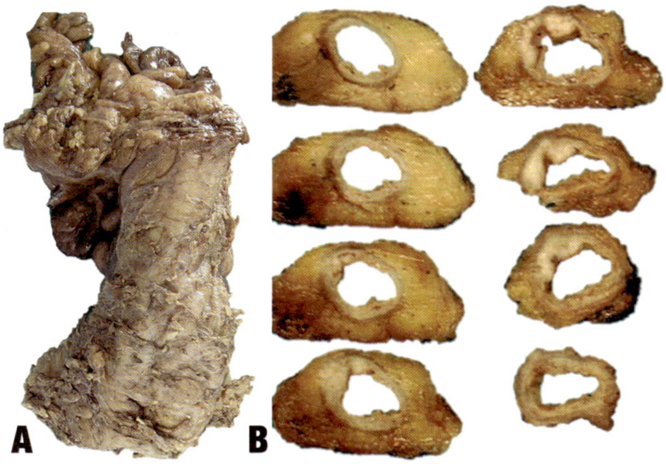

Incomplete TME

FIGURE 11.189. This image shows an incomplete TME with an irregular external surface, little bulk to the mesorectum, and defects to the muscularis propria.

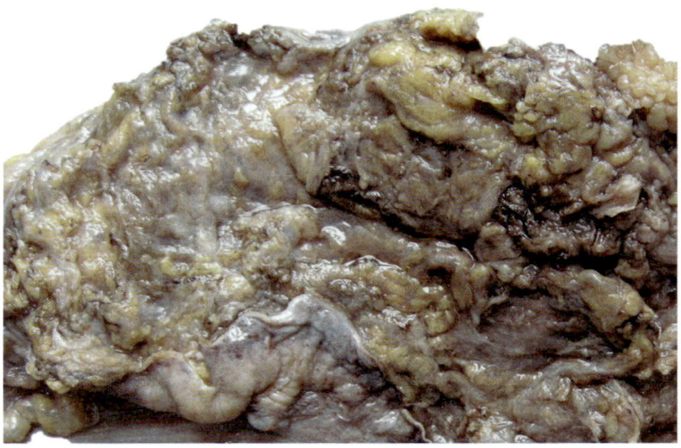

Nearly complete and incomplete TME

FIGURE 11.190. The nearly complete TME in (A) shows a defect in the mesorectum > 0.5 cm in depth, but not down to the muscularis propria. Image (B) shows an incomplete TME with a defect extending to the muscular layer.

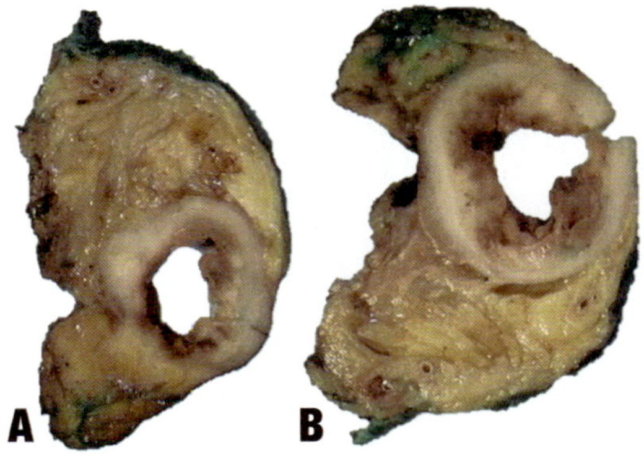

Complete TME

FIGURE 11.191. In (A), note the full bulk of the mesorectum with a smooth outer contour. Image (B) shows the lymph node, grossly identified near the radial resection margin inked black. The involvement of nodes by the tumor at the resection margin is an unfavorable prognostic sign.

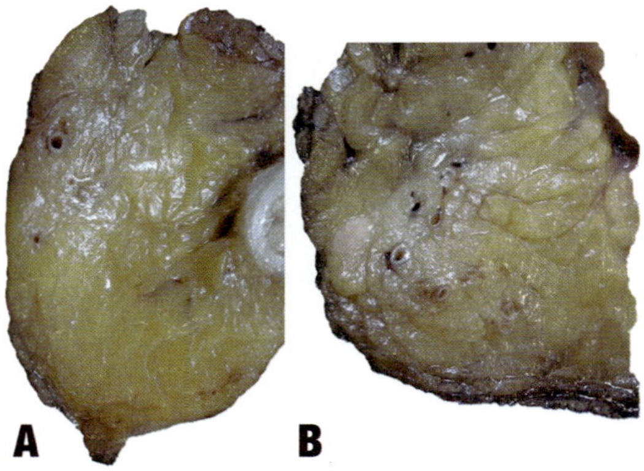

Inking TME specimen

FIGURE 11.192. Image (A) shows formalin-soaked gauze placed in the remaining lumen. Images (B) and (C) show the LAR specimen inked: image (B) shows the green anterior radial margin and blue serosa; image (C) shows the black posterior radial margin.

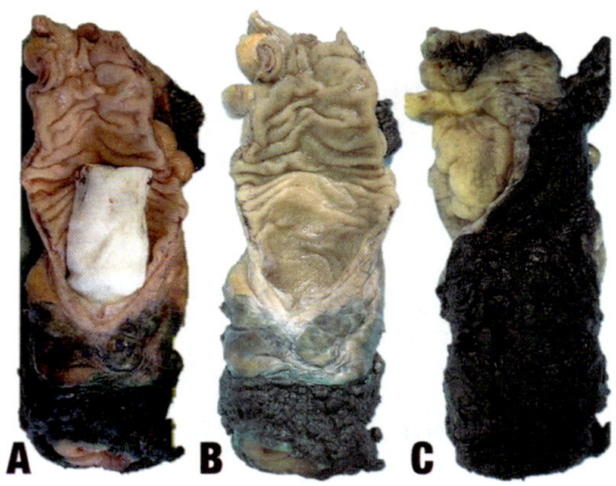

Cross-sections of TME specimen

FIGURE 11.193. These TME cross-sections are placed in order, from distal (bottom right) to proximal (top left). Targeted and systematic sampling is performed on cross-sections, focusing on the tumor's depth of invasion, lymph nodes, and margins, and on mapping the areas sampled for correlation with histological findings.

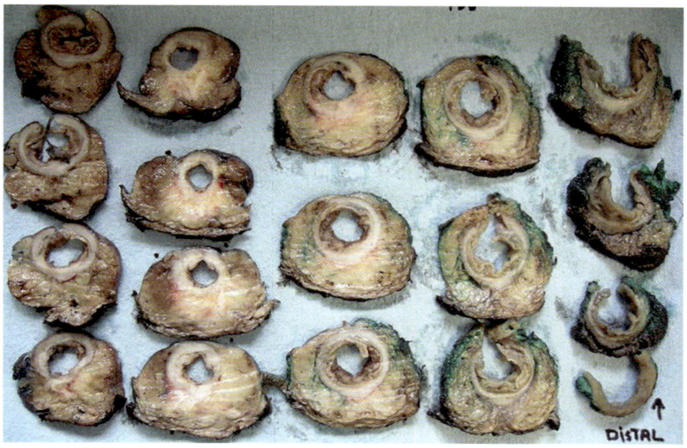

Neuroendocrine tumor of the colon and rectum

Although most cancers in the colon and rectum are adenocarcinomas, other types of tumors may also occur, such as tumors with neuroendocrine differentiation. The behavior of neuroendocrine tumors is variable, and in part depends on the grade of the tumor, assessed by mitotic count and Ki-67 index. Malignancy, however, is confirmed by the presence of metastasis.

FIGURE 11.194. Image (A) shows an LAR of a bulky specimen. Cross-sections in (B) show that the tumor invades extensively into the pericolorectal fat and has lymph node metastases, a malignant feature. On histology, this tumor had neuroendocrine differentiation.

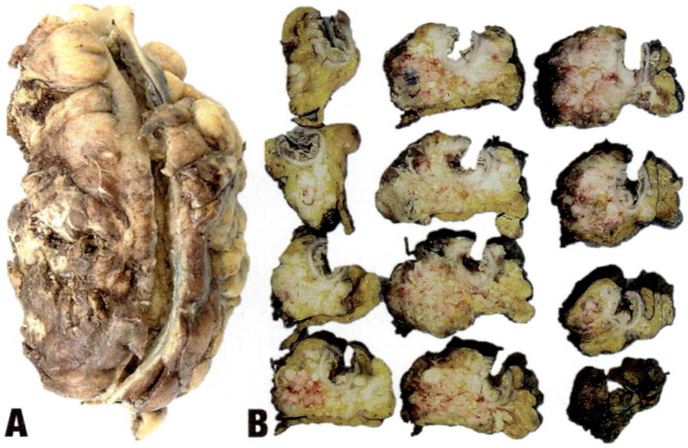

Mesenchymal Tumors of the Colon and Rectum

Gastrointestinal stromal tumor (GIST)

GISTs are mesenchymal tumors derived from interstitial cells of Cajal, the pacemaker cells of the GI tract. Approximately 5% of all GISTs arise in the colon and rectum. The behavior of colorectal GISTs depends on tumor size and mitotic count.

FIGURE 11.195. This image shows a fleshy tumor with hemorrhage and focal necrosis. Note the invasion into the overlying mucosa, reported to be a malignant feature.

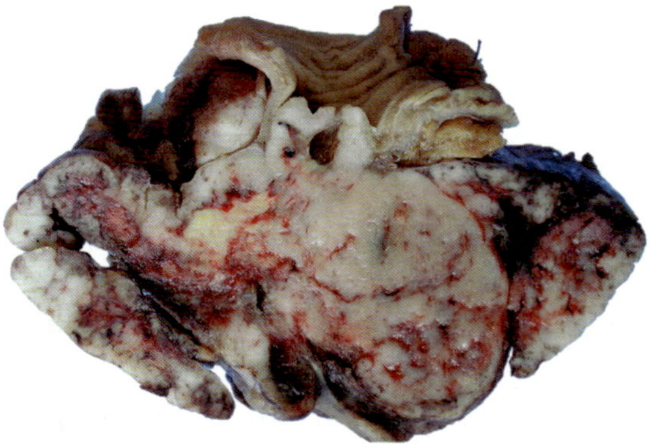

Submucosal lipoma

Submucosal lipomas are also mesenchymal tumors of the gastrointestinal tract. They are benign neoplasms composed of mature adipose tissue. They can cause intussusception.

FIGURE 11.196. This resected large bowel segment shows a solitary, spherical, smooth, yellow nodule with an intact overlying mucosa. The lipoma was sectioned to show the lobulated fatty tissue at the center of this lesion.

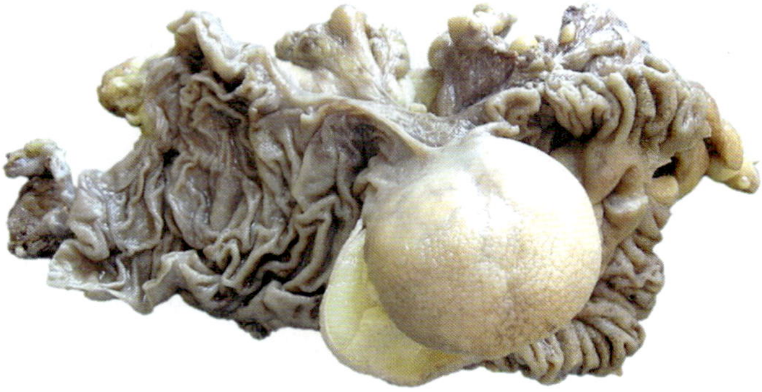

Neoplasms of the Anus

Squamous cell carcinoma (SCC) of the anus

SCC is the most common carcinoma of the anus. They are usually associated with high-risk human papillomavirus (HPV) infection.

FIGURE 11.197. In this image, note the ulcerative SCC straddling the dentate line.

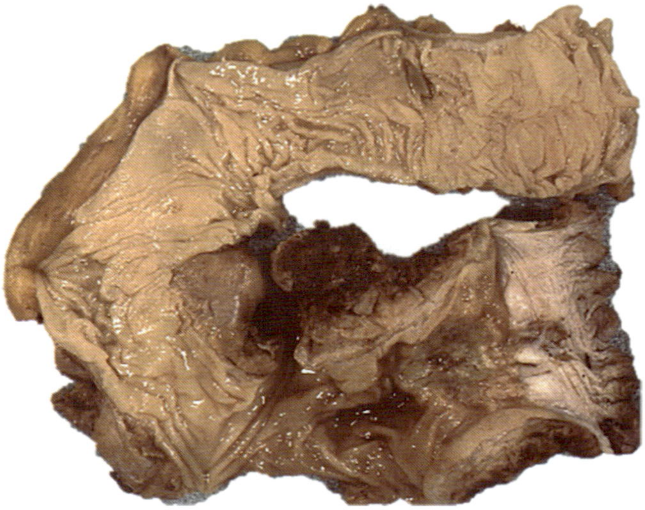

FIGURE 11.198. In these serial cross-sections of an anorectal specimen, arranged from proximal (top left) to distal (bottom right), the most distal section is the anal skin. Note the white, infiltrative tumor involving the muscularis propria and the perirectal adipose tissue.

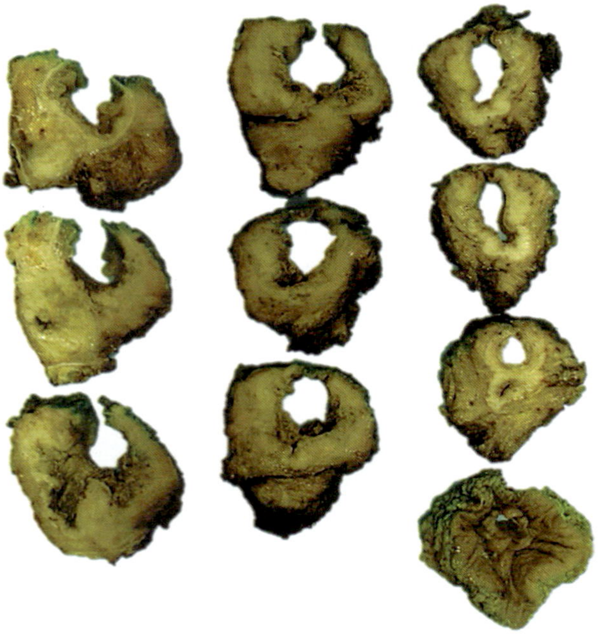

Primary anal malignant melanoma

Anal melanoma is a rare, aggressive disease. The anus is a less common primary site of melanoma than the skin or retina. Sometimes, anorectal melanoma may be confused with a hemorrhoid. Confirmation of the tumor type often requires immunohistochemistry. These aggressive tumors are typically positive for S100, melan-A (MART-1), and HMB45.

FIGURE 11.199. This image shows an abdominoperineal resection containing a large pigmented mass.

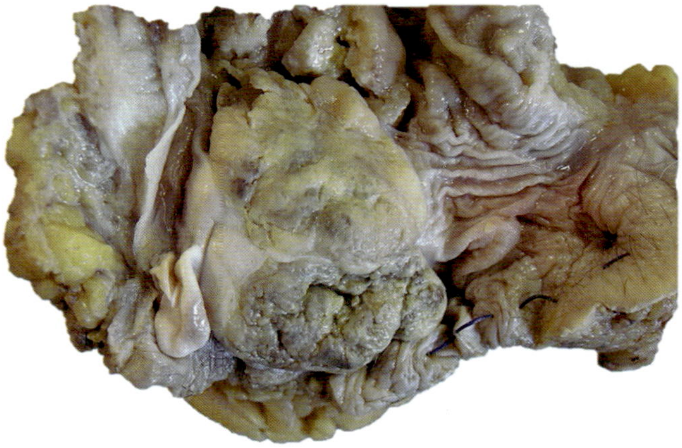

Appendix

REFERENCE: NORMAL APPENDIX

The appendix is a blind-ended, tube-like structure extending from the cecum. The appendix has no known function.

FIGURE 11.200. This image shows a normal appendix (bottom), cecum, ascending colon, ileocecal valve, and terminal ileum (right).

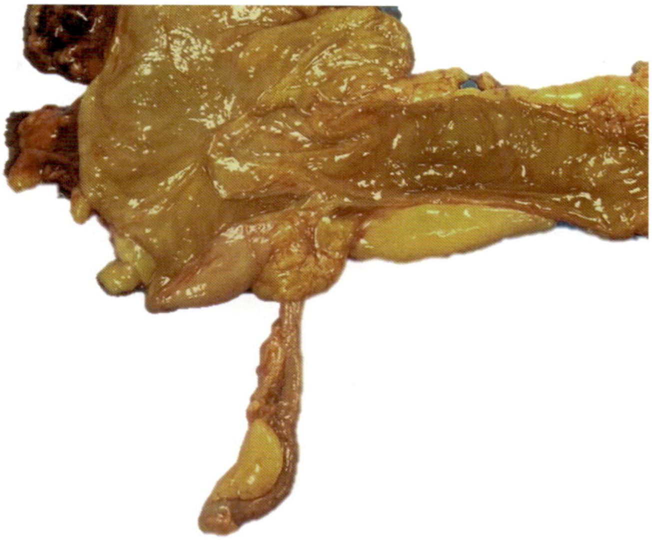

Nonneoplastic Diseases of the Appendix

Appendicitis

Appendicitis is a common cause of acute abdominal pain. It is usually initiated by blockage of the lumen by a fecalith, which results in increased pressure and local ischemia, then bacterial overgrowth and subsequent inflammation. Severe cases of acute appendicitis show transmural necrosis and rupture of the wall.

FIGURE 11.201. This image shows a congested appendix with fibrinopurulent exudate and hemorrhage focally identified on the serosal surface of the appendix.

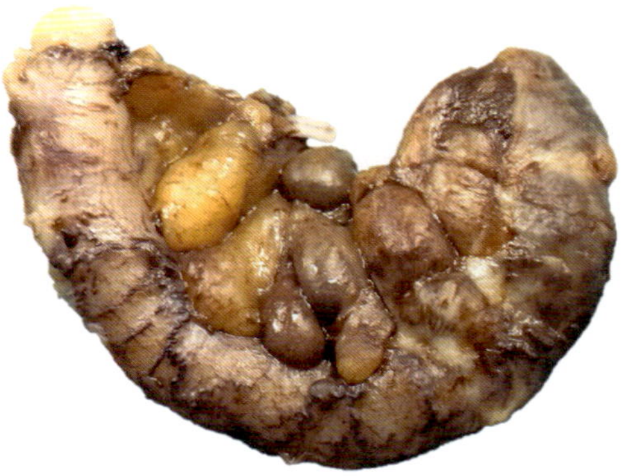

GRANULOMATOUS APPENDICITIS

The differential diagnosis of this uncommon entity includes infection (*Yersinia, M. tuberculosis*, etc.), delayed appendectomy, Crohn disease (in about 10% of cases), and idiopathy.

FIGURE 11.202. This image shows the thick wall of the appendix, which raised the surgeon's suspicion for a neoplasm intraoperatively.

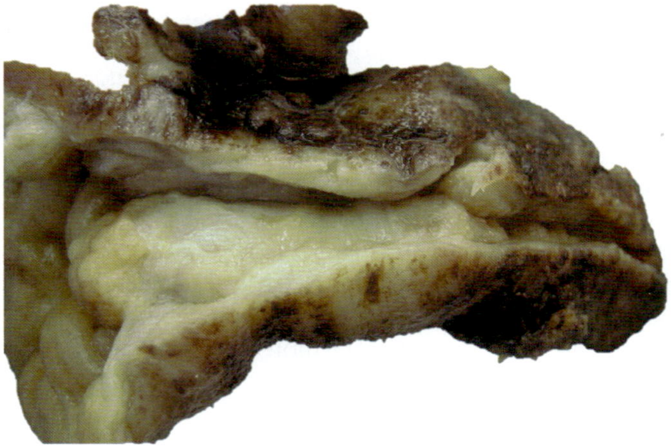

Diverticulosis of the appendix

Appendiceal diverticulosis is characterized by outpouching of the mucosa through the appendiceal wall. The diverticula may be acquired due to increased intraluminal pressure or may be congenital. The disease is uncommon and usually asymptomatic. The diverticula may, however, become inflamed. Appendiceal diverticulitis has an increased risk of perforation.

FIGURE 11.203. In this image, the outpouching of appendiceal mucosa is best illustrated in the 2 cross-sections at the lower left.

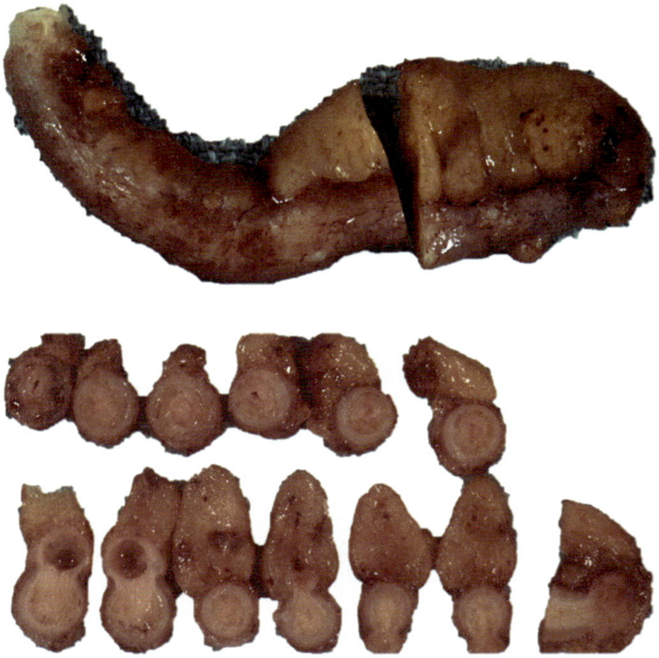

Neoplasms of the Appendix

Neuroendocrine tumor (NET) of the appendix

NET is the most common tumor of the appendix. On immunohistochemistry, these tumors express the neuroendocrine markers synaptophysin and chromogranin. Most appendiceal NETs are low grade and have traditionally been termed carcinoids. Goblet cell carcinoids of the appendix are the exception: they are aggressive and may evolve into high-grade adenocarcinoma. In fact, the new WHO classification (2019) renamed goblet cell carcinoid to be goblet cell adenocarcinoma. A right hemicolectomy is indicated if a NET is > 2 cm, is of goblet cell type, or involves the margin, mesoappendix, or lymph nodes.

FIGURE 11.204. The NET in this image is at the distal end of the appendix. It is causing wall thickening and has a yellow-gray cut surface.

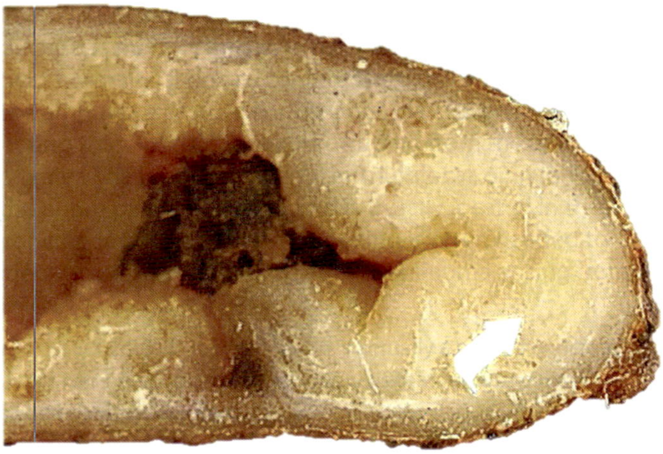

Primary appendiceal adenocarcinoma

This is a rare epithelial malignancy of the appendix. Histological types include intestinal, mucinous, signet ring cell, and mixed adenoneuroendocrine carcinoma.

FIGURE 11.205. This image shows an enlarged appendix with a white solid tumor obliterating its lumen.

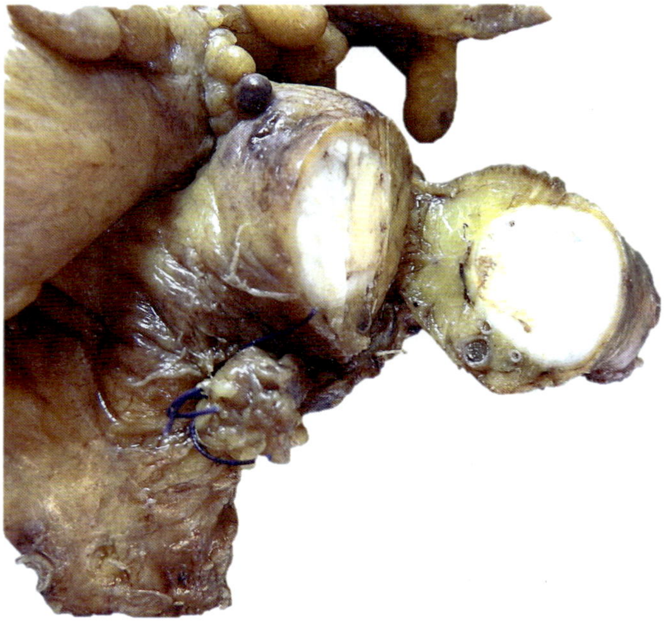

APPENDICEAL ADENOCARCINOMA INVOLVING THE TERMINAL ILEUM

Because of its proximity to the terminal ileum and cecum, direct extension from an appendiceal primary tumor to these sites may occur. Careful examination for the tumor epicenter and any precursor epithelial in situ lesion may help determine the primary origin of the malignancy.

FIGURE 11.206. This right hemicolectomy specimen was cut longitudinally and shows a white tumor infiltrating mainly into the external aspect of the terminal ileum with an involved lymph node. The ileal mucosa is relatively intact. This favors direct extension from an appendiceal tumor rather than a primary ileal tumor.

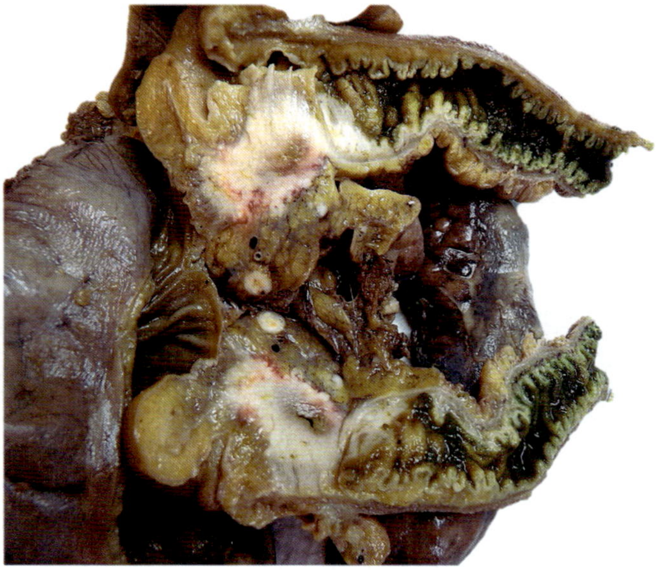

Mucocele

Mucocele is a clinical or gross term used to describe a dilated appendix filled with mucin. It is not a pathologic diagnosis. Some mucocele may be due to an underlying inflammatory process; most are now thought to be neoplastic. When mucin is identified grossly within an appendix, the entire appendiceal specimen should be examined histologically to search for underlying neoplastic epithelium. As well, the resection margin status needs to be reported.

FIGURE 11.207. This image shows a dilated appendix filled with mucin.

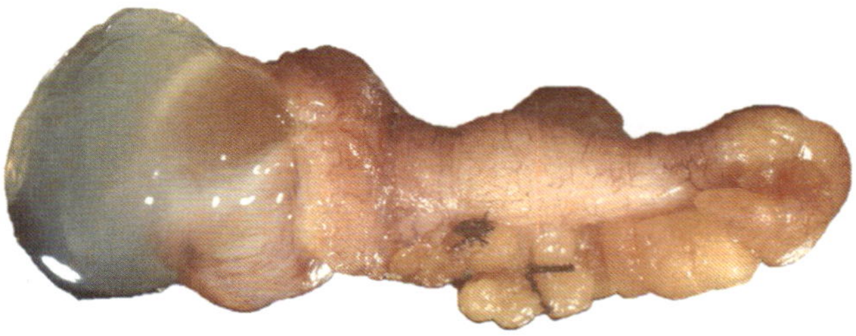

Low-grade appendiceal mucinous neoplasm (LAMN)

The nomenclature for mucin-producing tumors of the appendix has evolved and still remains controversial. Most are low-grade appendiceal mucinous neoplasms (LAMNs). Although LAMNs are considered low-grade tumors, they may spread to the ovaries and peritoneum. When they spread to the peritoneum, pseudomyxoma peritonei (PMP) may develop. High-grade infiltrating tumors are instead called mucinous adenocarcinoma.

FIGURE 11.208. These images show examples of LAMN with mucin filling the appendiceal lumen.

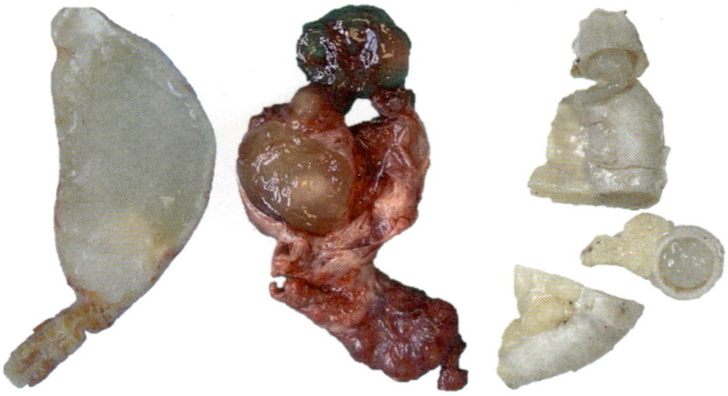

FIGURE 11.209. In image (A), the resected appendix specimen is enlarged. Note in (B) the gelatin-like mucin content of the cyst on opening.

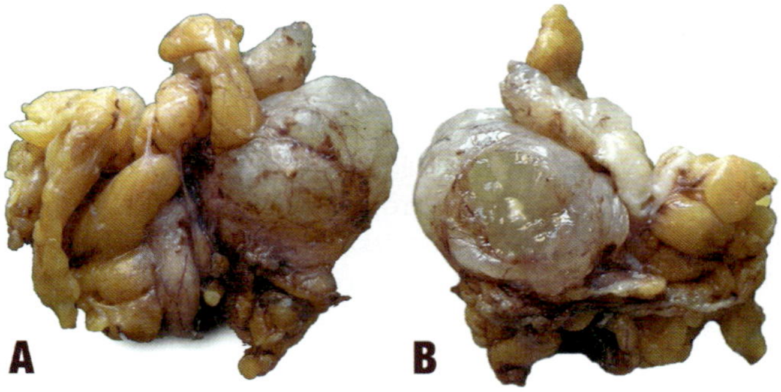

FIGURE 11.210. This image shows a resected specimen that consists of the right colon, cecum, and the cystically dilated appendix, opened to show excrescences on the inner surface of this LAMN.

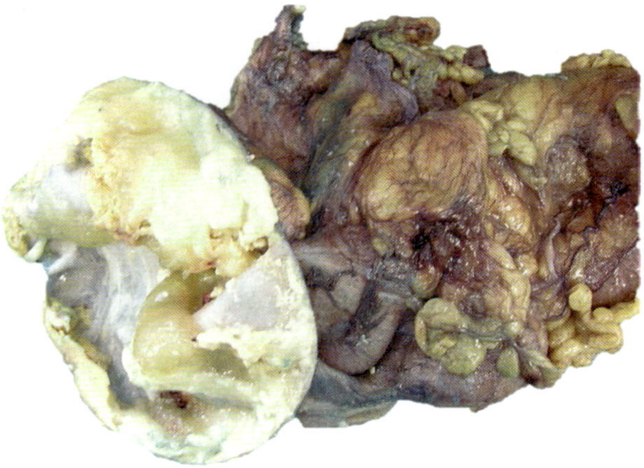

Pseudomyxoma peritonei (PMP)

When the appendiceal wall is perforated by LAMN, the neoplastic cells may enter and spread throughout the abdomen, and lead to the development of pseudomyxoma peritonei (PMP). PMP is a clinical condition characterized by gelatinous mucin filling the abdominal cavity. This gelatinous mucinous ascites may be so abundant that it may compress and damage abdominal organs. Patients with PMP, and concomitant mucinous tumors of the appendix and ovaries, usually have the primary tumor in the appendix; the ovary is usually secondarily involved.

FIGURE 11.211. Image (A) shows a vague, but still identifiable, appendix structure. Images (B) and (C) show the gelatinous mucin in the abdominal cavity.

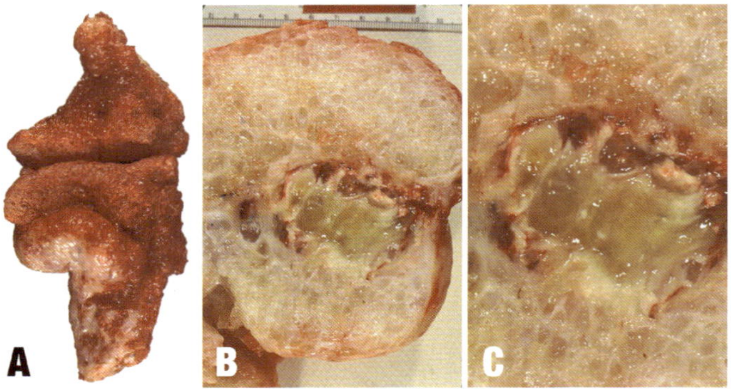

Benign multicystic peritoneal mesothelioma (BMPM)

BMPM is also called benign cystic mesothelioma and benign peritoneal cysts. It can be unilocular or multilocular, and free floating or attached to the serosa of an organ. On histology, the lining of the cysts demonstrates bland mesothelium. BMPM is a rare tumor that often recurs after resection, but rarely metastasizes.

FIGURE 11.212. Image (A) shows the smooth external surface of a benign peritoneal cyst. The cut section in (B) shows a multiloculated cystic lesion. The cysts were filled with clear serous-type fluid.

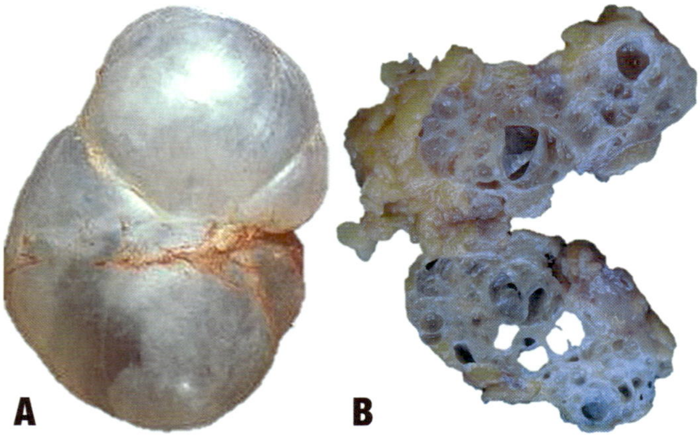

Leiomyomatosis peritonealis disseminata

Leiomyomatosis peritonealis disseminata is a rare disorder characterized by multiple smooth muscle tumors or nodules disseminated throughout the omental and peritoneal surfaces. It is a benign disease of unknown etiology that usually occurs in women of reproductive age. The tumor may originate from the mesentery, the omentum, or even the peritoneum. It is not always accompanied by uterine leiomyomas and can occur after menopause.

FIGURE 11.213. This image shows nodules due to leiomyomatosis peritonealis disseminata.

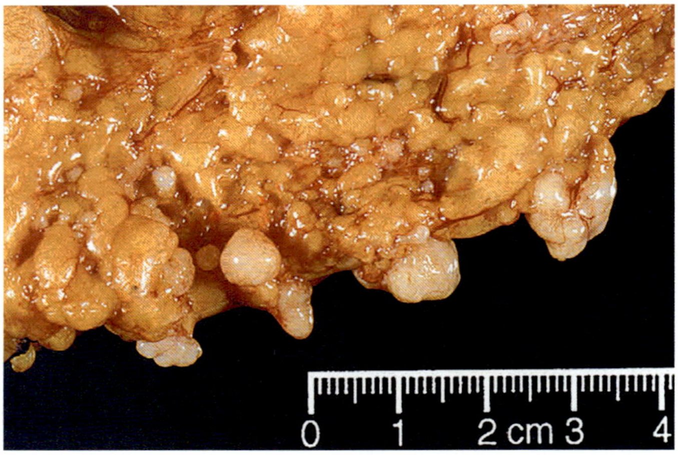

ACKNOWLEDGMENTS

We would like to acknowledge the valuable contributions of Dr. Vincent Falck, Dr. Olga Aleynikova, the late Dr. Esther Lamoureux, and the late Dr. John Lough, and the technical help of R. Gilot, E. Griss, A. Hossain, L. Korneichyuk Pasyuk, M. Mikhael, and E. Yaney.

REFERENCES

Goldblum JR, Lamps LW, McKenney JK, Myers JL. *Rosai and Ackerman's surgical pathology*. 11th ed. Philadelphia: Elsevier; 2018.

Kumar V, Abbas AK, Aster J. *Robbins and Cotran pathologic basis of disease*. 9th ed. Philadelphia: Elsevier Saunders; 2015.

Lester SC. *Manual of surgical pathology*. 3rd ed. Philadelphia: Elsevier Saunders; 2010.

Mills SE, Greenson JK, Hornick JL, Longacre TA, Reuter VE, editors. *Sternberg's diagnostic surgical pathology*. 6th ed. Philadelphia: Wolters Kluwer Health; 2015.

Odze RD, Goldblum JR. *Surgical pathology of the GI tract, liver, biliary tract, and pancreas*. 3rd ed. Philadelphia: Elsevier Saunders; 2015.

WHO Classification of Tumours Editorial Board, editors. *WHO classification of tumours. Digestive system tumours*. 5th ed. Lyon, France: IARC Press; 2019.

12

Liver and Gallbladder Diseases

RENÉ P. MICHEL, YU SHI, VICTORIA MARCUS, ZU-HUA GAO

Liver

REFERENCE: NORMAL LIVER

FIGURE 12.1. This anterior view of a normal liver shows the right lobe and left lobes. The Couinaud classification separates the lobes based on functional vascular and biliary anatomy, not the falciform ligament (arrow).

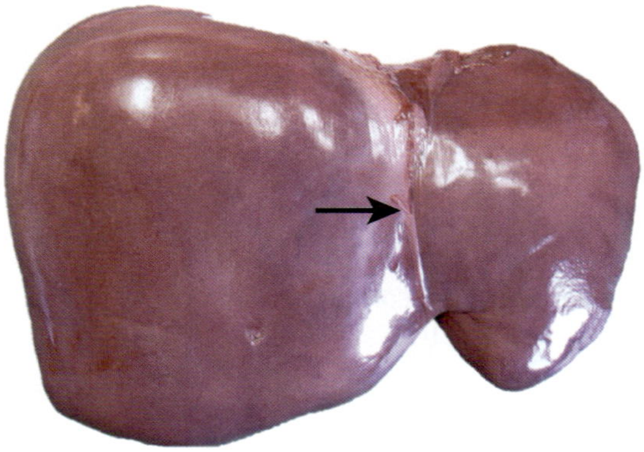

FIGURE 12.2. This is a posterior view, rotated upwards, of a normal liver. The gallbladder is attached to the inferior liver between the right and the quadrate lobes. The porta hepatis (white arrow) beside the gallbladder contains the hepatic artery, portal vein, and common bile duct. Below the porta hepatis lies the caudate lobe, also known as the posterior hepatic segment I (**), and above it lies the quadrate lobe (*). The black arrow points to the inferior vena cava.

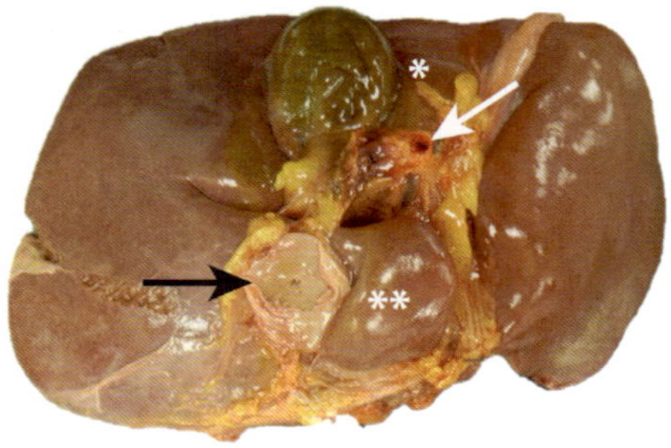

FIGURE 12.3. A transverse slice of a normal liver after formalin fixation shows a slightly variegated, light brown, uniform appearance. The capsule is smooth and glistening. At the hilum, the portal vein is visible (arrow).

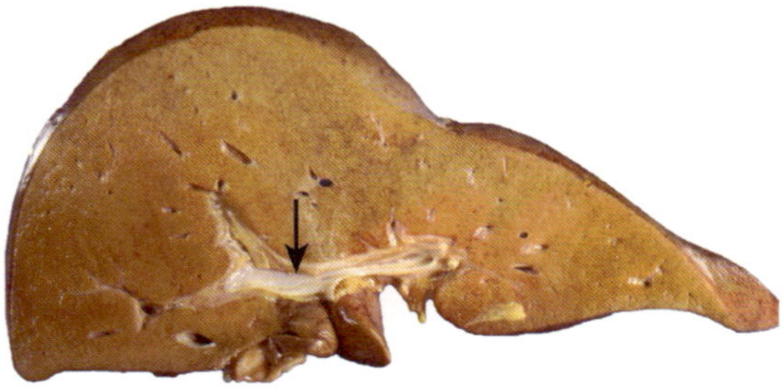

Nonmalignant Diseases of the Liver

Fatty liver

Fatty liver can be caused by alcohol intake or non-alcohol-related diseases such as obesity and drugs.

FIGURE 12.4. In this fatty liver specimen, notice the yellow color due to abundant lipid accumulation in hepatocytes.

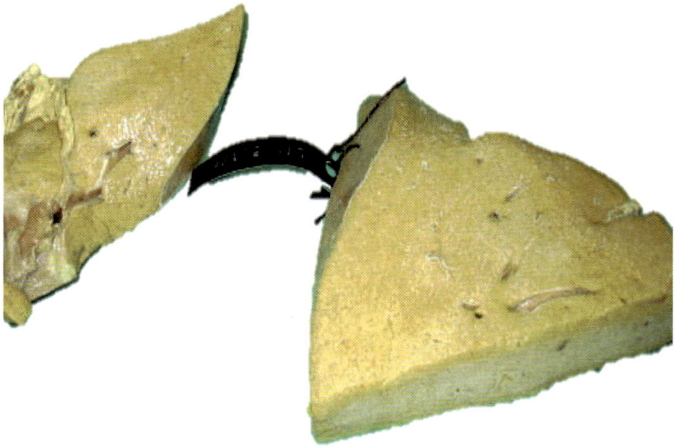

Courtesy of Dr. Vincent Falck

Congenital hepatic fibrosis

Congenital hepatic fibrosis is an autosomal recessive disorder caused by mutations of the *PKHD1* gene that encodes the protein fibrocystin (also called polyductin). The principal symptoms are related to portal hypertension and hepatosplenomegaly leading to ascites, abdominal distention, and respiratory compromise. The associated bile duct abnormalities may also result in cholangitis. The macroscopic appearance mirrors the microscopic alterations that show prominent portal-to-portal bridging fibrosis. True cirrhosis is usually absent because of the absence of prominent hepatocyte regenerative nodules.

FIGURE 12.5. Images (A) and (B) show cross-sections of a liver with portal-to-portal bridging fibrosis without regenerative nodules.

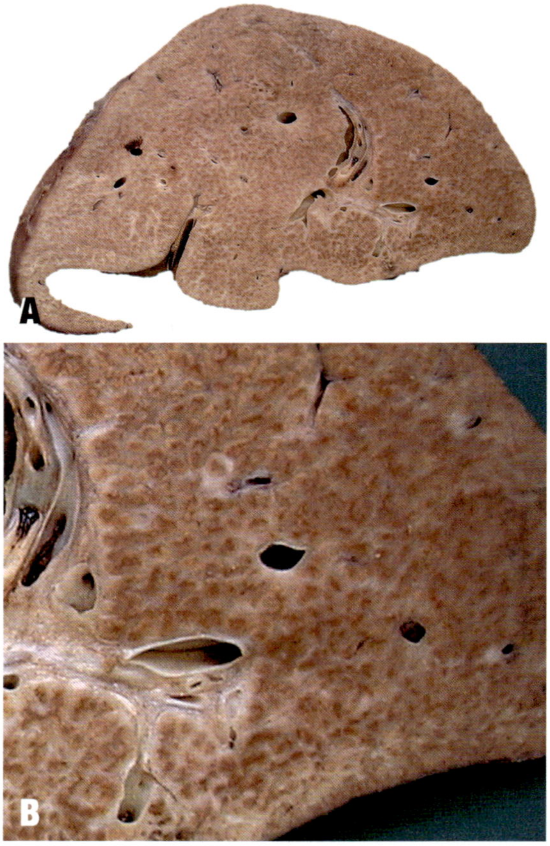

Simple hepatic cyst

Simple hepatic cyst is a common, nonneoplastic liver lesion with no malignant potential.

FIGURE 12.6. This resected liver segment shows multiple sections of a single, thin-walled, subcapsular cyst.

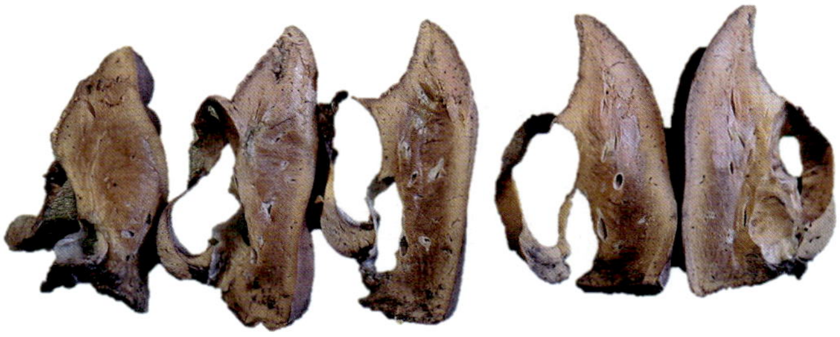

Adult polycystic liver disease

Adult polycystic liver disease is a rare autosomal dominant disease frequently accompanied by autosomal dominant polycystic kidney disease (ADPKD). Most cases are related to mutations of the *PKD1* gene that encodes the polycystin 1 protein. Although liver failure rarely occurs in these patients, kidney failure is frequent. About 20% of patients experience symptoms related to enlargement and may require surgery.

FIGURE 12.7. In (A), part of a resected liver shows multiple large, confluent, contiguous cysts of variable size. A closer view in (B) shows the cysts are interspaced by normal liver parenchyma. The smooth lining of the cysts is composed of a single layer of epithelial cells, which can be seen on light microscopy.

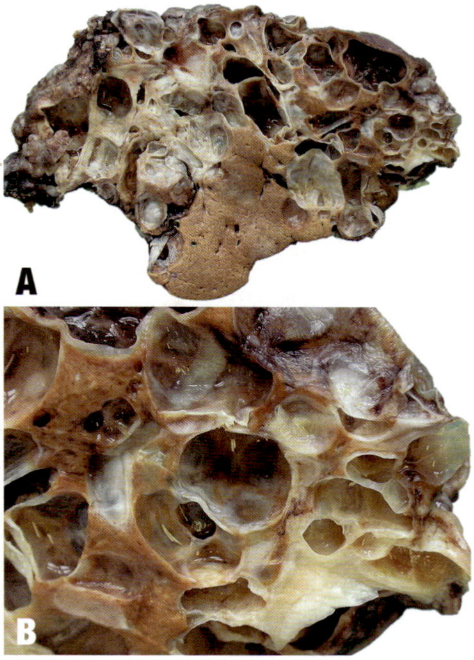

FIGURE 12.8. The resected liver in (A) is enlarged and has a smooth, tense capsule with numerous subcapsular cysts. The cross-section in (B) reveals many cysts of variable size filled with clear or straw-colored fluid.

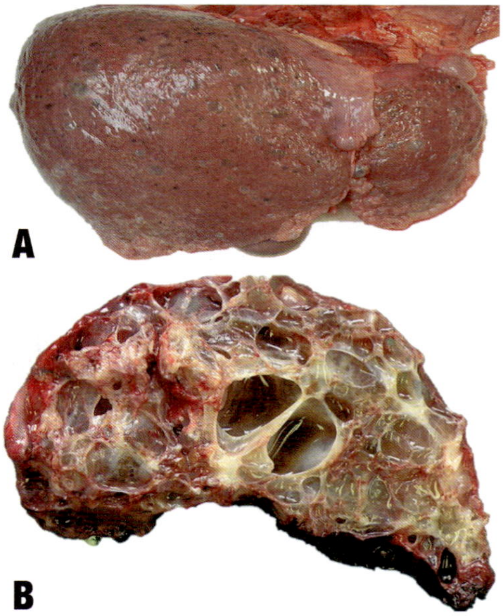

Bile duct cyst

Bile duct cyst is a type of simple hepatic cyst with no malignant potential. The cyst is lined by a single layer of flat or cuboidal epithelium on a fibrous stroma and contains clear, serous fluid.

FIGURE 12.9. This resected liver segment shows a large cyst with yellow-green patches of bile.

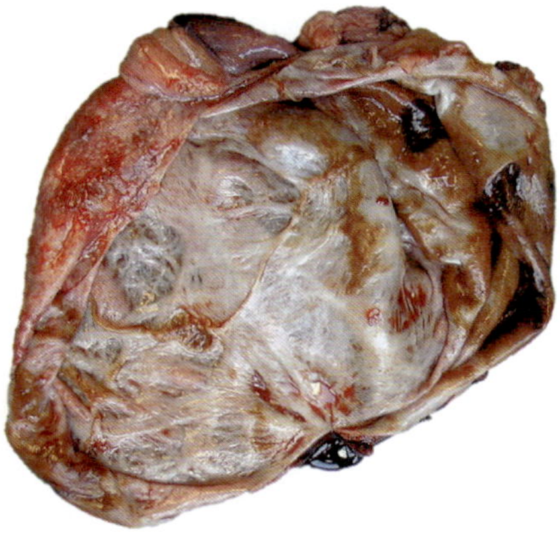

Hydatid cyst

Hydatid disease is caused by the tapeworm *Echinococcus*, most commonly *E. granulosus,* which usually results in unilocular disease. It is less commonly caused by *E. multilocularis,* which produces multilocular hydatidosis, a condition with a mortality rate of 80% if left untreated.

UNILOCULAR HYDATID CYST

FIGURE 12.10. Image (A) shows a unilocular hydatid cyst of *E. granulosus* containing numerous daughter cysts. Note the multilayered cyst wall composed of: the outer laminated acellular membrane (white arrow); the transparent germinal membrane with nuclei on microscopy (black arrow); and the protoscolices, budding from the germinal membrane. There was minimal inflammatory reaction to the cyst. Image (B) shows a fresh specimen of a unilocular hydatid cyst in a patient from a country near the Mediterranean. No definite organisms were identified.

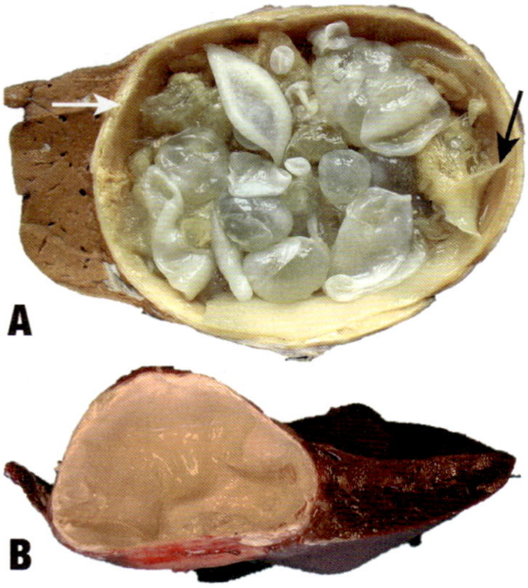

MULTILOCULAR HYDATID CYST

FIGURE 12.11. This image shows a resected multilocular hydatid cyst containing variably sized cysts with intact or partially intact cyst wall.

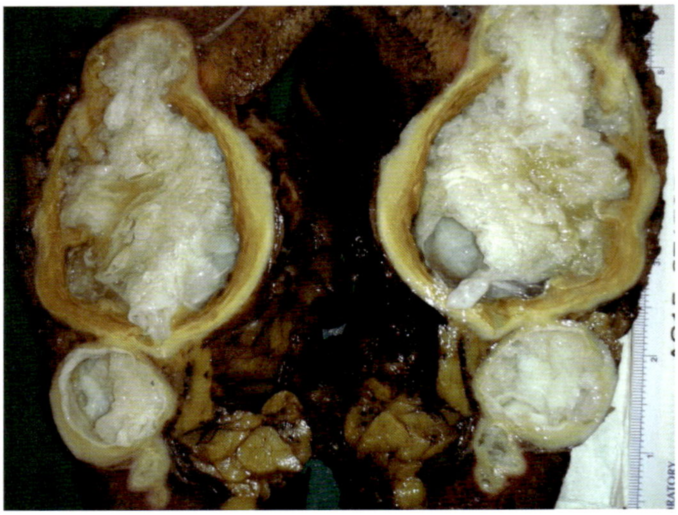

Liver amoeba abscess

Liver amoeba abscess is the involvement of liver tissue by trophozoites of *Entamoeba histolytica*. The liver abscess is due to necrosis.

FIGURE 12.12. This image shows an abscess cavity that contains chocolate-colored blood clots and necrotic tissue.

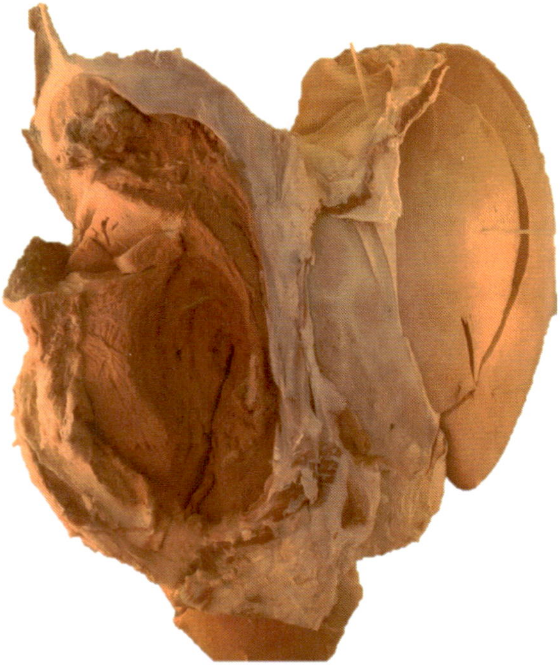

Acetaminophen toxicity

The mechanisms leading to hepatic damage are complex and multifactorial, involving CYP2E1 metabolism, oxidative stress, and individual susceptibility, among other factors. About 10% of patients with acetaminophen overdose present with liver failure and a subset of these require transplantation.

FIGURE 12.13. This image shows an example of a liver with submassive necrosis due to acetaminophen toxicity. Notice the pale yellow areas of necrosis scattered throughout the liver parenchyma.

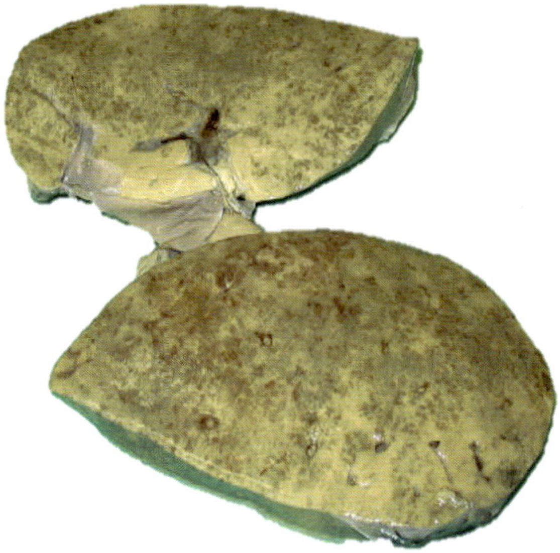

Courtesy of Dr. Vincent Falck

FIGURE 12.14. This is a case of acetaminophen overdose with fulminant liver failure requiring transplantation. The liver shows uniform green discoloration due to marked cholestasis and prominent centrilobular and bridging necrosis (inset). The relatively spared parenchyma is red-brown.

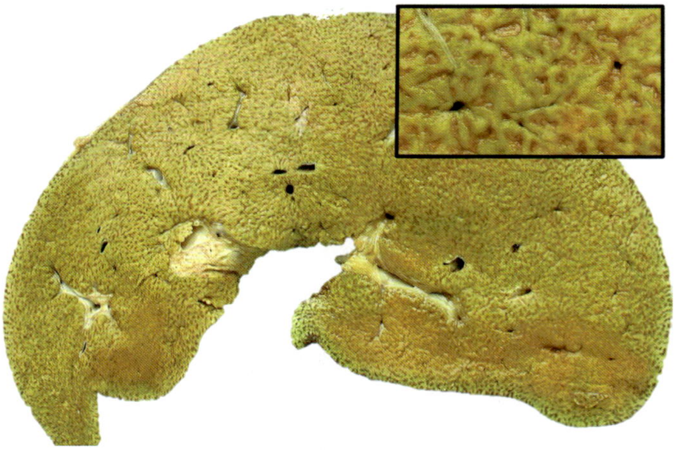

Hemochromatosis

Hemochromatosis is caused by excessive iron absorption. It can be hereditary, due to mutation of the *HFE* gene, or secondary, due to blood transfusion or hemolysis.

FIGURE 12.15. Notice the rusty brown color quite typical of iron overload in the liver.

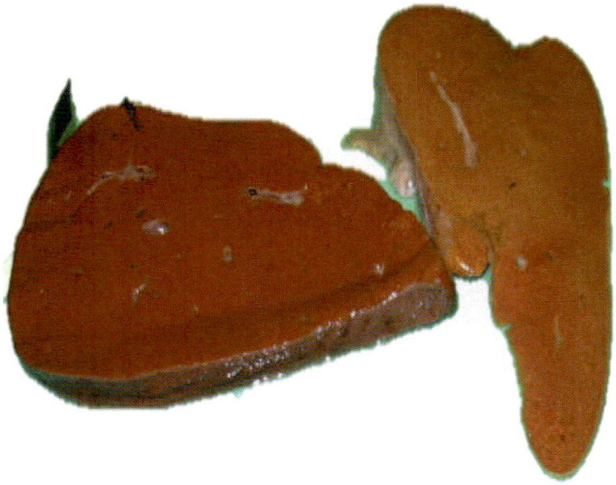

Courtesy of Dr. Vincent Falck

Congestive hepatopathy

Congestive hepatopathy is caused by a variety of cardiac or pulmonary conditions resulting in an increased central venous pressure, including right ventricular cardiac failure, severe pulmonary hypertension, tricuspid regurgitation, and hepatic venous obstruction caused by thrombi or Budd-Chiari syndrome.

FIGURE 12.16. These images show complete (A) and close-up (B) views of fresh liver with areas of prominent centrilobular congestion and hemorrhage interspersed with foci of more intact, paler parenchyma.

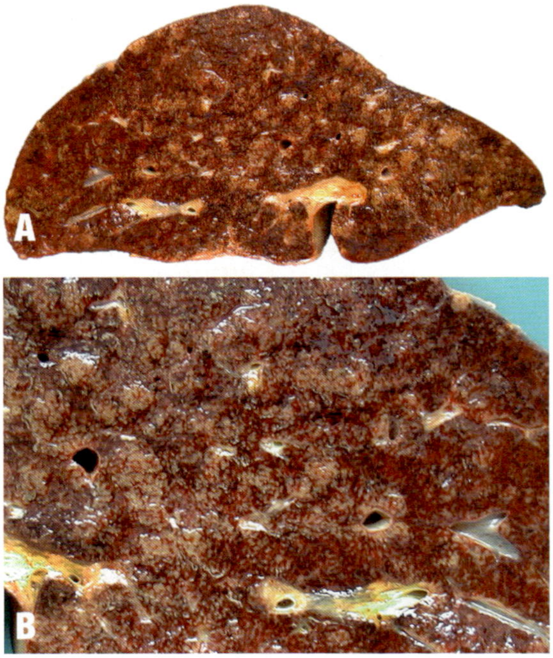

Budd-Chiari syndrome

Budd-Chiari syndrome has multiple etiologies including hypercoagulable states, malignancies (particularly myeloproliferative neoplasms), infections, and drugs.

FIGURE 12.17. Image (A) shows a native liver that was removed pretransplant for Budd-Chiari syndrome. In (B), a close-up view shows the mottled pattern with congested and hemorrhagic centrilobular areas alternating with preserved (predominantly periportal) areas.

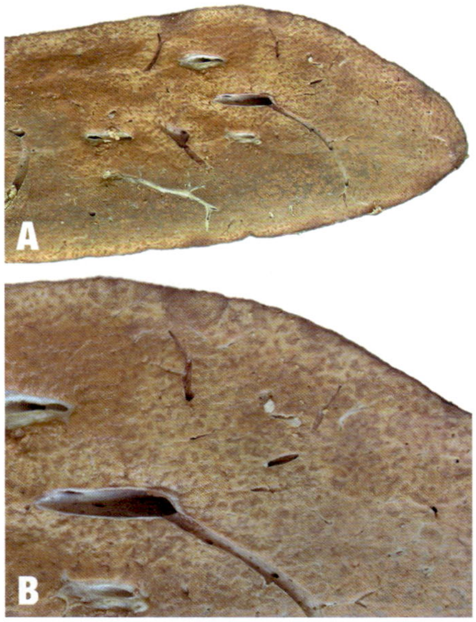

Portal vein thrombosis

The incidence of portal vein thrombosis is proportional to the severity of liver disease, ranging from less than 1% in compensated cirrhosis to between 7.4% and 16% in advanced disease. Its prevalence in patients undergoing transplantation is 5% to 16%. Pathogenetic factors include stasis, hypercoagulability, and endotoxemia.

FIGURE 12.18. Image (A) shows a native liver with thrombosis of the portal vein, resected pretransplant for incomplete cirrhosis due to hepatitis C. Note the fine septal fibrosis and early regenerating nodules. A closer view in (B) illustrates lamination of the thrombus and early hepatocyte regenerative nodules.

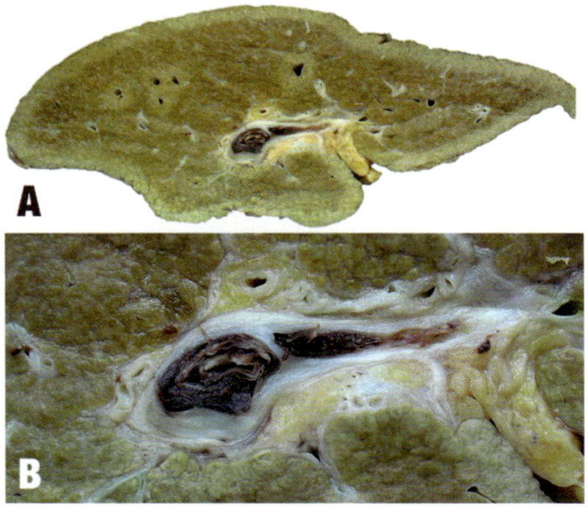

Cirrhosis

Cirrhosis is defined by diffuse involvement of the liver, fibrous septa, and regenerative nodules. The term *cirrhosis* comes from the Greek κιρρός (*kirros*), meaning "orange-yellow" or "tawny," which corresponds to the color of a cirrhotic liver (normal liver color is brown-red). Cirrhosis can be classified by morphology into micronodular, macronodular, and mixed patterns. However, a classification based on etiology is currently more meaningful in terms of diagnosis, therapy, and prognosis.

LIVER CIRRHOSIS DUE TO HEPATITIS B

In patients with chronic hepatitis B, progression to cirrhosis depends on the extent of viral replication and of histologic liver damage. The prominent necroinflammatory process associated with hepatitis B most frequently results in macronodular cirrhosis.

FIGURE 12.19. Image (A) shows cirrhosis due to hepatitis B: note the diffuse, predominantly macronodular pattern and marked cholestasis. In (B), a closer view shows large nodules divided into smaller nodules by fine fibrous septa.

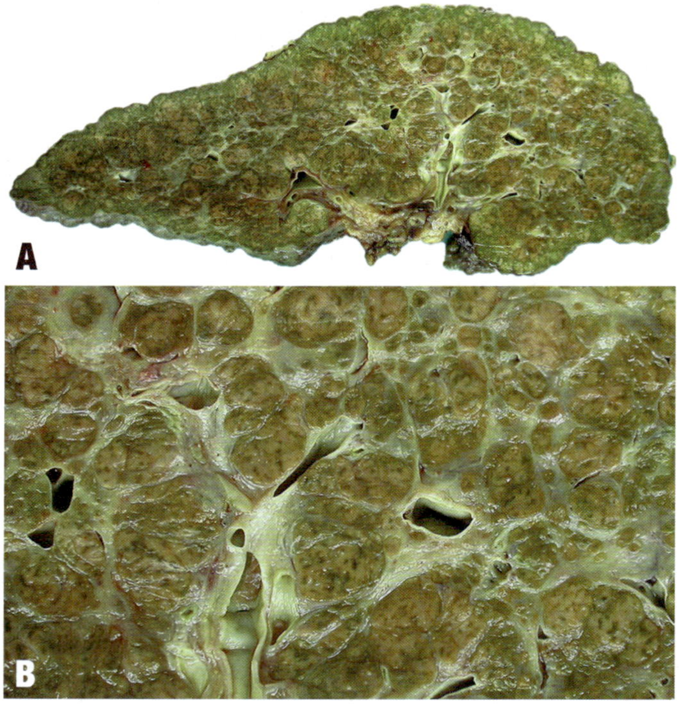

CIRRHOSIS DUE TO HEPATITIS C

In contrast to hepatitis B, cirrhosis in hepatitis C is a relatively late development, occurring in 20% to 40% of patients with follow-up of 10 to 20 years. Hepatitis C is the indication for 20% to 30% of liver transplants.

FIGURE 12.20. A whole slice of a liver specimen in (A) shows prominent cholestasis with bile-stained, variable-sized, regenerative nodules separated by variably wide pale fibrous septa. The closer view in (B) shows regenerative nodules separated by fibrous septa. The generally smaller size of the regenerative nodules in hepatitis C compared with hepatitis B can be attributed to milder necroinflammatory activity.

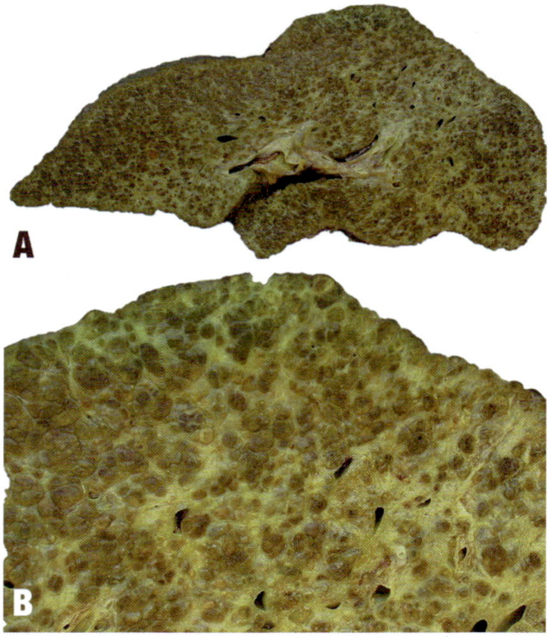

FIGURES 12.21. This liver shows relative regularity of the regenerating nodules, but heterogeneity of discoloration. In particular, the orange nodules refer back to the Greek origin of the term *cirrhosis,* noted above.

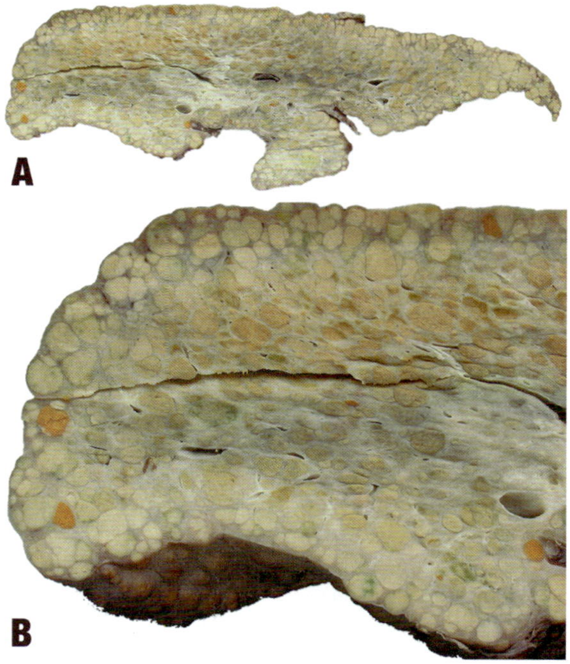

FIGURE 12.22. These images show an overall (A) and a closer view (B) of a native liver in a patient with cirrhosis due to hepatitis C with prominent regenerative nodules, of which some showed mild dysplasia. No carcinoma was found. Note the variegated color in several of the nodules, which should prompt sampling for microscopic examination.

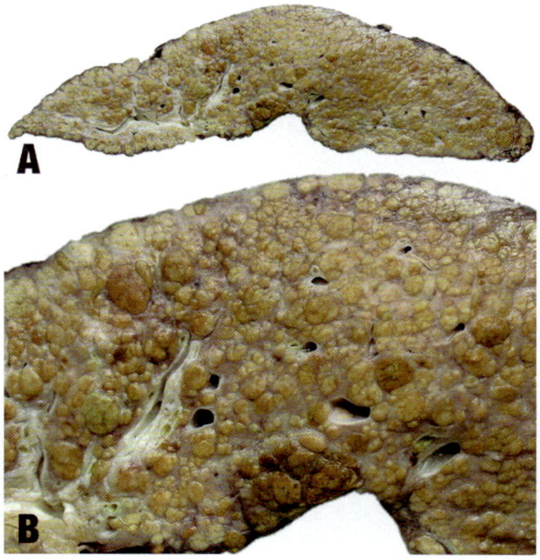

AUTOIMMUNE HEPATITIS (AIH) AND CIRRHOSIS

AIH is an uncommon cause of chronic hepatitis. It usually occurs in young women between the age 15 and 40 years. Findings in the blood include increased IgG level and a number of specific antibodies, such as: antinuclear antibody (ANA); anti–smooth muscle antibody (SMA); liver–kidney microsomal antibodies (LKM-1, LKM-2, LKM-3); and anti-soluble liver antigen and liver–pancreas antigen (SLA/LP). If left untreated, AIH can progress to cirrhosis.

FIGURE 12.23. Image (A) shows cirrhosis secondary to AIH: note the irregular, mixed micro- and macronodular pattern, and the variably wide fibrous septa (which are more prominent on the left side of the image). Note also the thrombosed portal vein (arrow). A closer view in (B) shows regenerative nodules and thrombus in the portal vein.

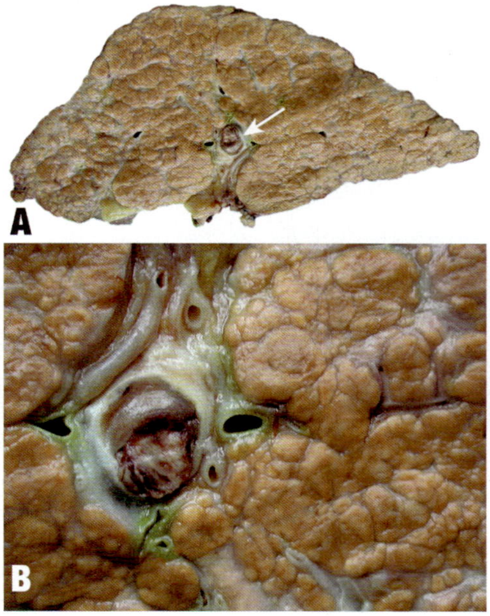

CIRRHOSIS FROM PRIMARY BILIARY CHOLANGITIS (PBC)

PBC is an autoimmune disease of middle-aged women (the female-to-male ratio is 9:1) characterized by florid ductal lesions composed of dense portal lymphoid aggregates and ductal centric granulomas. Most patients (more than 90%) have antimitochondrial antibodies against pyruvate dehydrogenase complex (PDC-E2), an enzyme complex found in the mitochondria. PBC can lead to cirrhosis of the liver, liver failure, cholangiocarcinoma, and hepatocellular carcinoma.

FIGURE 12.24. These images show an overall (A) and a close-up (B) view of a native liver transplanted for primary biliary cholangitis (PBC). Note the predominantly micronodular pattern of pale regenerative nodules with prominent intervening bile staining.

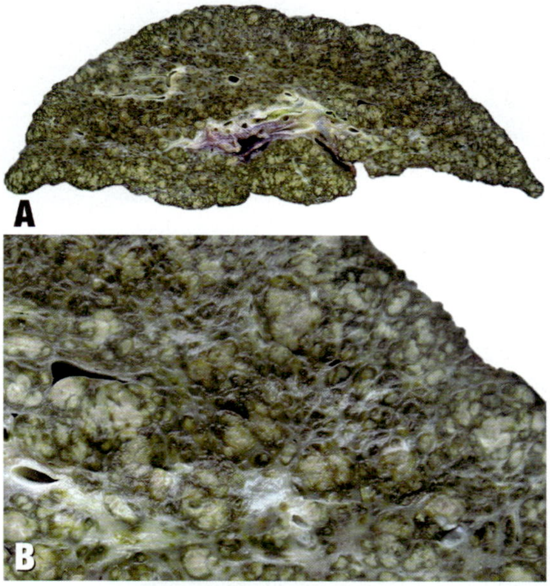

PRIMARY SCLEROSING CHOLANGITIS (PSC) AND BILIARY CIRRHOSIS

PSC is a chronic cholestatic liver disease characterized by bile duct fibrosis and stricturing. Inflammation and fibrosis of bile ducts and the liver cause impaired bile flow and progressive liver dysfunction.

FIGURE 12.25. This image shows a thickened, diseased large duct wall due to PSC.

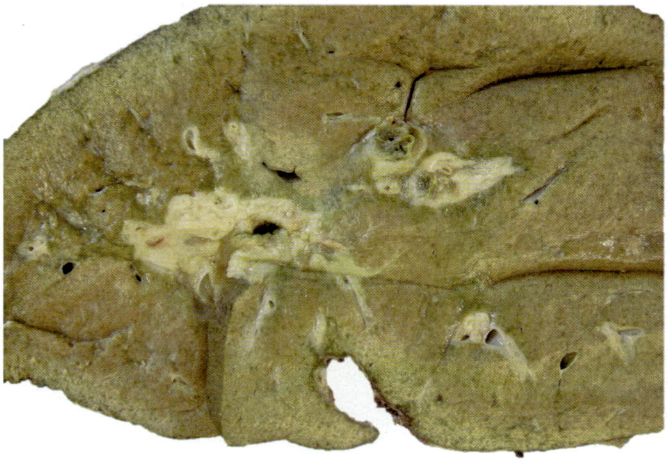

FIGURE 12.26. These images show an overall (A) and closer (B) view of a slice of native liver pretransplant with marked cholestasis and nodular regeneration. Dense fibrosis is evident in the top right subcapsular area.

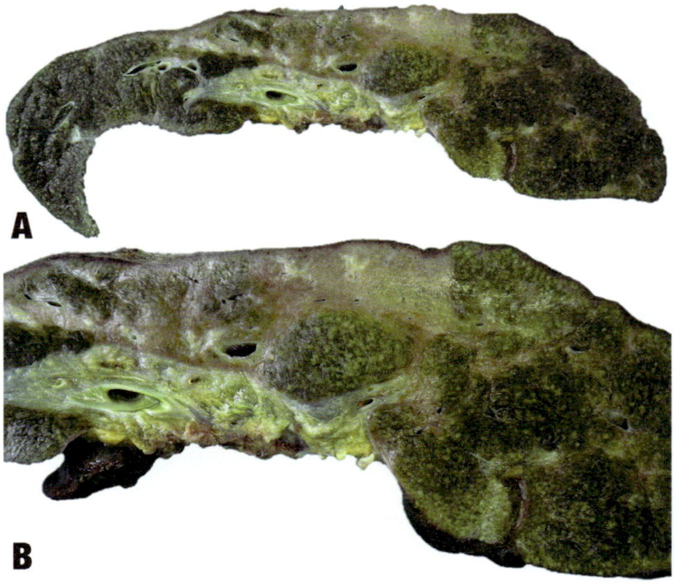

FIGURE 12.27. This liver shows marked green discoloration, large irregular regenerative nodules, dilated bile ducts filled with inspissated bile and stones (lower right), and an area of dense fibrosis (upper left). Due to the heterogeneity of bile duct involvement, the pattern of fibrosis and regeneration can show marked variation from area to area.

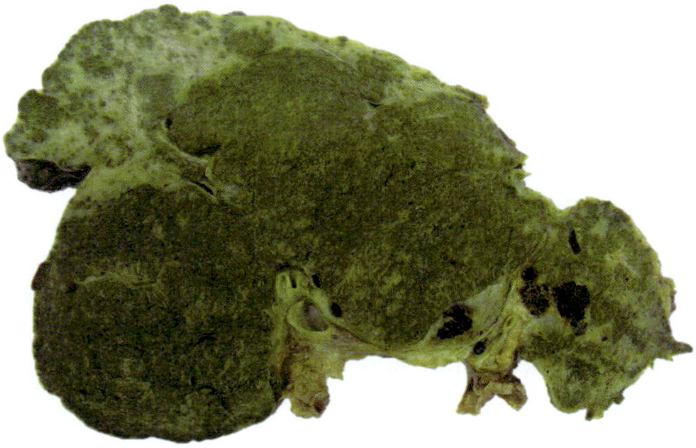

FIGURE 12.28. In this case, the liver contains smaller regenerative nodules with typical green discoloration.

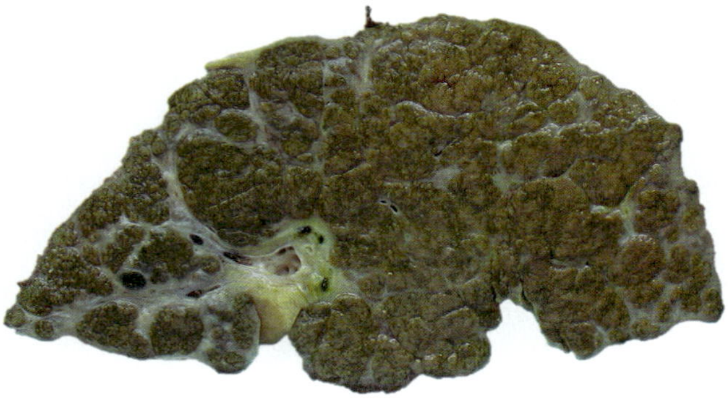

FIGURE 12.29. This image shows cirrhosis secondary to PSC in a patient with inflammatory bowel disease (IBD). The images show an overall (A) and closer (B) view of large regenerative nodules of biliary cirrhosis and marked intervening fibrosis surrounding the bile ducts. Note the central dilated bile duct (arrow). Approximately 75% of patients with PSC have IBD, most often ulcerative colitis.

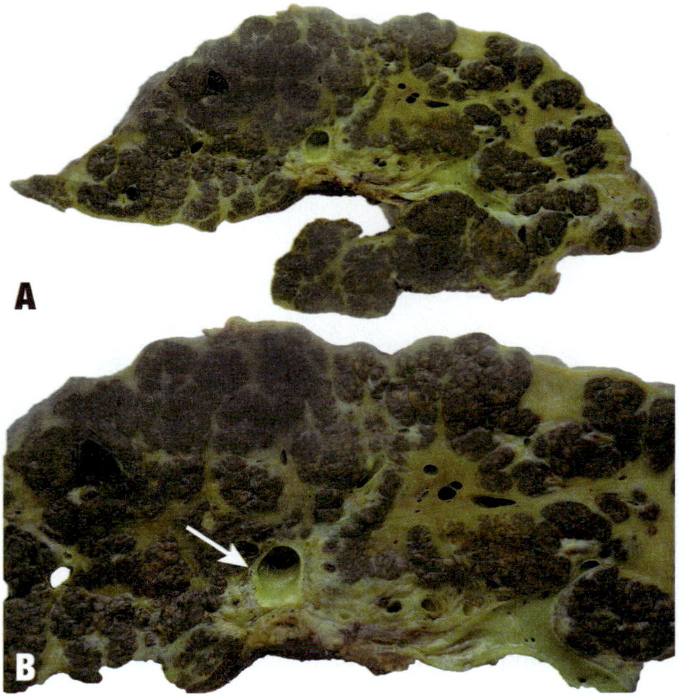

LANGERHANS CELL HISTIOCYTOSIS (LCH) AND CIRRHOSIS

LCH is a rare clonal disorder of Langerhans cells expressing S100, CD1a, and CD207/langerin. It has a range of clinical manifestations, from isolated bone lesions to multisystem disease. In the liver, LCH has a predilection for the bile ducts, which explains the ensuing biliary cirrhosis. Transplantation is a good option for patients with severe or progressive disease.

FIGURE 12.30. This case showed a characteristic pattern of biliary cirrhosis that had features of secondary sclerosing cholangitis on microscopy. The large central nodules are regenerative without bile discoloration. There was no carcinoma and no residual LCH.

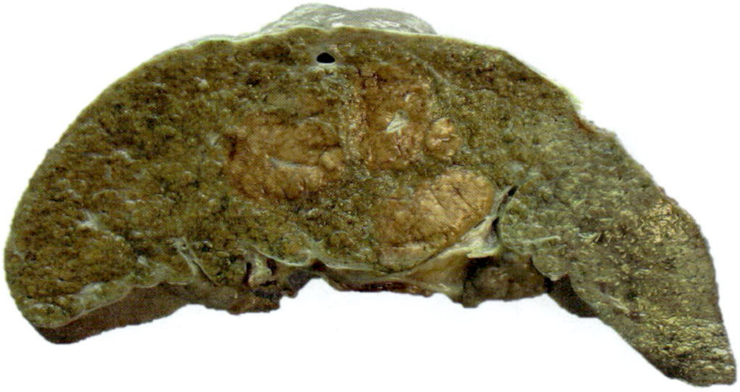

ALCOHOLIC CIRRHOSIS

Alcoholic cirrhosis is the major cause of liver disease in Western countries. Cirrhosis is part of the spectrum of alcoholic fatty liver disease (AFLD) that also includes steatosis, steatohepatitis, and hepatocellular carcinoma (HCC). Although steatosis will develop in any individual who consumes a large quantity of alcohol over a long period of time, only 15% to 20% of chronic alcohol users develop hepatitis or cirrhosis.

FIGURE 12.31. This image shows incomplete alcoholic cirrhosis with prominent portal vein thrombosis (arrows). Note the characteristic midzonal and centrilobular congestion and necrosis of the hepatocytes.

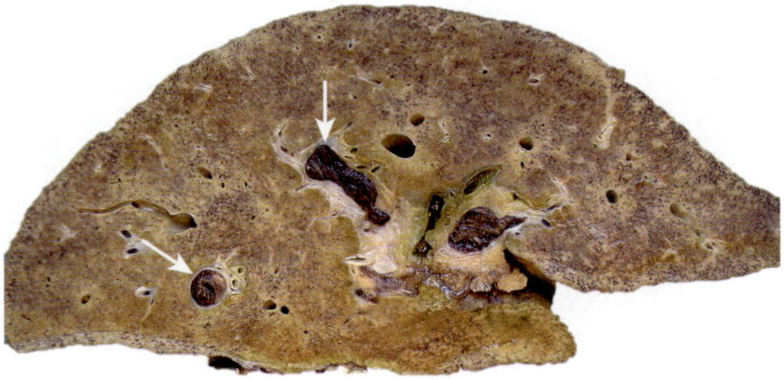

NONALCOHOLIC STEATOHEPATITIS (NASH) AND CIRRHOSIS

Histologically, NASH is characterized by steatosis, lobular inflammation, and ballooning degeneration of the hepatocytes. Compared with alcoholic hepatitis, NASH also has a relative paucity of well-formed Mallory–Denk bodies. About 20% of patients with NASH progress to cirrhosis.

FIGURE 12.32. This image shows a small, firm liver with a characteristic micronodular (nodule < 3 cm in diameter) cirrhosis.

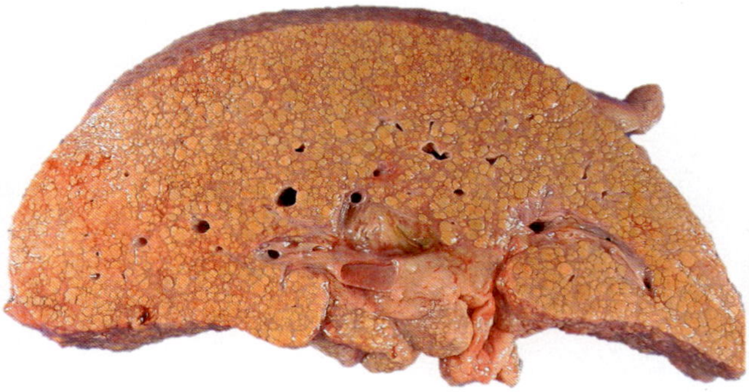

FIGURE 12.33. Image (A) shows micronodular cirrhosis due to NASH. Note the uniform yellow-orange-brown discoloration. A closer view in (B) of a liver edge shows nodules bulging from the surface of the liver, separated by retracted scar tissue.

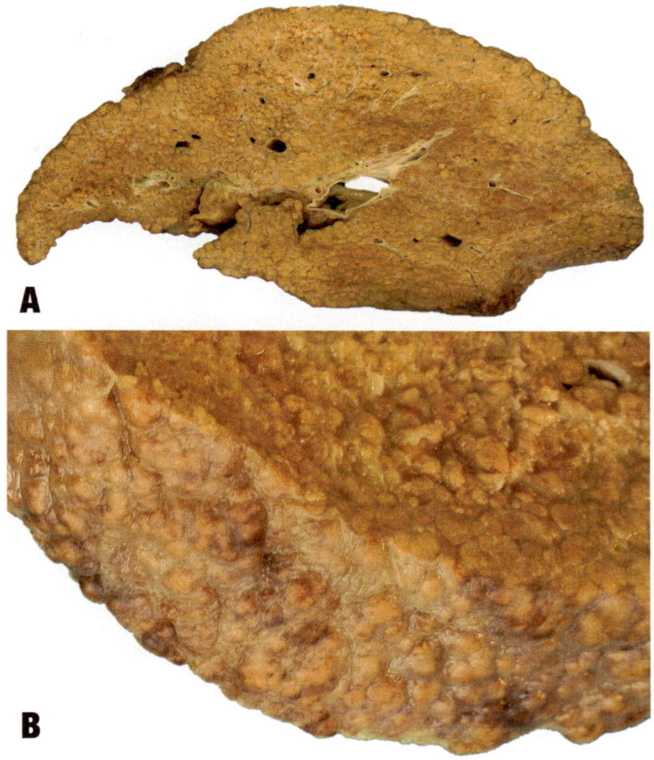

FIGURE 12.34. In (A), cirrhosis due to NASH shows a diffuse predominantly micronodular pattern. A closer view in (B) shows portal vein thrombosis in the hilum.

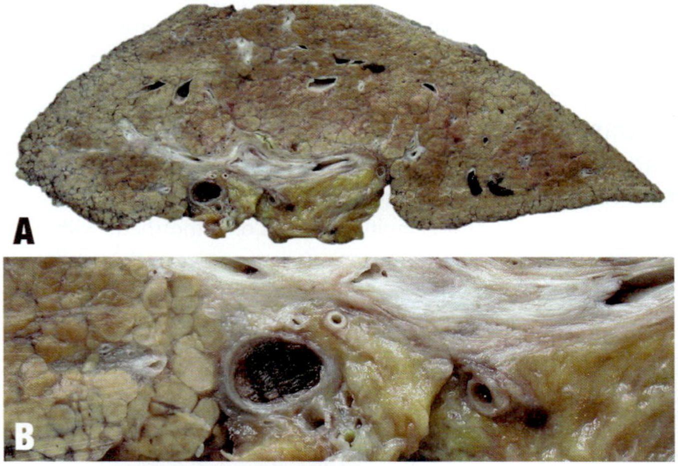

FIGURE 12.35. This image (A) shows micronodular cirrhosis due to end-stage alcoholic liver disease. The close-up view (B) is of small, regenerative nodules separated by fine bands of fibrosis. Although the micronodular pattern is characteristic of alcohol-related etiology, it is by no means pathognomonic.

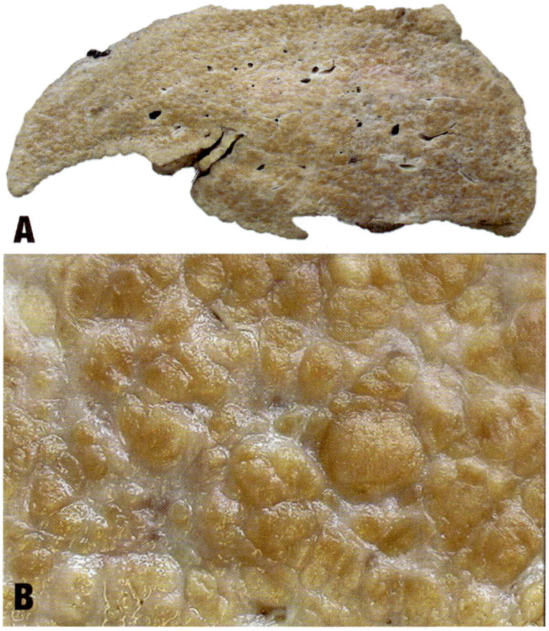

CARDIAC CIRRHOSIS

Cardiac cirrhosis is a rare complication of chronic heart failure. Most patients with heart failure do not progress to this advanced stage, but rather have bridging fibrosis between centrilobular and portal areas. Severe fibrosis and complete cirrhosis tend to occur in settings of superimposed portal vein thrombosis, Budd-Chiari syndrome, and other contributing factors such as ischemia, drugs, and viral hepatitides.

FIGURE 12.36. Image (A) shows a native liver with cardiac cirrhosis secondary to long-standing heart failure. The liver was removed at the time of a double heart and liver transplantation. A closer view in (B) shows multifocal areas of hemorrhage with variably prominent fibrous septa and regenerative nodules.

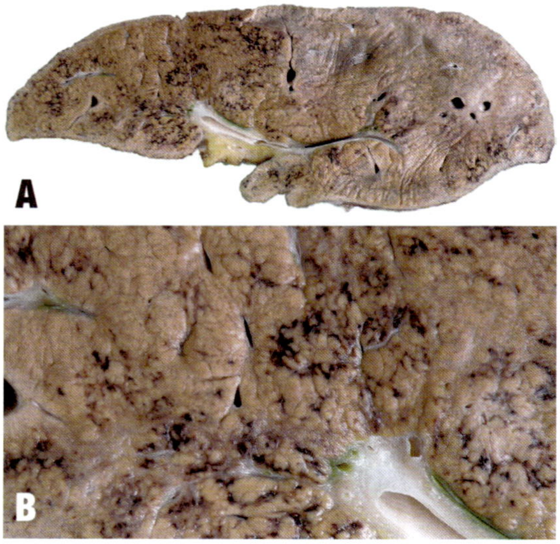

CRYPTOGENIC CIRRHOSIS

Most cases of cryptogenic cirrhosis were later found to be due to NASH in patients with various manifestations of the metabolic syndrome. The diagnosis of cryptogenic cirrhosis should be reserved for livers in which an exhaustive search for potential etiologies has failed.

FIGURE 12.37. This image shows a liver resected pretransplant for cryptogenic micronodular cirrhosis. Note the markedly distorted right and left lobes with coarse, small-to-medium, regenerative nodules. The gallbladder is visible in lower left of image.

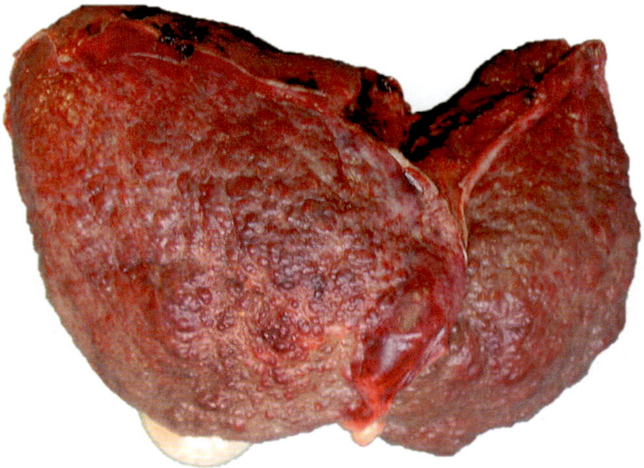

FIGURE 12.38. Image (A) shows a slice of the liver shown in Figure 12.37, emphasizing the uniform, micronodular pattern of cirrhosis. Image (B) shows a close-up of part of that slice, including the capsular surface with protruding nodules.

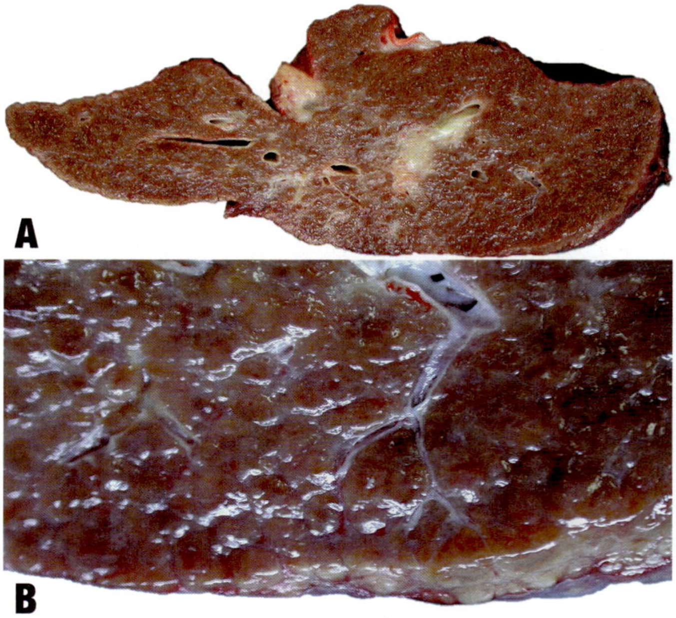

PROMINENT MACRONODULAR CIRRHOSIS DUE TO A COMBINATION OF HEPATITIS B AND ALCOHOL

FIGURE 12.39. The specimen in (A) demonstrates prominent macronodular cirrhosis due to both hepatitis B and alcohol. Large nodules with prominent cholestasis are separated by variably wide bands of dense fibrosis. A closer view in (B) reveals large nodules subdivided into small and medium-sized nodules, emphasizing the disorganization and heterogeneity of the process.

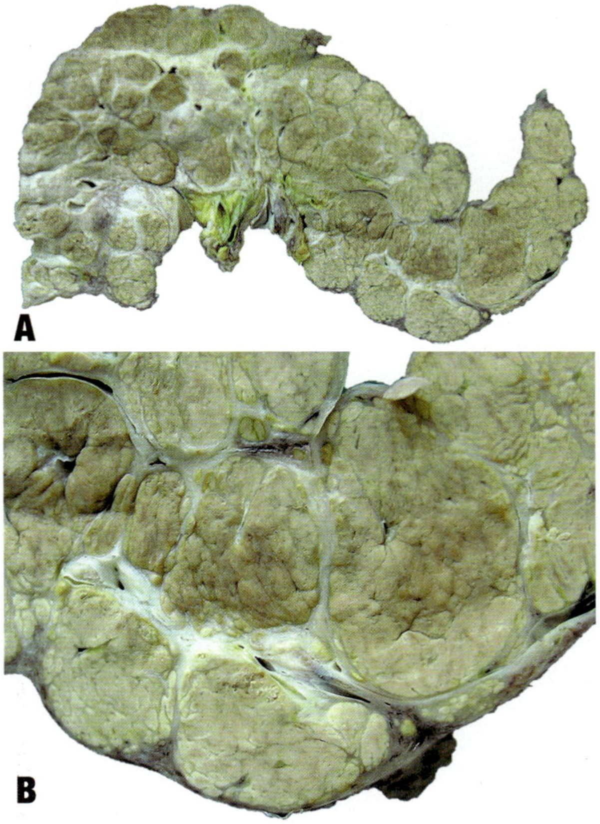

FIGURE 12.40. A magnetic resonance image from the patient in Figure 12.39 outlines findings that mirror those of the macroscopic specimen.

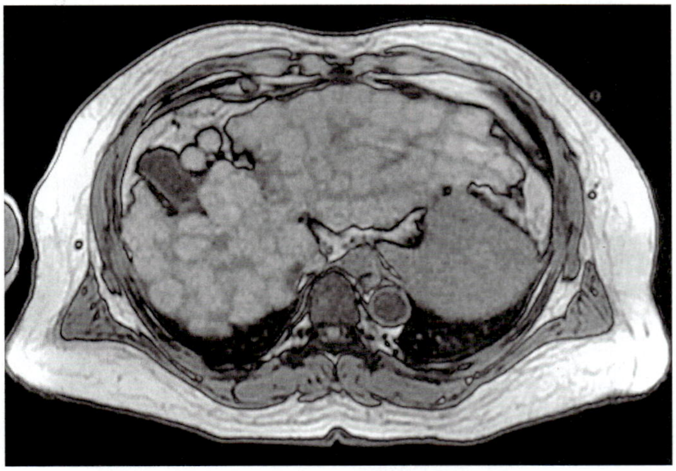

CIRRHOSIS DUE TO A COMBINATION OF NONALCOHOLIC STEATOHEPATITIS (NASH) AND HEPATITIS C

It is well known that NASH and hepatitis C act in concert to increase the incidence of cirrhosis.

FIGURE 12.41. Image (A) shows mixed micronodular and macronodular cirrhosis due to both NASH and hepatitis C. Image (B) shows prominent regenerating nodules; no carcinoma was found, despite these nodules.

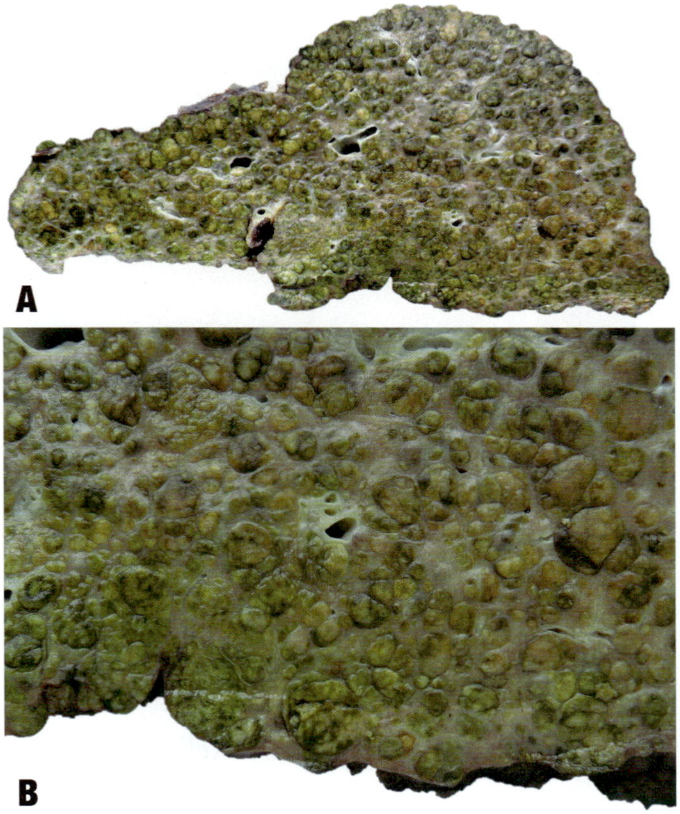

Amyloidosis of the liver

The liver is frequently involved in primary amyloidosis (amyloid light-chain associated with plasma cell neoplasms), in secondary amyloidosis of chronic inflammation (due to amyloid A), and in the hereditary and familial forms. The classic macroscopic appearance of "lardaceous" liver may occur with severe involvement. Microscopically, the deposits may be vascular or sinusoidal in the space of Disse. Hepatocytes become atrophic or disappear altogether due to compression.

FIGURE 12.42. A cross-section of this liver shows a yellow-brown color with a firm consistency.

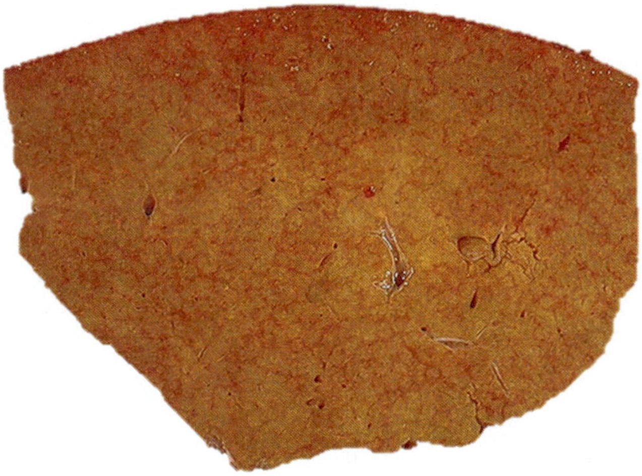

Focal nodular hyperplasia (FNH)

Focal nodular hyperplasia (FNH) is a nonneoplastic lesion that occurs most commonly in women. It is, however, unrelated to contraceptive drugs. The pathogenesis implicates hyperperfusion resulting from anomalous arteries.

FIGURE 12.43. A formalin-fixed partial liver resection shows a well-circumscribed nodule with a characteristic central stellate fibrous scar.

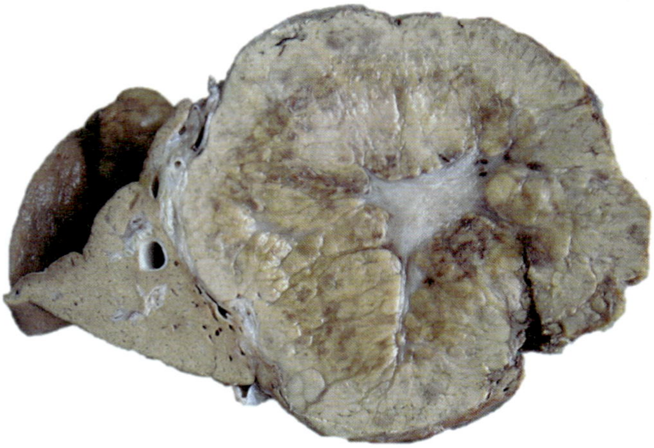

FIGURE 12.44. A fresh liver at autopsy shows FNH close to a central vein in a background of normal liver. Note the subtle central stellate fibrous area.

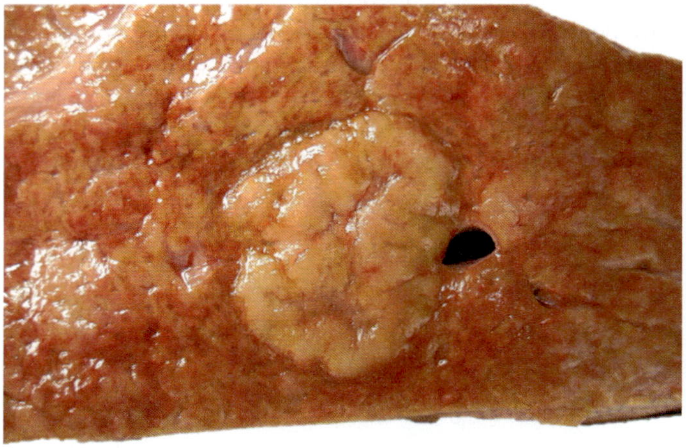

FIGURE 12.45. This image shows 2 adjacent nodules of FNH with focal hemorrhage.

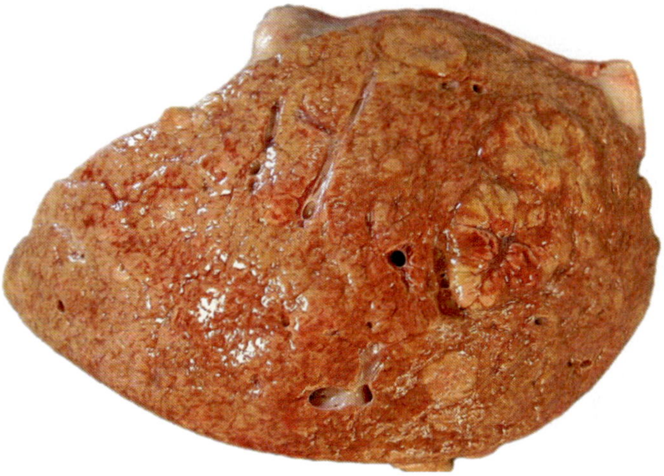

FIGURE 12.46. This image shows a closer view of a resected FNH. Note the thick, fibrous septa that subdivide the mass into multiple segments.

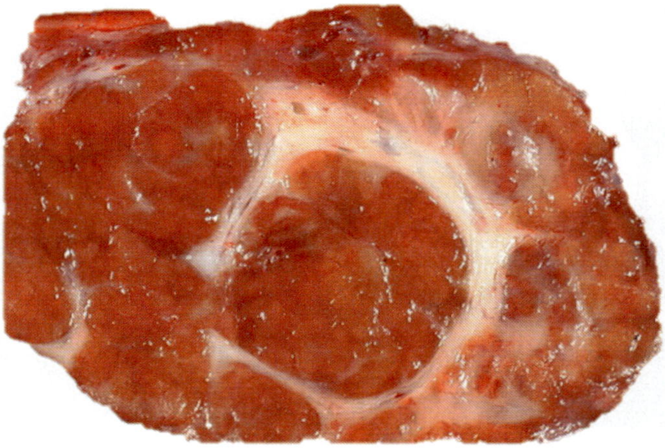

Liver hemangioma

Hemangioma is the most common benign liver lesion with an estimated prevalence ranging from 3% to 20%. Most are < 5 cm in diameter and patients are asymptomatic. Histologically, these are cavernous hemangiomas.

FIGURE 12.47. This image shows a large, solitary, well-demarcated, blood-filled mass with a central area of fibrosis.

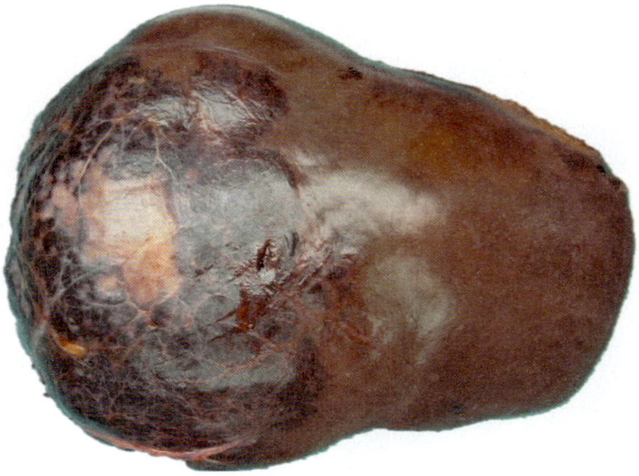

FIGURE 12.48. Although generally well circumscribed, this hemangioma (B) has an irregular, infiltrative pattern and is large (12 cm). A closer view in (C) shows the dark red, spongy appearance characteristic of liver hemangioma.

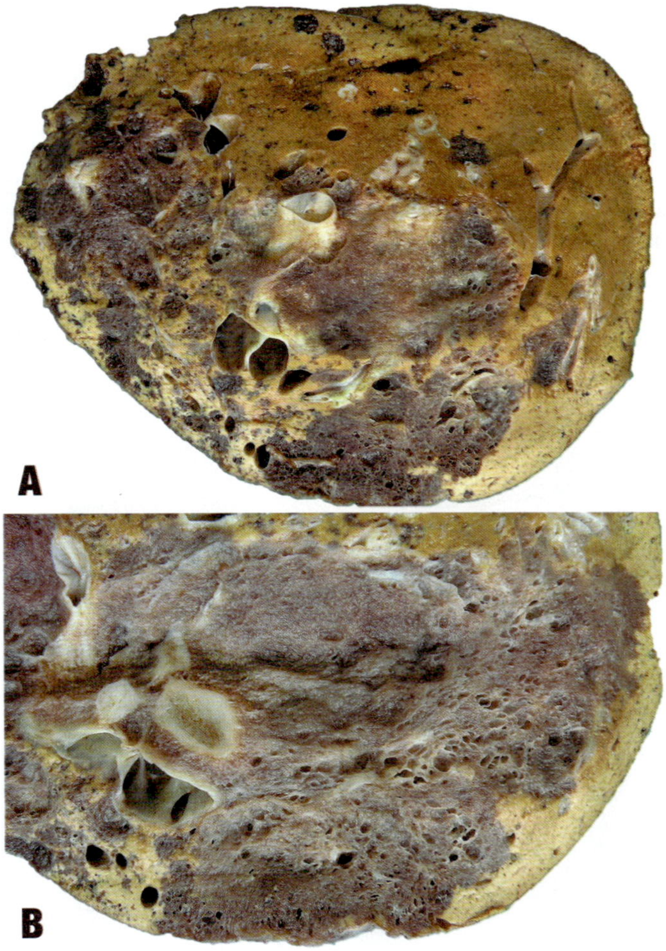

Hepatocellular adenoma (HCA)

HCA is a benign liver cell neoplasm that arises in noncirrhotic livers. It tends to occur in women taking oral contraceptives, although it has other associations and may also arise in men. The tumor is usually resected to prevent or treat acute intratumoral or intraperitoneal bleeding or, rarely, malignant transformation. Recent studies divide liver cell adenomas into 4 subtypes: *HNF1α*-mutated HCA; inflammatory HCA; β-catenin–mutated HCA; and unclassified HCA. Each subtype has distinctive histopathological features and associated prognoses.

FIGURE 12.49. This image shows a ruptured HCA of 6 cm in maximum diameter.

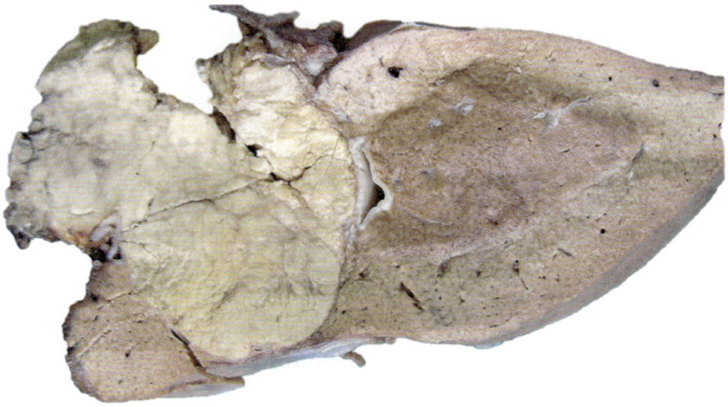

FIGURE 12.50. A subcapsular, well-demarcated tumor bulges from under the surface of the left lobe.

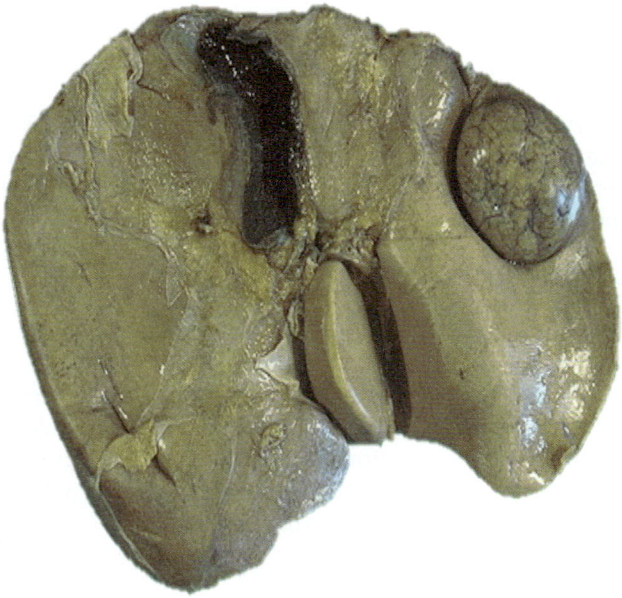

Courtesy of Dr. Vincent Falck

FIGURE 12.51. A partial resection of a liver shows a subcapsular, well-circumscribed, yellow mass close to the inked resection margin.

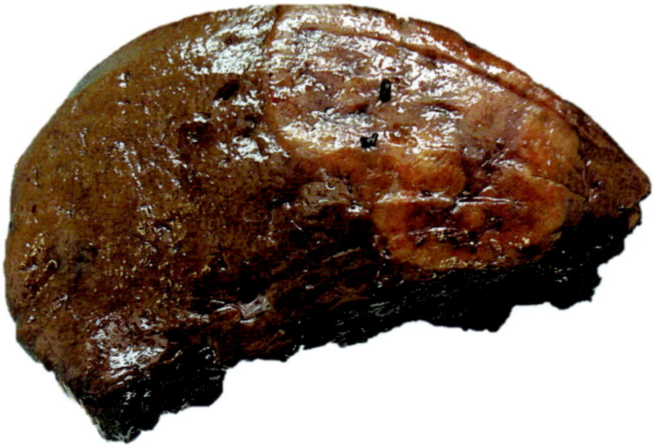

Liver mesenchymal hamartoma

Mesenchymal hamartomas are rare, benign tumors of young children (younger than 2 to 3 years). Patients generally present with respiratory distress or abdominal enlargement due to the large liver mass. Histologically, these tumors demonstrate mixed normal hepatocytes and bile ducts in myxoid fibrous stroma. Patients may exhibit high serum levels of α fetoprotein (AFP).

FIGURE 12.52. This partial liver resection depicts a well-circumscribed, cystic mass with myxoid fluid contents.

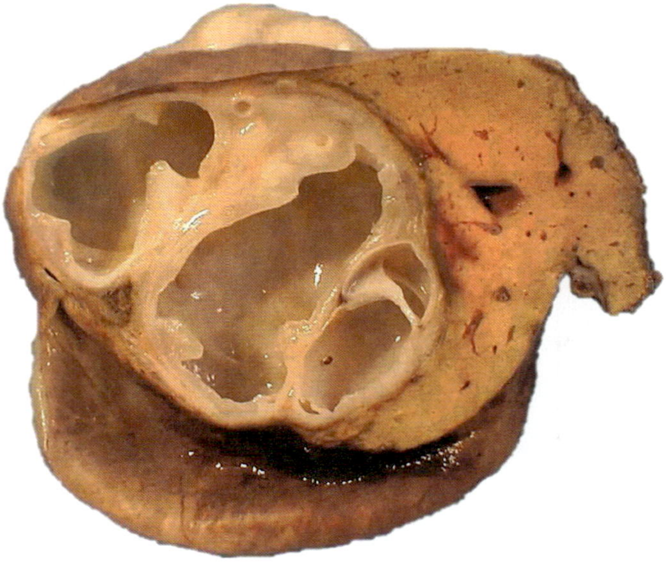

Liver Cancer

Hepatocellular carcinoma (HCC)

HCC develops in 2.4% of patients with chronic hepatitis B annually. The development of HCC is the result of repeated liver injury and regeneration, and a direct oncogenic effect of the hepatitis B virus.

CIRRHOTIC LIVER WITH SUSPICION OF HCC

Note that as the size of nodules in cirrhosis increases, the probability of dysplasia or carcinoma rises. Nodules < 2 cm are more likely benign; those > 2 cm are more likely malignant. It is important to sample all suspicious nodules for microscopic examination. There is a 15% to 30% error rate in the preoperative diagnosis of HCC compared with pathologic assessment of the explanted liver.

FIGURE 12.53. Image (A) shows cirrhosis due to hepatitis C with 1 large nodule suspicious for HCC. The closer view in (B) shows the large nodule has the same color as the surrounding parenchyma. This was, in fact, a large regenerative nodule, not a carcinoma.

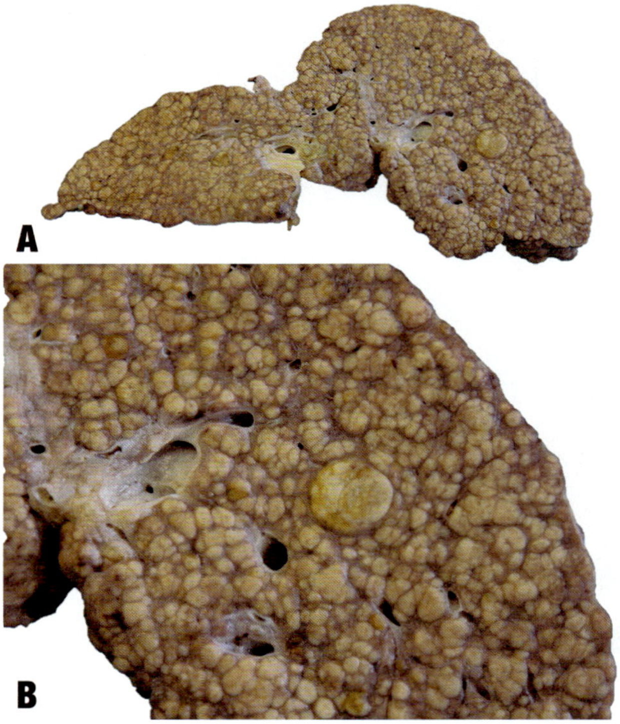

FIGURE 12.54. This is an example of cirrhosis due to NASH. On a background of micronodular cirrhosis, several large nodules are present, of which at least 1 is > 1 cm. There was no HCC.

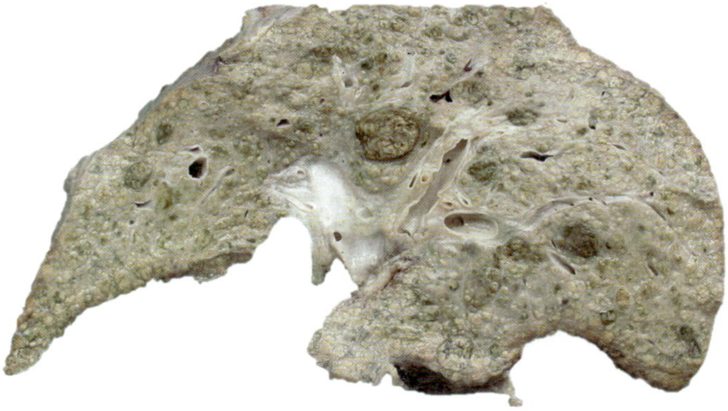

HCC AND HEPATITIS B–ASSOCIATED CIRRHOSIS

The HCCs that occur in hepatitis B–associated cirrhosis are often multifocal and associated with dysplastic nodules.

FIGURE 12.55. This image shows segment IV of the liver resected for an HCC located under the capsule (top). Inked resection margins are free of tumor. Note the pale, vaguely greenish lesion with a small satellite near the capsule; the surrounding liver showed mild steatosis and fibrosis (stage 3 out of 4). In general, HCCs < 5 cm in diameter are amenable to local resection, but this depends on other associated factors.

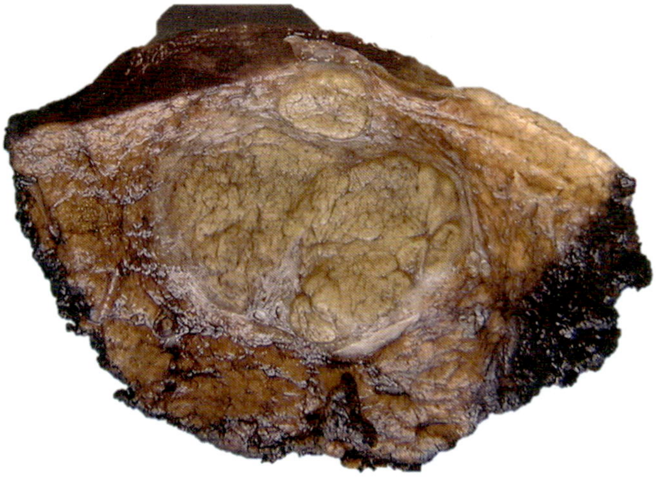

FIGURE 12.56. This image shows an HCC arising in a cirrhotic liver secondary to hepatitis B. It is a well-circumscribed white tumor in the right lobe.

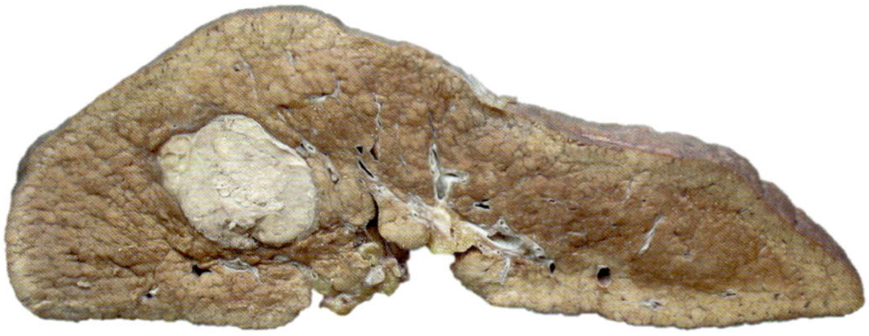

FIGURE 12.57. In this image, note the predominantly macronodular pattern of the cirrhosis (i.e., nodules > 3 mm) and the large, bulging HCC (top left).

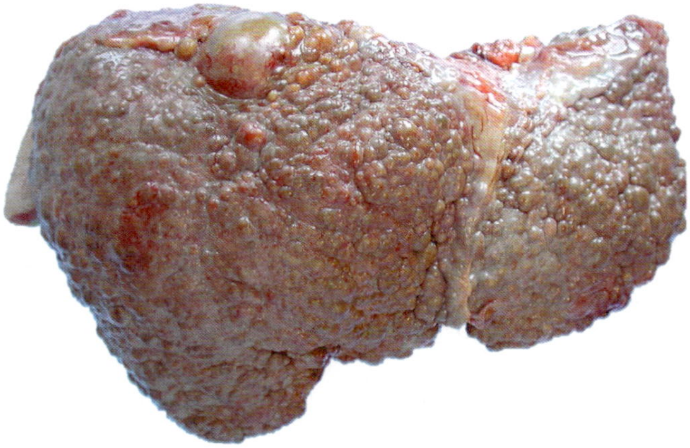

FIGURE 12.58. This image shows an HCC present at the top center of a specimen on a background of macronodular cirrhosis. The tumor is necrotic due to embolization.

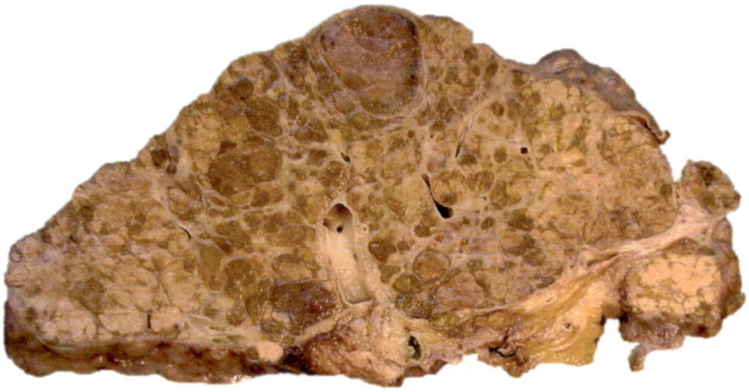

HEPATITIS B–ASSOCIATED HCC WITHOUT CIRRHOSIS

In North America, about 85% of HCCs arise in the context of cirrhosis and 15% arise in livers without cirrhosis, although many of noncirrhotic livers have at least some fibrosis. In the setting of chronic hepatitis B, 0.5% of HCCs occur without cirrhosis.

FIGURE 12.59. This image shows a large, poorly differentiated HCC on a background of hepatitis B without cirrhosis (but with fibrosis stage 2 of 4 on the Batts–Ludwig grading scale).

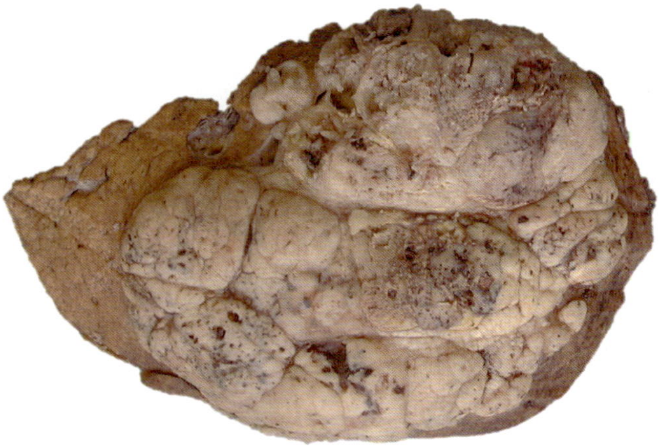

FIGURE 12.60. This image shows an HCC in a noncirrhotic liver. The tumor shows a variegated, bile-stained, pale yellow-and-green pattern clearly demarcated from the surrounding brown parenchyma.

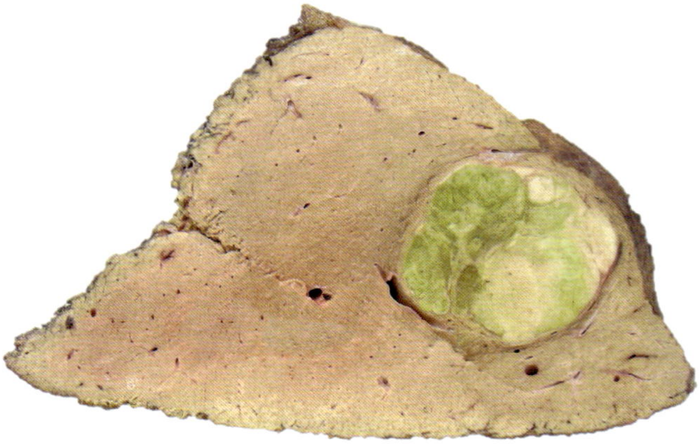

HCC WITH HEPATITIS C–ASSOCIATED CIRRHOSIS

Unlike hepatitis B, the risk of HCC in chronic hepatitis C is strongly linked to the presence of cirrhosis. In cirrhosis due to hepatitis C, the annual incidence of HCC is 1% to 7%.

FIGURE 12.61. Image (A) shows a native liver — explanted for cirrhosis due to combined hepatitis C and hemochromatosis — with a 1.2-cm HCC (arrow) and several regenerative nodules with dysplasia. Image (B) gives a close-up of the main nodule showing a distinctly different color than surrounding brown liver.

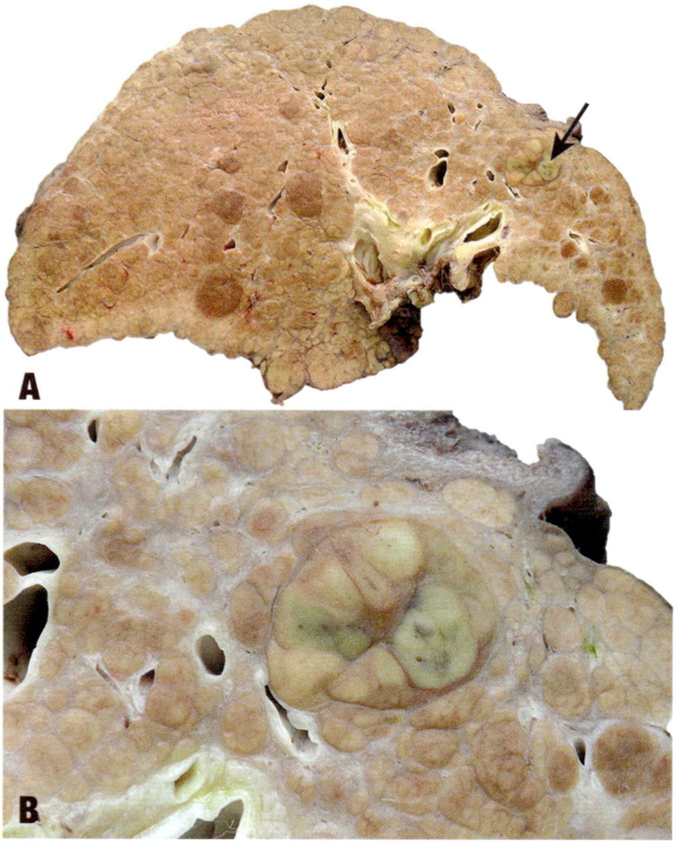

FIGURE 12.62. Image (A) shows a native liver with cirrhosis due to hepatitis C; a small (0.7 cm), well-to-moderately differentiated HCC is present (top center). Image (B) gives a closer view of this lesion. Note the contrast of the pale tumor on the surrounding tawny nodules.

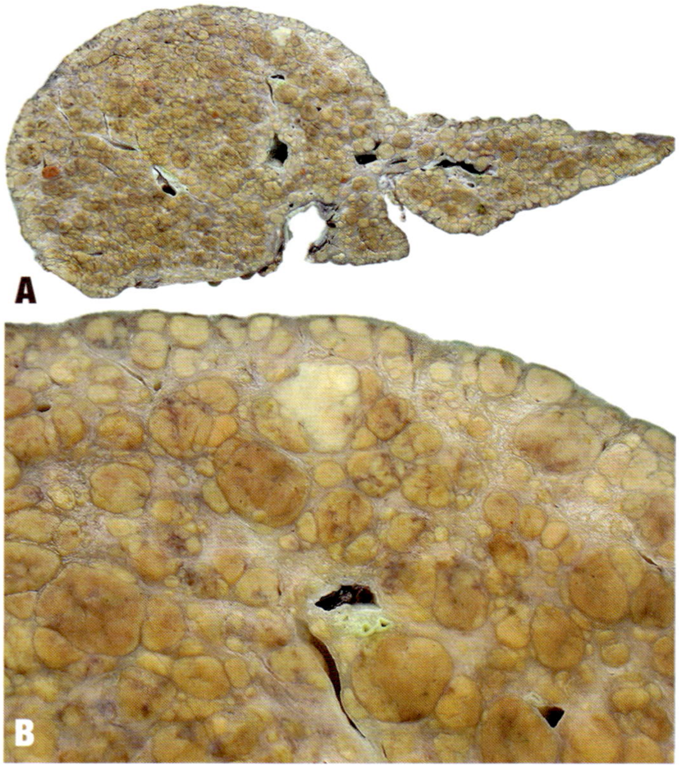

FIGURE 12.63. This is a native liver with cirrhosis due to hepatitis C; it has several HCCs of variable size, concentrated particularly in the right tip and upper left of the specimen. The other nodules would have to be assessed individually to determine whether they are regenerative or malignant. No vascular invasion was found.

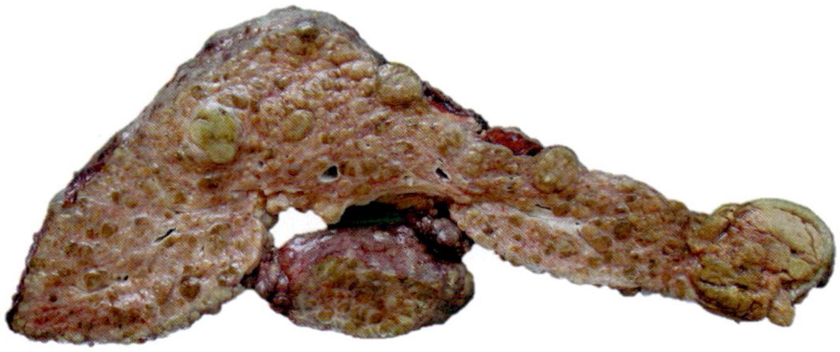

FIGURES 12.64. Image (A) gives a closer view of Figure 12.63, showing it to be a partly necrotic friable HCC. Smaller nodules in (B) show multilobulated and variegated discoloration.

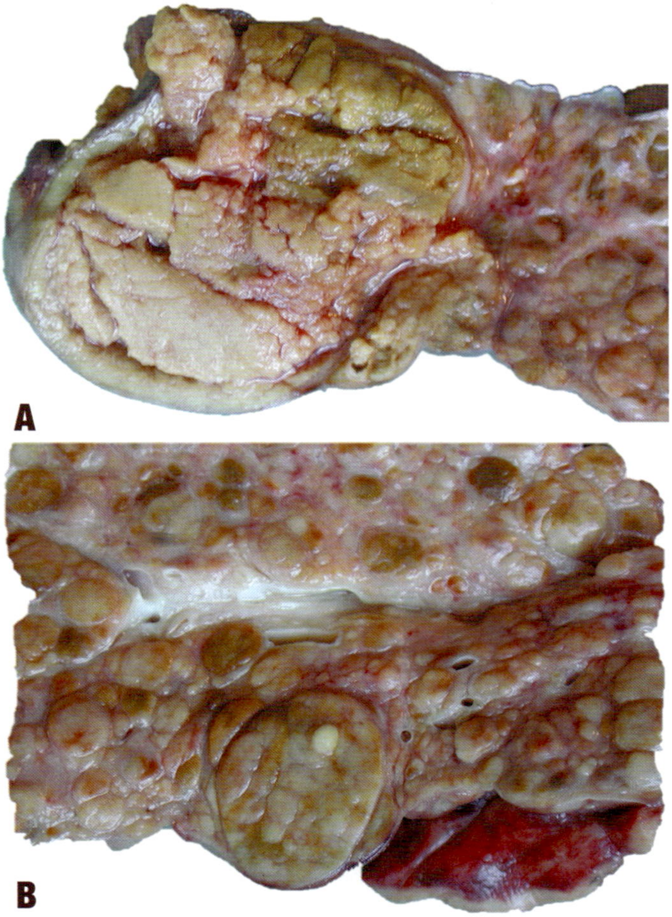

FIGURE 12.65. This image shows a poorly differentiated HCC, 8.5 cm maximum diameter, arising in a patient with chronic hepatitis C, stage 3 out of 4. There is 1 main mass with adjacent smaller extensions; the main mass invaded bile ducts and the diaphragm, but not vessels. Note the finely nodular pattern of the background liver.

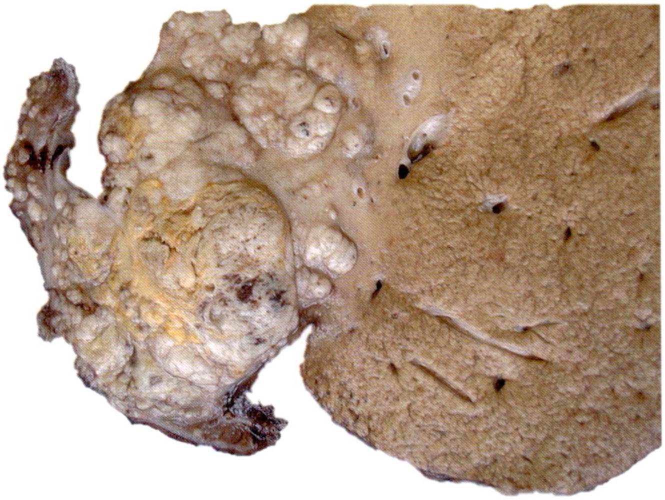

HCC AND STEATOHEPATITIS

FIGURE 12.66. Image (A) shows a native liver with cirrhosis due to steatohepatitis and a large multifocal HCC with numerous satellite lesions. Image (B) gives a closer view: note the yellow-brown coloration of the nonneoplastic liver due to the steatosis. Note also the fine, fibrous septa and regenerative nodules.

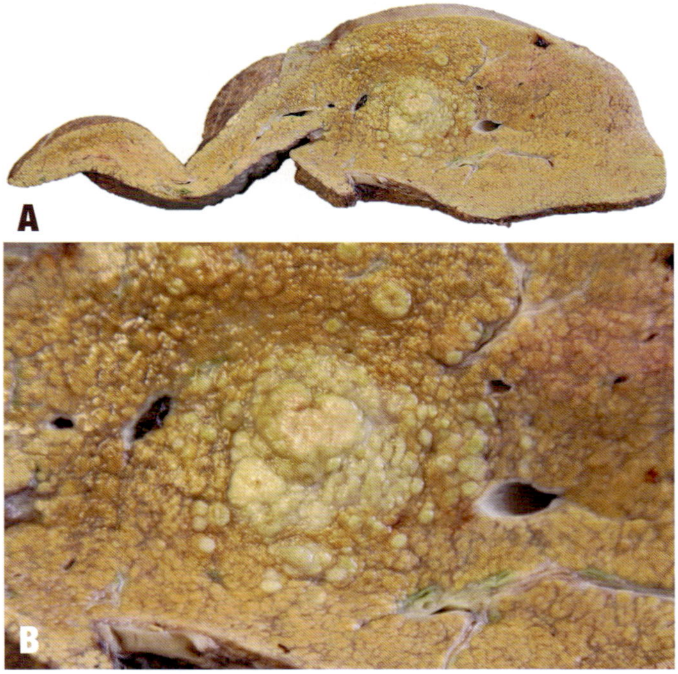

FIGURE 12.67. These images show a resected liver (segments VI to VIII) specimen, both fresh (A) and fixed (B), with a single HCC. The large (10.5 cm in maximum diameter), well-circumscribed tumor appears paler than the surrounding liver parenchyma. The nonneoplastic liver showed steatosis involving 20% of hepatocytes with portal and periportal fibrosis. There was no cirrhosis.

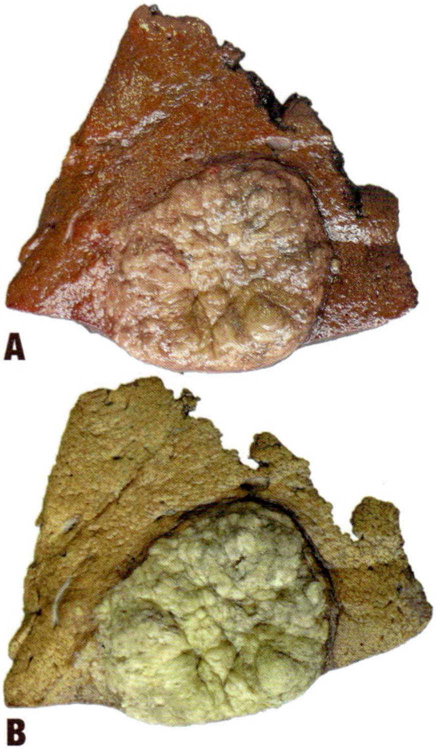

HCC AND CIRRHOSIS SECONDARY TO NASH

FIGURES 12.68. This image shows a liver with cirrhosis secondary to NASH, and a mix of large, regenerative nodules and HCCs. This image illustrates the potential difficulty in distinguishing HCCs from the background of regenerating macronodules of cirrhosis. In (A), note the predominantly macronodular pattern of the cirrhosis. In (B), note the similar color of the HCC to the surrounding nodules; in this case, size is the factor that clearly distinguishes the HCC from the rest of the specimen.

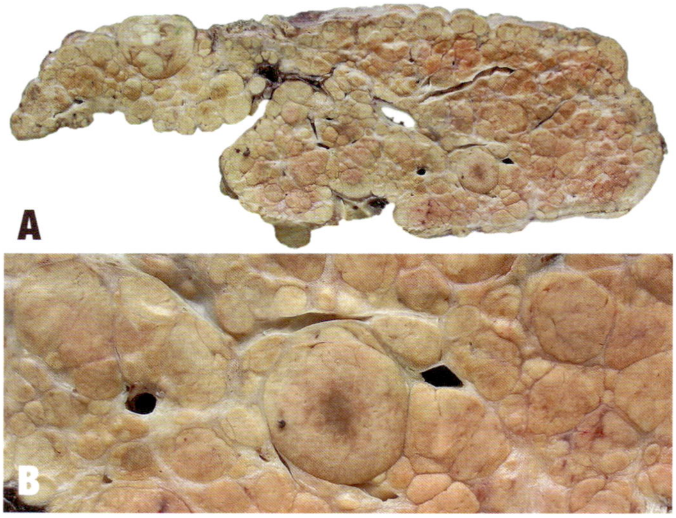

FIGURES 12.69. These images show a larger nodule from the liver pictured in Figure 12.68: (A) another slice and (B) a closer view. The nodule proved to be HCC.

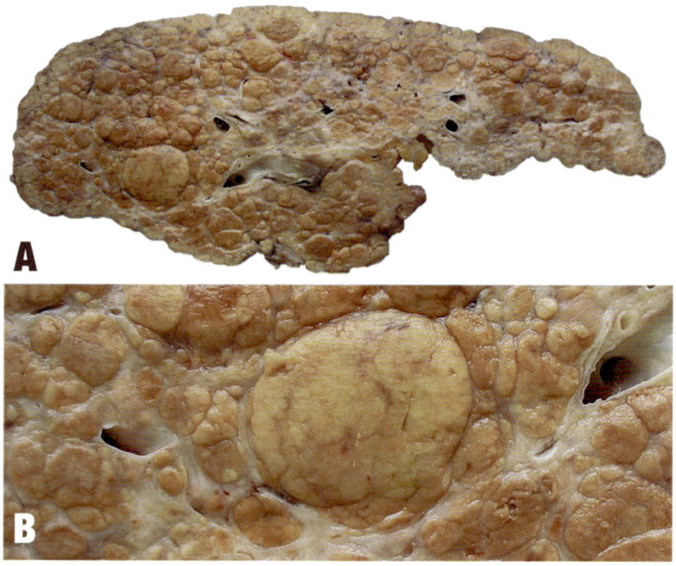

HCC POST–EMBOLIZATION THERAPY

Embolization therapy reduces the size of an HCC to enable resection or transplantation. The normal hepatic parenchyma is supplied mostly by the portal venous system, whereas the carcinoma is supplied by the hepatic artery. Embolization via the hepatic artery can selectively destroy the tumor.

FIGURE 12.70. This image shows a large, poorly differentiated HCC in a resected right lobe; the lesion is 12.5 cm in maximum diameter. Note the variegated appearance with extensive, pale yellow necrosis and hemorrhage secondary to the embolization.

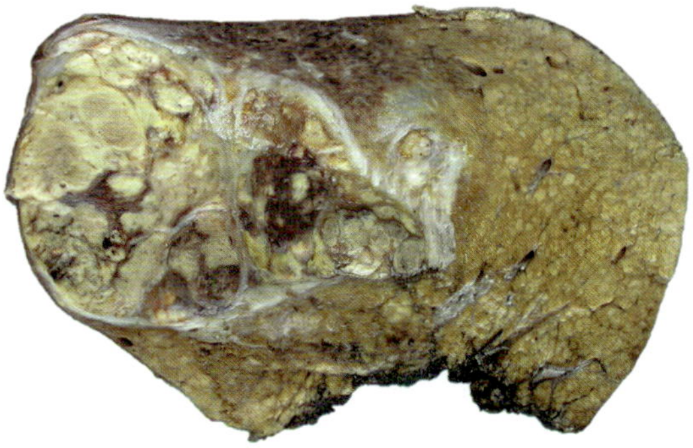

HCC POSTCHEMOTHERAPY

FIGURE 12.71. Overall (A) and close-up (B) of a cirrhotic liver with multiple HCCs in both lobes. Note the variegated, pale green discoloration of the tumor nodules. The patient had received neoadjuvant chemotherapy causing necrosis of some of the nodules (arrow).

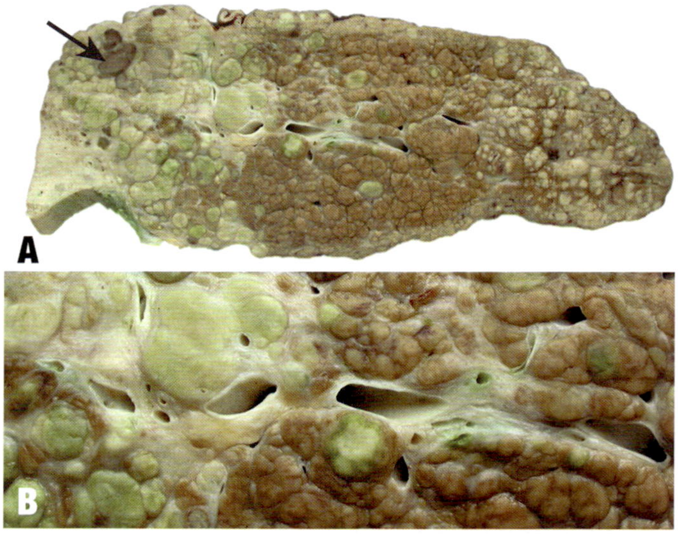

HCC WITH UNUSUAL GROSS APPEARANCE

FIGURE 12.72. This image shows multiple tan-white tumors of variable size that mimic metastatic carcinoma, neuroendocrine tumor, or cholangiocarcinoma.

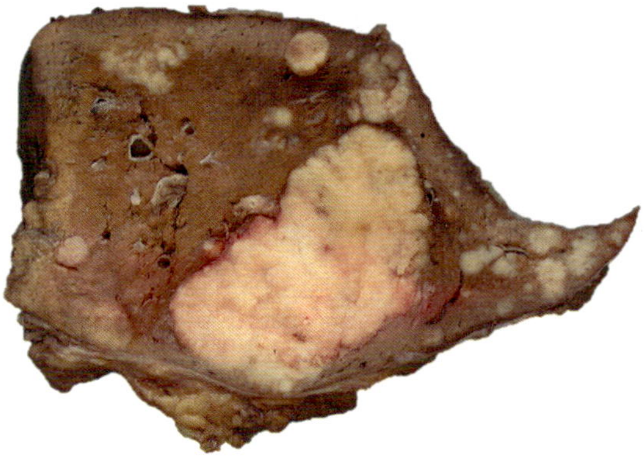

HCC IN A CIRRHOTIC LIVER SECONDARY TO HEMOCHROMATOSIS

The incidence of HCC in hemochromatosis is about 8% to 10%.

FIGURE 12.73. This liver is dark brown due to iron overload; the cirrhosis is mixed macro- and micronodular. The HCC is 4 cm in maximum diameter (white arrow). An attached adrenal gland is present in this hepatectomy specimen (red arrow).

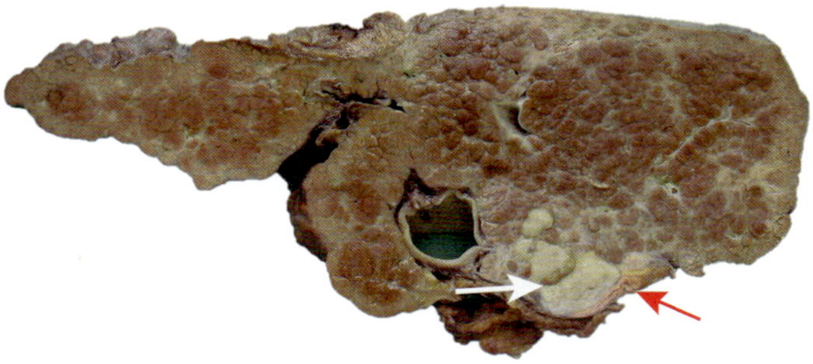

FIBROLAMELLAR HCC

Fibrolamellar carcinoma is a rare type of HCC arising in noncirrhotic livers and more common in young patients. The prognosis is similar to HCCs in noncirrhotic livers, but better than HCCs in cirrhotic livers.

FIGURE 12.74. This image shows a well-circumscribed, lobulated tumor with a central white, radiating, fibrous scar. This appearance overlaps with that of focal nodular hyperplasia, but the bile-related greenish discoloration may help in the distinction.

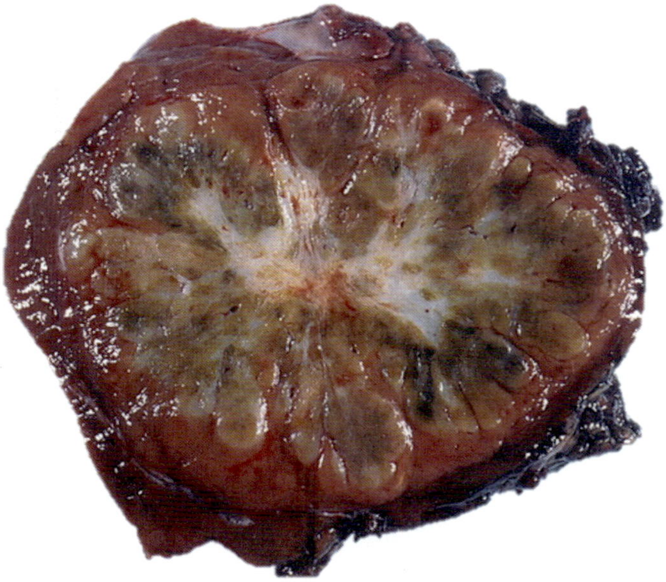

Combined HCC and cholangiocarcinoma

Combined HCC and cholangiocarcinomas comprise about 5% of hepatic carcinomas.

FIGURE 12.75. Image (A) shows mixed micro- and macronodular cirrhosis due to hepatitis C with mixed hepatocellular and cholangiocarcinoma. Note the intravascular tumor thrombus (arrow). A closer view in (B) of another area of the liver shows an intravascular thrombus.

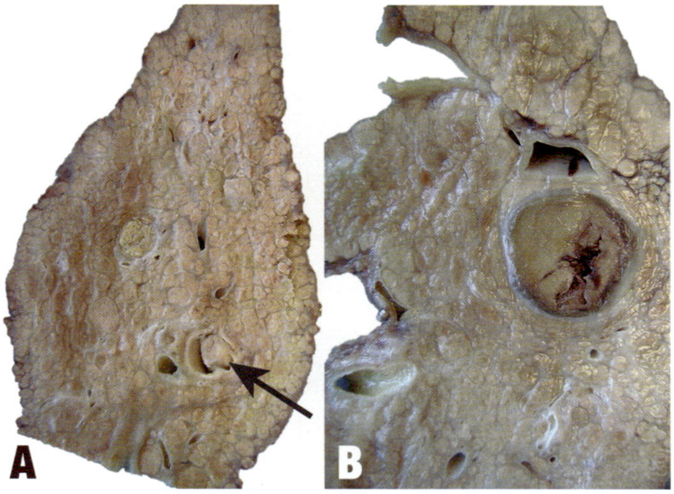

Cholangiocarcinoma

Cholangiocarcinomas arise from bile duct epithelium. Known risk factors include primary sclerosing cholangitis; infection with the parasitic liver flukes *Opisthorchis viverrini* or *Clonorchis sinensis*; congenital liver malformations; and exposure to Thorotrast (thorium dioxide).

FIGURE 12.76. This image shows a large, white mass — the cholangiocarcinoma — near the hilar area in the background of an otherwise noncirrhotic liver. The green color of liver parenchyma is likely due to cholestasis caused by obstruction of the bile ducts.

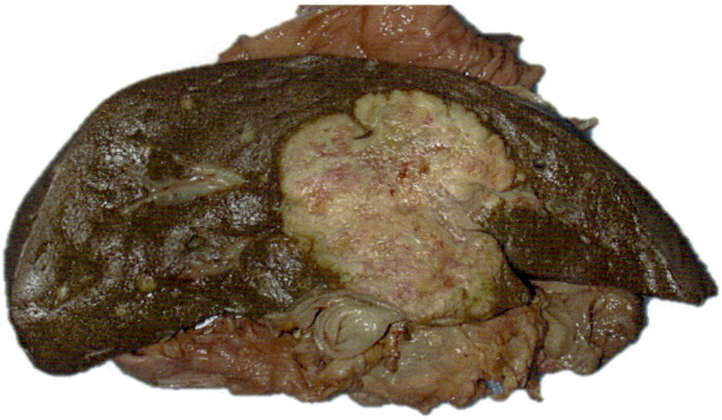

INTRAHEPATIC CHOLANGIOCARCINOMA

Although cholangiocarcinoma is an epithelial malignancy of bile duct origin, some authors prefer to restrict the term to only those lesions arising in intrahepatic bile ducts, because they behave more aggressively than those of extrahepatic bile duct origin.

FIGURE 12.77. This partially resected liver shows infiltrative white tumor growing along the intrahepatic duct and extending to the hilum. The background liver is not cirrhotic.

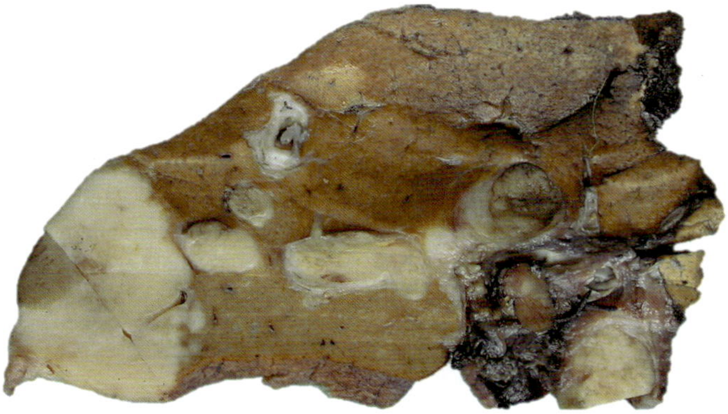

KLATSKIN TUMOR (PERIHILAR OR HILAR CHOLANGIOCARCINOMA)

Klatskin tumor (the eponym for perihilar or hilar cholangiocarcinoma) is a cholangiocarcinoma arising at the bifurcation of the common bile duct into left and right hepatic ducts. This type of tumor has a better prognosis than intrahepatic or peripheral cholangiocarcinomas, probably because it is more often amenable to local resection or transplantation.

FIGURE 12.78. Serial sections of this partial liver resection illustrate an infiltrative white tumor in the hilar area and along the intrahepatic duct. The background liver has no cirrhosis.

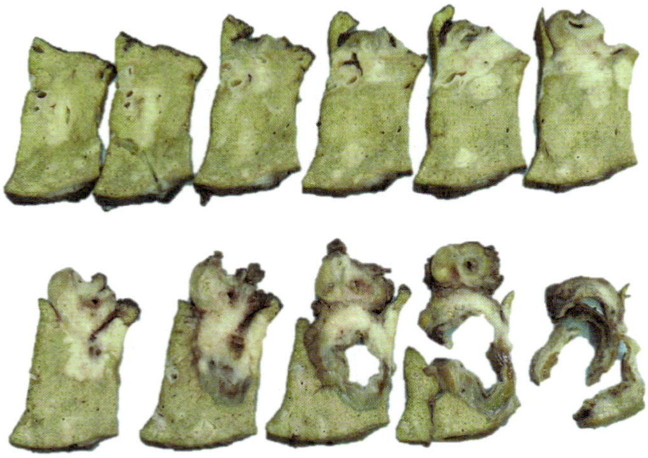

Embryonal (or undifferentiated) sarcoma of the liver

Embryonal sarcomas typically present in children aged 6 to 10 years as rapidly growing cystic masses. Although their prognosis has traditionally been poor, significant improvements have been achieved with combined surgery and chemotherapy.

FIGURE 12.79. This image shows a cystic tumor with necrosis and blood clot. It is separated from the adjacent liver parenchyma by a fibrous pseudocapsule.

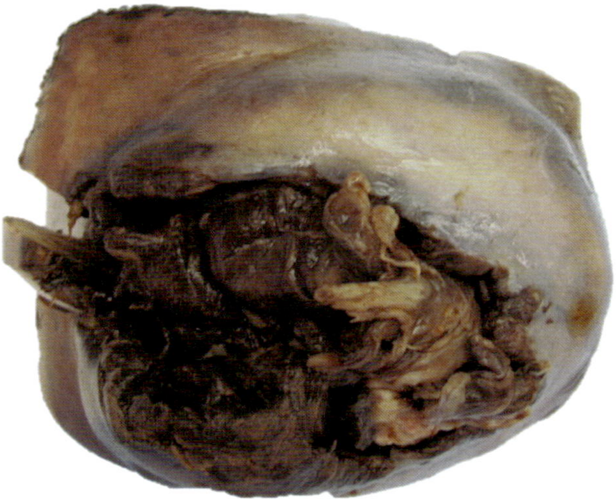

Courtesy of Dr. Van Hung Nguyen

Primary hepatic malignant fibrous histiocytoma (MFH)

MFHs are extremely rare. Storiform–pleomorphic, myxoid, giant cell, and inflammatory variants have been described. The precise origin of MFH cells has been disputed and the concept of fibrohistiocytic differentiation has been challenged. Note that the World Health Organization (WHO) advocates a new name for this entity: undifferentiated pleomorphic sarcoma.

FIGURE 12.80. This large MFH is partly viable (white fleshy cut surface, upper left), and partly necrotic (variegated area, lower right).

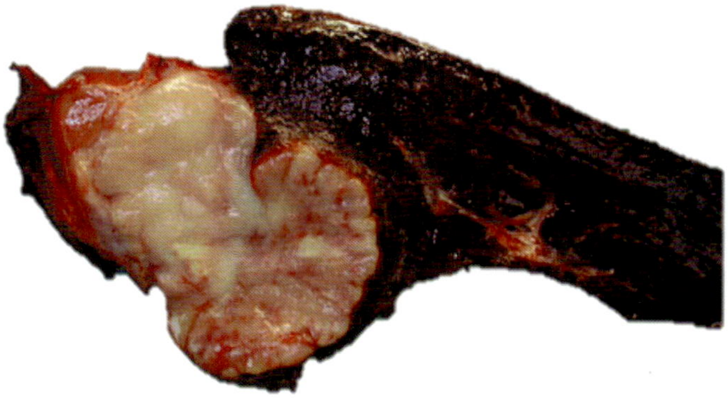

Angiosarcoma of the liver

Hepatic angiosarcomas are rare vascular endothelial cell malignancies; about 10 to 20 cases occur each year in the United States. They have been linked to several environmental carcinogens, including vinyl chloride monomer, arsenic-containing insecticides, and Thorotrast, among others.

FIGURE 12.81. This large tumor bulges from the capsule and extends deep into the parenchyma, with extensive hemorrhage and necrosis. There is no clear demarcation between the nonneoplastic parenchyma and the tumor, because the malignant endothelial cells can travel along the sinusoids far beyond the apparent edge of the mass.

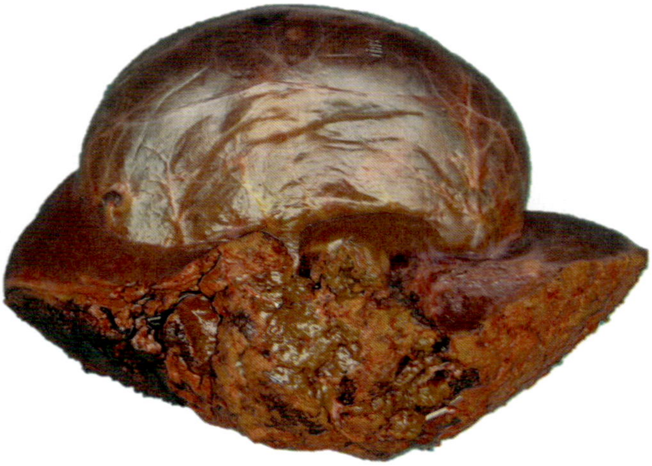

FIGURE 12.82. This partial resection (note the inked resection margin, lower left) shows a well-circumscribed lesion with extensive necrosis and focal hemorrhage.

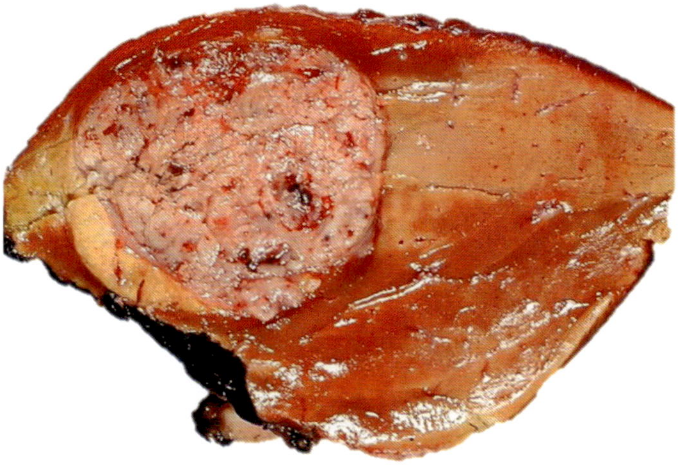

Hepatoblastoma

Hepatoblastoma is the most common hepatic tumor in neonates and young children, with a mean age of 18 months. Histologically, it is divided into 2 main types: epithelial and mixed epithelial–mesenchymal. Up to 90% of patients have elevated AFP. Patients may have other associated congenital abnormalities, such as cleft palate, macroglossia, and absence of the right adrenal gland, among others. If the tumor is resectable, the mainstay of therapy is surgery; however, neoadjuvant chemotherapy has substantially improved 5-year survival for larger, initially unresectable tumors.

Metastasis to the liver

The most common primary sites of metastases to the liver are the colon and rectum, breast, and lung.

METASTATIC COLORECTAL CARCINOMA

The liver is the most common site of metastasis for colorectal carcinoma: about 50% to 60% of patients with colorectal carcinoma develop liver metastases. These metastases may be multiple, and either synchronous (about one-third of cases) or metachronous (about two-thirds of cases). The survival of patients with metastatic colorectal carcinoma has risen from below 10% to, currently, 25% to 40%. This improvement comes from combining surgery with neoadjuvant and adjuvant chemotherapy, or embolization therapy. It means that many resected liver metastases are partially or subtotally necrotic on pathologic examination.

FIGURE 12.83. This image shows a single, well-circumscribed, subcapsular mass with extensive pale yellow necrosis and few foci of hemorrhage on a background of normal liver tissue.

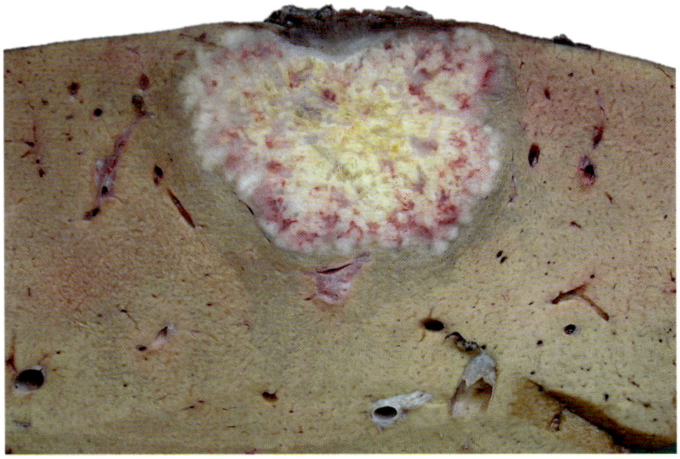

FIGURE 12.84. This image shows part of a right lobe of a liver with a single, subcapsular, irregular, pale metastasis, well away from a jagged inked resection margin (lower right).

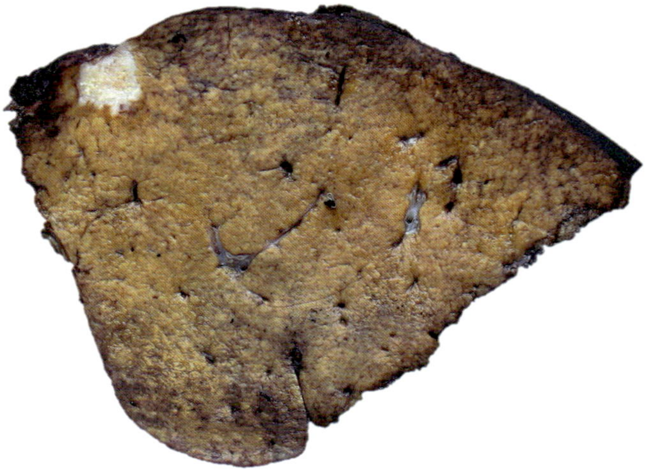

FIGURE 12.85. Slices of a resection specimen show a large, pale, multinodular, partly hemorrhagic mass. The inked resection margin (arrow) is free of the carcinoma.

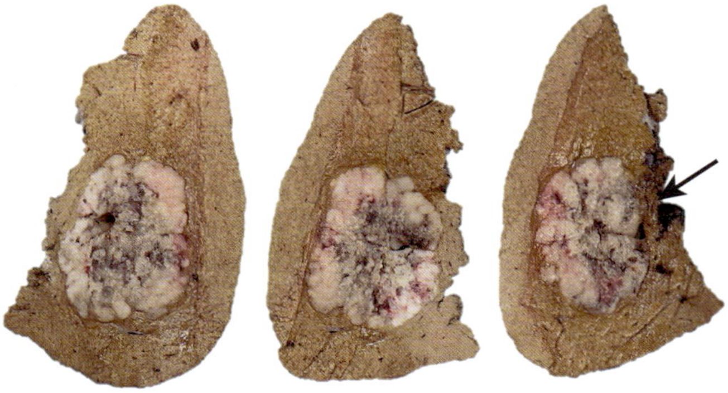

FIGURE 12.86. This image shows a slice of a partial liver resection for metastatic colorectal carcinoma following neoadjuvant chemotherapy with oxaliplatin. The carcinoma (subcapsular, lower right) is largely necrotic. The background parenchyma illustrates typical features of "blue liver syndrome" with sinusoidal obstruction leading to centrilobular congestion, hemorrhage, and hepatocyte necrosis.

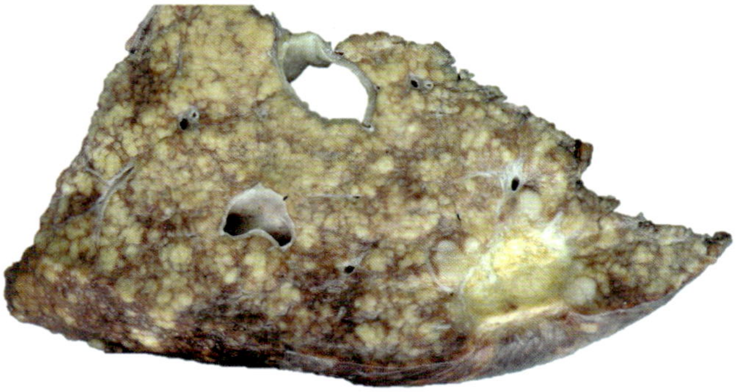

FIGURE 12.87. This image shows another example of metastatic colorectal carcinoma following chemotherapy. This patient was treated with oxaliplatin for 12 weeks prior to liver resection. There are multiple metastases. In this close-up view, the background liver shows nodular regenerative hyperplasia (NRH), a condition characterized by a vague nodularity resulting from the collapse of parenchyma between centrilobular areas with increased reticulin staining and without fibrosis. NRH arises from the acute damage caused by chemotherapy.

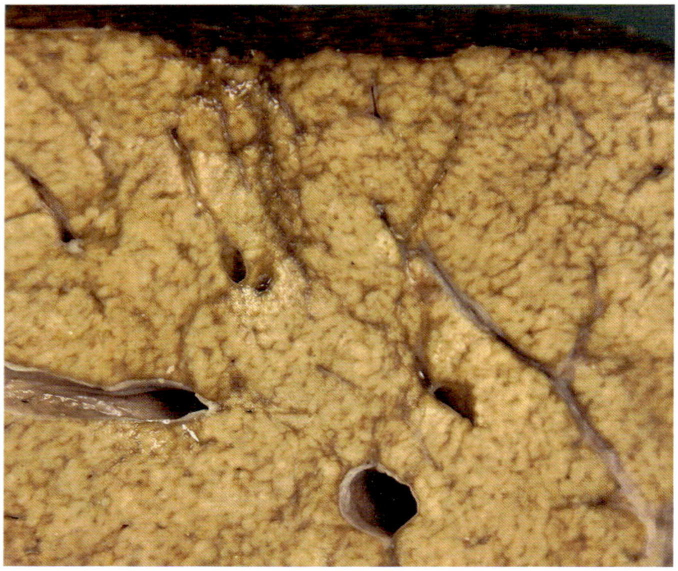

LIVER INVOLVED BY DIFFUSE LARGE B-CELL LYMPHOMA

FIGURE 12.88. The surface of the left lobe has an umbilicus-like, whitish lesion, which is a characteristic gross appearance of lymphoma involving the liver.

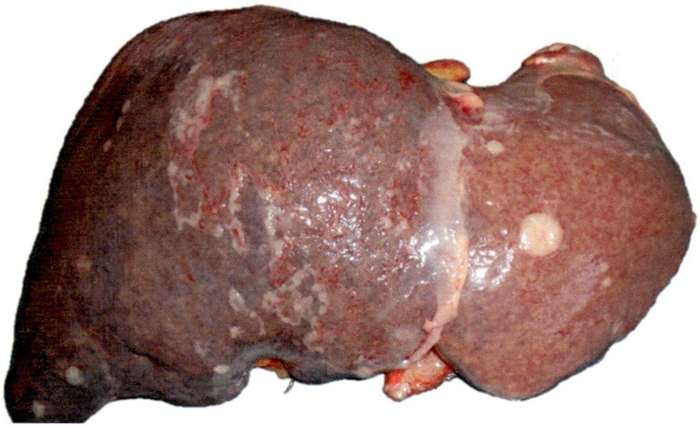

METASTATIC PULMONARY SMALL CELL CARCINOMA

Unlike patients with other metastatic malignancies to the liver, the aggressiveness of lung cancer precludes surgical resection and patients are generally treated with chemotherapy.

FIGURE 12.89. The outer surface of the fresh autopsy liver in (A) shows multiple metastases from a pulmonary small cell carcinoma. In (B), a slice of the liver shows several white nodules with focal hemorrhage.

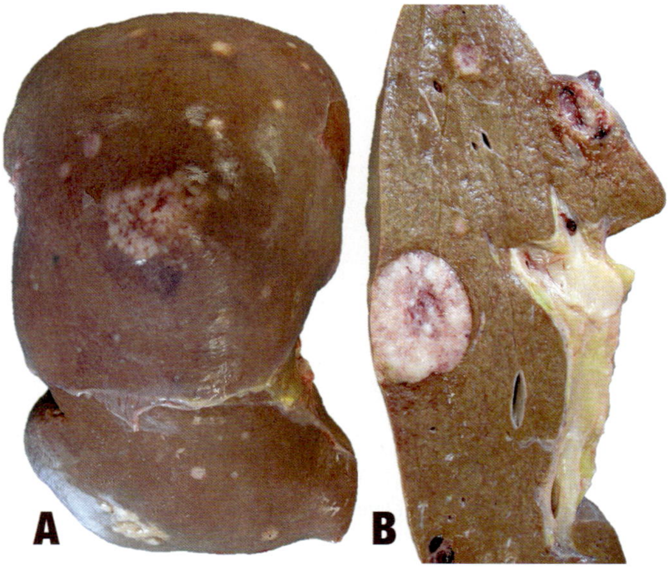

METASTATIC NEUROENDOCRINE TUMOR

FIGURE 12.90. This partial liver resection shows 2 pale and multilobular tumors. There were 8 tumors in all in this specimen.

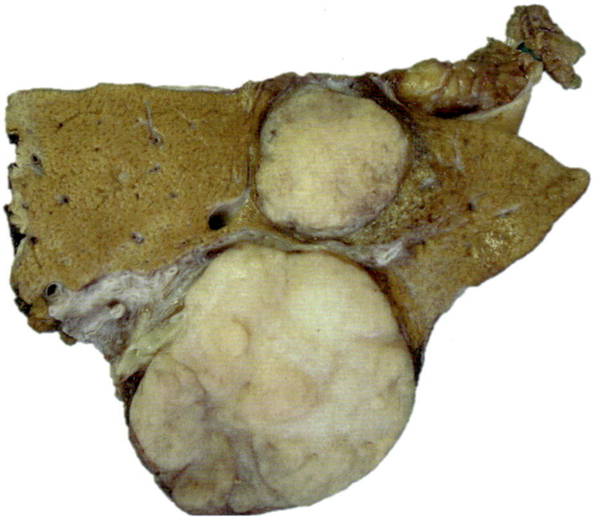

FIGURE 12.91. This image shows a partial resection of a liver studded with multiple nodules of metastatic neuroendocrine carcinoma.

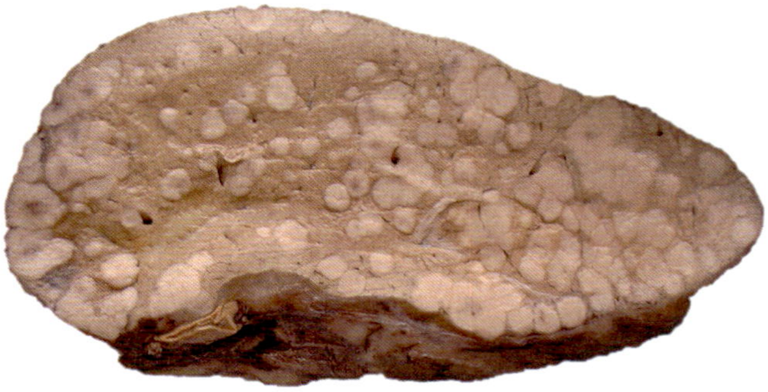

METASTATIC GASTROINTESTINAL STROMAL TUMOR (GIST)

Metastases to the liver are a common occurrence in GISTs. They are typically treated with a combination of surgery, tyrosine kinase inhibitors, and, if needed, radiofrequency ablation or transarterial chemoembolization.

FIGURE 12.92. In this example, note the bulging, pale, tan mass about 4 mm from the closest inked resection margin (right lateral).

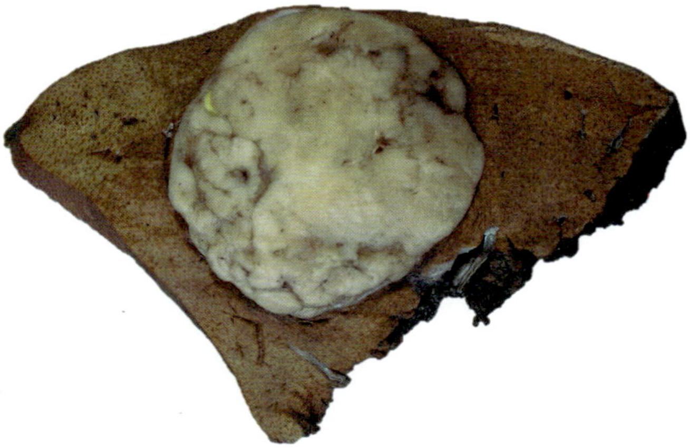

METASTATIC LEIOMYOSARCOMA

Soft tissue sarcomas are complicated by liver metastases in 25% to 40% of cases despite the initially adequate appearance of local therapy. The aim of resection is to eradicate all the disease, with negative margins.

FIGURE 12.93. This partial liver resection is from an 87-year-old male with metastatic leiomyosarcoma (maximum diameter 19 cm). Note the well-circumscribed mass with prominent lobulation and focal hemorrhages.

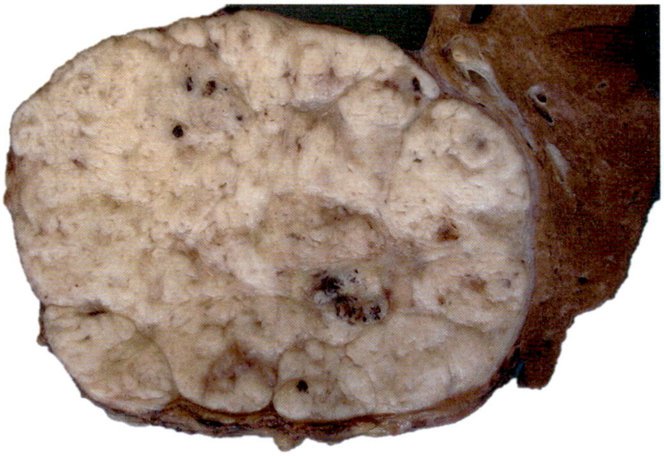

Liver Transplantation

Hepatectomy

FIGURE 12.94. These images show a whole slice (A) and closer view (B) of a hepatectomy pretransplant with relatively large regenerative nodules surrounded by markedly bile-stained fibrous septa.

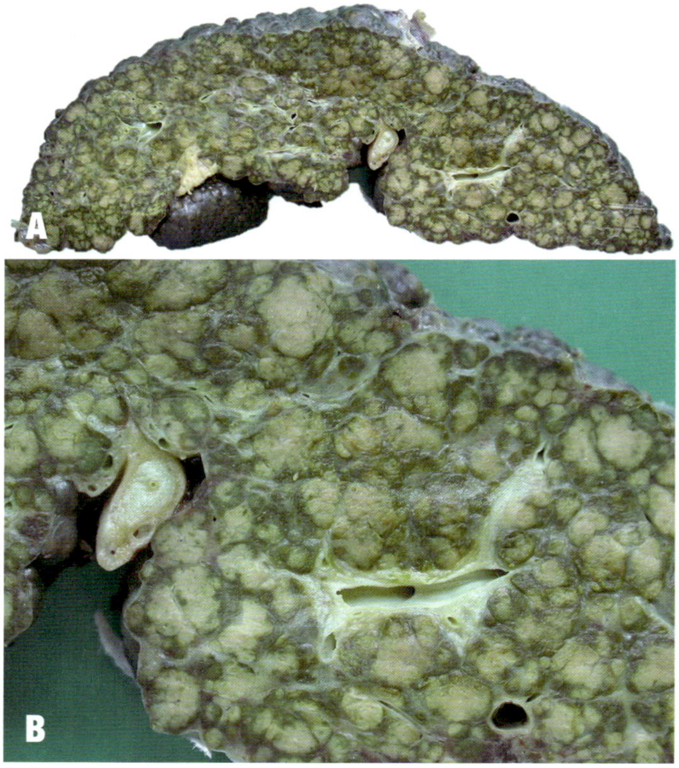

Transplant complications

STEATOSIS OF THE DONOR LIVER

Moderate (30% to 60%) or severe (more than 60%) macrovesicular steatosis in a donor liver is the major contraindication to liver transplantation, because it portends either a difficult postoperative recovery or primary graft failure.

FIGURE 12.95. This image shows marked steatosis in a fresh, unused donor liver, as indicated by its uniform orange-brown discoloration.

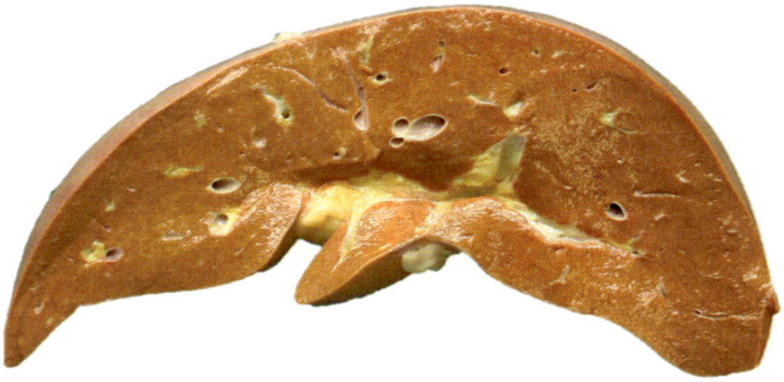

FIGURE 12.96. This donor liver with marked steatosis (more than 80% of hepatocytes) was not used for transplantation. Note the irregular fractures (A) attesting to the friability of the liver. Image (B) shows intense yellow discoloration. There was no fibrosis.

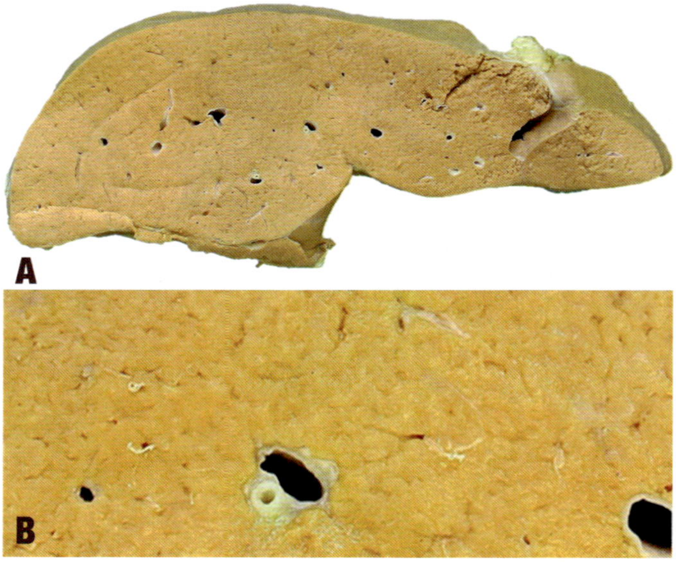

HEPATIC ARTERY THROMBOSIS FOLLOWING LIVER TRANSPLANT

Posttransplant hepatic artery thrombosis is the most frequent vascular complication of transplantation. It is divided into early (less than 1 month posttransplantion) and late (more than 1 month posttransplantion). Although the current incidence of hepatic artery thrombosis is less than 10%, this complication continues to account for significant morbidity, frequently requiring retransplantation and increasing the risk of mortality.

FIGURE 12.97. The liver in (A) was removed because of extensive infarctions that are visible at the periphery and around the large green central necrotic bile duct. A closer view in (B) highlights the liver parenchyma with cholestasis and necrosis in a "nutmeg" pattern adjacent to the infarction.

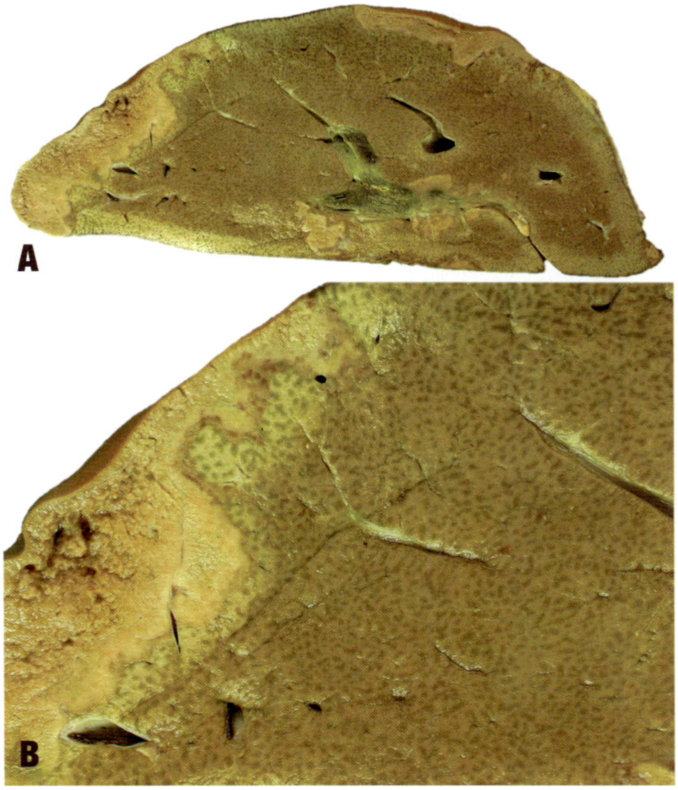

FIGURE 12.98. This posttransplant liver shows a large infarction and secondary abscess following hepatic arterial thrombosis.

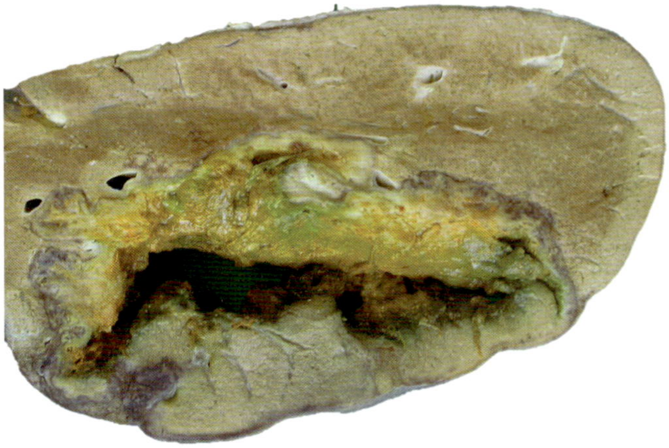

FIGURE 12.99. These images show posttransplantion hepatic artery thrombosis with ischemic cholangiopathy. Since the blood supply to the bile duct comes entirely from the hepatic artery, bile ducts undergo ischemic necrosis when hepatic artery thrombosis occurs. In (A), note the marked green discoloration, indicative of cholestasis, and prominent pale infarctions. Image (B) gives a close-up of an infarcted hilar area (lower center).

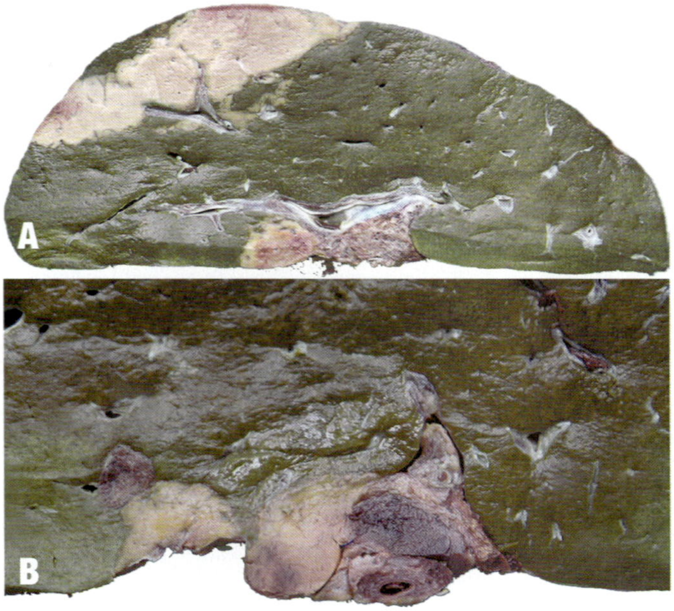

PRIMARY NONFUNCTION POSTTRANSPLANT

Primary nonfunction is defined as severe liver dysfunction incompatible with allograft survival. It is at the most advanced end of the spectrum of ischemia or reperfusion injury. It can result from vascular lesions (principally thrombosis of the hepatic artery or portal vein), or from to severe donor-related issues, including steatosis. Urgent retransplantation is required.

FIGURE 12.100. This liver was removed shortly following transplantation. Note the diffuse green discoloration and infarctions (large on top, medium at left edge, and tiny at bottom right). A large hilar lymph node is also necrotic (arrow).

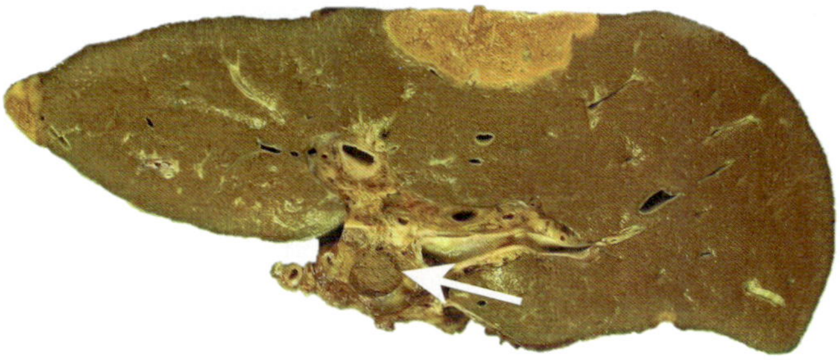

FIGURE 12.101. This image shows a liver allograft removed due to hepatic artery thrombosis. It was photographed prior to formalin fixation. Note the clear demarcation between the infarcted left lobe and the viable right lobe.

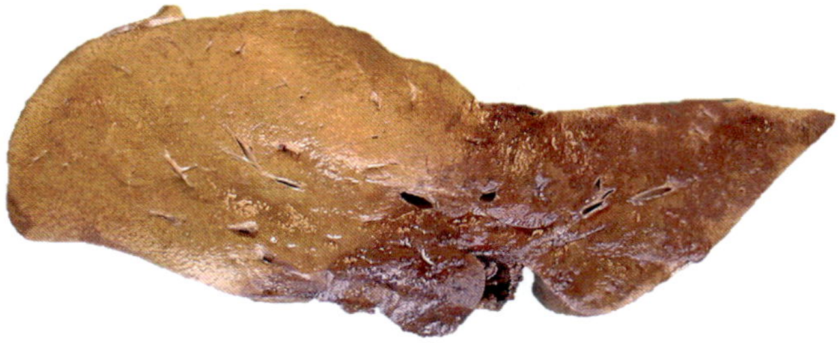

FIGURE 12.102. This image shows primary graft nonfunction shortly following transplantation. The nonfunction was due to severe hepatic arterial atherosclerosis and portal vein thrombosis. The graft was removed soon after transplantation. In (A), note the prominent cholestatic pattern and thrombosed portal vein in the hilum. A closer view in (B) shows thrombus, and emphasizes a fine nodular pattern of bile-stained congestive hepatopathy caused by necrosis of centrilobular hepatocytes.

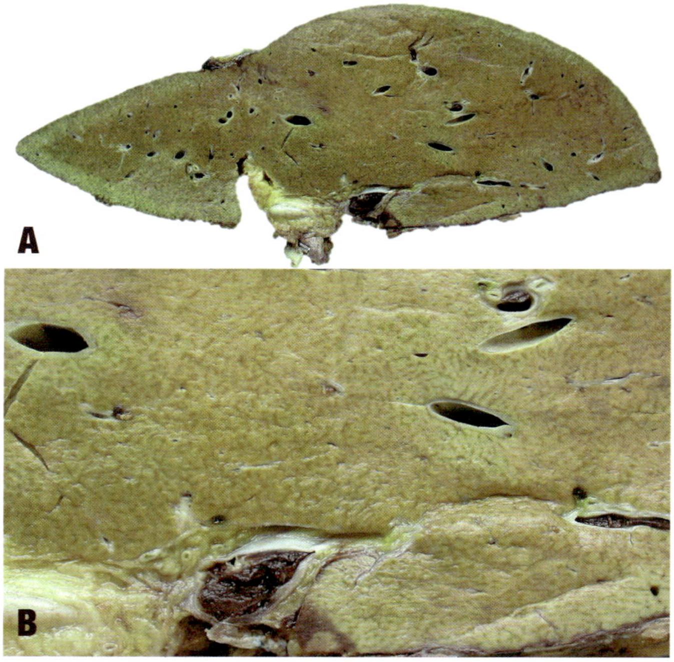

POSTTRANSPLANT ISCHEMIC CHOLANGIOPATHY

The small size of the hepatic artery renders anastomosis at the time of transplantation difficult. The exquisite sensitivity of the bile duct to ischemia explains the dreaded complication of ischemic cholangiopathy that frequently requires retransplantation. Affected medium-to-large-sized bile ducts can show multifocal or diffuse nonanastomotic strictures and dilatations filled with inspissated bile, sludge, casts, and stones.

FIGURE 12.103. This is an example of posttransplant ischemic cholangiopathy secondary to hepatic arterial and portal venous thrombosis, and to recurrent hepatitis C with incomplete cirrhosis. Note in (A) the fine nodular parenchymal pattern and dilated hilar bile ducts with inspissated bile. A closer view in (B) shows dilated bile ducts, fine fibrous septa, and early regenerating nodules of hepatocytes.

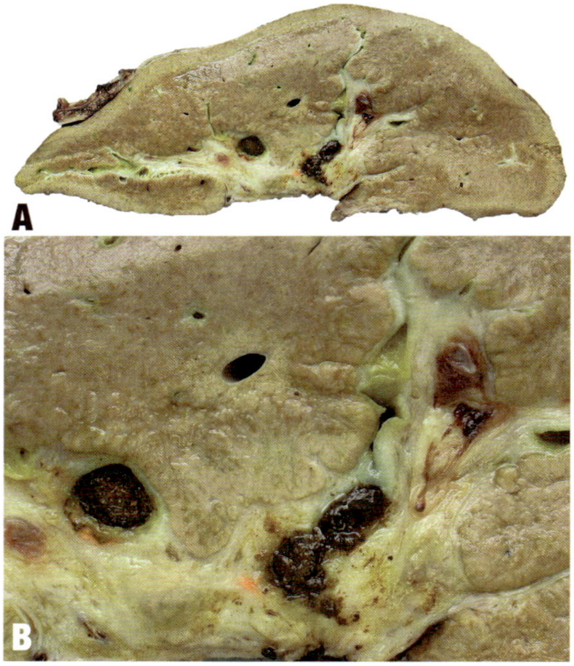

FIGURE 12.104. This image shows an example of ischemic cholangiopathy secondary to prior hepatic artery thrombosis. Note the inspissated bile in large ducts (arrows) surrounded by variably wide, bile-stained zones of cholestasis. The background liver has the "nutmeg" pattern of chronic passive congestion and cholestasis.

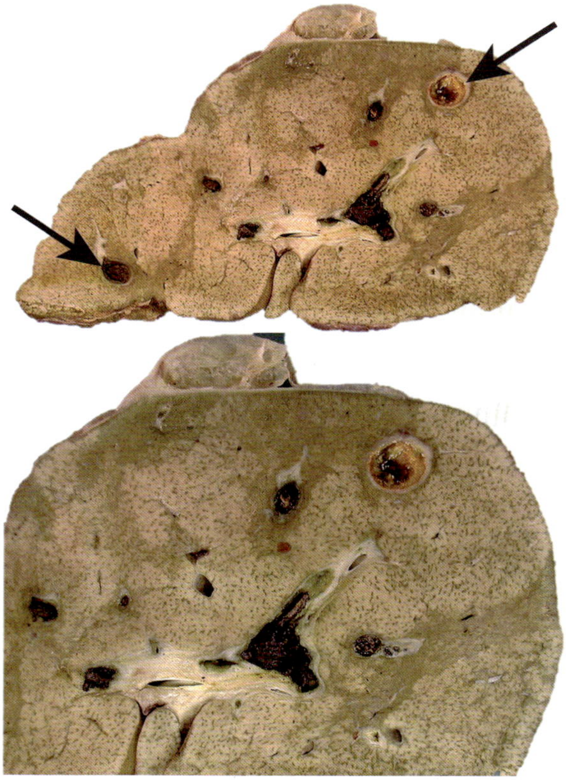

POSTTRANSPLANT CIRRHOSIS SECONDARY TO HEPATITIS C

Cirrhosis develops in about 10% to 30% of patients transplanted for hepatitis C. Among the variant patterns of recurrence, fibrosing cholestatic hepatitis is the most likely to progress to cirrhosis.

FIGURE 12.105. Image (A) shows cirrhosis in a liver 12 years posttransplant, secondary to recurrent hepatitis C. A closer view in (B) shows regenerative nodules of variable size on a greenish cholestatic and fibrotic background. There was no carcinoma in this patient.

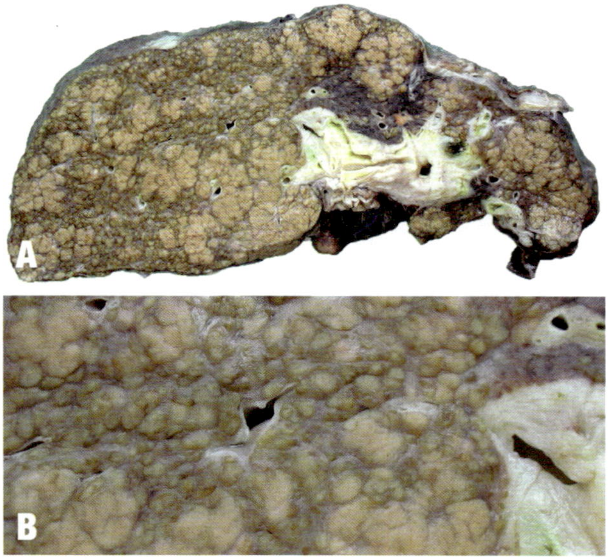

FIGURE 12.106. Image (A) shows posttransplant recurrence of hepatitis C with marked cholestasis and cirrhosis. There was also chronic rejection with foam cell arteriopathy. A closer view in (B) shows the micronodular pattern of cirrhosis with marked cholestasis.

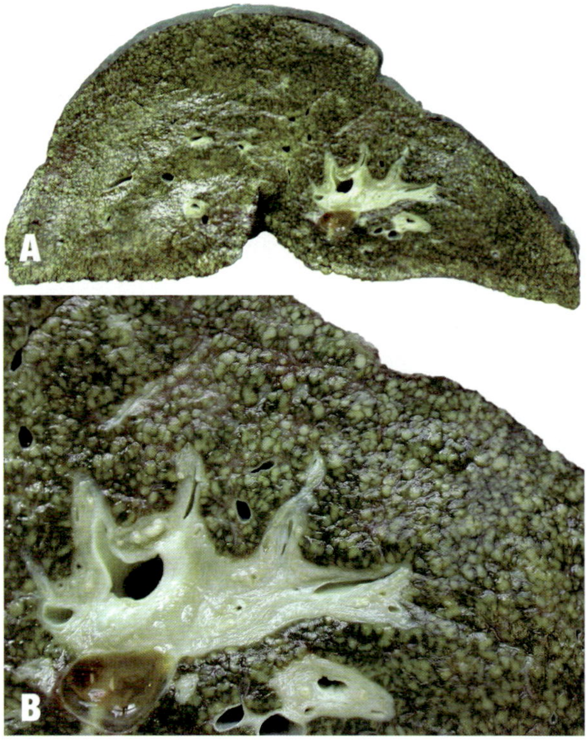

Failed liver transplant

FIGURE 12.107. This is a liver transplant that was removed prior to retransplantation. Multiple processes were responsible for the liver failure, including extrahepatic biliary obstruction, chronic rejection with abnormal bile ducts, and arteriopathy. The patient's original disease was cirrhosis due to NASH. The slice in (A) shows a markedly bile-stained liver with irregularly distributed partial fibrous septa without definite regenerative nodule formation. A closer view of another slice in (B) shows the metal mesh stent of the transjugular intrahepatic portosystemic shunt (TIPS) in the portal vein, inserted to reduce the elevated portal venous pressure.

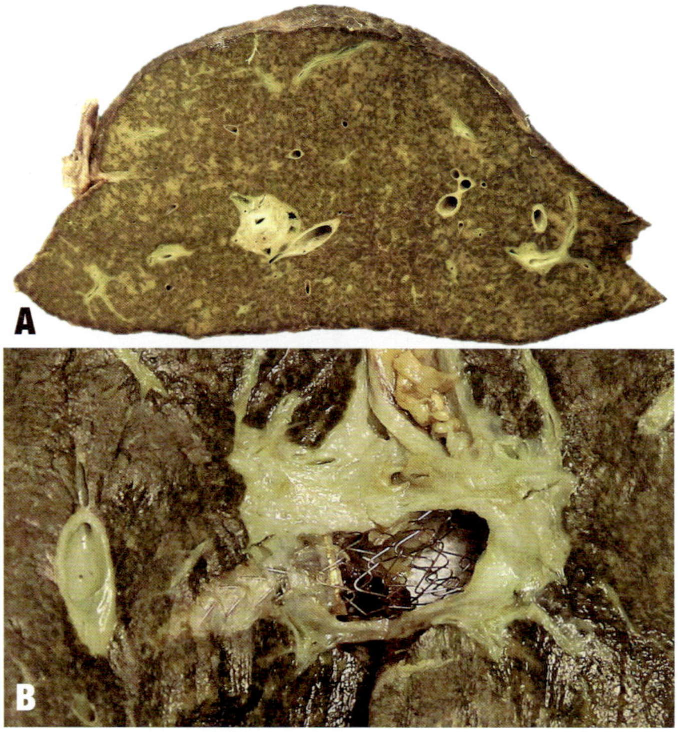

Gallbladder

REFERENCE: NORMAL GALLBLADDER

FIGURE 12.108. The gallbladder is a small muscular bag-like structure that sits just under the liver. It stores and concentrates bile before releasing it into the duodenum via the common bile duct. Anatomically, the gallbladder is divided into 3 sections: the fundus, body, and neck. The neck tapers to become the cystic duct, which unites with the common hepatic duct to form the common bile duct. At the junction of the neck and the cystic duct, the gallbladder wall forms a mucosal fold known as Hartmann pouch, where gallstones commonly get stuck.

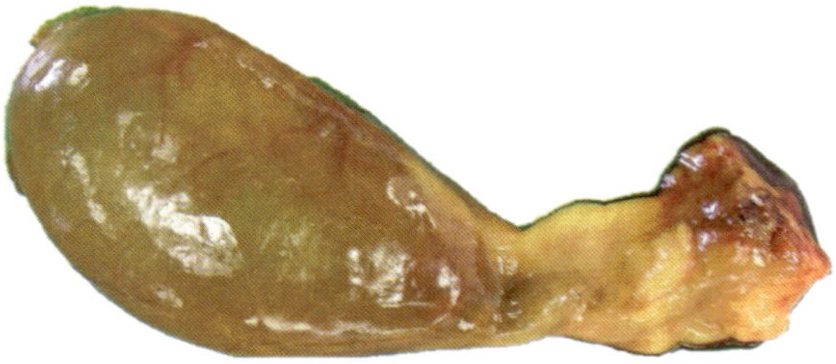

Nonneoplastic Diseases and Benign Neoplasms of the Gallbladder

Gallbladder with cysts

Nonneoplastic cysts in the gallbladder may be congenital or acquired. Congenital cysts are rare, and may be accompanied by other malformations of the biliary or vascular tree. Acquired cysts are more common, and are due to partial or complete obstruction of bile outflow.

FIGURE 12.109. This resected gallbladder shows multiple cysts filled with viscous, black-green bile. The cyst wall is fibrotic, with variable thickness and yellow cholesterol deposit.

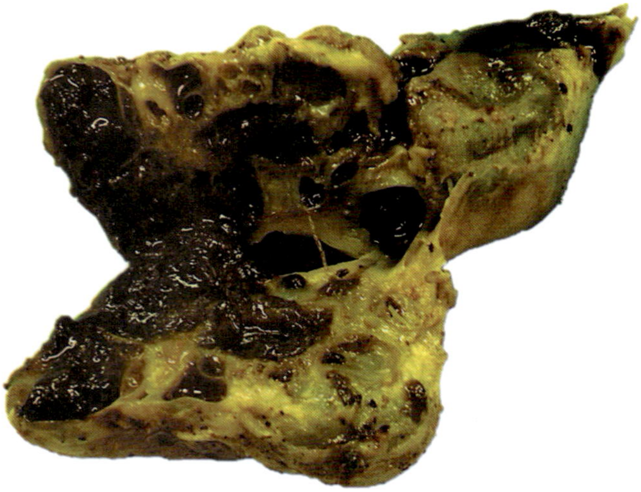

Cholesterolosis of the gallbladder

Cholesterolosis of the gallbladder, also called "strawberry gallbladder," results from an abnormal accumulation of cholesterol esters mainly in macrophages within the lamina propria of the gallbladder. It has no known clinical significance.

FIGURE 12.110. The mucosal surface of this gallbladder, carpeted with white dots, mimics the surface of a strawberry.

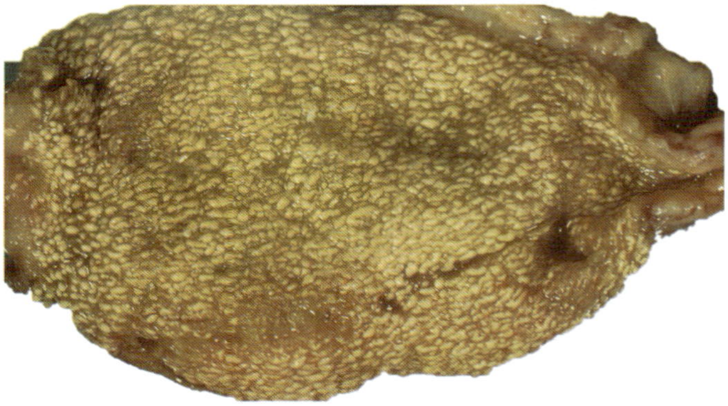

Cholelithiasis and cholecystitis

CHOLELITHIASIS (GALLSTONES, CALCULI)

There are 2 types of gallstones: cholesterol stones (more common) containing more than 50% crystalline cholesterol monohydrate, and pigment stones composed of bilirubin calcium salts. The clinical presentation of acute cholecystitis is characterized by right upper quadrant pain due to inflammation of the gallbladder, which usually results from a gallstone (calculus) obstructing the cystic duct.

FIGURE 12.111. The gallbladder in (A) contains numerous faceted cholesterol stones, 1 of which is firmly wedged in the neck. Image B shows a gallbladder containing many pigment stones.

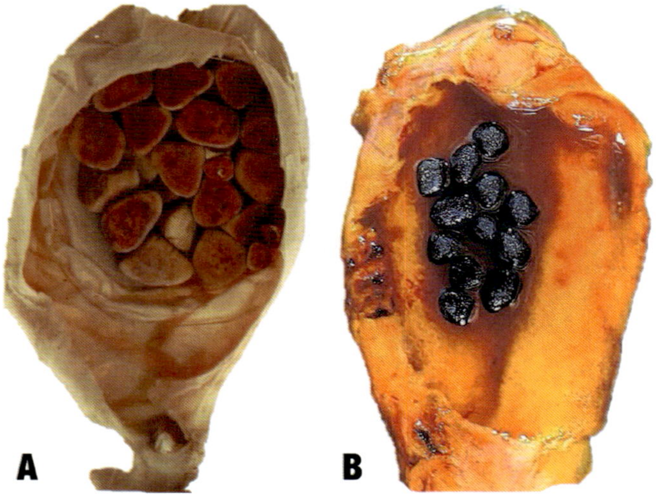

ACUTE CALCULOUS CHOLECYSTITIS

FIGURE 12.112. This image shows a gallstone (calculus) obstructing the cystic duct.

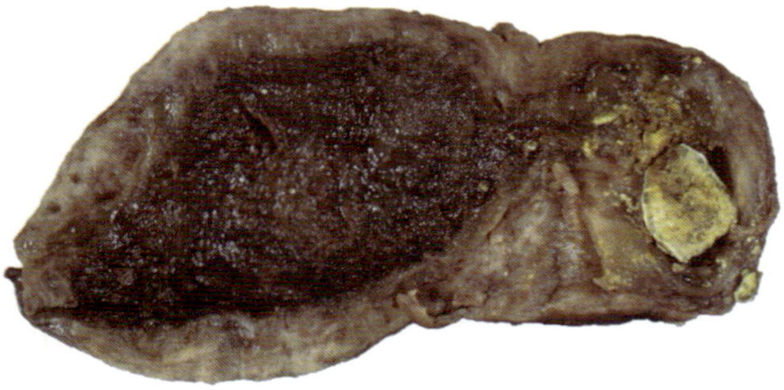

ACUTE GANGRENOUS CHOLECYSTITIS

There are many complications of acute cholecystitis including gallbladder gangrene (extensive full-thickness necrosis), rupture and/or perforation, abscess, fistula formation, and superimposed infection. Cholecystectomy is indicated.

FIGURE 12.113. This image shows a cholecystectomy due to gangrenous cholecystitis.

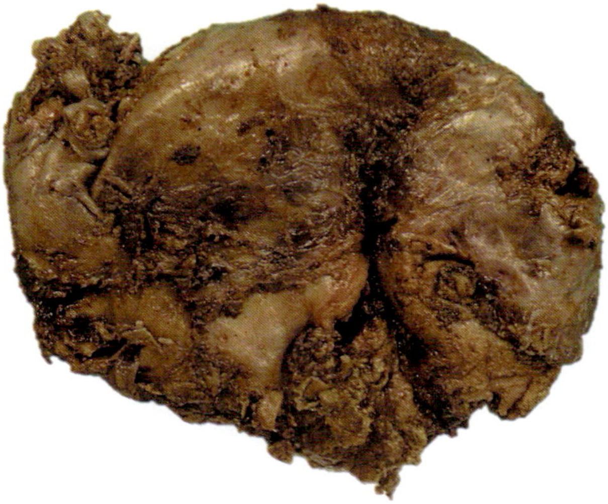

GALLSTONE CAUSING SMALL BOWEL OBSTRUCTION

This is a rare complication of acute cholecystitis. A large gallstone may erode through the gallbladder wall, into the lumen of the adjacent small bowel, then travel down the bowel to finally become lodged, often in the terminal ileum, and cause small bowel obstruction.

FIGURE 12.114. This image illustrates a 3-cm cholesterol gallstone that caused so-called gallstone ileus.

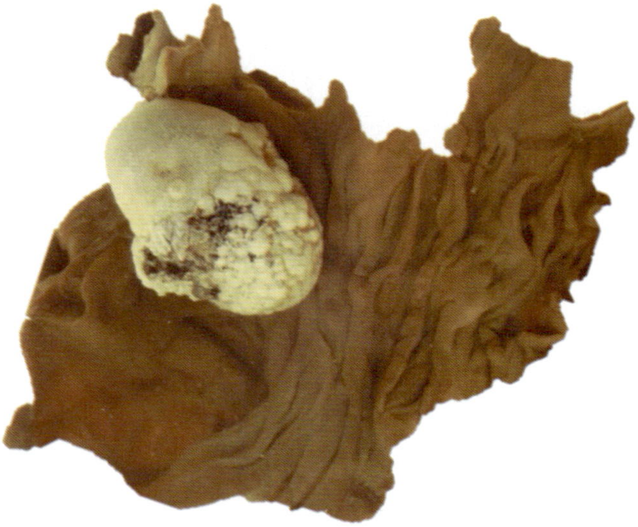

CHRONIC CHOLECYSTITIS AND CHOLELITHIASIS

Recurrent intermittent obstruction by gallstones, resulting in increased gallbladder pressure, leads to herniation of the mucosa into the muscle layer. Compared to acute cholecystitis, chronic cholecystitis is more commonly seen in a resected gallbladder (cholecystectomy) specimen, because the majority of cholecystectomies are performed after recovery of the acute episode.

FIGURE 12.115. This gallbladder with chronic cholecystitis shows typical wall thickening.

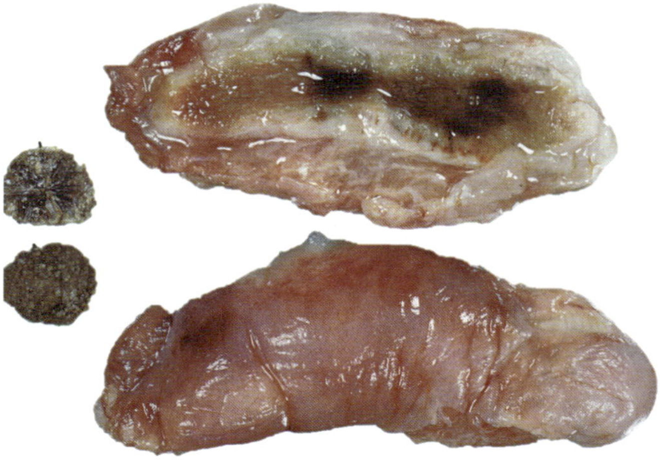

FIGURE 12.116. Note the thick gallbladder wall and the rough mucosa.

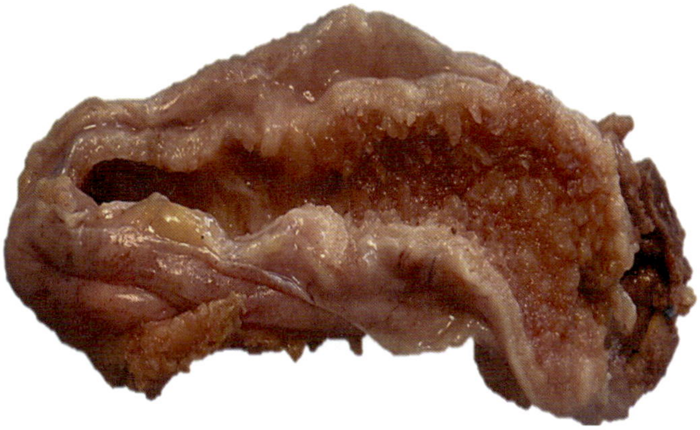

Cholesterol polyp

Cholesterol polyps are the most common type of gallbladder polyp. They are essentially areas with marked cholesterolosis. Cholesterol polyps are benign with no malignant potential.

FIGURE 12.117. This image shows cholesterol polyps in a gallbladder with background cholesterolosis (or "strawberry gallbladder").

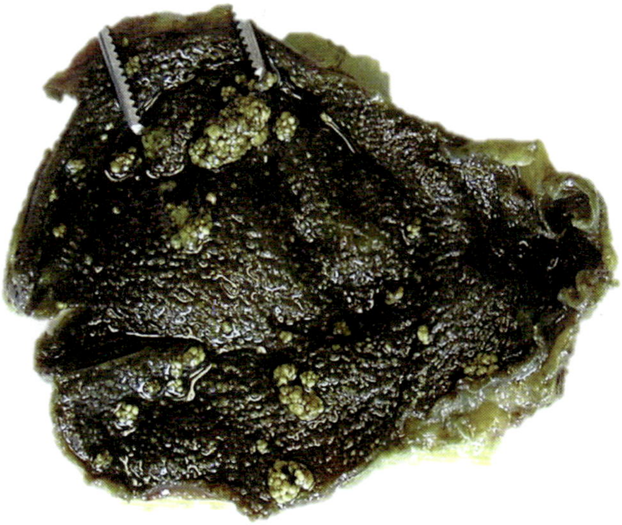

Adenomyoma of gallbladder

Adenomyomas are usually solitary and located at the fundus. They are characterized by marked mucosal invagination into a thickened muscular wall. If diffuse, the term *adenomyomatosis* is preferred.

FIGURE 12.118. This image shows a tumor-like lesion at the fundus that has a cystic cut surface due to mucosa invagination.

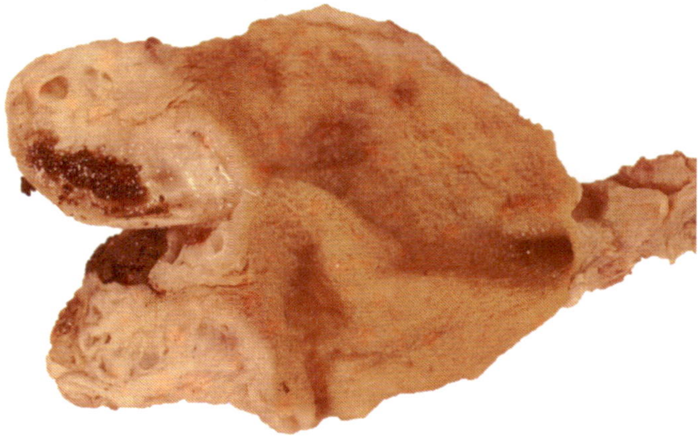

Gallbladder adenoma

Also called intracholecystic papillary tubular neoplasm (ICPN), gallbladder adenoma is premalignant. It shows at least low-grade dysplasia (i.e., intraepithelial neoplastic proliferation).

FIGURE 12.119. In this image, 2 whitish papillary lesions are present on the mucosal surface.

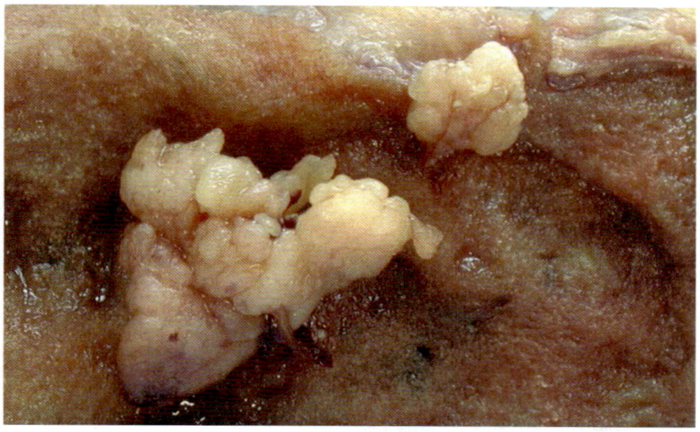

Gallbladder with dysplasia

Dysplasia may be polypoid or flat, low grade or high grade. Flat dysplasia may not be grossly identifiable. Extensive sampling of the gallbladder in cases of dysplasia is needed to exclude an associated adenocarcinoma.

FIGURE 12.120. In this image, the mucosa appears a bit irregular, but no obvious mucosa lesion is present by gross examination. The diagnosis of flat low-grade dysplasia was made on histology.

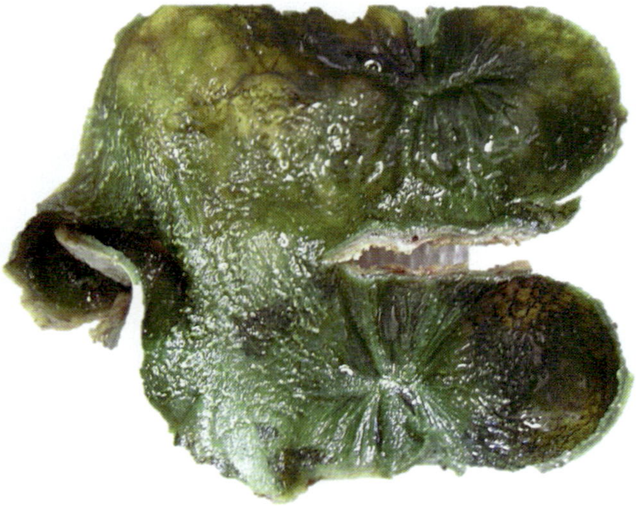

Gallbladder Cancer

Gallbladder adenocarcinoma

Gallbladder cancer is more common in elderly women, and is strongly associated with cholelithiasis. Approximately 1% of cholecystectomies performed for gallstones contain cancer. The majority of gallbladder cancer is adenocarcinoma. Gallbladder adenocarcinoma is the most common malignancy of the extrahepatic biliary tract.

FIGURE 12.121. In this image, the mucosa contains a sessile polypoid mucosal lesion.

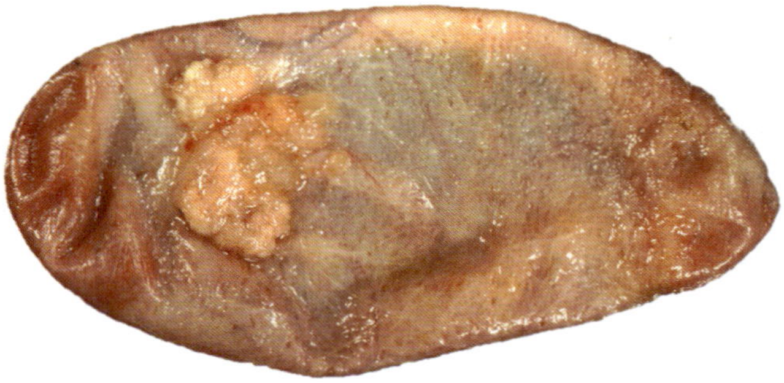

FIGURE 12.122. This gallbladder contains a large exophytic tumor that partially fills the lumen.

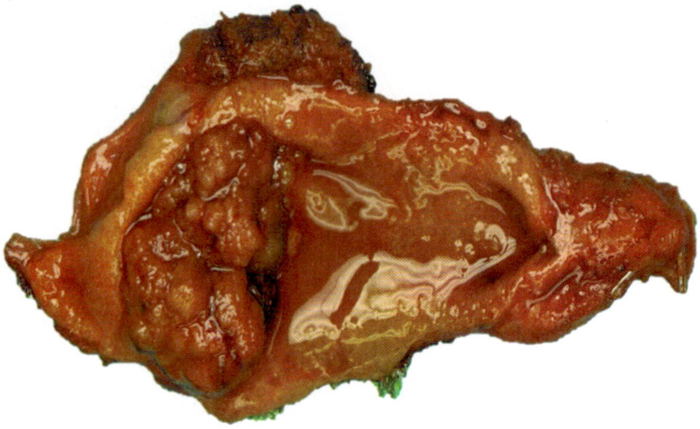

ADVANCED GALLBLADDER ADENOCARCINOMA

This epithelial malignancy of the gallbladder is often discovered at an advanced stage and may already show invasion into the liver at presentation.

FIGURE 12.123. In this case, the gallbladder was resected en bloc with some adjacent liver (seen at the top of image). The gallbladder shows a large multinodular mass that had focally invaded into the liver.

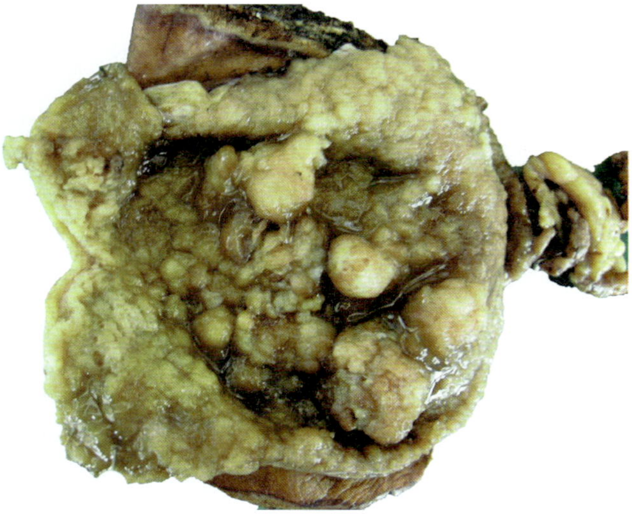

FIGURE 12.124. This example shows direct invasion into the liver, and a metastatic nodule away from the main tumor. Gallbladder cancers are usually firm and whitish because they elicit a prominent desmoplastic response.

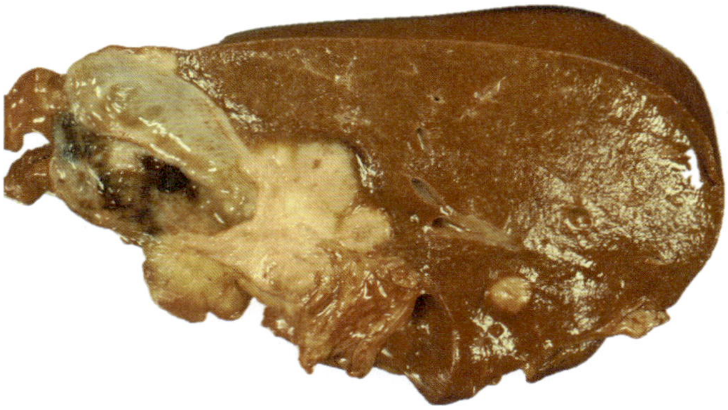

Common bile duct carcinoma

Unlike gallbladder cancer, which is more common in females, bile duct cancer (also called distal cholangiocarcinoma) has no gender predilection. It is morphologically identical to intrahepatic (peripheral) and perihilar (Klatskin) cholangiocarcinoma. Risk factors for common bile duct carcinoma include primary sclerosing cholangitis and liver fluke infections. Gallstones have no clear association. Cholangiocarcinoma overall has a poor prognosis.

FIGURE 12.125. This specimen consists of a Whipple resection with the duodenum, distal stomach, head of pancreas, and distal common bile duct. The probe is placed through the ampulla of Vater. Note the wall thickening and the dilatation of the common bile duct.

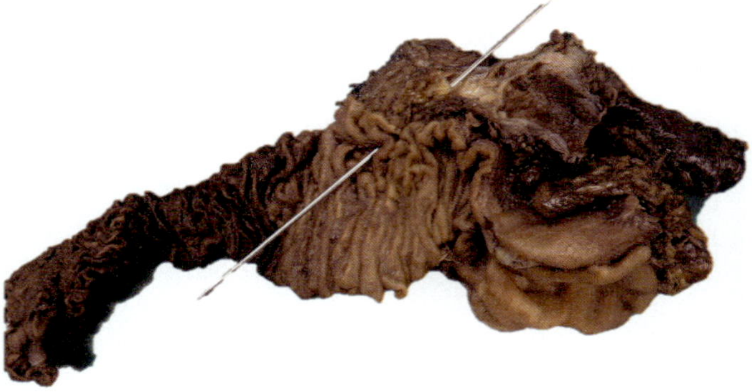

FIGURE 12.126. In this image, a dilated distal common bile duct was opened and shows a neoplasm growing into the lumen.

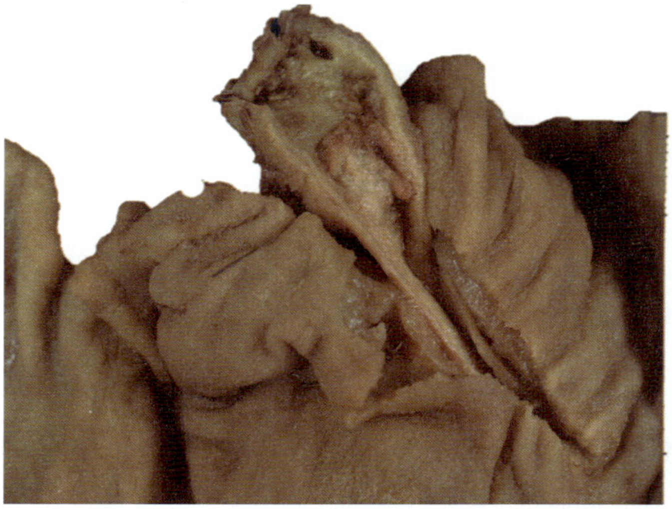

REFERENCES

Bosman FT, Carneiro F, Hruban RH, Theise ND, editors. *WHO classification of tumors of the digestive system*. 4th ed. Lyon, France: IARC Press; 2010.

Burt AD, Portman BC, Ferrell LD. *MacSween's pathology of the liver*. 5th ed. Philadelphia: Elsevier Churchill Livingstone; 2007.

Kumar V, Abbas AK, Fausto N, Aster J. *Robbins and Cotran pathologic basis of disease*. 8th ed. Philadelphia: Saunders/Elsevier; 2010.

Lester SC. *Manual of surgical pathology*. 2nd ed. Philadelphia: Elsevier Churchill Livingstone; 2006.

Michel RP, Berry GJ, editors. *Pathology of transplantation: a practical diagnostic approach*. Switzerland: Springer; 2016. https://doi.org/10.1007/978-3-319-29683-8

Mills SE, Carter D, Greenson JK, Reuter VE, Stoler MH, editors. *Sternberg's diagnostic surgical pathology*. 5th ed. Philadelphia: Lippincott Williams & Wilkins; 2010.

Odze RD, Goldblum JR, Crawford JM. *Surgical pathology of the GI tract, liver, biliary tract, and pancreas*. Philadelphia: Saunders/Elsevier; 2004.

Rosai J. *Rosai and Ackerman's surgical pathology*. 10th ed. Edinburgh, NY: Mosby/Elsevier; 2011.

13

Pancreas Diseases

VICTORIA MARCUS, YU SHI, ZU-HUA GAO

REFERENCE: NORMAL PANCREAS

FIGURE 13.1. The pancreas is a vital organ involved in digestion and the production of hormones such as insulin. This image shows a normal pancreas with duodenum. It is a tan-yellow lobulated organ composed of the uncinate process, head, neck, body, and tail. The pancreatic head is surrounded by the duodenum, which drains the common bile duct (probe A) and the pancreatic duct (probe B) via an opening at the ampulla of Vater. The bile and the pancreatic enzymes from these ducts help digest the food in the intestine.

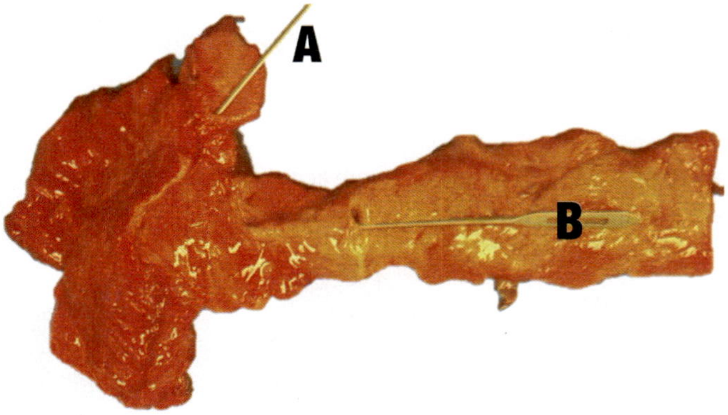

Annular pancreas

This rare congenital condition is characterized by pancreatic tissue abnormally surrounding the second part of the duodenum. Annular pancreas may lead to small bowel obstruction.

FIGURE 13.2. This image shows an example of annular pancreas. The pencil demonstrates the abnormal ring of pancreatic tissue.

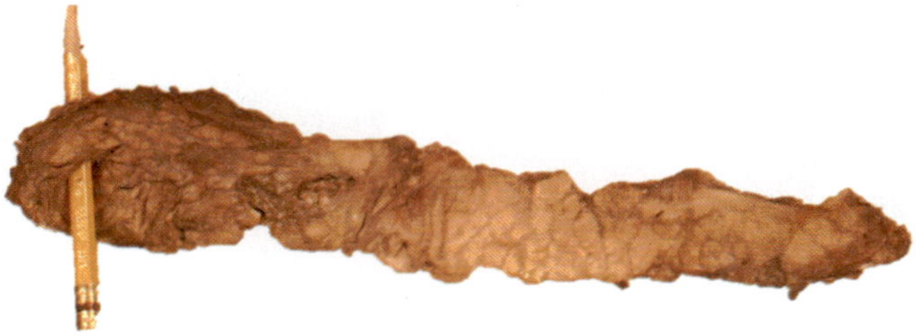

Accessory spleen within the pancreas

Accessory spleens are present in about 10% of the population and may be located in the pancreas. These may be congenital or they may be due to trauma to the spleen. Accessory spleens are nonneoplastic.

FIGURE 13.3. In this image, the encapsulated beefy-red spleen tissue is surrounded by normal yellowish pancreas tissue.

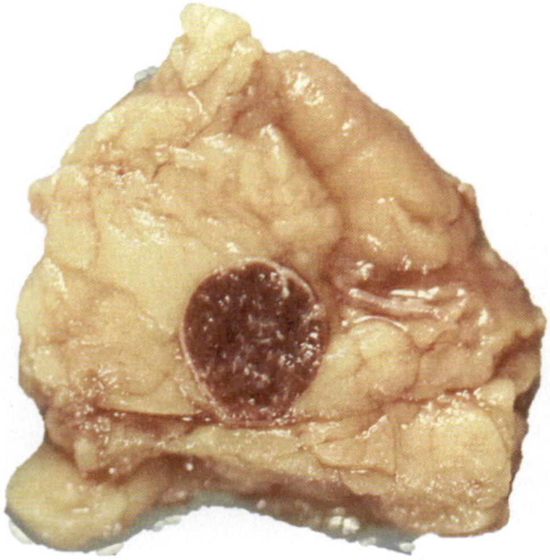

Hematochromatosis

Hereditary hemochromatosis is an autosomal recessive condition characterized by iron accumulation in various organs including the pancreas, liver, and heart. It leads to to organ damage. Excess iron causes brown pigmentation of the tissue. Involvement of the pancreas may lead to diabetes.

FIGURE 13.4. This pancreas in a patient with hereditary hemochromatosis appears dark brown due to iron accumulation (A) compared to a more yellowish normal pancreas (B).

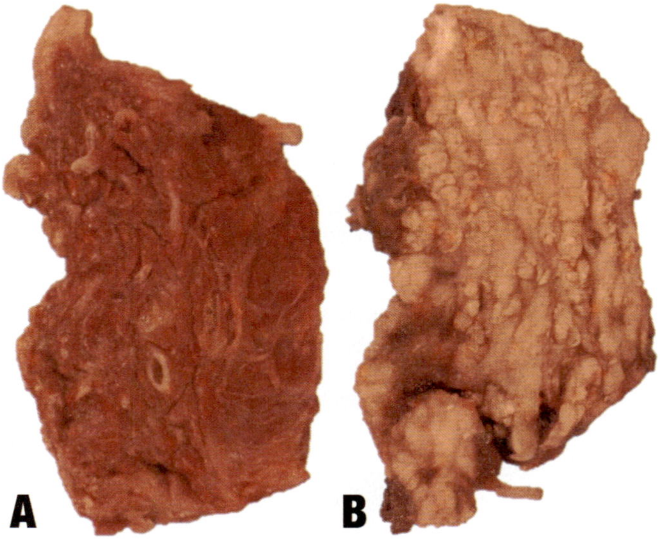

Acute pancreatitis

Patients with acute pancreatitis typically present with sudden-onset severe upper-abdominal (epigastric) pain radiating to the back. The 2 main risk factors for acute pancreatitis are gallstones and excess alcohol. Clinical and radiological scoring systems are available to help predict the severity of acute pancreatitis and guide therapy. Severe forms of acute pancreatitis can be life-threatening, and usually require hospitalization, intensive medical care, and close monitoring.

FIGURE 13.5. This image shows an early, mild form of acute pancreatitis. Most of the pancreatic parenchyma appears edematous. Focal necrosis is present.

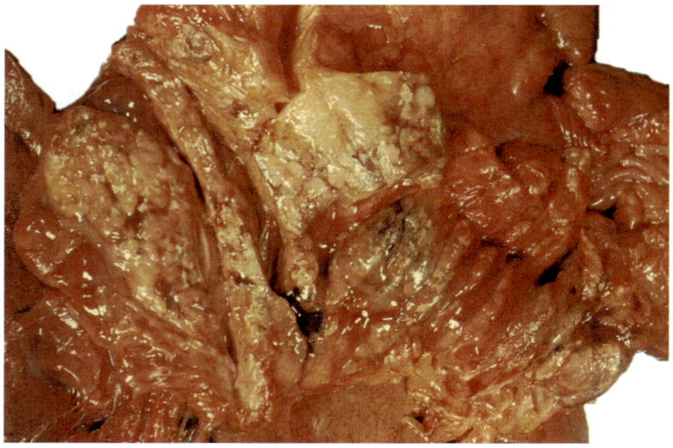

FIGURE 13.6. This image shows a severe form of acute pancreatitis with extensive hemorrhage and necrosis.

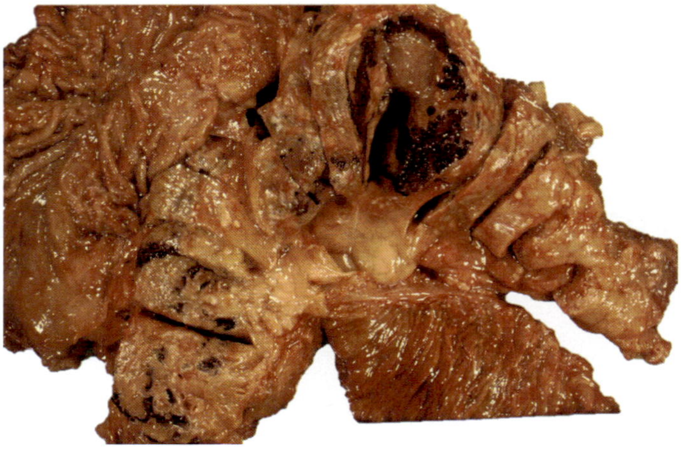

FIGURE 13.7. These cross-sections of a pancreas show necrosis and hemorrhage of the pancreatic parenchyma, indicating a severe form of acute pancreatitis.

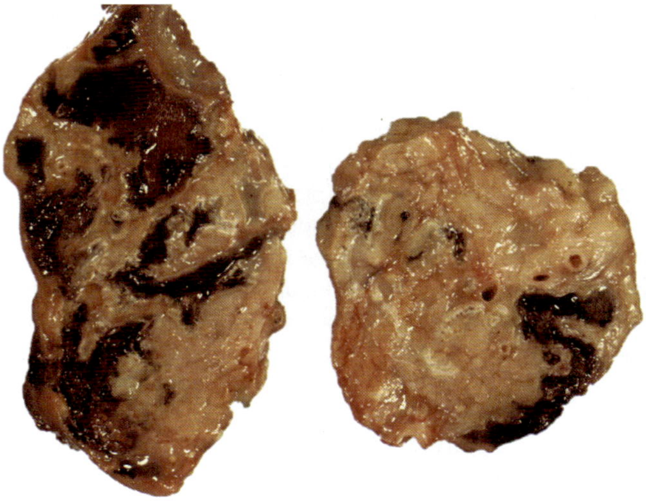

FIGURE 13.8. This image of severe acute pancreatitis shows extensive necrosis

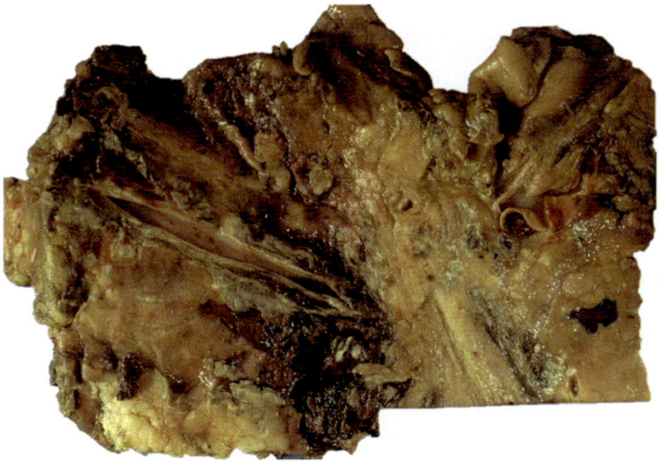

FIGURE 13.9. This image is from an autopsy performed to confirm cause of death. It shows a pancreas autodigested by its own pancreatic enzymes, leading to parenchymal necrosis and hemorrhage.

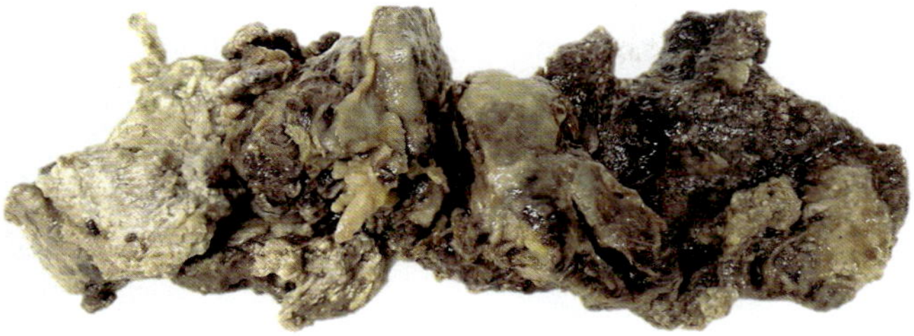

Chronic pancreatitis

Chronic pancreatitis is an irreversible process that usually results from repeated episodes of acute pancreatitis, and is characterized by fibrosis and loss of the pancreatic parenchyma. Irreversible damage to the acinar cells and islet cells with replacement by fibrosis leads to pancreatic exocrine and endocrine insufficiency, respectively. The resulting clinical presentation includes malabsorption (with steatorrhea) and diabetes mellitus. Chronic pancreatitis may sometimes be confused with pancreatic neoplasm due to its firm consistency on gross examination.

FIGURE 13.10. This image shows a white, rubbery pancreas due to extensive fibrosis.

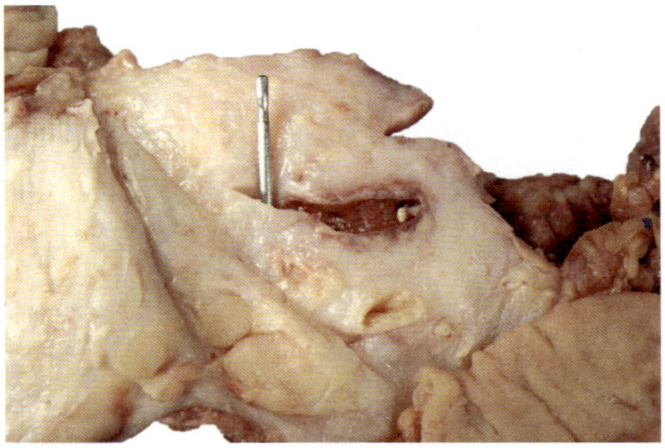

FIGURE 13.11. This image shows chronic pancreatitis with an intraductal stone. The resected pancreas demonstrates fibrosis, calcifications, loss of lobulation, and a dilated pancreatic duct blocked by the stone.

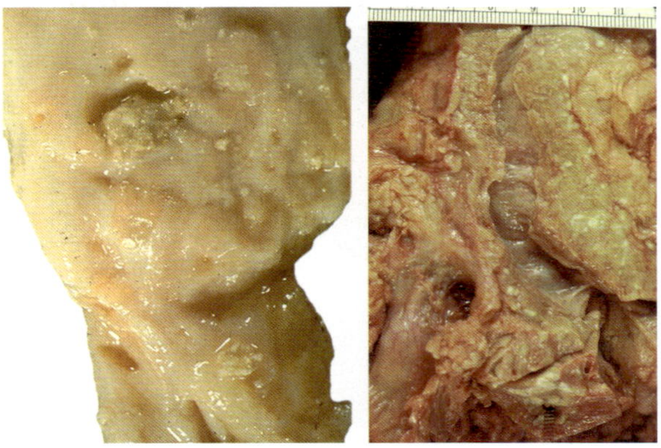

IGG4-RELATED AUTOIMMUNE PANCREATITIS (LYMPHOPLASMACYTIC SCLEROSING PANCREATITIS)

IgG4-related autoimmune pancreatitis is a distinct form of chronic pancreatitis that is associated with other increasingly recognized IgG4-related diseases. It is characterized by fibrosis and numerous IgG4-positive plasma cells. It may form a firm mass, which may mimic cancer in its clinical, radiological, and macroscopic presentation. This entity usually responds to steroid therapy and does not require resection.

FIGURE 13.12. This resected pancreas appears firm and rubbery with a fleshy cut surface that grossly could mimic a malignancy.

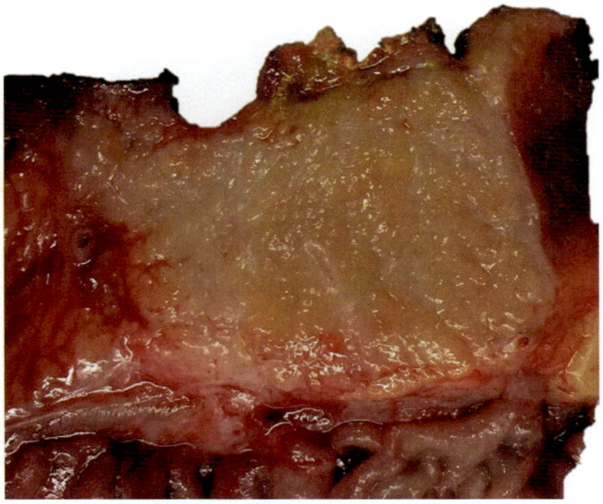

Pancreatic pseudocyst

Pseudocysts are the most common cystic lesion in the pancreas. Pancreatic pseudocysts are fluid-filled collections rich in necrotic tissue, pancreatic enzymes, and blood, and are surrounded by granulation tissue and fibrosis; they have no epithelial lining. Pseudocysts result from autodigestion of the pancreas by pancreatic enzymes, and may be a complication of acute or chronic pancreatitis.

FIGURE 13.13. The pseudocyst on the superior part of this pancreas shows an irregular shape and variation of wall thickness. The remaining pancreas tissue has features of chronic active pancreatitis.

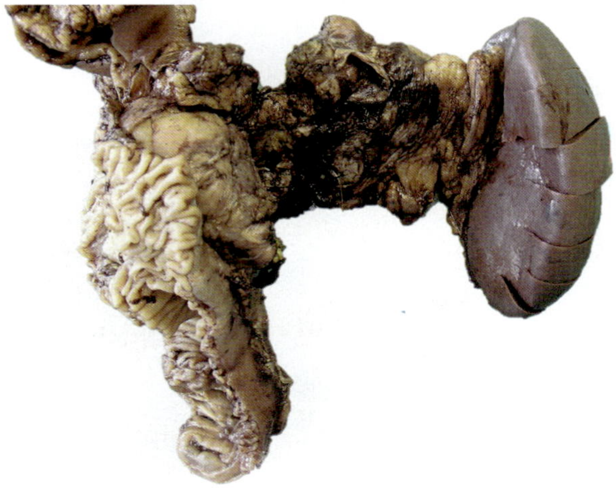

Hydatid cyst of the pancreas

Hydatid cyst of the pancreas, a very rare disease, is caused by infection from a tapeworm of *Echinococcus* genus. Tapeworm eggs are shed in the stool of a host organism (usually a dog); the disease is spread to humans through ingestion of the eggs via contact with the infected stool.

FIGURE 13.14. This specimen consists of the pancreas tail and the spleen (right, serially sectioned). There is a large mass in the pancreatic parenchyma, which, on cut section, revealed a cystic lesion.

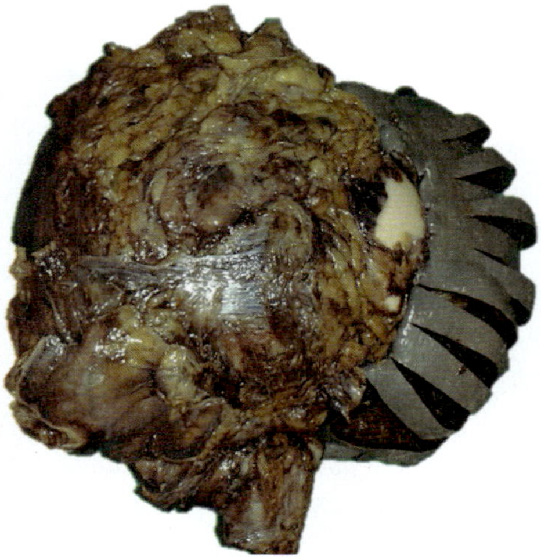

Serous cystadenoma of the pancreas

MICROCYSTIC SEROUS CYSTADENOMA

Serous cystadenomas usually occur in women aged 60 to 70 years. The lesions are almost always benign and may occur anywhere in the pancreas. Microcystic serous cystadenoma is the more common type of serous cystadenoma.

FIGURE 13.15. This image shows a pancreatic lesion composed of characteristic small cysts with delicate thin walls and filled with serous fluid.

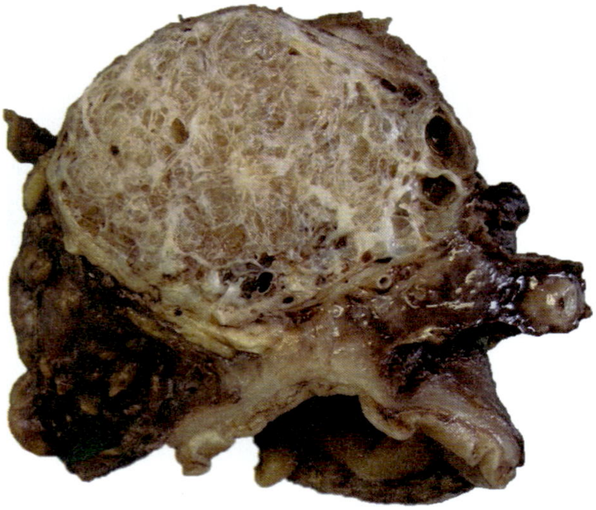

FIGURE 13.16. This example is from the tail of the pancreas (note the spleen, right). The photo was taken around the time of surgery and shows the fresh specimen without formalin fixation.

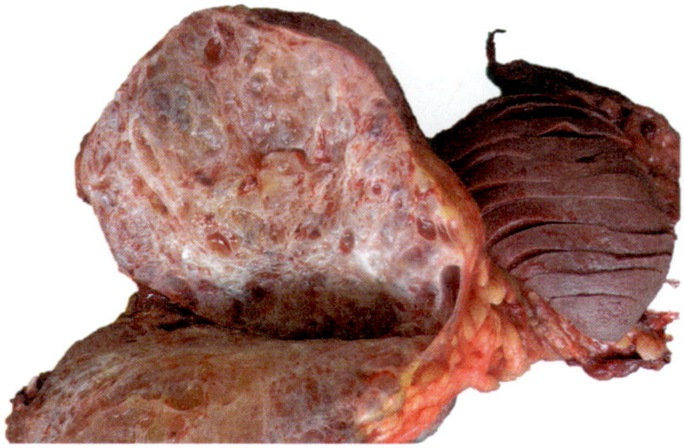

FIGURE 13.17. This patient underwent a Whipple procedure to resect the tumor in the head of the pancreas. The specimen was bisected into anterior and posterior aspects, and demonstrates the tumor in relationship to the head of the pancreas and the duodenum. The pancreas shows a well-circumscribed tumor containing numerous thin-walled cysts of variable size and focal fibrous scarring.

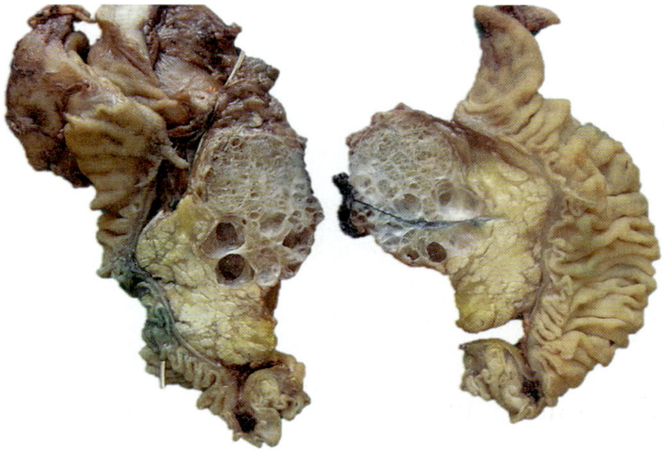

OLIGOCYSTIC (MACROCYSTIC) SEROUS CYSTADENOMA

Although most serous cystadenomas are composed of numerous small cystic spaces, oligocystic serous cystadenoma is characterized by larger and less numerous cysts. There is no difference in prognosis from the usual variant.

FIGURE 13.18. This image shows oligocystic serous cystadenoma of the pancreas. The cysts contained serous fluid. Note the smooth, shiny internal surface of the cysts.

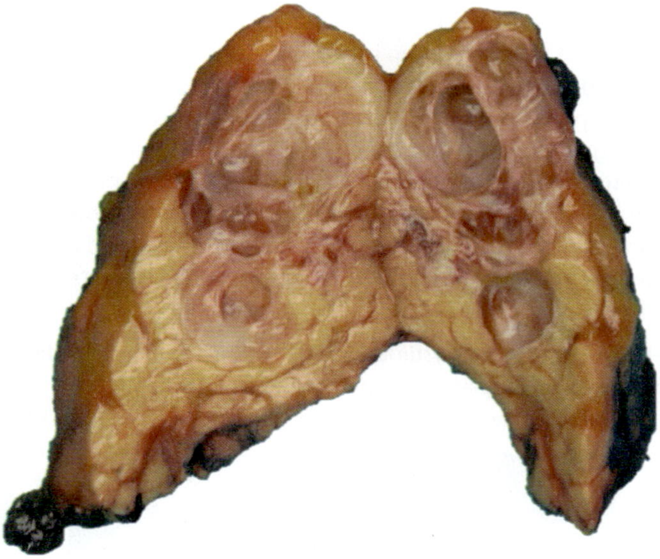

SOLID SEROUS CYSTADENOMA

The solid variant of pancreatic serous cystadenoma is rare and may be confused with neuroendocrine tumor. This misdiagnosis could lead to overtreatment. Solid serous cystadenoma is characterized by a solid pattern of growth with cytological features of serous microcystic adenoma.

FIGURE 13.19. This image of the pancreas shows a well-circumscribed solid tumor with no obvious cysts, necrosis, or hemorrhage.

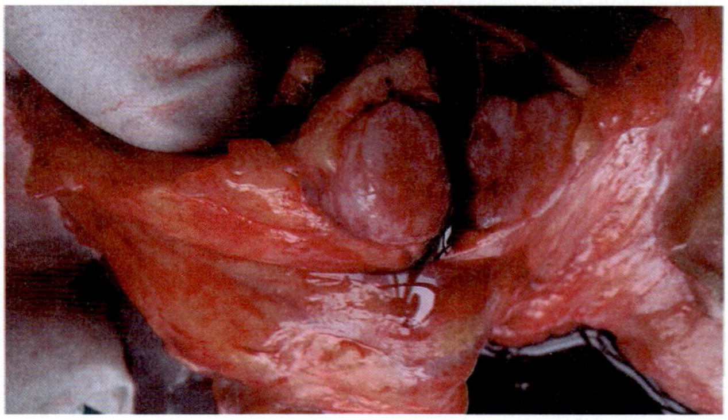

Von Hippel–Lindau disease (VHL) and associated pancreatic serous cystic neoplasm

Patients with VHL may develop 1 or more pancreatic serous cystadenoma. VHL is also associated with neuroendocrine tumors of the pancreas, pheochromocytoma, renal cell carcinoma, and hemangioblastoma.

FIGURE 13.20. This specimen was bisected longitudinally to demonstrate the cystic lesions.

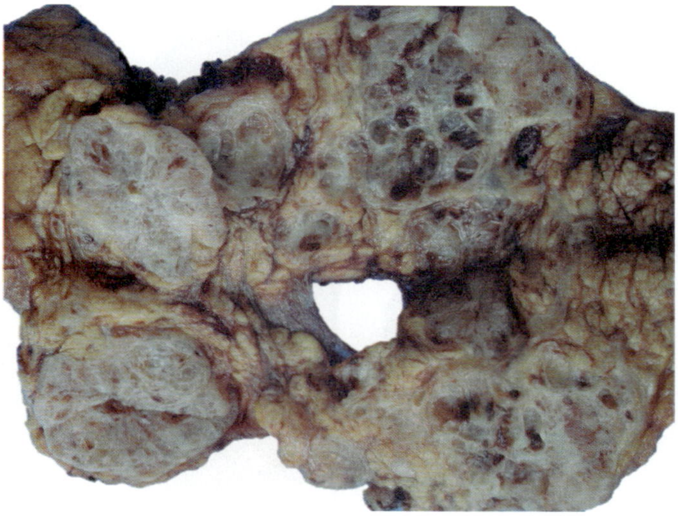

Mucinous cystic neoplasm (MCN) of the pancreas

MCN of the pancreas nearly always arises in perimenopausal women and usually occurs in the tail of the pancreas. The cystic lesions are usually between 6 cm and 10 cm in size, and consist of multiloculated cysts containing thick mucin. The cyst wall classically contains ovarian-type stroma under the epithelial lining. MCNs do not communicate with the pancreatic ductal system. On histology, MCNs are lined by neoplastic, mucin-producing, columnar epithelial cells.

FIGURE 13.21. This resected specimen consists of the pancreatic tail and spleen. The cyst is multiloculated and thick walled.

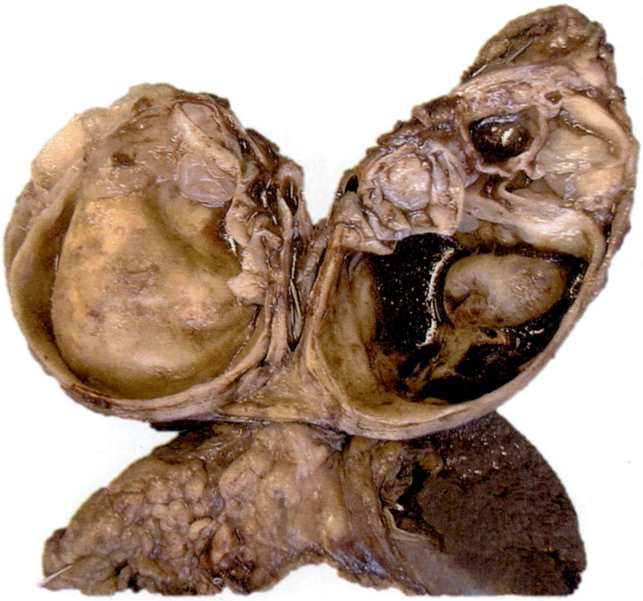

FIGURE 13.22. These images show the cyst before and after it was opened to remove the mucinous contents.

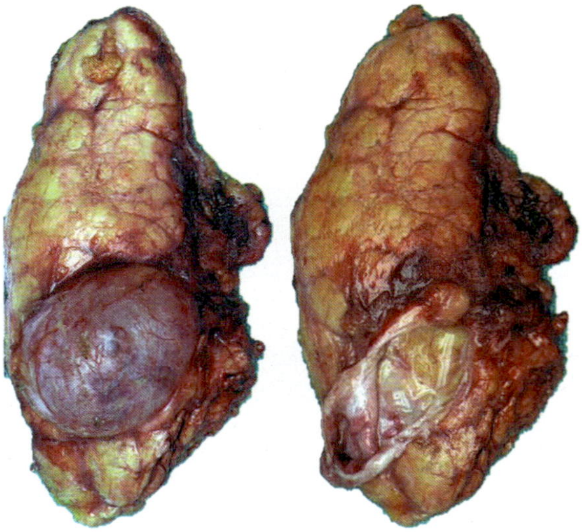

FIGURE 13.23. The MCN in this image appears multilocular and shows a thick wall.

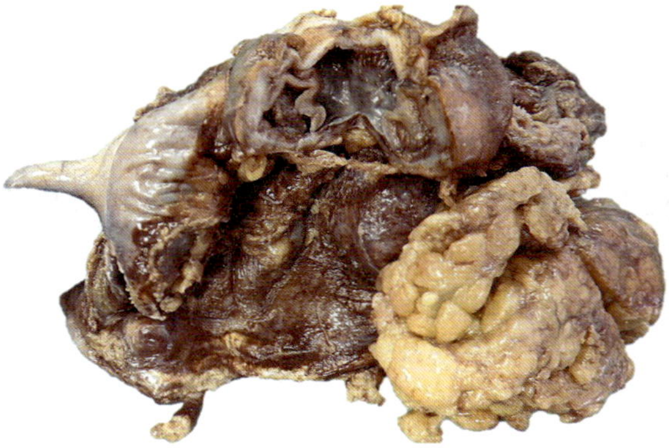

MUCINOUS CYSTIC NEOPLASM (MCN) OF THE PANCREAS WITH INVASIVE ADENOCARCINOMA

MCN can be a precursor lesion of pancreatic adenocarcinoma. Sometimes, the malignant lesion is small and involves only a small part of the cystic lesion. Therefore, all MCNs must be extensively sampled to exclude the possibility of adenocarcinoma.

FIGURE 13.24. This MCN in the tail of the pancreas had an adenocarcinoma identified only on histology.

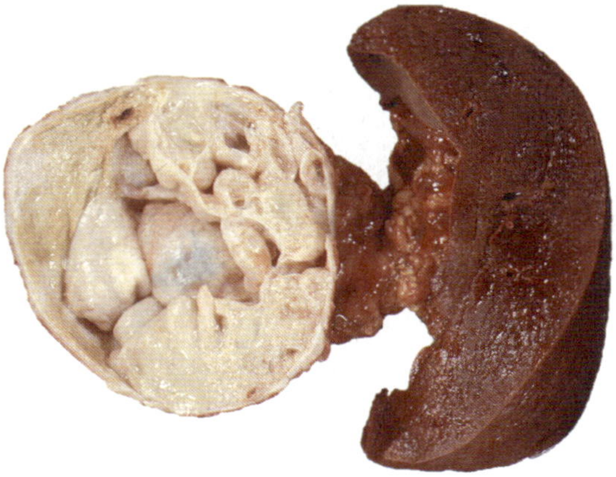

Intraductal papillary mucinous neoplasm (IPMN) of the pancreas

IPMN is typically an intraductal, grossly visible (> 1 cm) lesion involving the main pancreatic duct and/or its branch ducts. It is more common in men. Given that the pancreatic duct normally drains its contents into the duodenum via the ampulla, an astute endoscopist may suspect IPMN upon noting thick viscous mucin protruding from the ampulla of Vater. The lesion may be focal, multifocal, or involve the entire pancreatic duct, and is usually located in the pancreatic head. Extensive sampling is often needed to identify or exclude invasive adenocarcinoma arising from IPMN.

FIGURE 13.25. This cystic lesion is actually a dilated pancreatic duct lined by neoplastic mucinous cells that form papillary structures and secrete mucin.

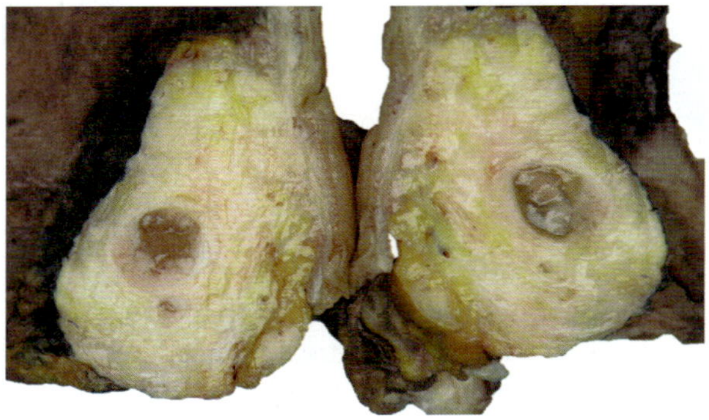

FIGURE 13.26. This image shows a total pancreatectomy specimen with attached duodenum and spleen that is nearly entirely involved by IPMN. Note the diffusely, cystically dilated, tortuous main duct, which was filled with mucin preresection.

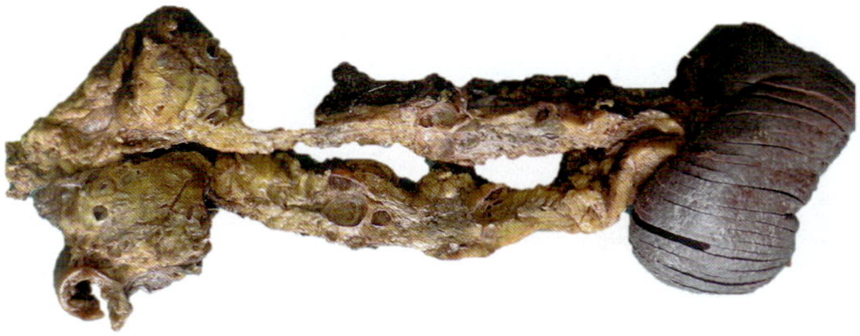

FIGURE 13.27. This image shows IPMN involving the main pancreatic duct in the head of a pancreas. At the center of the image, the dilated pancreatic main duct is visible, with glistening papillary projections into the lumen.

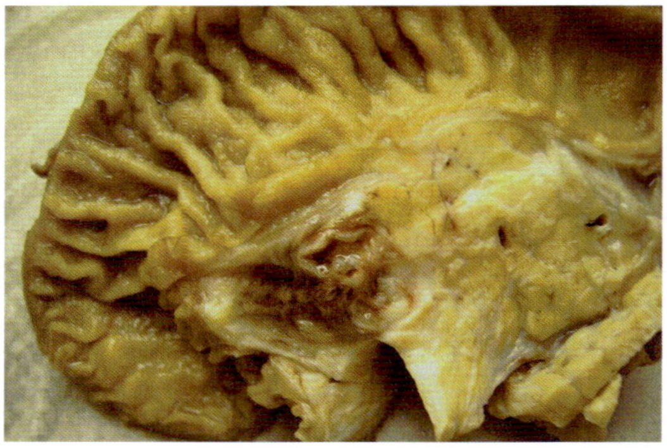

Intraductal tubulopapillary neoplasm (ITPN) of the pancreas

ITPN is a rare, newly recognized entity. It is described as an intraductal epithelial neoplasm of the main pancreatic duct, forming papillary and tubular structures, with high-grade dysplasia but no copious mucin production. It is classified as a separate entity from IPMN.

FIGURE 13.28. Serial sections of this resected pancreas show a solid tumor obstructing the dilated pancreatic duct, with no overt mucin production.

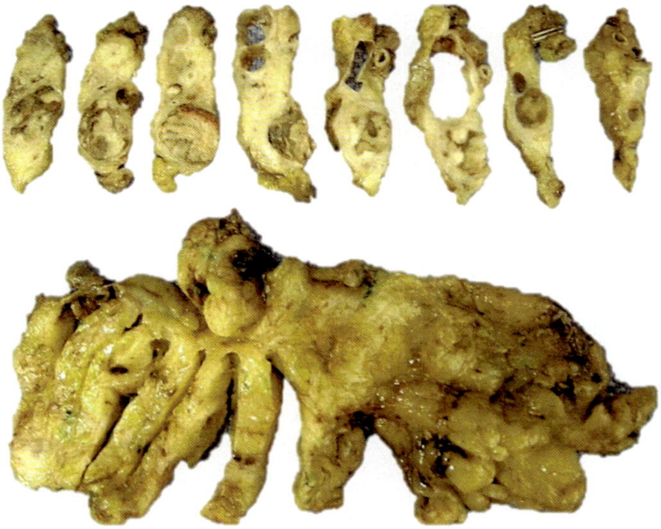

Invasive ductal adenocarcinoma of the pancreas

Invasive ductal adenocarcinoma is among the most aggressive solid tumors and is the most common malignancy of the pancreas. It primarily occurs in older adults (aged 60 to 80 years). It is associated with smoking, obesity, and hereditary diseases such as hereditary pancreatitis, *BRCA* mutation, Lynch syndrome, and Peutz–Jeghers syndrome, among others. There are 3 precursor lesions to invasive ductal adenocarcinoma: pancreatic intraepithelial neoplasia (PanIN), IPMN, and MCN. The genes involved in progression to cancer include K-*ras*, *p16/CDKN2A*, *TP53*, and *SMAD4*. The 5-year survival for patients with invasive ductal adenocarcinoma of the pancreas is approximately 5% overall.

FIGURE 13.29. Note the white, fibrous cancer mass (CA) at the head of the pancreas. Its relation to the pancreatic duct (PD), common bile duct (BD), and ampulla of Vater (AV) is illustrated.

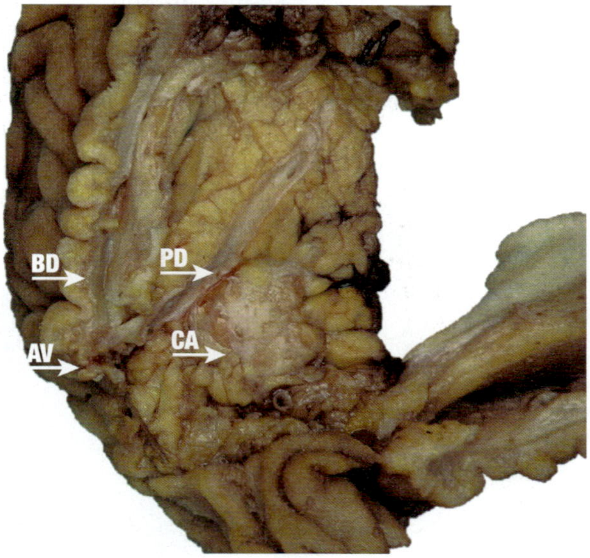

FIGURE 13.30. These serial sections of a resected pancreas show a solid white tumor invading the pancreatic parenchyma with involvement of a round lymph node.

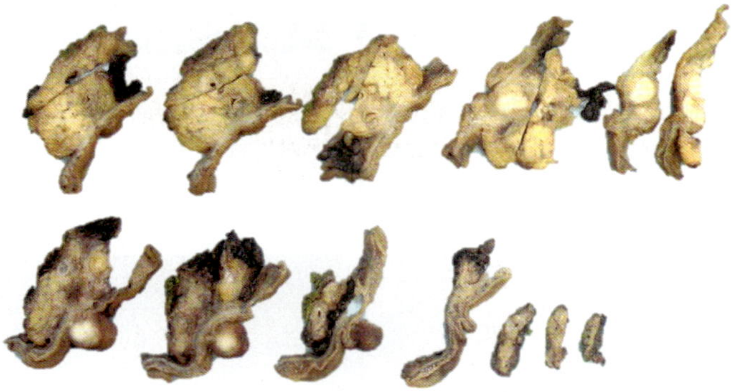

FIGURE 13.31. This image shows a firm, whitish tumor infiltrating the head of a pancreas. Green ink was used to identify the ampulla of Vater and the common bile duct.

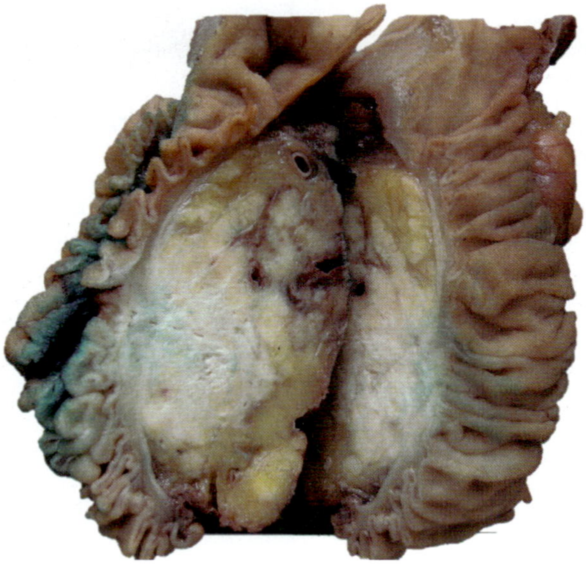

INVASIVE DUCTAL ADENOCARCINOMA ARISING FROM AN IPMN IN THE HEAD OF THE PANCREAS

Tumors in the pancreatic head generally present earlier than those in the tail, because they may impinge on the common bile duct and cause jaundice.

FIGURE 13.32. This Whipple resection shows the head of the pancreas with a white tumor diffusely infiltrating the parenchyma surrounding the cystically dilated and tortuous duct of an IPMN.

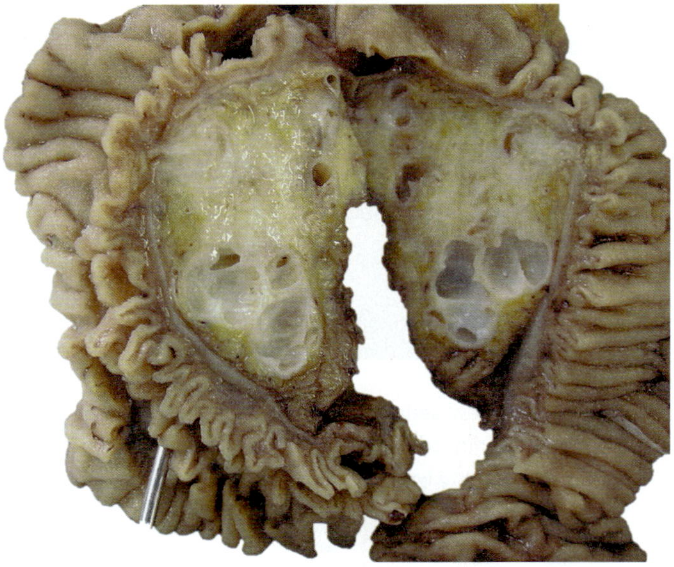

FIGURE 13.33. This close-up shows an invasive ductal adenocarcinoma that has arisen from IPMN in the head of a pancreas. Note the white fibrous tumor infiltrating the head of the pancreas.

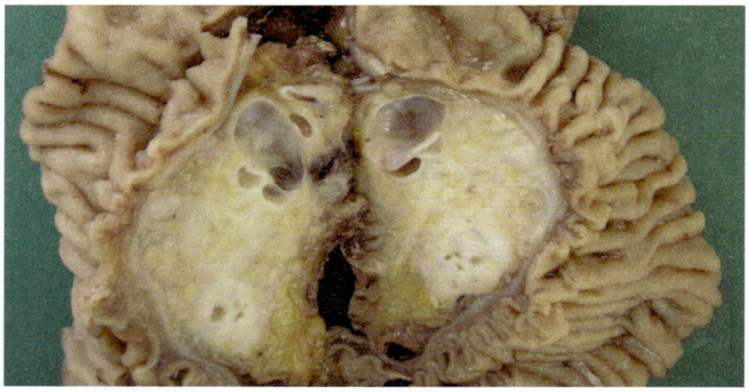

INVASIVE DUCTAL ADENOCARCINOMA OF THE DISTAL PANCREAS

Tumors in the distal pancreas usually present late, after invasion of adjacent organs.

FIGURE 13.34. In this distal pancreatectomy and splenectomy specimen, the tail of the pancreas shows a whitish tumor diffusely infiltrating the parenchyma.

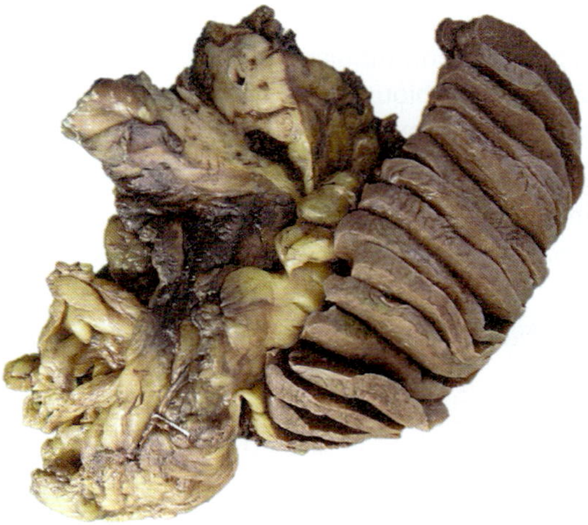

FIGURE 13.35. This resected specimen consists of the distal pancreas and spleen. The tail of the pancreas shows a white tumor diffusely infiltrating the parenchyma but sparing the spleen.

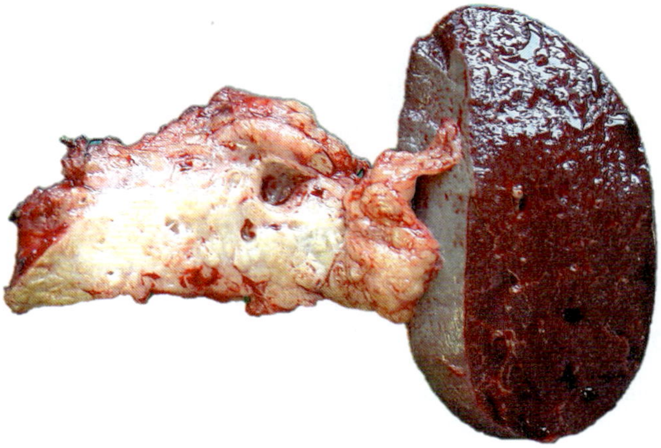

INVASIVE DUCTAL ADENOCARCINOMA — STAGE T3

FIGURE 13.36. This Whipple resection shows a pancreatic tumor infiltrating the duodenal wall. According to the TNM (tumor–lymph node–metastasis) staging system, this type of invasion beyond the pancreas is stage T3.

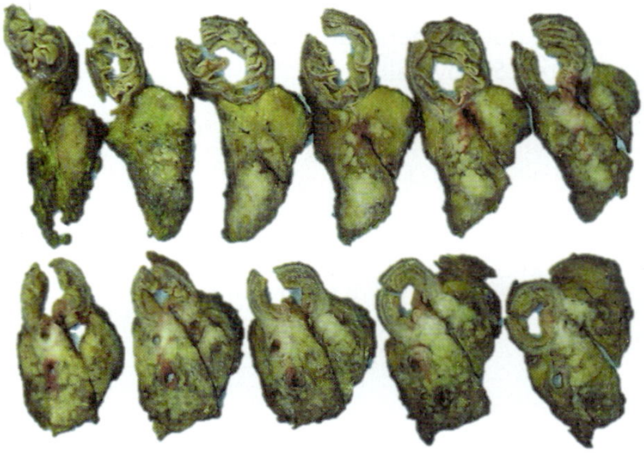

Neuroendocrine tumor (NET) of the pancreas

Unlike invasive ductal adenocarcinoma, NET is usually well circumscribed and may appear encapsulated. NETs, such as insulinomas, may be functional and secrete enough hormone to lead to symptoms. They may be benign or behave aggressively. Even when malignant, pancreatic NETs grow more indolently than ductal adenocarcinomas. Pancreatic NET may be sporadic or may arise in certain hereditary syndromes, such as multiple endocrine neoplasia (MEN) type 1, von Hippel Lindau syndrome, and tuberous sclerosis. The neuroendocrine differentiation of the tumor is confirmed by immunohistochemistry for synaptophysin and chromogranin. In the absence of a clear malignant feature such as nodal or distant metastasis, the assessment of prognosis in pancreatic NETs takes into consideration tumor size, mitotic count, Ki-67 proliferation index, vascular invasion, and local invasion.

FIGURE 13.37. The well-circumscribed solid mass in this distal pancreatectomy specimen shows a typical yellowish, fine cut surface.

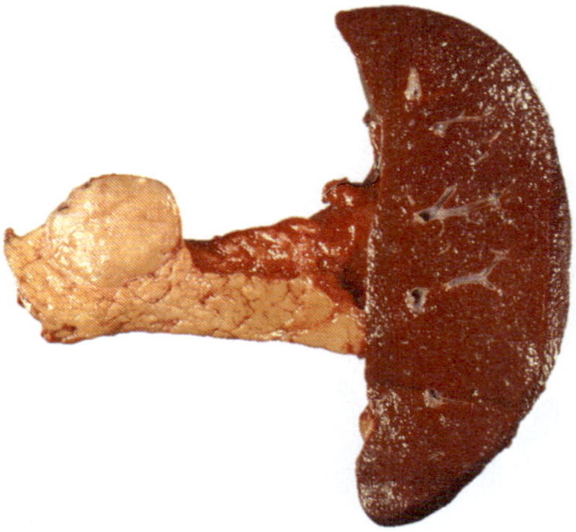

FIGURE 13.38. In this image, note the well-circumscribed pancreatic neoplasm with a yellow-brown homogenous cut surface.

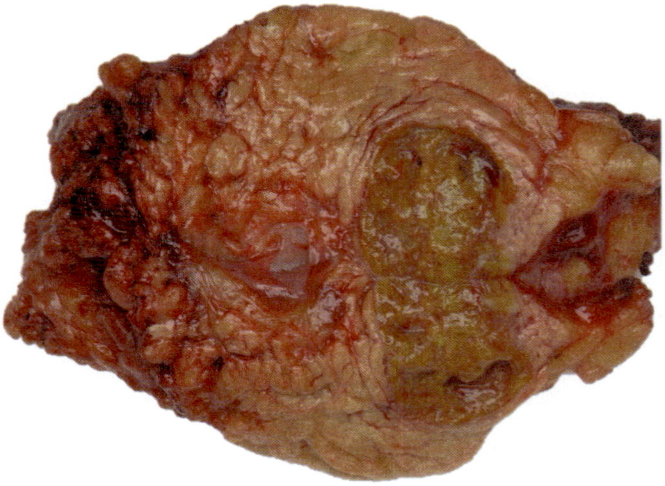

FIGURE 13.39. Images (A) and (B) show tumors with tan-yellow, homogenous cut surfaces. The tumors are well circumscribed and appear encapsulated.

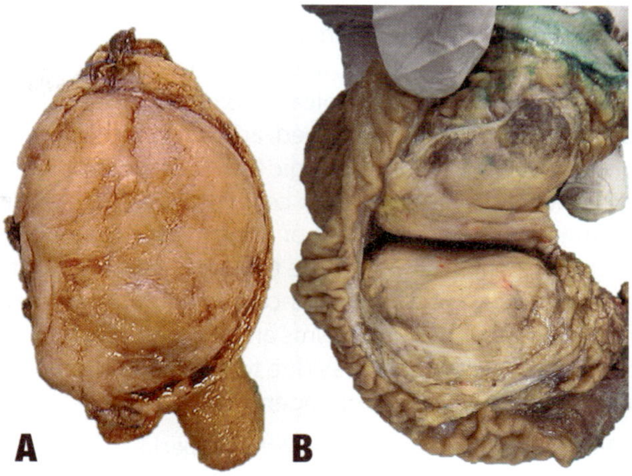

FIGURE 13.40. This example shows a more hemorrhagic, darker neoplasm. It is well circumscribed and surrounded by a capsule.

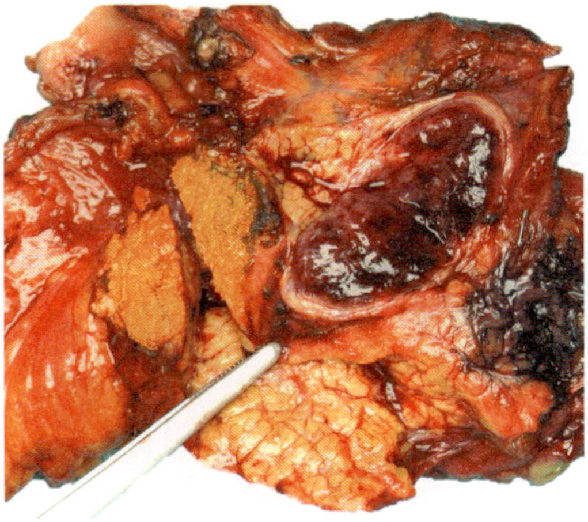

MALIGNANT NEUROENDOCRINE TUMOR (NET) OF THE PANCREAS

FIGURE 13.41. The malignant NET in (A) had numerous liver metastases, shown in (B).

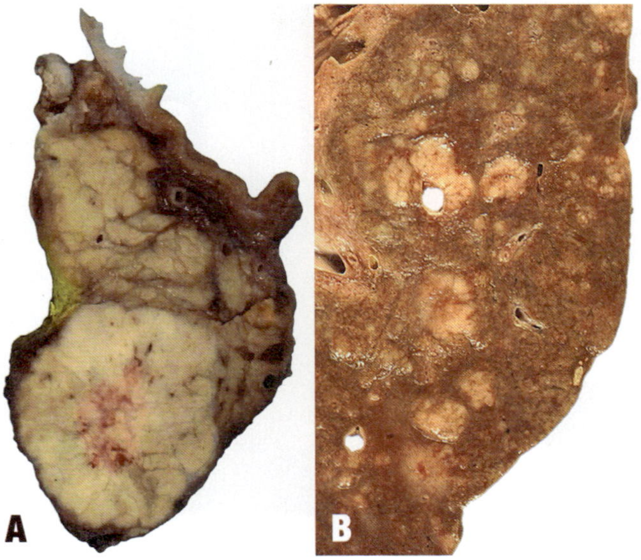

Solid pseudopapillary neoplasm of the pancreas

This is a rare, low-grade malignancy of the pancreas, occurring mainly in young females. It may be locally invasive, but is not usually metastatic, and therefore can be cured by wide resection. Macroscopically, solid pseudopapillary neoplasms are well circumscribed, and have both solid and cystic areas with hemorrhagic foci. Microscopically, they show solid sheets of tumor cells with pseudopapillary structures created by drop-out of noncohesive tumor cells. Immunohistochemistry for these tumors is variable, but they characteristically show nuclear ß-catenin immunostaining. Solid pseudopapillary neoplasms are associated with activation of the Wnt pathway due to an acquired activating mutation of the ß-catenin oncogene.

FIGURE 13.42. This distal pancreatectomy specimen demonstrates a pale tumor with focal hemorrhage. The tumor almost completely replaces the tail of the pancreas, but does not involve the spleen.

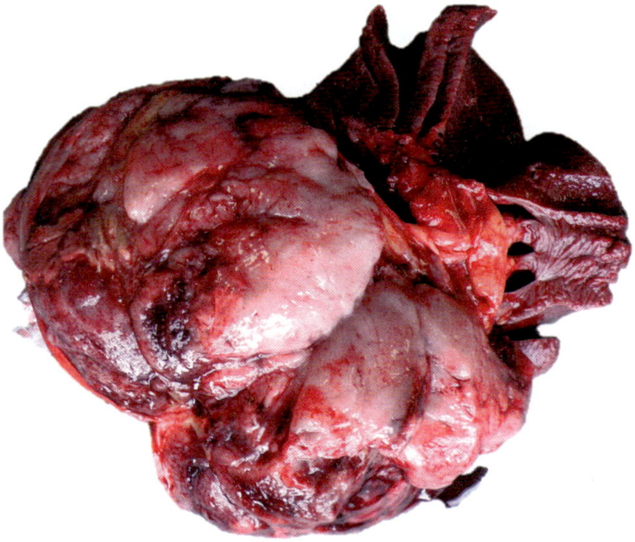

FIGURE 13.43. This tumor shows distinct solid and cystic areas with focal hemorrhage.

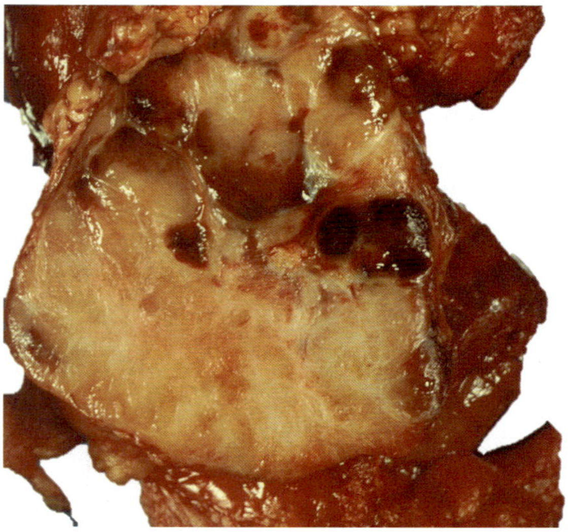

FIGURE 13.44. This tumor appears predominantly cystic with papillary projections into the cystic cavity. The cyst is formed due to tissue necrosis and hemorrhage. The papillary structure represents the viable tumor tissue.

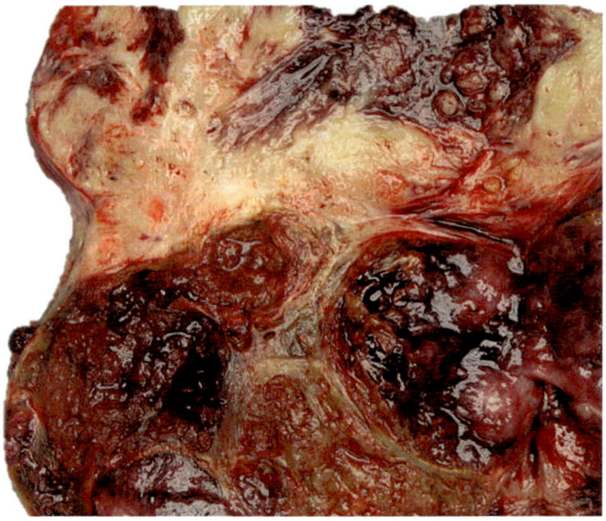

Pancreas with metastatic renal cell carcinoma (RCC)

Although the pancreas is rarely involved by metastasis from other sites, RCC is the most common primary tumor causing pancreatic metastasis.

FIGURE 13.45. These serial sections of a pancreas show a well-circumscribed, variegated tumor with hemorrhage and necrosis.

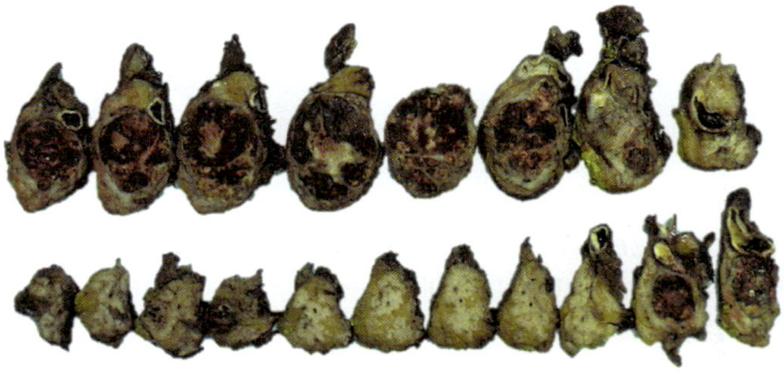

REFERENCES

Bosman FT, Carneiro F, Hruban RH, Theise ND, editors. *WHO classification of tumours of the digestive system*. 4th ed. Lyon, France: IARC Press; 2010.

Kumar V, Abbas AK, Fausto N, Aster J. *Robbins and Cotran pathologic basis of disease*. 9th ed. Philadelphia: Saunders/Elsevier; 2015.

Lester SC. *Manual of surgical pathology*. 3rd ed. Philadelphia: Elsevier Churchill Livingstone; 2010.

Mills SE, Carter D, Greenson JK, Hornick JL, Longacre TA, Reuter VE, editors. *Sternberg's diagnostic surgical pathology*. 6th ed. Philadelphia: Wolters Kluwer Health; 2015.

Odze RD, Goldblum JR. *Surgical pathology of the GI tract, liver, biliary tract, and pancreas*. 3rd ed. Philadelphia: Saunders/Elsevier; 2015.

Rosai J. *Rosai and Ackerman's surgical pathology*. 10th ed. Edinburgh, NY: Mosby/Elsevier; 2011.

14

Diseases of the Kidney, Bladder, and Male Genital Organs

FADI BRIMO, DUC-VINH THAI, PYLYP ZOLOTAROV, SARAH-JEANNE PILON, OLUYOMI AJISE, JENNIFER MERRIMEN

Kidney

Fetal lobulation

Fetal lobulation is considered a normal variant of kidneys in adults, and should be distinguished from renal cortical scarring.

FIGURE 14.1. Note the lobulated appearance of the kidneys. These are remnants of fetal lobulation that occasionally persist into adult life.

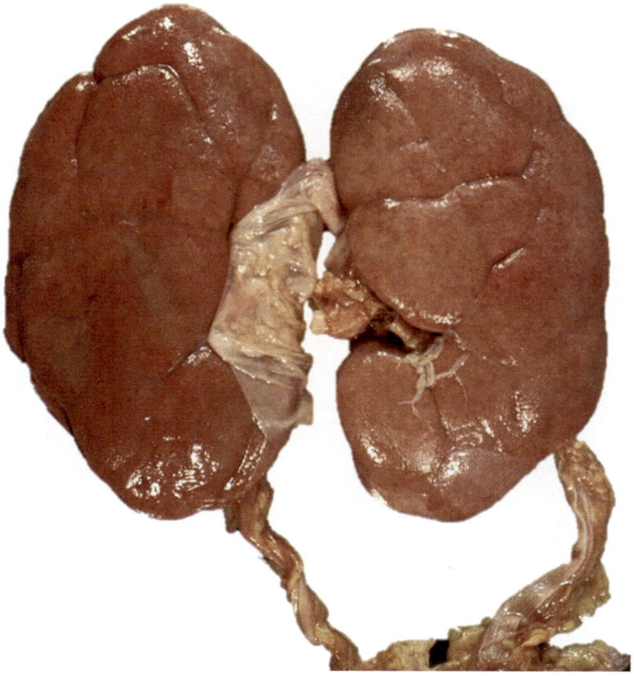

Double ureters

Duplication of ureters can occur from aberrant development of the ureteric bud. They are usually asymptomatic, but, rarely, can cause recurrent urinary tract infections.

FIGURE 14.2. This image of the urinary tract of a full-term female anencephalic fetus shows kidneys with double ureters and marked fetal lobulation.

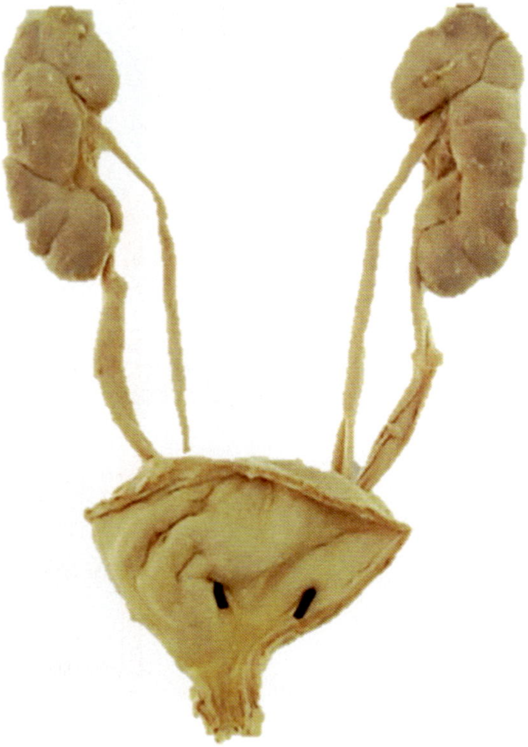

Kidney with double collective system

This anomaly, in which a single renal parenchyma is drained by 2 pyelocaliceal systems, is also called duplex kidney. This condition can be unilateral or bilateral, and can be associated with a variety of congenital genitourinary tract abnormalities. Most patients are asymptomatic: genitourinary tract abnormalities are generally detected incidentally on imaging for other reasons.

FIGURE 14.3. This image shows a kidney drained by 2 pyelocaliceal systems located at the upper and lower poles of the kidney.

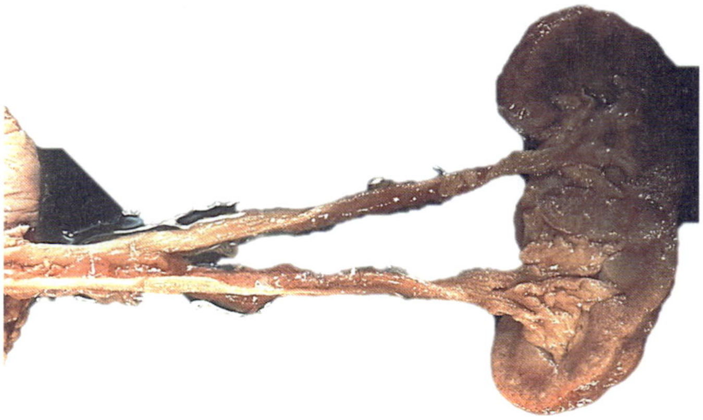

Hydroureter

Structural anomalies of the ureter may be congenital or acquired. Hydroureter is a dilatation and elongation of the ureter with increased tortuosity leading to increased risk of urinary flow obstruction and secondary pyelonephritis.

FIGURE 14.4. This image shows a dilated ureter (arrow).

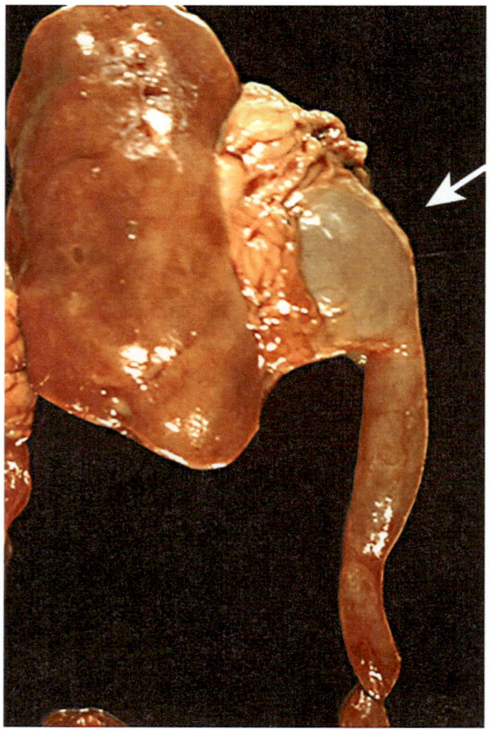

Horseshoe kidney

Horseshoe kidney — along with agenesis of the kidney, hypoplasia, and ectopic kidneys — is among a collection of significant congenital renal anomalies that may account for more than 20% of pediatric chronic kidney disease. Horseshoe kidney is a rare congenital anomaly. The horseshoe shape of the kidneys is due to the fusion of independent metanephric blastema during the second gestational month, which prevents the normal rotation of the kidney during embryogenesis. It has a male predominance and an incidence that ranges from 1:350 to 1:1800. Horseshoe kidney is usually an incidental finding on plain radiographs, or is found during postmortem examination.

FIGURE 14.5. The horseshoe shape of the kidney in this postmortem is due to the fusion of the lower poles of the kidney.

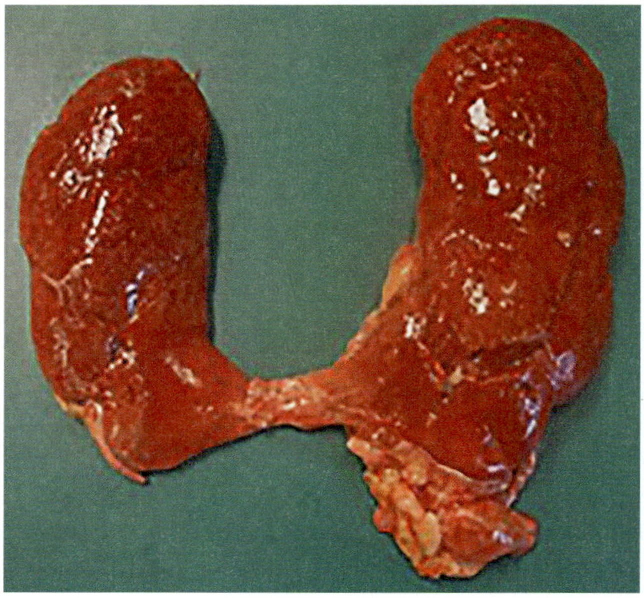

FIGURE 14.6. These kidneys are connected at their lower poles, and the left ureter has an abnormal course. The isthmus of this horseshoe kidney was at the pelvic brim.

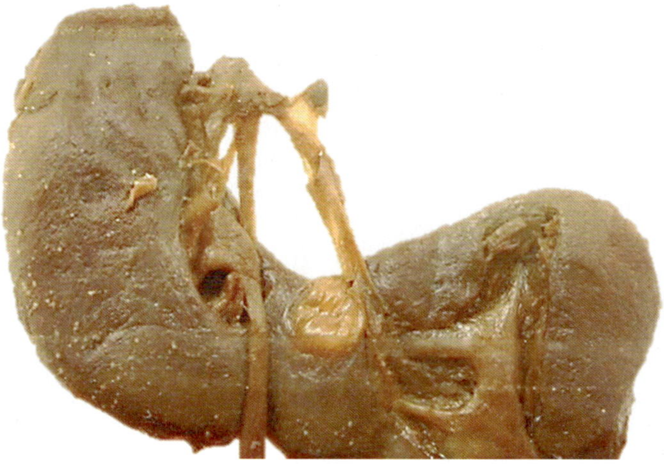

Allograft rejection

Allograft rejection may be due to antibody-mediated rejection, T-cell mediated rejection, chronic allograph nephropathy, nephrotoxicity from immunosuppressive drugs, viral infections, and recurrence of renal disease.

FIGURE 14.7. The cut surface of this kidney is hemorrhagic, brown, and friable-to-soft due to necrosis of the tissue post–allograft rejection.

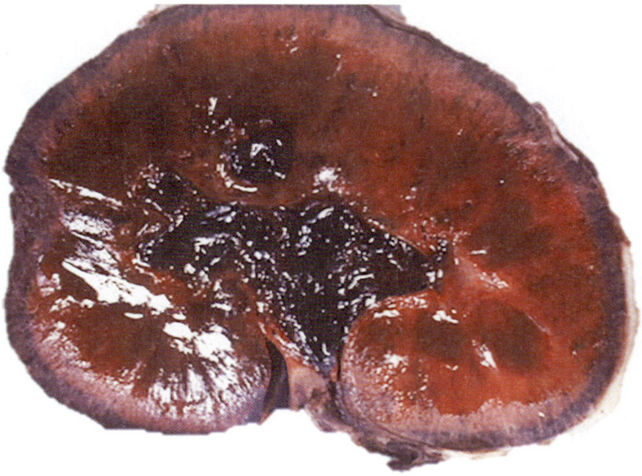

Xanthogranulomatous pyelonephritis

Xanthogranulomatous pyelonephritis is an uncommon variant of chronic pyelonephritis due to an infection (e.g., *Escherichia coli*) or renal stones. This disease can be easily mistaken for clear cell–type (conventional) renal cell carcinoma (RCC).

FIGURE 14.8. The cut surface of this kidney shows xanthogranulomatous inflammation involving the calyces and renal pelvis. In addition, there are some yellow, irregularly shaped, firm staghorn calculi lodged within the renal pelvis.

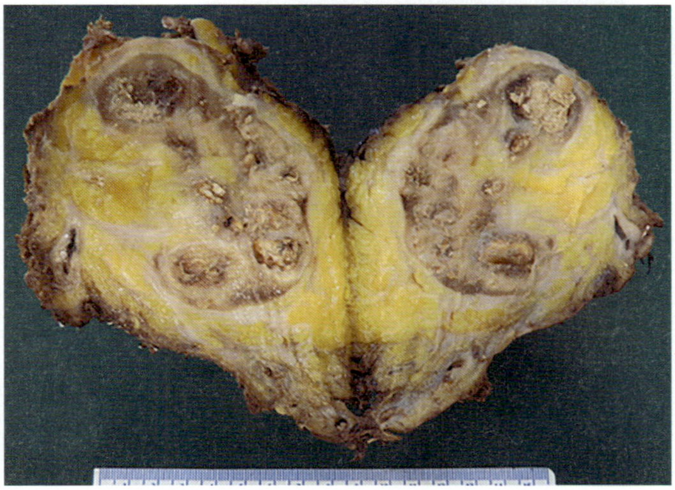

Multiple multilocular cysts of the kidney

Simple renal cysts are very common and are usually benign. Multiloculated cysts may be benign, but may also represent cystic renal tumors such as cystic clear cell RCC, cystic clear cell papillary RCC, and multilocular cystic renal neoplasm of low malignant potential, among others.

FIGURE 14.9. This image shows several cysts in the upper pole of a kidney, some of which are multiloculated.

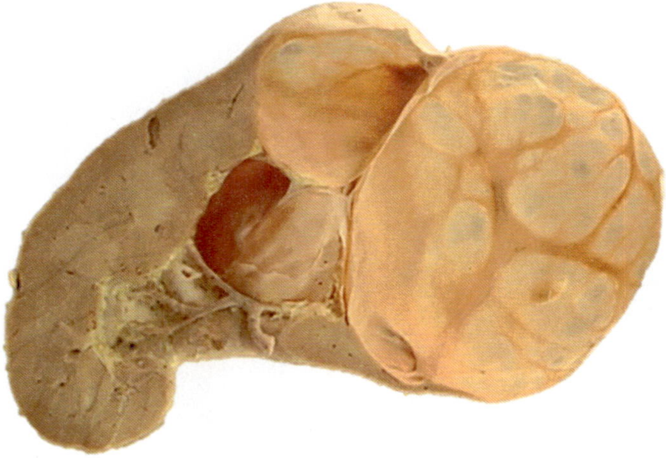

Autosomal-recessive polycystic kidney disease (ARPKD)

This a rare condition affecting both the kidneys and liver, and results from a range of mutations in the *PKHD1* gene. Multiple cysts develop starting from birth over the course of life, replacing the parenchyma and leading to renal failure.

FIGURE 14.10. This image shows an enlarged kidney with multiple cysts and a staghorn calculus.

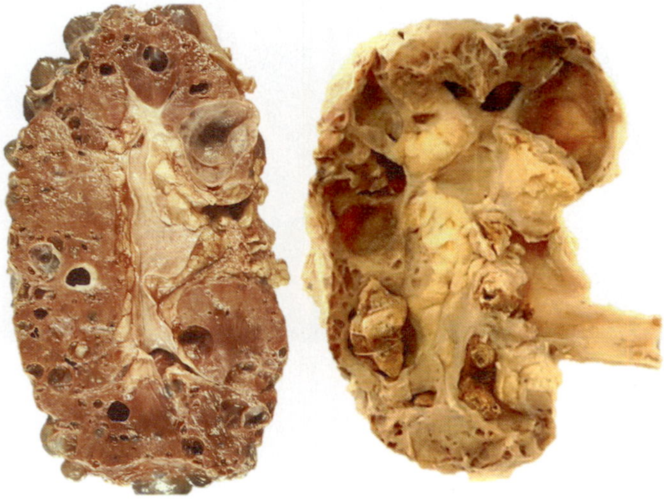

Autosomal-dominant polycystic kidney disease (ADPKD)

This is a frequent genetic cause of end-stage renal disease. It is a common inherited disorder and is usually due to mutations in gene coding for polycystin 1 and 2 by the *PKD1* and *PKD2* genes.

FIGURE 14.11. These kidneys are enlarged because of cysts of variable size replacing the entire parenchyma.

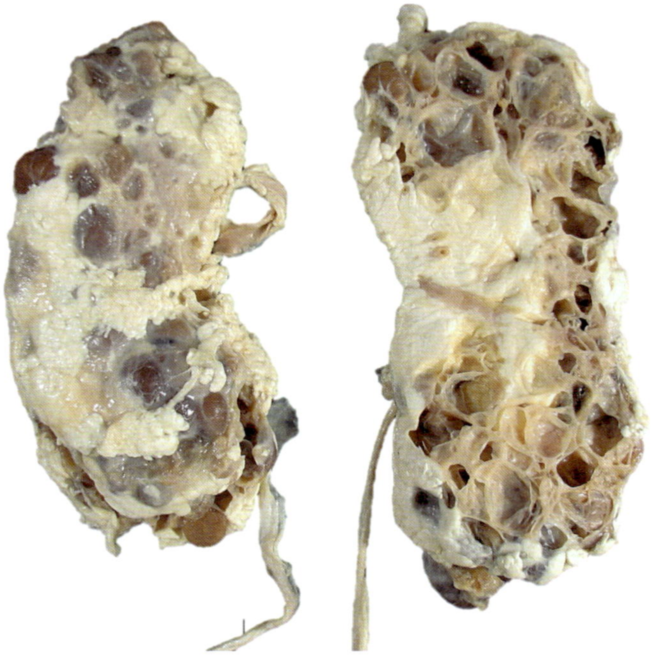

FIGURE 14.12. This magnified view of the kidney shown in figure 14.11 shows multiple variable sized cysts separated by fibrous septa.

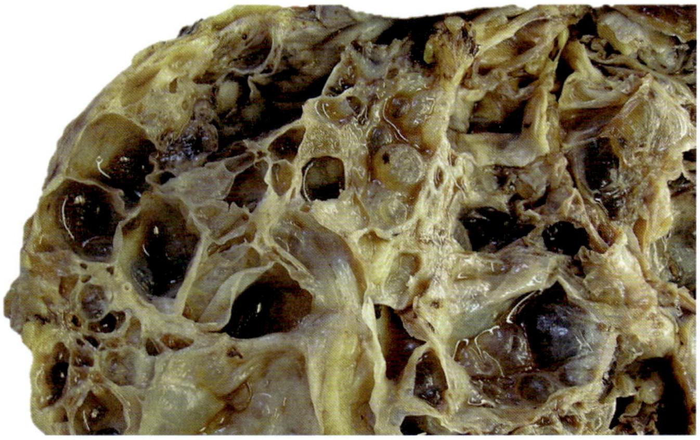

FIGURE 14.13. Note the enlarged kidneys and the presence of a large number of cysts of variable sizes.

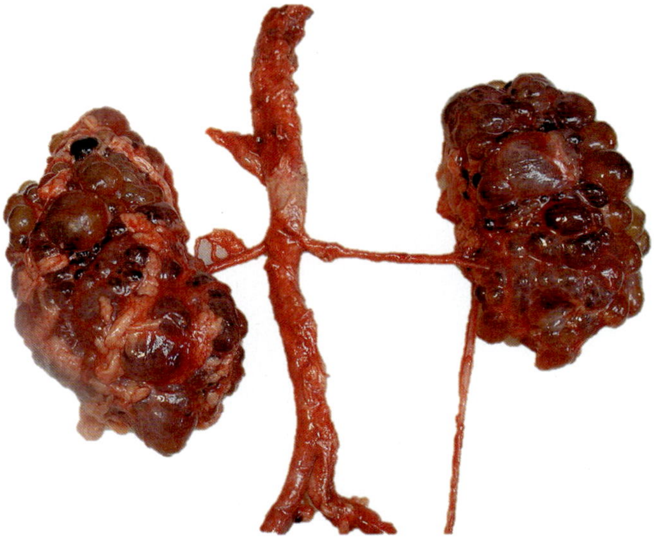

Oncocytoma

Oncocytomas are benign renal neoplasms with male predominance that primarily affect adults. They may be asymptomatic or may present with hematuria, flank pain, or a palpable mass. Oncocytomas usually appear as solid tumors with a homogenous mahogany brown color. In some cases, the lesion may be tan-to-pale in color. In up to a third of cases, oncocytomas show a central, stellate scar.

FIGURE 14.14. On this cut section of a partial nephrectomy, the tumor appears well circumscribed and nonencapsulated. This lesion has the classic appearance of a solid tumor with homogenous mahogany brown color and central scar.

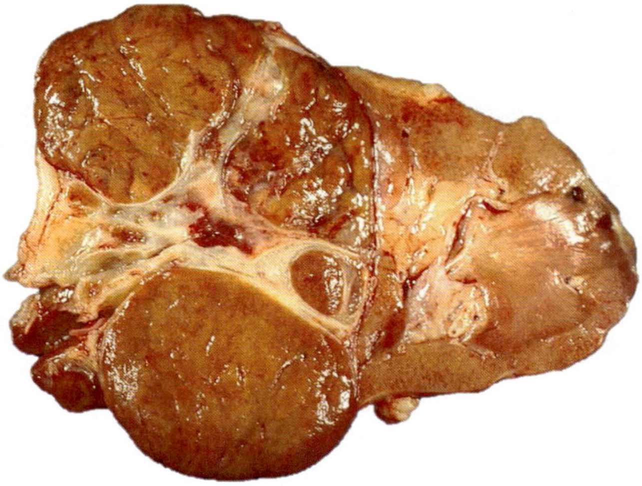

FIGURE 14.15. This image shows an oncocytoma with tan-to-pale coloring, which is less common than mahogany brown coloring. Oncocytomas with this coloring may be mistaken for chromophobe RCC.

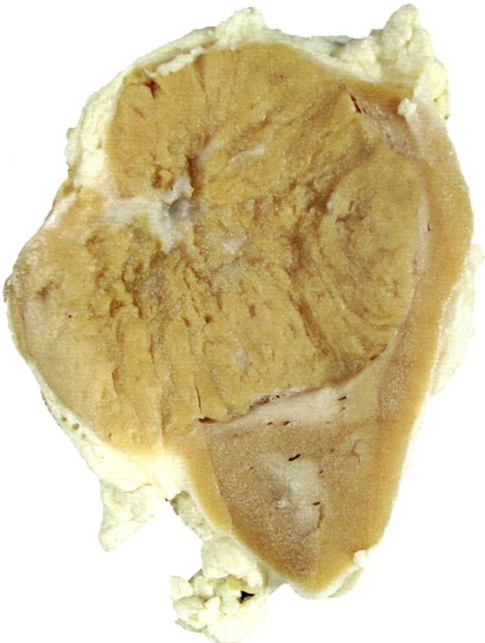

FIGURE 14.16. In this example, the tumor has a solid homogenous appearance with a dark brown color and no central scar.

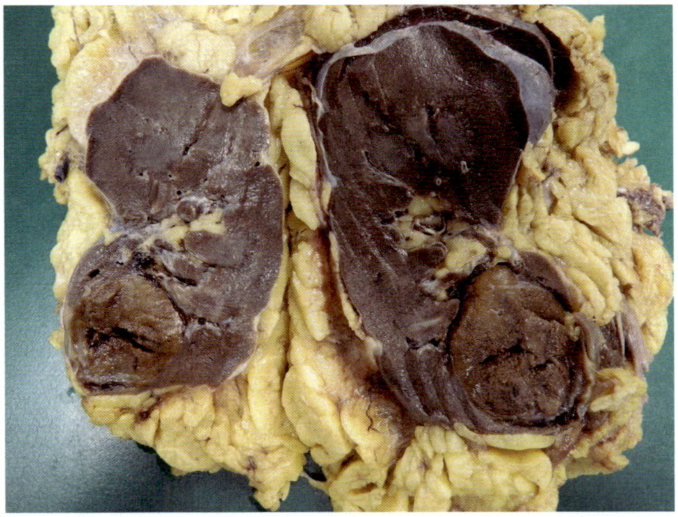

Mixed epithelial stromal tumor (MEST)

MESTs are biphasic tumors composed of epithelial elements, usually in the form of cysts of variable sizes mixed with expansile stromal elements forming solid nodules. MESTs grossly resemble cystic nephromas. Cystic nephromas, however, are composed of multiple noncommunicating, thin-walled cysts in the absence of solid mural nodules, hemorrhage, and necrotic areas.

FIGURE 14.17. This MEST shows both solid and cystic areas. Expansile stromal elements forming thickened septa or solid nodules (arrow) are also visible.

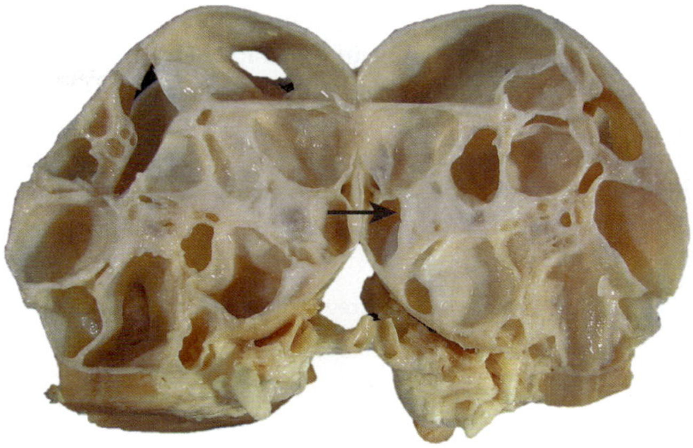

Echinococcal (hydatid) cyst

Hydatidosis may rarely involve the kidneys and can easily be mistaken for a cystic tumor clinically and macroscopically.

FIGURE 14.18. This cyst has a unilocular configuration and is lined by an easily detached membrane showing polypoid structures, which microscopically display the typical features seen in hydatid cyst, including protoscolices and hooklets.

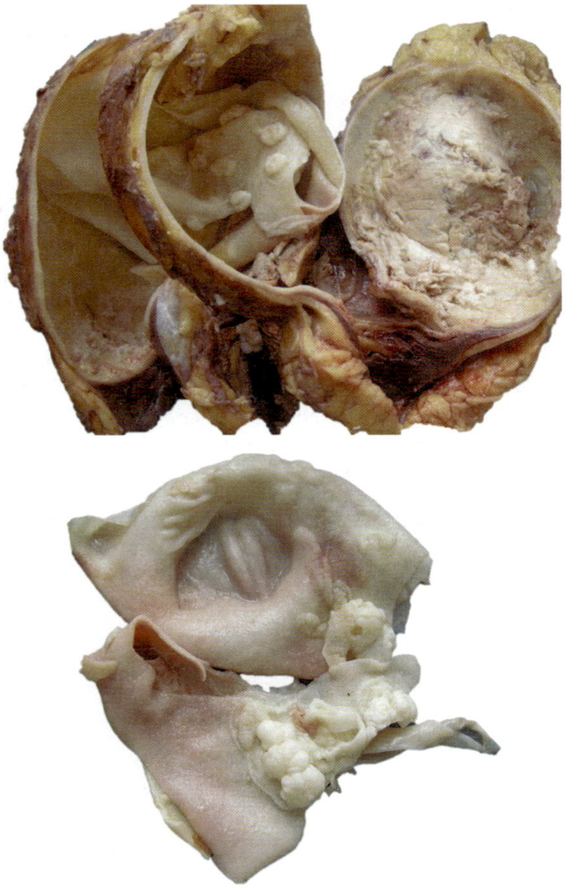

Clear cell (conventional) renal cell carcinoma (RCC)

Clear cell RCC accounts for 80% of RCCs and has metastatic potential. The most common genetic abnormality is loss of the short arm of chromosome 3, which harbors the von Hippel–Lindau (VHL) gene. Although most RCCs present as well-circumscribed, rounded, and solitary masses, some may occur as multiple infiltrative nodules. Findings of necrosis, hemorrhage, and calcifications are common. "Fish flesh" white areas may suggest sarcomatoid differentiation and should be sampled.

FIGURE 14.19. This cut surface reveals the characteristic golden-yellow color with areas of necrosis and hemorrhage.

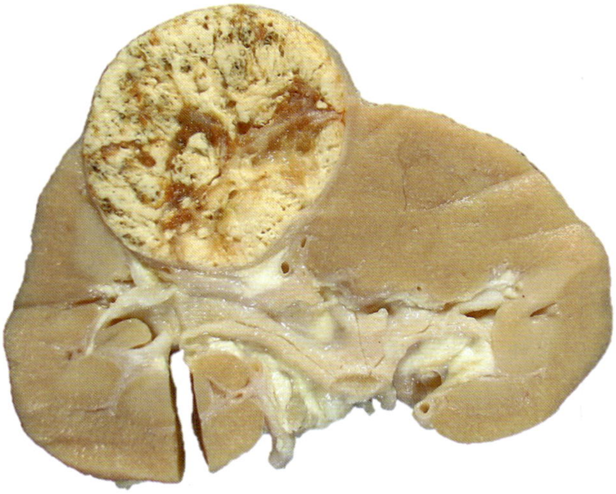

RCC WITH EXTRARENAL SPREAD

The most common route of extrarenal spread is invasion of the renal hilum and renal vein, but some tumors may also invade the perirenal adipose tissue. Even in the absence of macroscopic involvement, it is recommended to routinely sample the hilar region.

FIGURE 14.20. This very large tumor almost entirely replaces the renal parenchyma and shows invasion of the renal vein. Note the renal vein tumor thrombus in the left upper corner.

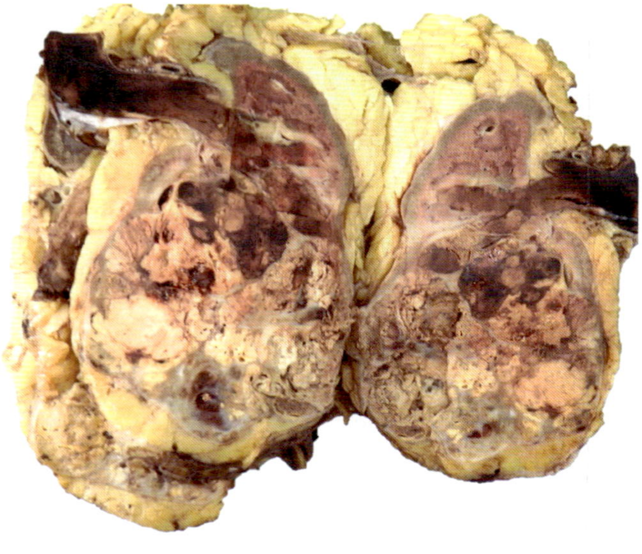

FIGURE 14.21. This very large tumor almost entirely replaces the renal parenchyma with invasion of the renal vein.

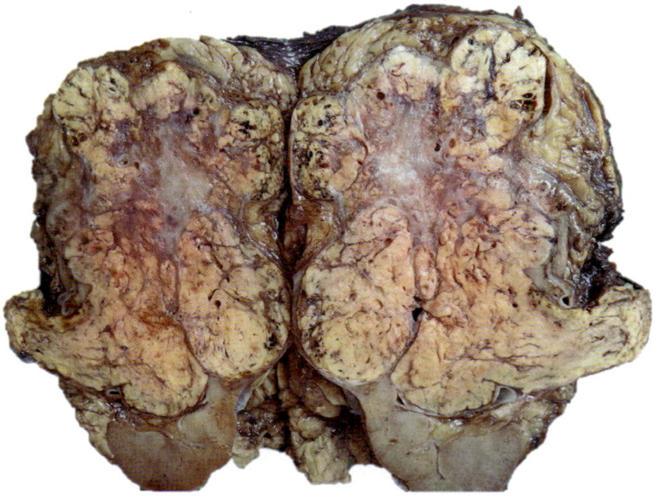

FIGURE 14.22. This large tumor replaces most of the renal parenchyma and shows gross invasion of the renal vein (arrow).

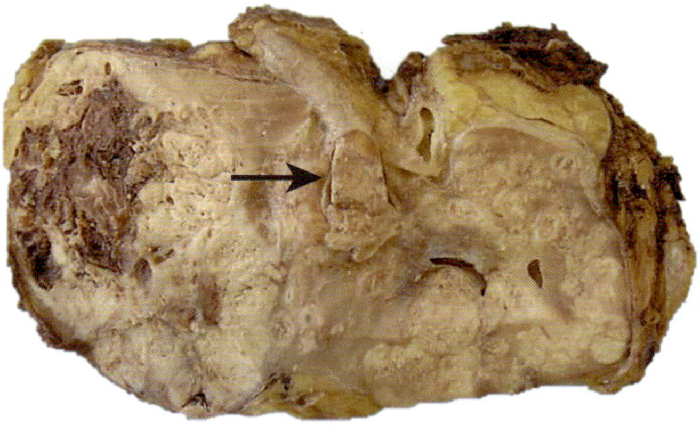

FIGURE 14.23. This image shows a tumor invading the perirenal adipose tissue (arrow).

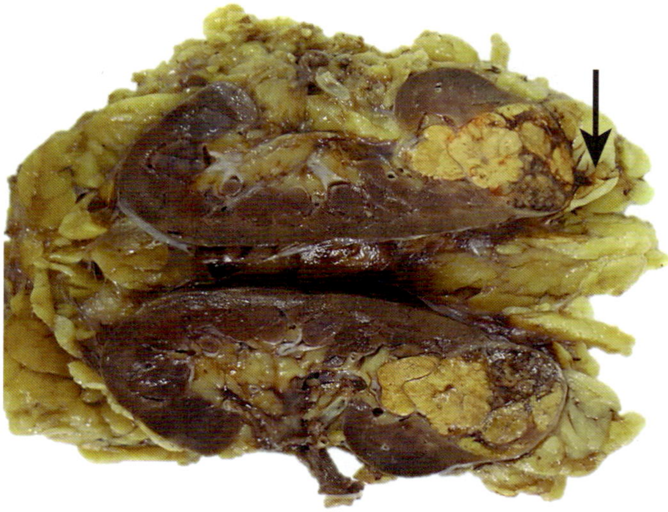

FIGURE 14.24. This tumor invades the hilar adipose tissue (arrowhead, left) and the perirenal adipose tissue (arrowhead, right). The "fish flesh" white areas (arrow) may suggest sarcomatoid differentiation and should be sampled.

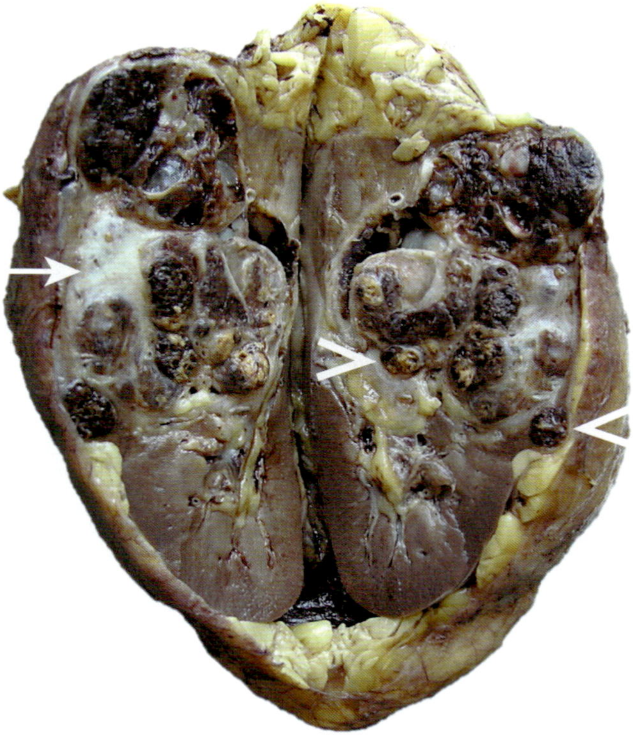

FIGURE 14.25. Although tumors showing hilar adipose tissue invasion are generally > 5 cm, smaller tumors can occasionally invade the hilum as seen in this image (arrow).

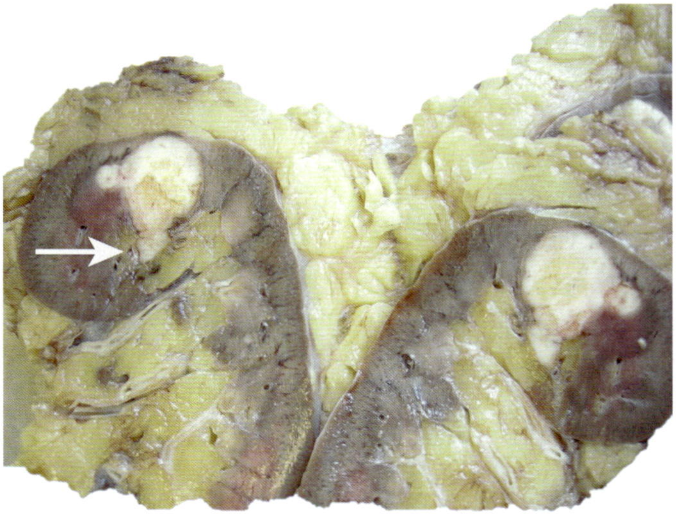

CLEAR CELL RCC WITH TUMOR THROMBUS

In cases of clear cell RCC involving tumor thrombus, care should be taken not to overinterpret the tip of the thrombus as a positive surgical margin. Instead, the distal end of the vein wall is considered the true renal vein margin.

FIGURE 14.26. This clear cell RCC invades the renal vein and forms a tumor thrombus. Note the tip of the thrombus (arrow) and the distal end of the vein wall (arrowheads).

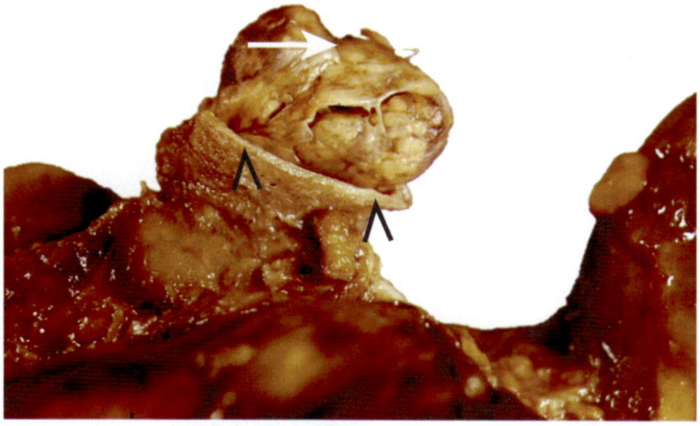

CLEAR CELL RCC WITH CYSTIC CHANGES

Cystic changes are a common finding in clear cell RCC and are usually due to the presence of necrosis and secondary degenerative changes. Tumors with extensive cystic changes may raise the possibility of cystic renal neoplasms, such as cystic nephroma and multilocular cystic renal neoplasm of low malignant potential.

FIGURE 14.27. This is a clear cell RCC showing extensive cystic degeneration.

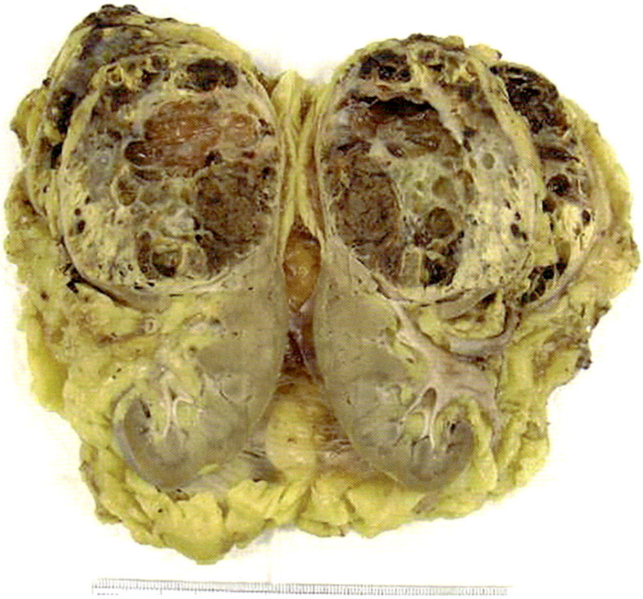

CLEAR CELL RCC ARISING IN THE SETTING OF AUTOSOMAL DOMINANT POLYCYSTIC KIDNEY DISEASE (ADPKD)

ADPKD increases the risk of developing renal tumors, which include papillary adenoma, papillary carcinoma, clear cell RCC, and clear cell papillary RCC, among others. Therefore, radical nephrectomies performed in the setting of polycystic kidney disease should be carefully examined for any solid areas: these should be sampled to exclude tumoral processes.

FIGURE 14.28. Image (A) shows a kidney from a patient with ADPKD with multiple small cysts; a small clear cell RCC is also present (arrow). Image (B) gives a closer view of the same tumor.

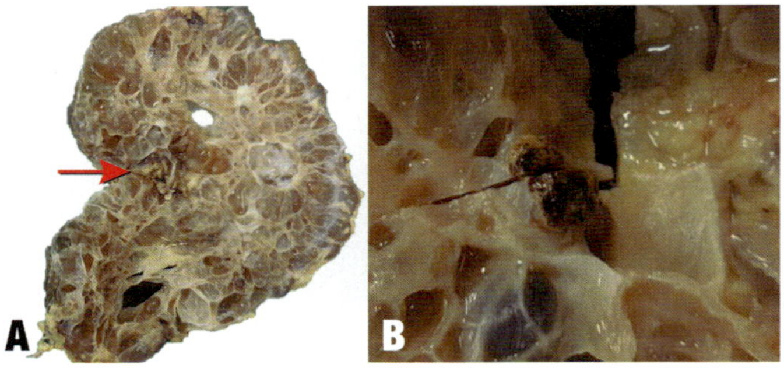

Multilocular cystic renal neoplasm of low malignant potential

This tumor has an excellent prognosis and can be distinguished from cystic clear cell RCC (which has metastatic potential) by the following: absence of solid, grossly discernible, expansile nodules of clear cells; low-grade cytological features; and absence of necrosis, vascular invasion, or sarcomatoid differentiation. Generous sampling is recommended before making this diagnosis.

FIGURE 14.29. This multilocular cystic renal neoplasm is composed of multiple cysts and shows no expansile or solid nodules.

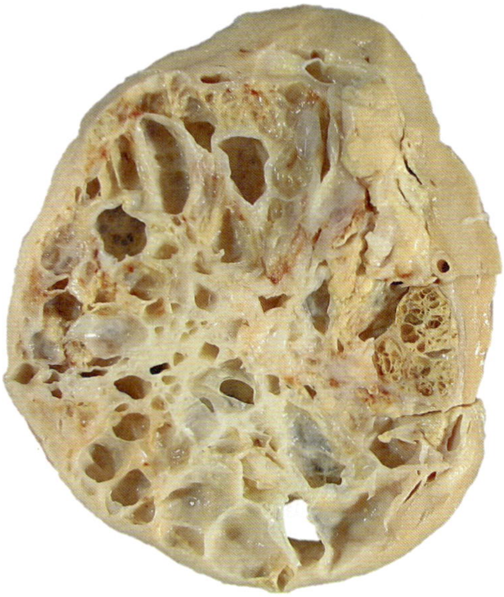

Papillary renal cell carcinoma

This common type of RCC has distinct histological types: type 1 and type 2. Type 2 tumors have a larger size, higher grade, and worse prognosis than type 1 tumors.

FIGURE 14.30. Macroscopically, this papillary RCC is well circumscribed, and is surrounded by a fibrous capsule. It has a characteristic friable appearance, and ranges in color from beige to red depending on the extent of intratumoral hemorrhage and necrosis.

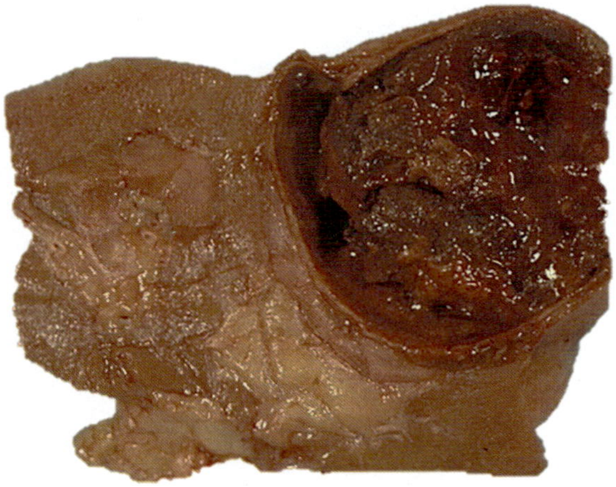

FIGURE 14.31. This tumor has a tan color and shows cystic degeneration.

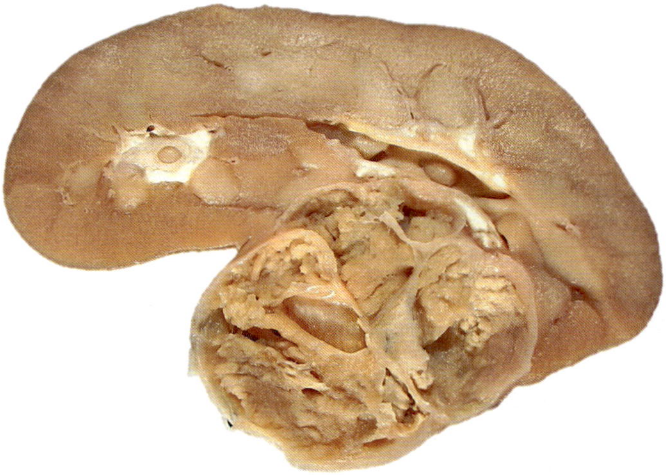

Chromophobe renal cell carcinoma (ChRCC)

ChRCC is generally confined to the kidney and usually has a favorable prognosis. In rare cases, the tumor can show extrarenal extension and metastasis.

FIGURE 14.32. This well-circumscribed tumor shows a solid cut surface and a homogeneous light brown color.

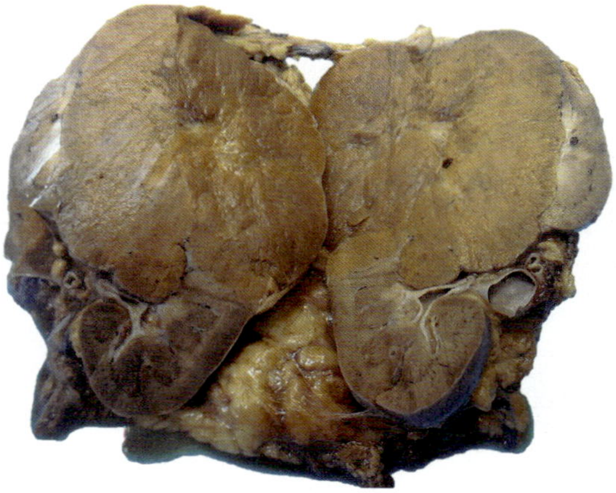

FIGURE 14.33. This ChRCC shows a solid cut surface. It has a homogeneous light brown color and focal areas of hemorrhage.

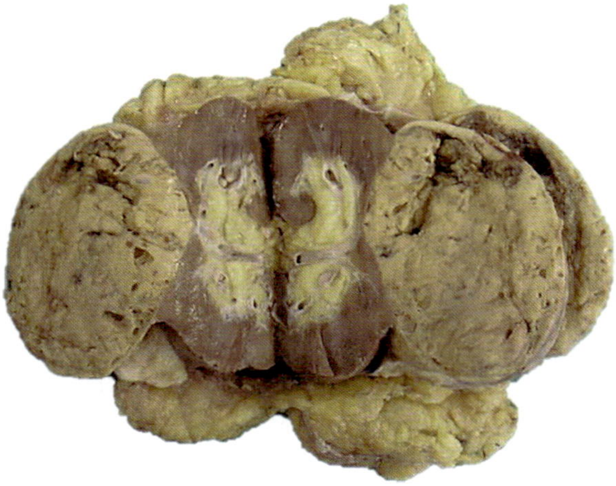

SARCOMATOID DIFFERENTIATION IN CHRCC

Although a sarcomatoid component may be associated with almost any type of RCC, chromophobe RCC has a high proclivity for harboring such a component.

FIGURE 14.34. This image shows a white, "fish flesh" nodule (arrow) of pure sarcomatoid component arising within an otherwise typical ChRCC (arrowhead).

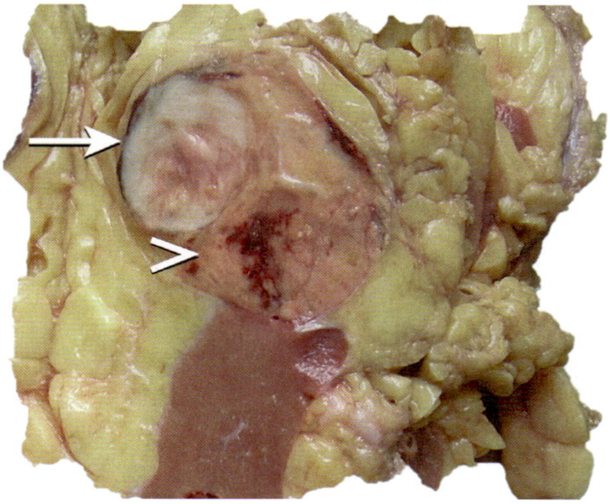

Acquired cystic kidney disease–associated RCC

The risk of RCC increases significantly in the setting of acquired cystic kidney disease. In fact, acquired cystic kidney disease–associated RCC is the most common subtype of RCC in end-stage kidneys. Other types of RCC seen in this setting include papillary, clear cell (conventional), and clear cell papillary RCC.

FIGURE 14.35. The cut surface of this bisected kidney shows multiple cortical cysts of variable sizes and an atrophic cortex. A well-circumscribed, brown, necrotic tumor is present at the superior pole. Distinguishing this tumor from papillary RCC may be difficult macroscopically.

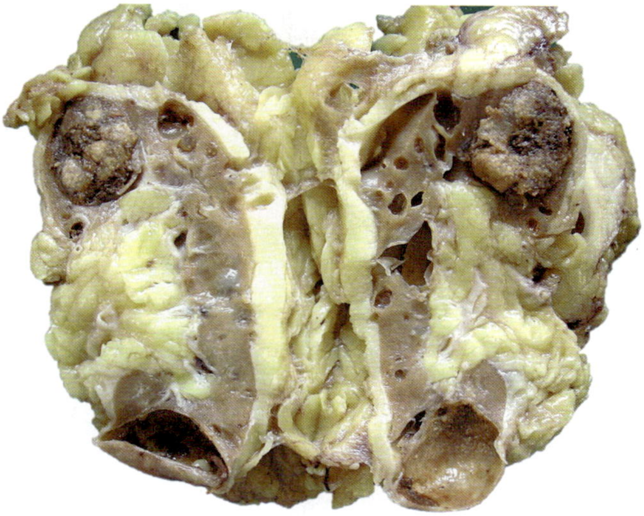

Clear cell papillary RCC

This newly recognized and generally indolent variant of RCC arises sporadically, or in the context of end-stage renal disease and von Hippel–Lindau syndrome. These tumors are often small, encapsulated, and confined within the kidney, and have a solid and cystic cut surface. Necrosis is typically absent.

FIGURE 14.36. This image shows a solid and partly cystic tumor. There is a thick, fibrous pseudocapsule with the cystic cavity (inferior aspect of tumor) adjacent to this pseudocapsule.

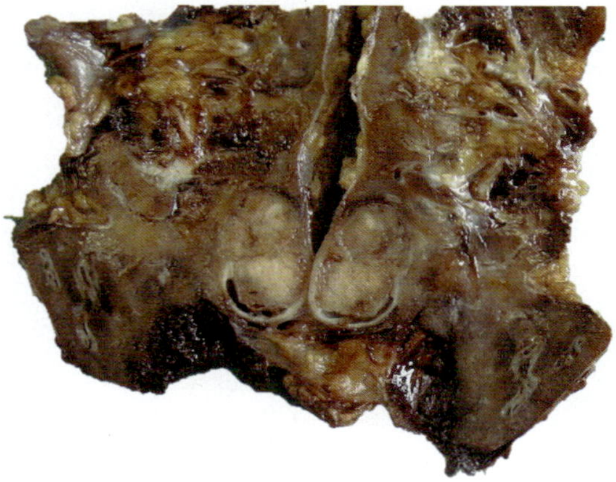

Urothelial carcinoma

Urothelial carcinoma is estimated to be the ninth most common cancer worldwide. It affects males more than females, and occurs across a wide age range, with a mean age of occurrence in the mid-60s. It usually presents with hematuria. The most common risk factors for this type of carcinoma include tobacco use and occupational exposure to carcinogens. *Schistosoma haematobium* is a known infectious cause of urothelial carcinoma.

INVASIVE UROTHELIAL CARCINOMA OF THE RENAL PELVIS

FIGURE 14.37. This image shows the cut surface of a bisected kidney, revealing a large, white-to-beige, variegated tumor with papillary fronds filling the pelvic calyceal system and invading into the renal parenchyma.

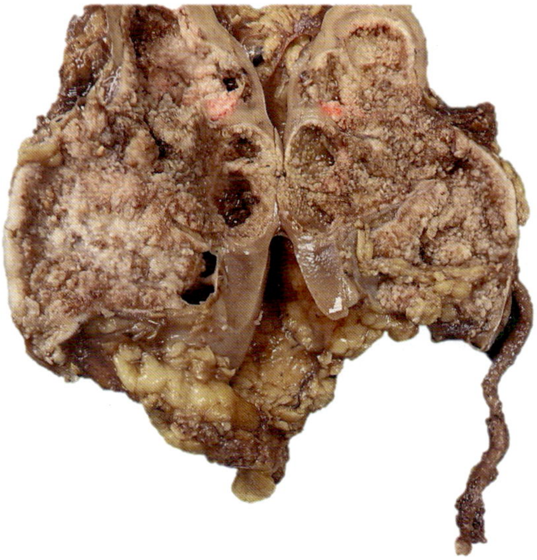

UPPER-TRACT INVASIVE UROTHELIAL CARCINOMA

FIGURE 14.38. This upper-tract invasive urothelial carcinoma shows intracalyceal and ureteral papillary components, and a solid invasive component invading the hilar adipose tissue and the renal parenchyma (arrow).

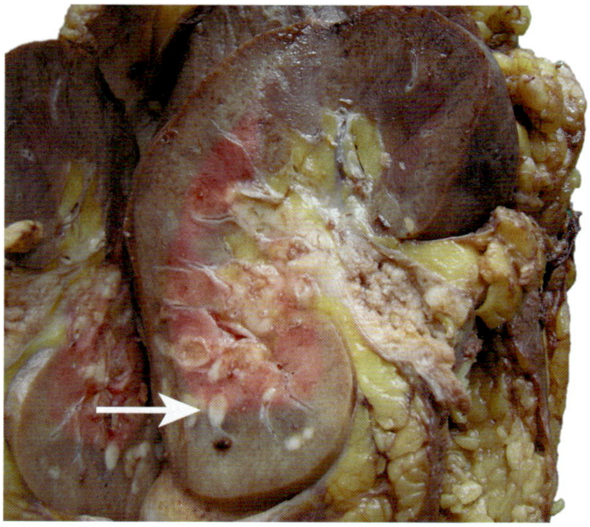

UPPER-TRACT NONINVASIVE UROTHELIAL CARCINOMA

FIGURE 14.39. This upper-tract noninvasive urothelial carcinoma shows an intracalyceal papillary component (arrow) in the absence of solid invasive components. Note the secondary calyceal dilatation secondary to obstruction.

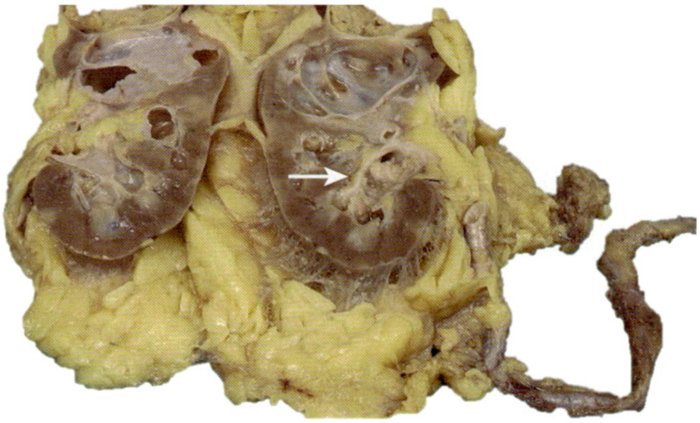

INVASIVE HIGH-GRADE URETERAL UROTHELIAL CARCINOMA OF THE URETER

FIGURE 14.40. Image (A) shows a left nephroureterectomy with invasive, high-grade ureteral urothelial carcinoma. The cut surface in (B) reveals a circumferential, solid, irregular, white tumor that almost entirely occludes the lumen and infiltrates the periureteric soft tissue.

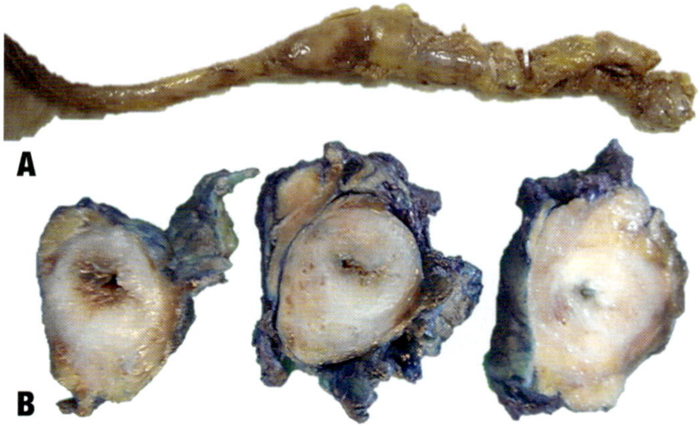

Bladder

REFERENCE: NORMAL BLADDER

FIGURE 14.41. As seen here, the bladder has an inverted pyramid shape. The superior portion (the dome) is covered with peritoneum. The trigone (triangular region at the base) is located between the ureteral orifices laterally and the urethra inferiorly. The neck (most distal part) opens into the urethra.

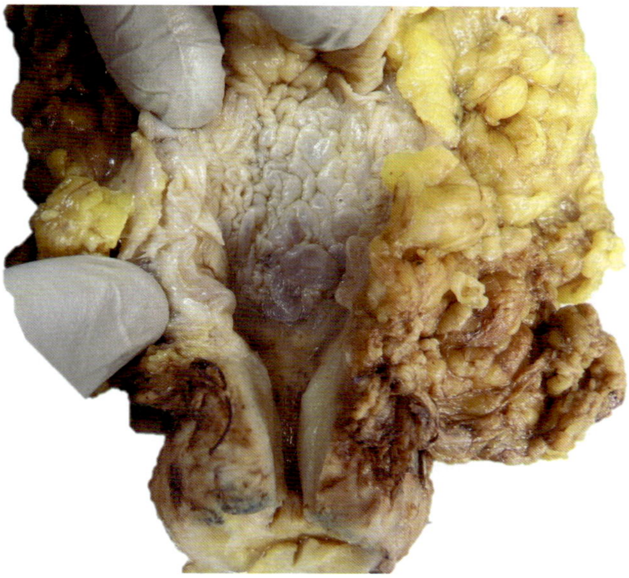

Hemorrhagic cystitis

This severe type of cystitis is usually related to chemotherapy, radiotherapy, or infection. It may be mistaken for a necrotic tumor because of its cystoscopic or macroscopic appearance.

FIGURE 14.43. The entire bladder mucosa appears hemorrhagic and necrotic.

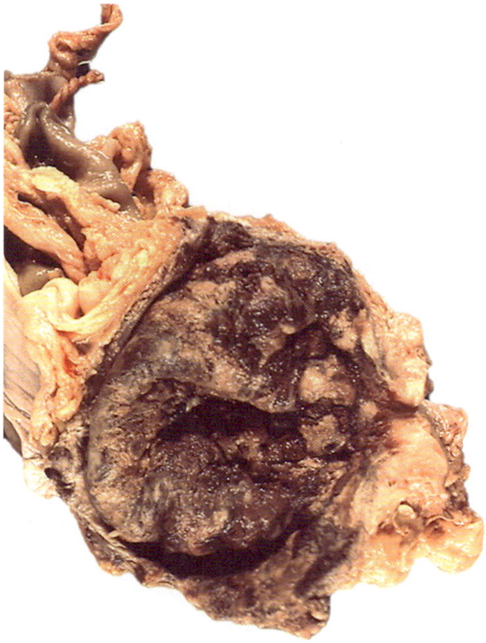

Acquired diverticulum

Bladder diverticula are common, and tend to arise from increased intravesical pressure secondary to an obstruction distal to a diverticulum. They commonly occur at the dome of the bladder, and close to the ureteral and urethral orifices. The presence of a diverticulum can lead to stone formation, infections, and carcinoma.

FIGURE 14.42. This diverticulum and bladder are connected via a narrow orifice that traverses the inner muscularis propria layer. The mucosa near a diverticulum is usually hyperemic or ulcerated, and the muscularis propria is hypertrophic. The diverticular wall shows a thinned or absent layer of muscularis propria.

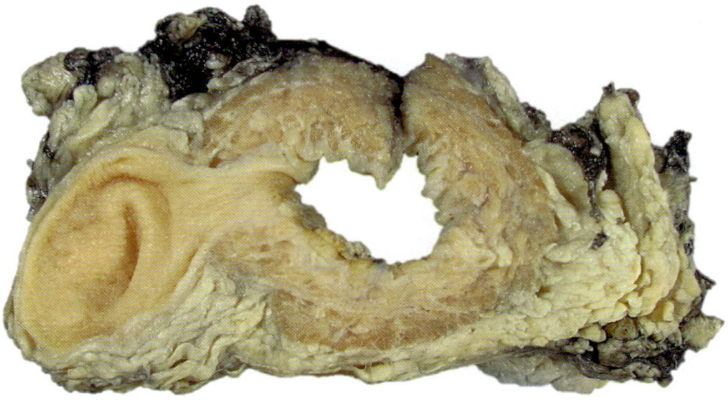

Papillary urothelial neoplasm

Papillary urothelial neoplasms are divided into the following categories: papilloma; urothelial neoplasm of low-malignant potential; and low- or high-grade papillary urothelial carcinoma.

FIGURE 14.44. The large size and the multifocality of the neoplasms in both (A) and (B) are consistent with a diagnosis of papillary urothelial carcinoma.

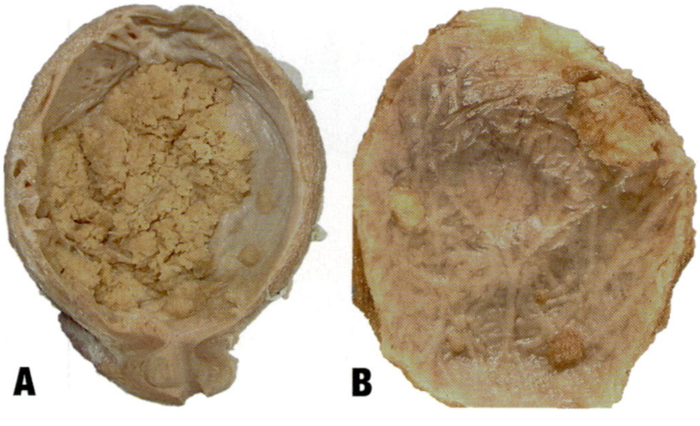

Invasive urothelial carcinoma

Approximately 30% of urothelial carcinoma presents with invasive disease. Invasive urothelial carcinoma can be focal or multifocal, but usually presents as a single mass. It can be polypoid, sessile, or ulcerative. It is usually solid, whitish-gray, and infiltrative. Sessile lesions are more commonly associated with papillary tumors.

FIGURE 14.45. This sessile mass involves the left lateral and posterior bladder walls.

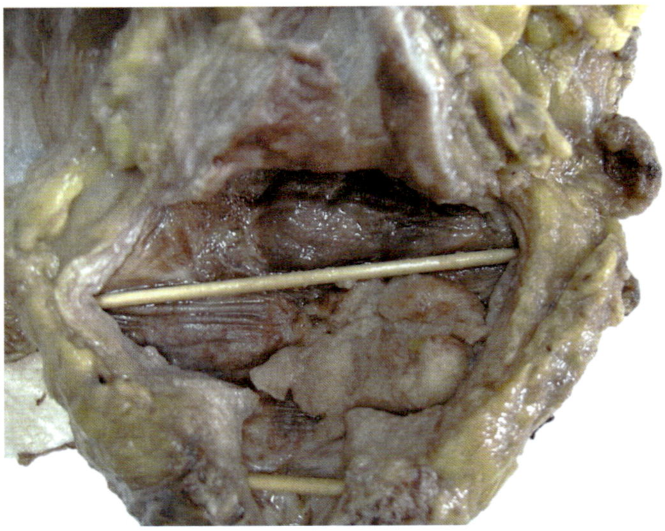

FIGURE 14.46. This is a large, polypoid tumor with a sessile component and necrosis filling the entire bladder cavity.

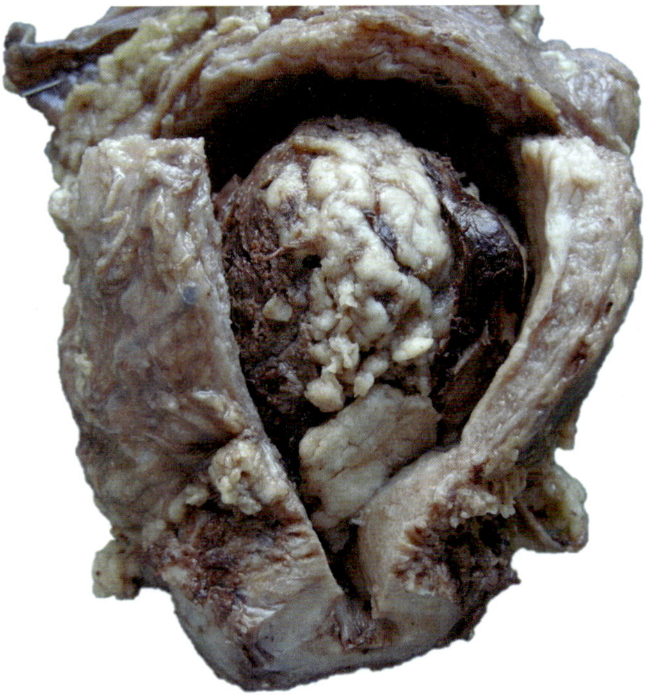

FIGURE 14.47. This image shows a large, invasive tumor with papillary and sessile components.

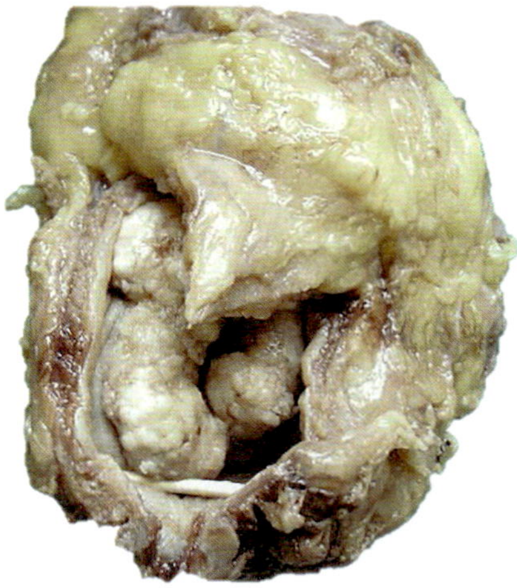

INVASIVE UROTHELIAL CARCINOMA INVADING PERIVESICAL ADIPOSE TISSUE

A tumor with macroscopic invasion of the perivesical adipose tissue is considered stage pT3b according to the American Joint Committee on Cancer (AJCC) staging manual (8th edition).

FIGURE 14.48. In this image of a bisected bladder, note the white, solid mass infiltrating the bladder wall and the perivesical adipose tissue.

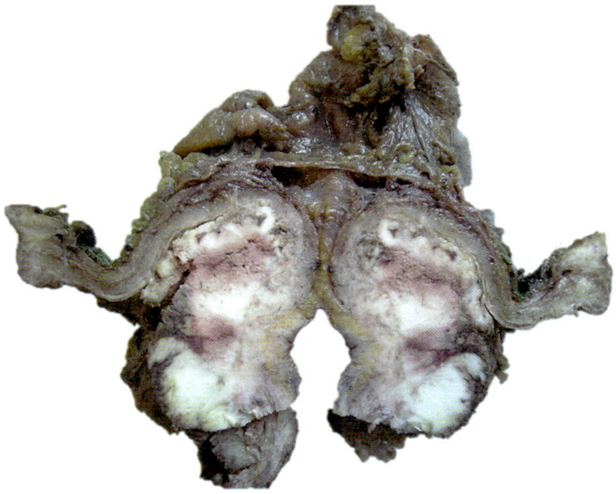

FIGURE 14.49. This invasive urothelial carcinoma is infiltrating the bladder wall and the perivesical adipose tissue (arrows).

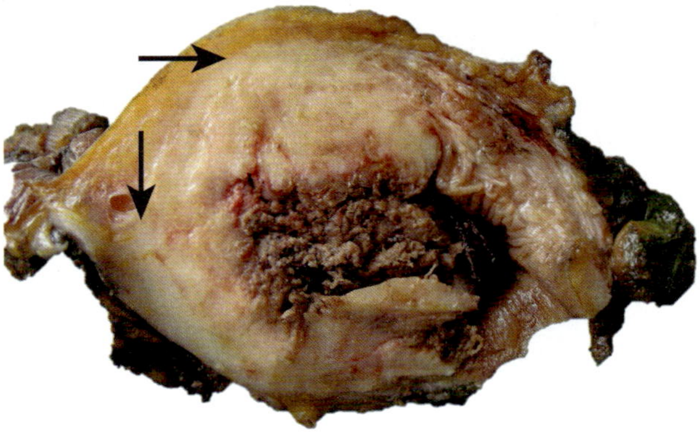

Testis

Testicular infarction

TESTICULAR INFARCTION SECONDARY TO TESTICULAR TORSION

Typically, untreated testicular torsion results in hemorrhage and infarction of the entire testis and epididymis.

FIGURE 14.50. This image shows hemorrhage and infarction of an entire testis and epididymis secondary to testicular torsion. The testis has a dusky purple and hemorrhagic appearance.

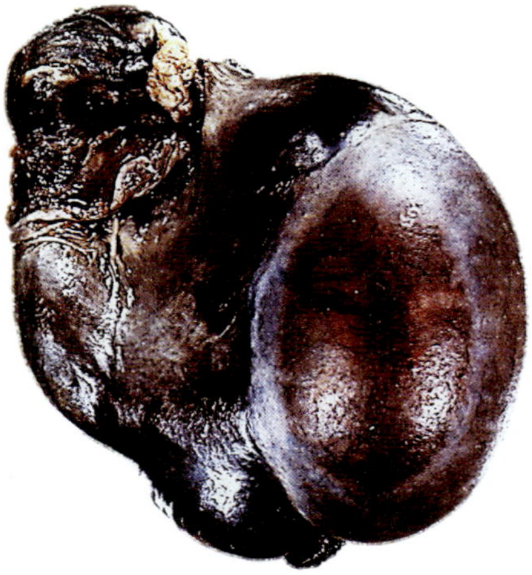

LOCALIZED TESTICULAR INFARCTION

Localized testicular infarction may result from testicular torsion, or from other causes that range from traumatic to vasculitic (e.g., vasculitis, thromboembolic events).

FIGURE 14.51. This image shows a localized testicular infarction secondary to testicular torsion with associated necrosis and hemorrhage of the epididymis.

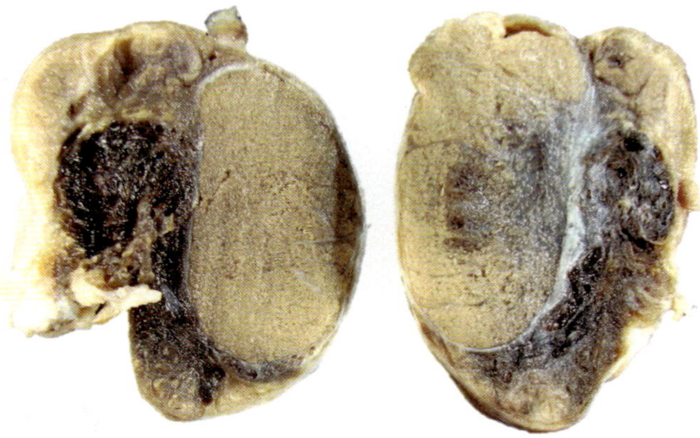

Epididymal cyst (spermatocele)

Epididymal cysts are cystic dilatations of the rete testis or the head of the epididymis. They can be unilocular or multilocular with cysts up to several centimeters in diameter. The cysts are thin walled, translucent, and filled with sperm. If an epithelial lining is identified histologically, these lesions are called spermatocele.

FIGURE 14.52. This image shows a testis with multiple thin-walled cysts.

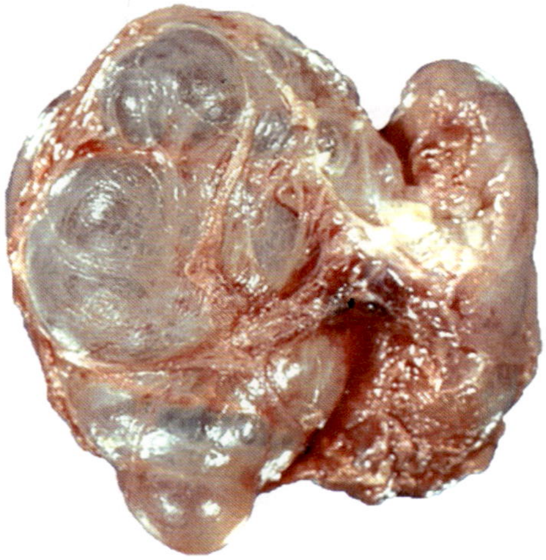

Epididymitis

Epididymitis most commonly has infectious origins, and may or may not be accompanied by orchitis.

FIGURE 14.53. This testis is uninvolved, and the epididymis shows a white, irregular pseudotumor mass (arrow) with white, chalky areas of necrosis suggestive of caseous necrosis. Histologically, necrotizing granulomatous inflammation was present, and the diagnosis of tuberculous epididymitis was confirmed by tissue culture.

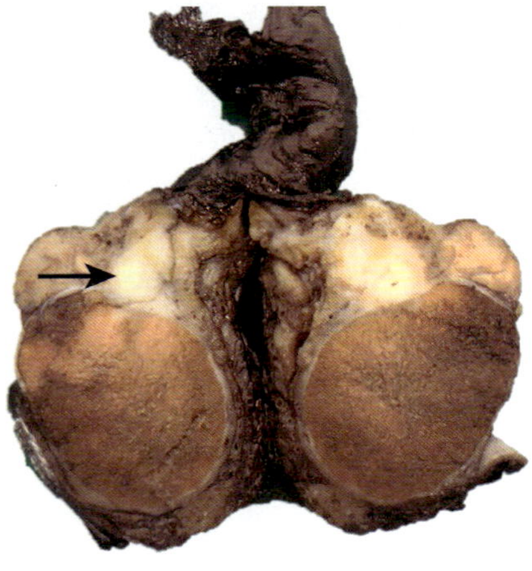

Infectious epididymoorchitis

Typical findings of infectious epididymoorchitis include: irregular, white, necrotic pseudotumor mass; areas of hemorrhage and necrosis; and cystic degeneration. These findings may be clinically and macroscopically mistaken for paratesticular or testicular tumors.

FIGURE 14.54. In this image, the epididymis and testis are involved by an irregular, white, necrotic pseudotumor mass with areas of hemorrhage, necrosis, and cystic degeneration.

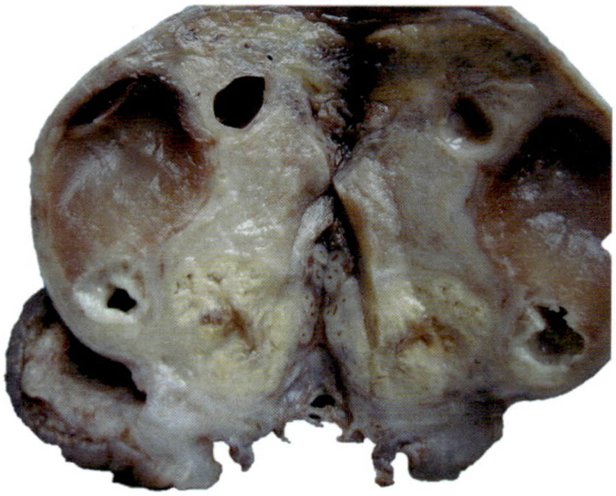

Epidermoid cyst (epidermal inclusion cyst)

Epidermoid cysts are benign, squamous, epithelial-lined cysts that may be as large as 10 cm, but mostly measure < 2 cm in their greatest dimension. On cut surface, these are well-circumscribed masses with thin walls. They contain keratin, which characteristically looks like yellow curd material.

FIGURE 14.55. This image shows a thin-walled cyst that is completely filled with keratin debris.

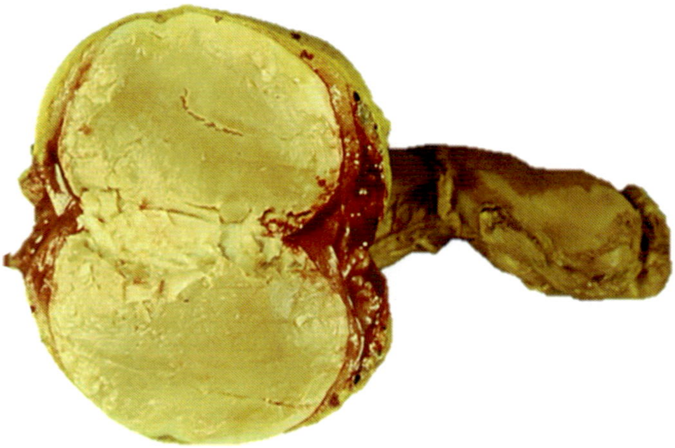

Pure seminoma

Seminoma typically has a solid multilobulated homogeneous appearance and white color. Hemorrhage and necrosis are usually absent, but are sometimes (rarely) seen macroscopically.

FIGURE 14.56. This tumor is circumscribed, nodular, and has a gray-white appearance that bulges from the cut surface of the testis. It occupies a large percentage of the testicular parenchyma.

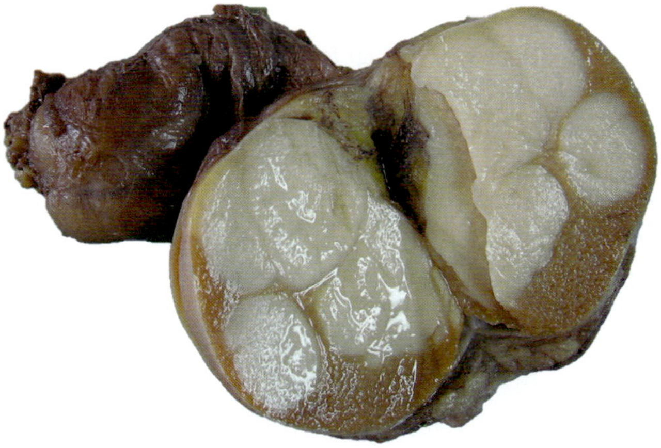

FIGURE 14.57. Note, in this image, the lobulated, white, nodular tumor confined within the testicular parenchyma.

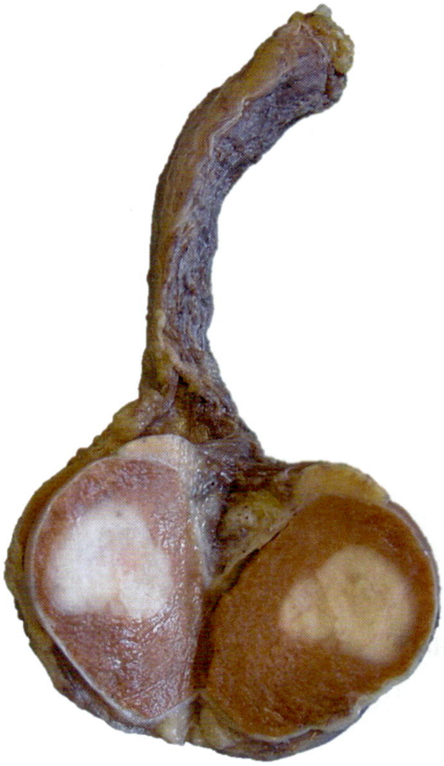

PURE SEMINOMA WITH CENTRAL HEMORRHAGE

Central hemorrhage is an uncommon but acceptable finding in pure seminoma. Hemorrhagic foci should be sampled to exclude a nonseminomatous component.

FIGURE 14.58. This tumor nodule shows central hemorrhage.

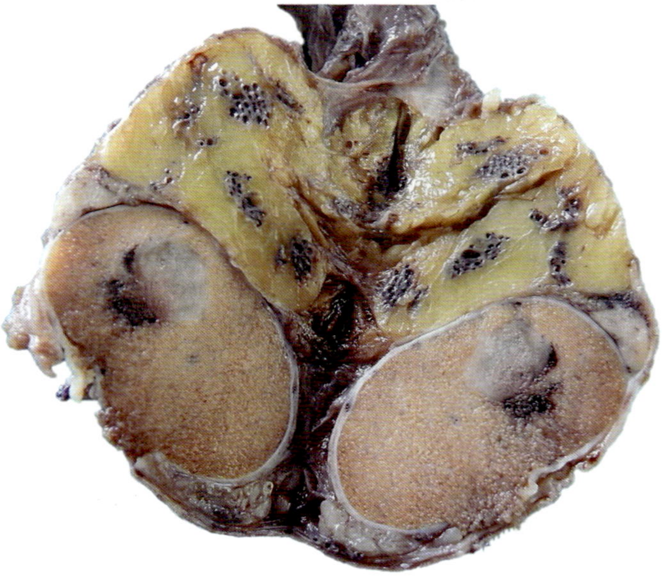

Pure testicular teratoma

Cystic structures within a testicular tumor usually indicate dilated glandular elements within a teratomatous component, but can also indicate a yolk sac tumor component.

FIGURE 14.59. Note the solid multilobulated tumor with scattered cystic areas almost entirely replacing the testis.

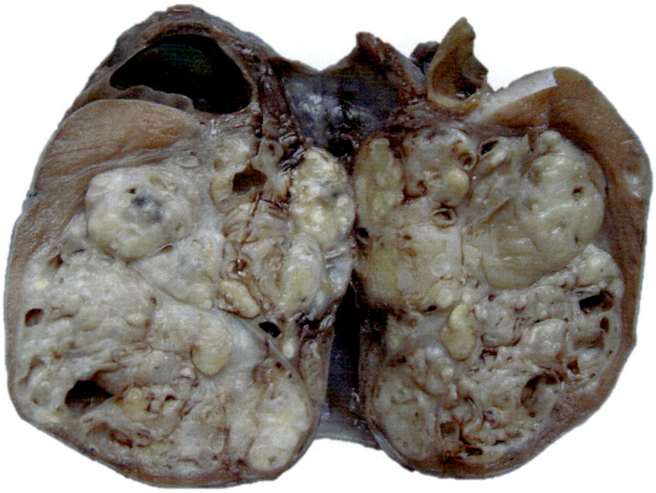

Mixed germ cell tumor

Except in cases of pure seminoma, testicular germ cell tumors most commonly occur as a combination of testicular germ cell tumor types. These tumors are heterogenous in gross appearance, depending on the specific tumor components and their percentage of involvement.

FIGURE 14.60. This tumor is composed of seminoma in the form of white, solid, homogeneous nodules (top), and teratoma in the form of fluid-filled cysts (bottom).

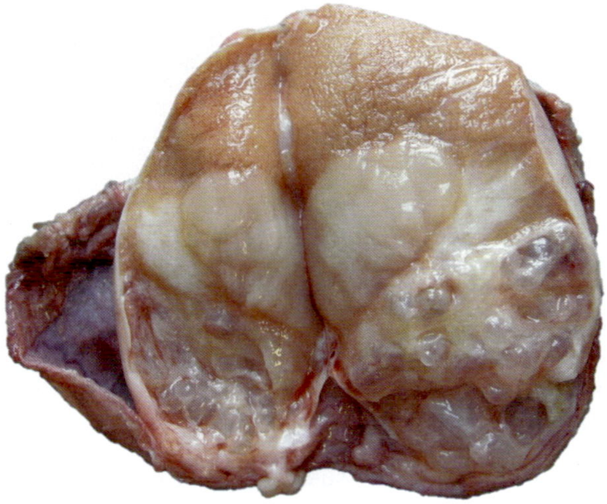

FIGURE 14.61. This image shows a tumor with alternating seminomatous and nonseminomatous components. The seminoma is composed of peripheral, lobulated, homogeneous, white foci. The nonseminomatous component has central, irregular, heterogeneous, and necrotic foci. The nonseminomatous component is embryonal carcinoma.

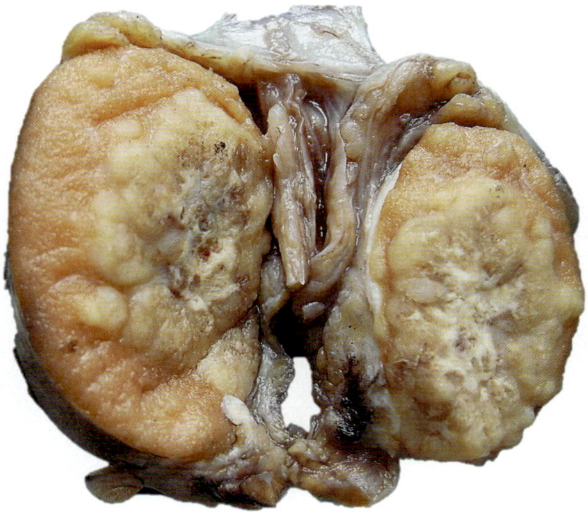

FIGURE 14.62. This tumor is composed of seminoma, which is the white, solid, homogeneous nodule (bottom), and embryonal carcinoma, which is the hemorrhagic and necrotic nodule (top). Ill-defined, whitish, fibrotic areas (arrow) are also visible, where tumor regression has occurred. Histologically, these areas show fibrosis and an absence of tumor cells.

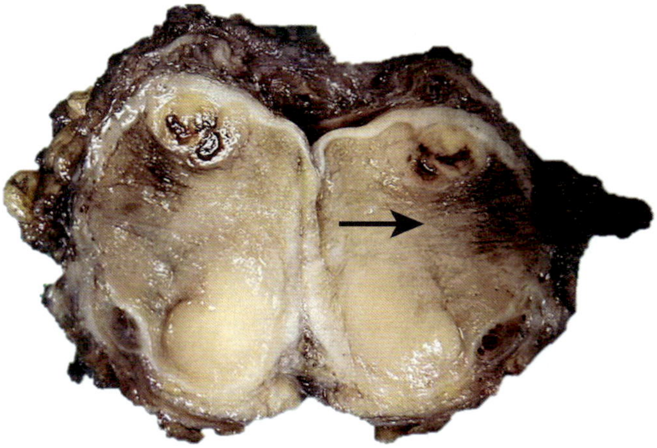

MIXED GERM CELL TUMOR WITH PROMINENT CHORIOCARCINOMA COMPONENT

FIGURE 14.64. Note, in this image, the extensive areas of hemorrhage within the tumor.

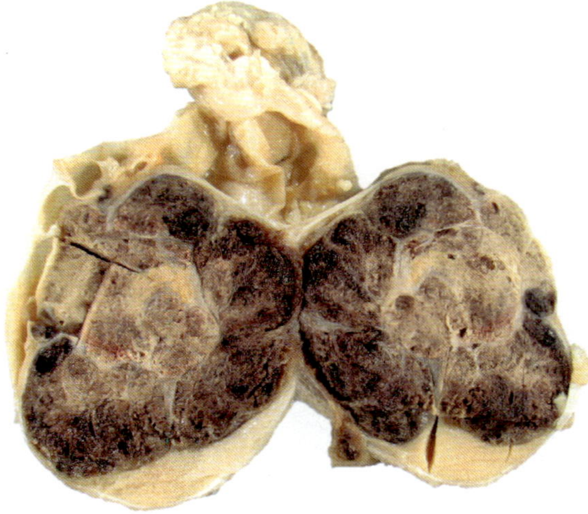

MIXED GERM CELL TUMOR INVADING THE HILAR SOFT TISSUE

Invasion of the hilar soft tissue is associated with more advanced disease and a higher risk of metastases. Therefore, the hilar region should be routinely sampled in orchiectomy specimens.

FIGURE 14.63. This mixed germ cell tumor is invading the hilar soft tissue (arrow). It is composed primarily of seminoma in the form of white, solid, homogeneous nodules; it also includes a minor component of teratoma, in the form of small, cystic structures.

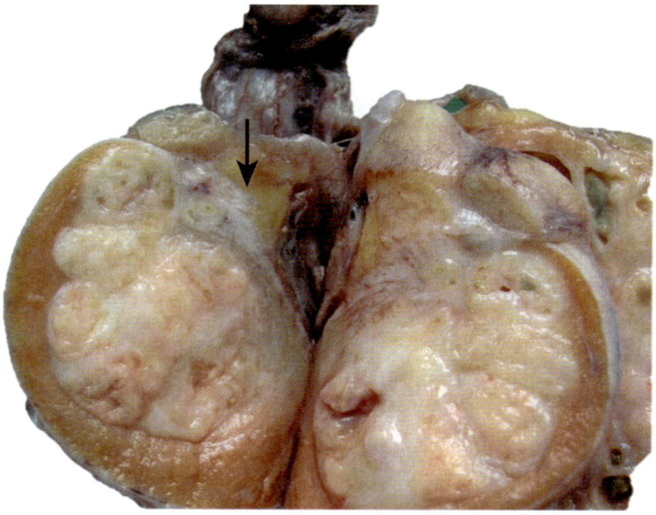

MIXED GERM CELL TUMOR INVADING THE SPERMATIC CORD

Spermatic cord invasion is considered stage pT3 according to the AJCC staging manual (8th edition).

FIGURE 14.65. This tumor infiltrates the hilar region and extends superiorly to involve the spermatic cord (arrow). Note the heterogeneous tumor cut surface, and the presence of hemorrhagic and necrotic foci, which usually indicate a component of embryonal carcinoma or choriocarcinoma.

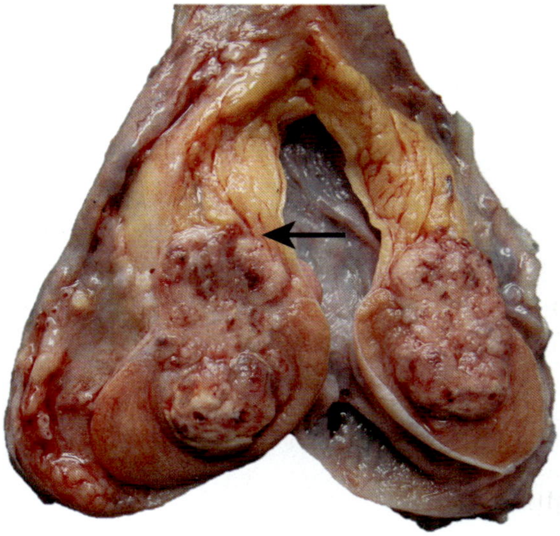

Metastasis

Metastatic tumors represent a very small minority of testicular tumors. They can be solitary or multiple, and they can involve the testis or the paratesticular region. Most are metastatic prostatic adenocarcinomas. Typically, patients have a history of prior malignancy, and the age of presentation is more than 50 years. Areas of lymphovascular invasion are typically present. The possibility of metastasis should be considered when a testicular tumor has atypical morphology for a primary tumor, and when the age of presentation is after age 40 (germ cell tumors typically present before age 40).

METASTATIC SARCOMATOID RENAL CELL CARCINOMA TO THE TESTIS

FIGURE 14.66. This image shows 1 well-defined solid tumor with a white, fleshy appearance that could easily be mistaken for primary testicular germ cell tumor.

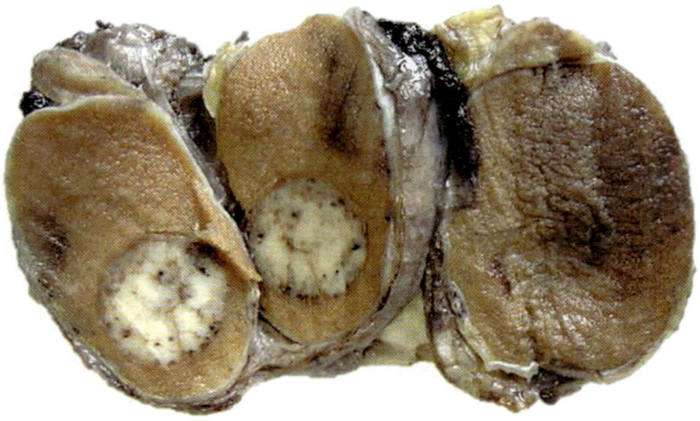

Paratesticular fibrous pseudotumor

These rare, benign, and mass-forming lesions appear as paratesticular solid fibrous masses that typically do not involve the testicular parenchyma. Histologically, they are composed of reactive fibroblasts or myofibroblasts in a variably inflammatory background.

FIGURE 14.67. This image shows white, firm, rubbery, and markedly thickened paratesticular tissue forming a mass.

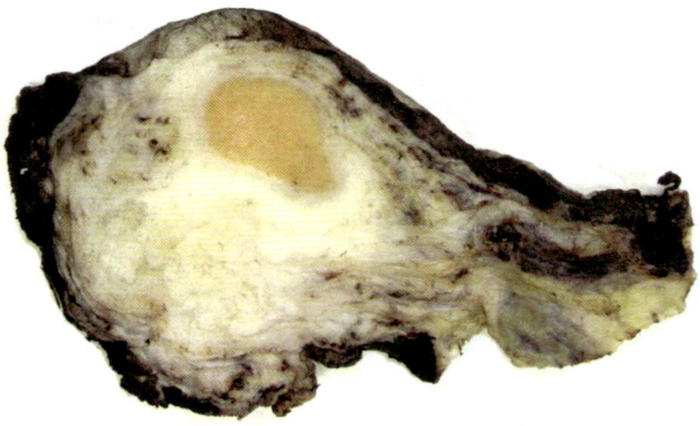

Malignant mesothelioma of the paratestis

FIGURE 14.68. This image shows 2 white, solid tumor nodules attached to the tunica albuginea with infiltration into the testicular parenchyma and the paratesticular adipose tissue (arrows). The differential diagnosis in this case was adenomatoid tumor. Although both lesions are composed of mesothelial cells, the presence of invasion of the surrounding tissue and nuclear atypia (histologically) are consistent with malignant mesothelioma.

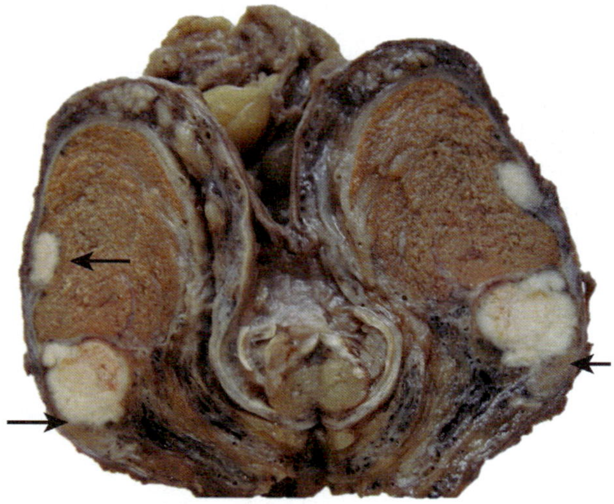

Adenomatoid tumor

Adenomatoid tumor is a benign lesion that appears as a solitary, well-circumscribed, white, fibrous, and solid nodule attached to the head or tail of the epididymis, or attached to the tunica albuginea. Most are < 2 cm; in rare cases, they reach larger sizes.

FIGURE 14.69. Note the well-circumscribed, firm, white nodule in the lower left.

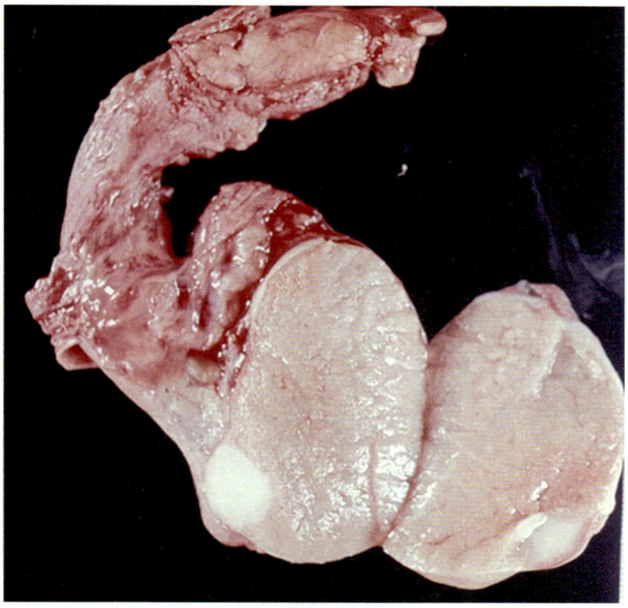

Prostate

Benign prostatic hyperplasia (BPH)

BPH is the most common benign prostate condition in men older than 50 years. In BPH, nodular proliferation of benign prostatic epithelial and stromal elements occurs in the prostatic tissue surrounding the urethra (transitional zone). It can lead to a variety of urinary symptoms. In severe and long-standing cases, urinary obstruction leads to urine retention, hydronephrosis, and infection.

FIGURE 14.70. This images shows BPH nodules occupying almost the entire prostate gland.

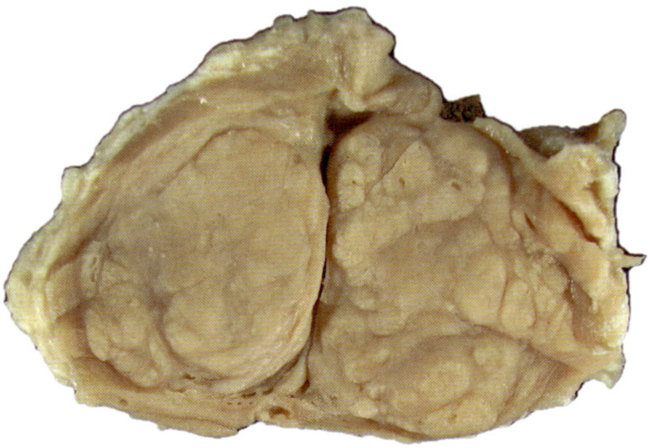

HYDRONEPHROSIS SECONDARY TO BPH

FIGURE 14.71. This image shows hydronephrosis secondary to BPH. Note the enlarged nodular prostate obstructing the bladder neck (bottom). Prominent trabeculation and thickening of the bladder wall, and dilated ureters and renal pelvis, are also present.

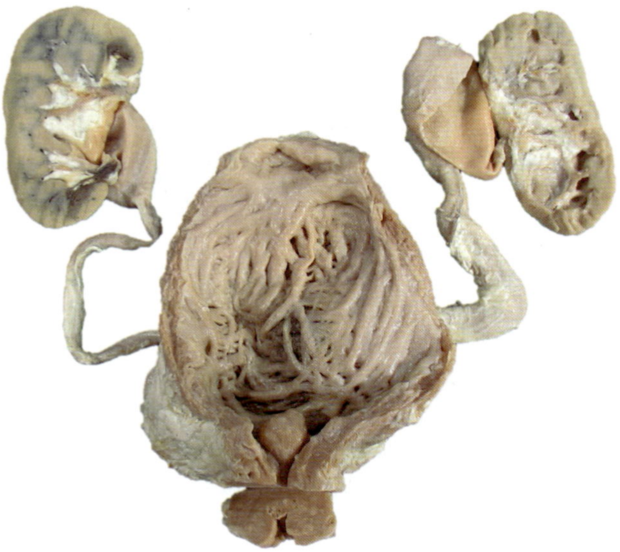

Prostatic adenocarcinoma

Prostatic adenocarcinoma is usually difficult to discern macroscopically. Typically, the peripheral zone is affected, but multifocality is very common.

FIGURE 14.72. In this image, cancer foci appear solid and white (arrow), contrasting with the normal spongy appearance of the prostate. On cross-sections, the prostate is oriented by the following: 1) seminal vesicles posteriorly; 2) flat shape posteriorly; and 3) the urethra, which forms an arrow-shaped structure that points anteriorly.

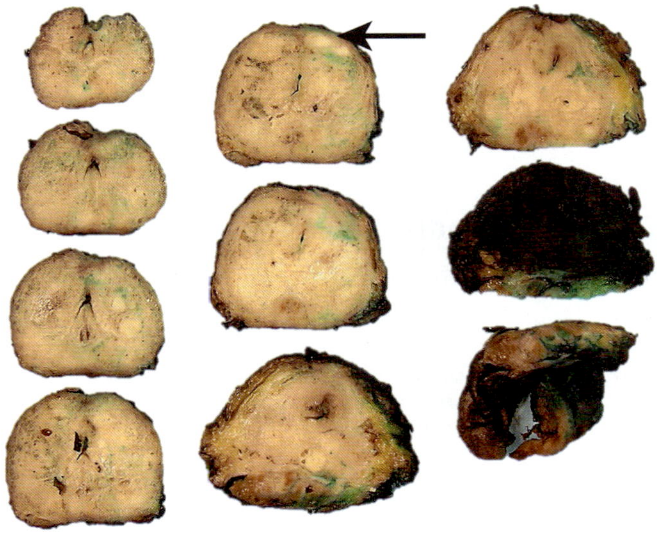

FIGURE 14.73. This cancer forms a large, white, solid nodule mainly affecting the transitional periurethral zone.

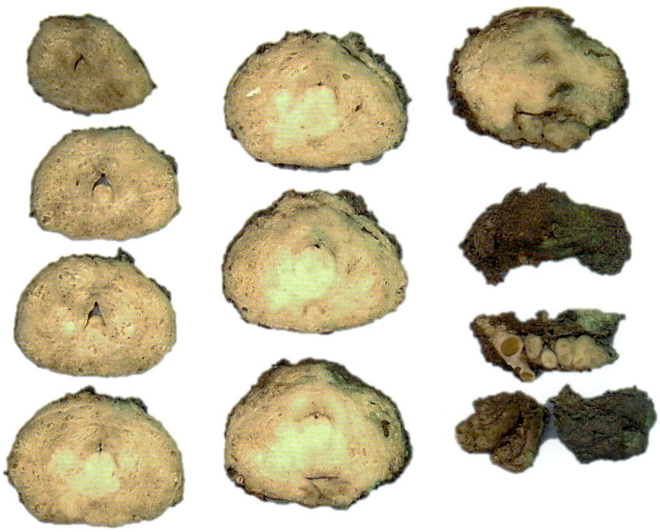

FIGURE 14.74. This cancer forms a large, white, solid nodule involving the posterior aspect of the right lobe.

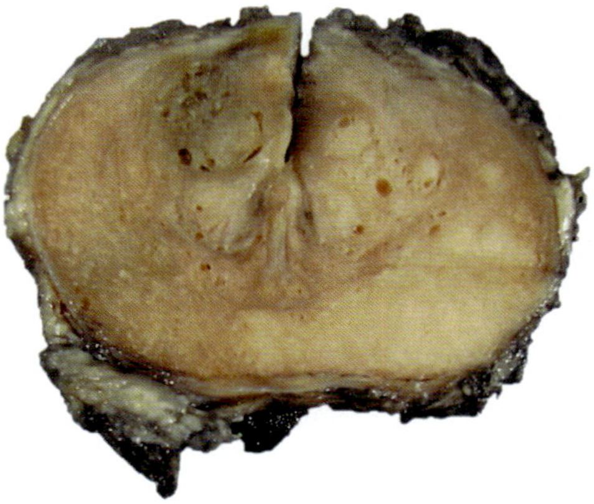

PROSTATE ACINAR ADENOCARCINOMA

FIGURE 14.75. In this image, note the irregular, white, solid areas in contrast to the benign, spongy-looking prostatic tissue.

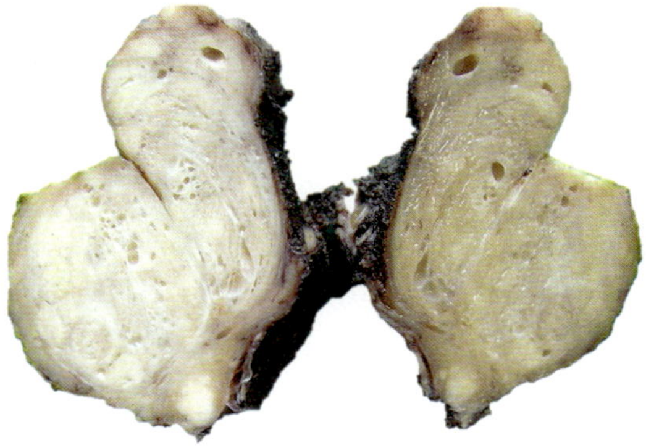

Penis

Penile squamous cell carcinoma (SCC)

The most common risk factors for penile SCC include lack of circumcision, phimosis, poor hygiene, HPV infection, smoking, and chronic balanitis. The glans is the most common site of involvement, followed by the foreskin.

FIGURE 14.76. This apical view of the glans shows a white, cauliflower-like tumor involving the foreskin and the glans.

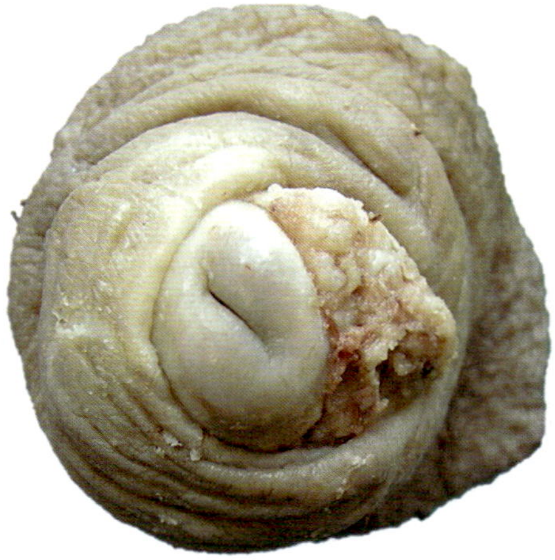

WARTY-VARIANT PENILE SCC

The warty variant and basal variant of penile SCC are the most common subtypes of HPV-related penile SCC.

FIGURE 14.77. In (A), the glans and the distal shaft are involved by a large, polypoid cauliflower tumor. The cut section in (B) reveals the verruciform appearance of the surface tumor component and the significant degree of tissue invasion. The tumor invades the corpus spongiosum and part of the corpus cavernosum (arrow), and totally replaces the urethra. Histologically, this tumor showed cytoplasmic clearing and koilocytotic nuclear changes, consistent with the diagnosis of warty variant of SCC.

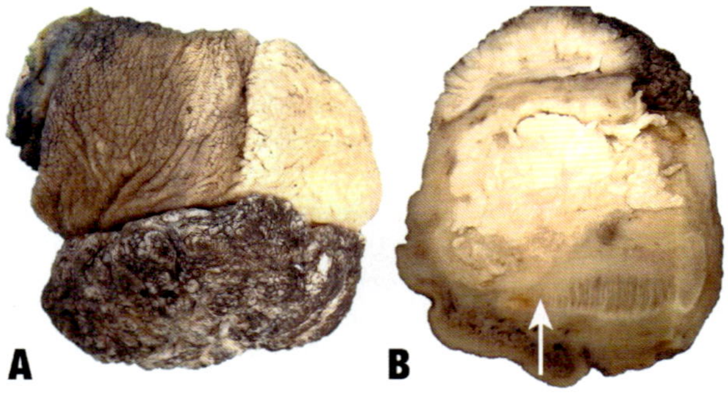

FIGURE 14.78. The exophytic tumor component shows a verruciform growth pattern. The invasive component forms white, solid areas invading the corpus spongiosum and corpus cavernosum.

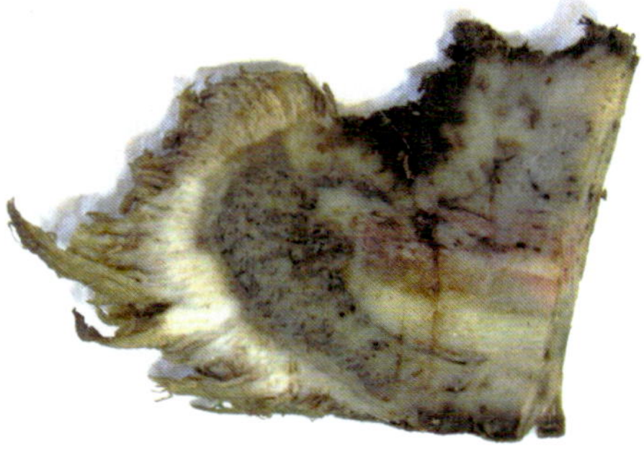

BASALOID-VARIANT PENILE SCC

The most common subtypes of HPV-related penile SCC are the basaloid variant and the warty variant

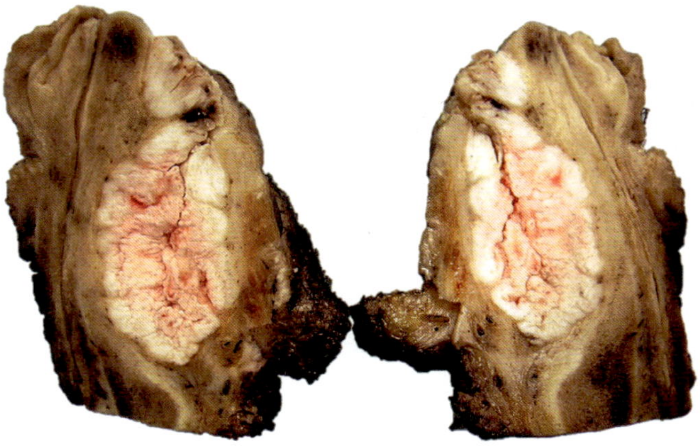

FIGURE 14.79. This partial penectomy shows a large, whitish tumor invading the foreskin, the glans, and the shaft in the presence of a minimal exophytic tumor component. This vertical pattern of growth is typical of the basaloid or sarcomatoid variants of penile SCC.

ACKNOWLEDGMENTS

We would like to thank the valuable contributions of Dr. A. Nahal and the technical help of R. Gilot, E. Griss, A. Hossain, L. Korneichyuk Pasyuk, M. Mikhael, and E. Yaney.

REFERENCES

Amin MB, Edge SB, editors. *AJCC cancer staging manual*. 8th ed. Chicago: Springer; 2018.

Amin M, Grignon D, Srigley J, Eble J. *Urological pathology*. 1st ed. Philadelphia: Wolters Kluwer Health/Lippincott Williams & Wilkins; 2014.

Bostwick DG, Cheng L. *Urologic surgical pathology*. Philadelphia: Saunders/Elsevier; 2014.

Epstein J, Netto G. *Differential diagnosis in surgical pathology genitourinary system*. Philadelphia: Wolters Kluwer Health/Lippincott Williams & Wilkins; 2014.

Epstein J, Reuter V, Amin M. *Biopsy interpretation of the bladder*. 3rd ed. Philadelphia: Wolters Kluwer; 2017.

Grasso M. *Ureteropelvic junction obstruction* [Medscape Website]. 2015 Jan 30 [accessed 2016 Mar]. Available from: http://emedicine.medscape.com/article/450785-overview#a7.

Humphrey PA, Moch H, Cubilla AL, Ulbright TM, Reuter VE. The 2016 WHO classification of tumours of the urinary system and male genital organs—part B: prostate and bladder tumours. Eur Urology. 2016;70(1):106–119. https://doi.org/10.1016/j.eururo.2016.02.028.

Khan AN. *Duplicated collecting system imaging* [Medscape Website]. 2015 Dec 27 [accessed 2016 Mar]. Available from: http://emedicine.medscape.com/article/378075-overview.

Klimas R, Bennett B, Gardner WA. Prostatic calculi: a review. Prostate. 1985;7(1):91–96.

Krueger GRF, Buja LM, editors. *Atlas of anatomic pathology with imaging: a correlative diagnostic companion*. London: Springer; 2013. p. 316. https://doi.org/10.1007/978-1-4471-2846-5.

Kumar V, Abbas AK, Aster JC. *Robbins and Cotran pathologic basis of disease*. Philadelphia: Saunders/Elsevier; 2014.

Lack EE, Kozakewich HPW. Embryology, developmental anatomy and selected aspects of non-neoplastic pathology. In: Lack EE, editor. *Pathology of the adrenal glands*. New York: Churchill Livingstone; 1990. p. 1–74.

Lester SC. *Manual of surgical pathology*. Philadelphia: Saunders/Elsevier; 2010.

Megyeri J, Varga J. Prostatic infarction. Int Urol Nephrol. 1975;7(4):315–319.

Mills SE, Carter D, Greenson JK, Hornick JL, Longacre TA, Reuter VE, editors. *Sternberg's diagnostic surgical pathology*. 6th ed. Philadelphia: Wolters Kluwer Health; 2015.

Moore K, Persaud T. *The developing human: clinically oriented embryology*. Philadelphia: WB Saunders; 2003.

Pernick N. *Chronic cystitis*. [PathologyOutlines Website]. 2016 Mar 23 [cited 2016 Mar]. Available from: http://www.pathologyoutlines.com/topic/bladderchroniccystitis.html.

Petersen RO, Sesterhenn I, Davis CJ. *Urologic pathology*. Philadelphia: Wolters Kluwer Health/Lippincott Williams & Wilkins; 2009.

Rafael J. *Spermatic cord torsion* [PathologyOutlines Website]. 2014 Jan 14 [accessed 2016 Mar]. Available from: http://www.pathologyoutlines.com/topic/testistorsion.html.

Rafael J. *Spermatic granuloma (epididymitis nodosa)* [PathologyOutlines Website]. 2014 Jan 14 [accessed 2016 Mar]. Available from: http://www.pathologyoutlines.com/topic/testisepidspermgran.html.

Rodriguez MM. Congenital anomalies of the kidney and the urinary tract (CAKUT). Fetal Pediatr Pathol. 2014;33(5–6):293–320.

Rosai J. *Rosai and Ackerman's surgical pathology*. 10th ed. Edinburgh: Mosby/Elsevier; 2011.

Roychowdhury M. *Hemorrhagic cystitis* [PathologyOutlines Website]. 2016 May 11 [accessed 2016 Jun]. Available from: http://www.pathologyoutlines.com/topic/bladderhemorrhagiccystitis.html.

Stocker JT, Dehner LP, Husain AN. *Stocker and Dehner's pediatric pathology*. Philadelphia: Wolters Kluwer Health/Lippincott Williams & Wilkins; 2011.

Tickoo S, Chen Y, Zynger D. *Biopsy interpretation of the kidney and adrenal gland*. 1st ed. Philadelphia: Wolters Kluwer; 2016.

Turki AL. *Testis and epididymis, general, atrophy* [PathologyOutlines Website]. 2013 Apr 14 [accessed 2016 Mar]. Available from: http://www.pathologyoutlines.com/topic/testisatrophy.html.

Turki AL. *Testis and epididymis, germ cell tumors, choriocarcinoma* [PathologyOutlines Website]. 2013 Apr 21 [accessed 2016 Mar]. Available from: http://www.pathologyoutlines.com/topic/testischorio.html.

Turki AL. *Testis and epididymis, germ cell tumors, embryonal carcinoma* [PathologyOutlines Website]. 2013 Apr 21 [accessed 2016 Mar]. Available from: http://www.pathologyoutlines.com/topic/testisembryonal.html.

Turki AL. *Testis and epididymis, germ cell tumors, mixed germ cell tumors* [PathologyOutlines Website]. 2013 Apr 21 [accessed 2016 Mar]. Available from: http://www.pathologyoutlines.com/topic/testisnsgctgeneral.html

Turki AL. *Testis and epididymis, germ cell tumors, teratoma* [PathologyOutlines Website]. 2013 Apr 21 [accessed 2016 Mar]. Available from: http://www.pathologyoutlines.com/topic/testisteratoma.html.

Williamson S. *Infectious testicular lesions*. [PathologyOutlines Website] Tuberculosis (Edinb). 2013;20 [accessed 2016 March]. Available at http://www.pathologyoutlines.com/topic/testisinfectious.html.

Williamson S. *Non-neoplastic testicular lesions, hydrocele* [PathologyOutlines Website]. 2013 Apr 12 [accessed 2016 Mar]. Available from: http://www.pathologyoutlines.com/topic/testishydrocele.html.

Williamson S. *Sarcomatoid renal cell carcinoma* [PathologyOutlines Website]. 2012 Jun 30 [accessed 2016 Mar]. Available from: http://www.pathologyoutlines.com/topic/kidneytumormalignantrccsarcoma.html.

Zhou M, Cristina MG. *Genitourinary pathology*. Philadelphia: Saunders/Elsevier; 2015.

15

Gynecological Diseases

TUYET NHUNG TON NU, MANUELA PELMUS, ZARI DASTANI, LARA RICHER

Vulva

Vulvar squamous cell carcinoma (SCC)

Vulvar SCC is the most common vulvar malignancy and represents approximately 3% of female genital cancers. It develops via 1 of 2 pathways: the human papillomavirus (HPV)–dependent pathway (seen in young, smoking patients), or the p53 or Rb protein alteration pathway (seen in older women, and associated with chronic inflammation, such as lichen sclerosus and lichen planus). The precursor of the HPV-dependent pathway is high-grade squamous intraepithelial lesion (HSIL) or vulvar intraepithelial neoplasia (VIN). HPV-positive carcinoma is often basaloid and warty (condylomatous). The precursor of the p53-dependant pathway is differentiated-type VIN, and the associated carcinomas are keratinizing. The most common sites of involvement are the labia majora and minora. Staging of vulvar SCC has implications for prognosis and recurrence. According to the American Joint Committee on Cancer (AJCC) staging manual (8th edition), primary SCCs are staged as:

Stage I — tumor is limited to the vulva or perineum;

Stage II — tumor extends to the adjacent perineal structures without lymph node involvement;

Stage III — tumor has regional lymph node metastasis; and

Stage IV — tumor extends to the proximal two-thirds of the urethra or vagina, the bladder mucosa, and/or the rectal mucosa; or is fixed to the pelvic bone; or has fixed or ulcerated regional lymph node metastasis; or has distant metastasis.

FIGURE 15.1. Image (A), shows a hemivulvectomy with a large, tan, and nodular mass extending from the left labium majora. The cut surface in (B) shows the tumor penetrating into the underlying tissue. The yellow tissue is fat.

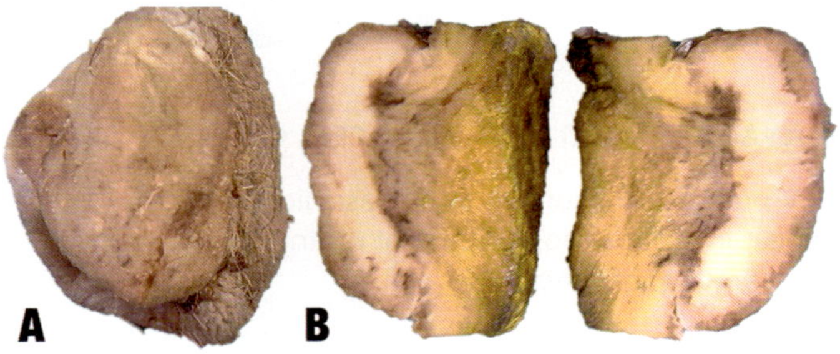

FIGURE 15.2. The hemivulvectomy in (A) displays an ulcerated lesion with raised edges. In (B), note the ulcer at the center with white, elevated edges.

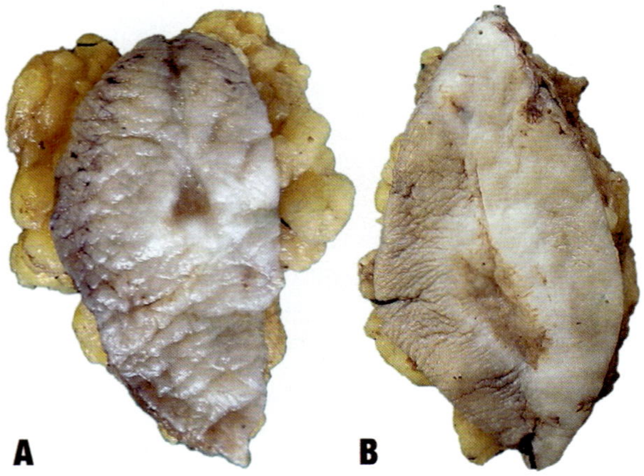

FIGURE 15.3. This vulvectomy shows an exophytic tumor with an irregular, ulcerated surface. Note that the sutures were placed by surgeons to orient the specimen, and the blue dye was injected during the surgery to identify the sentinel lymph node.

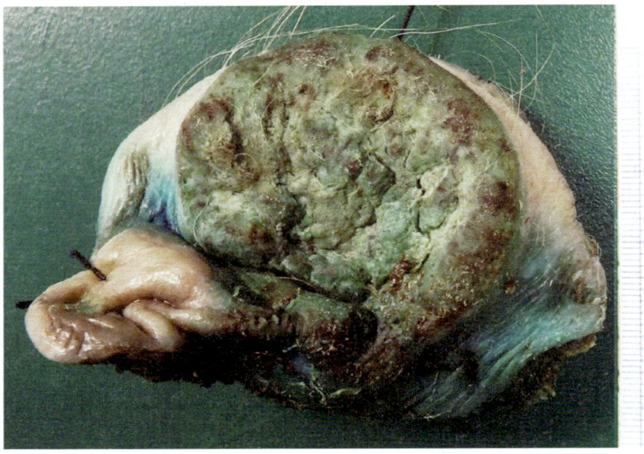

FIGURE 15.4. Note the large, ulcerated, and poorly delineated lesion in (A). In (B), there is a large nodular mass with raised borders involving the entire labia.

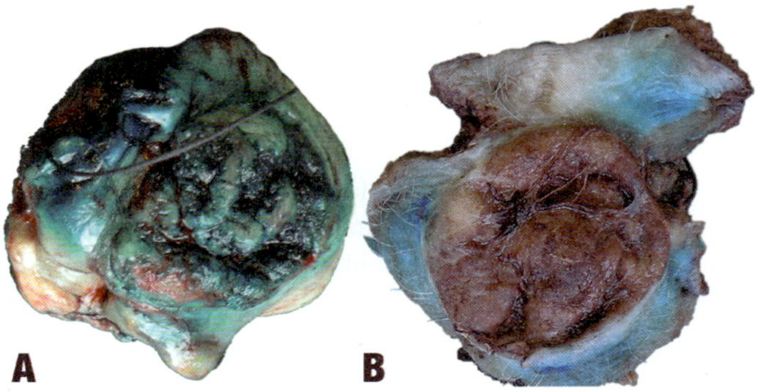

VULVAR BASALOID SQUAMOUS CELL CARCINOMA (SCC)

HPV-positive carcinoma is often basaloid; the gross appearance of basaloid SCC is not distinguishable from other variants of vulvar SCC.

FIGURE 15.5. This hemivulvectomy shows a brown, nodular, and exophytic mass extending from the surface of the vulva.

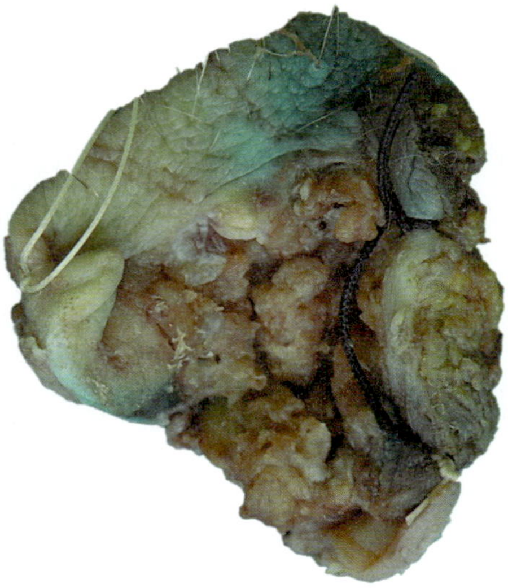

Vulvar squamous intraepithelial lesion (SIL)

High-grade SIL (HSIL) is the precursor lesion to the HPV-dependent pathway of SCC. Vulvar HSIL carries a significant clinical risk of SCC development if not treated.

FIGURE 15.6. The hemivulvectomy in (A) shows a vulvar high-grade SIL viewed from the superficial surface. The mass is tan to brown, polypoid, and ill defined. Image (B) shows a poorly defined, nodular, and white lesion on the labia minora. The blue tinge is due to sentinel-lymph-node mapping dye. Microscopy showed it was a high-grade SIL with foci of superficially invasive SCC.

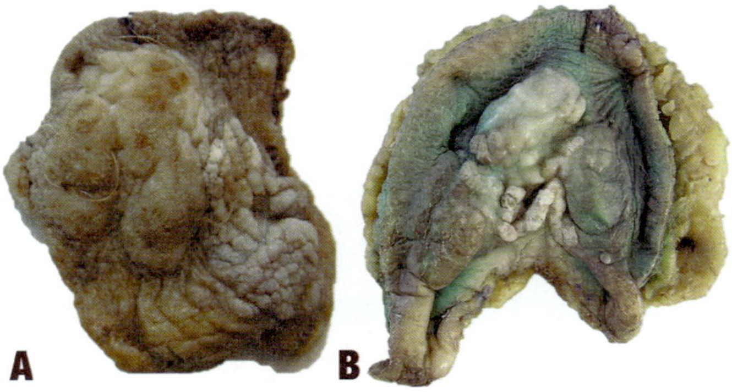

Vulvar verrucous carcinoma

Vulvar verrucous carcinoma is not associated with HPV or lichen sclerosus. It represents less than 1% of vulvar cancers.

FIGURE 15.7. This vulvectomy shows an exophytic tumor with irregular borders. Histologically, this tumor's rete ridges were bulbous with a pushing border. There was minimal atypia, abundant eosinophilic cytoplasm, and normal mitotic figures.

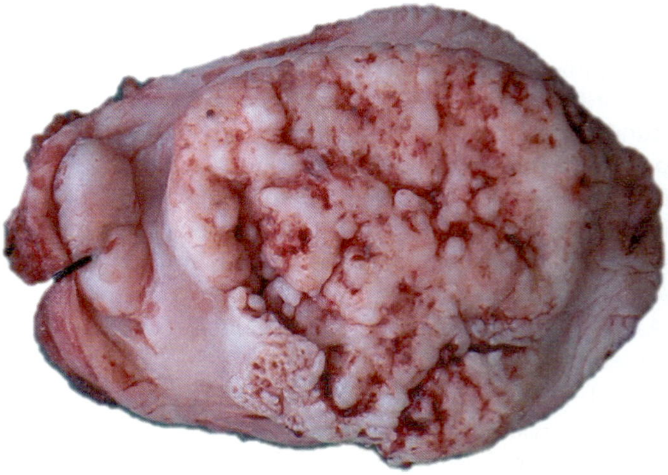

Extramammary Paget disease

Extramammary Paget disease represents less than 1% of vulvar neoplasms. It can be of pluripotent epidermal stem cell origin, or can occur secondary to underlying malignancy in 12% to 33% of cases. The genetic underpinnings of this disease are uncertain.

FIGURE 15.8. In this hemivulvectomy specimen, the surface of the skin appears erythematous and there is an ill-defined plaque in the upper part of the specimen (arrow).

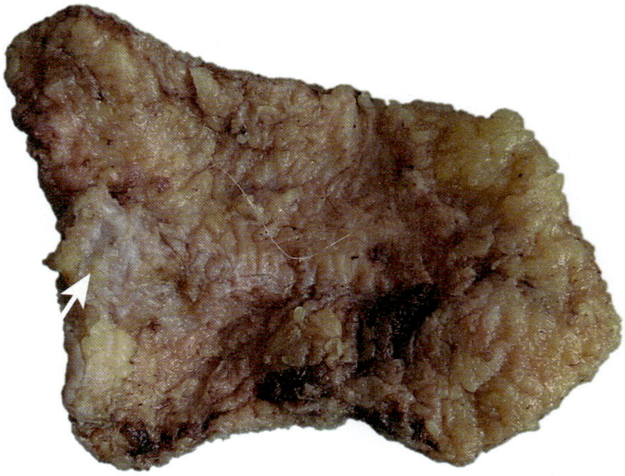

Vulvar adenoid cystic carcinoma

Microscopically, adenoid cystic carcinoma is characterized by a cribriform architectural pattern with infiltration in perineural spaces. Metastasis from another more common site of adenoid cystic carcinoma must be ruled out before making a diagnosis of primary vulvar adenoid cystic carcinoma.

FIGURE 15.9. In (A), a large, ill-defined mass is present in the center of the vulvectomy specimen. In (B), a cut opening of the specimen shows a poorly circumscribed and solid mass.

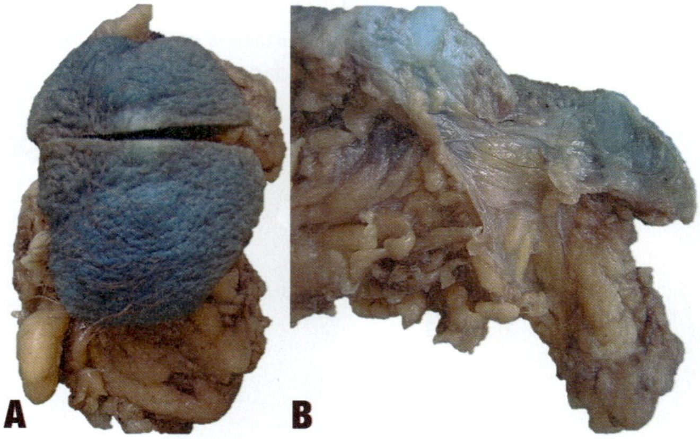

Vagina

Vaginal squamous cell carcinoma (SCC)

Vaginal carcinoma represents less than 2% of all gynecologic malignancies. SCC is the most common type, accounting for over 80% of invasive malignancy of the vagina. Risk factors for this SCC include HPV infection, smoking, previous gynecological malignancy, ethnicity, young age of first sexual intercourse, and multiple sexual partners.

FIGURE 15.10. Image (A) shows a uterus and upper vagina. A red and exophytic tumor is located in the upper part of the posterior vagina. A closer view in (B) highlights the exophytic appearance of this tumor.

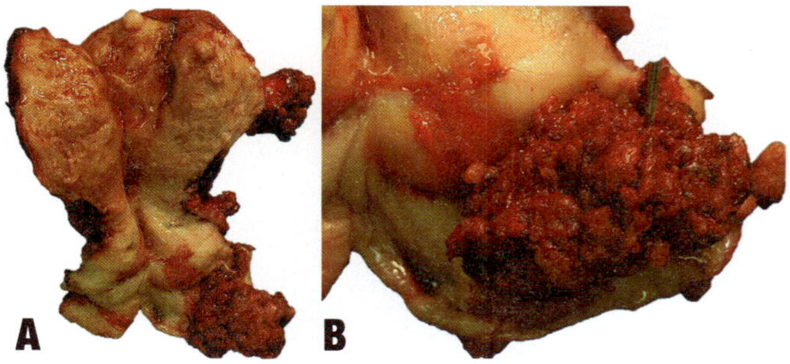

FIGURE 15.11. This image shows a hysterectomy and bilateral salpingo-oophorectomy. There are 3 distinct, raised, flat top lesions in the vagina (arrows).

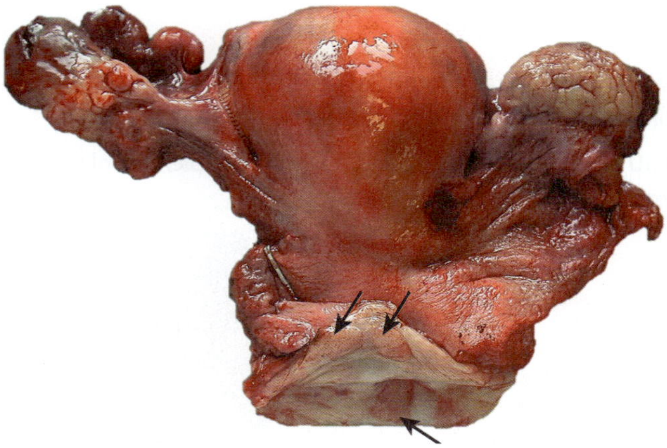

Vaginal malignant melanoma

Vaginal malignant melanoma is a rare type of mucosal melanoma, representing approximately 3% of vaginal tumors. The etiology remains unknown. Unlike in cutaneous melanoma, *BRAF* mutations are found in only 10% of mucosal melanomas. One-third of vaginal mucosal melanomas have an *NRAS* mutation. Typically, they are found in the lower third of the vagina, in contrast to SCCs, which are generally found in the superior vagina.

FIGURE 15.12. Image (A) shows a vagina with a large and pigmented polypoid lesion extending from the mucosa surface. In (B), a polypoid mass with a nodular surface is present in the vagina. It is erythematous with areas of darker pigmentation.

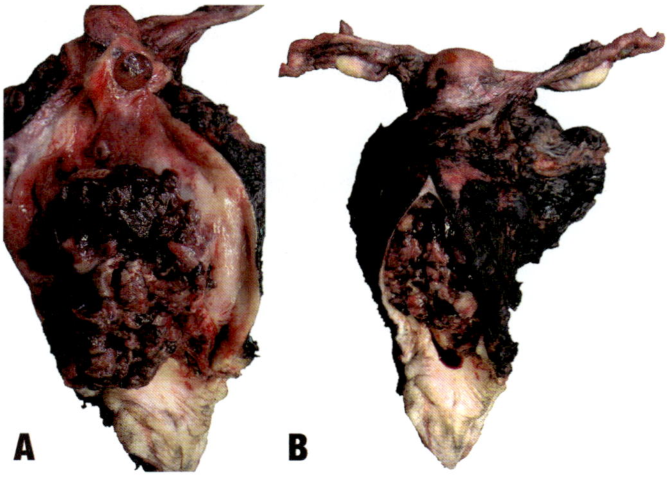

Uterine Cervix

Nabothian cyst

Nabothian cysts are common incidental findings that correspond to retention cysts of the cervical glands.

FIGURE 15.13. Images (A) and (B) show multiple, variably sized cysts filled with mucus in the cervix.

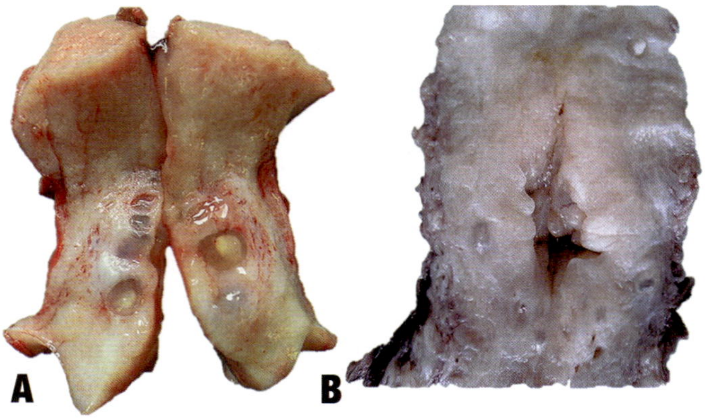

Endocervical polyp

FIGURE 15.14. The cut surface of this polypoid lesion shows numerous small retention cysts at the periphery. The stroma is pale yellow with hemorrhagic foci.

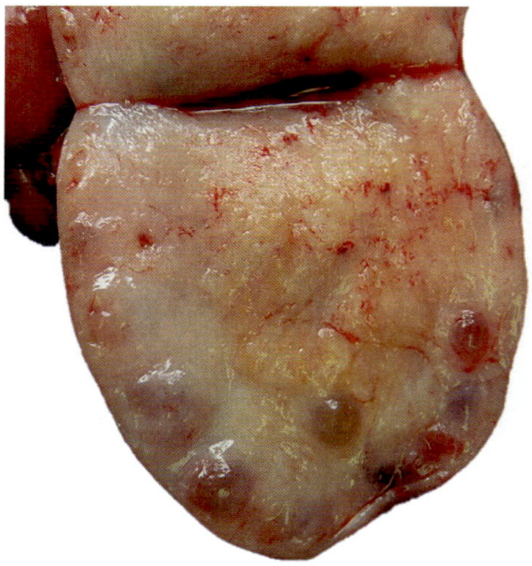

Lobular endocervical glandular hyperplasia

FIGURE 15.15. This hysterectomy shows mass-forming cystic structures of varying sizes located in the inner half of the cervix. The lesion is benign.

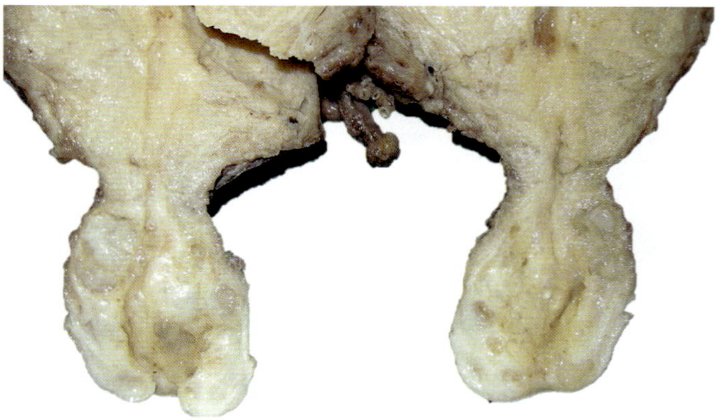

Cervical squamous cell carcinoma (SCC)

Cervical SCC develops from precancerous squamous intraepithelial lesions and is associated with HPV infection. Vaccination against high-risk HPV subtypes, now available, helps lower the risk of developing this cancer.

FIGURE 15.16. The trachelectomy in (A) shows a red, exophytic, and ill-defined mass involving the exocervix. In (B), opening the cervix revealed a red, nodular mass involving the endocervix and the cervical stroma. Image (C) shows an ulcerative, friable lesion extending from the external os.

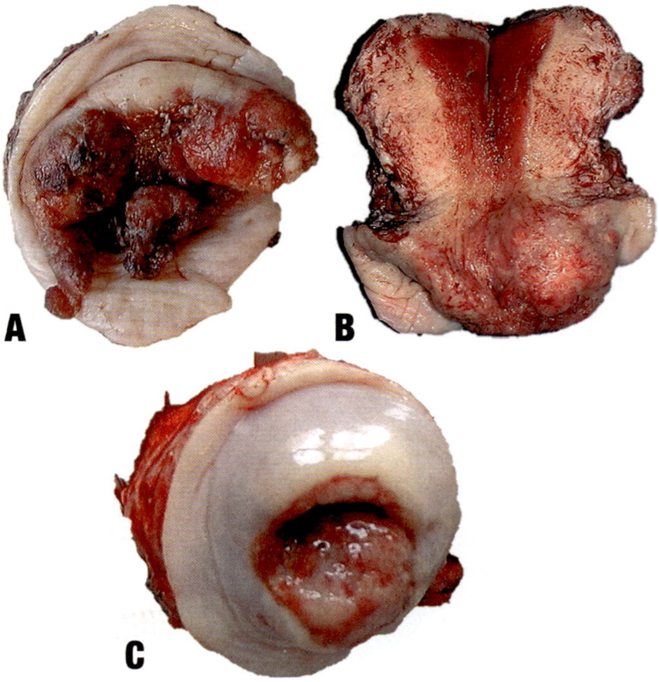

Endocervical adenocarcinoma

In developed countries, endocervical adenocarcinoma currently accounts for 10% to 25% of all carcinomas of the uterine cervix.

FIGURE 15.17. This hysterectomy specimen shows a large, nodular, hemorrhagic mass involving the entire endocervix and part of the endometrium.

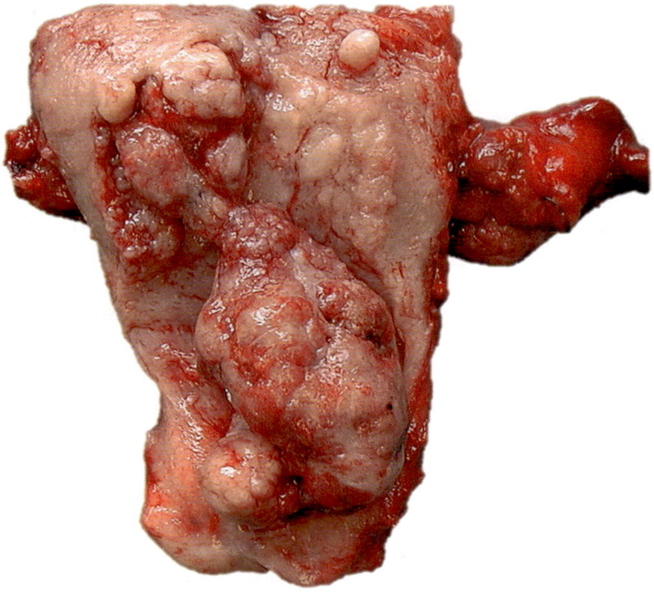

Leiomyosarcoma involving the cervix

FIGURE 15.18. The cervix in this trachelectomy specimen has been significantly distorted by a large, tan, fleshy, and polypoid mass with irregular borders.

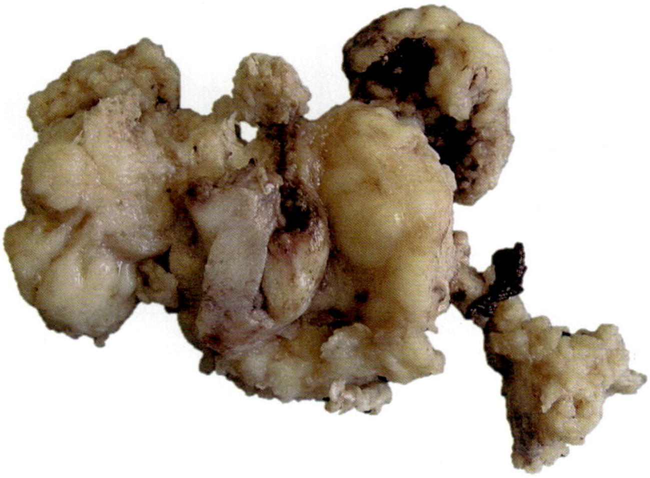

Uterus

REFERENCE: NORMAL UTERUS

FIGURE 15.19. This image shows a rear view of a normal uterus, normal bilateral ovaries, and normal fallopian tubes.

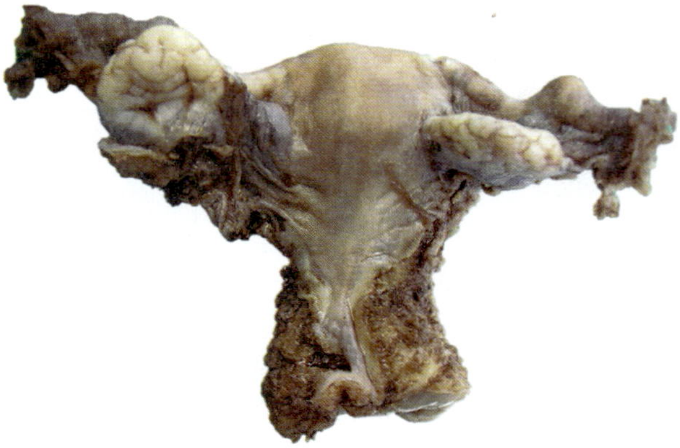

Endometriosis

Endometriosis is a condition in which endometrial tissue occurs at sites outside the uterine cavity (e.g., the uterosacral ligaments, uterine surface, ovaries, fallopian tubes, pelvic peritoneum, or pouch of Douglas). It is almost exclusively a disease of reproductive-age women. Patients may present with dyspareunia, secondary dysmenorrhea, pelvic pain, or infertility, or may be asymptomatic.

FIGURE 15.20. In these specimens, the serosa of the uterus shows thick, irregular hemorrhagic adhesions.

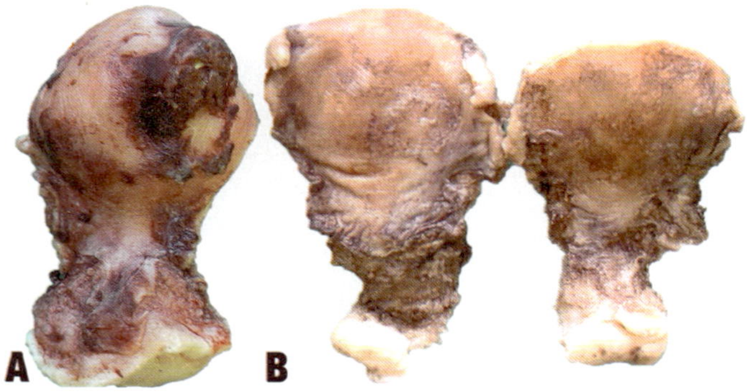

Adenomyosis

Adenomyosis is a nonneoplastic condition with nonspecific symptomatology, characterized by the presence of endometrial tissue within the body of the myometrium. Factors that play a role in the pathogenesis of adenomyosis include abnormality of the most superficial zone of myometrium ("junctional zone"), and hormonal and immune factors.

FIGURE 15.21. This uterus with adenomyosis is diffusely enlarged. The cut surface of the myometrium is markedly thickened with numerous small, blood-filled cysts.

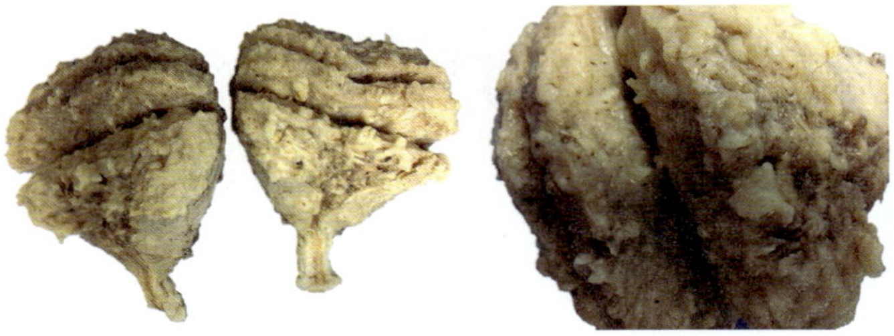

FIGURE 15.22. Image (A) shows a uterus with extensive adenomyosis. Brown spots within the body of the enlarged uterus are areas of endometrial bleeding within the myometrium. Image (B) shows multiple small cysts with areas of focal hemorrhage. The myometrium is markedly thickened.

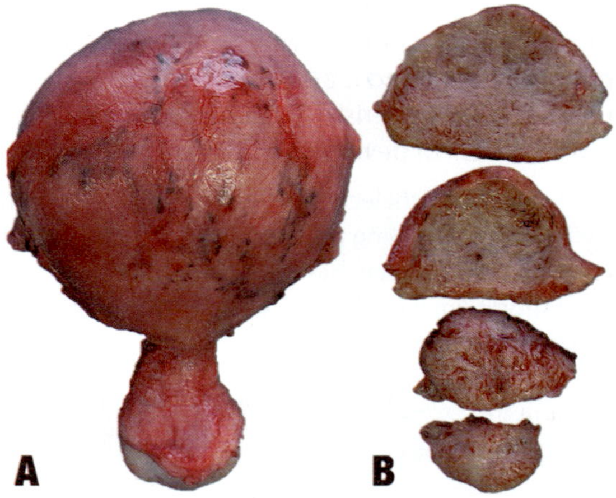

Endometrial polyp

Endometrial polyps are composed of a disorganized proliferation of benign endometrial glands and fibrous stroma with thick-walled blood vessels.

FIGURE 15.23. Image (A) shows a total abdominal hysterectomy and bilateral salpingo-oophorectomy. The exposed uterine cavity reveals multiple pedunculated polyps with a smooth, bosselated surface. Image (B) shows a large pedunculated polyp in a uterus.

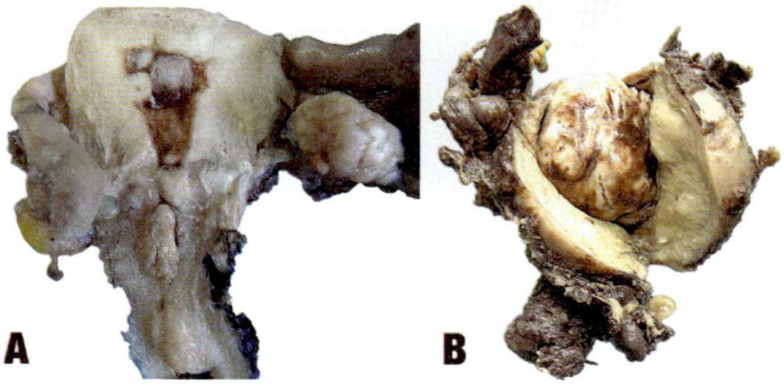

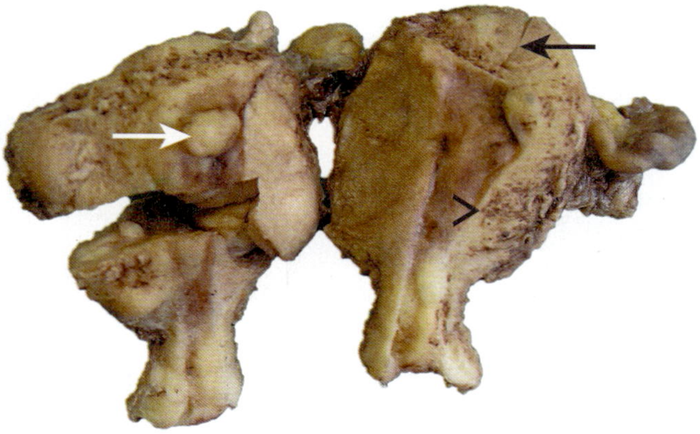

FIGURE 15.24. This uterus has multiple abnormalities, including a small sessile polyp in the uterine fundus (white arrow); an intramural leiomyoma (black arrow); and small, brown specks within the myometrium, which are adenomyosis (arrowhead).

ATYPICAL ENDOMETRIAL HYPERPLASIA

FIGURE 15.26. In this hysterectomy specimen, the endometrium is thickened with nodularity and hemorrhage. A diagnosis of atypical endometrial hyperplasia / EIN was confirmed microscopically.

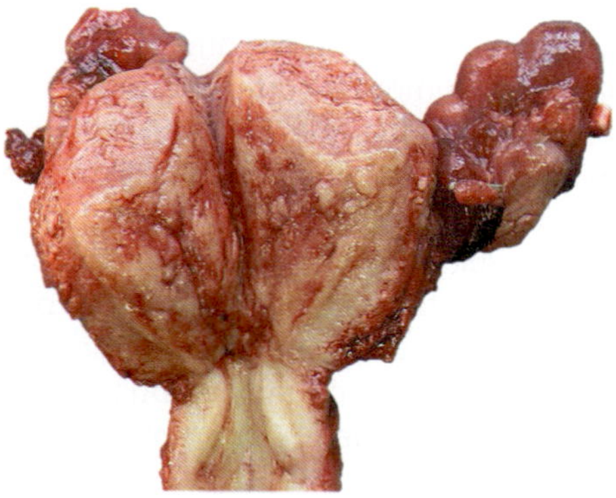

Endometrial hyperplasia

The World Health Organization (WHO) divides endometrial hyperplasia into 2 categories: hyperplasia without atypia, and atypical hyperplasia / endometrial intraepithelial neoplasia (EIN). Nonatypical hyperplasia is induced by an abnormal hormonal environment, usually unopposed estrogens. Atypical hyperplasia is a monoclonal proliferation of endometrial glands due to a risk factor of endogenous and exogenous hyperestrinism; patients are at high risk for endometrial cancer.

FIGURE 15.25. Image (A) shows a normal, smooth endometrium. Image (B) shows irregular thickening of the endometrium due to hyperplasia. Image (C) shows an endometrial carcinoma; the endometrium is diffusely thick, irregular, nodular, and friable.

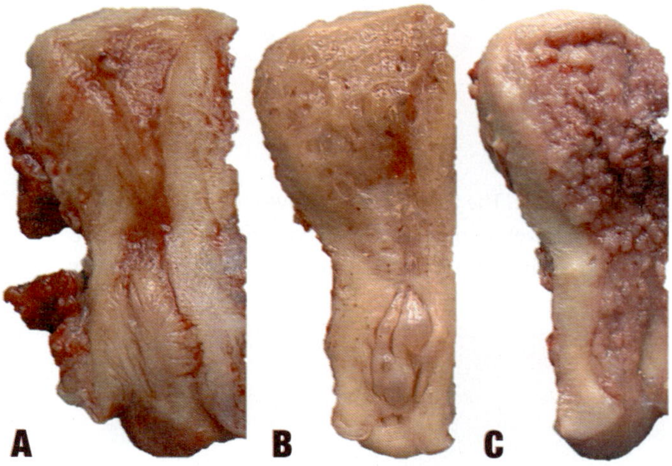

Polycystic ovary syndrome

Polycystic ovary syndrome (Stein–Leventhal syndrome) is characterized by anovulation, menstrual dysfunction, hyperandrogenism, and enlarged polycystic ovaries. The endometrium may demonstrate hyperplasia or endometrioid adenocarcinoma due to increased peripheral conversion of androgenic to estrogenic compounds.

ATYPICAL ENDOMETRIAL HYPERPLASIA IN A PATIENT WITH POLYCYSTIC OVARIAN DISEASE

FIGURE 15.27. The ovaries in (A) are bilaterally enlarged with a lobulated surface and a thick, white capsule. The endometrium is thickened and nodular. The cut surface of the ovaries in (B) shows multiple small follicles in a subcapsular location.

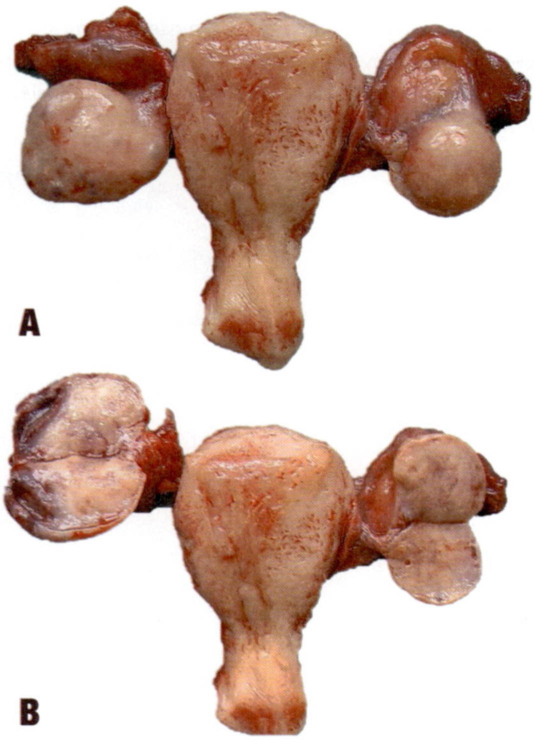

Endometrial adenocarcinoma

Endometrial carcinoma has 2 clinicopathologic types. Type I carcinoma, which represents 75% to 90% of cases, typically occurs in pre- and perimenopausal women in the setting of hyperestrogenism. Its precursor lesion is atypical hyperplasia / endometrial intraepithelial neoplasia (EIN) and, by histology, it presents as endometrioid carcinoma and its variants. The tumors are often low grade and show microsatellite instability, *PTEN* and *K-ras* mutations, and ß-catenin nuclear accumulation. Type II carcinoma represents 10% to 25% of cases. It is unrelated to estrogen stimulation, and typically occurs in postmenopausal women. Type II carcinoma is often high grade with poor prognosis. By histology, it presents as serous carcinoma, clear cell carcinoma, carcinosarcoma, or undifferentiated carcinoma. Molecular alterations include p53 abnormalities and loss of heterozygosity.

ENDOMETRIOID-TYPE ENDOMETRIAL ADENOCARCINOMA

FIGURE 15.28. Image (A) shows an extensive nodular and pink-to-tan tumor located in the uterine cavity and involving the endocervix. The tumors in (B) are located in the fundus, in the lower segment, and involve the cervix (arrows).

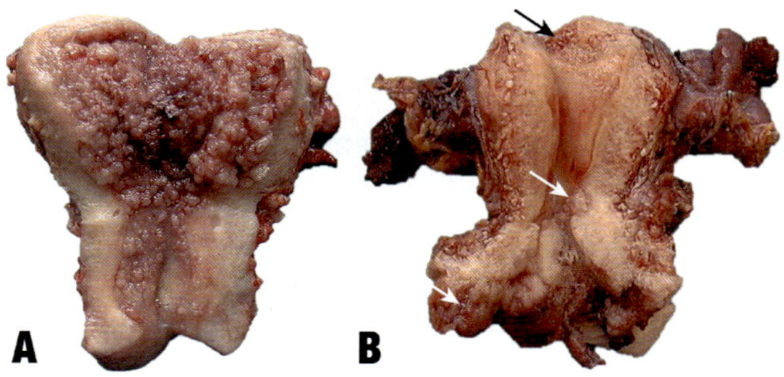

FIGURE 15.29. Image (A) shows a total hysterectomy and bilateral salpingo-oophorectomy with a mass in the fundus (sliced). In (B), the full thickness of the uterus shows a tumor invading over half of the myometrium depth.

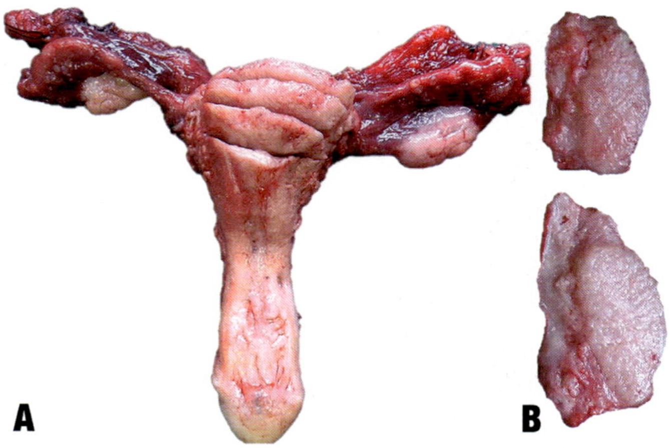

FIGURE 15.30. Image (A) shows a large tumor involving the entire endometrial cavity. In (B), the tumor is invading the outer half of the posterior myometrium (2 mm from the serosal surface). According to the International Federation of Gynecology and Obstetrics (FIGO) staging system, a tumor with invasion beyond 50% of the myometrium is stage IB.

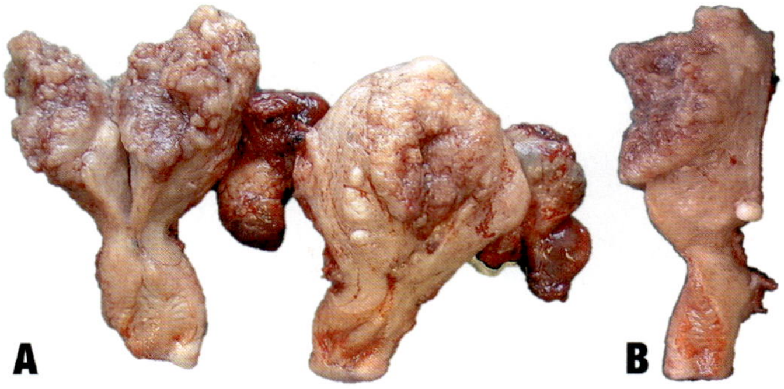

FIGURE 15.31. In (A), an endometrioid-type endometrial adenocarcinoma shows minimal myometrium invasion. Note the enlarged bilateral ovaries. The cut opening of bilateral ovaries in (B) shows features of polycystic ovary syndrome with multiple subcortical, small, follicular cysts.

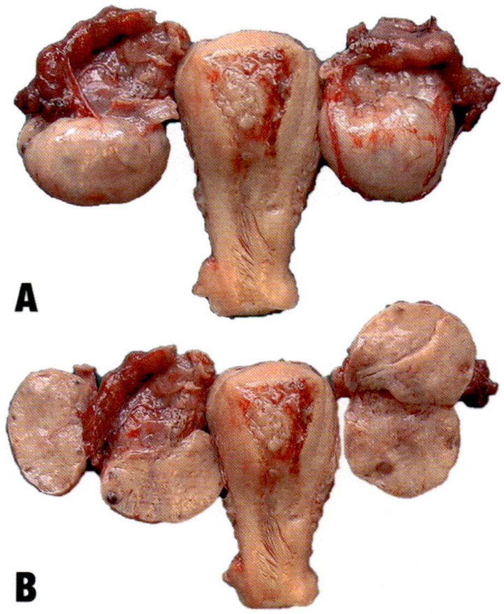

FIGURE 15.32. The tumor in (A) involves most of the uterine cavity and lower uterine segment, and extends to the upper endocervix. The cut surface in (B) shows myometrial invasion.

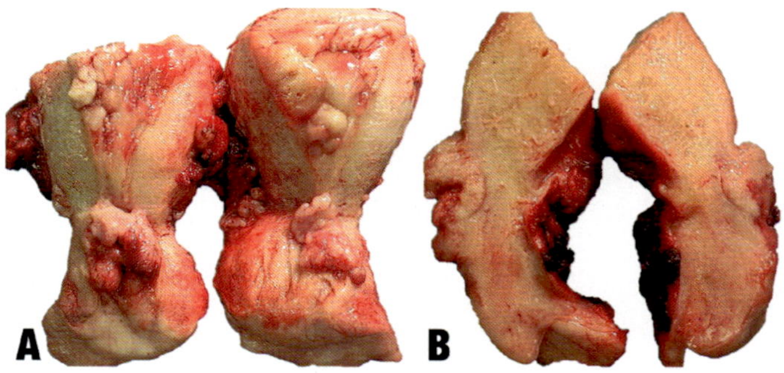

FIGURE 15.33. In (A), a large polypoid growth extends from the fundus of the uterine cavity. It is tan in color with small foci of hemorrhage. Image (B) shows an endometrioid adenocarcinoma within an endometrial polyp. The cut surface of the polyp displays solid cystic components with necrosis.

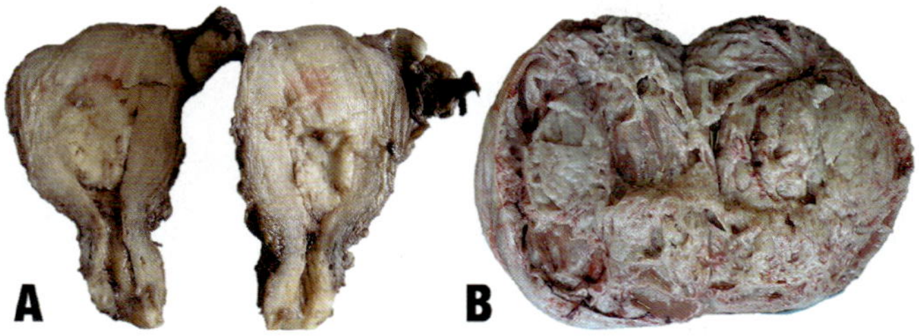

Endometrial carcinoma

The International Federation of Gynecology and Obstetrics (FIGO) developed a 3-tiered grading system for endometrial carcinoma based on the amount of solid, nonsquamous areas within a tumor. The WHO endorses this grading system. Grade 1 tumors show no more than 5% solid growth; grade 2 tumors show 6% to 50% solid growth; and grade 3 tumors show more than 50% solid growth.

TYPE I: ENDOMETRIAL ENDOMETRIOID ADENOCARCINOMA

FIGURE 15.34. In (A), an exophytic lesion is growing in a diffuse pattern and exhibiting necrosis. Microscopically, it is endometrial endometrioid carcinoma, FIGO grade 2. The endometrioid carcinoma in (B) was classified microscopically as FIGO grade 3.

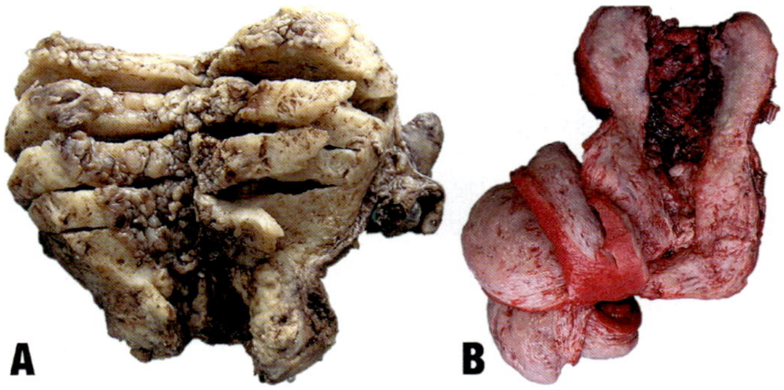

FIGURE 15.35. The endometrioid carcinoma in (A) was microscopically classified as a FIGO grade 3 exophytic growth. Images (B) and (C) show endometrial endometrioid adenocarcinoma with diffuse growth filling up the uterine cavity.

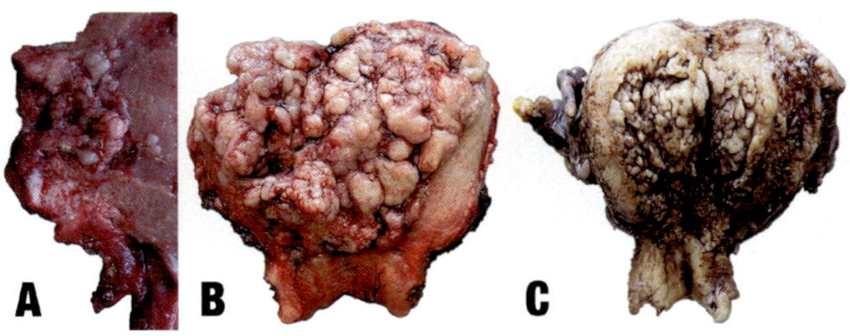

TYPE II: ENDOMETRIAL CARCINOMA

Type II endometrial carcinoma accounts for approximately 10% of all endometrial carcinomas. It typically occurs in postmenopausal women and has an aggressive clinical behavior.

FIGURE 15.36. Images (A) and (B) show type II endometrial clear cell carcinomas. In (A), an exophytic, tan, and nodular mass fills most of the endometrial cavity. Image (B) shows a clear cell carcinoma involving the entire endometrium, lower uterine segment, and cervix. Clear cell carcinoma is typically negative for estrogen receptor (ER) and progesterone receptor (PR).

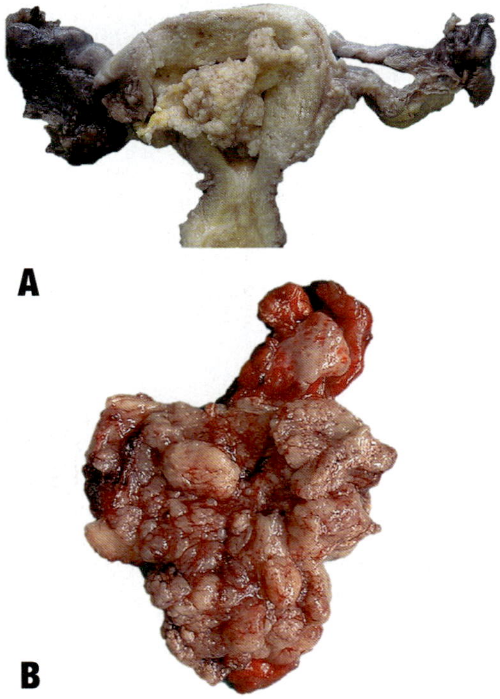

ENDOMETRIAL SEROUS CARCINOMA

Endometrial serous carcinoma accounts for 5% to 10% of endometrial carcinomas and is the prototype of type II tumors. The precursor lesion is serous endometrial intraepithelial carcinoma (EIC). Both lesions develop in an atrophic endometrium and can be confined to an endometrial polyp.

FIGURE 15.37. Image (A) shows 3 small foci (arrow) of confluent neoplastic glands on the surface of a polyp in the anterior endometrium. Microscopically, serous EIC was diagnosed. In (B), serous carcinoma involves the endometrial polyp.

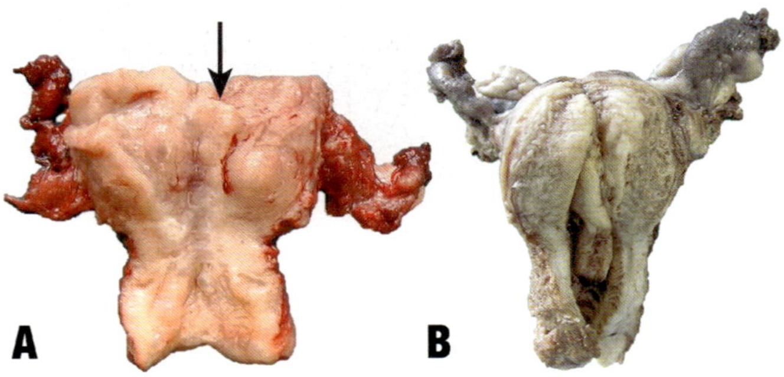

FIGURE 15.38. Image (A) shows a thickened endometrium with a nodular and papillary surface. Image (B) shows endometrial serous carcinoma with polypoid projections into the uterine cavity.

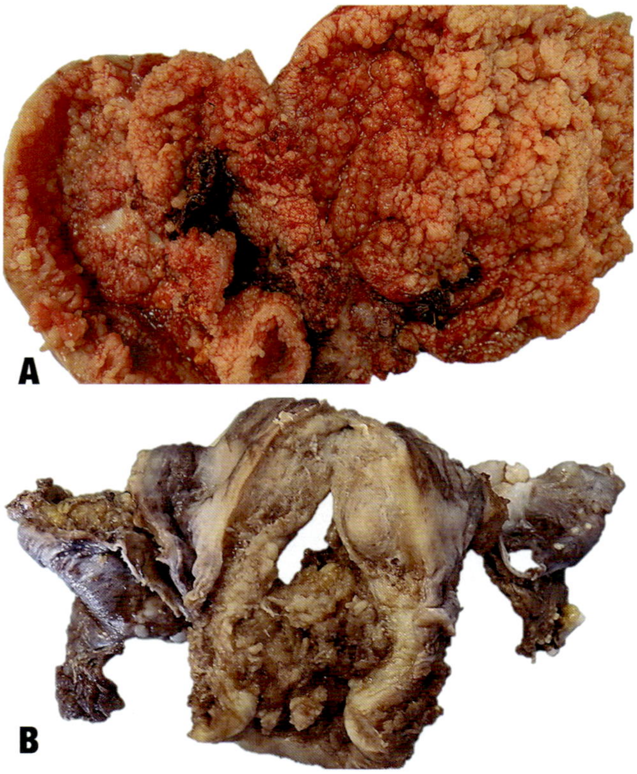

DEDIFFERENTIATED CARCINOMA OF THE ENDOMETRIUM

A dedifferentiated carcinoma is defined as a neoplasm with 2 components: a FIGO grade 1 or 2 endometrioid carcinoma, and an undifferentiated carcinoma. These lesions often confer a poor prognosis.

FIGURE 15.39. On microscopic examination, this large, polypoid intraluminal mass with hemorrhage and necrosis was consistent with dedifferentiated carcinoma of the endometrium.

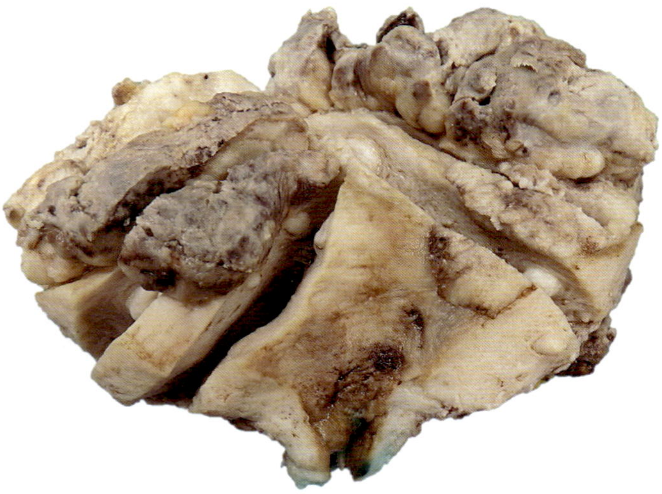

LARGE CELL NEUROENDOCRINE CARCINOMA (LCNEC) OF THE ENDOMETRIUM

LCNEC is a rare malignancy with an aggressive course.

FIGURE 15.40. Image (A) shows a solid tumor with a fleshy, yellow cut surface. In (B), an LCNEC invades the myometrium.

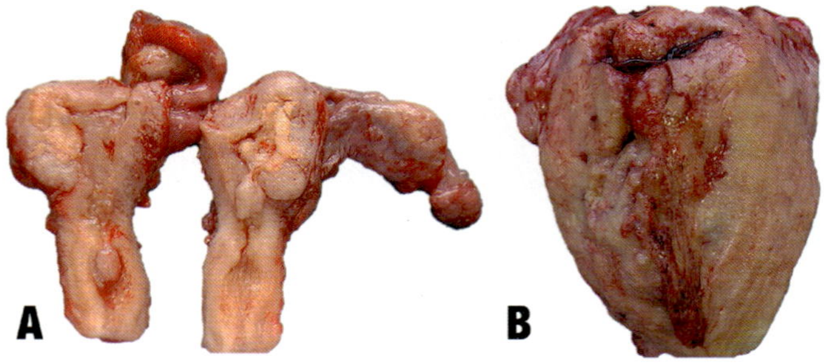

ENDOMETRIAL UNDIFFERENTIATED CARCINOMA

FIGURE 15.41. Image (A) shows a bulky tumor mass with necrosis. Image (B) shows another endometrial undifferentiated carcinoma; the cut surface shows tumor invasion through the uterine wall to surrounding tissue.

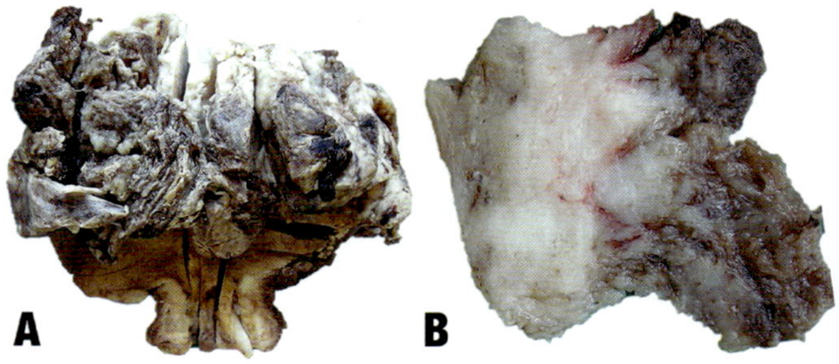

Endometrial carcinosarcoma

This neoplasm used to be called malignant mixed Müllerian tumor. The WHO renamed it carcinosarcoma in 2014, to reflect its character as a primary epithelial tumor that develops a mesenchymal component. The malignant mesenchymal component may include homologous or heterologous sarcomatous elements.

FIGURE 15.42. The tumors in (A) and (B) appear as polypoid lesions protruding into the uterine cavity. Necrosis is present in (A).

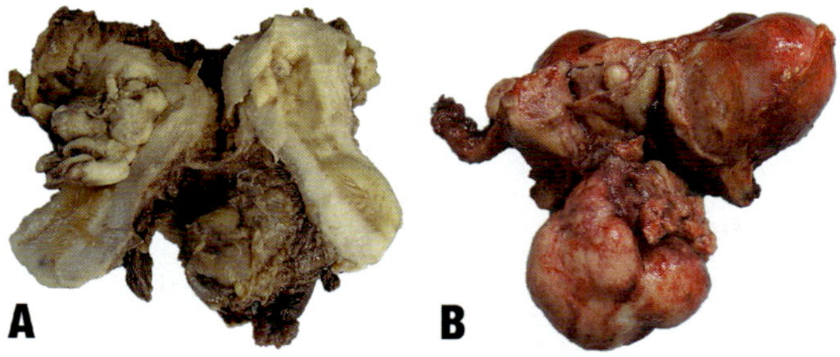

FIGURE 15.43. These images show a uterus with endometrial carcinosarcoma. The tumor not only protrudes into the uterine lumen, but also invades into the outer half of the myometrium toward the right side of the fundus. The deepest tumor is located 1.5 mm from uterine serosa.

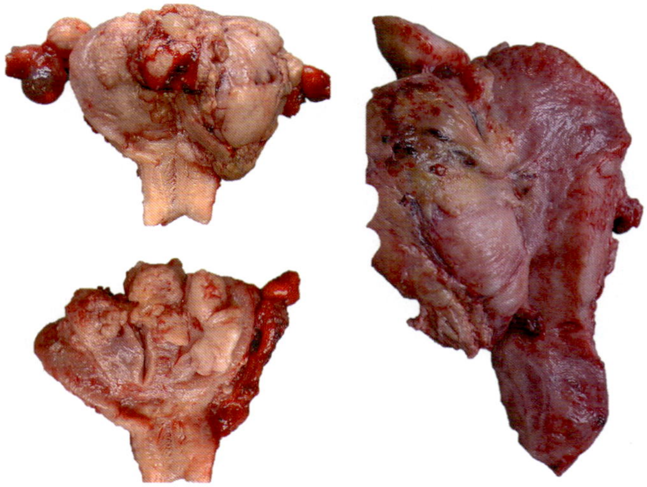

FIGURE 15.44. Image (A) shows an endometrial carcinosarcoma (6 cm) with invasion into the inner third of the myometrium. Image (B) shows a cut surface of the same specimen.

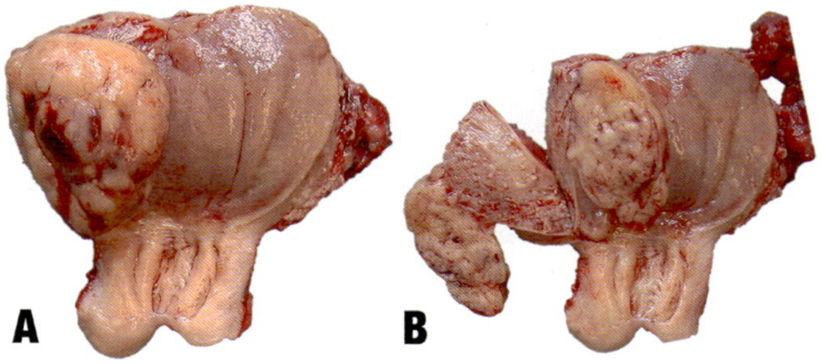

CARCINOSARCOMA POST-NEOADJUVANT CHEMOTHERAPY

FIGURE 15.45. Image (A) shows a carcinosarcoma post-neoadjuvant chemotherapy with residual ulcerated tumor in the cervix. There is no evidence of residual tumor in the endometrium. Image (B) gives a high magnification of the malignant tumor in (A).

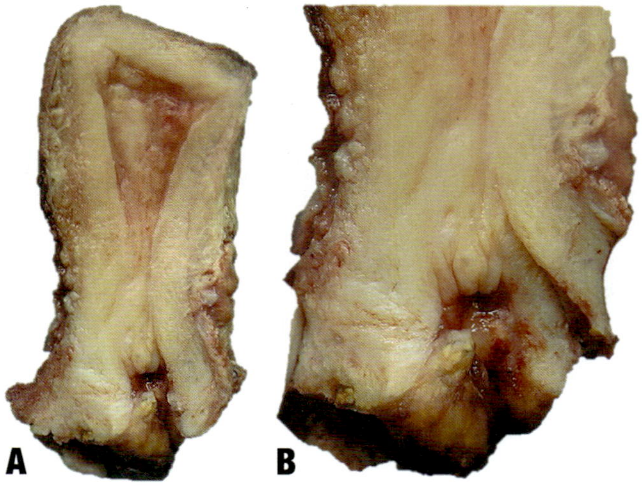

Uterine leiomyoma

Leiomyomas (or fibroids) are benign smooth muscle tumors of the uterus.

FIGURE 15.46. Image (A) shows uterine leiomyomas: multiple well-circumscribed, spherical, and tan masses of varying sizes are present in submucosal, intramural, and subserosal locations. Image (B) shows a uterine leiomyoma (20 cm) in the anterior wall with degenerative changes.

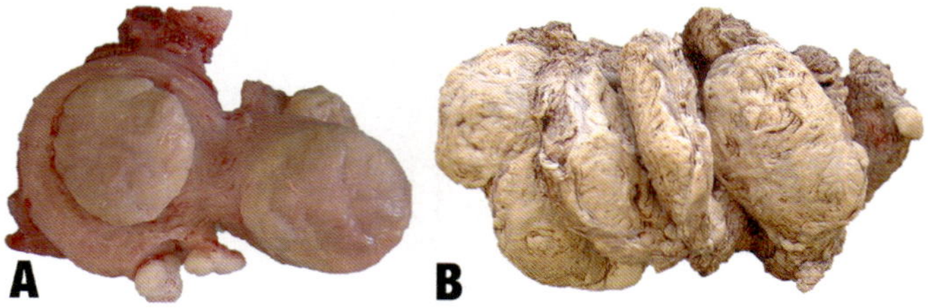

FIGURE 15.47. A large (18 cm), well-defined, white, and pedunculated mass with small foci of hemorrhage extends from the uterus. The cut surface has the characteristic features of a leiomyoma with a whorled pattern and bulging appearance.

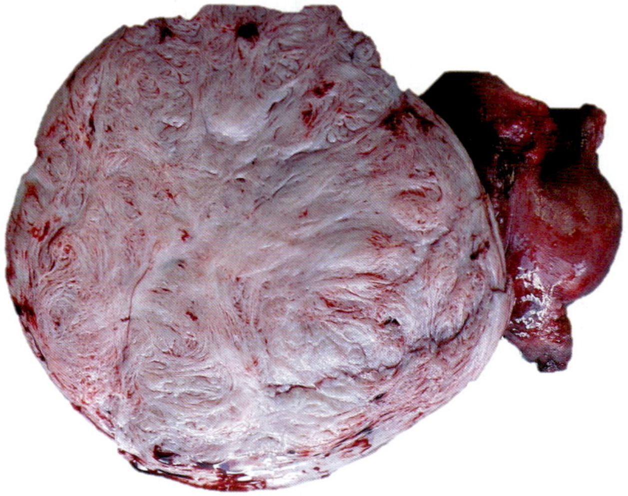

FIGURE 15.48. These images show uteruses with multiple leiomyomas.

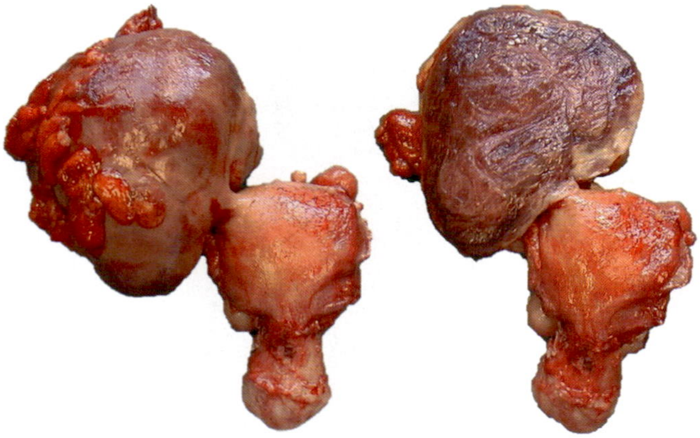

FIGURE 15.49. The myomectomy in (A) shows a leiomyoma with degenerative changes including hyalinization, cystification, and focal calcifications. For the leiomyoma in (B), note the endometrium with tamoxifen-related diffuse cystic change.

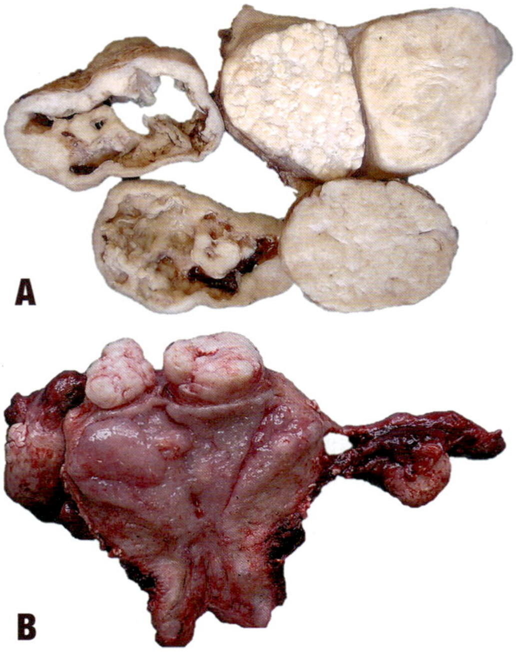

FIGURE 15.50. The hysterectomy specimen in (A) shows an intrauterine device (IUD) within the uterine cavity. Note that the endometrium appears congested. Image (B) shows a uterus with multiple well-circumscribed and tan nodules, and a whorled appearance on cut section. The nodules are benign smooth muscle tumors called leiomyomas found in the subserosa, submucosa, and intramural locations of the uterus. An IUD is present within the uterine cavity.

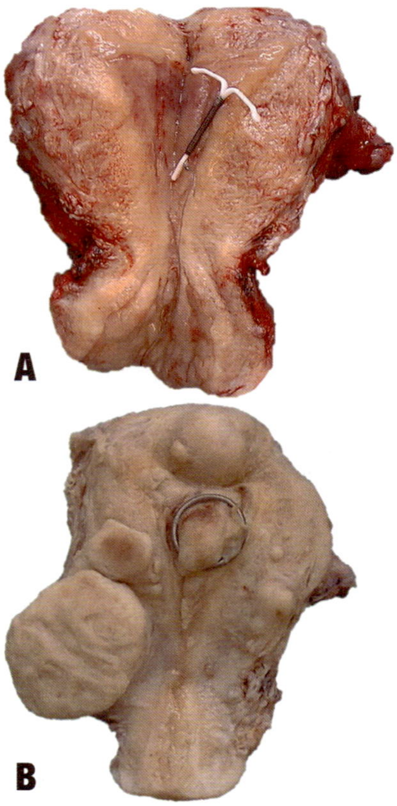

SUBMUCOSAL LEIOMYOMA

FIGURE 15.51. Image (A) shows a large submucosal leiomyoma forming a polypoid mass protruding into the uterine lumen (blue arrows). The myometrium shows features consistent with previous uterine artery embolization (black arrows): multifocal, intravascular, foreign-body material. Image (B) shows higher magnification of the myometrium.

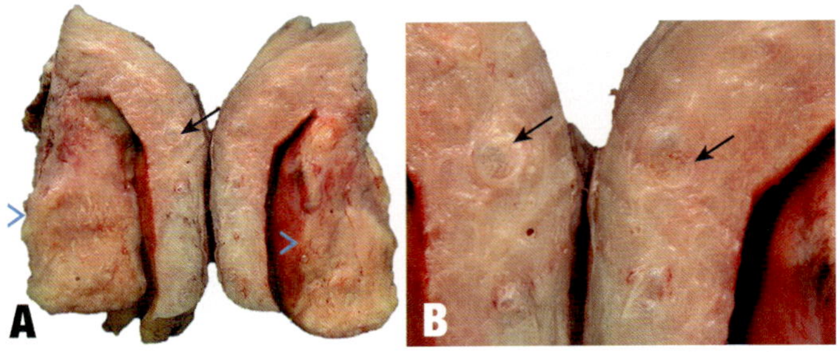

LIPOLEIOMYOMA

FIGURE 15.52. This image shows uterine leiomyomata in intramural and subserosal locations. The largest lesion measures 5 cm.

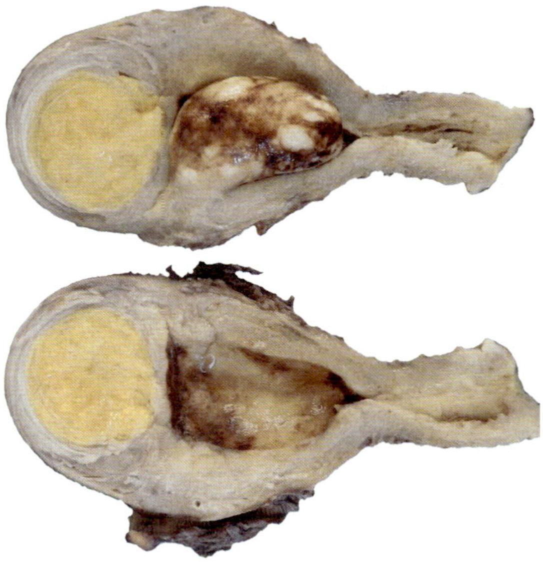

FIGURE 15.53. A well-circumscribed lesion with a mostly yellow appearance corresponds to a mature adipose tissue component.

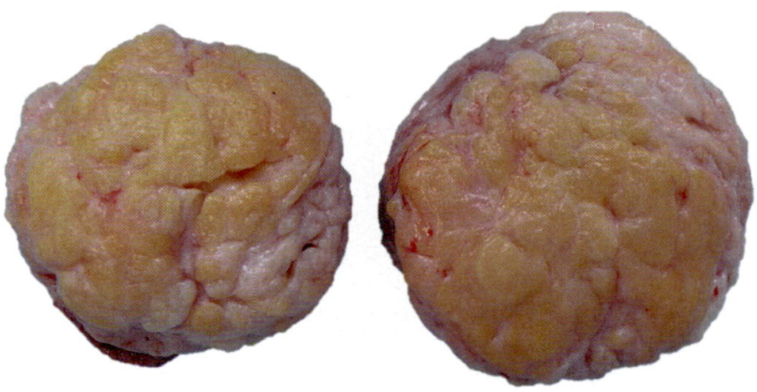

FIGURE 15.54. Image (A) shows a bulge tumor in a submucosal and intramural location. The cut surface in (B) shows that the bulging mass has a heterogeneous surface composed of yellow adipose tissue and lighter smooth muscle tissue with a whorled appearance.

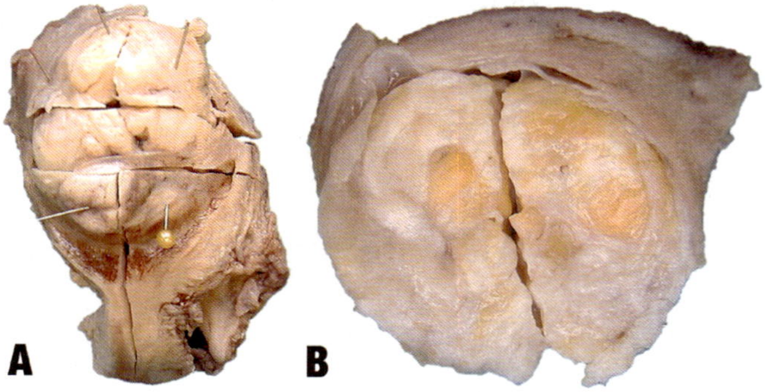

ADENOLIPOLEIOMYOMA

Adenolipoleiomyoma contains benign Müllerian-type glands, and smooth muscle and adipose tissue. It is considered a hamartomatous lesion.

FIGURE 15.55. Image (A) shows a 4.3-cm, tan, intramural, and subserosal lesion located in the lower uterine segment and upper endocervix. The mass has a mildly polypoid appearance and is well circumscribed. The lesion in (B) has a yellow cut surface with slit-like spaces and glistening mucoid areas.

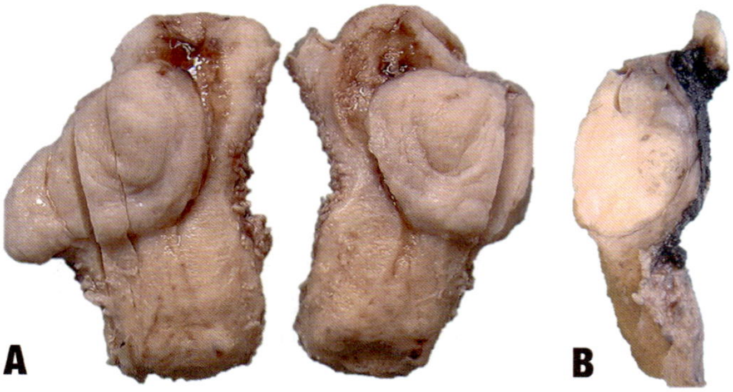

Intravenous leiomyomatosis

Intravenous leiomyomatosis is a rare condition in which masses of benign smooth muscle proliferation are found within venous channels.

FIGURE 15.56. This image shows multiple tan-white hemorrhagic nodules of varying sizes, similar to a leiomyoma, located in the vascular lumen.

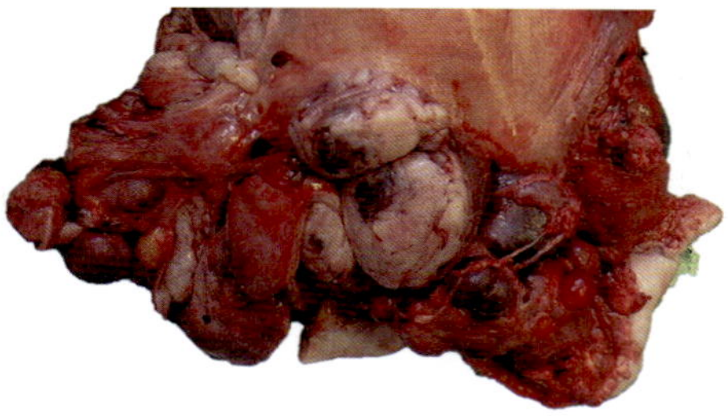

FIGURE 15.57. Images (A) and (B) demonstrate intravenous leiomyomatosis. Image (B) shows the lesion extending through the inferior vena cava to the atrium.

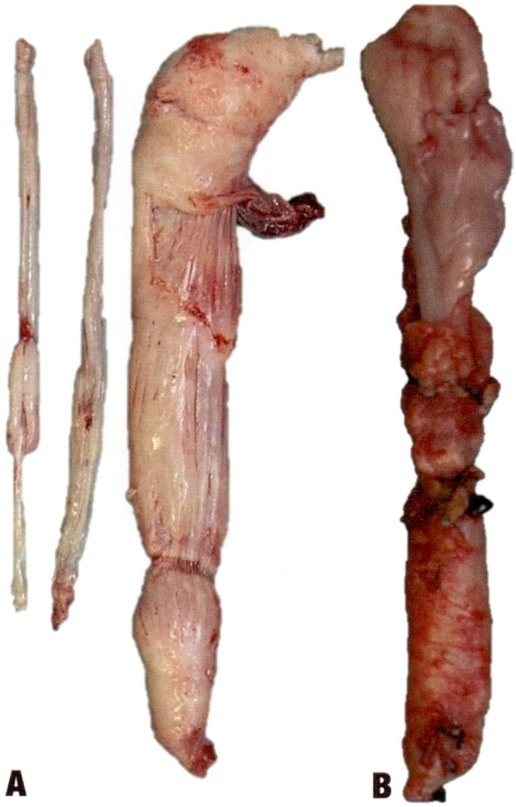

Smooth muscle tumor of uncertain malignant potential (STUMP)

This group of tumors shows features that preclude an unequivocal diagnosis of leiomyosarcoma. On gross examination, it is often impossible to differentiate leiomyoma from STUMP.

FIGURE 15.58. Image (A) shows a highly vascularized tumor with foci of interstitial hemorrhage. Focal microcystic degenerative changes are present. The cut surface in (B) shows areas of hemorrhage.

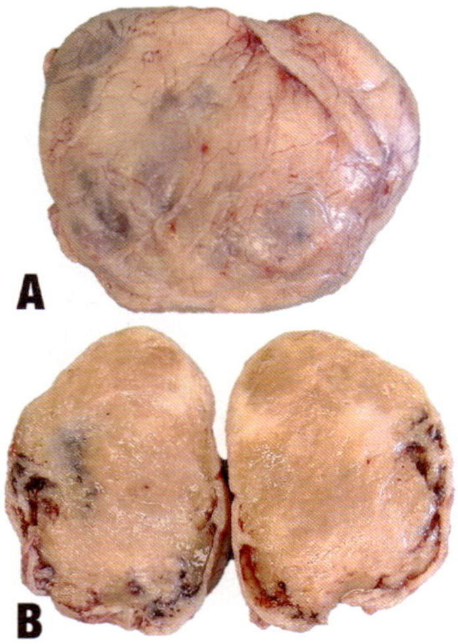

FIGURE 15.59. The STUMP in (A) shows a well-circumscribed and smooth-surfaced white nodule. Image (B) shows the cut surface of this specimen.

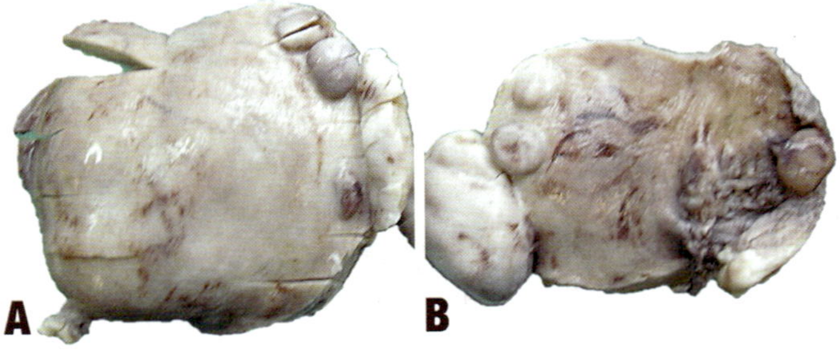

FIGURE 15.60. These images show a cut section (A) and external view (B) of a STUMP resembling a regular leiomyoma.

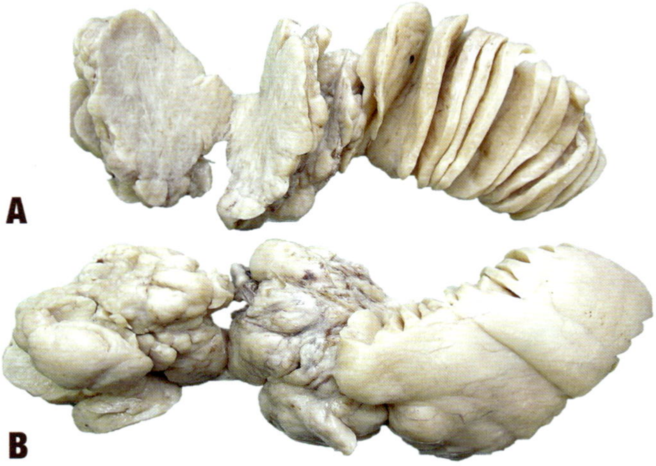

Uterine leiomyosarcoma

This malignant smooth muscle tumor represents the most common type of uterine sarcoma (more than 50%), but only 1% to 2% of all uterine malignancies. The presence of necrosis signals the possibility of malignancy in a uterine smooth muscle tumor.

FIGURE 15.61. Image (A) shows bulging, fleshy masses with areas of hemorrhage and necrosis. Image (B) shows a tan, irregularly shaped leiomyosarcoma with small areas of hemorrhage and necrosis arising mostly in the cervix.

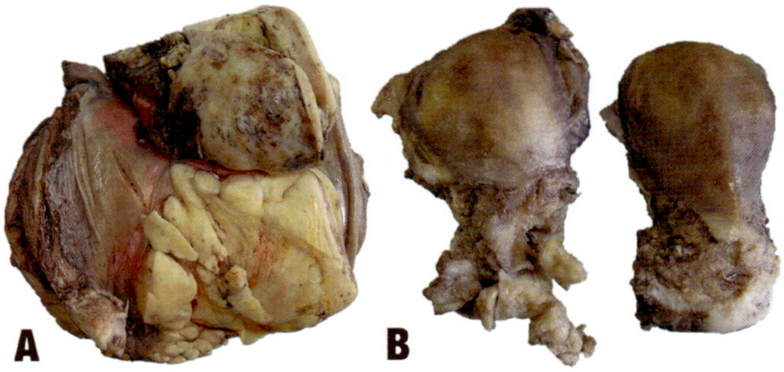

FIGURE 15.62. This image shows a bulging heterogeneous mass with extensive hemorrhage and necrosis.

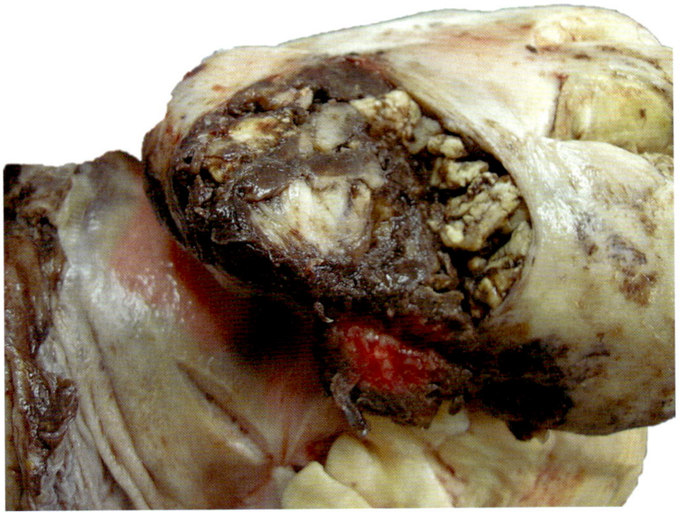

Endometrial stromal sarcoma

Endometrial stromal tumors are rare (fewer than 1% of all uterine tumors). According to the latest classification, endometrial stromal tumors are divided into 4 categories based on resemblance to proliferative-type endometrial stroma: endometrial stromal nodule (ESN); low-grade endometrial stromal sarcoma (LGESS); high-grade endometrial stromal sarcoma (HGESS); and undifferentiated uterine sarcoma (UUS).

LOW-GRADE ENDOMETRIAL STROMAL SARCOMA (LGESS)

FIGURE 15.63. In (A), the entire uterine body appears bulky due to diffuse invasion by a low-grade endometrial stromal sarcoma. Image (B) shows the cut surface of the same specimen, which demonstrates a characteristic fleshy and worm-like appearance.

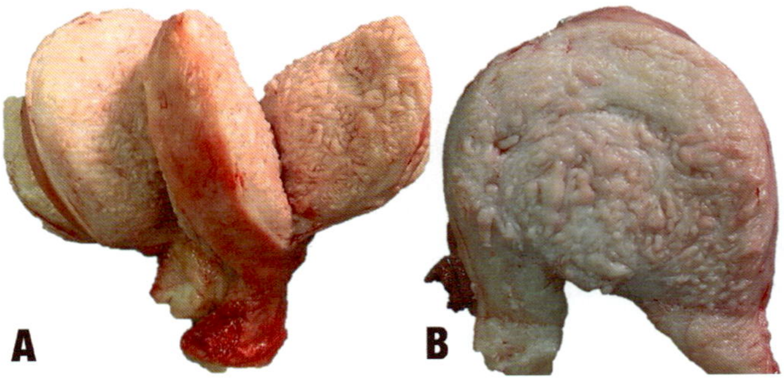

HIGH-GRADE ENDOMETRIAL STROMAL SARCOMA (HGESS)

FIGURE 15.64. Image (A) shows an HGESS forming a mass at the lower uterine segment. In (B), an HGESS extends to the rectum (right side of the image).

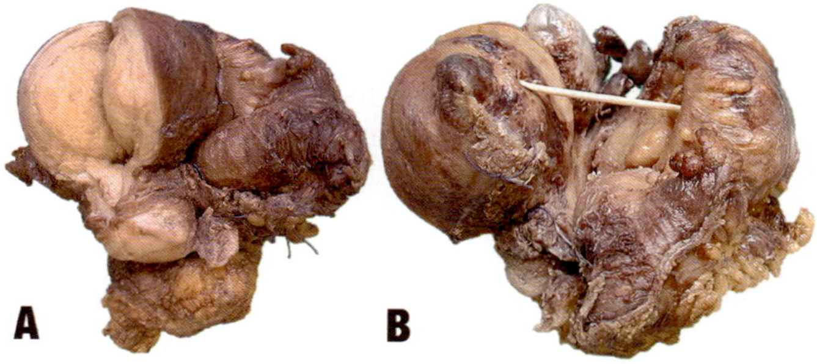

Uterine large B-cell lymphoma

Lymphoma of the uterine corpus is usually secondary to a lymphoma from another site. Patients have a poor prognosis.

FIGURE 15.65. This specimen of large B-cell lymphoma of the uterus shows a large, fleshy, and poorly demarcated polypoid mass.

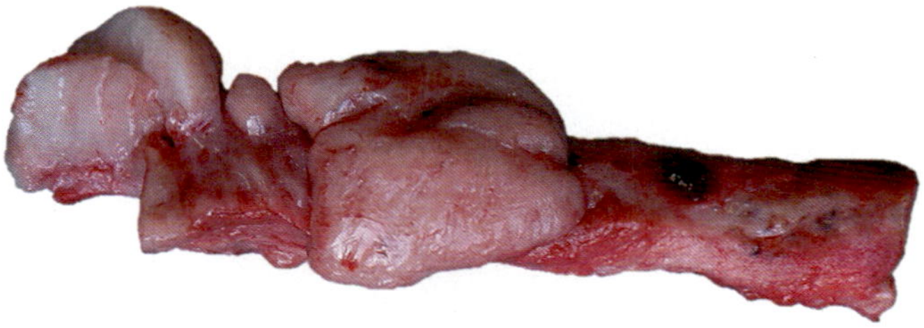

Fallopian Tube

Paratubal cyst

Paratubal cysts could be derived from a remnant of the Müllerian or Wolffian ducts, or they could originate in mesothelial cells. Those derived from the Müllerian ducts are the most common and include the hydatid cyst of Morgagni.

FIGURE 15.66. This specimen of a hysterectomy with bilateral salpingo-oophorectomy shows translucent cystic structures adjacent to a fallopian tube. These thin-walled cavities are filled with clear fluid.

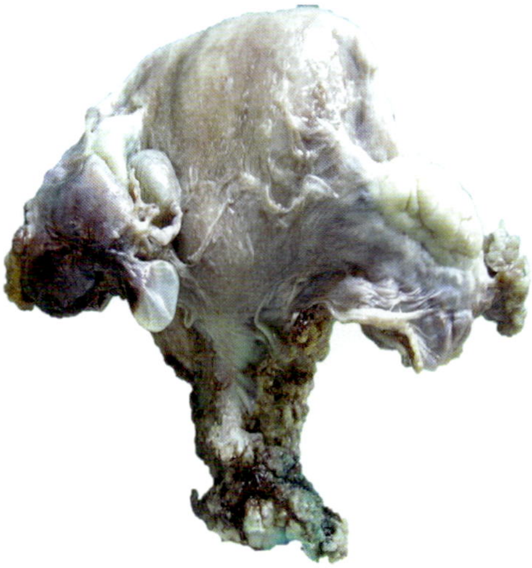

Salpingitis isthmica nodosa (SIN)

SIN consists of nodular swelling of the isthmic segment of the fallopian tube. It is associated with diverticula of the lumen and smooth muscle proliferation. It is a common cause of infertility.

FIGURE 15.67. These images show cross-sections of SIN with well-defined, white nodules measuring up to 2 cm. The central lumen is visible in some nodules (arrows).

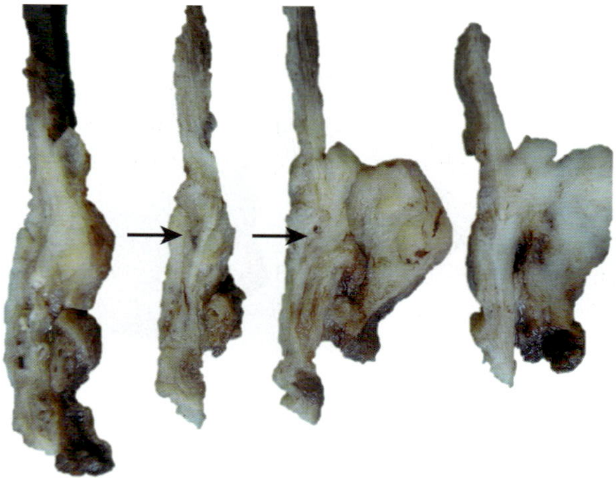

Hydrosalpinx

A hydrosalpinx results from severe inflammation and occlusion of the fimbriated end of a fallopian tube, and resorption of the exudate with replacement of pus by clear, serous fluid.

FIGURE 15.68. This image shows a severely distended fallopian tube containing serous fluid.

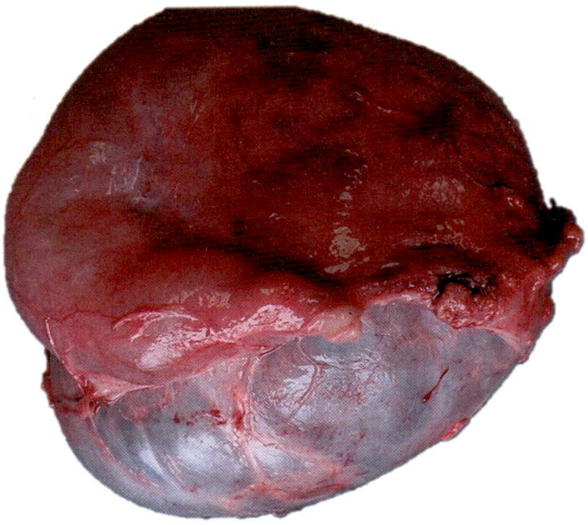

Paratubal endometriosis

Retrograde flow of menstrual debris through the fallopian tubes is considered the primary cause of tubal endometriosis. It affects 0.6% to 11% of women during their reproductive years. Tubal endometriosis is a common cause of infertility.

FIGURE 15.69. This image shows extensive dark-to-chocolate brown nodules on the serosa of the fallopian tubes.

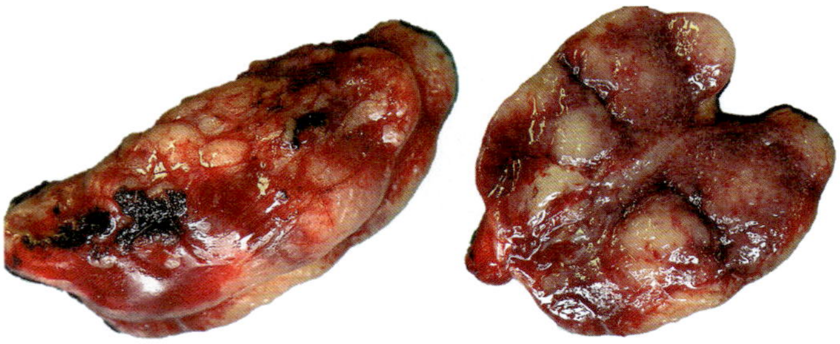

High-grade serous carcinoma of the fallopian tube

This is the most common type of tubal carcinoma and is histologically identical to other high-grade pelvic serous carcinomas.

FIGURE 15.70. In image (A), the fallopian tube shows marked dilation and a dusky color. The ovary is partially covered by a lightly colored nodular mass. In (B), the cut surface of the specimen shows multiple white-to-yellow polypoid masses involving the ovary and fallopian tube.

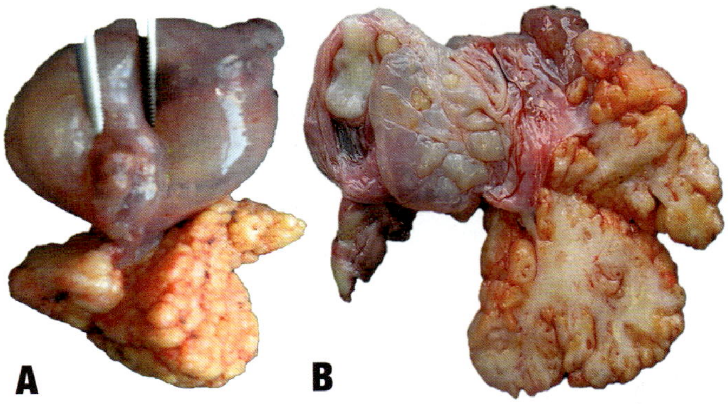

FIGURE 15.71. Image (A) shows a solid mass at the fimbriated end of a fallopian tube. Note the attached fallopian tube appears dilated and congested. In (B), the cut surface of the same specimen shows a solid, yellow-tan mass with small foci of hemorrhage connecting to the ovary and fimbria.

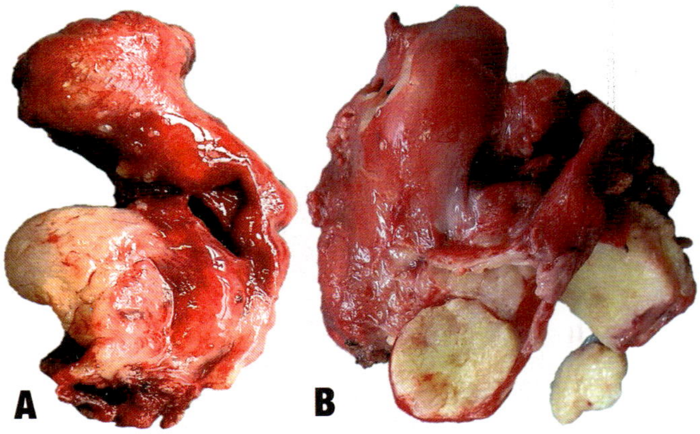

Ovary

Endometriosis

Endometriosis refers to the presence of endometrial glands and/or stroma outside the uterine cavity. The ovaries are common sites of endometriosis. There are 2 main theories of endometriosis: the transplantation theory and the metaplastic theory. The transplantation theory suggests that endometrial cells are implanted at ectopic sites through retrograde flow through the lumen of the fallopian tubes into the pelvic peritoneal cavity. The metaplastic theory suggests an endometrial metaplasia of the peritoneal serosa.

FIGURE 15.72. In this image, the ovary appears as a large cystic mass filled with black-to-brown material. Fibrous adhesions with hemorrhage are visible on the surface of the ovary and fallopian tube.

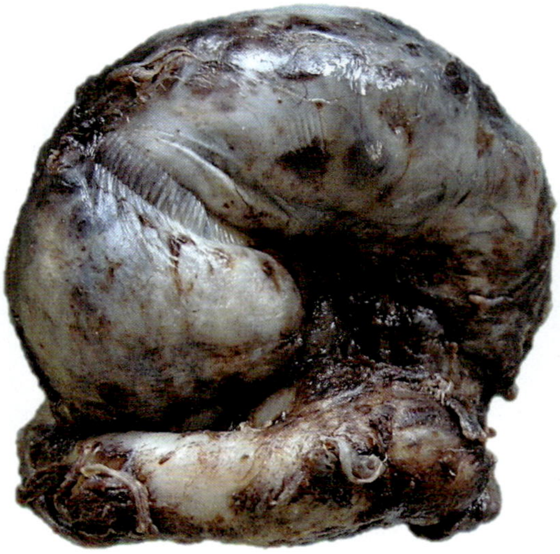

FIGURE 15.73. This image shows irregular areas of dark brown deposits on the serosa surface of an ovary and uterus.

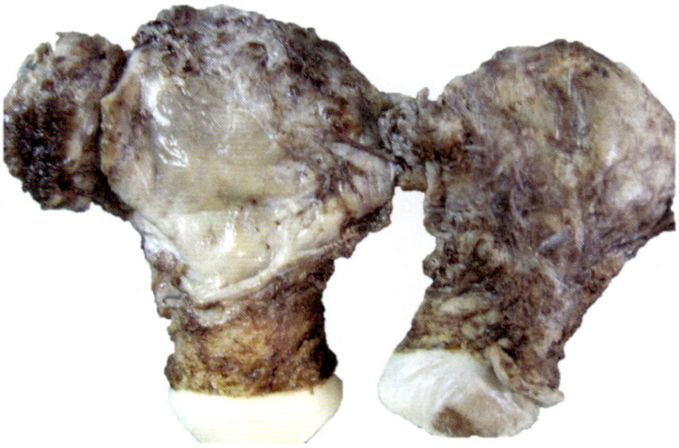

FIGURE 15.74. This image shows a large cystic mass of the ovary filled with dark brown material or "chocolate fluid."

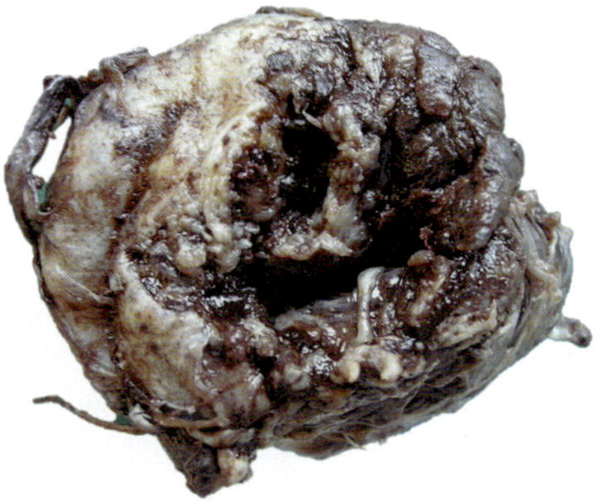

FIGURE 15.75. This dark brown cystic lesion of the ovary is consistent with endometriosis microscopically.

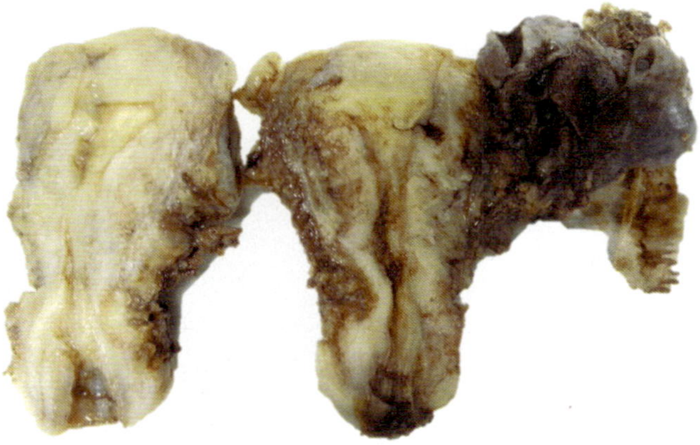

FIGURE 15.76. Image (A) shows a cyst between the uterus and rectum. In (B), the cut inner surface shows a large cystic mass filled with "chocolate" material.

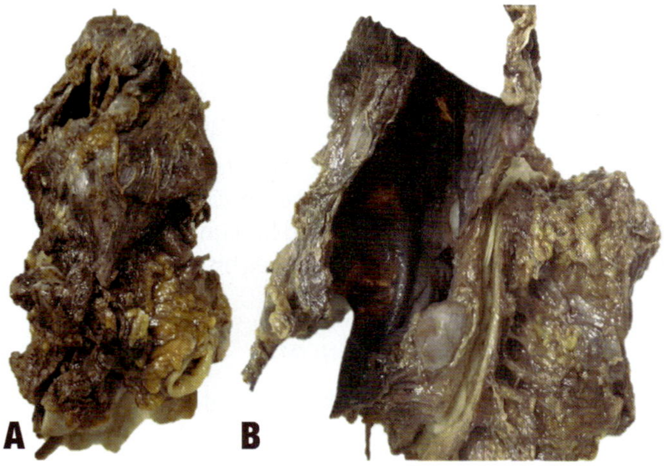

Corpus luteum cyst

These cysts are lined by luteinized granulosa and theca cells, and measure > 3 cm in diameter. These cysts are common, often asymptomatic, and found incidentally. On gross examination, endometriotic cysts are sometimes difficult to distinguish from corpus luteum cysts.

FIGURE 15.77. Image (A) shows a hysterectomy and unilateral salpingo-oophorectomy with a cystic mass extending from the left ovary. The wall of the mass appears slightly convoluted. Image (B) shows a magnified view of the cut surface of the same specimen. The mass is a unilocular, blood-filled cyst with a yellow-colored wall.

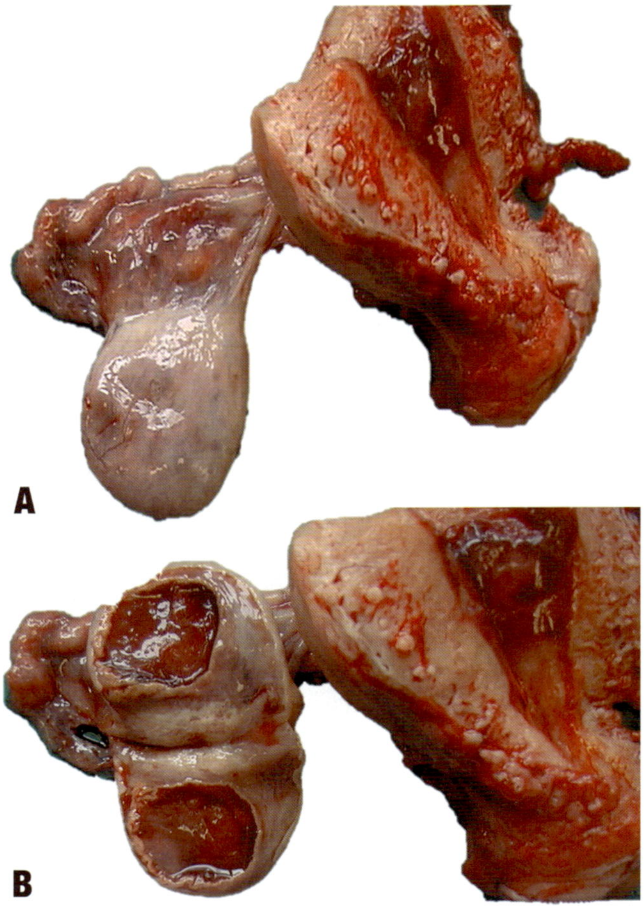

Ovarian serous tumor

Serous tumors represent 30% to 40% of all ovarian tumors. They are often bilateral. Sixty percent of cases are benign (cystadenoma), 10% are borderline, and 30% are malignant (serous carcinoma). Distinguishing benign, borderline, and malignant serous tumors requires histology, so tissue sampling is very important.

OVARIAN SEROUS CYSTADENOMA

A cutoff size of 1 cm distinguishes cortical inclusion cysts (< 1 cm) and serous cystadenoma (≥ 1 cm). The contents of serous cystadenoma are usually watery and clear or pale yellow, but are sometimes viscous and mucoid.

FIGURE 15.78. This ovarian cyst has a thin, smooth, and glistening wall without surface excrescences.

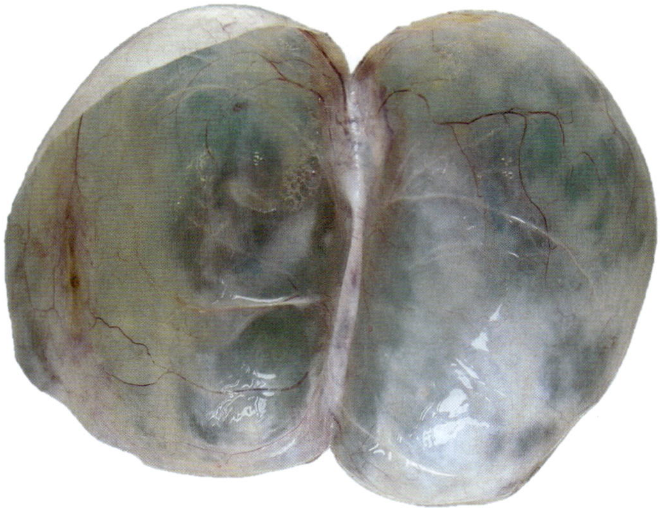

FIGURE 15.79. Image (A) shows a unilocular serous cystadenoma with a smooth, shiny surface. The cut inner surface in (B) shows the contents of the cyst, which are viscous and mucoid.

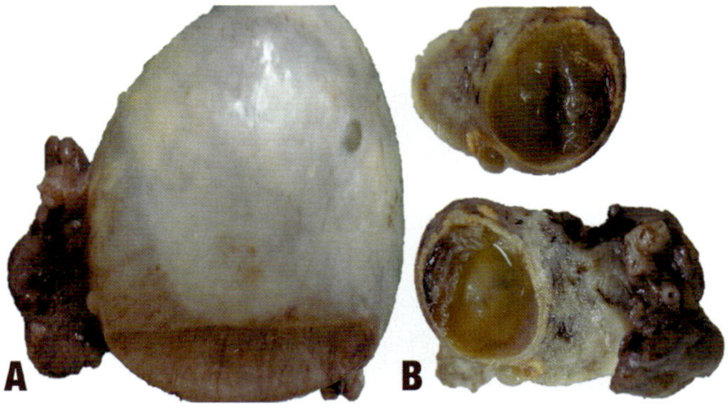

FIGURE 15.80. This hysterectomy with bilateral salpingo-oophorectomy shows a unilocular cyst with a smooth, shiny surface that occupies the majority of the ovary. Small endometrial polyps are also present.

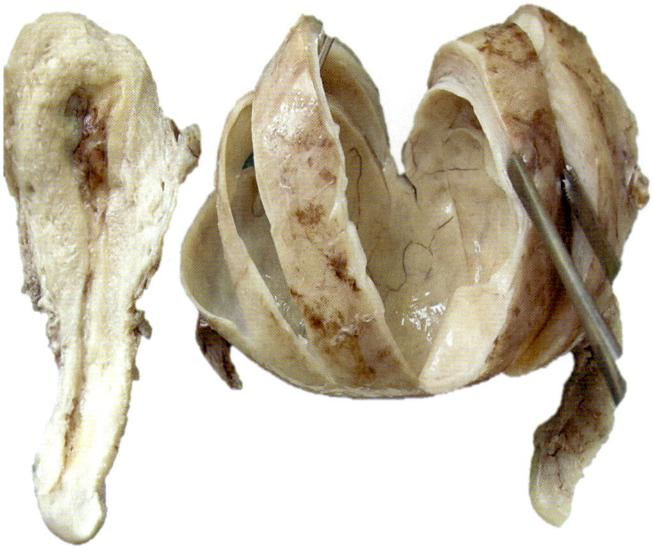

BILATERAL SEROUS CYSTADENOMA

FIGURE 15.81. Image (A) shows unilocular cysts with smooth and shiny surfaces. In (B), a cut opening of the same specimen shows that the inner surface is smooth.

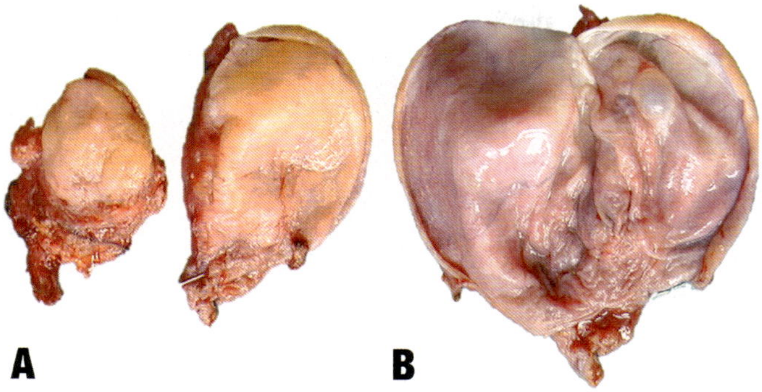

OVARIAN SEROUS CYSTADENOFIBROMA

Serous cystadenoma surrounded by fibrotic tissue (of variable amount) is called serous cystadenofibroma.

FIGURE 15.82. This image shows a serous cystadenofibroma in the context of uterine leiomyoma.

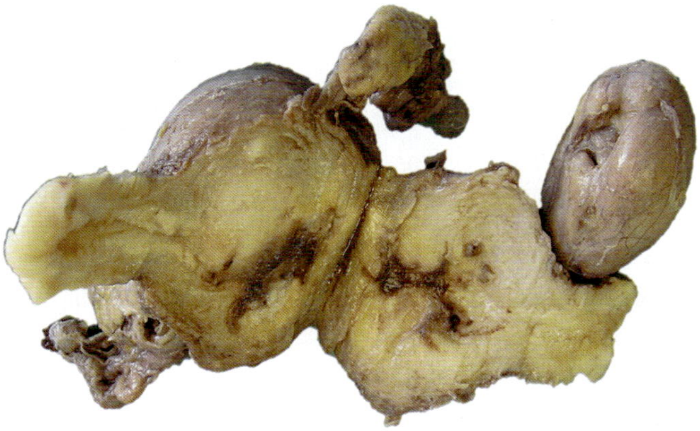

FIGURE 15.83. Images (A) and (B) show a serous cystadenofibroma. Note the extensive hemorrhagic infarction (arrows).

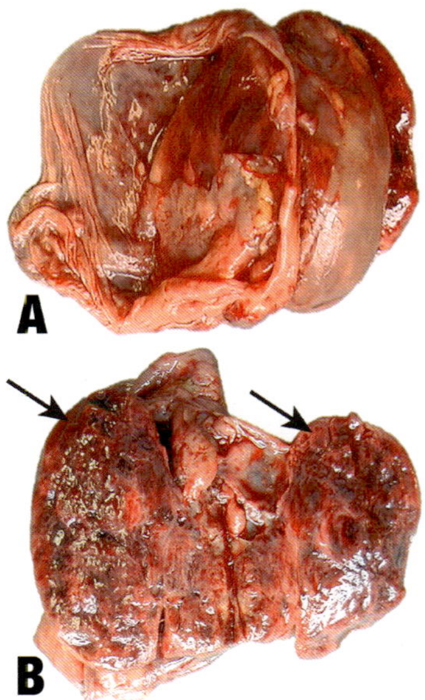

FIGURE 15.84. This serous cystadenofibroma consists of a multilocular cyst with a thick wall and small papillary projections (arrow). On histology, the projections had papillary architectures lined by nonstratified or stratified cuboidal-columnar cells. There was no nuclear atypia.

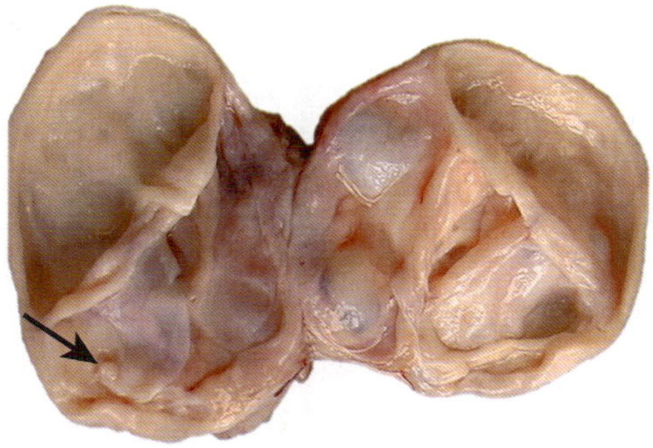

PAPILLARY SEROUS CYSTADENOMA AND CYSTADENOFIBROMA

FIGURE 15.85. This unilocular cyst has a thin wall and a focus of prominent exophytic papillary projections (arrow).

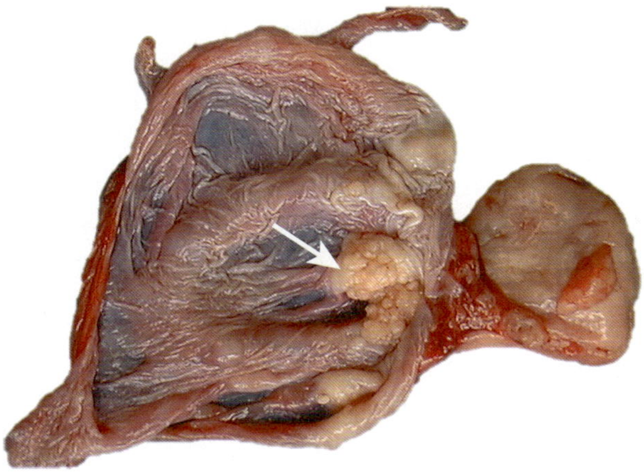

FIGURE 15.86. This image shows an ovarian cyst with prominent, white-to-tan, cauliflower-like, papillary projections.

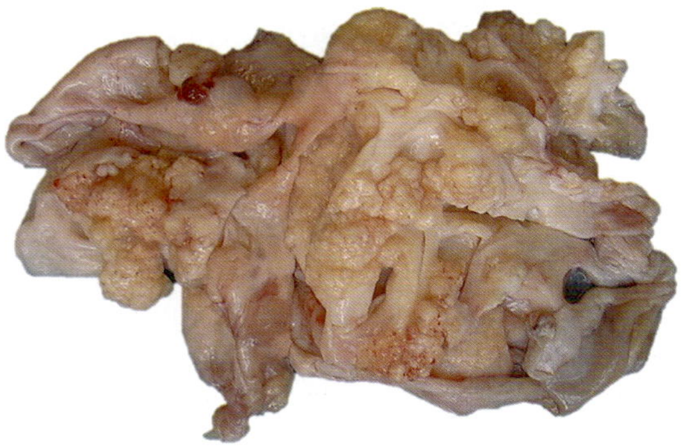

FIGURE 15.87. Image (A) shows a serous cystadenofibroma with edematous papillary projections on the inner surface (arrow). In (B), a serous cystadenofibroma shows small cysts mixed with solid areas.

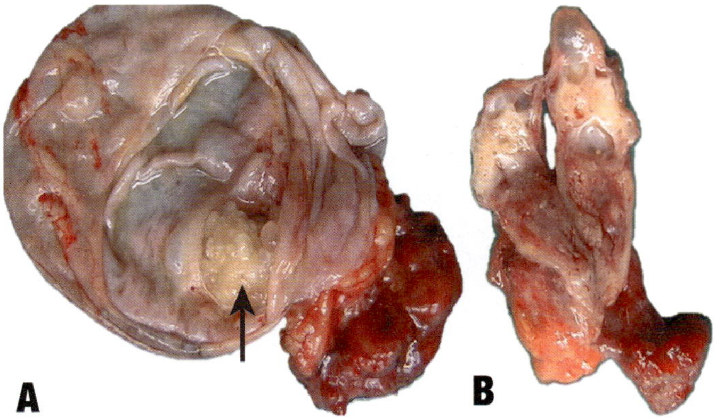

FIGURE 15.88. This serous cystadenofibroma shows focal epithelial proliferation. A large benign serous cystadenoma with limited focal epithelial proliferation (less than 1%) is present.

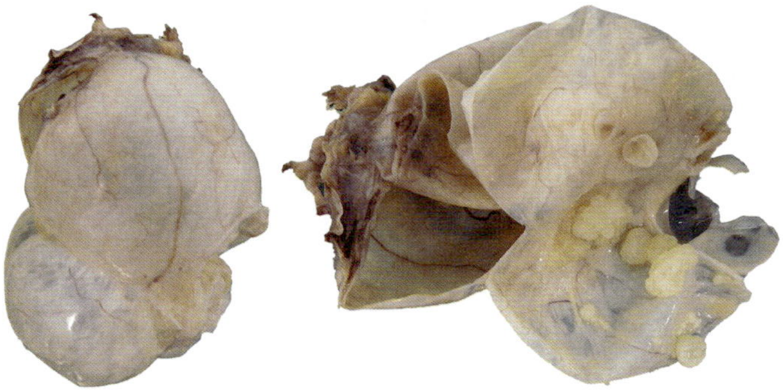

SEROUS BORDERLINE TUMOR / ATYPICAL PROLIFERATIVE SEROUS TUMOR

Approximately 10% to 15% of all ovarian serous tumors are classified as borderline. They occur at a mean age of 42 years and may present with extraovarian implants. In approximately 50% of cases, somatic mutations are found in the *K-ras* and *BRAF* genes. Histologically, the tumors are characterized by hierarchically dividing papillae covered by a nonstratified or stratified tubal-type epithelium with mild-to-moderate atypia.

FIGURE 15.89. This oophorectomy shows a large mass with a smooth but irregular external surface. The cut opening in (B) shows the cyst lining is velvety with a few small papillary projections.

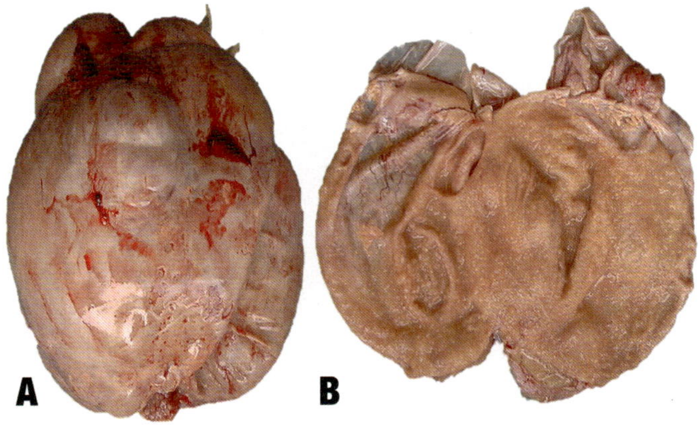

FIGURE 15.90. This image shows multiple fragments of a previously ruptured ovarian mass, and a multilobulated beige papillary lesion with a few solid areas (measuring approximately 2 cm in greatest dimension).

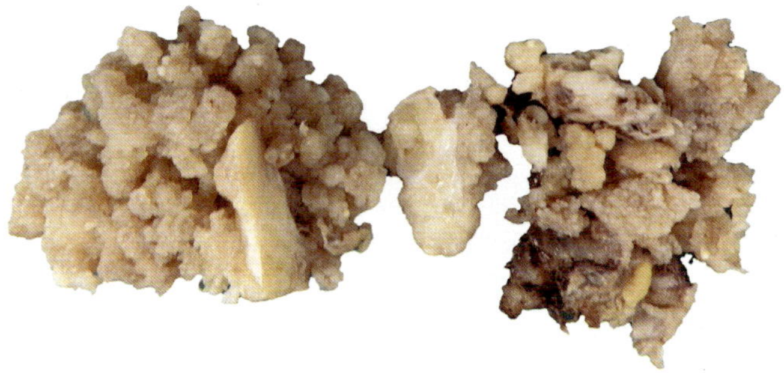

FIGURE 15.91. This image shows an ovarian cystic mass carpeted with papillary projections.

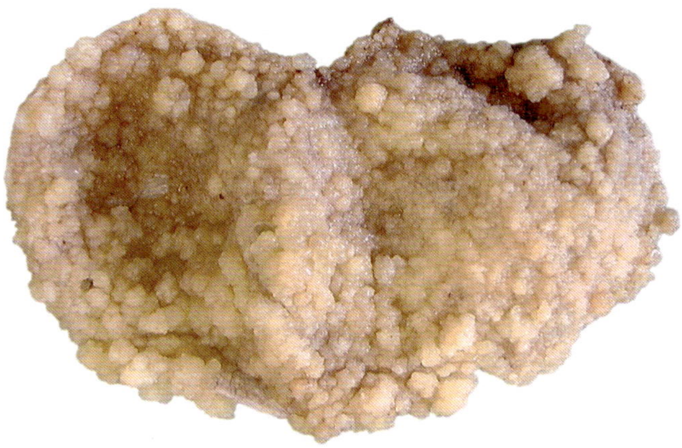

FIGURE 15.92. Image (A) shows an ovarian mass with an irregular external surface and adhesions. The cut opening in (B) shows a cystic mass containing prominent papillary growth within the cavity.

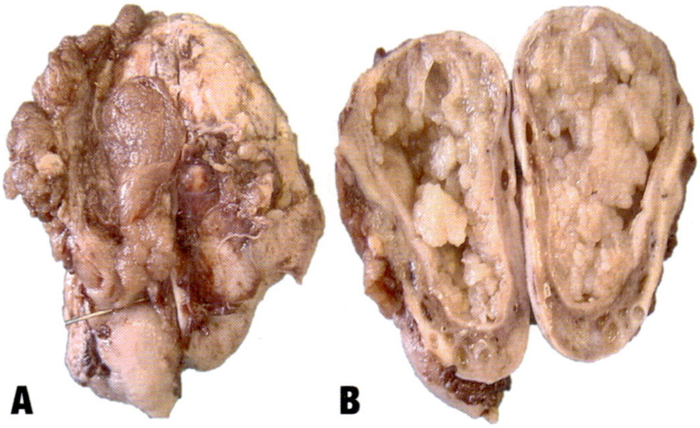

A B

OVARIAN LOW-GRADE SEROUS CARCINOMA

Low-grade serous carcinomas represent fewer than 5% of all ovarian carcinomas in industrialized countries. They are thought to develop from cystadenomas and borderline serous tumors, and often demonstrate *K-ras* and *BRAF* gene mutations. Clinically, these tumors are found in slightly younger women, as compared to high-grade serous carcinoma. Low-grade serous carcinomas do not respond well to conventional platinum-based chemotherapy.

FIGURE 15.93. In this surgical specimen, cystic masses with prominent papillary growths have replaced the ovary. No tumor necrosis is identified grossly.

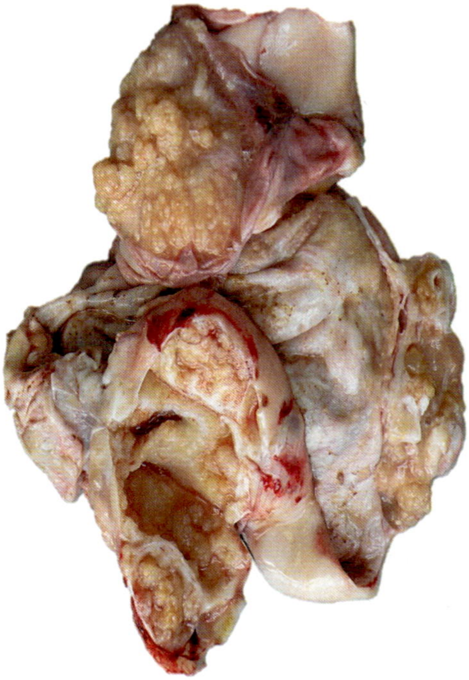

OVARIAN HIGH-GRADE SEROUS CARCINOMA (HGSC)

HGSCs are composed of cells with marked nuclear atypia and increased mitotic rate. The tumor cells are arranged in papillary, solid, slit-like, cribriform, or glandular patterns. They are thought to develop from fallopian tube epithelium, and are associated with *TP53*, *BRCA1* and *BRCA2* germ-line mutations. Patients have a poor prognosis. Serous tubal intraepithelial carcinomas (STICs) that develop in the distal fimbriated end are thought to be precursors for HGSC. STICs and related tumors classified as ovarian in origin have a clonal relationship: they have identical *TP53* mutations. Tumor stage is a significant predictor of prognosis in all serous carcinomas.

FIGURE 15.94. Images (A) and (B) show a bilateral ovarian HGSC. The outer surfaces of the ovaries contain papillary friable projections with necrosis and hemorrhage.

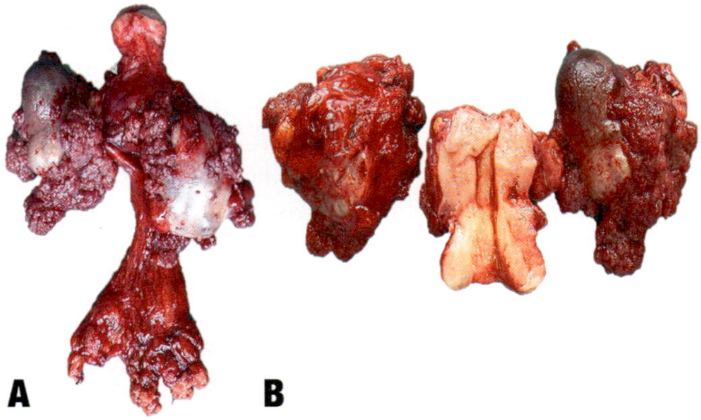

A B

FIGURE 15.95. This large cyst contains solid nodular growths with a heterogenous appearance and necrosis.

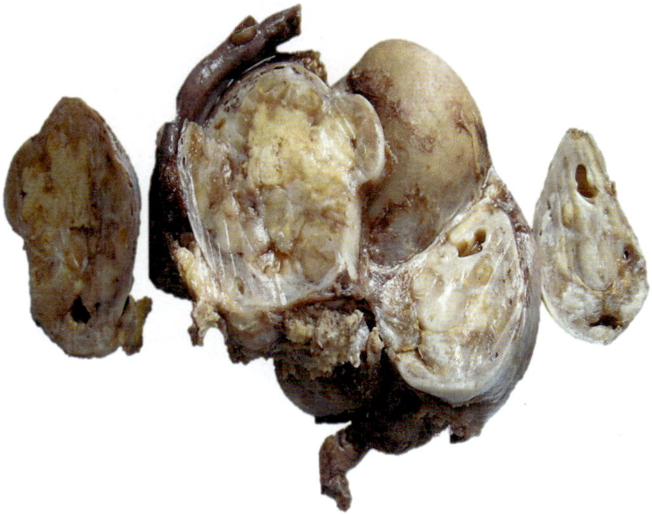

FIGURE 15.96. Image (A) shows nodular, papillary lesions on the outer surface of an ovary. The cut inner surface in (B) shows the ovary has been replaced by a solid, cystic mass. Areas of necrosis are present.

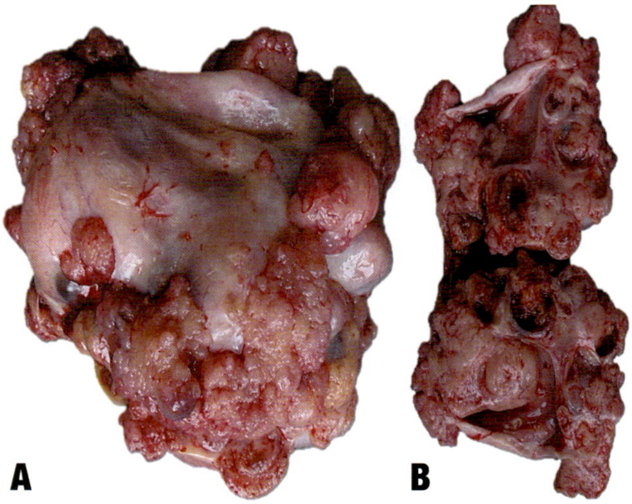

FIGURE 15.97. Image (A) shows a fallopian tube and ovary that are involved by a large cystic mass with a solid and papillary component. The cut surface in (B) shows a large and tan-yellow nodule in the cystic wall with multiple papillary projections on the inner surface of the cyst.

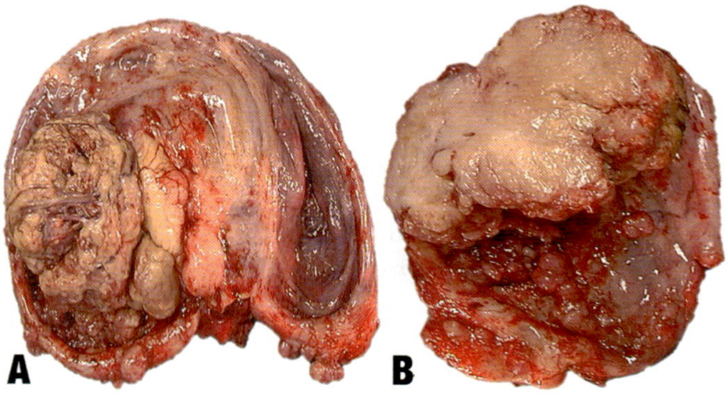

FIGURE 15.98. In (A), the ovary is completely replaced by a solid tumor with papillary projections on the serosal surface. In (B), the cut section of the tumor shows a fleshy surface with yellow areas of necrosis.

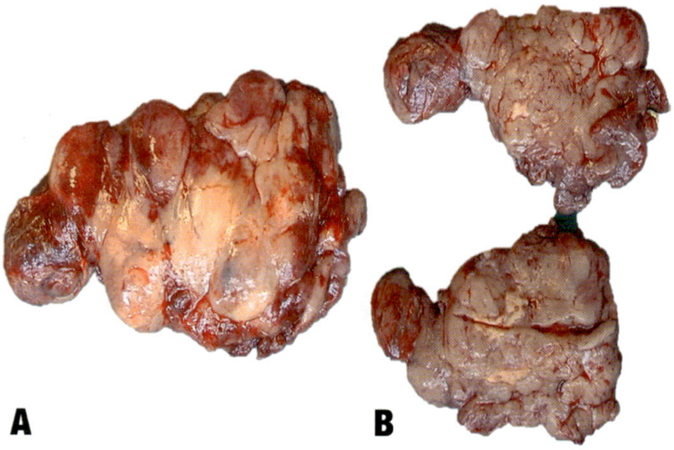

FIGURE 15.99. Image (A) shows a high-grade serous carcinoma almost completely replacing the omentum. Image (B) shows another high-grade serous carcinoma, which involves both ovaries and fallopian tubes.

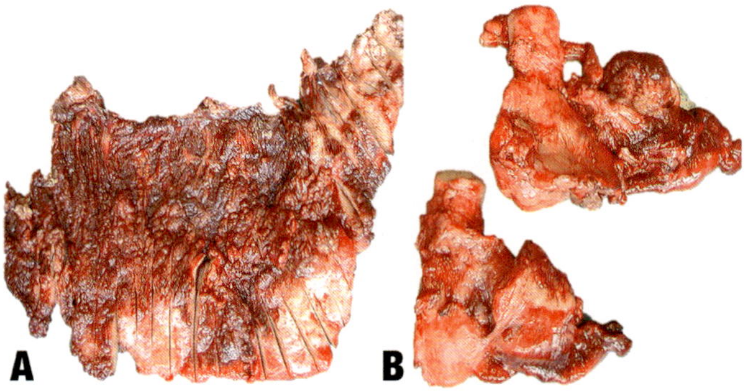

FIGURE 15.100. This high-grade serous carcinoma involves the peritoneum. The firm, hemorrhagic, multinodular surface of the peritoneum is consistent with malignancy.

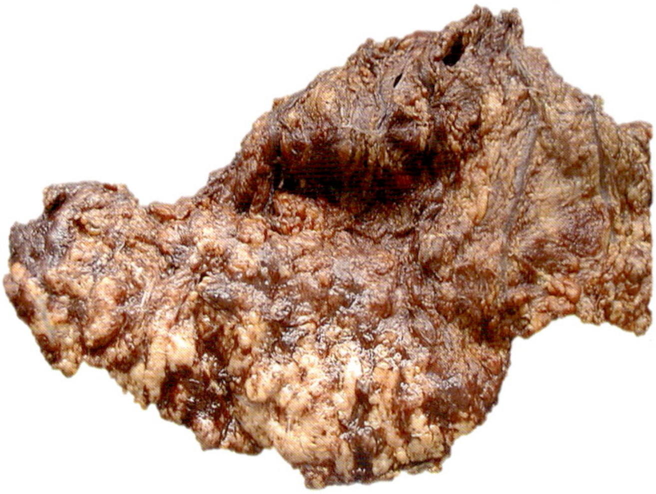

FIGURE 15.101. Image (A) shows a nodular mass that has involved the ovary and associated fimbria. On microscopy, the tumor was composed of predominantly high-grade serous carcinoma, with components of clear cell carcinoma and endometrioid carcinoma. In (B), the cut surface of the tumor shows solid and cystic components with small foci of necrosis.

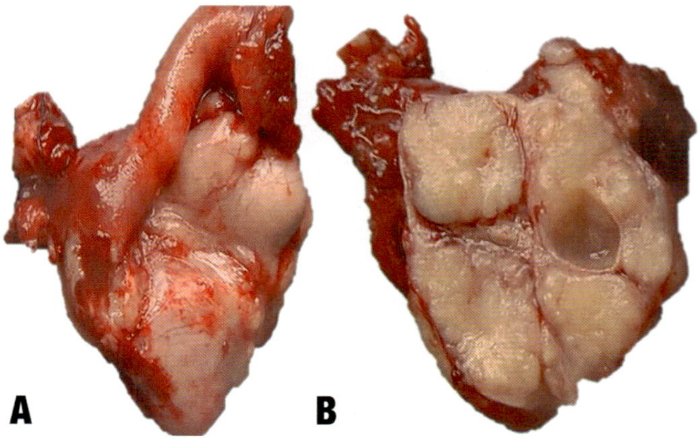

UNDIFFERENTIATED OVARIAN CARCINOMA

Grossly, it is difficult to distinguish the histologic subtypes of high-grade tumors, such as high-grade serous carcinoma, high-grade endometrioid carcinoma, poorly differentiated carcinoma, and so on.

FIGURE 15.102. In (A), an appendectomy specimen shows undifferentiated ovarian carcinoma extensively involving the serosa of appendix. Image (B) shows another undifferentiated ovarian carcinoma.

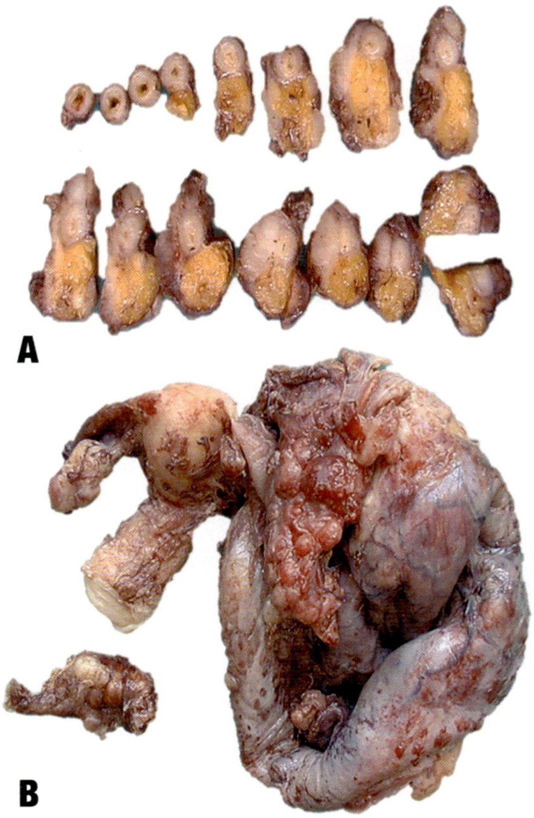

Ovarian mucinous cystadenoma

Approximately 36% of ovarian epithelial tumors are a mucinous histologic type. By definition, all mucinous tumors of the ovary have gastrointestinal-type cells. Approximately 75% are benign, 10% are borderline, and 15% are malignant. Benign tumors have a smooth lining; borderline and malignant mucinous tumors often have papillae and solid areas. Approximately 5% of primary mucinous tumors are bilateral. Mutations in the *K-ras* gene have been found in cases of ovarian mucinous tumor. These tumors are often large; careful extensive sampling is recommended for an accurate diagnosis.

FIGURE 15.103. Image (A) shows a left ovary with a mucinous cystadenoma. A unilocular cyst with smooth surface is extending from the ovary. Note, in (B), that the inner surface appears smooth without areas of thickening or protrusions.

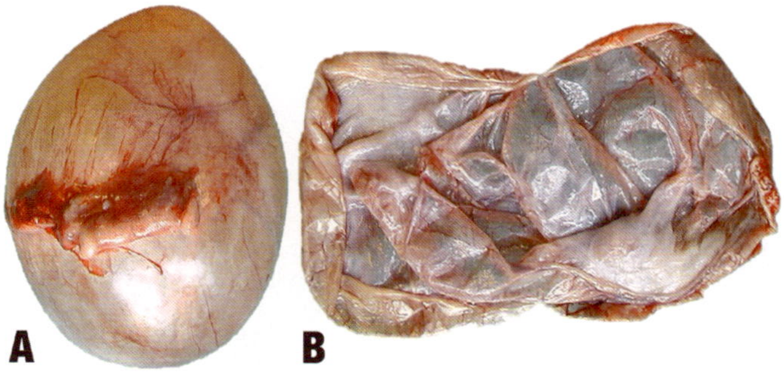

FIGURE 15.104. These bilateral ovarian mucinous cystadenomas are multilocular cysts with smooth lining. The cysts are collapsed.

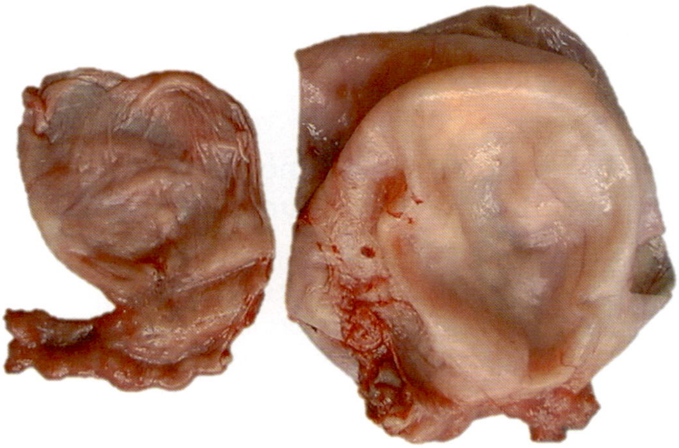

FIGURE 15.105. This multilocular cyst contains mucinous material and has a smooth lining wall. There is no solid area on cut section in either ovary.

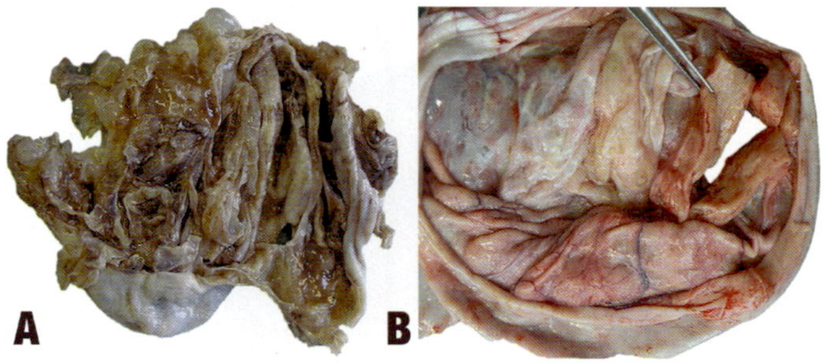

FIGURE 15.106. Ovarian cysts from 2 patients show thin and smooth cyst walls.

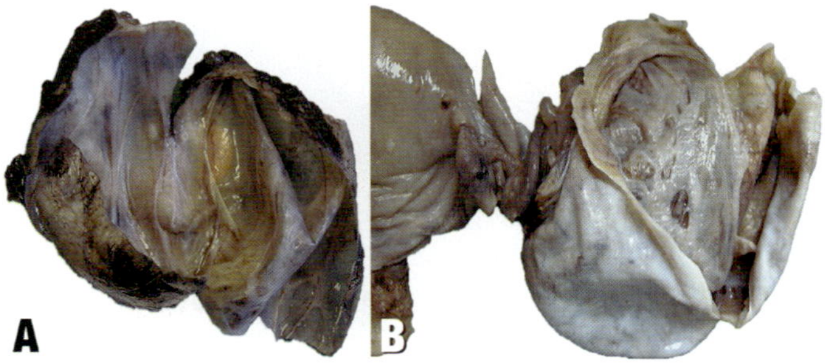

Ovarian mucinous cystadenofibroma

FIGURE 15.107. This image shows a large ovarian cystic mass. The mass contains a solid component with a yellow-to-white area of thickening of the cyst wall. Microscopically, the solid area is composed of fibrous stromal tissue.

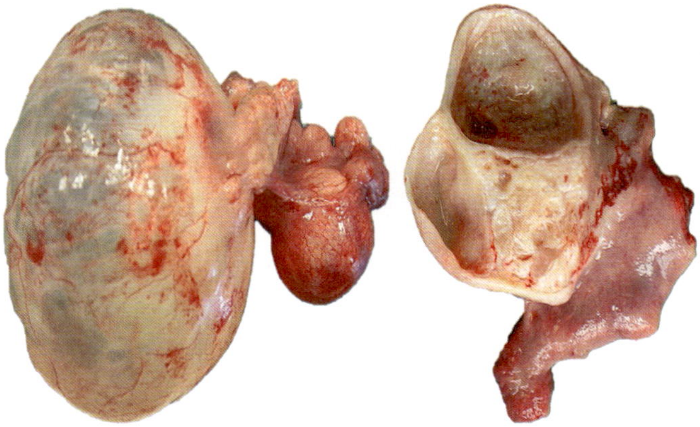

Mucinous borderline tumor / atypical proliferative mucinous tumor

Borderline tumors are distinguished by their cytological atypia, degree of proliferation, and lack of stromal invasion. Mucinous borderline ovarian tumors, less common than serous borderline tumors, have been associated with *K-ras* mutations. To qualify as borderline, a tumor must derive more than 10% of its epithelial volume from proliferative areas. Extensive sampling is key to distinguishing mucinous borderline tumor from mucinous carcinoma.

FIGURE 15.108. Image (A) shows a tan mass with a bosselated surface extending from the ovary. In (B), a cross-section of the same specimen shows a solid and cystic mass.

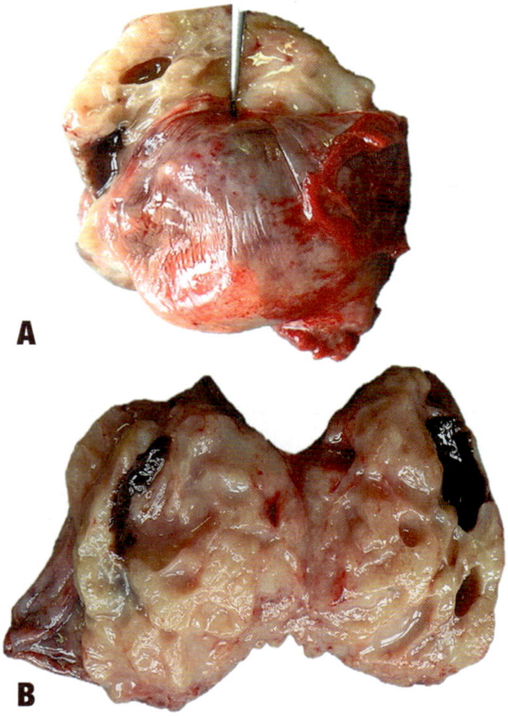

A

B

FIGURE 15.109. The wall of this cystic mass of the left ovary has a polypoid protrusion.

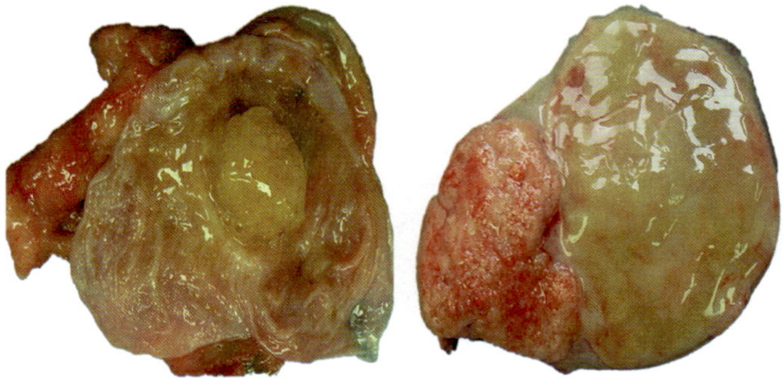

FIGURE 15.110. This image shows a multiloculated cystic lesion with a variably thick wall. Extensive sampling is needed to distinguish mucinous borderline tumor (in this case) from mucinous carcinoma.

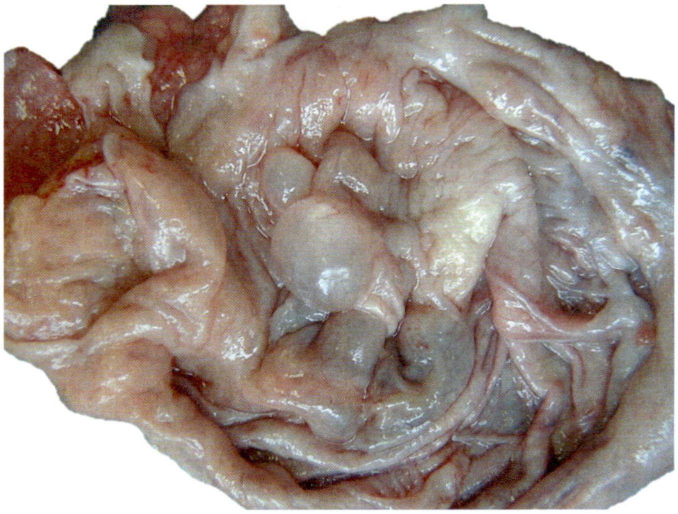

FIGURE 15.111. This mucinous borderline tumor of the ovary is a cystic lesion with multiple nodular projections on the inner surface of the cyst. It had extensive intraepithelial carcinoma by microscopy.

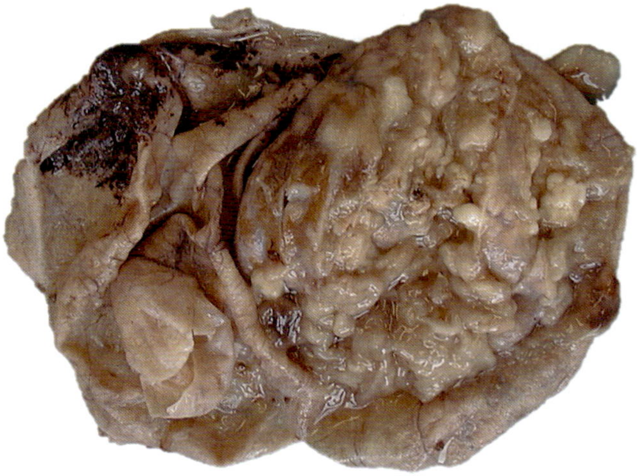

Low-grade appendiceal mucinous neoplasm

FIGURE 15.112. Images (A) and (B) show an appendix with a low-grade appendiceal mucinous neoplasm. This neoplasm has low-grade dysplasia and an associated mucocele, with rupture and spillage of acellular mucus within the muscular appendiceal wall and peritoneal outer surface. Images (C) and (D) show right-and-left-ovary (surface and cortex) mucinous cystic tumors, low-grade by histology, associated with pseudomyxoma peritonei. Pseudomyxoma peritonei is a clinical term for intraperitoneal deposits of extracellular mucin caused by rupture of an intraabdominal tumor, usually appendiceal low-grade mucinous tumor.

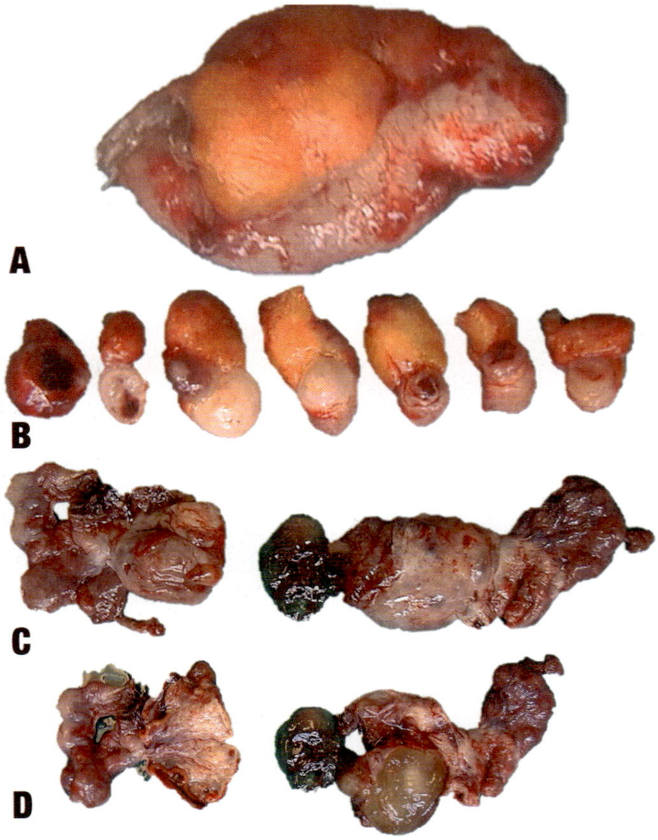

A B C D

Mucinous adenocarcinoma

Ovarian mucinous adenocarcinoma represents less than 10% of ovarian carcinomas. By definition, mucinous ovarian adenocarcinomas are composed of gastrointestinal-type cells. They can demonstrate an infiltrative or expansile pattern of invasion into the stroma. The possibility of metastasis from another site should be considered in all mucinous tumors, especially in those that involve both ovaries. Like its precursor borderline lesions, primary mucinous ovarian adenocarcinomas are associated with *K-ras* mutations.

FIGURE 15.113. Image (A) shows a right oophorectomy. The large mass has a smooth surface. Image (B) shows the inner surface, composed of multiple yellow-to-tan, solid, and papillary growths on the cystic wall.

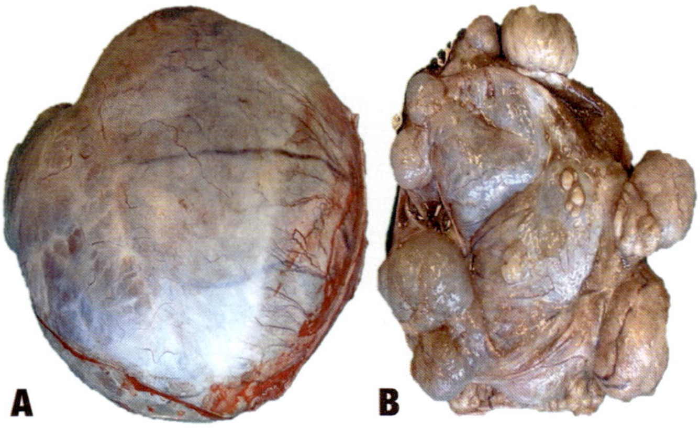

A B

FIGURE 15.114. A large cystic mass shows a heterogeneous appearance. The inner surface has small, intracystic, and papillary or polypoid protuberances. The diagnosis of mucinous adenocarcinoma is made on histology.

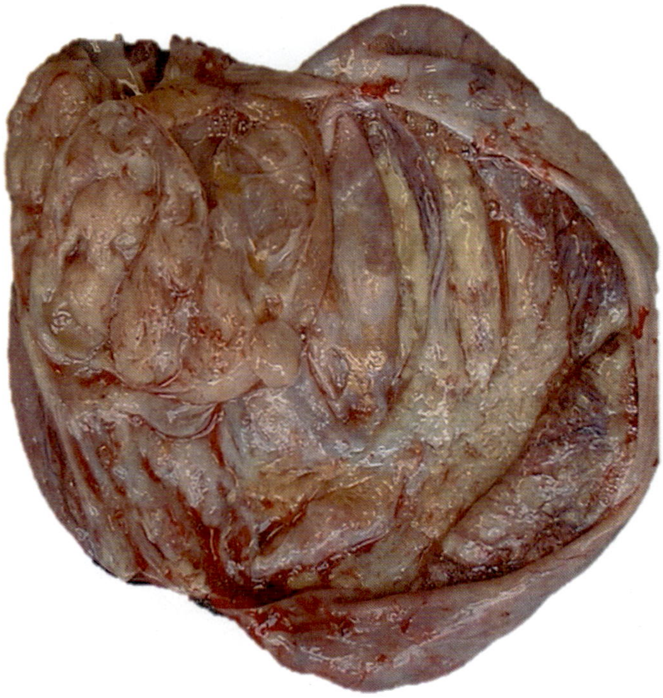

Ovarian endometrioid tumor

Endometrioid carcinoma of the ovary is a glandular epithelial tumor that grows in tubules, cribriform structures, and solid sheets. Histologically, it resembles uterine endometrioid carcinoma. This carcinoma represents approximately 10% to 15% of ovarian cancers, and is the second most common type of epithelial ovarian tumor. It is often found in a background of endometriosis, which may represent a precursor lesion. In 15% to 20% of cases, endometrioid carcinoma of the ovary occurs in conjunction with endometrial cancer. It could also occur as metastasis from endometrial endometrioid-type carcinoma. It is associated with microsatellite instability and mutations in *CTNNB1*, *ARID1A*, *PPP2R1A*, *p53*, *PIK3CA*, and *PTEN*.

OVARIAN ENDOMETRIOID CARCINOMA

Ovarian endometrioid carcinoma is graded by a 3-tiered system proposed by FIGO. The grading is similar to its uterine counterpart: FIGO grade 1 is defined as predominant glandular growth and up to 5% nonsquamous solid component; FIGO grade 2 is defined as 6% to 50% nonsquamous solid component; and FIGO grade 3 is defined as more than 50% nonsquamous solid component.

FIGURE 15.115. In (A), an ovarian tumor shows multiple friable, hemorrhagic nodules on the outer surface of an ovary. Image (B) shows an ovarian tumor with nodular, tan, solid areas interspersed with multiple cystic spaces.

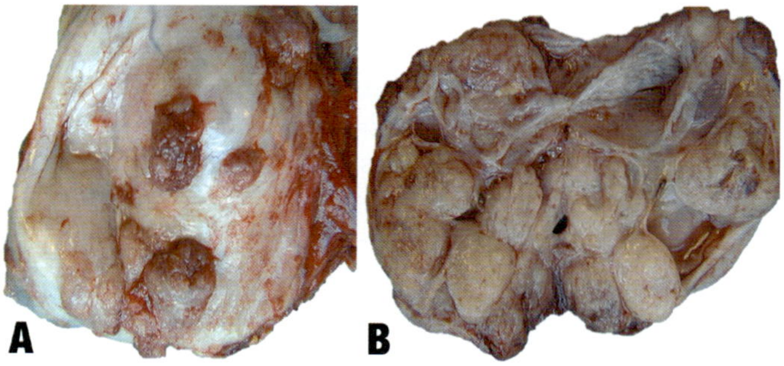

FIGURE 15.116. These images show a well-differentiated endometrioid carcinoma of the right ovary. The oophorectomy specimen shows a heterogeneous-appearing and well-circumscribed mass. It has fleshy, nodular, solid areas, and hemorrhagic and necrotic foci. By histology, it consisted of well-differentiated endometrioid carcinoma.

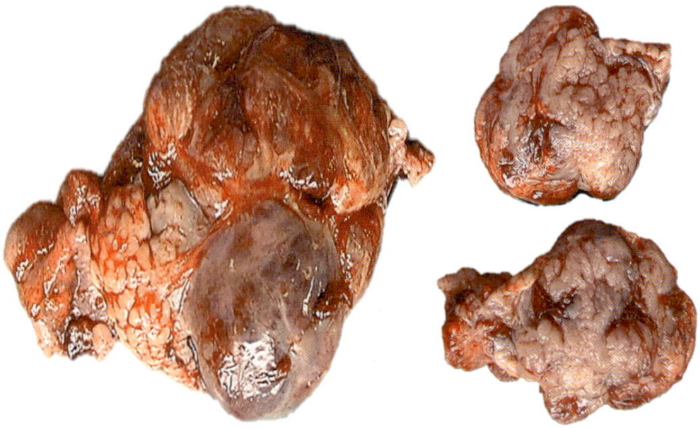

FIGURE 15.117. In (A), a multiloculated cystic lesion with papillary projections has replaced the ovary. Areas of hemorrhage and friable solid tissue with necrosis are visible. Image (B) shows a solid, cystic mass with necrosis and hemorrhage.

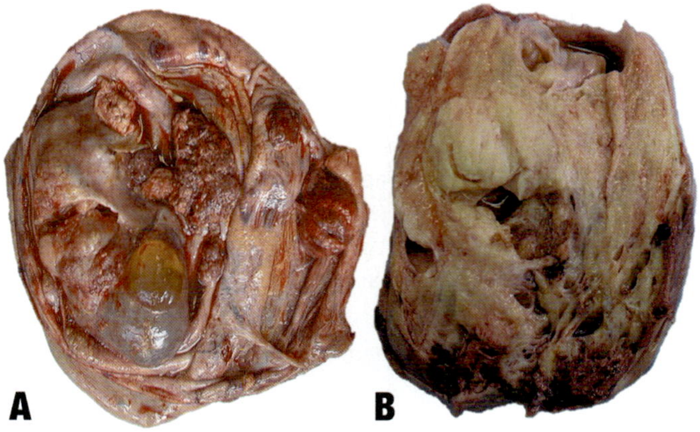

FIGURE 15.118. In (A), an external view of an ovary shows solid and cystic components. In (B), the cut opening of the solid areas appears nodular with necrosis and hemorrhage.

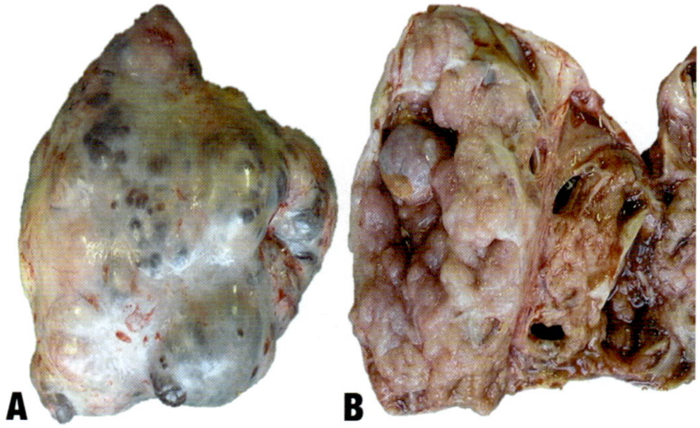

FIGURE 15.119. The ovary in (A) has been completely effaced by a well-circumscribed tumor containing a few visible cysts. In (B), the cut surface of the same specimen shows diffuse pink, exophytic, nodular, and fragile-appearing tumor tissue.

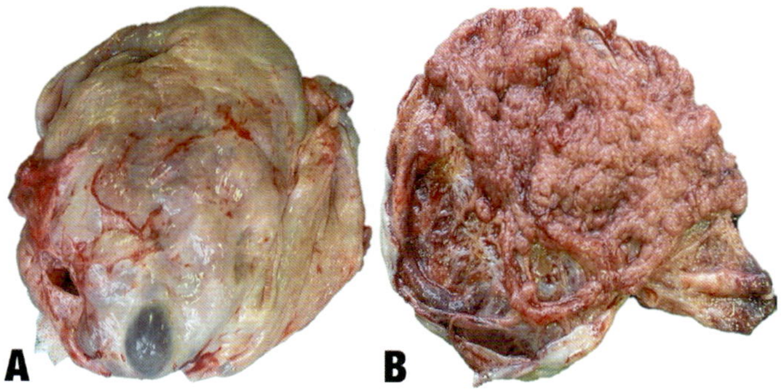

FIGURE 15.120. This image shows a well-circumscribed ovarian mass with hemorrhage on the outer surface. Small cystic areas are also visible.

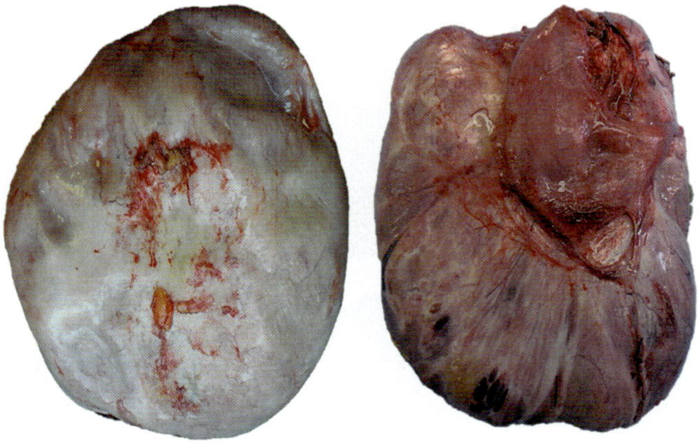

OVARY WITH ENDOMETRIOID CARCINOMA FIGO GRADE 3

FIGURE 15.121. This bisected ovarian endometrioid carcinoma specimen has a large heterogeneous mass with solid and cystic components. Areas of hemorrhage are present. On histology, it was endometrioid carcinoma FIGO grade 3.

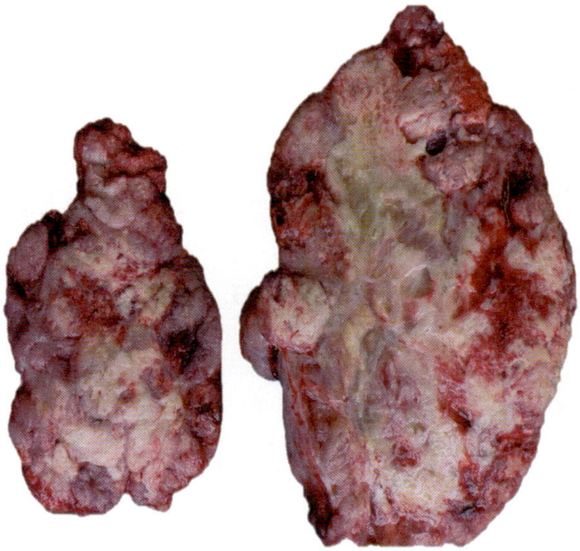

FIGURE 15.122. This is another example of a FIGO grade 3 endometrioid carcinoma. In (A), the ovary is replaced by a lobulated and well-circumscribed tumor mass with a smooth outer surface. The cut opening in (B) shows a fleshy, tan, and nodular mass with cystic components arising from the ovary.

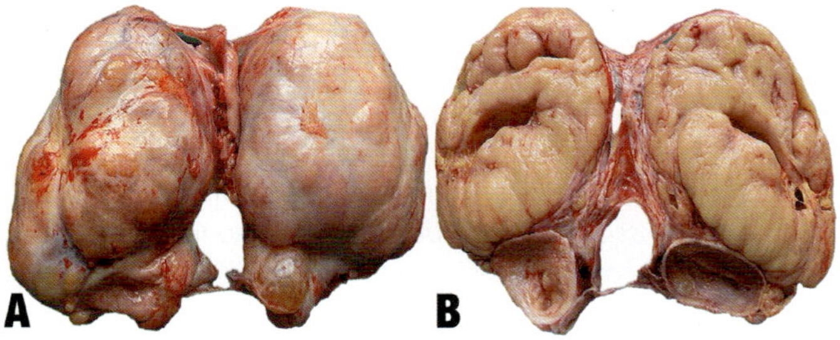

ENDOMETRIOID CARCINOMA INVOLVING OVARIES AND ENDOMETRIUM

In the context of ovarian endometrioid carcinoma and endometrial endometrioid carcinoma, the distinction between 2 synchronous primary tumors and a single metastatic tumor cannot always be made with certainty.

FIGURE 15.123. In (A), the ovary is completely replaced by a well-circumscribed solid and cystic mass. The solid component is tan and fleshy. Image (B) shows a tumor that involves the endometrium, protruding to the uterine cavity and invading into the myometrium (arrow).

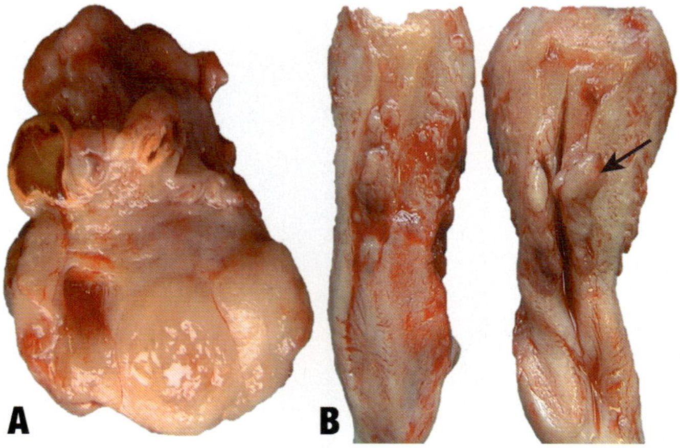

ENDOMETRIOID CARCINOMA OF THE LEFT ADNEXA

FIGURE 15.124. Image (A) shows an endometrioid carcinoma of the left adnexa. It is a large mass with exophytic projections extending from the left adnexa to the bowel and omentum. In (B), the cut surface of the same specimen is nodular and solid with tan, fleshy areas mixed with yellowish necrotic areas.

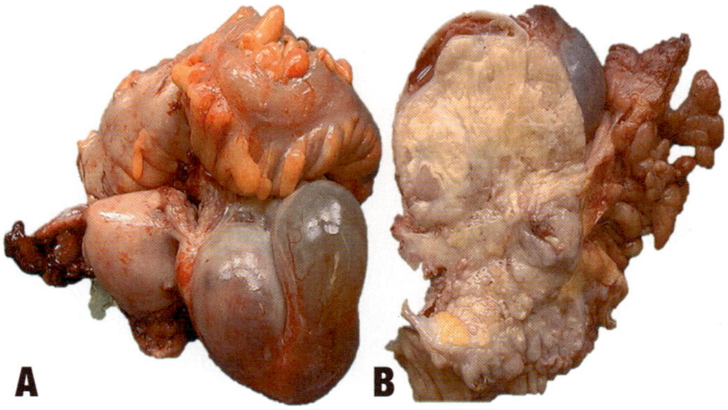

OVARIAN ENDOMETRIOID CARCINOMA ASSOCIATED WITH ENDOMETRIOTIC CYST

FIGURE 15.125. This cystic lesion of the ovary has a nodular solid area protruding from the inner surface of the cyst wall. The endometriotic cyst is filled with dark brown fluid.

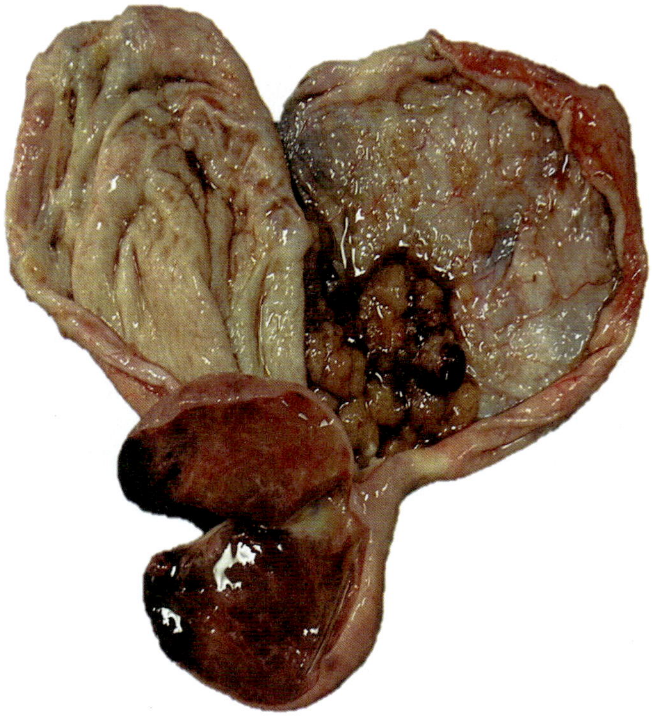

FIGURE 15.126. Image (A) shows a well-differentiated endometrioid carcinoma with squamous differentiation, arising within an endometriotic cyst. A polypoid nodule extends from an endometriotic cyst. Dark brown areas are also present. The cut surface in (B) shows the solid growth of this polypoid tumor.

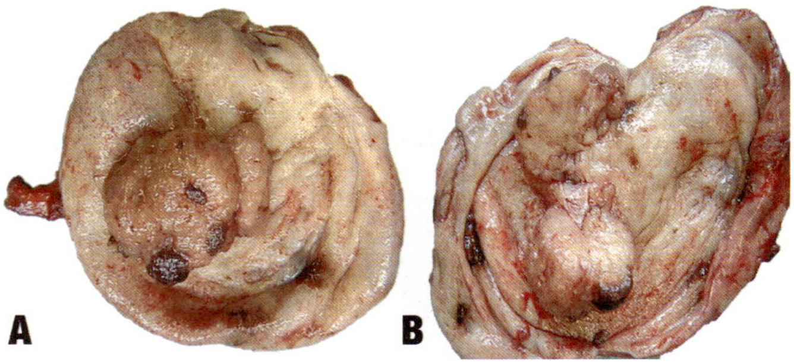

Malignant mixed epithelial tumor of the ovary

The WHO defines mixed epithelial ovarian tumors as involving at least 2 histologic subtypes, where the minor components account for at least 10% of the tumor on microscopic examination. Sampling of the tumor must be extensive to identify all the components.

FIGURE 15.127. This malignant mixed epithelial tumor of the ovary has a predominant high-grade serous carcinoma component. The ovary has been effaced by a solid and cystic mass.

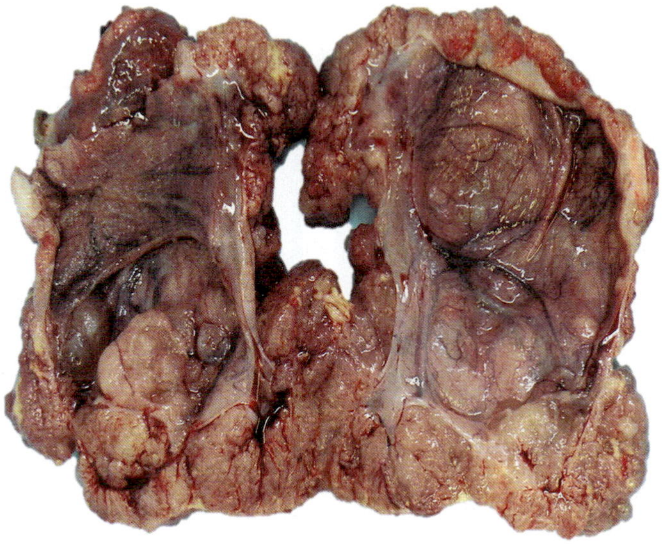

FIGURE 15.128. This image shows a cystic mass with a nodular and solid region. Note the large hemorrhagic foci in the solid component. Microscopic examination showed this to be a mixed high-grade serous carcinoma and well-differentiated endometrioid carcinoma.

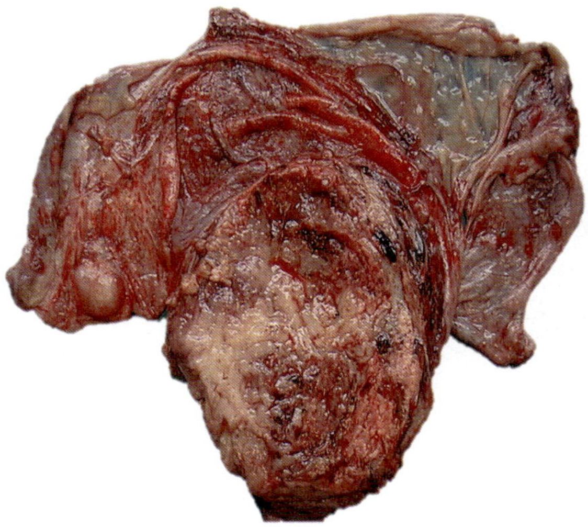

Ovarian clear cell carcinoma (CCC)

CCC accounts for fewer than 5% of all ovarian malignancies. It typically affects middle-aged women and is associated with endometriosis. It is relatively resistant to conventional platinum-based chemotherapy. CCC occurs in patients with Lynch syndrome, particularly those with *MSH2* mutations. *K-ras* and *PTEN* mutations are also involved. Clinically, CCC coincides with venous thromboembolism and paraneoplastic hypercalcemia more often than with other ovarian epithelial tumors. Grossly, CCC is typically unilateral with solid or solid and cystic components. On microscopic examination, it is composed of polyhedral or hobnail cells with clear and/or eosinophilic granular cytoplasm (containing glycogen). The tumors exhibit a variety of architectural patterns such as tubulocystic, solid, papillary, and (rarely) reticular. The reticular pattern could simulate yolk sac tumor.

FIGURE 15.129. The ovarian cystic mass in (A) has a solid polypoid projection in the inner layer of the cyst. In (B), the cut surface of the same specimen shows both solid and cystic components.

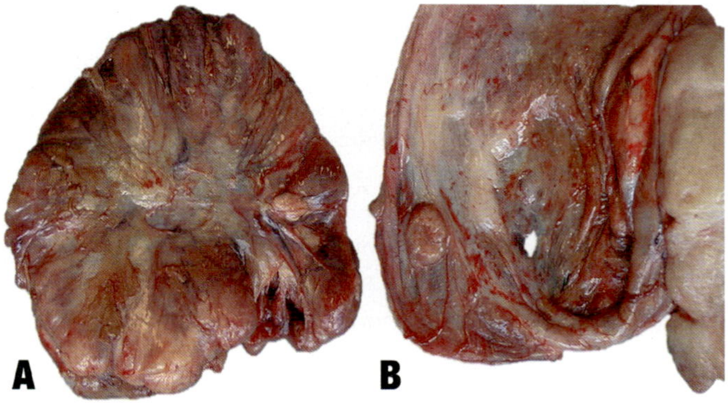

FIGURE 15.130. In (A), a multilobulated mass with an irregular surface occupies the entire ovary. The cut surface in (B) shows a heterogeneous, solid, and cystic lesion with foci of hemorrhage.

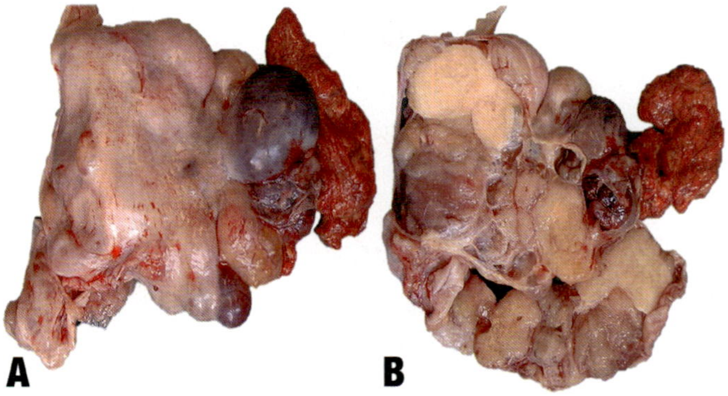

FIGURE 15.131. Image (A) shows a bulging mass with a smooth surface. Image (B) shows that the mass is solid and mostly composed of fleshy tan tissue.

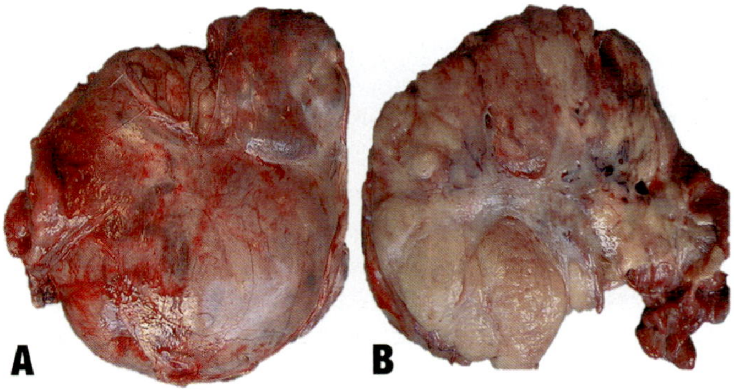

FIGURE 15.132. In (A), the cut section of a tumor shows solid and cystic components. The solid component is polypoid and nodular, protruding into the lumen. In (B), a cross-section of a solid area of the same tumor shows solid, tan-white tissue.

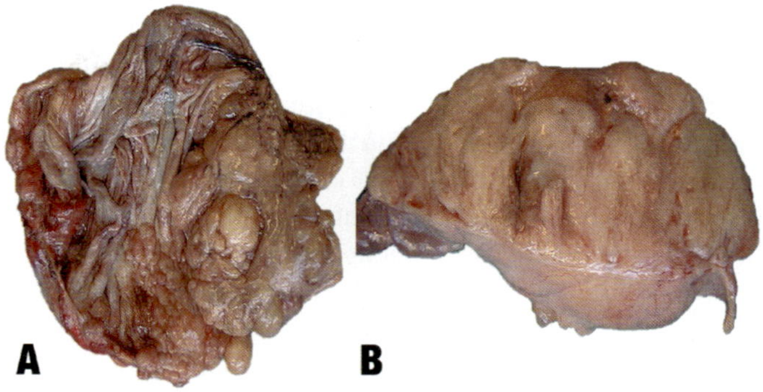

FIGURE 15.133. This total hysterectomy and bilateral salpingo-oophorectomy show CCC of the right ovary associated with endometriosis involving the left ovary and uterine serosa. The right ovarian tumor has a predominantly cystic appearance. Red-to-brown deposits are visible on the serosa of the uterus and on the left ovary — a finding consistent with endometriosis.

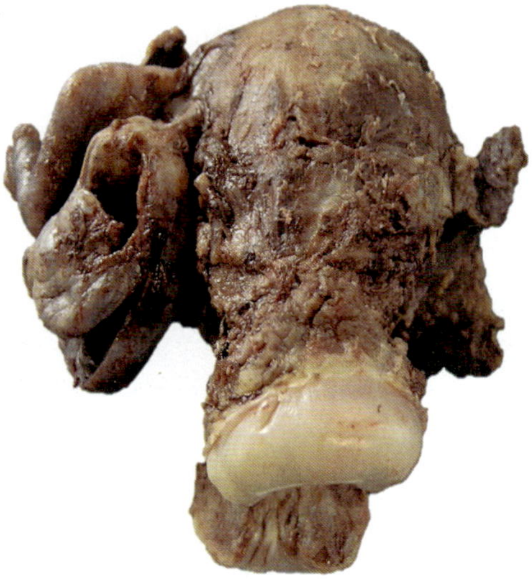

FIGURE 15.134. In (A), a total hysterectomy with bilateral salpingo-oophorectomy shows an irregular, solid mass in the left adnexa (arrow) and a white nodule (corresponding to a leiomyoma) on the uterine wall. The cut surface in (B) shows a dark brown, solid tumor in the ovary, and a small leiomyoma into myometrium.

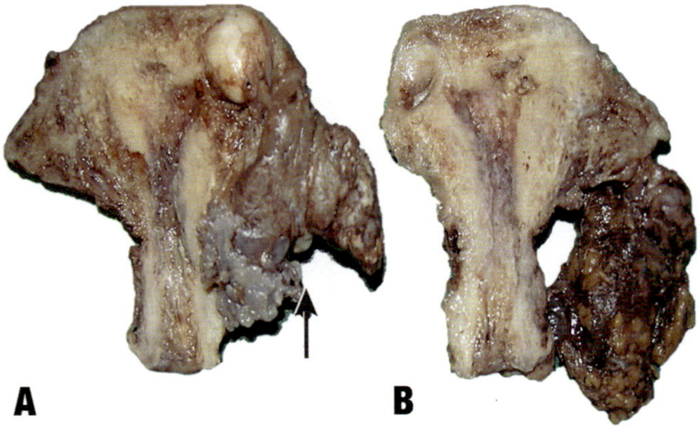

Ovarian transitional cell (Brenner) tumor

This group of neoplasms accounts for approximately 1% to 3% of ovarian epithelial neoplasms. Histologically, Brenner tumor cells resemble the transitional cells of the urothelium. They are round or polygonal in shape, with distinct cell membrane and oval nuclei with longitudinal grooving ("coffee bean" appearance). This group of neoplasms includes Brenner tumor (the most frequent subtype representing approximately 99% of this group); borderline Brenner tumor / atypical proliferative Brenner tumor (less than 1%); and malignant Brenner tumor (less than 1%).

BENIGN BRENNER TUMOR

Benign Brenner tumors are asymptomatic and typically found incidentally in the ovaries.

FIGURE 15.135. This image shows a solid, sharply circumscribed, yellow-tan mass.

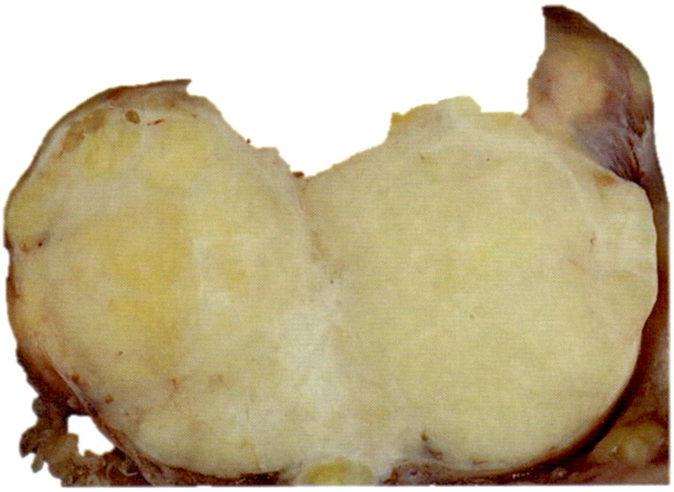

BORDERLINE BRENNER TUMOR / ATYPICAL PROLIFERATIVE BRENNER TUMOR

Unlike benign Brenner tumors, borderline Brenner tumors are associated with the loss of *CDKN2A*, a tumor suppressor gene. This mutation therefore may represent the mechanism of progression from benign to borderline Brenner tumors. *CDKN2A* gene loss has also been found in mucinous ovarian tumors, which may explain why mucinous cystadenomas sometimes occur with borderline Brenner tumors in an ovary. *K-ras* and *PIK3CA* gene mutations may also be implicated.

FIGURE 15.136. This image shows a borderline Brenner tumor associated with a mucinous cystadenoma. On cross-section, the tumor had a multicystic lesion with a tan-to-yellow and ill-defined solid component present on the inner cyst wall surface (arrow).

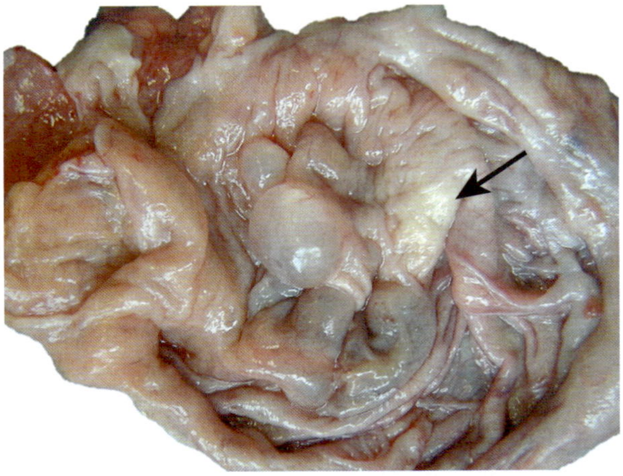

FIGURE 15.137. In (A), an oophorectomy specimen presents a well-circumscribed, firm tumor with smooth surface. The sectioned surface in (B) shows a lobulated, solid tumor that is pale yellow-to-white in color.

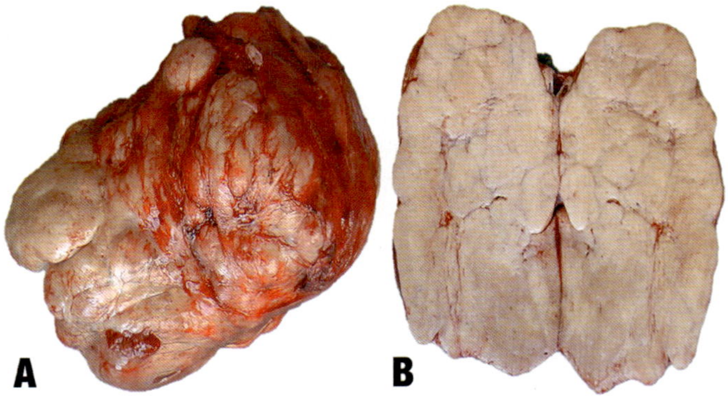

MALIGNANT BRENNER TUMOR

These tumors are large with a median size of 16 cm to 20 cm. Approximately 12% of cases are bilateral.

FIGURE 15.138. This cut section of an ovarian mass reveals a cystic tumor with solid, mural, white-to-yellow nodules.

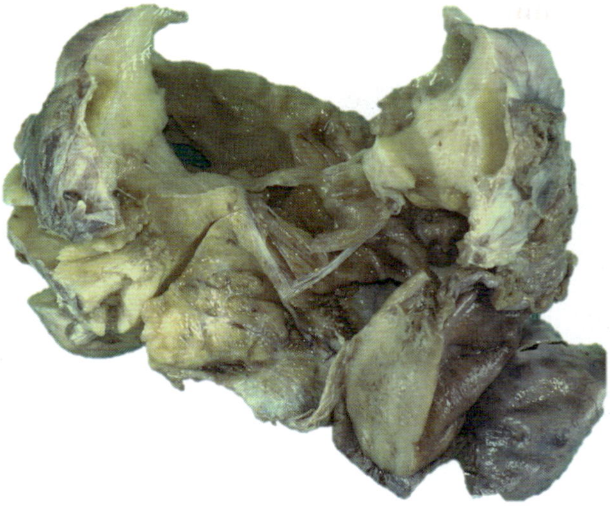

Ovarian germ cell tumor

Germ cell tumors account for 30% of primary ovarian tumors. Most (approximately 95%) are benign dermoid cysts (mature cystic teratoma). The vast majority of malignant forms occur in children and young adults. Around 90% of malignant germ cell tumors occur in a pure form; 10% contain 2 or more types.

OVARIAN EPIDERMOID CYST

These rare cystic lesions are lined by keratinizing squamous epithelium in the absence of other teratomatous elements. They may originate from the ovarian surface epithelium or from the rete ovarii.

FIGURE 15.139. In this specimen, the cyst has a smooth wall and is filled with creamy contents.

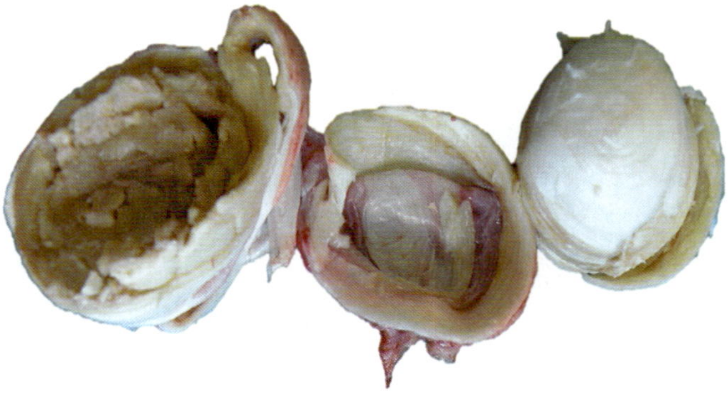

FIGURE 15.140. This image shows a confined cystic structure in the ovary filled with yellow-white creamy material.

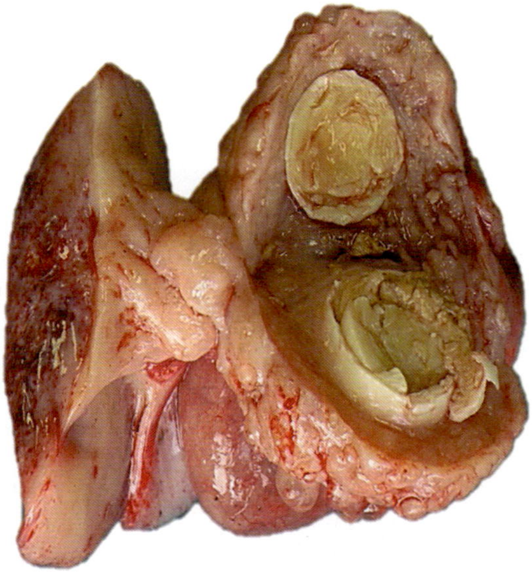

MATURE CYSTIC TERATOMA (DERMOID CYST)

These lesions are defined by the presence of tissues derived from at least 2 of the 3 embryonic layers (ectoderm, mesoderm, and endoderm). Derivatives of the ectoderm are the most common tissues present. Dermoid cysts are believed to be derived from primordial germ cells.

FIGURE 15.141. This oophorectomy specimen shows a cystic lesion with abundant hair, sebaceous material, and solid mural nodules (called Rokitansky protuberance).

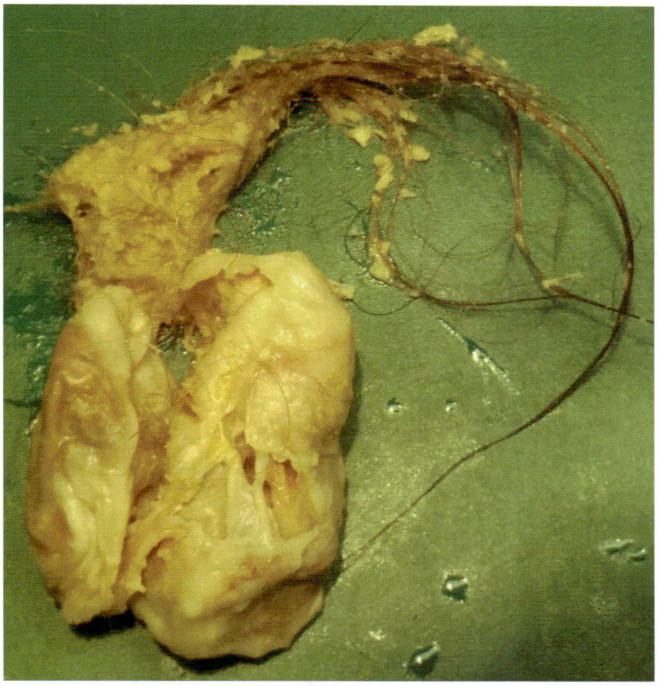

FIGURE 15.142. This image shows an ovarian cystic mass filled with sebaceous material and hair. The lesion is adherent to the omentum.

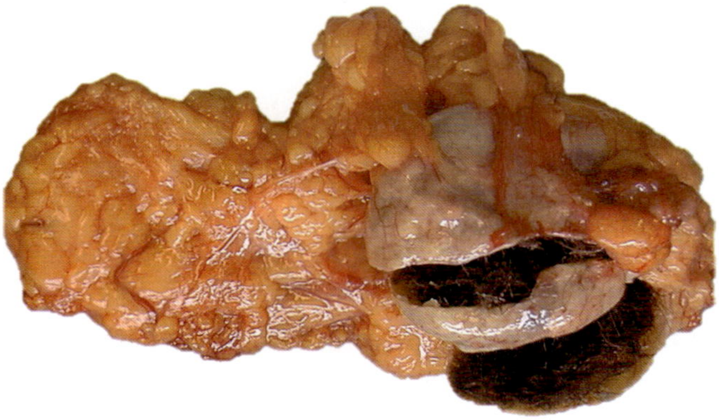

FIGURE 15.143. In (A), a round, well-circumscribed cyst has a smooth and glistening outer surface. The cut surface in (B) shows a multiloculated cyst with a soft, white-to-tan solid component.

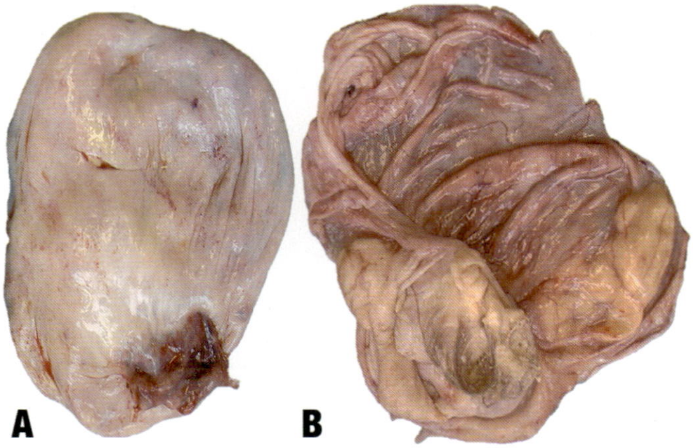

FIGURE 15.144. Image (A) shows the outer surface of a cystic mass, which appears heterogeneous and discontinuous, with darker brown areas mixed with lighter background tissue. The inner surface in (B) shows a cystic lesion with hair, sebaceous material, and solid mural nodules.

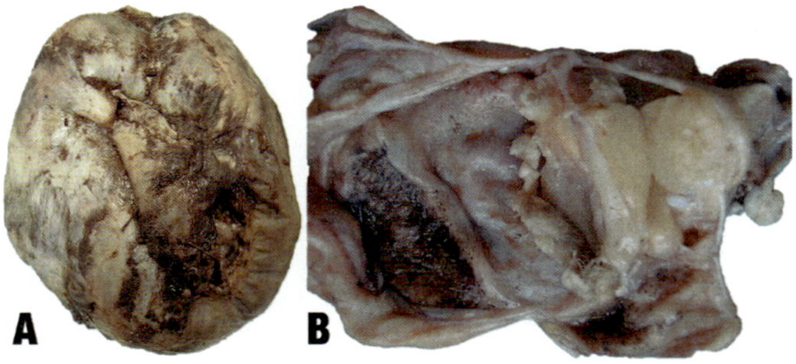

FIGURE 15.145. This cystic lesion is filled with heterogeneous tissue. Several poorly formed teeth are present (arrow).

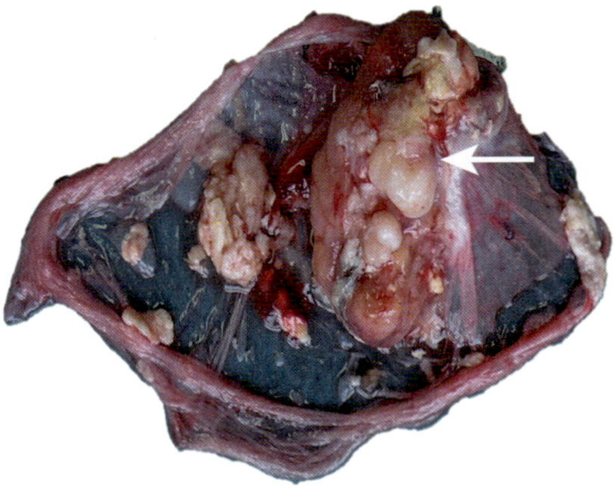

OVARIAN THECOMA

Thecomas are stromal tumors composed of lipid-containing cells resembling theca cells (see ovarian sex cord–stromal tumors, in this chapter).

FIGURE 15.146. The superior part of this ovarian tumor (a thecoma) is characterized by a well-circumscribed, solid mass with a yellow, lobulated cut surface (arrow). Beneath the thecoma is a dermoid cyst characterized by a cystic structure filled with sebaceous material and hair.

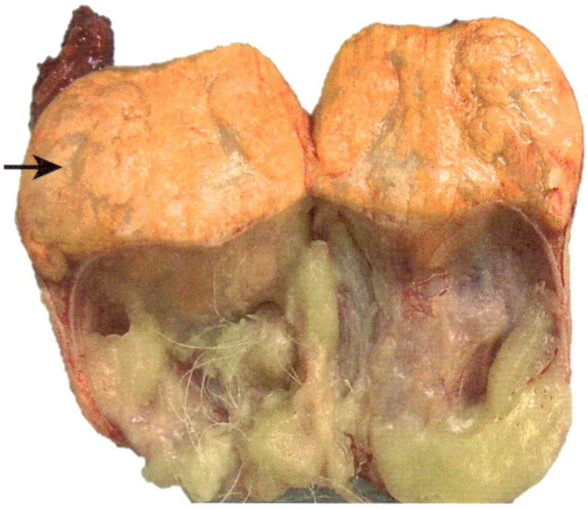

STRUMA OVARII

Struma ovarii is the most common form of monodermal teratoma and represents approximately 3% of all ovarian teratomas. Usually, struma ovarii occurs in a pure form. Rarely, it is associated with a dermoid cyst; occurs as a component of a stromal carcinoid; or is mixed with mucinous cystadenomas or Brenner tumors. Struma ovarii is defined by the presence of thyroid tissue comprising more than 50% of the overall mass. Occasionally, patients may present with hyperthyroidism. Most tumors are unilateral and range from 0.5 cm to 10 cm in diameter.

FIGURE 15.147. This well-defined mass with a solid appearance contained thyroid tissue on microscopic examination. The lesion is associated with a mature cystic teratoma (dermoid cyst) filled with creamy material (arrow).

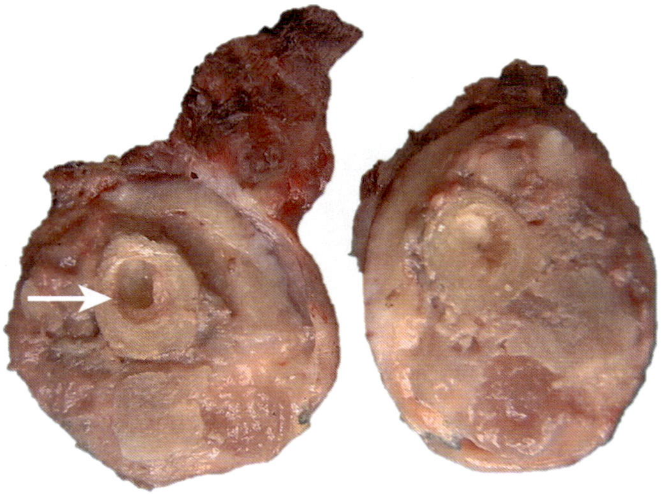

FIGURE 15.148. This image shows a multilocular cystic mass filled with gelatinous fluid.

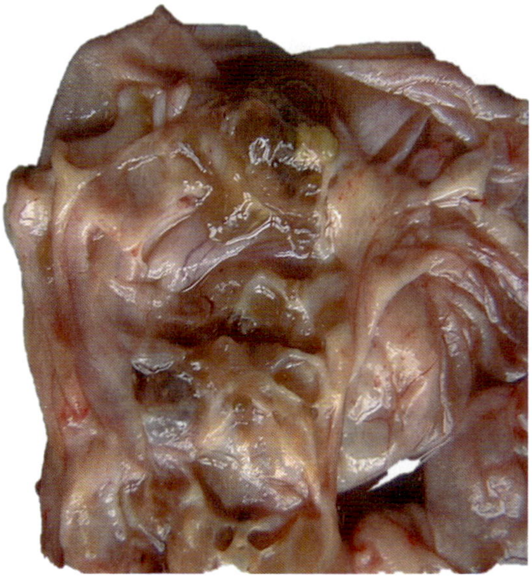

IMMATURE TERATOMA

The WHO defines an immature teratoma as a teratoma containing immature elements. The most common immature element is neuroepithelium. The tumors are graded based on the amount of immature neuroepithelium they contain; the histologic grade dictates their treatment. In grade 1 tumors, the immature neuroepithelium present in any 1 slide should not exceed 1 LPF (low-power field, or 40-times magnification). In grade 2 tumors, immature neuroepithelium is present in 1 to 4 LPF/slide. In grade 3 tumors, immature neuroepithelium is present in more than 4 LPF/slide.

FIGURE 15.149. The cystic lesion of this ovary has multiple tan foci of soft tissue, which corresponded to immature neural tissue on microscopy.

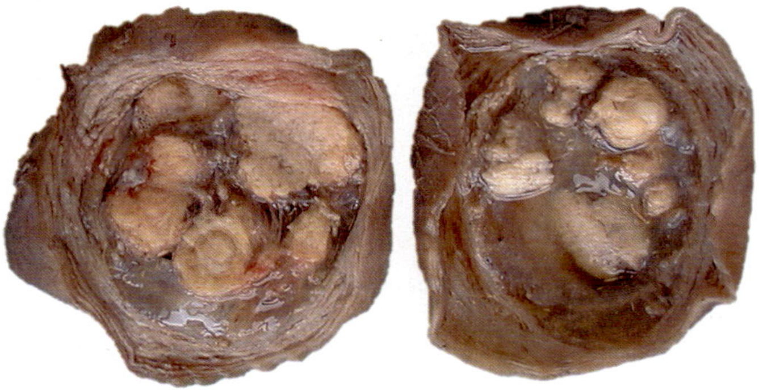

FIGURE 15.150. This tumor is predominantly multicystic and contains a few solid areas. On histology, it was grade 1 immature teratoma.

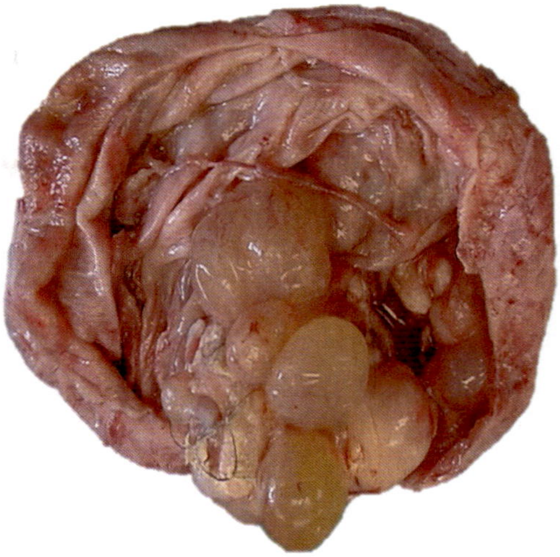

FIGURE 15.151. The outer surface of the tumor in (A) appears mostly light gray, but is variegated. No tumor invasion of the surface is present. In (B), the cut inner surface of the same specimen shows multiple yellow-to-brown nodules within a cystic cavity. By microscopy, these nodules consist of immature neural tissue in 5 LPF/slide.

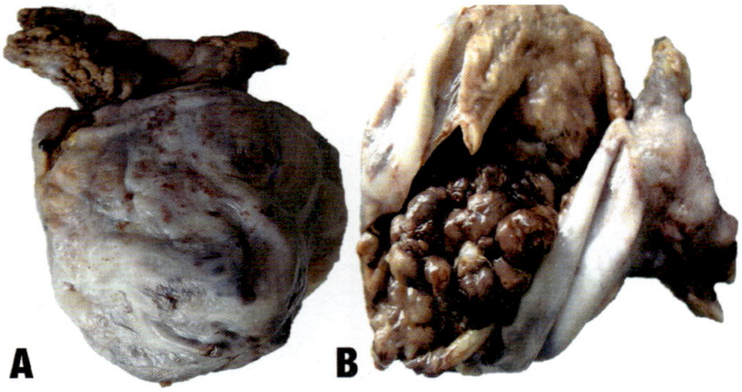

A B

FIGURE 15.152. Image (A) shows a well-defined mass with a smooth surface. The cut surface in (B) shows the tumor to be mostly solid. On microscopy, the tumor contained an abundance of immature neuroectodermal tissue.

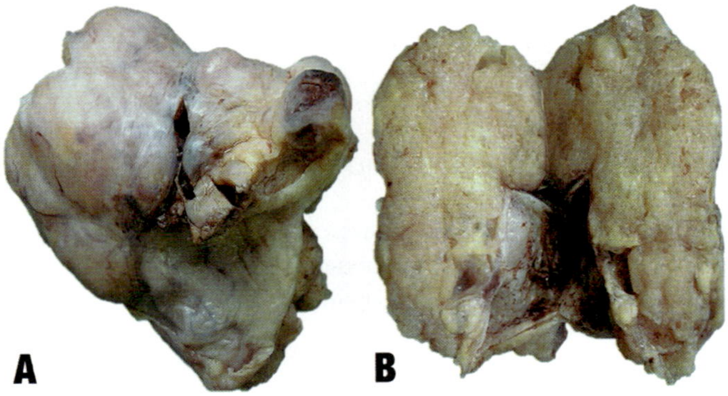

A B

DYSGERMINOMA

Dysgerminoma is a common malignant germ cell tumor of the ovary: it represents 1% to 2% of all ovarian cancers. The tumor occurs almost exclusively in children and young women, and almost all patients have elevated serum levels of lactic dehydrogenase (LDH).

FIGURE 15.153. This image shows a tumor with cystic necrotic areas and solid, white viable tumor tissue with hemorrhage in the periphery.

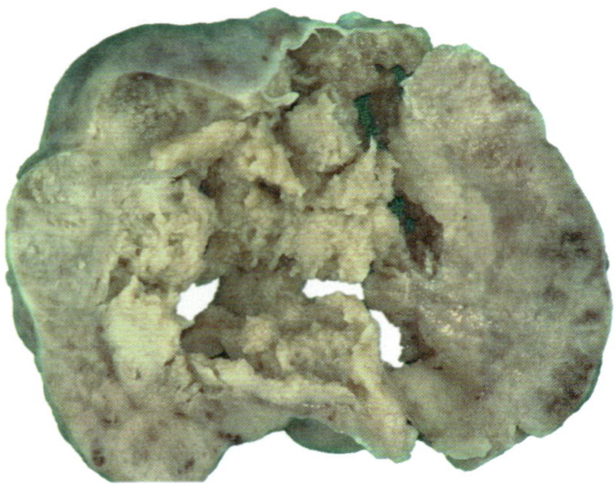

YOLK SAC TUMOR (YST; PRIMITIVE ENDODERMAL TUMOR)

YSTs are germ cell tumors that may have features of endodermal differentiation, or derivatives of extraembryonal and embryonal somatic tissues. They usually occur in children and young adults, and consistently produce elevated serum levels of α fetoprotein (AFP). It is a highly malignant tumor and all patients need chemotherapy.

FIGURE 15.154. Image (A) shows a large, soft, variegated, and well-encapsulated mass. The cut surface in (B) appears gray-to-yellow and trabeculated with areas of hemorrhage, necrosis, and cystic degeneration.

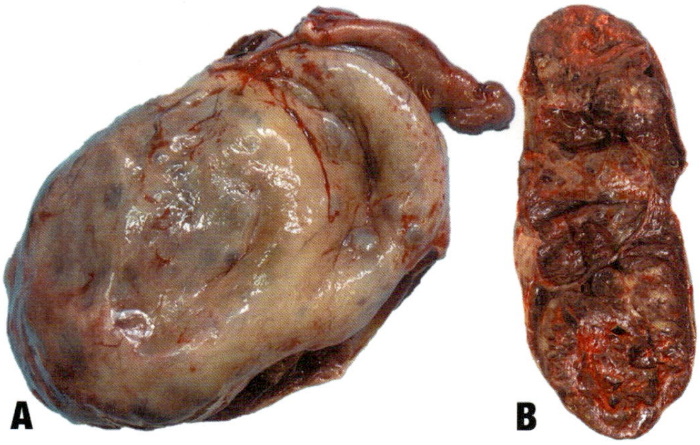

YOLK SAC TUMOR POSTCHEMOTHERAPY

FIGURE 15.155. This image shows a yolk sac tumor postchemotherapy (bisected). The tumor presents solid and cystic areas with fibrosis secondary to chemotherapy.

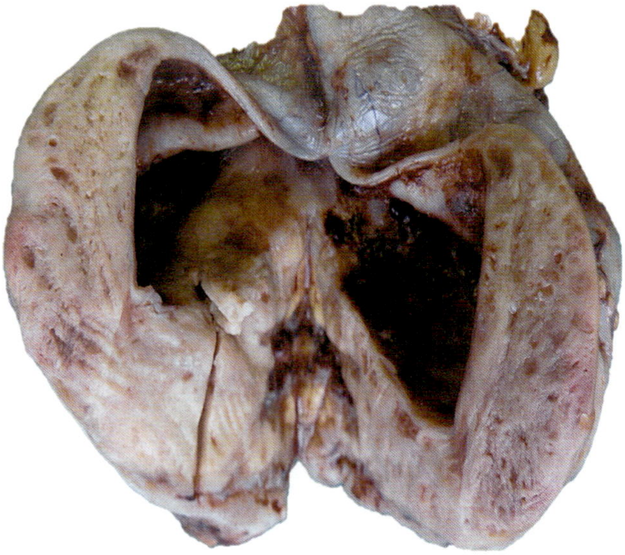

OVARIAN MALIGNANT MIXED GERM CELL TUMOR

Dysgerminomas and yolk sac tumors are the tumors most commonly seen in combination.

FIGURE 15.156. The ovarian malignant mixed germ cell tumor in (A) has a smooth surface and congested blood vessels. The cut surface in (B) appears highly heterogeneous. It is mostly tan-to-yellow and solid, with foci of cystic degeneration and hemorrhage. Histologically, it consisted of dysgerminoma and yolk sac tumor.

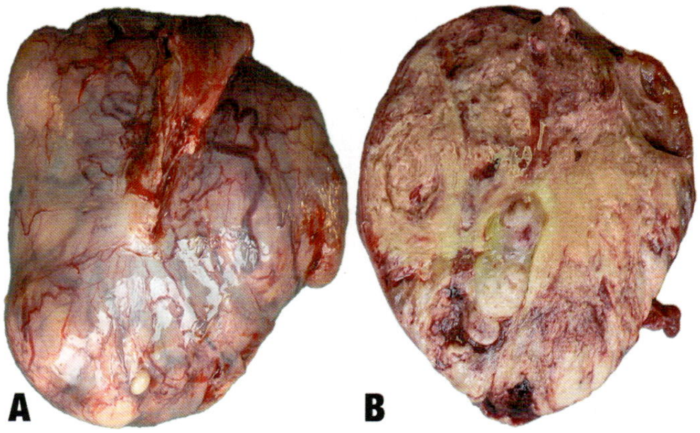

SQUAMOUS CELL CARCINOMA (SCC)

SCC of the ovary is rare. It occurs in conjunction with mature cystic teratomas, endometriosis, mucinous ovarian neoplasms, Brenner tumors, epidermoid carcinoma, and carcinosarcoma.

FIGURE 15.157. This oophorectomy specimen shows multiple cystic cavities with foci of hemorrhage on the cyst wall. Microscopic examination revealed SCC arising from the wall of a mature cystic teratoma (dermoid cyst).

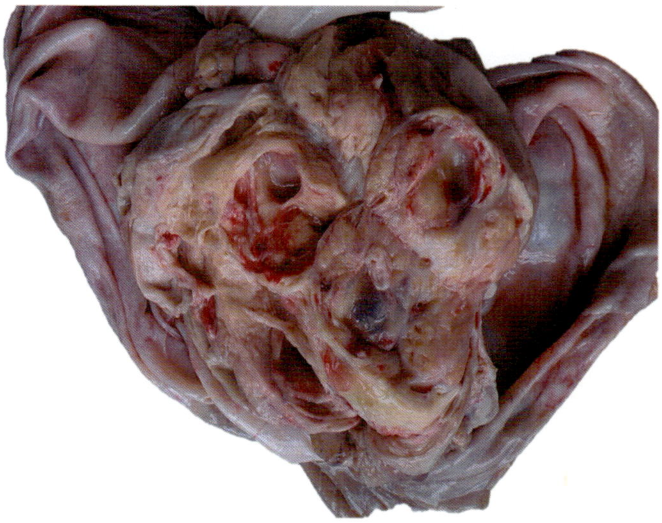

Ovarian sex cord–stromal tumors

Sex cord–stromal tumors account for approximately 8% of ovarian tumors and can be associated with endocrine manifestations. They are classified by cell type: granulosa cells, theca cells, Sertoli cells, Leydig cells, fibroblasts, and cells with nonspecific differentiation.

OVARIAN FIBROMA

Ovarian fibromas are benign tumors that represent 4% of ovarian tumors. They are hormonally inert and generally cause symptoms related to their mass effect. In a small percentage of cases, patients develop ascites and pleural effusions, which is known as Meigs syndrome. Ovarian fibromas are also associated with Gorlin syndrome (nevoid basal cell carcinoma syndrome). In this context, tumors are more likely to be bilateral, calcified, and seen at younger ages (younger than 30 years). These lesions have abnormalities in chromosome 12.

FIGURE 15.158. Image (A) shows an ovary replaced by a firm mass with a smooth, lobulated surface. In (B), the cut surface of the lesion is white and homogenous. No areas of hemorrhage or necrosis are visible.

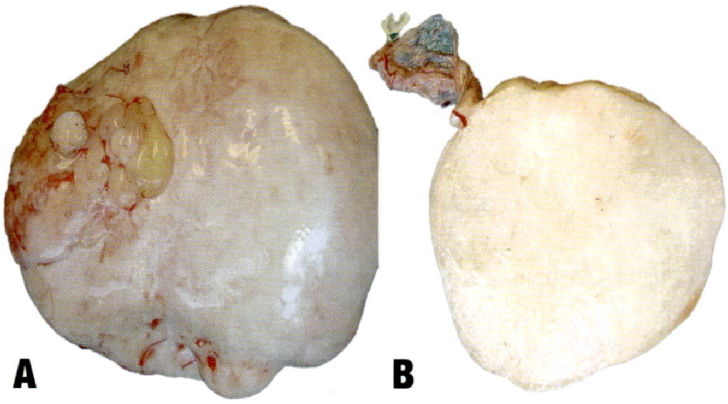

A B

FIGURE 15.159. A well-defined and firm mass shows white-to-yellow, edematous areas and focal cystic degeneration.

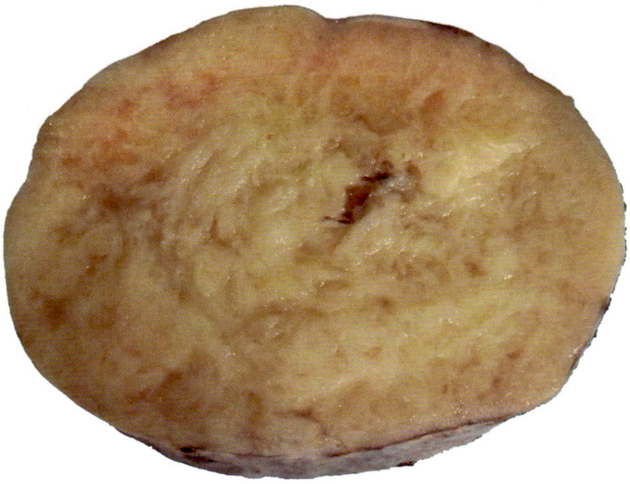

FIGURE 15.160. The cut surface of this ovarian fibroma displays yellow-to-white, firm tissue with cystic degeneration and small hemorrhagic foci.

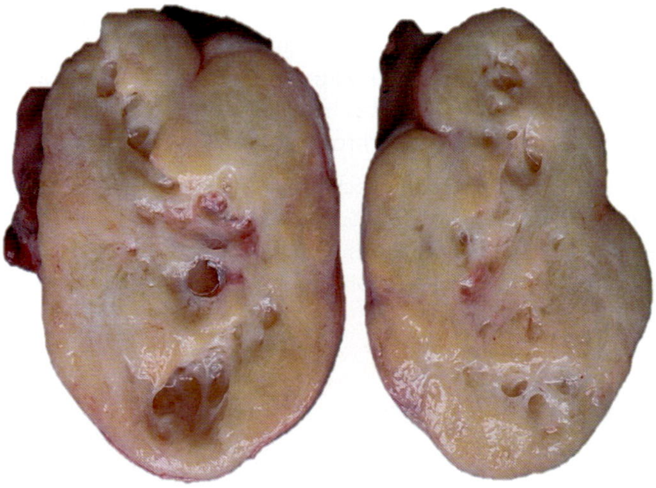

CELLULAR FIBROMA OF THE OVARY

A cellular fibroma refers to a fibroma with increased cellularity, scant collagen, mild nuclear atypia, and more than 4 mitoses per 10 HPF (high-power field). These tumors tend to be larger and softer than regular fibromas. They can range in color from white to yellow to tan.

FIGURE 15.161. The oophorectomy in (A) shows a well-circumscribed mass with a smooth surface. Areas of edema and hemorrhagic infarction are visible. In (B), a rear view shows darker red areas of hemorrhagic infarction mixed with remaining white, solid tumoral tissue.

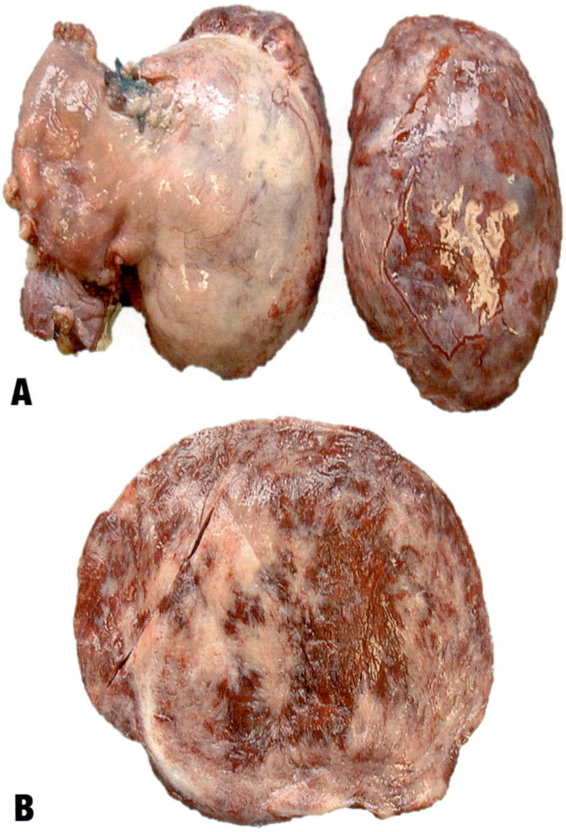

A

B

FIBROTHECOMA

Ovarian fibrothecomas account for 3% to 4% of all ovarian tumors. They are usually unilateral (90% of cases). They occur both in pre- and postmenopausal women. Histologically, they are characterized by the presence of collagen-producing fibrous tissue and lipid-rich theca cells. Thecomas, fibrothecomas, and fibromas have all been associated with trisomy and tetrasomy of chromosome 12.

FIGURE 15.162. The oophorectomy in (A) shows a well-demarcated mass measuring 10.5 cm and with an extensive hemorrhagic infarction. In (B), the cut surface of this infarcted mass appears very heterogeneous with multiple foci of hemorrhage and with cystic degeneration.

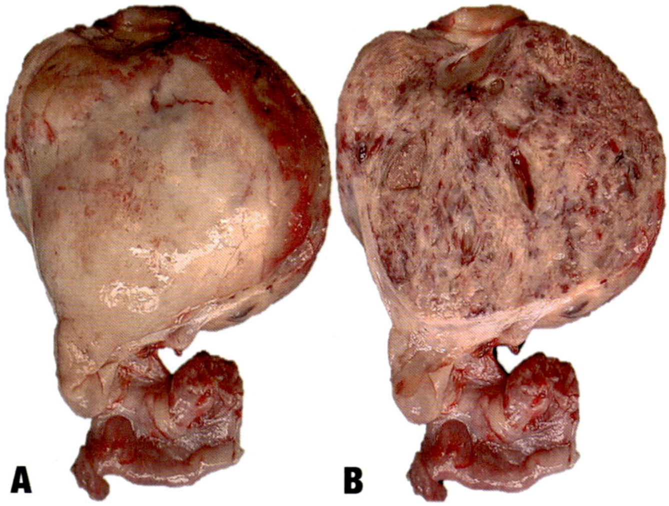

FIGURE 15.163. Image (A) shows an ovary replaced by a solitary, smooth, and firm mass. In (B), the cut surface of the tumor appears heterogeneous in color with oval patches of more yellow tissue against a lighter white-to-pink background.

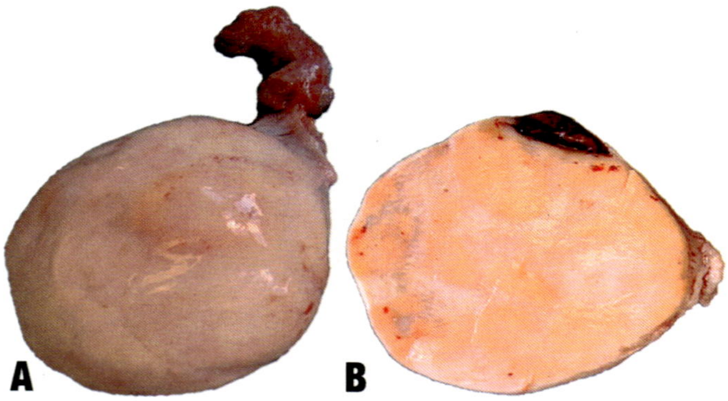

FIGURE 15.164. Image (A) shows a smooth multinodular mass occupying the ovary. The cut surface in (B) appears solid with heterogeneous white-to-tan areas.

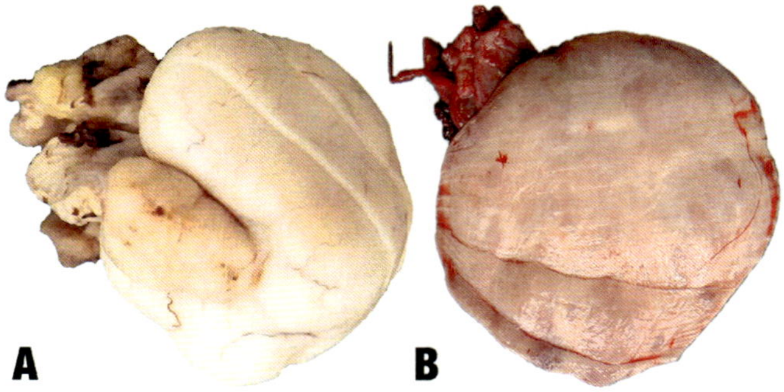

FIGURE 15.165. In (A), a smooth multinodular mass has replaced the ovary. The cut surface in (B) is solid and heterogeneous with areas of yellow tissue on a background of white tissue.

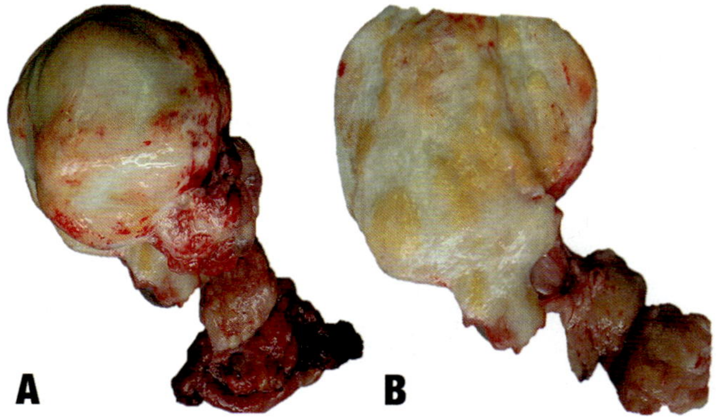

FIGURE 15.166. Image (A) shows an ovary replaced by a well-circumscribed, lobulated, and solid mass with a yellow hue. In (B), the cut surface shows solid, yellow tissue rich in theca cells mixed with lighter white tissue rich in fibrous cells.

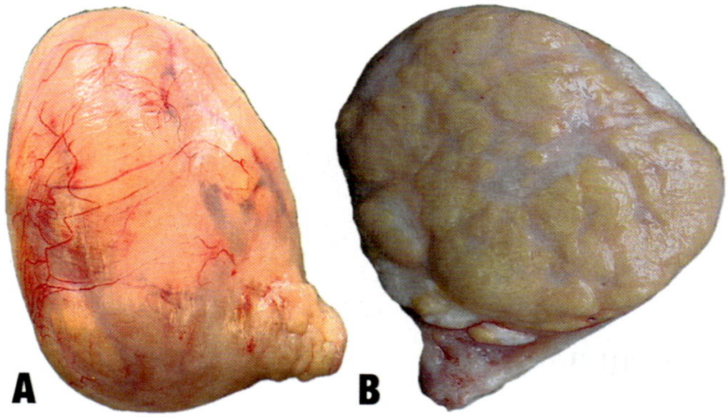

THECOMA

Ovarian thecomas are stromal tumors composed of lipid-containing cells resembling theca cells, lutein cells, and fibroblasts. Thecomas are unilateral in 97% of cases.

FIGURE 15.167. In this oophorectomy specimen, the ovaries have an irregular shape with deposits of yellow material on their outer surfaces.

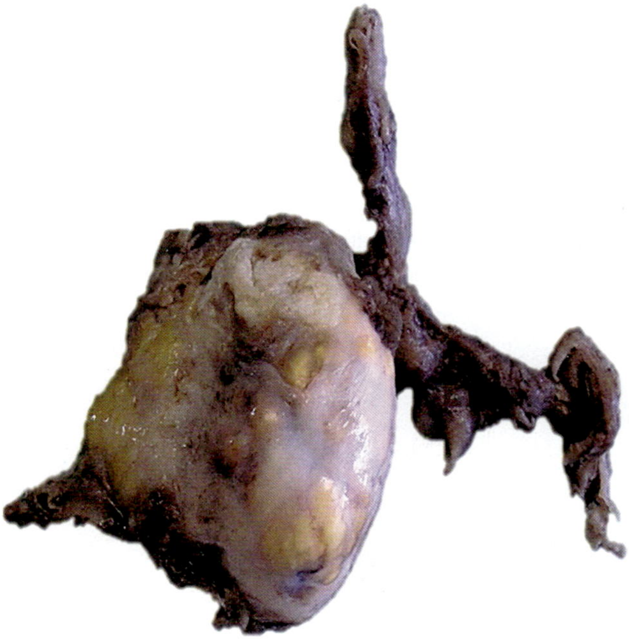

FIGURE 15.168. Image (A) shows an oophorectomy that has been serially sectioned and inked. There is a well-circumscribed, lobulated, and solid mass. The cut surface in (B) shows yellow-and-white tissue mixed with yellow tissue. A circular nodule of brown material (a focal hemorrhage) is visible in the inferior aspect of the ovary.

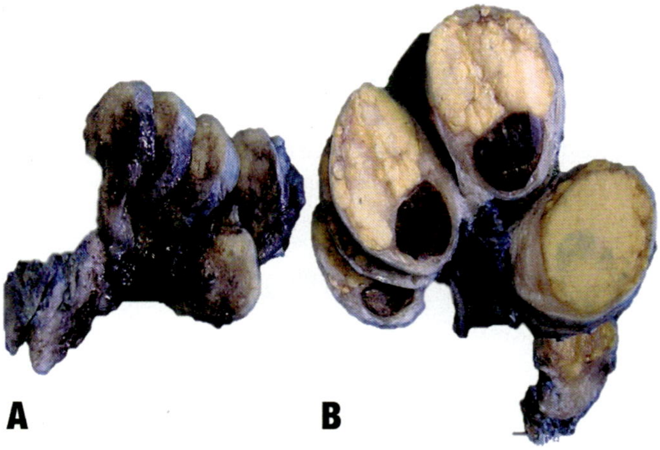

FIGURE 15.169. This image shows a well-demarcated, solid, and yellow left ovarian mass. The attached fallopian tube is dilated.

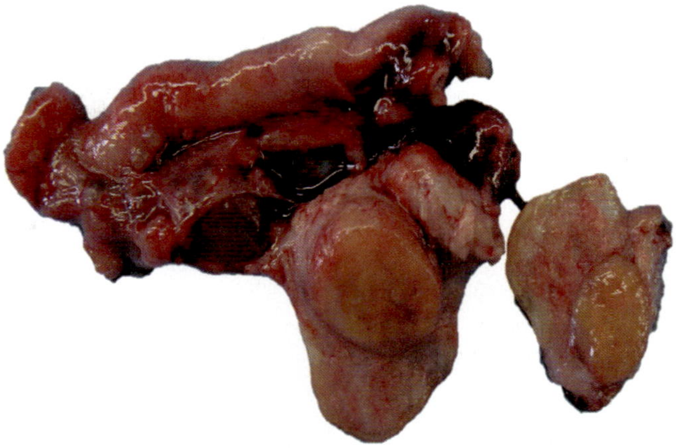

ADULT GRANULOSA CELL TUMOR

Granulosa cell tumor (GCT) represents 2% to 5% of ovarian cancers. It has 2 clinicopathologic subtypes: adult and juvenile. The adult form occurs more often in middle-aged and postmenopausal women. The juvenile form occurs mainly in children and younger women. The pathogenesis of ovarian GCT is not yet known, but may relate to hyperestrogenism.

FIGURE 15.170. This oophorectomy shows a well-circumscribed yellow mass that has solid and cystic areas and hemorrhagic foci.

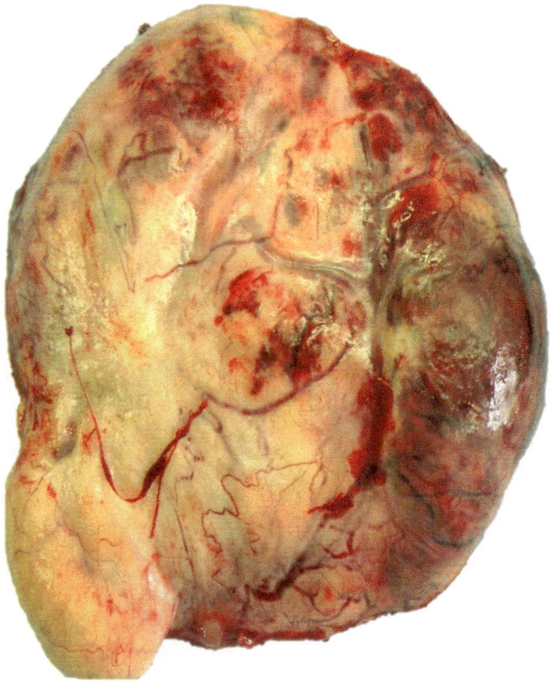

FIGURE 15.171. This image shows an adult GCT with fibrothecomatous background. The bisected oophorectomy shows a well-defined solid mass confined to the ovary. The cut surface of the tumor appears nodular with a few small foci of cystic degeneration and hemorrhage. Otherwise, the background appears solid with tan-to-yellow components consistent with a fibrothecomatous background.

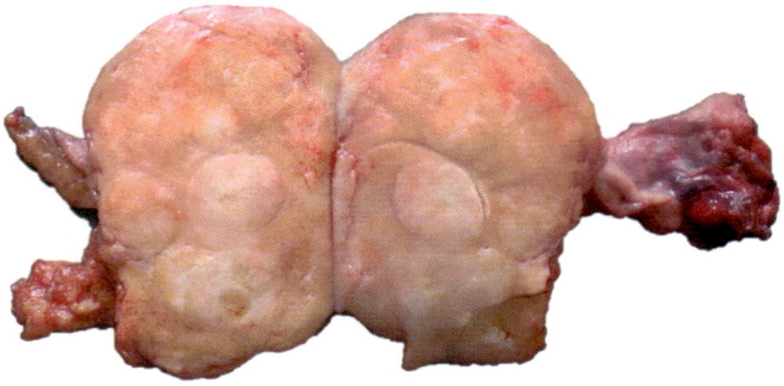

LEYDIG CELL TUMOR

These benign tumors account for 20% of steroid cell tumors and derive from Leydig cells, which are normally located in the ovarian hilus (hilus cell tumors) or, rarely, develop within the ovarian stroma (nonhilar subtype). Microscopically, the tumors comprise nests of polygonal, eosinophilic Leydig cells and fibrinoid necrosis of blood vessel walls. Reinke crystals may or may not be present in cell cytoplasm. The tumors are often androgenic, thereby causing virilization in patients.

LEYDIG CELL TUMOR (HILUS CELL TUMOR)

FIGURE 15.172. This oophorectomy specimen has a small, well-circumscribed, and yellow-reddish solid mass at the center of the ovary.

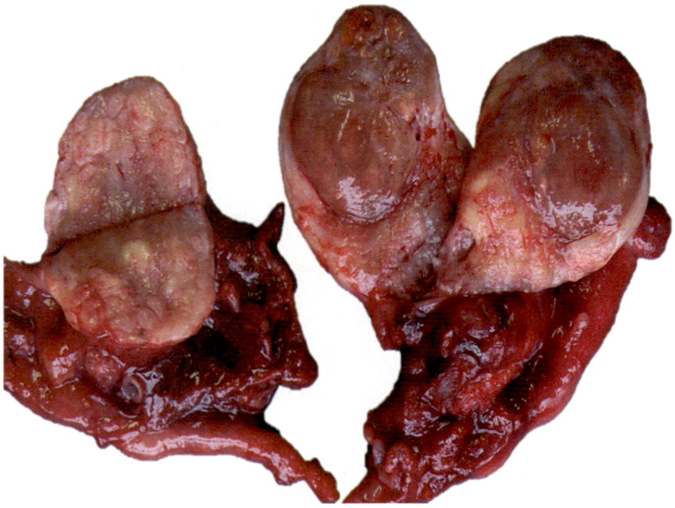

SERTOLI–LEYDIG CELL TUMOR

Ovarian Sertoli–Leydig tumors are rare: they account for less than 0.1% of ovarian neoplasms. They can secrete androgens, which causes virilization in 40% to 60% of patients. Other tumors of this category can be nonfunctioning or secrete estrogens. Histologically, these tumors are divided into well-differentiated, intermediate, or poorly differentiated subtypes, based on the degree of tubular differentiation of the Sertoli cell component and the quantity of spindle cell gonadal stroma. The histologic subtype correlates with clinical behavior. Some ovarian Sertoli–Leydig cell tumors have been associated with *FOXL2* and *DICER* mutations.

FIGURE 15.173. These images show an example of the poorly differentiated (sarcomatoid) subtype. The oophorectomy in (A) shows a circumscribed yellow mass with solid and cystic areas. The cut surface in (B) shows a yellow lobulated solid tumor.

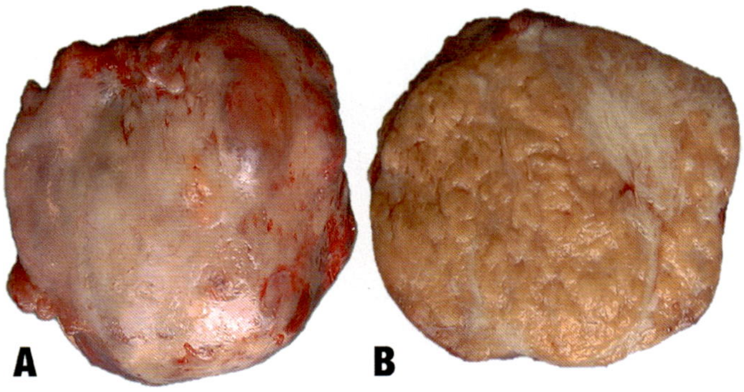

OVARIAN SEX CORD TUMOR

Ovarian sex cord tumors are rare tumors characterized by the presence of simple or complex annular tubules. These tumors may be associated with Peutz–Jeghers syndrome or be sporadic. When associated with Peutz–Jeghers syndrome, the tumors tend to be smaller, hormonally inert, and bilateral with calcifications. When sporadic, the tumors tend to be larger, unilateral, and without calcification; they may produce estrogen.

FIGURE 15.174. On the cut surface of this oophorectomy specimen, the tumor appears uniformly yellow and solid with annular tubules.

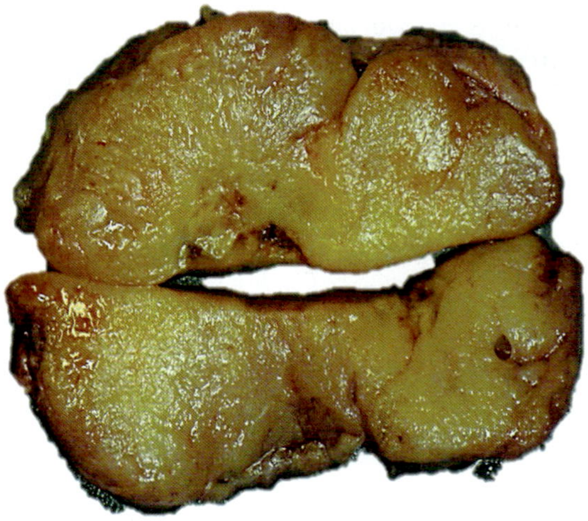

CARCINOSARCOMA OF THE OVARY

This tumor accounts for less than 4% of ovarian cancers and has a poor prognosis. It was formerly called malignant mixed Müllerian tumor. The WHO renamed it carcinosarcoma in 2014, because it is a primary epithelial tumor that has developed a mesenchymal component. The malignant mesenchymal component may include homologous or heterologous sarcomatous elements (e.g., chondrosarcoma, rhabdomyosarcoma).

FIGURE 15.175. The cut surface of this oophorectomy specimen displays an ill-defined, lobulated, heterogeneous mass composed of solid and cystic areas.

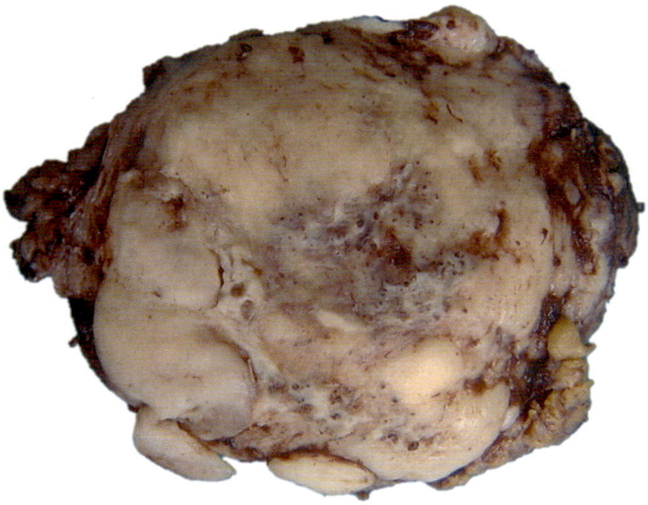

Ovarian metastasis

The proportion of malignant ovarian tumors that are of metastatic origin differs by geographic region. In Western countries, ovarian metastatic tumors occur in 3% to 15% of cases; this proportion rises to 21% to 30% in Eastern countries. Carcinomas of the colon, stomach, breast, and endometrium are the most frequent sites of origin for ovarian metastatic tumors. Tumors spread to the ovary by several routes: the hematogenous-lymphatic pathway; the transtubal and/or transperitoneal pathway; or by direct extension. Grossly, some features that suggest metastatic ovarian tumors include: bilaterality and multinodularity of the tumor; smaller size (< 10 cm) than primary neoplasms; involvement of the ovarian surface; presence of lymphovascular invasion and desmoplastic reaction; unusual histology and clinical history; and, in some cases, extensive extraovarian spread.

METASTATIC BREAST CARCINOMA TO THE OVARY

Metastases from the breast generally form solid masses and are found bilaterally in 60% to 80% of cases. Lobular carcinoma has a greater tendency for ovarian metastasis than ductal breast carcinoma.

FIGURE 15.176. Images (A) and (B) show diffuse ovarian involvement by a nodular, mostly solid mass with focal cystic and hemorrhagic areas.

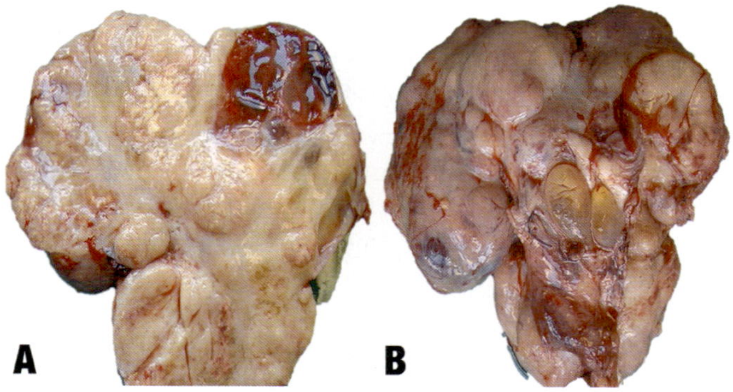

FIGURE 15.177. This cut surface shows white, tan, and yellow solid tissue with a few small cystic structures.

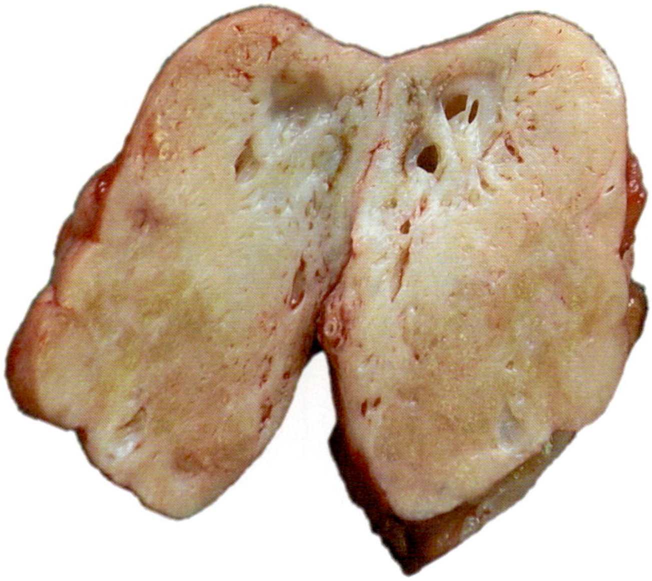

FIGURE 15.178. Image (A) shows the outer surface of an ovarian mass, which appears heterogeneous. In some areas, red, friable tissue invades the capsule. Necrosis is also present. In (B), the cut surface of the ovary has a heterogeneous appearance. It is mostly solid and tan-to-yellow with areas of hemorrhage and necrosis.

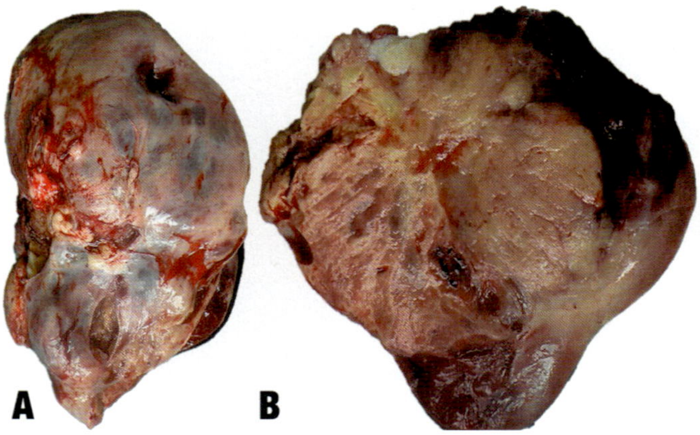

METASTATIC MUCINOUS ADENOCARCINOMA TO THE OVARY

Metastases originating from the gastrointestinal tract, pancreatic–biliary system, uterine cervix, or lung may closely simulate primary ovarian carcinoma. Metastatic colorectal adenocarcinoma is a common secondary ovarian tumor.

FIGURE 15.179. Image (A) shows the outer surface of a large tumor, which is irregular and mostly smooth with hemorrhagic foci of different sizes. The cut surface in (B) reveals a multilocular cystic tumor with focal mucinous and small tan nodules.

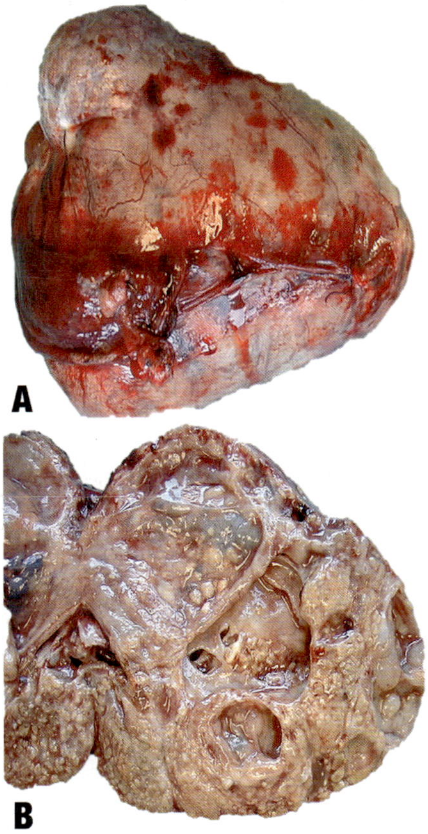

FIGURE 15.180. In this oophorectomy specimen, the tumor appears solid and cystic with areas of hemorrhage and necrosis.

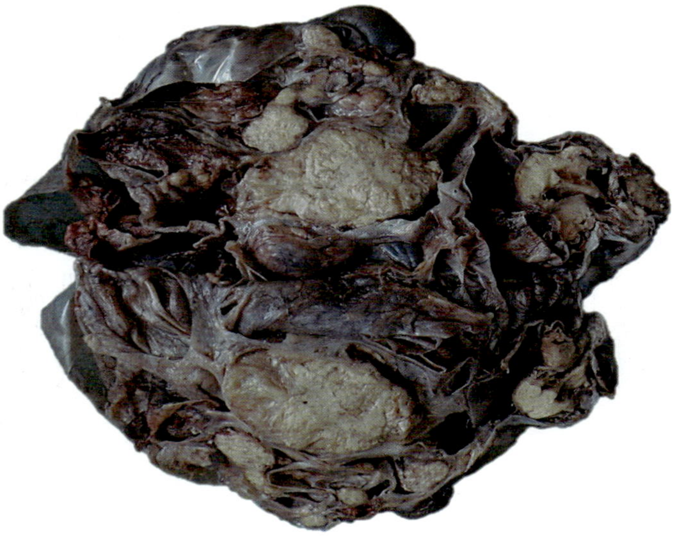

FIGURE 15.181. The ovary in (A) is completely replaced by a yellow-tan tumor with a cyst (lower part of specimen). In (B), the cut surface of the tumor appears mostly solid with some cystic areas.

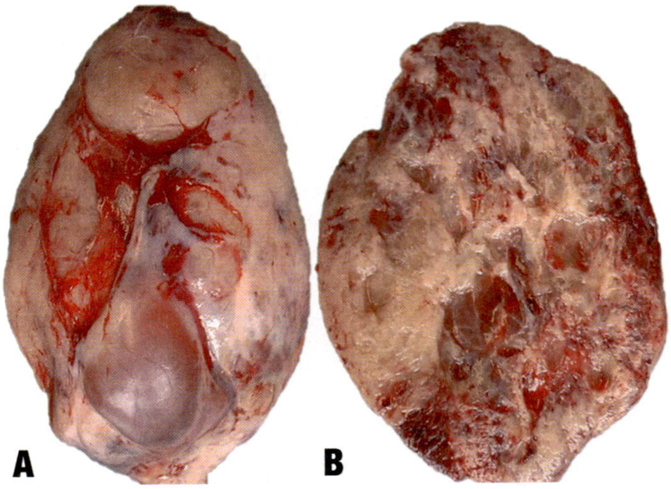

KRUKENBERG TUMOR

Krukenberg tumor is a metastatic adenocarcinoma composed of signet ring cells, most frequently originating from gastric carcinoma. The resulting ovarian tumors are bilateral in 60% to 80% of cases.

FIGURE 15.182. In (A), a tan-to-white, nodular solid mass has replaced the ovary. In (B), the cut opening of the solid tumor shows a uniform, white-pale surface with small foci of hemorrhage.

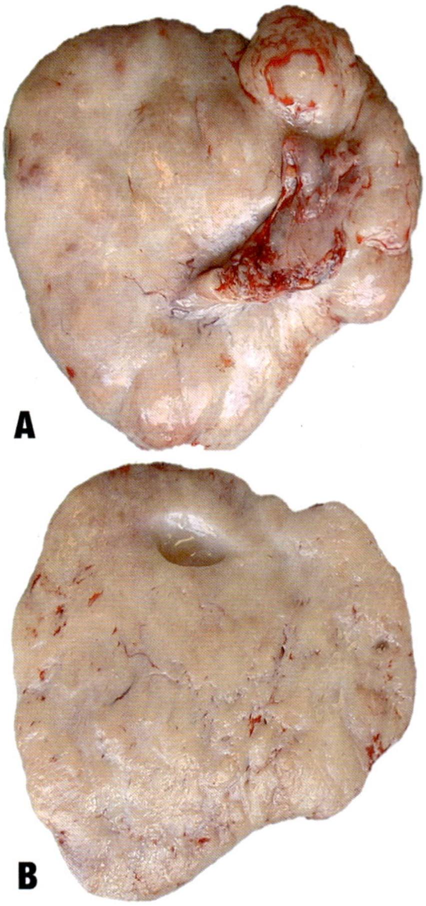

FIGURE 15.183. The ovary is replaced by a solid, variegated, ill-defined tumor with central necrosis.

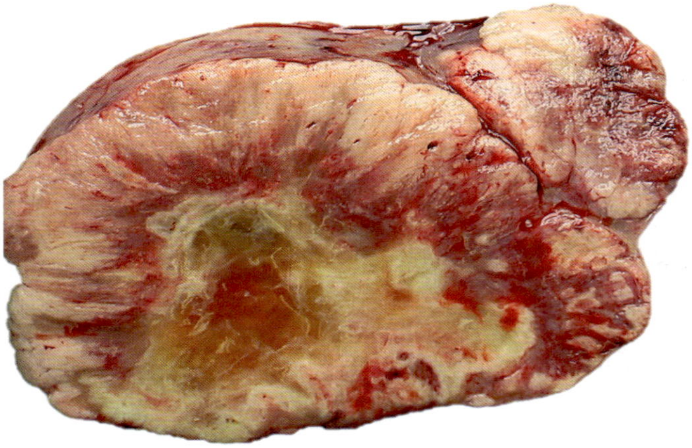

FIGURE 15.184. Image (A) shows a multinodular, white tumor with a smooth capsule. In (B), the cut opening of the tumor shows a homogeneous white-tan surface with hemorrhagic areas.

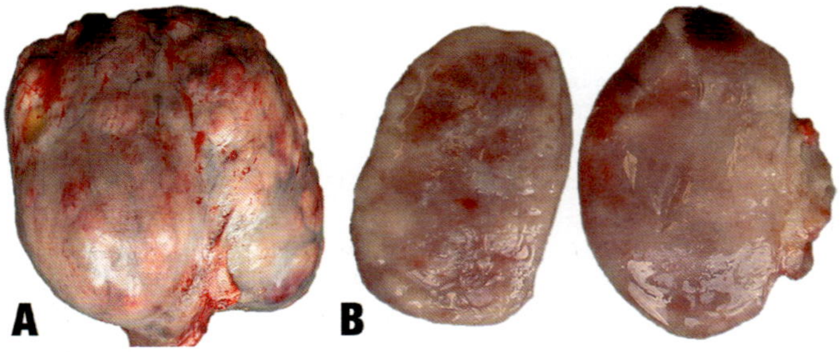

METASTATIC UTERINE CARCINOSARCOMA TO THE OVARY

FIGURE 15.185. Image (A) shows a multinodular, irregular, and friable mass that originated in the uterus and has involved the fallopian tube and ovary. In (B), the cut section of the ovarian tumor shows prominent white-to-yellow, solid masses and hemorrhagic foci.

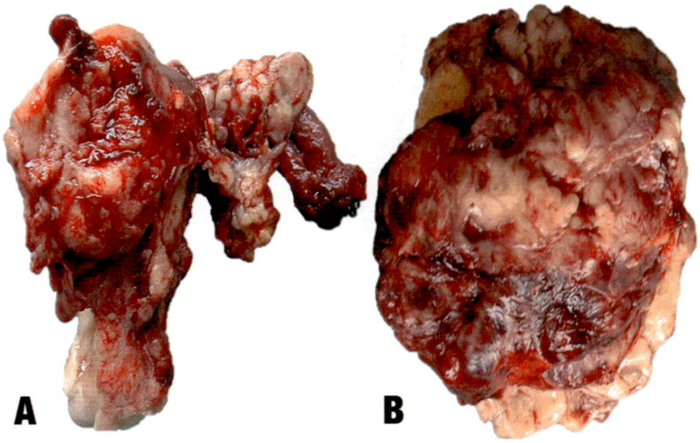

FIGURE 15.186. This hysterectomy with bilateral salpingo-oophorectomy shows an aggressive tumor extending from the uterus to the ovary, fallopian tube, and uterine serosa. One ovary is completely replaced by a large, multinodular lesion with surface hemorrhage and adhesions. Metastatic tumoral tissue with red, granular appearance is also present on uterine serosa.

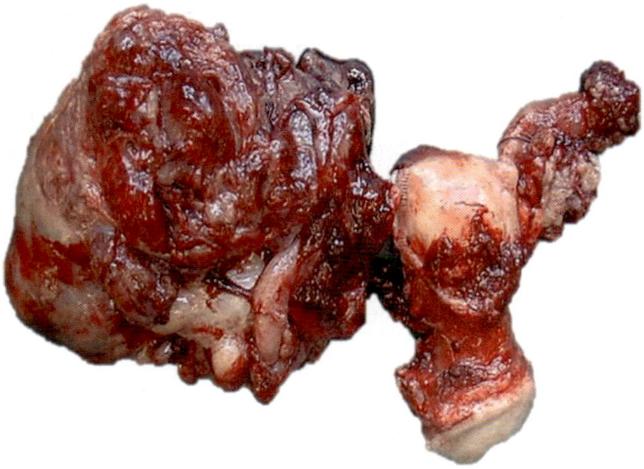

METASTATIC MELANOMA

Ovarian involvement is present in approximately 20% of melanoma cases and most primary tumors originate in the skin.

FIGURE 15.187. This oophorectomy specimen shows multiple black-to-brown nodules of varying sizes budging onto the serosa surface.

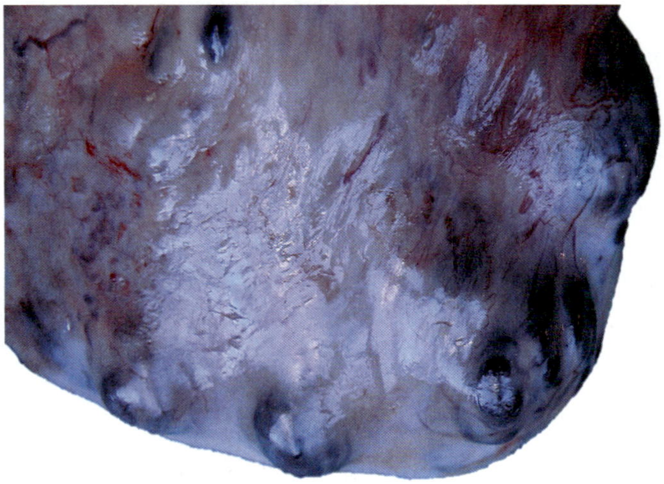

ACKNOWLEDGMENTS

We would like to thank the valuable contributions of Dr. Jocelyne Arseneau, Dr. Manon Auger, Dr. Atilla Omeroglu, and Dr. Lili Fu, and the technical help of R. Gilot, E. Griss, A. Hossain, L. Korneichyuk Pasyuk, M. Mikhael, and E. Yaney.

REFERENCES

Chen R, Yu Z, Zhang H, Ding J, Chen B. Primary malignant lymphoma of the uterus and broad ligament: a case report and review of literature. OncoTargets Ther. 2015;8:265–268. https://doi.org/10.2147/OTT.S78171. Medline:25674001

Cuatrecasas M, Catasus L, Palacios J, Prat J. Transitional cell tumors of the ovary: a comparative clinicopathologic, immunohistochemical, and molecular genetic analysis of Brenner tumors and transitional cell carcinomas. Am J Surg Pathol. 2009;33(4):556–567. https://doi.org/10.1097/PAS.0b013e318188b84c. Medline:19033864

Felix AS, Weissfeld JL, Stone RA, et al. Factors associated with type I and type II endometrial cancer. Cancer Causes Control. 2010;21(11):1851–1856. https://doi.org/10.1007/s10552-010-9612-8. Medline:20628804

Hart WR. Mucinous tumors of the ovary: a review. Int J Gynecol Pathol. 2005;24(1):4–25. Medline:15626914

Kuhn E, Ayhan A, Shih IeM, Seidman JD, Kurman RJ. The pathogenesis of atypical proliferative Brenner tumor: an immunohistochemical and molecular genetic analysis. Mod Pathol. 2014;27(2):231–237. https://doi.org/10.1038/modpathol.2013.142. Medline:23887305

Kurman RJ, Carcangiu ML, Herrington CS, Young RH, editors. WHO classification of tumours of the female reproductive organs. 4th ed. Lyon: IARC Press; 2014.

Lacey JV Jr, Ioffe OB, Ronnett BM, et al. Endometrial carcinoma risk among women diagnosed with endometrial hyperplasia: the 34-year experience in a large health plan. Br J Cancer. 2008;98:45–53. https://doi.org/10.1038/sj.bjc.6604102. Medline:18026193

Leung SW, Yuen PM. Ovarian fibroma: a review on the clinical characteristics, diagnostic difficulties, and management options of 23 cases. Gynecol Obstet Invest. 2006;62(1):1–6. https://doi.org/10.1159/000091679. Medline:16498263

McCluggage WG. A practical approach to the diagnosis of mixed epithelial and mesenchymal tumours of the uterus. Mod Pathol. 2016;29(Suppl 1):S78–S91. https://doi.org/10.1038/modpathol.2015.137. Medline:26715175

McCluggage WG. New developments in endocervical glandular lesions. Histopathology. 2013;62(1):138–160. https://doi.org/10.1111/his.12012. Medline:23134447

McConechy MK, Ding J, Senz J, et al. Ovarian and endometrial endometrioid carcinomas have distinct CTNNB1 and PTEN mutation profiles. Mod Pathol. 2014;27(1):128–134. https://doi.org/10.1038/modpathol.2013.107. Medline:23765252

Montoriol PF, Mons A, Da Ines D, Bourdel N, Tixier L, Garcier JM. Fibrous tumours of the ovary: aetiologies and MRI features. Clin Radiol. 2013;68(12):1276–1283. https://doi.org/10.1016/j.crad.2013.07.005. Medline:23937826

Morice P, Leary A, Creutzberg C, Abu-Rustum N, Darai E. Endometrial cancer. The Lancet. 2016;387(10023):1094–1108. https://doi.org/10.1016/S0140-6736(15)00130-0.

Morice P, Uzan C, Fauvet R, Gouy S, Duvillard P, Darai E. Borderline ovarian tumour: pathological diagnostic dilemma and risk factors for invasive or lethal recurrence. Lancet Oncol. 2012;13(3):e103–e115. https://doi.org/10.1016/S1470-2045(11)70288-1. Medline:22381933

Nocito AL, Sarancone S, Bacchi C, Tellez T. Ovarian thecoma: clinicopathological analysis of 50 cases. Ann Diagn Pathol. 2008;12(1):12–16. https://doi.org/10.1016/j.anndiagpath.2007.01.011. Medline:18164409

Oliva E, Young RH. Endocrine pathology of the ovary: in tribute to Robert E Scully, MD. Endocr Pathol. 2014;25:102–19. https://doi.org/10.1007/s12022-013-9285-4.

Rio Frio T, Bahubeshi A, Kanellopoulou C, et al. *DICER1* mutations in familial multinodular goiter with and without ovarian Sertoli-Leydig cell tumors. JAMA. 2011;305(1):68–77. https://doi.org/10.1001/jama.2010.1910. Medline:21205968

Roth LM, Czernobilsky B. Perspectives on pure ovarian stromal neoplasms and tumor-like proliferations of the ovarian stroma. Am J Surg Pathol. 2011;35(3):e15–e33. Medline:21317704

Roth LM, Talerman A. Recent advances in the pathology and classification of ovarian germ cell tumors. Int J Gynecol Pathol. 2006;25(4):305–320. https://doi.org/10.1097/01.pgp.0000225844.59621.9d. Medline:16990705

Soslow RA. Histologic subtypes of ovarian carcinoma: an overview. Int J Gynecol Pathol. 2008;27(2):161–174. https://doi.org/10.1097/PGP.0b013e31815ea812. Medline:18317227

Soslow RA. Practical issues related to uterine pathology: staging, frozen section, artifacts, and Lynch syndrome. Mod Pathol. 2016;29(Suppl 1):S59–S77. https://doi.org/10.1038/modpathol.2015.127. Medline:26715174

Ueda Y, Enomoto T, Kimura T, Yoshino K, Fujita M, Kimura T. Two distinct pathways to development of squamous cell carcinoma of the vulva. J Skin Cancer. 2011;2011:1-7. https://doi.org/10.1155/2011/951250. Medline:21188235

Young RH. Sex cord-stromal tumors of the ovary and testis: their similarities and differences with consideration of selected problems. Mod Pathol. 2005;18(Suppl 2):S81–S98. https://doi.org/10.1038/modpathol.3800311. Medline:15502809

16

Diseases of the Lymph Nodes and Spleen

DUC-VINH THAI, ZU-HUA GAO

Lymph Nodes

Reactive lymph node

There are 500 to 600 lymph nodes in the human body, usually ranging from 0.2 cm to 2 cm in diameter. They are bean- or kidney-shaped, and play an important role in the immune system. They can become quite enlarged and swollen in response to infection or inflammation.

FIGURE 16.1. This reactive lymph node is round with a pink-to-brown homogenous cut surface.

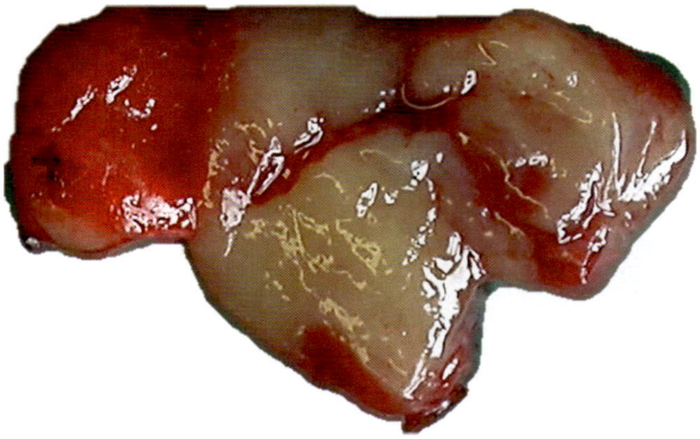

Castleman disease

Castleman disease, also called giant lymph node hyperplasia, is a rare lymphoproliferative disorder of unknown etiology. Clinically, Castleman disease may either be localized to a single lymph node (unicentric) or occur systemically (multicentric). Surgical removal usually cures the unicentric form. The multicentric form usually occurs in immunocompromised, HIV-positive patients, and is often associated with lymphoma and Kaposi sarcoma.

FIGURE 16.2. On cut surface, this lymph node is enlarged, solid, and beefy-red due to vascular congestion.

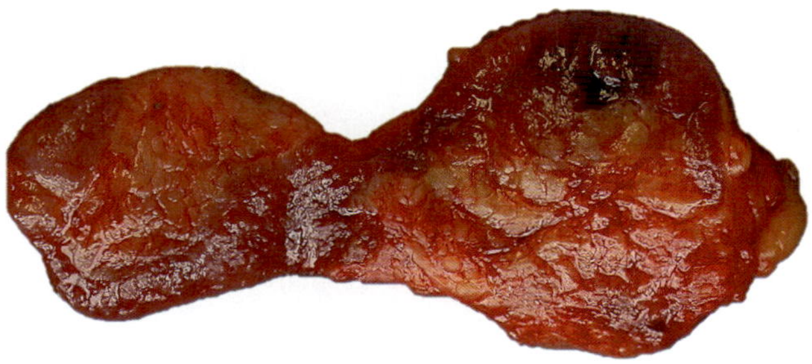

Sézary disease

Sézary disease is a type of cutaneous T-cell lymphoma characterized by a triad of features: erythroderma; generalized lymphadenopathy; and the presence of clonal neoplastic T-cells with cerebriform nuclei (Sézary cells) in skin, lymph nodes, and peripheral blood.

FIGURE 16.3. This enlarged inguinal lymph node with Sézary disease shows completely effaced lymph node architecture by large tumor nodules with a fish-flesh white cut surface.

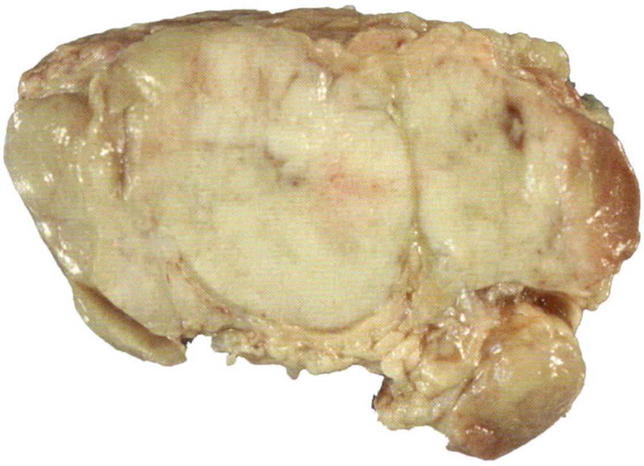

Mucosa-associated lymphoid tissue (MALT) lymphoma

MALT lymphoma is a type of marginal zone lymphoma. The most common genetic mutation in pulmonary MALT lymphoma is t(11;18)(q21;q21). The disease usually follows an indolent course.

FIGURE 16.4. This image shows lung extranodal MALT lymphoma. On cut surface, the lung is infiltrated by a solid, fleshy, homogenous, beige (cream-colored) mass. The mass abuts the visceral pleural, but does not invade through it. The tumor surrounds and compresses airways and vessels.

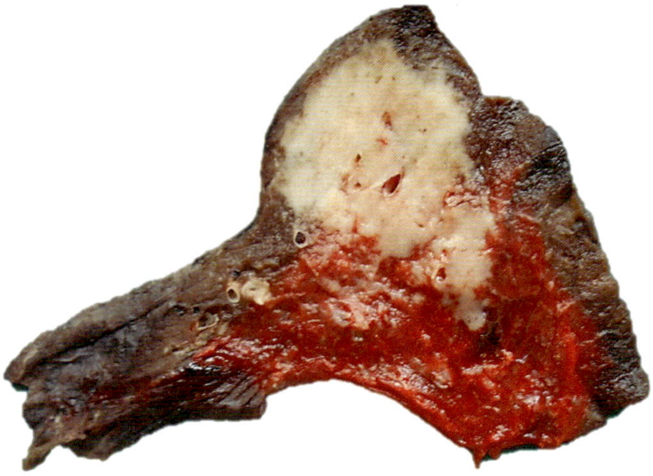

Follicular lymphoma

Follicular lymphoma is the most common type of non-Hodgkin lymphoma. Clinically, follicular lymphoma occurs in older adults with generalized lymphadenopathy. The typical genotype of follicular lymphoma is t(14;18) that leads to *BCL2-IgH* fusion gene. Follicular lymphoma is considered indolent because of its excellent prognosis even without chemotherapy.

FIGURE 16.5. Images (A) to (D) show lymph nodes that, on cut surface, appear enlarged and homogenously beige with small nodules bulging out from the cut surface.

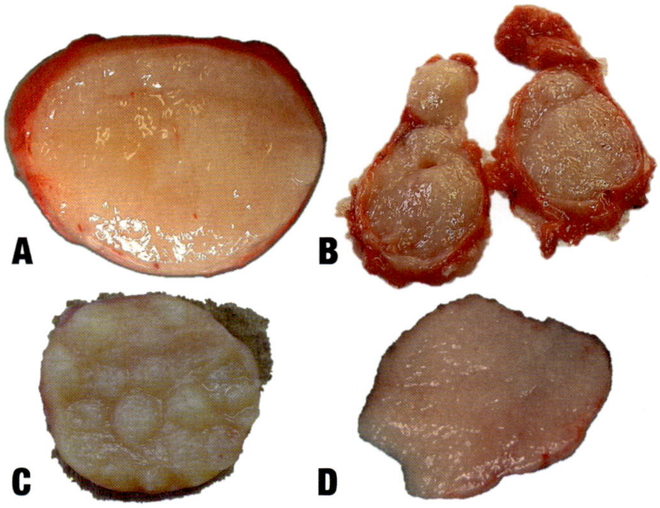

EXTRANODAL FOLLICULAR LYMPHOMA

Rarely, primary follicular lymphoma may affect the gastrointestinal tract, the breast, and the testis, which may cause local symptoms. Extranodal involvement may also occur as part of widespread nodal disease.

FIGURE 16.6. This image shows a small bowel opened along the antimesenteric side. The small bowel predominantly shows preserved circumferential mucosal folds. However, near the bowel's midpoint, the mucosa is edematous and raised by a submucosal mass. This mass leads to partial luminal obstruction with dilatation of the proximal bowel. Note the difference of the lumen size proximal and distal to the obstruction.

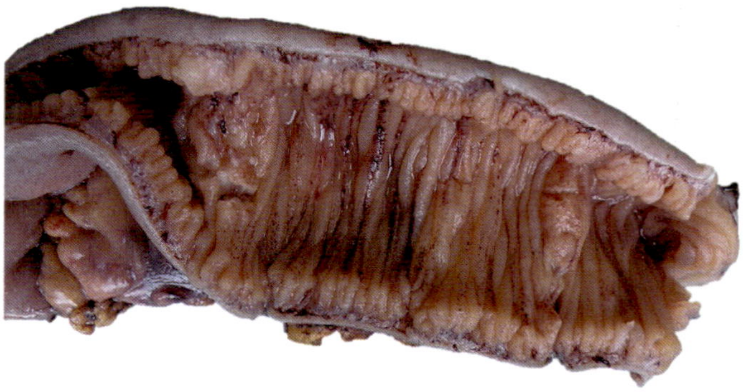

Diffuse large B-cell lymphoma (DLBCL)

DLBCL is an aggressive type of lymphoma that presents with rapidly growing lymphadenopathy. Many genetic alterations occur in this lymphoma, including *BCL6*, *BLC2*, and *MYC*.

FIGURE 16.7. This image shows a right clavicular lymph node with DLBCL. On the external surface in (A), the lymph node appears enlarged with variegated beige to red capsule. On the cut surface in (B), the lymph node shows a homogenous, beige-fleshy color.

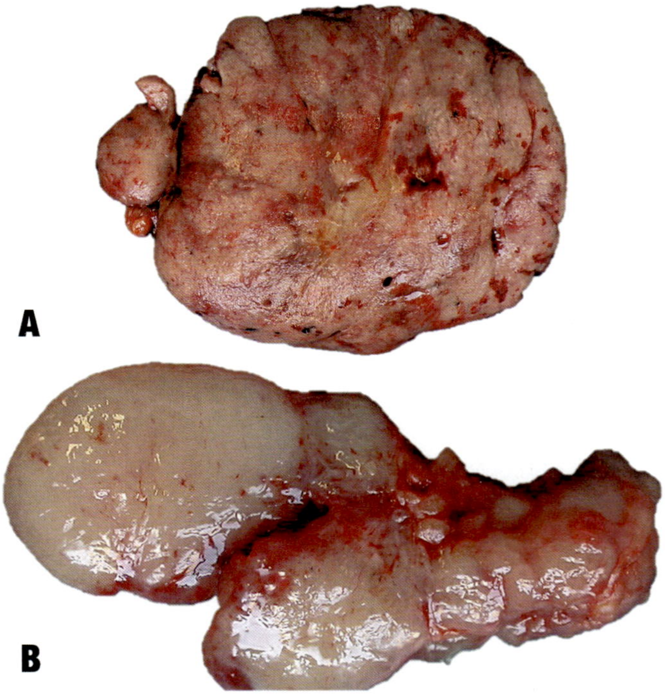

Multiple myeloma

Multiple myeloma is the most common plasma cell neoplasm. Clinically, it may present with the "CRAB" symptoms: hyper**c**alcemia, **r**enal failure, **a**nemia, and **b**one lesions (lytic lesions with possible pathologic fracture).

FIGURE 16.8. This image shows multiple myeloma involving the right clavicular lymph node. On cut surface, the lymph node is round and enlarged with effacement of the normal architecture by a solid beige mass.

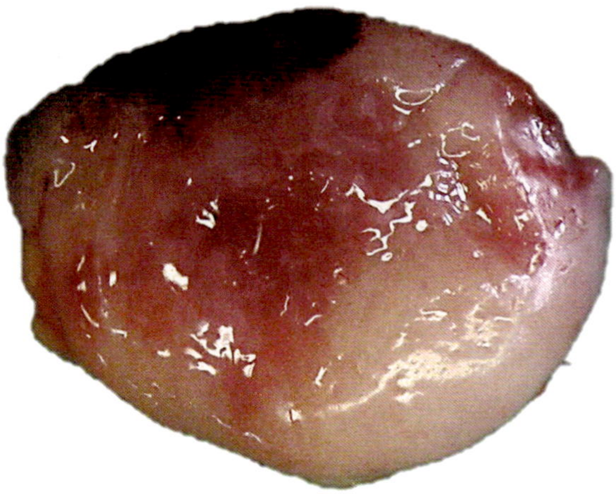

Nodular sclerosing Hodgkin lymphoma

Hodgkin lymphoma is a distinct group of lymphomas that share certain characteristics, including involvement of lymph nodes, spread of disease to anatomically contiguous lymph nodes, and presence of Reed–Sternberg cells, among others. There are 5 subtypes of Hodgkin lymphoma: the nodular sclerosing, mixed cellularity, lymphocyte-rich, and lymphocyte depletion subtypes (the classic subtypes), and the lymphocyte predominance subtype. The nodular sclerosing subtype is the most common form of Hodgkin lymphoma, and it is the easiest subtype to recognize on gross examination.

FIGURE 16.9. Image (A) shows the cut surface of a lymph node enlarged with a vague nodular surface. These nodules are separated by dense, white tissue that is consistent with fibrosis. Image (B) shows another case: the cut surface after serial sectioning shows a lymph node with multiple well-circumscribed, beige nodules separated by fibrosis (sclerosis).

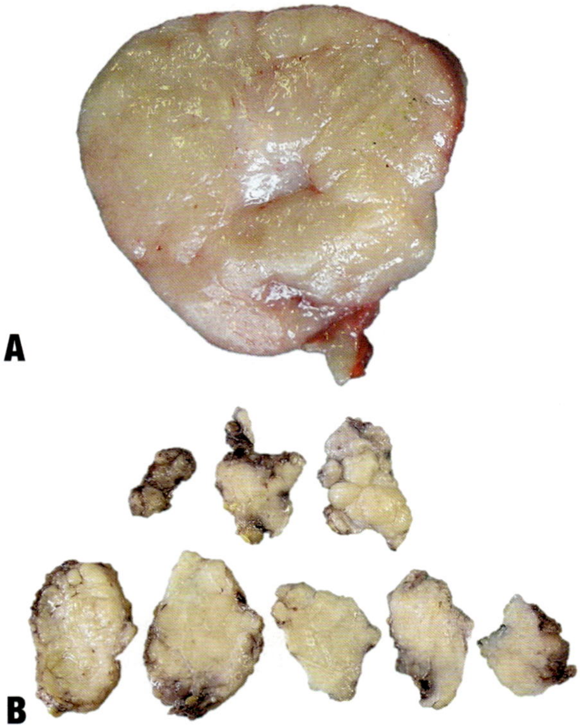

Spleen

REFERENCE: NORMAL SPLEEN

The spleen is the largest lymphatic organ in the human body: it normally weighs between 125 g and 195 g. It plays an essential role in immune response to blood-borne antigens. Various pathologies may affect the spleen, including splenomegaly, neoplasms, congenital anomalies, and ruptures. The splenic parenchyma is composed of red pulp (venous sinuses) and white pulp (lymphoid tissue).

FIGURE 16.10. Image (A) shows a lateral view of the spleen. Image (B) shows a medial view of the spleen with its hilum. A smooth peritoneal layer covers the bean-shaped organ.

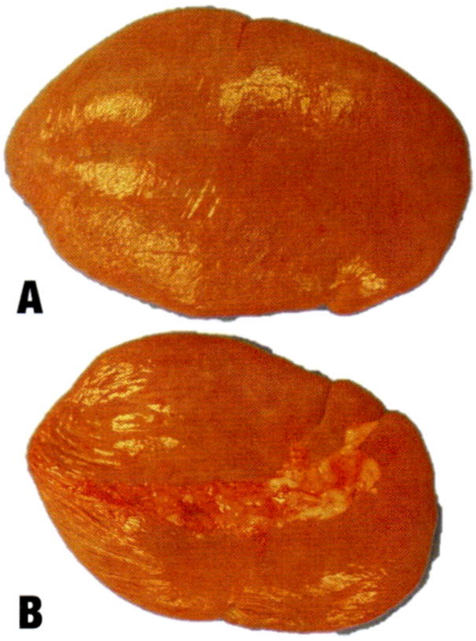

Accessory spleen

Accessory spleens are histologically and functionally identical to normal spleens. They can occur at any site within the abdomen, and are detected in up to 35% of postmortem examinations. They become clinically relevant when they contribute to certain hematologic disorders, such as immune thrombocytopenia (ITP).

FIGURE 16.11. The cut surface of this specimen shows a deep red, highly vascular structure similar to a normal spleen.

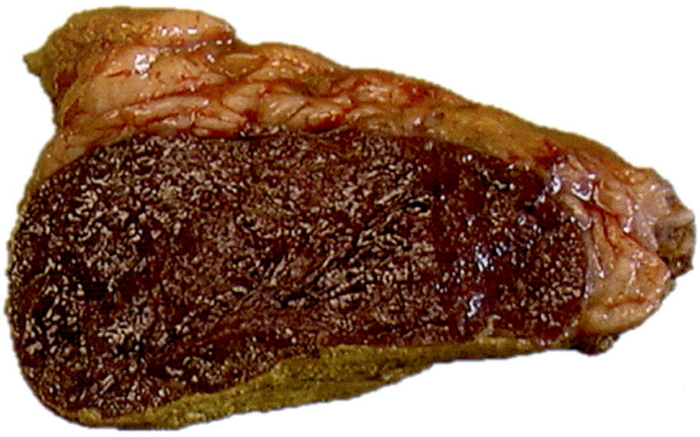

Primary epithelial splenic cyst

Primary epithelial splenic cysts are benign cysts with an epithelial lining that stains positive for carcinoembryonic antigen (CEA) and cancer antigen 19-9 (CA 19-9). They can grow large and require surgical removal. Primary splenic cysts constitute 10% of all nonparasitic cysts of the spleen, and can be divided into congenital, neoplastic, traumatic, and degenerative types. Usually they are asymptomatic and found incidentally on ultrasound examination of the abdomen in pediatric and adolescent age groups. They can rupture, become infected, or bleed. Differential diagnosis should include neoplastic conditions.

FIGURE 16.12. As seen in this image, epithelial (primary) splenic cysts are thin-walled cysts with marked trabeculations that may be solitary or, less commonly, multiple.

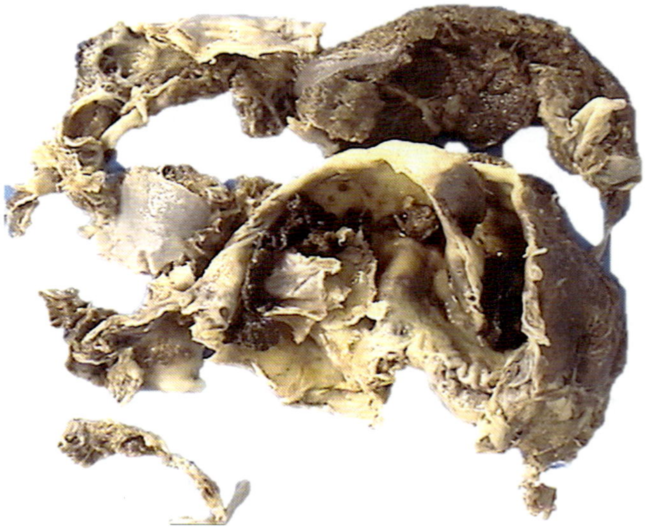

Primary mesothelial cyst of the spleen

Primary mesothelial cysts of the spleen, also called solitary splenic lymphangioma, are benign cysts that occur in the context of trauma.

FIGURE 16.13. This image shows a large, unilocular cyst arising from the spleen. These cysts typically have a glistening inner surface. On microscopic examination, this cyst was lined by cuboidal cells that stained positive for pankeratin (AE1-AE3) and calretinin, consistent with a mesothelial layer.

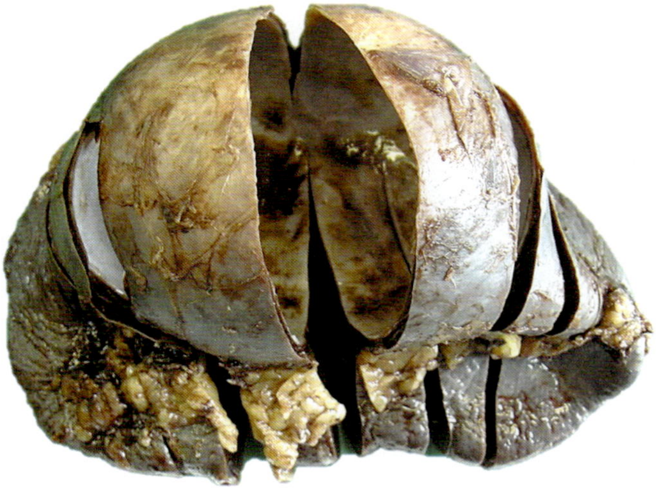

Splenic laceration

Splenic ruptures may be secondary to trauma (usually blunt trauma). Because the spleen is a reservoir of blood, splenic ruptures often lead to dramatic intraperitoneal hemorrhage that requires emergency splenectomy to prevent death.

FIGURE 16.14. Images (A) and (B) show the external surface of a spleen with multiple lacerations through the splenic capsule into the parenchyma.

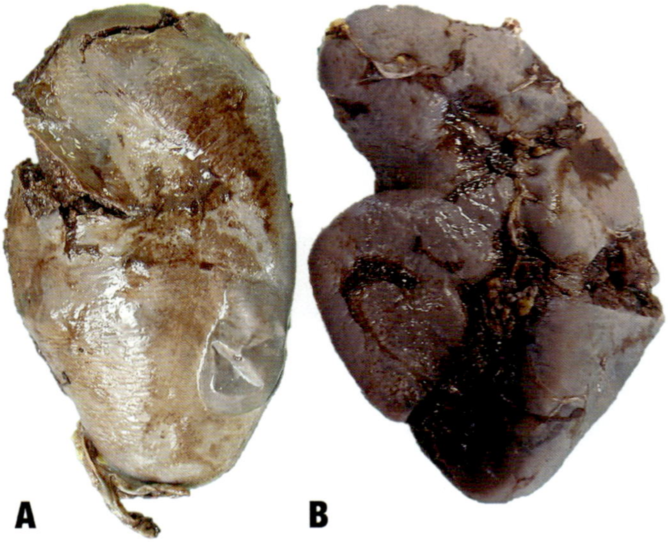

Thrombotic thrombocytopenic purpura

Thrombotic thrombocytopenic purpura is a disorder of the coagulation system, leading to extensive clotting in small blood vessels. It may be acquired or inherited, and is characterized by fever, splenomegaly, thrombocytopenia, microangiopathic hemolytic anemia, transient neurologic deficits, and renal failure.

FIGURE 16.15. Image (A) shows an enlargement of splenic white pulp secondary to thrombotic thrombocytopenic purpura. Hyperplasia of white pulp is considered a reactive process. Image (B) shows a cross-section that reveals an increased number of white pulp nodules secondary to follicular hyperplasia.

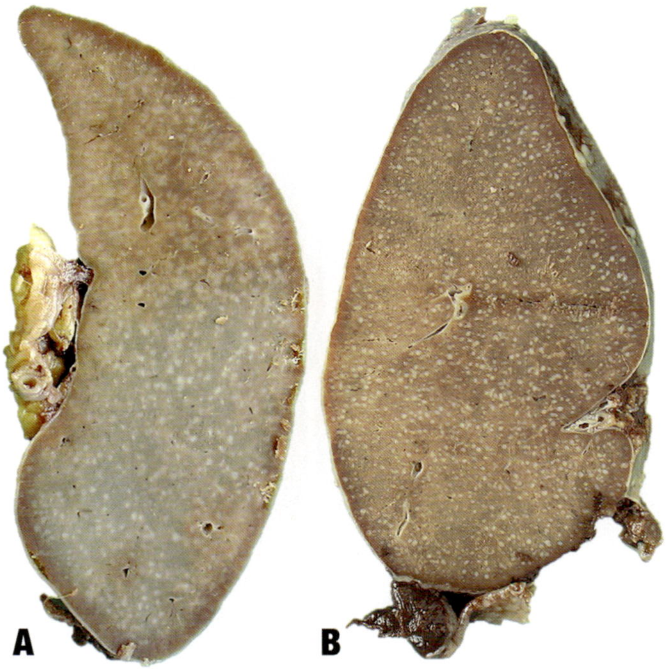

Sickle cell disease and hemangioma

Sickle-cell disease is a common hereditary hemoglobinopathy caused by a mutation in β-globin. This mutation leads to red blood cell distortion and ischemic damage of tissue. It has an autosomal recessive pattern of inheritance.

Hemangiomas are the most common primary neoplasia of the spleen. They are often < 2 cm. Hemangiomas are usually clinically silent, but they can be associated with anemia, thrombocytopenia, and consumption coagulopathy (Kasabach–Merritt syndrome).

FIGURE 16.16. These images show sickle cell disease and hemangioma present in 1 patient. The spleen appears atrophic due to autoinfarction. The cut surface of the spleen reveals discrete, red, soft nodules at the lower part of the specimen, which proved to be hemangioma on histological examination.

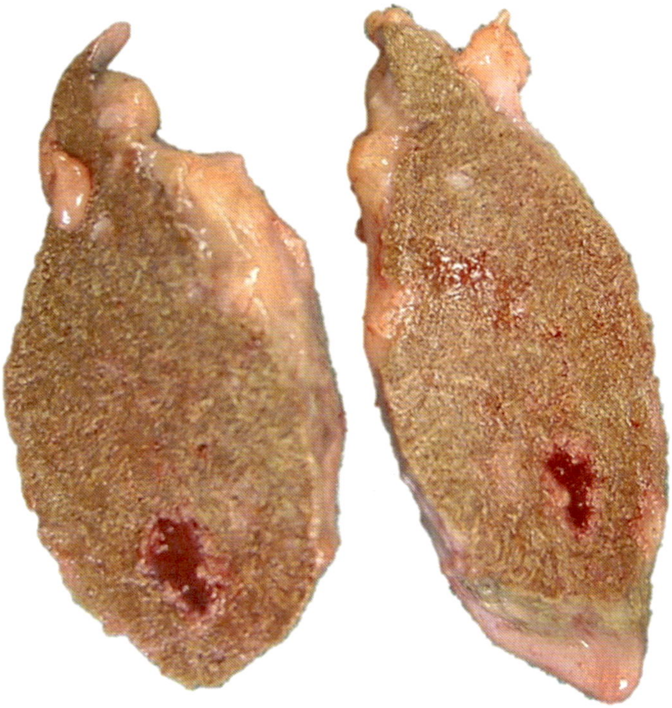

Infectious mononucleosis

Epstein–Barr virus (EBV) infection can cause infectious mononucleosis and certain lymphomas. The infection itself may affect the lymph nodes, liver, and spleen. EBV-infected spleens are especially vulnerable to rupture.

FIGURE 16.17. Image (A) shows a lateral view of a large soft, fleshy, congested spleen from a patient with infectious mononucleosis. Image (B) shows a medial view.

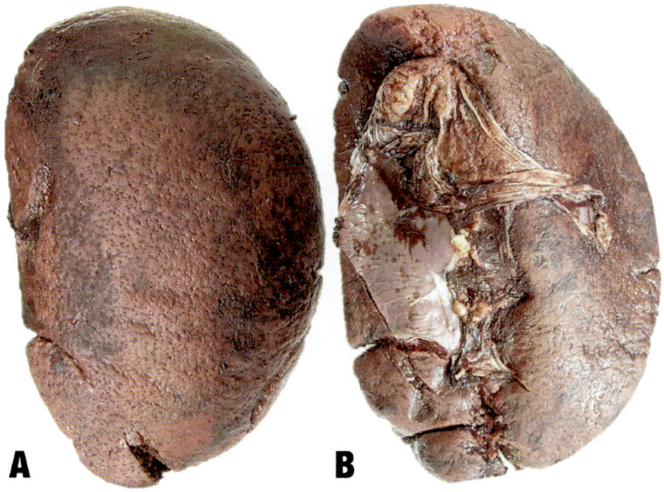

Sclerosing angiomatoid nodular transformation

Sclerosing angiomatoid nodular transformation of the spleen is a benign, reactive process caused by the pathologic increased stromal proliferation of splenic red pulp. Cases may be asymptomatic, or present as splenomegaly or with abdominal pain.

FIGURE 16.18. This image shows multiple prominent nodules of red pulp that are vaguely arranged in a lobular architecture surrounded by a fibrous shell.

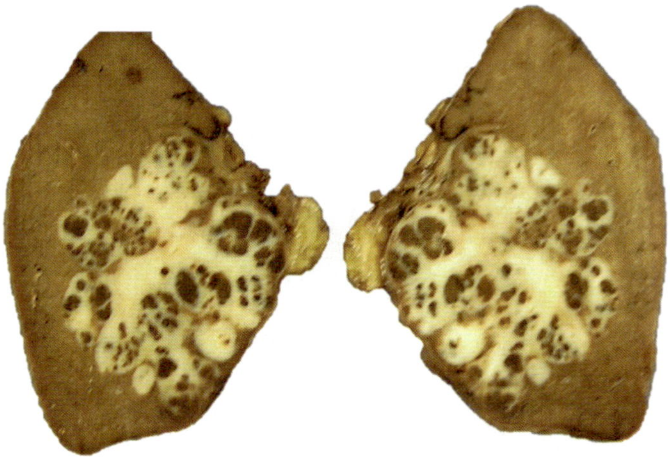

Spleen congestion

Splenomegaly and congestion can result from reactions to systemic diseases (e.g., infection) or from hematological disorders (e.g., thrombocytopenia). The most common cause of spleen congestion is portal hypertension.

FIGURE 16.19. These images show an enlarged spleen with a beefy-red cut surface.

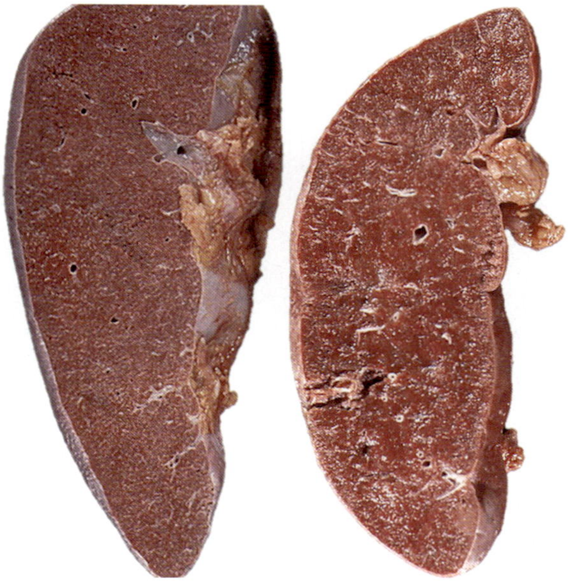

Spleen infarction

Any factor that compromises the splenic artery can cause infarction. These factors include trauma, thromboembolization due to atherosclerosis, hematological disorders, and others.

FIGURE 16.20. These images show infarcted tissue that is necrotic. The triangular distribution of the infarcted area is due to the compromised circulation of the artery feeding that area.

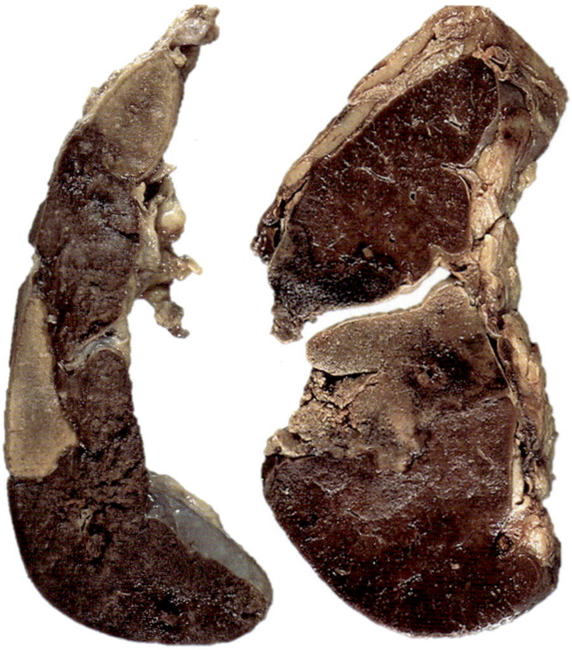

Perisplenitis

Perisplenitis is an incidental finding at autopsy and is usually associated with portal hypertension.

FIGURE 16.21. This image shows thick, fibrous plaques coating the splenic surface.

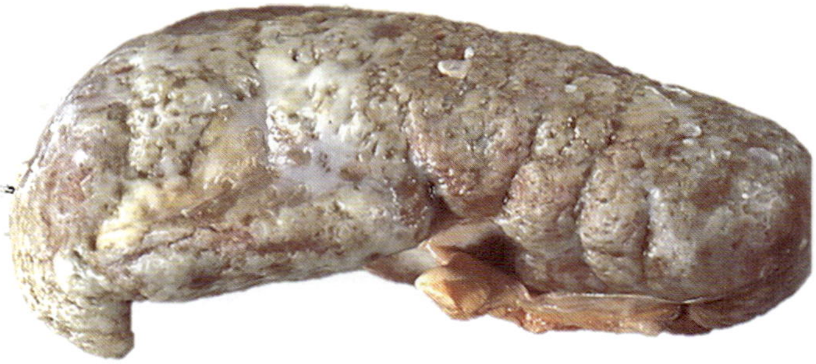

Malakoplakia

Malakoplakia is a rare granulomatous disease due to an acquired defect in phagocytic function. It commonly arises in the setting of *Escherichia coli* infection, and commonly occurs in the genitourinary tract. Histologically, it is characterized by numerous macrophages containing laminated calcified concretions called Michaelis–Gutmann bodies.

FIGURE 16.22. This image shows a distinct lesion with central necrosis in the spleen.

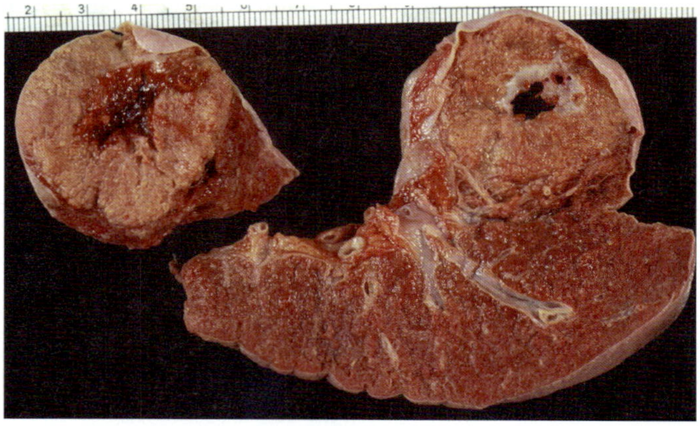

Splenic diffuse large B-cell lymphoma (DLBCL)

Lymphoma is the most common malignant tumor of the spleen. The 2 most common primary splenic tumors are DLBCL and splenic marginal zone lymphoma. DLBCL is a highly aggressive type of lymphoma.

FIGURE 16.23. This image shows 3 irregular, fleshy-colored tumors of variable size invading the splenic parenchyma. One tumor is transgressing the capsule. Histologic examination demonstrated atypical large B cells.

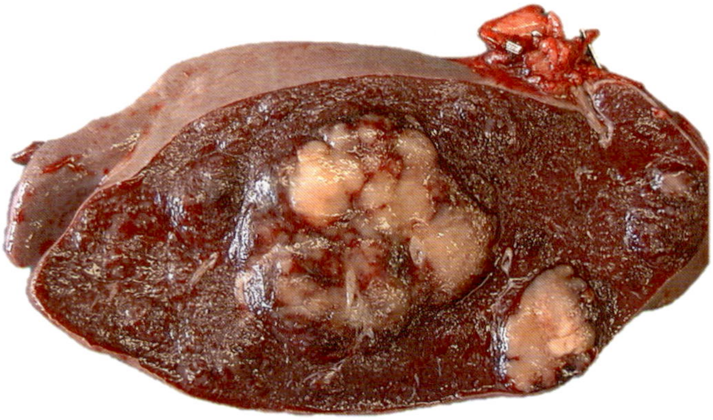

Acute myeloid leukemia (AML)

AML is a type of cancer in which the bone marrow makes abnormal myeloblasts (a type of white blood cell), red blood cells, or platelets. Spleen enlargement in AML can result from compensation for bone marrow failure, or from direct infiltration by tumor cells.

FIGURE 16.24. This image shows spleen enlargement from direct infiltration by tumor cells in AML.

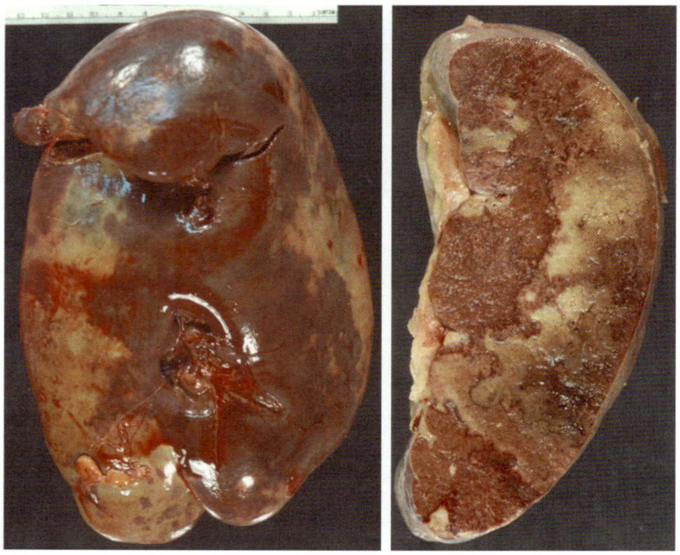

Metastasis to the spleen

Common metastases to the spleen include carcinomas arising from the lung, gastrointestinal tract, breast, and ovary, or from melanoma. Splenic metastases, however, rarely cause clinical symptoms.

FIGURE 16.25. This image shows a well-circumscribed, large, beige tumor with a necrotic center within the splenic parenchyma. Histologic examination confirmed that it was a metastatic carcinoma from the lung.

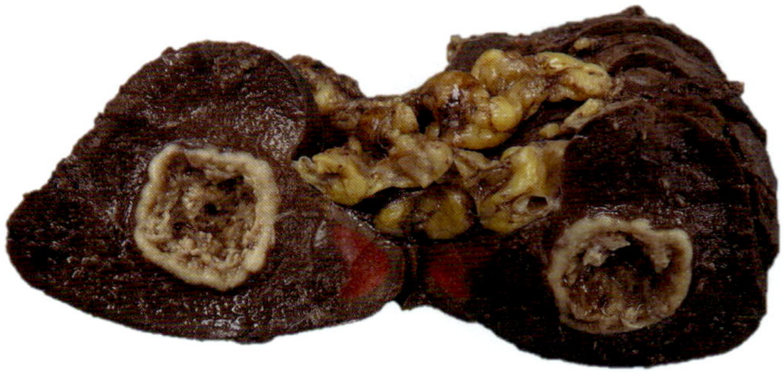

ACKNOWLEDGMENTS

We would like to thank Dr. R. Michel, Dr. R. Amre, and Dr. D. Haegert for their valuable contributions. We would also like to thank R. Gilot, E. Griss, A. Hossain, L. Korneichyuk Pasyuk, M. Mikhael, and E. Yaney for their technical help.

REFERENCES

Kumar V, Abbas AK, Aster JC. *Robbins and Cotran pathologic basis of disease*. 9th ed. Philadelphia: Saunders/Elsevier; 2015.

Lester SC. Chapter 27: Spleen. *Manual of surgical pathology*. 3nd ed. Philadelphia: Elsevier Churchill Livingstone; 2010. p. 517–528

Mills SE, Carter D, Greenson JK, Hornick JL, Longacre TA, Reuter VE, editors. *Sternberg's diagnostic surgical pathology*. 6th ed. Philadelphia: Wolters Kluwer Health; 2015.

Ovalle WK, Nahirney PC. *Netter's essential histology*. 2nd ed. Philadelphia: Saunders/Elsevier; 2013.

Rosai J. *Rosai and Ackerman's surgical pathology*. 10th ed. Edinburgh, NY: Mosby/Elsevier; 2011.

Travis WD, Brambilla E, Burke AP, Marx A, Nicholson AG. *WHO classification of tumours of the lung, pleura, thymus and heart*. Lyon, France: IARC Press; 2015.

17

Diseases of the Placenta and Fetus

MOY FONG CHEN, LIFENG GU

Placenta

True knot

FIGURE 17.1. Image (A) shows the placenta of a stillbirth with a true knot and vascular compromise. Image (B) shows a true knot with no vascular sequela.

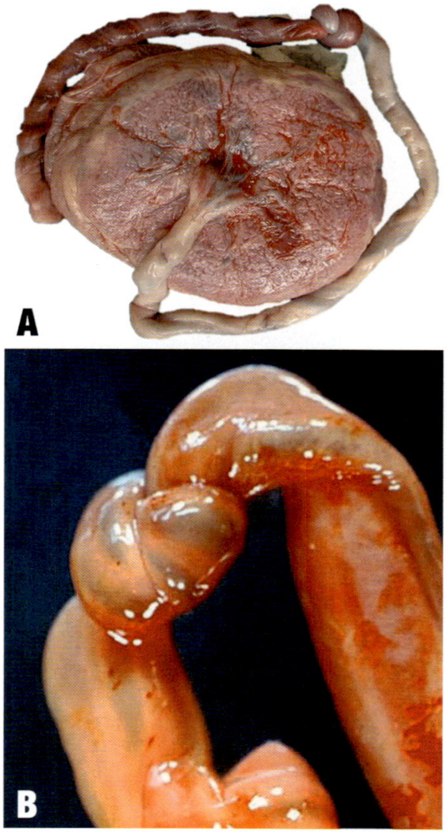

Thrombosis in the cord

FIGURE 17.2. This image shows thrombosis in the cord (arrow).

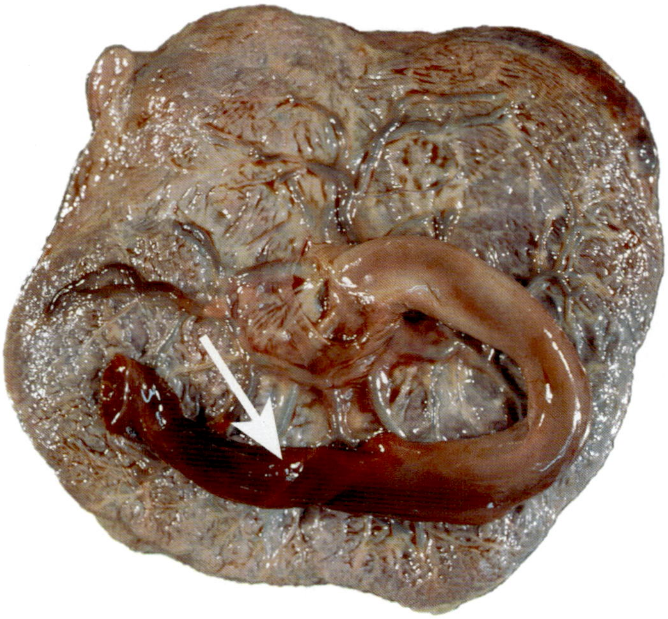

Velamentous insertion of the cord

Velamentous insertion of the cord could result in rupture or thrombosis.

FIGURE 17.3. This image shows velamentous insertion of the cord.

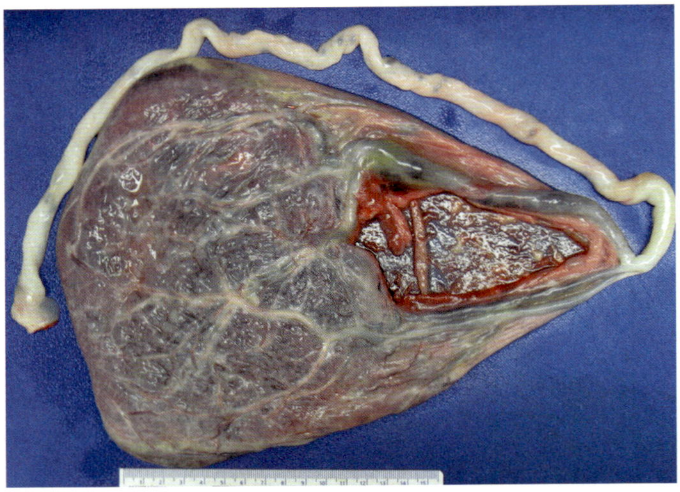

Circummarginate placenta

Circummargination usually has no particular associated changes in the placenta.

FIGURE 17.5. This image of a circummarginate placenta shows surface chorionic vessels foreshortened from the margin of the chorionic plate.

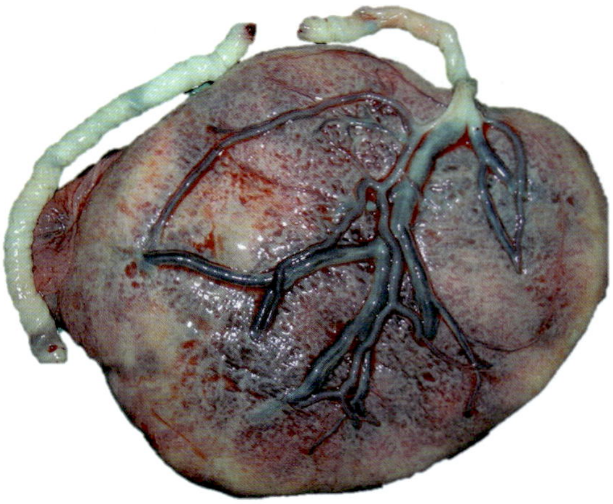

Circumvallate placenta

Circumvallate placenta often shows marginal retroplacental thrombosis or hemorrhage.

FIGURE 17.4. This gross specimen shows a circumvallate placenta with a ring of membranes on the fetal surface.

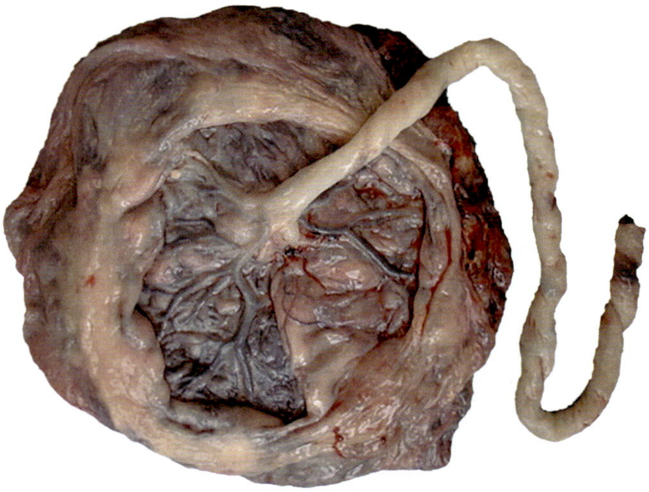

Severe chorioamnionitis

Severe chorioamnionitis is often a complication of the premature rupture of membranes.

FIGURE 17.6. In this example of severe chorioamnionitis with a history of prolonged premature rupture of membranes, note the opaque fetal surface.

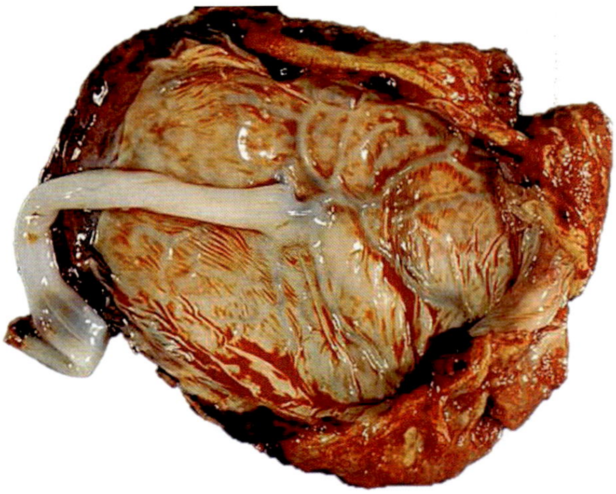

Amnion nodosum

Amnion nodosum is an amniotic surface phenomenon with decreased amniotic fluid.

FIGURE 17.7. Image (A) shows a stippled and granular fetal surface (amnion nodosum) in a case of severe oligohydramnios. Image (B) gives a close-up view of the same specimen.

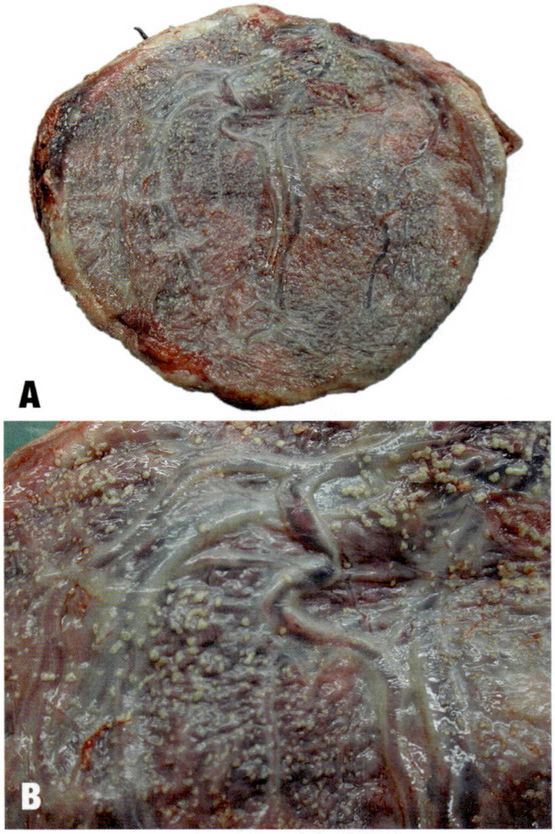

Meconium-stained placenta

Meconium-stained placenta is a sign of fetal distress.

FIGURE 17.8. This image shows a placenta with a green fetal surface.

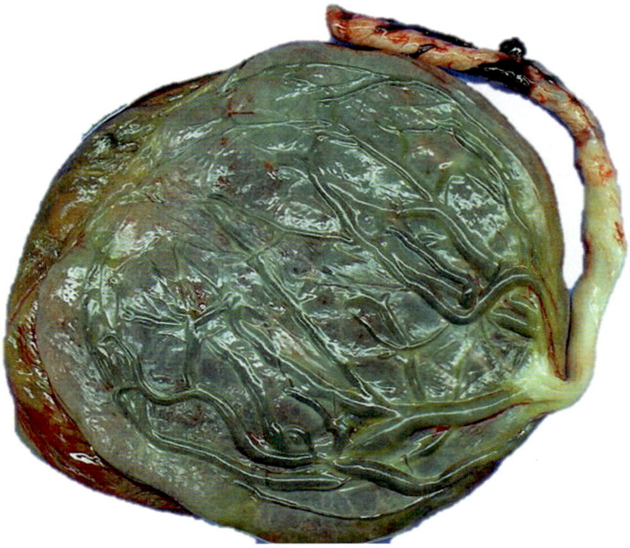

Subchorionic thrombohematoma presenting as a cyst (Breus mole)

FIGURE 17.9. This is a subchorionic cyst on the surface of the placenta filled with organized blood clots.

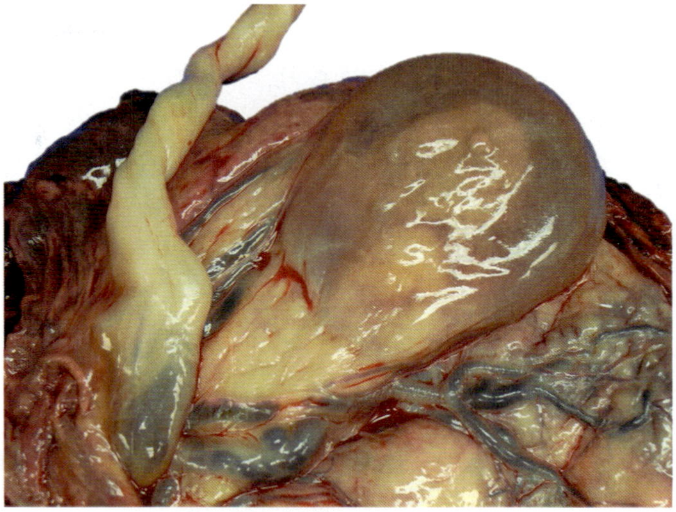

Villous infarction

Typically, remote villous infarctions appear pale, and recent villous infarctions appear red.

FIGURE 17.10. Image (A) shows the maternal surface of a placenta with multiple pale lesions. In (B), serial cut surfaces show pale and red lesions.

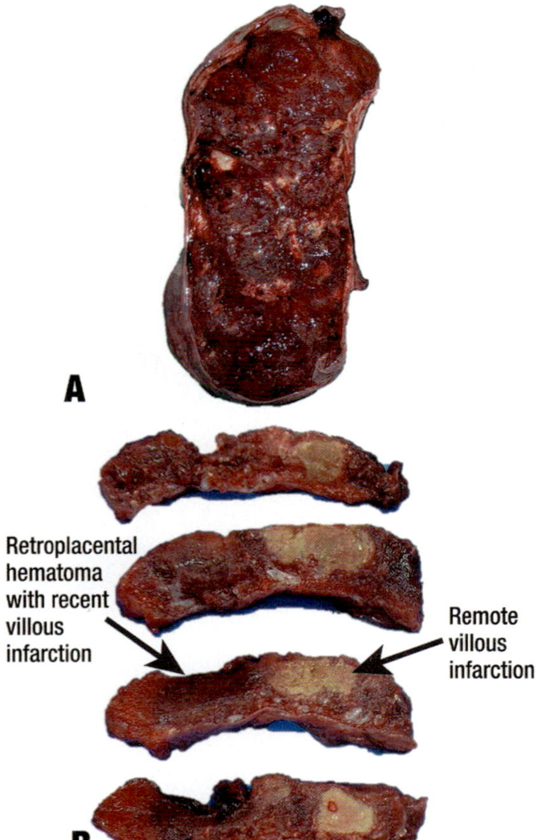

Thrombotic fetal vasculopathy

Thrombotic fetal vasculopathy has been associated with the late development of cerebral palsy.

FIGURE 17.11. Image (A) shows a close-up view of a thrombotic chorionic vein. In (B), thrombotic chorionic vessels appear pale on the surface. They were firm to the touch.

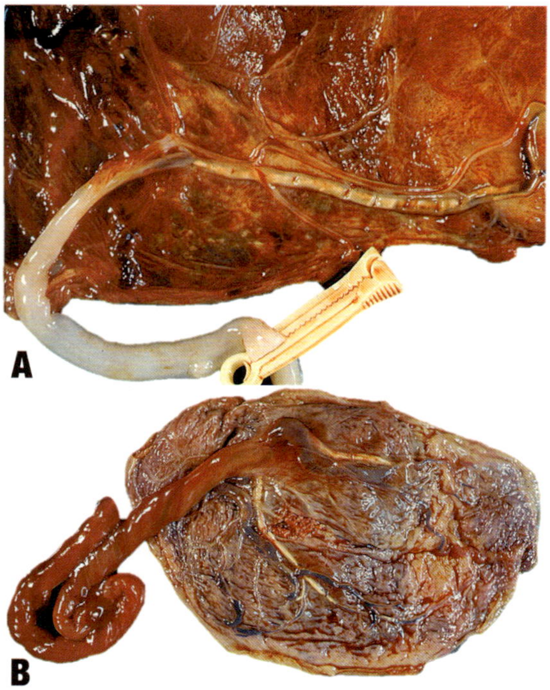

Chorangioma

Chorangioma is a benign hemangioma of the placenta. Small tumors have no clinical significance; large tumors can shunt blood across the tumor, and are associated with congestive heart failure, polyhydramnios, and premature delivery.

FIGURE 17.12. This image shows a well-circumscribed red homogeneous mass. Microscopy revealed proliferation of small vessels lined by benign endothelium.

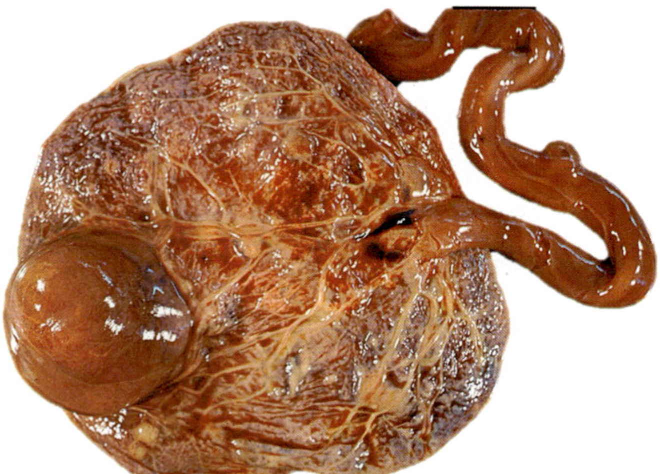

Hydropic placenta and fetal anemia

Hydropic placenta can be a manifestation of fetal anemia.

FIGURE 17.13. The pale and hydropic placenta in (A) correlates with an anemic and hydropic fetus, and can be a manifestation of parvovirus infection. Image (B) shows an example of fetal hydrops.

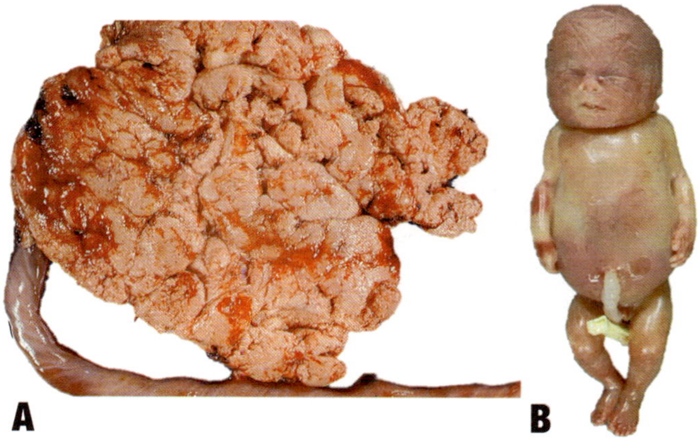

Massive intervillous fibrin

Massive intervillous fibrin, when extensive, can cause placental insufficiency.

FIGURE 17.14. This image shows the maternal surface of a placenta with pale and firm lesions (arrows).

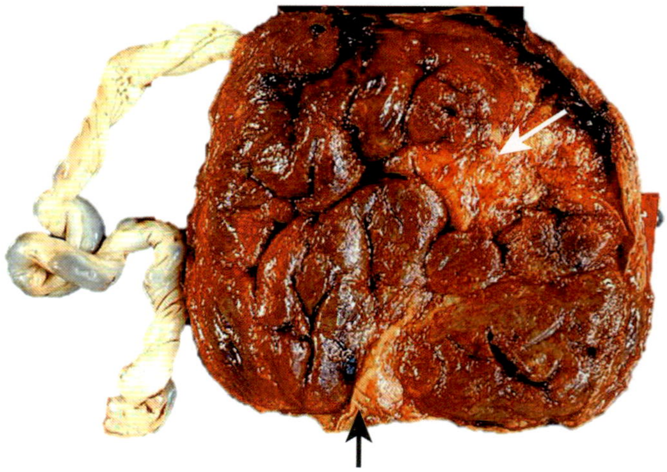

Unusual molar change

FIGURE 17.15. This specimen shows an unusual partial mole in a twin placenta. Note the grape-like tissue (arrow) indicating molar changes.

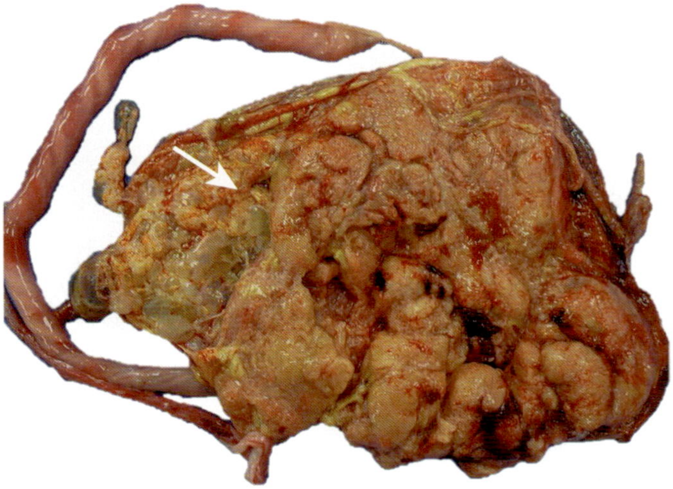

Mesenchymal dysplasia

FIGURE 17.16. The prominent sausage-like superficial vessels visible in this image are a clue to mesenchymal dysplasia of the placenta.

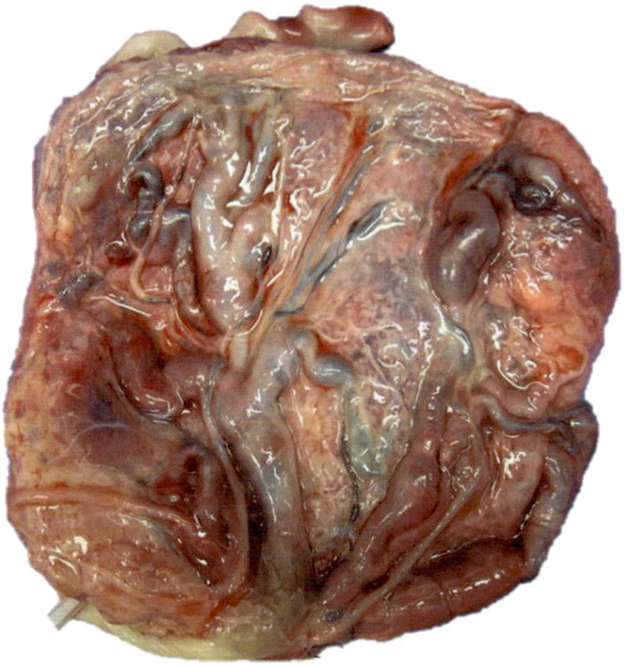

Placenta abruption

Retroplacental hematoma is typically seen in acute cases of abruption. Placental abruption is a common cause of asphyxia of the newborn.

FIGURE 17.17. Image (A) shows a retroplacental hematoma. Image (B) shows pleural and epicardial petechial hemorrhages, which are typically seen in cases of asphyxia of the newborn.

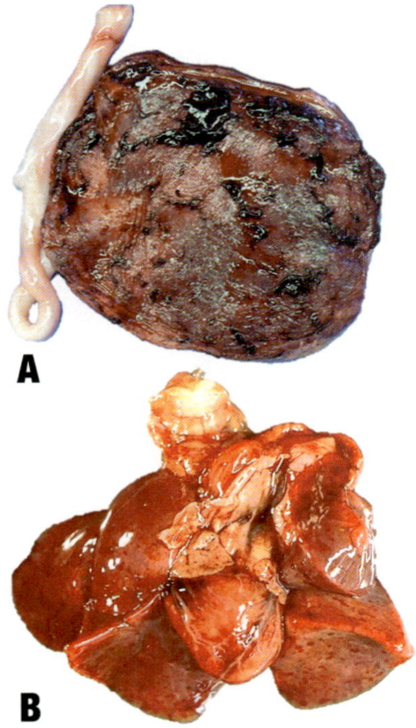

Maternal floor infarction

Maternal floor infarction is a cause of placental insufficiency and can recur in subsequent pregnancies.

FIGURE 17.18. Image (A) shows a cerebriform maternal surface. Image (B) shows a corrugated maternal (decidual) surface, which correlates with lesions of maternal floor infarction.

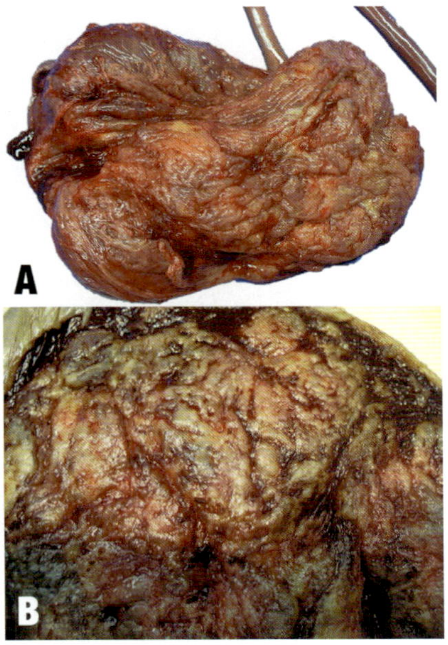

Fused dichorionic diamniotic placenta

Dichorionic placenta can occur in monozygotic (identical) or dizygotic twins.

FIGURE 17.19. This image shows a fused dichorionic diamniotic placenta with a thick septum.

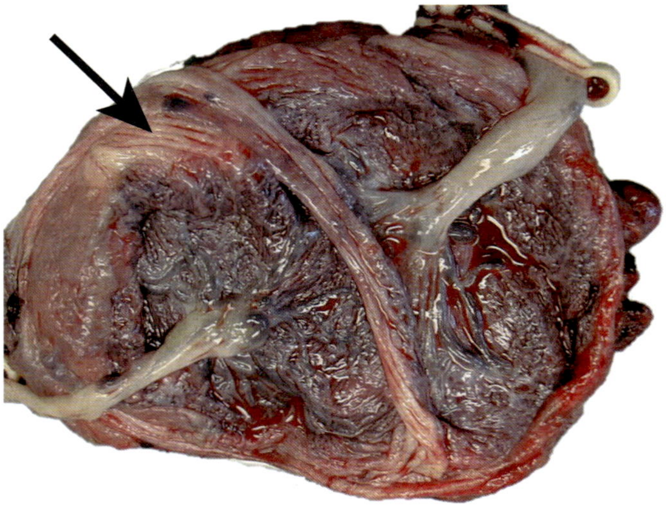

Monochorionic monoamniotic placenta

A monochorionic monoamniotic placenta is always monozygotic.

FIGURE 17.21. Notice the absence of a septum in this placenta.

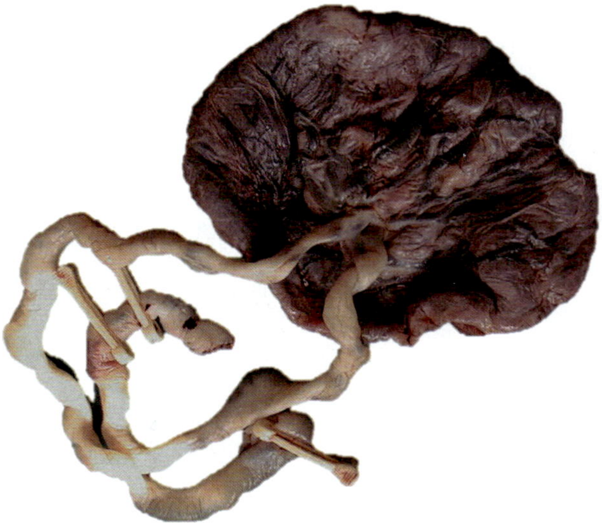

Monochorionic diamniotic placenta

Monochorionic diamniotic placentas occur exclusively in monozygotic (identical) twins. In twin–twin transfusion syndrome, arteriovenous shunts are present in the twin fetal circulation; these preferentially increase blood flow to 1 twin leading to underperfusion of the other twin. Severe forms of the disease can be lethal to 1 or both twins.

FIGURE 17.20. Image (A) shows a fetal surface with vessels crossing the septum (arrow). In (B), a maternal surface with unequal perfusion shows a dark red area on the right belonging to the recipient twin in a case of twin–twin transfusion syndrome.

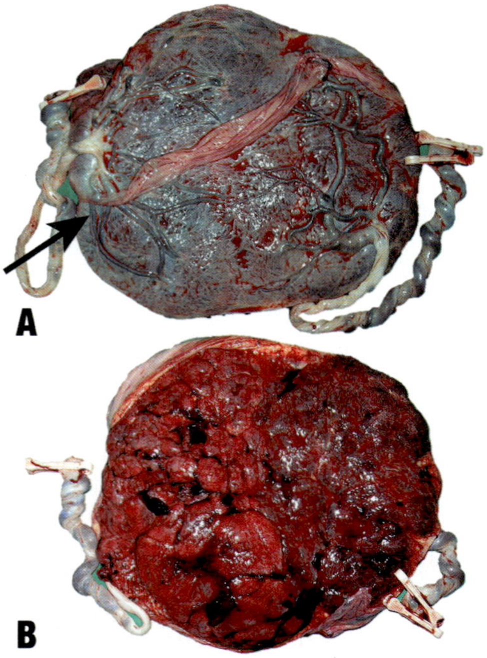

Fetus papyraceus

Fetus papyraceus occurs in multiple pregnancy when a fetus with early intrauterine demise becomes mummified. When the death happens very early (less than 8 weeks old), it can be absorbed into the placenta or become an amorphous mass.

FIGURE 17.22. Image (A) shows a case of fetus papyraceus with a mummified fetus and sclerotic placenta in the context of monochorionic diamniotic twins. Image (B) shows an amorphous mass in the placenta due to early death.

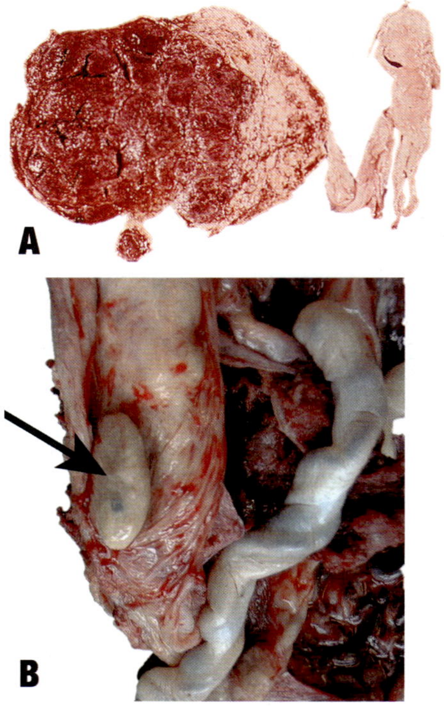

Fetus

Fetal Malformations

Trisomy 21 (Down) syndrome

Trisomy 21 (Down) syndrome is the most common chromosomal disorder; it occurs in 1 per 700 births. Characteristic features are: brachycephaly (short head); flat facial profile with oblique palpebral fissures and epicanthic folds; microtia and thickened nuchal folds; congenital heart defects; umbilical hernia; intestinal stenosis; hypotonia; simian crease; and a gap between the first and second toe. Affected children have intellectual disability, and are also 10 to 20 times more likely to develop leukemia.

FIGURE 17.23. Image (A) shows a thickened nuchal fold. Image (B) shows a specimen with brachycephaly and small ears.

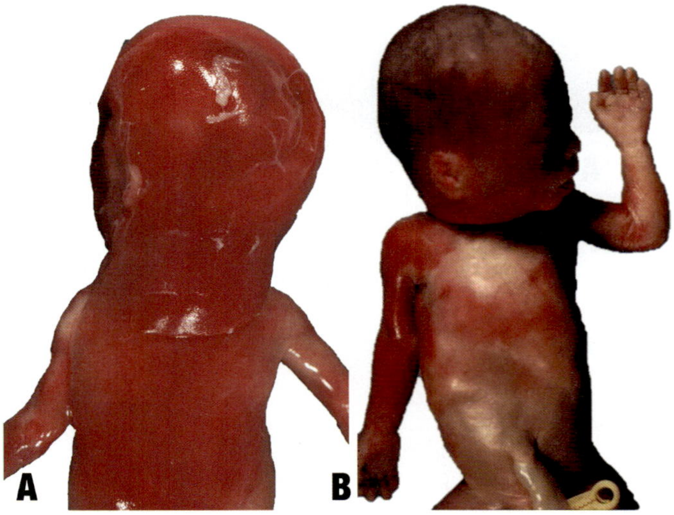

FIGURE 17.24. Image (A) shows a simian crease of the hand. Image (B) shows an example of persistent common atrioventricular canal (arrow), a congenital heart malformation.

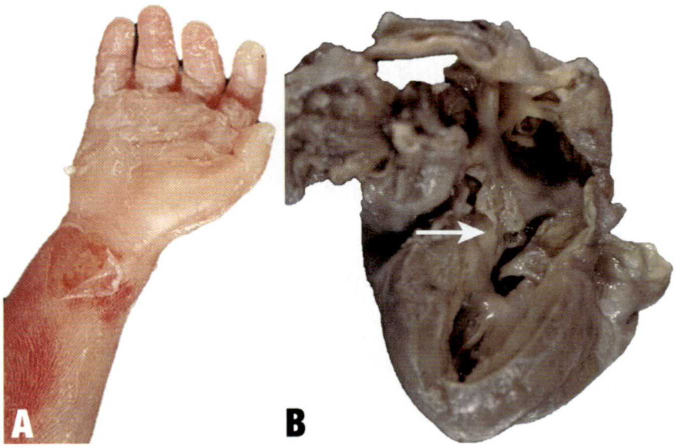

Trisomy 18 (Edwards) syndrome

Trisomy 18 (Edwards) syndrome occurs in 1 per 8000 births. It is associated with advanced maternal age, and can present with a constellation of features, such as craniofacial abnormalities (misshapen ears, prominent occiput, micrognathia, short neck); cardiac and renal defects; gastrointestinal defects (e.g., hernias and omphalocele); limited hip abduction; overlapping fingers; and rocker-bottom feet. Most infants succumb in the first year of life.

FIGURE 17.25. These images show fetuses with features of trisomy 18 (Edwards) syndrome: (A) omphalocele; and (B) micrognathia and misshapen ear lobules.

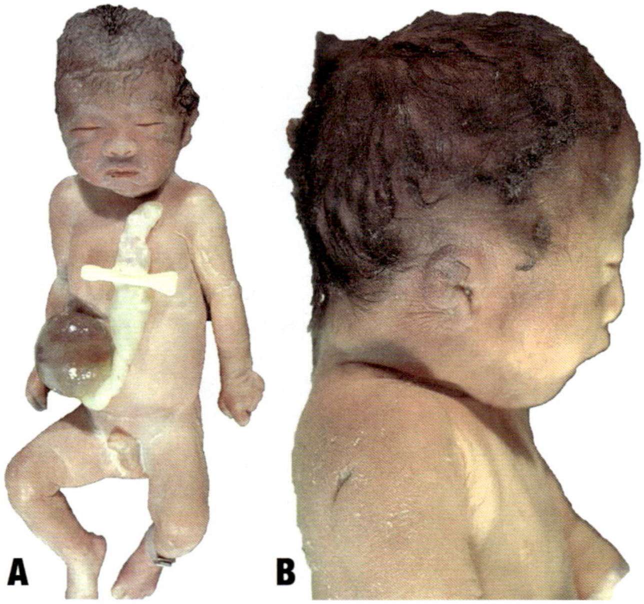

FIGURE 17.26. This image shows a case of trisomy 18 (Edwards) syndrome with a ventricular septal defect, a congenital heart malformation.

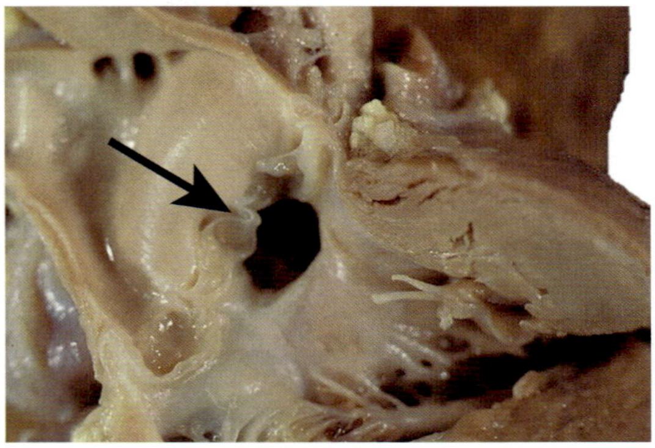

FIGURE 17.27. Images (A) and (B) show trisomy 18 (Edwards) syndrome specimens with (A) club foot and (B) rocker-bottom foot.

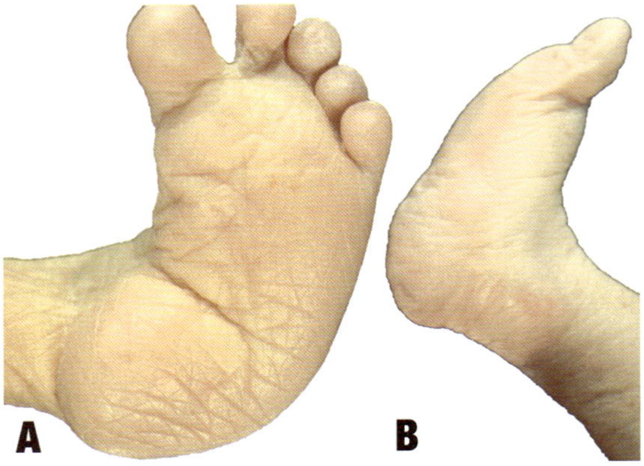

FIGURE 17.28. A fetus with trisomy 18 (Edwards) syndrome shows overlapping fingers with a prominent flexed index finger.

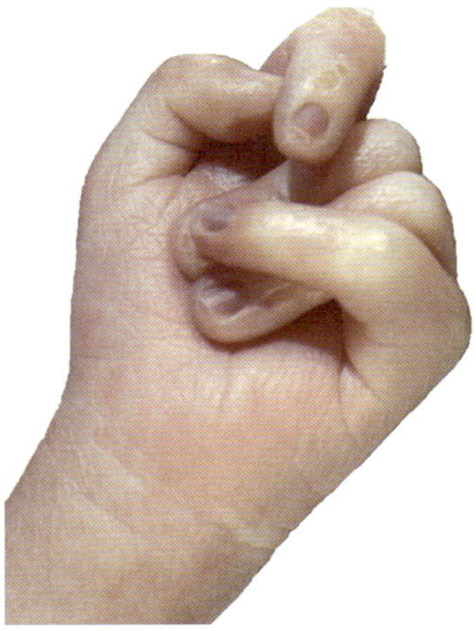

Trisomy 13 (Patau) syndrome

Trisomy 13 (Patau) syndrome occurs in 1 per 15 000 births and is associated with advanced maternal age. It causes severe malformations, including microcephaly and holoprosencephaly; cardiac and renal defects; cleft lip and palate; umbilical hernia; polydactyly; and rocker-bottom feet. Most infants succumb in the first year of life.

FIGURE 17.29. These images show fetuses with trisomy 13 (Patau) syndrome. Image (A) shows a midline cleft lip and palate, and hypotelorism. Image (B) shows cyclopia, an extreme form of midline facial defect.

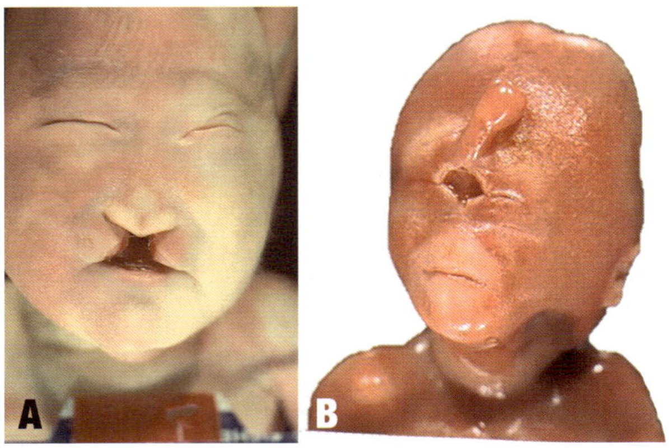

FIGURE 17.30. Images (A) and (B) show trisomy 13 (Patau) syndrome fetuses with holoprosencephaly, which encompasses a spectrum of malformations distinguished by incomplete separation of the cerebral hemispheres across the midline.

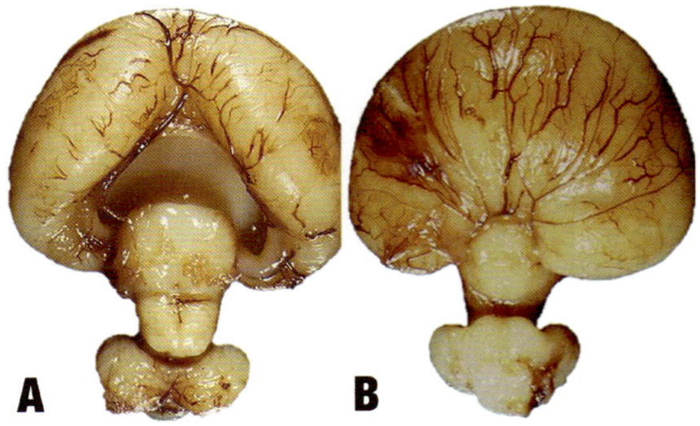

FIGURE 17.31. These images of trisomy 13 (Patau) syndrome fetuses display cardiac defects: (A) bicuspid aortic valve defect (arrow), and (B) atrial septal defect.

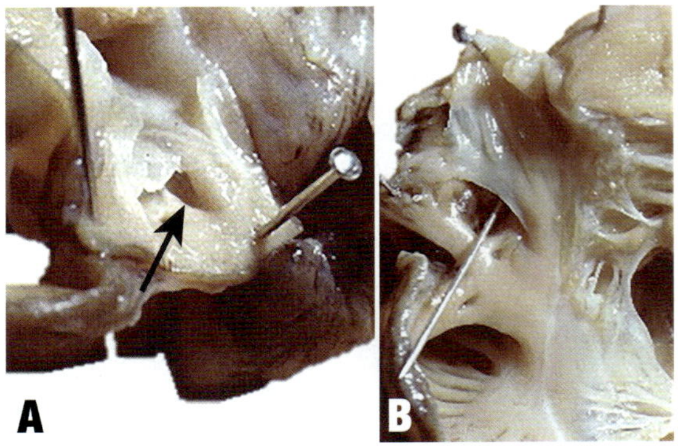

FIGURE 17.32. These images show polydactyly (extra digits) in (A) the hand and (B) the foot.

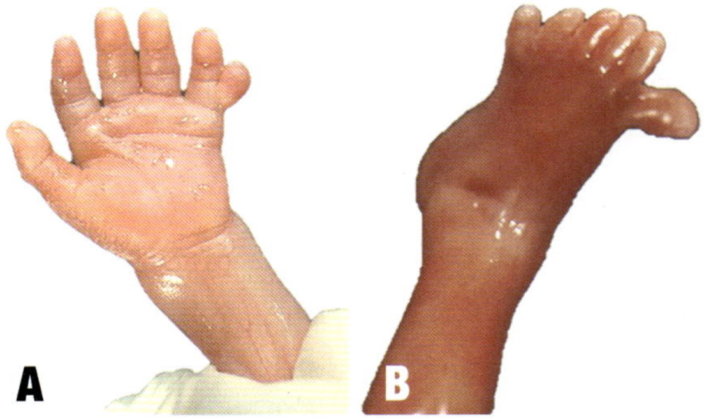

FIGURE 17.33. This image shows an example of cutis aplasia, a typical scalp defect seen in trisomy 13 (Patau) syndrome.

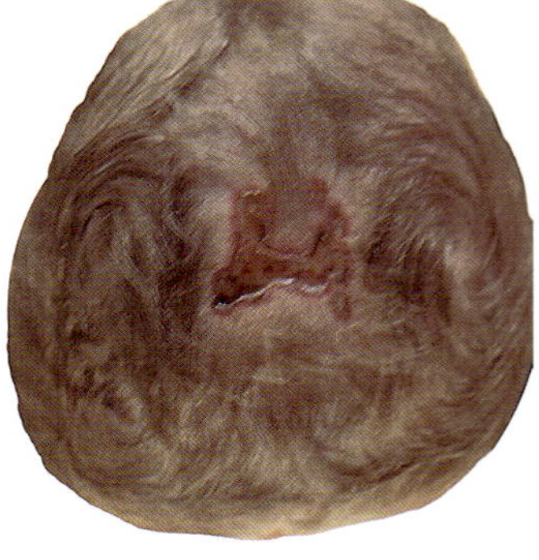

Turner syndrome

Turner syndrome results from partial or complete monosomy of the short arm of the X chromosome. It occurs in 1 per 3000 female births. Characteristic features are short stature, widely spaced nipples, cystic hygroma, coarctation of the aorta, streak ovaries, pigmented nevi, and peripheral lymphedema. Horseshoe kidney is another possible defect, and occurs in 15% of Turner syndrome cases.

FIGURE 17.34. Image (A) shows horseshoe kidney in a case of Turner syndrome. Image (B) shows preductal coarctation of the aorta (arrow).

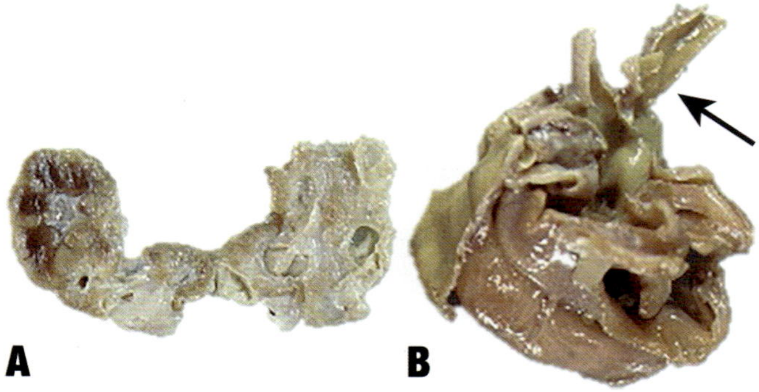

FIGURE 17.35. Images (A) and (B) demonstrate cystic hygroma, which occurs in the posterior triangle of the neck.

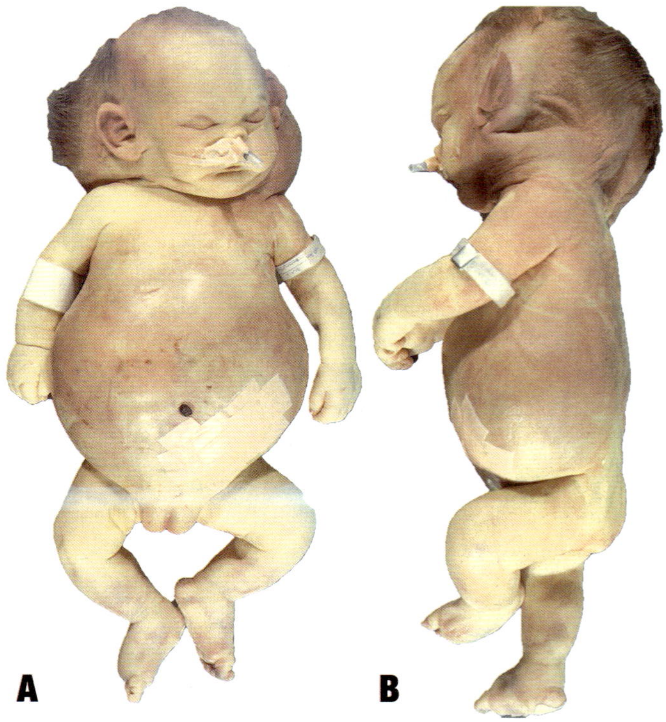

FIGURE 17.36. Images (A) and (B) show a fetus with hydrops fetalis and cystic hygroma, which occur in the posterior triangle of the neck.

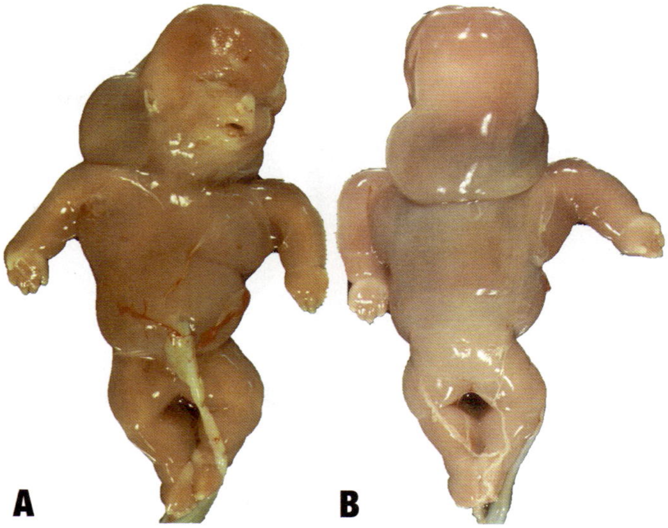

Triploidy

Triploidy (with 69,XXX; 69,XXY; or 69,XYY karyotypes) occurs in 1% of conceptions. Affected fetuses rarely survive past the first trimester. Growth restriction and major malformations (renal, cardiac, and brain) can occur. Syndactyly of the third and fourth digits of the hand is a characteristic feature. Triploidy can be associated with placental partial hydatidiform mole.

FIGURE 17.37. Image (A) shows a triploid female. Image (B) shows syndactyly of the third and fourth digits of the right hand and right foot.

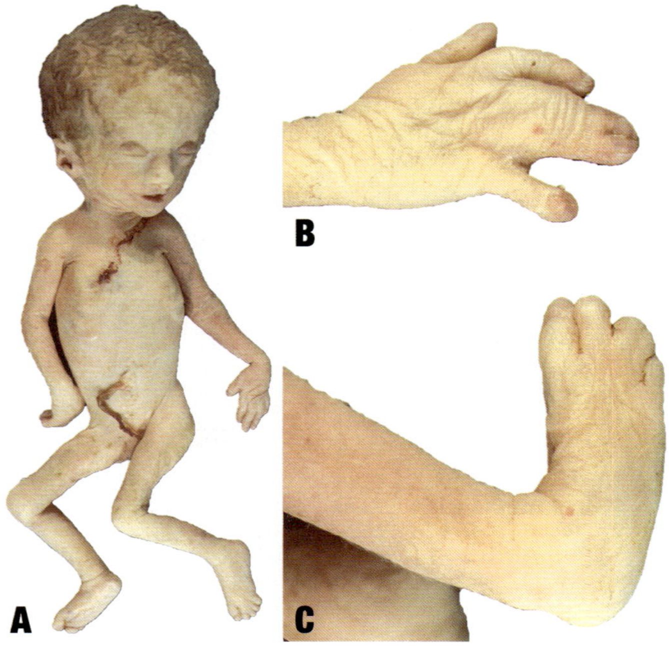

FIGURE 17.38. Image (A) shows another case of syndactyly in the third and fourth digits in the context of triploidy 69,XXX. Image (B) shows the double bubble sign due to atresia of distal duodenum.

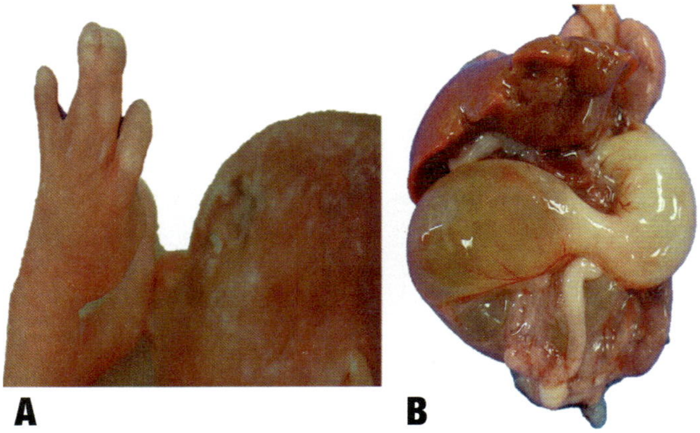

B courtesy of Dr. Eugenia Ducharne Asuaje

Neural tube defects

Neural tube defects encompass defects of primary neural tube closure (anencephaly and myelomeningocele), and mesodermal defects with herniation of neural tube tissue (encephalocele and meningocele). Folic acid supplement during pregnancy decreases, but does not eliminate, the incidence of these malformations.

ANENCEPHALY

Anencephaly occurs when the rostral end of the neural tube fails to close, resulting in a missing portion of brain, skull, and scalp.

FIGURE 17.39. This image shows an example of anencephaly. Note the lack of cranium with a residue of brain tissue.

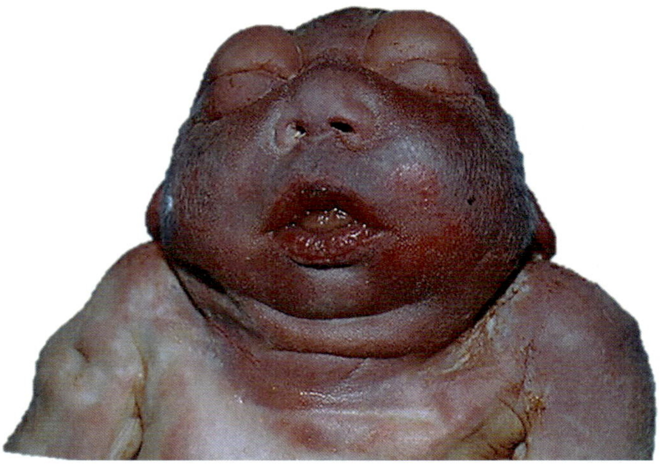

MENINGOCELE AND ENCEPHALOCELE

Meningocele is the herniation of meninges through a defect of the bony spine. Encephalocele is the herniation of brain tissue through a defect in the skull.

FIGURE 17.40. Image (A), an example of meningocele, shows a cystic mass covered by skin and containing cerebrospinal fluid (CSF). Image (B) shows an encephalocele specimen.

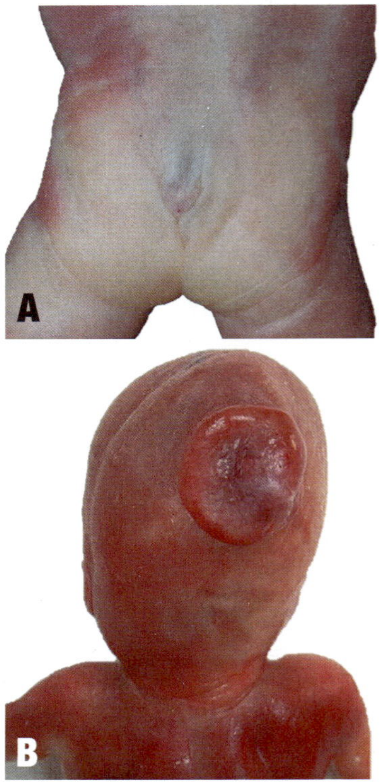

MYELOMENINGOCELE

In myelomeningocele, the caudal neural tube fails to fuse, leading to a defective open canal containing spinal cord tissue. Myelomeningocele is the most common condition associated with Arnold–Chiari malformation, in which deformities of the posterior fossa cause the cerebellar vermis to herniate through the foramen magnum, resulting in CSF obstruction and hydrocephalus.

FIGURE 17.41. Images (A) and (B) show examples of myelomeningocele. In (B), the specimen shows an open lesion with vascular connective tissue and disorganized neural tissue.

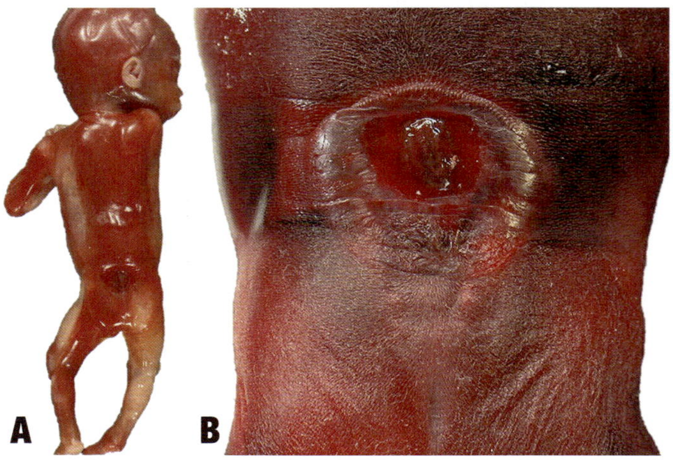

FIGURE 17.42. These images give examples of (A) myelomeningocele and (B) associated hydrocephalus. Note also the extended lower limbs.

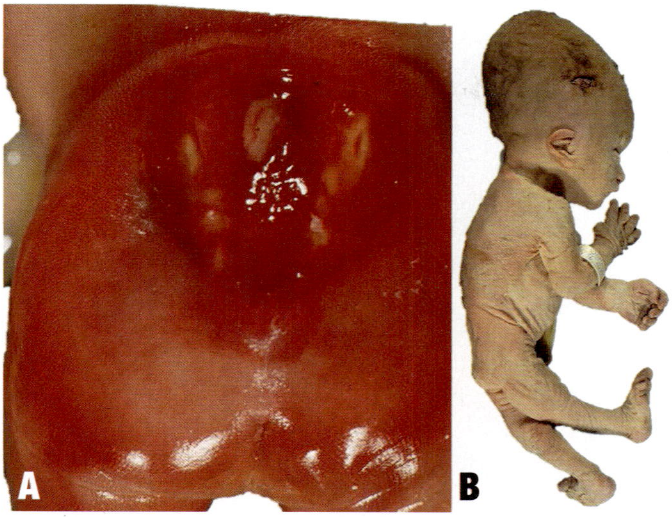

Potter syndrome and Potter sequence

Potter syndrome and Potter sequence designate the group of findings associated with oligohydramnios and renal failure. Potter syndrome results from renal agenesis. Potter sequence, by contrast, results from renal hypoplasia, renal cystic disease, or obstructive uropathy. Affected infants have aging Potter facies with dehydrated wrinkled skin, prominent epicanthal folds, flattened nose, recessed chin, and low-set ears. Positional deformities such as bowed legs and club feet also occur. Lung hypoplasia secondary to oligohydramnios can lead to pulmonary failure.

FIGURE 17.43. This image shows Potter facies. Note the dry skin and small chest.

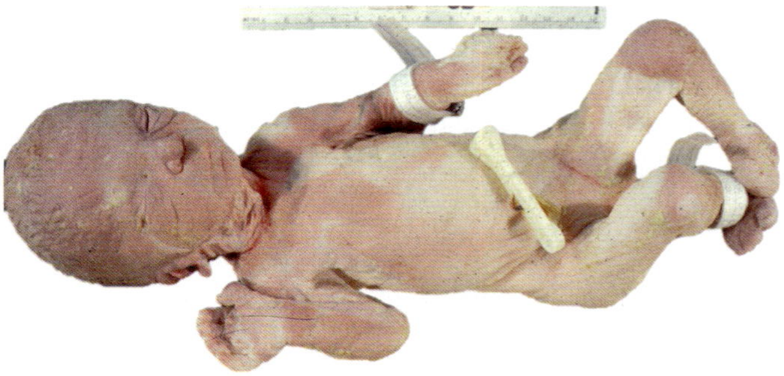

FIGURE 17.44. These images show (A) autosomal recessive polycystic kidney disease, and (B) left renal agenesis and right multicystic renal dysplasia in association with Potter sequence.

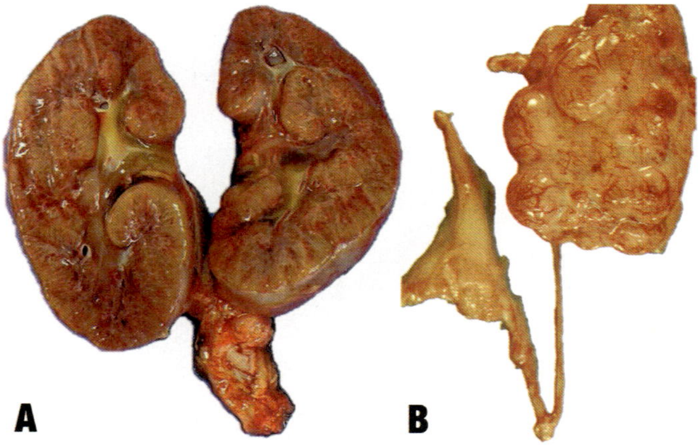

FIGURE 17.45. These images show Potter sequence fetuses with (A) wrinkled dehydrated skin; (B) bilateral renal aplasia; and (C) hypoplasia of the lungs.

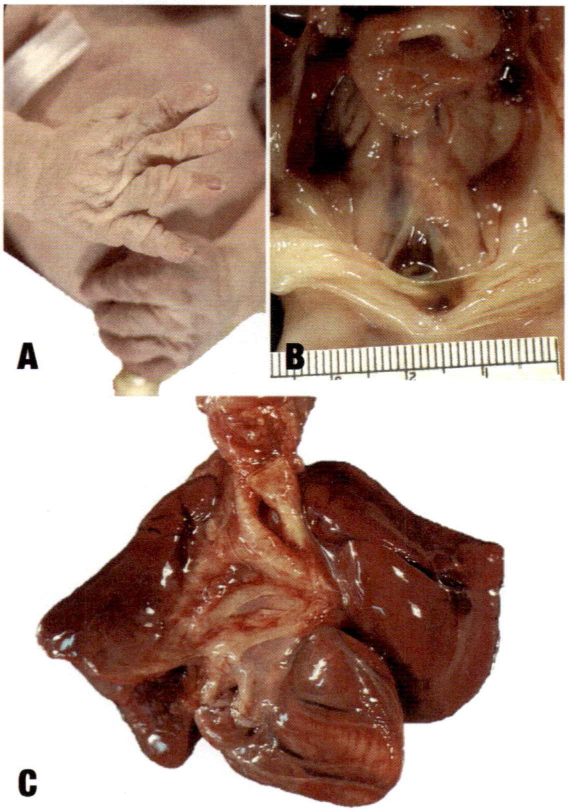

Anhydramnios

Anhydramnios — complete or near-complete lack of amniotic fluid — can occur in fetal renal tract anomalies and preterm premature rupture of membranes.

FIGURE 17.46. This image shows a fetus in a sac with a complete lack of amniotic fluid.

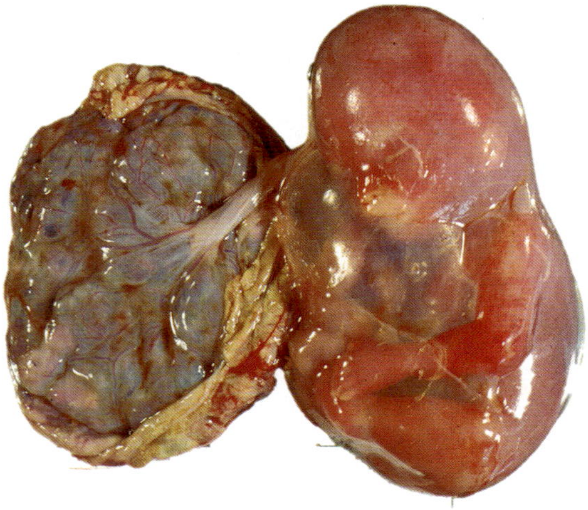

FIGURE 17.48. This image shows urethral stenosis with a markedly dilated bladder and cystic kidneys in a case of prune belly syndrome.

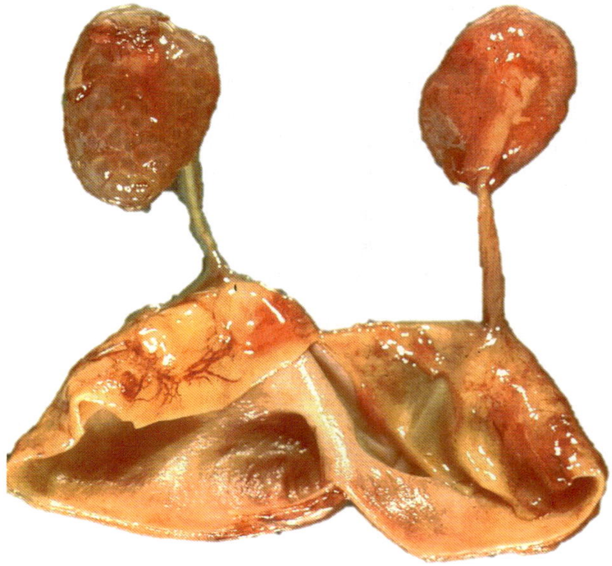

Prune belly (Eagle–Barrett) syndrome

Prune belly (Eagle–Barrett) syndrome mainly affects males, with an incidence of 1:30 000 to 1:40 000 live male births. Urinary tract defects (more specifically urethral obstructions) cause: hydroureter and hydronephrosis; degenerated abdominal muscles and wrinkled abdominal skin (much like a drying prune); and cryptorchidism (undescended testes). Secondary oligohydramnios also causes pulmonary hypoplasia and Potter facies.

FIGURE 17.47. Image (A) shows Potter facies and a bell-shaped chest due to bilateral lung hypoplasia. Image (B) shows prune belly and cryptorchidism.

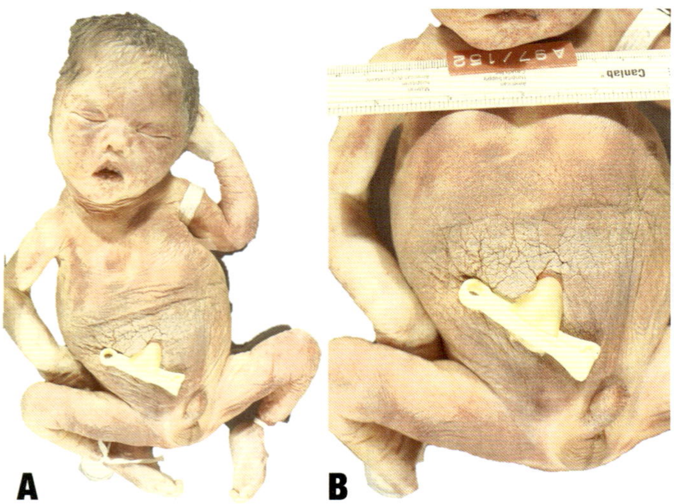

Achondroplasia

Achondroplasia is the most common skeletal dysplasia that causes dwarfism. It is an autosomal dominant disease, caused by gain-of-function mutations in *FGFR3*, whose main effect is suppression of cartilage growth. Patients have shortened proximal extremities, enlarged head with frontal bossing, and depression of the root of the nose; the trunk is of normal length. Usually, the condition does not affect survival, intelligence, or fertility. On microscopy, achondroplasia demonstrates no abnormal bone growth at the metaphysis of long bones, which contrasts with other bone dysplasias.

FIGURE 17.49. This fetus has extremely short limbs, a small chest, and a relatively large head and short neck.

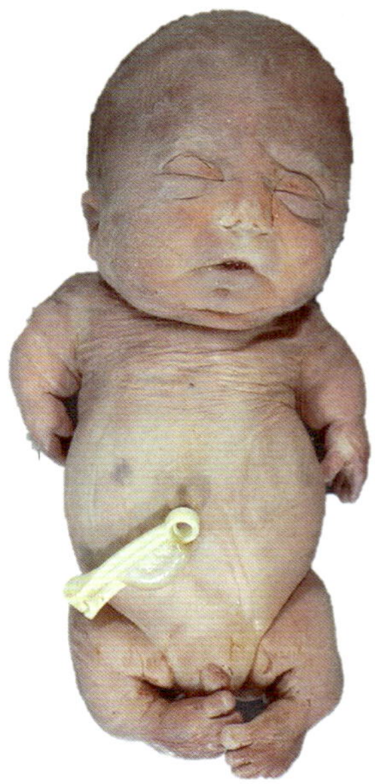

Thanatophoric dysplasia

Thanatophoric dysplasia is a lethal autosomal dominant disorder caused by a mutation in the *FGFR3* gene at 4p16.3. Affected patients have a characteristic form of dwarfism, with a short and bell-shaped thorax, a disproportionately large skull, prominent forehead, prominent eyes, a flat nasal bridge, and extremely short limbs. On microscopy, thanatophoric dysplasia demonstrates abnormal bone growth at the metaphysis of long bones.

FIGURE 17.50. Image (A) shows a case of thanatophoric dysplasia. The radiography in (B) shows a narrow thorax, short ribs, small iliac bone, short and broad long bones, and wide intervertebral spaces.

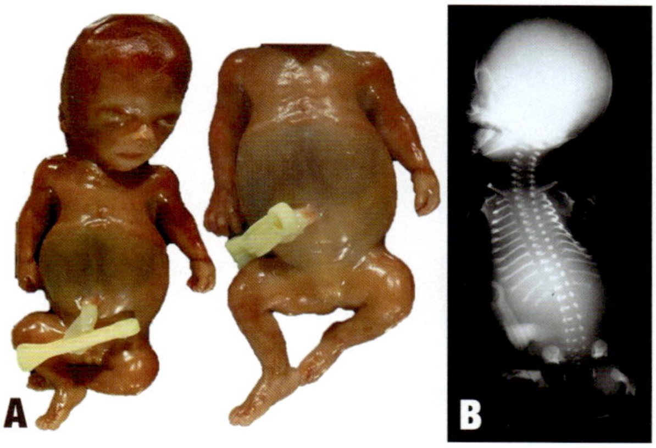

Osteogenesis imperfecta (OI)

OI is a group of inherited disorders due to defective synthesis of collagen type I. The main result is bone fragility with multiple fractures. Seven types of OI have been described, of varying severity. Type II is a lethal form with multiple congenital fractures; it is the most common form encountered in the perinatal period. Other types of OI may have extraskeletal manifestations such as blue sclera, hearing loss, and small teeth.

FIGURE 17.51. Image (A) shows an infant with short limbs with multiple bone fractures. Image (B) shows continuously beaded ribs due to multiple fractures. Image (C) shows multiple fractures of femur and tibia.

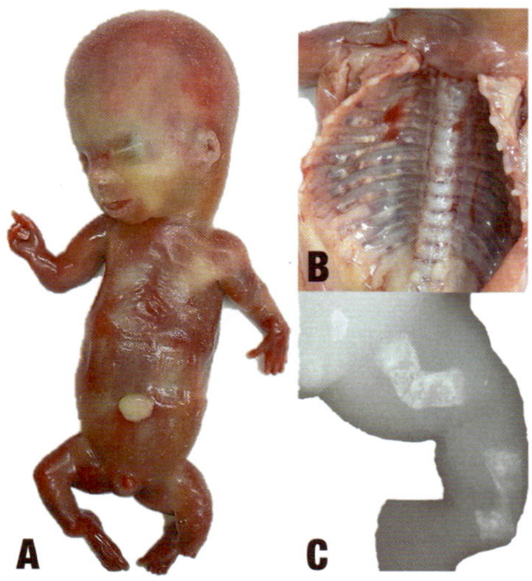

Diastrophic dysplasia

Diastrophic dysplasia is a rare autosomal recessive disease of cartilage and bone development due to mutations in the *SLC26A2* gene. The disorder manifests itself as short stature, arms, and legs; club foot; "hitchhiker" thumbs; abnormally curved spine; cleft palate; and ear anomalies.

FIGURE 17.52. Image (A) shows an example of dwarfism with short limbs. Image (B) shows the characteristic "hitchhiker" thumb. Image (C) shows a specimen with club foot.

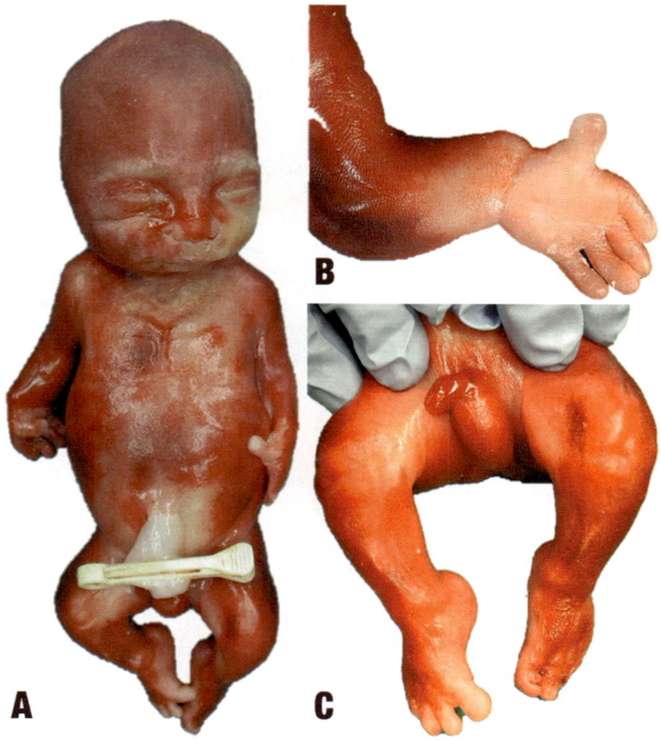

FIGURE 17.53. These images show features associated with diastrophic dysplasia: (A) micrognathia (arrow), and (B) cleft palate (arrow).

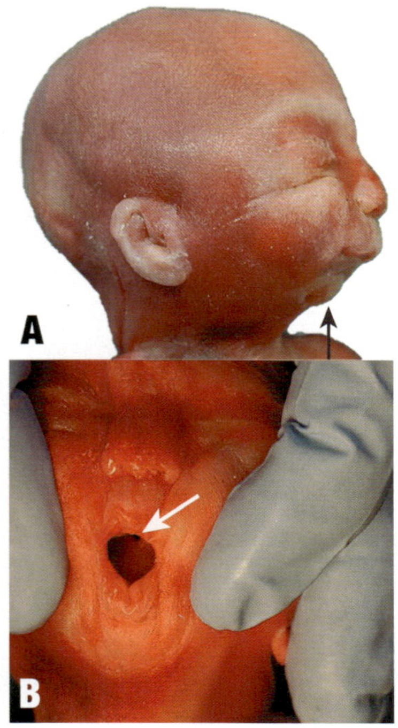

Fetal Membrane Disorders

Amniotic band syndrome

Amniotic bands, or constriction bands, are caused by rupture of the amniotic sac: fetal membranes from the sac form bands that can surround, compress, or adhere to fetal body parts. The bands result in disruption (extrinsic disturbance in morphogenesis) of a fetal organ or body region. The incidence of amniotic band syndrome is estimated as 1 per 70 spontaneous abortions, and 1 per 1300 to 2000 births.

FIGURE 17.54. This image shows disrupted fetal head growth from amniotic bands.

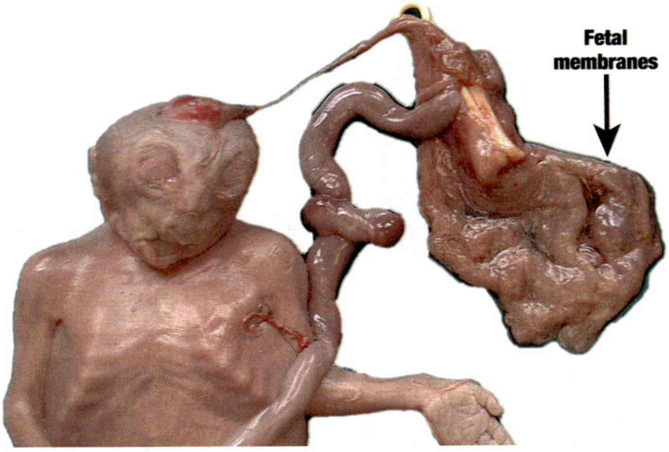

FIGURE 17.55. This image shows the sequelae of amniotic bands wrapping around the face, disrupting facial structure growth and resulting in cleft lip and palate.

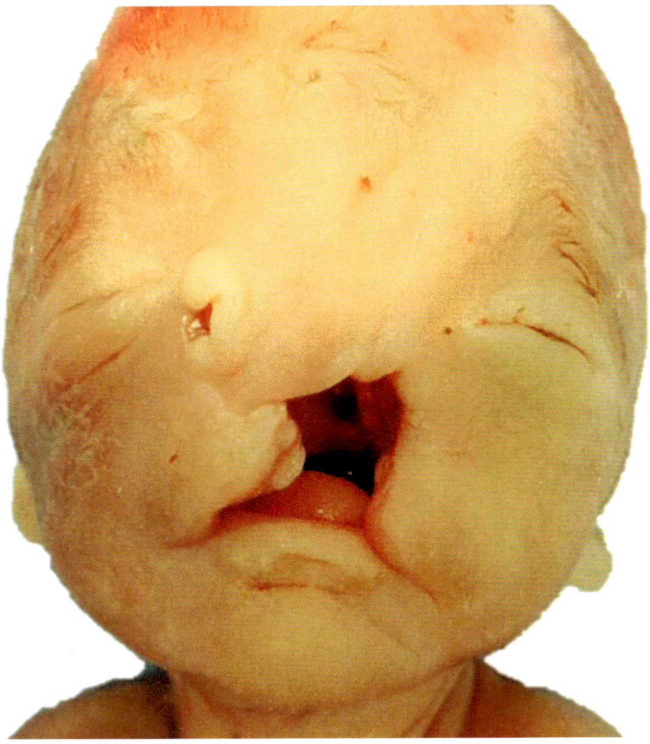

FIGURE 17.56. In (A), bands encircle the right wrist and result in a right hand amputation. Image (B) shows amniotic bands wrapping around the fingers, causing multiple amputations.

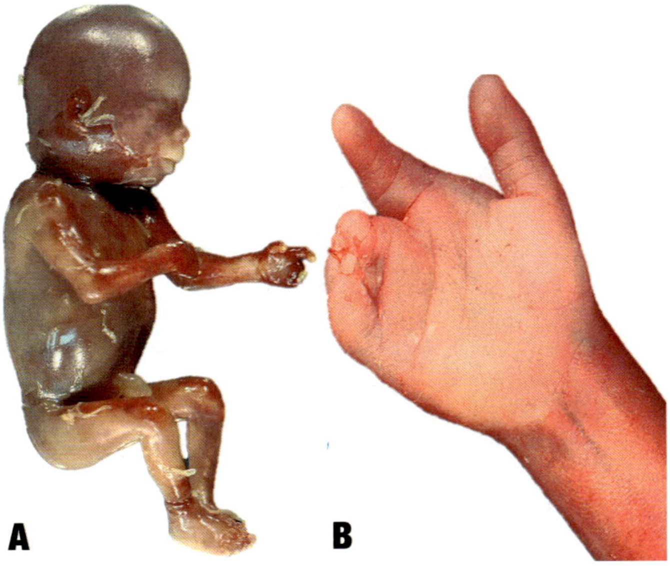

FIGURE 17.57. This image shows bands that wrap around the head and partially decapitate the fetus.

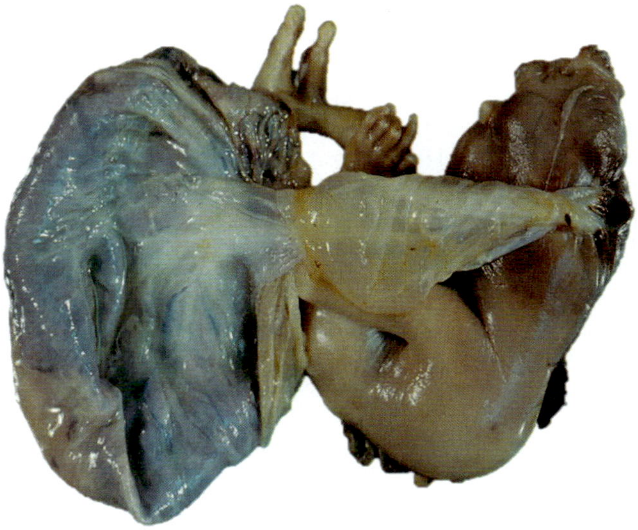

VATER/VACTERL association

VATER/VACTERL association gets its name from a group of nonrandom co-occurring malformations: **v**ertebral anomalies, **a**nal atresia, **c**ardiovascular anomalies, **t**racheoesophageal fistula, **e**sophageal atresia, **r**enal and/or radial anomalies, and **l**imb anomalies. It is of unknown etiology. It occurs in 16 per 100 000 live births, and most commonly affects infants of diabetic mothers. The detection of any defect within this group warrants investigation for the other defects.

FIGURE 17.58. These images show possible findings in VATER/VACTERL association: (A) a short neck and left radial hypoplasia, (B) anal atresia, and (C) oligodactyly.

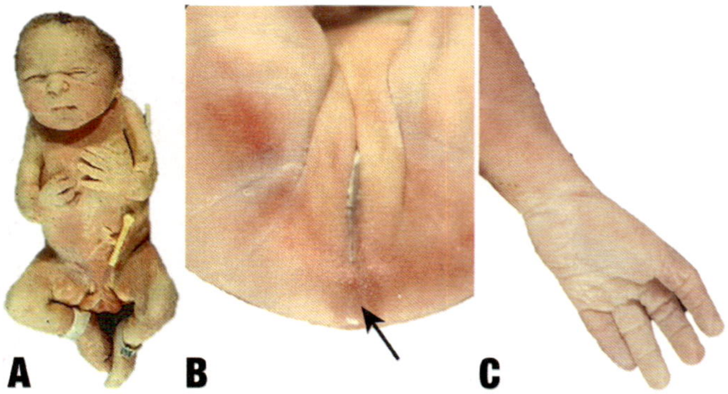

FIGURE 17.59. These images show other VATER/VACTERL association findings: (A) tracheoesophageal fistula (arrow points to esophageal atresia); (B) multiple limb defects (in this case, hypoplasia/aplasia of the radius, hands with flexion deformity and oligodactyly, and club feet); and (C) renal defect (horseshoe kidneys).

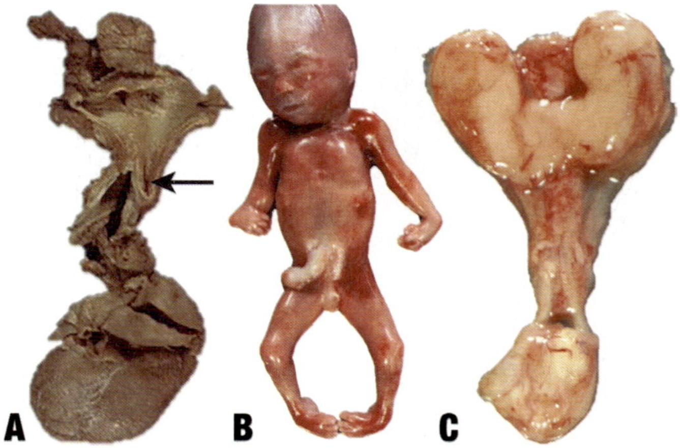

Congenital high airway obstruction syndrome (CHAOS)

CHAOS is a rare disease that involves fetal airway obstruction due to laryngeal or tracheal atresia, subglottic stenosis, laryngeal cyst, or laryngeal web. Secondary changes include enlarged lungs, hydrops with ascites, flattened or everted diaphragms, dilated distal airways, and mediastinal compression. Many affected fetuses die in utero or are stillborn. Prenatal ultrasound diagnosis, detailed fetal assessment, and adequate postnatal intervention for establishing airways are key to survival.

FIGURE 17.60. These images show examples features associated with CHAOS: (A) fetus with severely distended abdomen, and (B) laryngeal subglottic atresia (arrow).

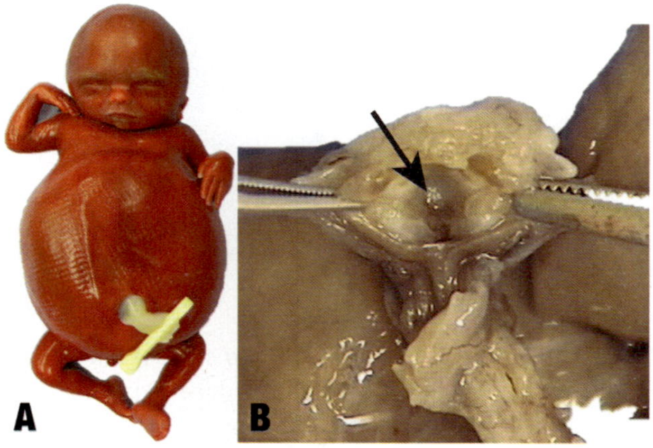

FIGURE 17.61. These images show other features associated with CHAOS: (A) pulmonary hyperplasia, with (B) everted diaphragm (arrow).

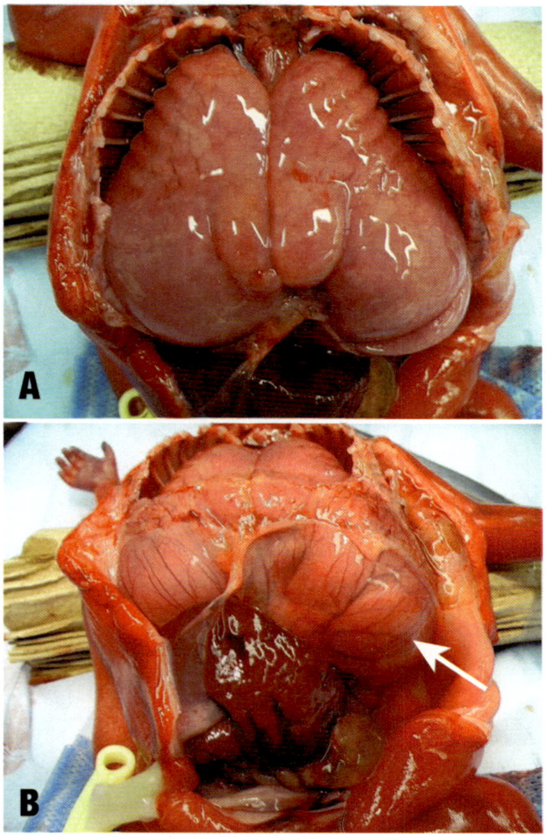

CHARGE syndrome

CHARGE syndrome occurs in 1 per 8500 to 10 000 births. Its name is an acronym for the defects found in the syndrome: **c**oloboma (including cataract), **h**eart defect, choanal **a**tresia, **r**etarded growth, and **g**enital and **e**ar abnormalities. Mutations in the *CHD7* gene account for more than half of cases. Diagnosis relies on identification of major features (coloboma, choanal stenosis or atresia, and cranial nerve and middle/inner ear abnormalities) and minor features (heart defects, developmental problems, cleft lip and/or palate, hypogonadism, tracheoesophageal fistula, and facial asymmetry).

FIGURE 17.62. Images (A) and (B) show an eye displaying cataract.

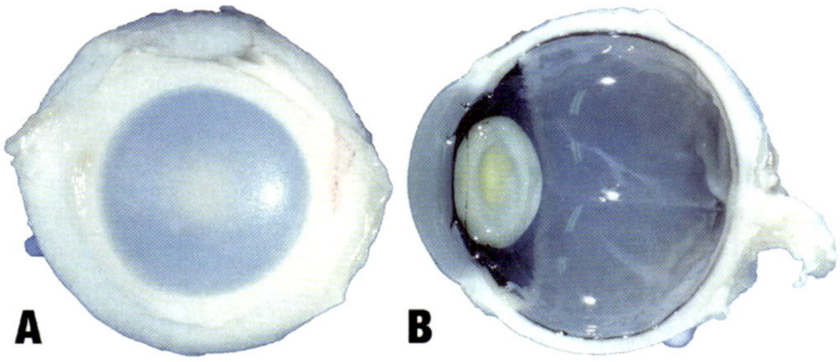

FIGURE 17.63. Image (A) shows a pointed nose tip with choanal stenosis. Image (B) shows an example of arrhinencephaly, the absence of olfactory bulbs (arrows). Both of these are findings in CHARGE syndrome.

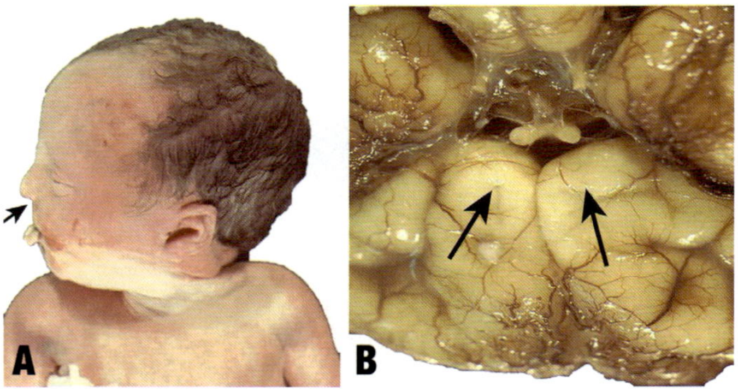

FIGURE 17.64. This image shows a ventricular septal defect (arrow), which is a minor feature of CHARGE syndrome.

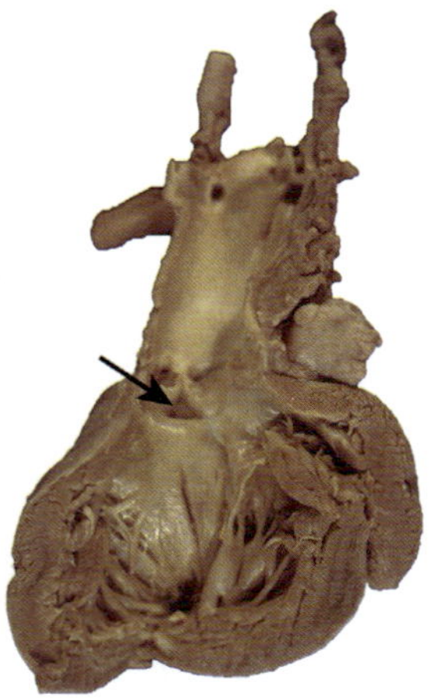

Meckel–Gruber syndrome

Meckel–Gruber syndrome is a rare and lethal autosomal recessive disease characterized by a triad of findings: occipital encephalocele, large polycystic kidneys, and postaxial polydactyly. Genetic mapping to 12 genetic loci (*MKS1* to *MKS12*) suggests genetic heterogeneity. Other findings include liver fibrotic or cystic changes, CNS malformations, and orofacial cleft.

FIGURE 17.65. Image (A) shows a fetus with an enlarged abdomen due to bilaterally large kidneys. An associated facial midline defect is also present. Image (B) gives a direct view of the enlarged kidneys.

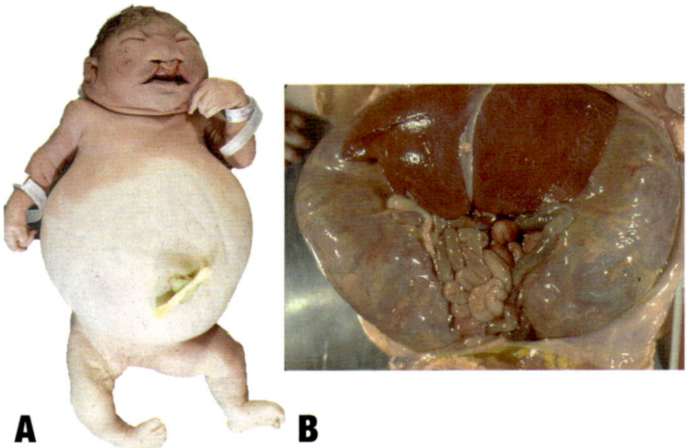

FIGURE 17.66. These images show findings linked to Meckel–Gruber syndrome: (A) polycystic kidneys, (B) postaxial polydactyly of the feet, and (C) occipital encephalocele.

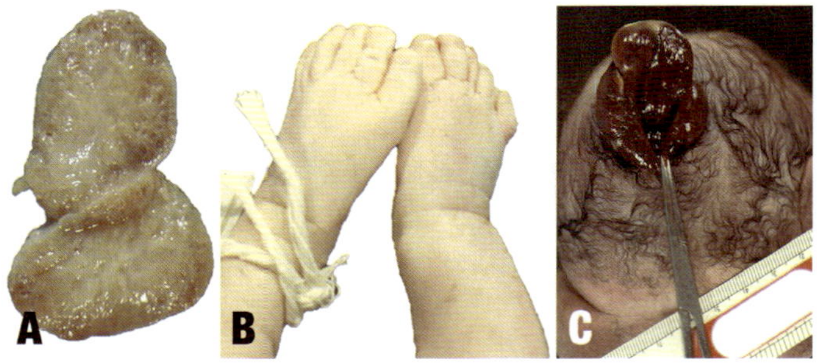

Fraser syndrome

Fraser syndrome is a rare autosomal recessive condition with mutations in the *FRAS1*, *FREM2*, or *GRIP1* genes; these mutations prevent formation of the *FRAS/FREM* complex in the basement membrane of the skin, leading to blister formation during development. The blisters cause cryptophthalmos (malformed eyes covered by skin) and cutaneous syndactyly (fusion of the skin between digits). Other findings in the syndrome include genital anomalies, ear anomalies, renal hypoplasia or agenesis, and laryngeal stenosis or atresia.

FIGURE 17.67. These images show (A) cryptophthalmos and (B) cutaneous syndactyly in association with Fraser syndrome.

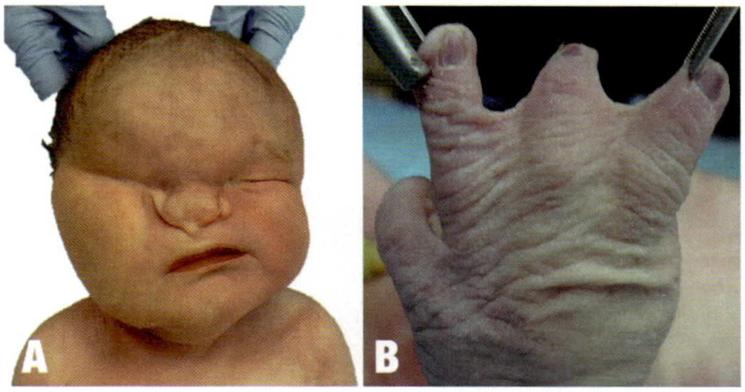

FIGURE 17.68. These images show other anomalies associated with Fraser syndrome: (A) an ear anomaly and (B) laryngeal atresia (arrow).

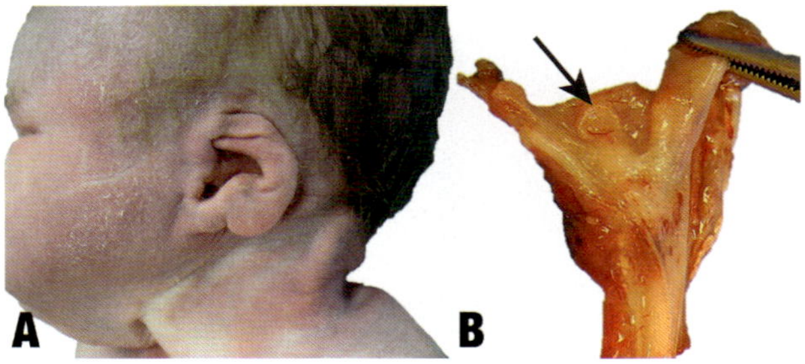

Caudal regression syndrome

Caudal regression syndrome, or sacral agenesis or hypoplasia, is a congenital disorder that impairs the development of the lower (caudal) half of the body. It occurs in 1 to 2.5 per 100 000 newborns (but 1 per 350 infants born to diabetic mothers). The lower spine and spinal cord may be misshapen or missing; the pelvic bone and femur bones are underdeveloped. Variable genitourinary tract abnormalities (renal agenesis, bladder exstrophy, hypospadia, and rectovaginal fistula) and gastrointestinal tract abnormalities (malrotation and imperforate anus) may occur.

FIGURE 17.69. These images show extreme forms of caudal regression syndrome, characterized by a mermaid-like caudal half of the body. Image (A) shows sacral hypoplasia and (B) shows sacral agenesis.

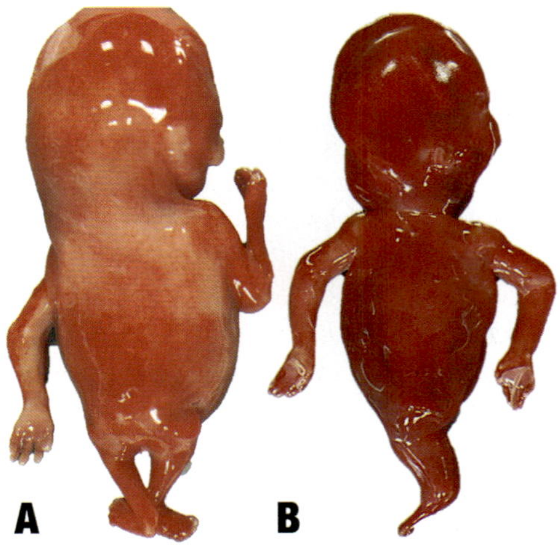

Congenital pulmonary airway malformation (CPAM)

CPAM is a rare hamartomatous disease. There are 5 types of CPAM with variably sized cysts and different microscopic cell linings. Type 0 features small, firm lungs and acinar dysplasia. Type 1 usually features multiple large (> 10 cm) cysts, and ciliated columnar-to-pseudostratified tall and mucogenic cells. Type 2 features multiple cysts (up to 2 cm) and ciliated cuboidal-to-columnar cells. Type 3 features bulky, firm masses with small cysts (< 0.5 cm) and ciliated cuboidal cells. Type 4 features large cysts (up to 10 cm) and flattened epithelial cells. Type 0 is incompatible with life; types 1 and 2 are the most common; type 4 can resemble pleuropulmonary blastoma, a childhood malignant tumor of the lung.

FIGURE 17.70. Image (A) shows an enlarged right lower lobe due to CPAM. Image (B) shows the diminutive left lung from the same patient. (Image labels: RUL: right upper lobe; RLL: right lower lobe; LUL: left upper lobe; LLL: left lower lobe.)

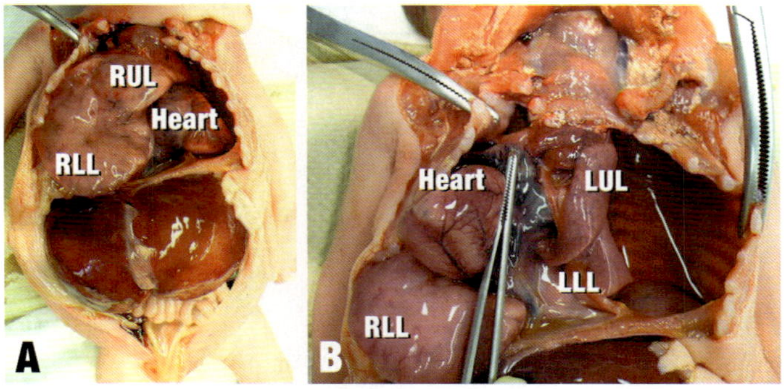

FIGURE 17.71. This image shows hydrops resulting from heart and vein compression by an enlarged lung associated with CPAM.

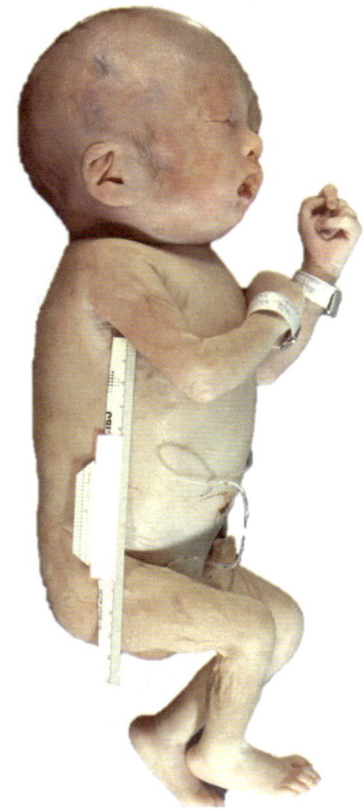

Diaphragmatic hernia

Diaphragmatic hernia occurs in 1 per 2000 to 5000 births. The diaphragm defect, usually located in the posterolateral aspect and more commonly left sided, allows abdominal contents to herniate into the thoracic cavity, causing pulmonary hypoplasia. Infants with large hernia may present with severe respiratory distress at birth. With surgical repair and supportive extracorporeal membrane oxygenation (ECMO), survival rates can reach 75% to 95%.

FIGURE 17.72. This image shows the stomach and part of the intestine herniating into the left side of the chest cavity (arrow).

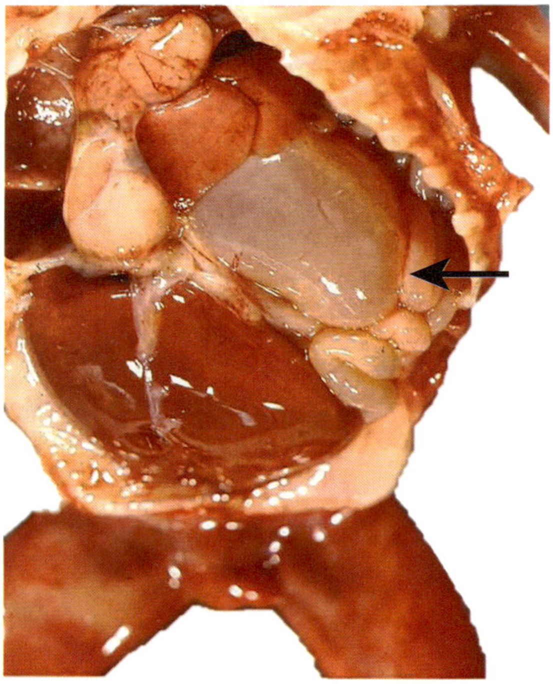

Meckel diverticulum

Meckel diverticulum is the most common true diverticulum, consisting in a blind outpouching of all 3 layers of the small bowel wall. It occurs due to failed involution of the vitelline duct. Meckel diverticulum follows the "rule of 2s": it occurs in 2% of the population, is found within 2 feet of the ileocecal valve, is 2 inches long, is 2 times as common in males, and is symptomatic by age 2. Microscopy may show a normal small bowel, or ectopic pancreatic or gastric tissue.

FIGURE 17.73. In this specimen, note a protrusion from the bowel segment.

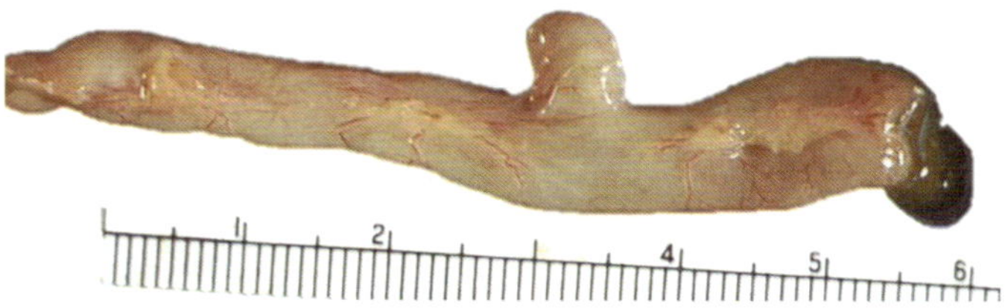

Enteric duplication cyst

Enteric duplication cyst results from abnormal recanalization of the gastrointestinal tract. It can be associated with vertebral anomalies.

FIGURE 17.74. This image shows cystic structures in the thoracic cavity in proximity to the diaphragm and liver.

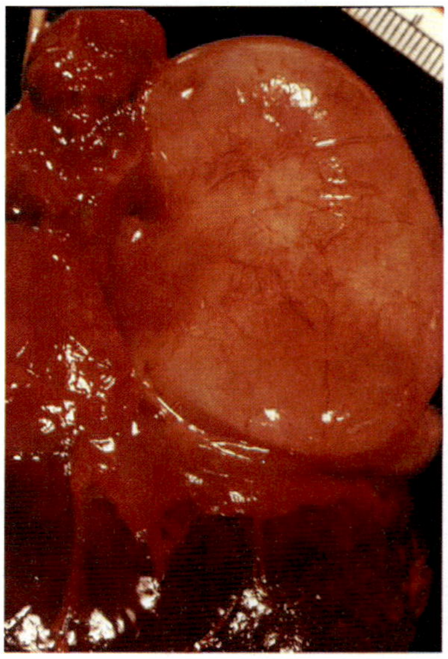

Gastroschisis

Gastroschisis is the incomplete closure of all layers of the abdominal wall, resulting in herniation of abdominal organs.

FIGURE 17.75. This image shows extrusion of small and large bowel, the tip of the spleen, and the right ovary and fallopian tube. Unlike omphalocele, there is no membrane overlying the herniated contents.

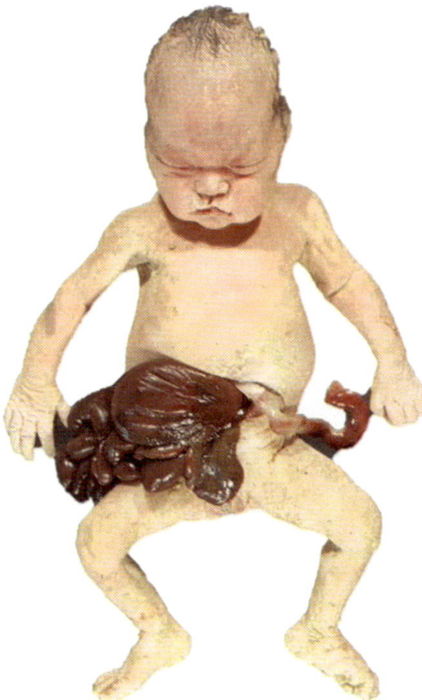

Omphalocele

Omphalocele is the incomplete closure of abdominal wall musculature that results in herniation of abdominal contents. The hernia is covered by a thin membrane on which the umbilical cord inserts. This condition is often associated with other birth defects, such as chromosomal abnormalities, congenital diaphragmatic hernia, and cardiac defects.

FIGURE 17.76. These images show (A) the external appearance of a fetus with omphalocele and (B) the herniated organs.

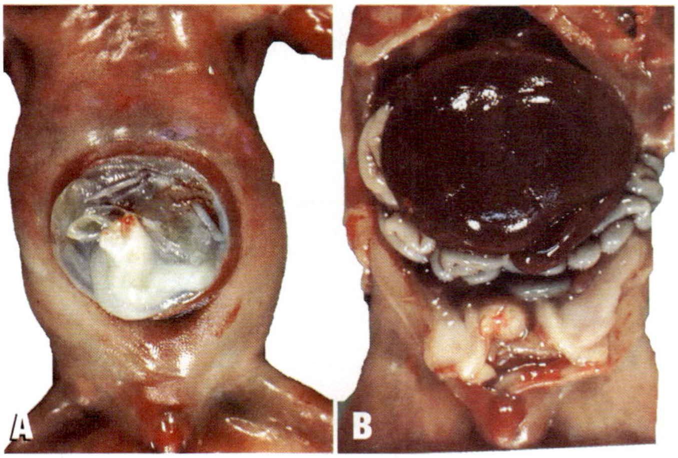

Intrauterine growth restriction (IUGR)

IUGR manifests as asymmetrical growth, with a head of relatively normal or large size and a small body. The causes include, among others, preeclampsia, multiple pregnancies, maternal malnutrition, and maternal smoking.

FIGURE 17.78. Note the relatively large head in this specimen.

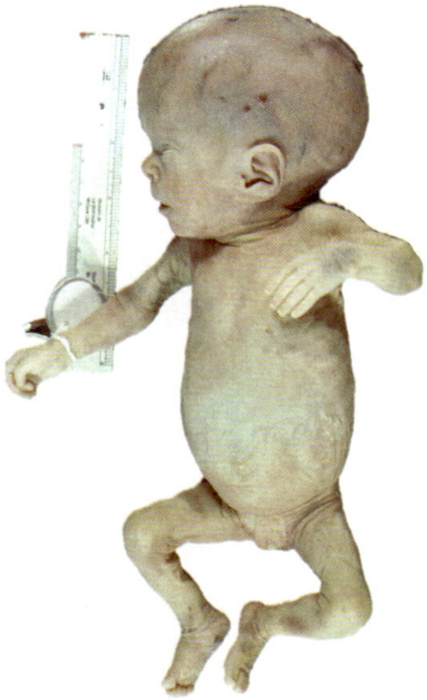

Hyaline membrane disease of prematurity

FIGURE 17.77. This image shows nonaerated and congested lungs with a liver-like appearance. Microscopy showed hyaline membrane disease.

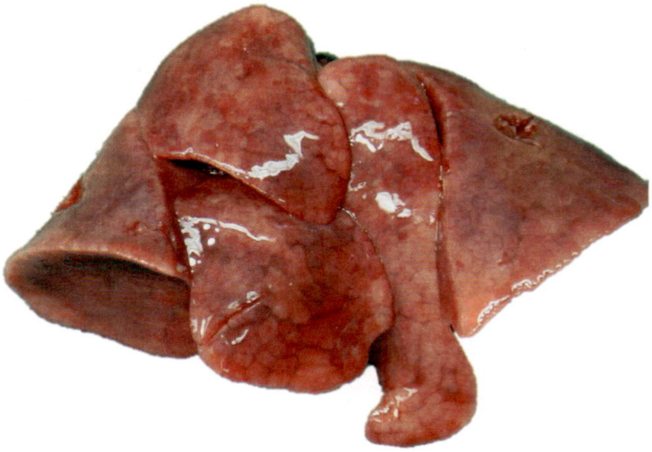

Fetal macrosomia

Major malformations occur in 6% to 10% of infants born to mothers with diabetes mellitus. Maternal hyperglycemia can induce a state of hyperinsulinemia in the fetus, which manifests as fetal macrosomia (more than 90th percentile for gestational age, or > 4 kg for babies brought to term) with enlarged organs and increased body fat and muscle mass. Other findings in infants born to mothers with diabetes mellitus include impaired fetal growth, respiratory distress syndrome, electrolyte abnormalities, polycythemia-related thrombotic events, cardiac malformations, neural tube defects, and renal abnormalities.

FIGURE 17.79. Image (A) shows fetal macrosomia. Image (B) shows multiple infarcted organs (adrenal glands, kidney, and testes) due to thrombotic events.

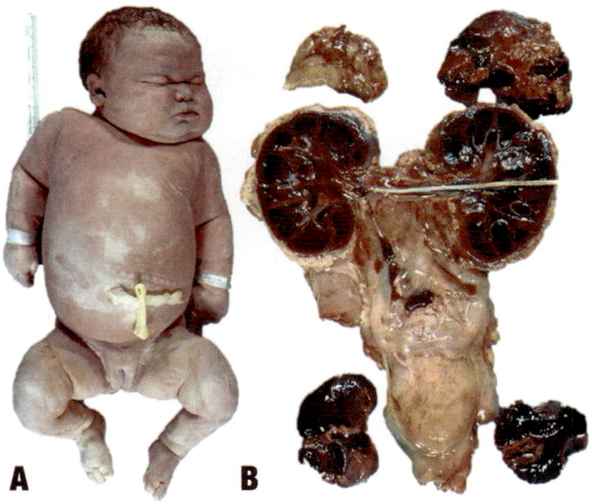

TORCH complex

The most important transplacental perinatal infections are the TORCH complex (**to**xoplasma, **r**ubella, **c**ytomegalovirus, **h**erpesvirus, and other infections such as *Treponema pallidum*). The infections may have similar clinical and pathological manifestations. Infants affected in early gestation present with growth restriction, mental retardation, congenital cataracts, and cardiac anomalies. Infants affected in late gestation may develop encephalitis, chorioretinitis, hepatosplenomegaly, pneumonia, or myocarditis.

FIGURE 17.80. This image shows a fetus with disseminated cytomegalovirus infection.

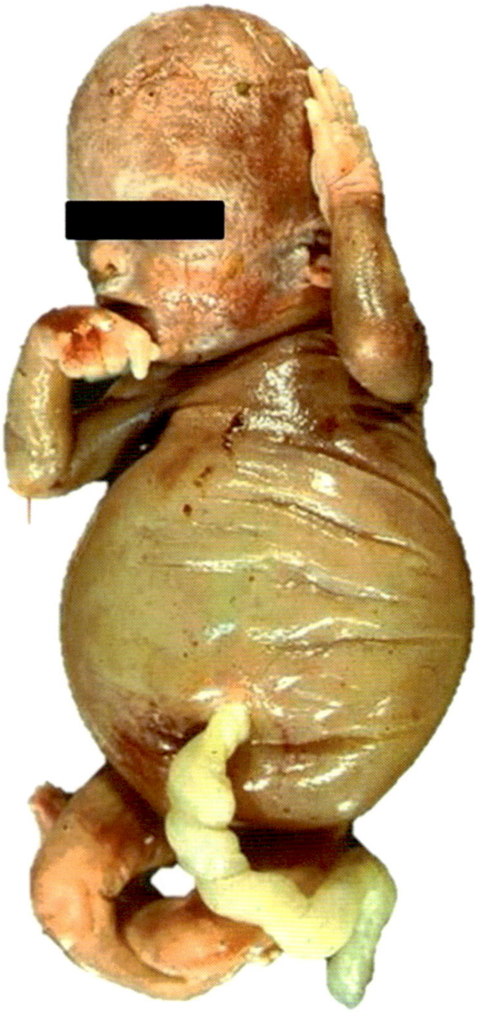

Varicella-zoster virus *(Varicellavirus,* chickenpox)

Varicella-zoster virus is a herpesvirus that can be transmitted to the fetus by the transplacental route and cause disseminated infection.

FIGURE 17.81. This image shows a case of congenital varicella-zoster infection with an erythematous vesicular rash in a dermatome distribution.

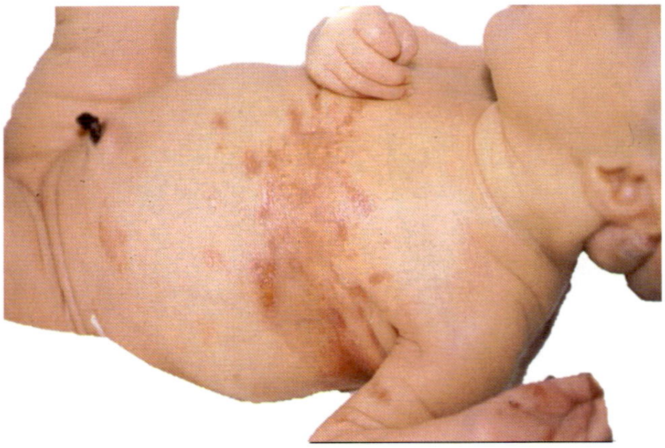

Syphilis

Syphilis is due to spirochete *Treponema pallidum* infection. It can be transmitted transplacentally, causing congenital syphilis. Untreated syphilis results in intrauterine death in 25% of cases and in perinatal death in another 25% of cases.

FIGURE 17.82. Image (A) shows hydrops fetalis with maceration and congested cord due to syphilis. Image (B) shows a pale placenta. Microscopic exam revealed severe erythroblastosis and focal mild chronic villitis. There is also focal acute funisitis.

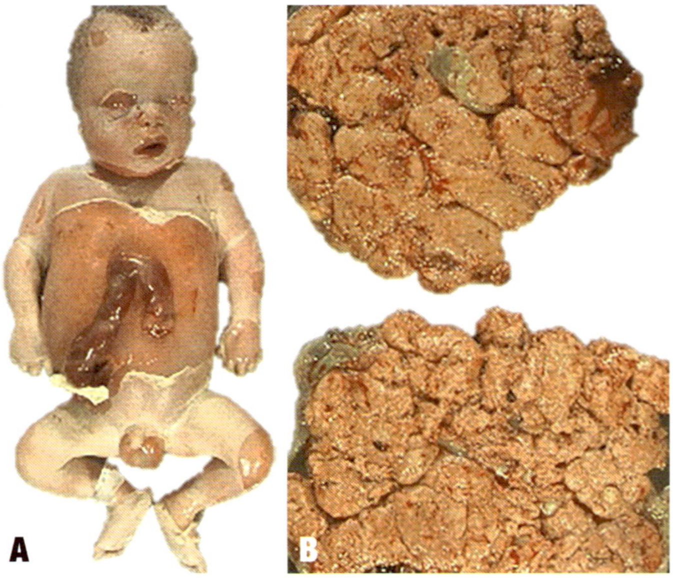

Neonatal sepsis

Neonatal sepsis is a major cause of neonatal morbidity and mortality. Neonatal sepsis with early onset (occurring in the first 7 days after birth) is commonly seen in premature infants and is caused by maternal organisms such as group B streptococci or *Escherichia coli*, transmitted transplacentally or as ascending cervical infections. Neonatal sepsis with late onset (occurring between 8 and 90 days after birth) is environmentally acquired via colonization of the conjunctiva, skin, or gastrointestinal tract.

FIGURE 17.83. Image (A) shows hemorrhagic bronchopneumonia due to group B streptococci. Images (B) and (C) show purulent meningoencephalitis, also due to group B streptococci.

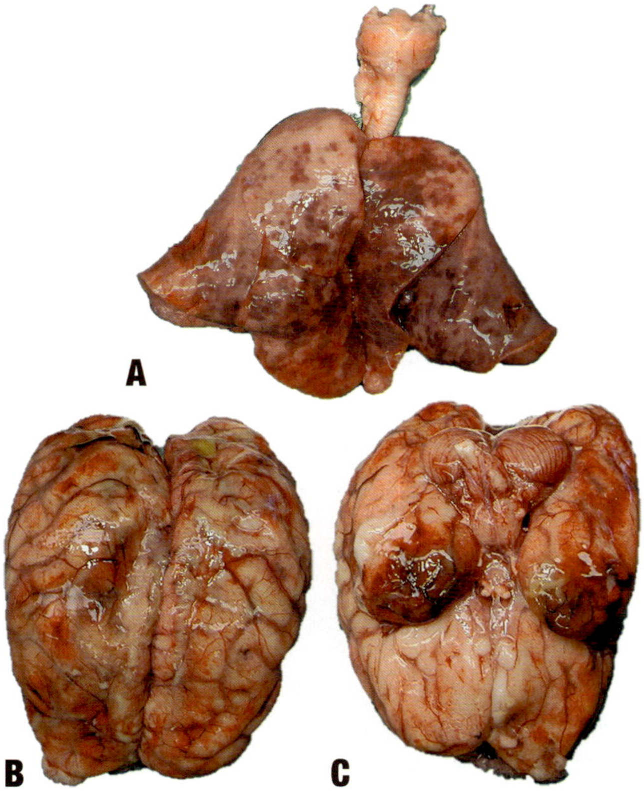

FIGURE 17.84. This image shows purulent meningoencephalitis due to disseminated *E. coli* infection.

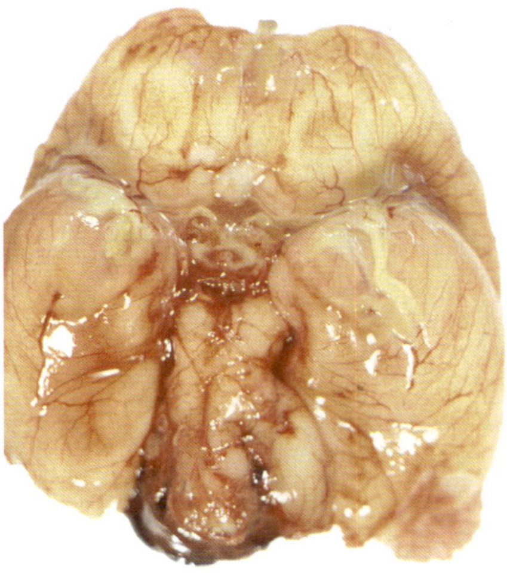

Peritonitis

Peritonitis is defined as inflammation of the serosal lining of the abdominal cavity. It has various causes in newborns; the most common causes are bacterial infection or bowel perforation.

FIGURE 17.85. Image (A) shows a case of peritonitis with copious pus. In this case, the peritonitis was caused by intrauterine *Candida* sepsis. Image (B) shows a close-up view of the same specimen.

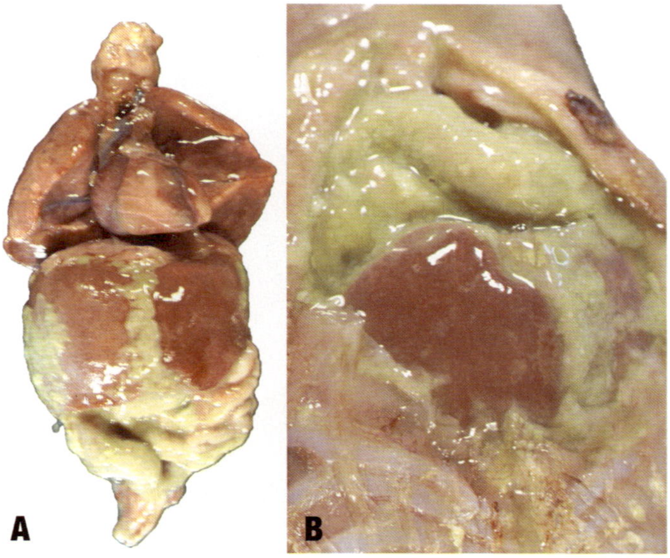

Hepatic necrosis

Hepatic necrosis may be due to ischemia, toxins, or infection.

FIGURE 17.86. This image shows septic shock causing hypoperfusion of the liver and resulting in ischemic necrosis.

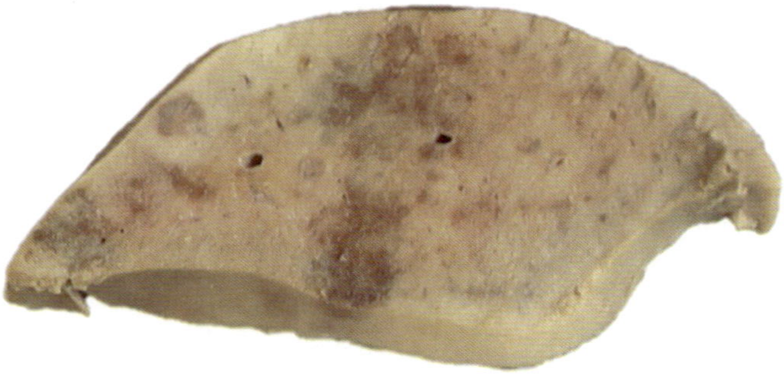

Cystic fibrosis (mucoviscidosis)

Cystic fibrosis, or mucoviscidosis, is an autosomal recessive disorder caused by mutations of the *CFTR* gene, and characterized by viscous mucoid secretions in the lungs, pancreas, liver, and gastrointestinal tract.

FIGURE 17.87. These images show cystic fibrosis–related findings: (A) lungs filled with mucoid material, and (B) fibrosis and bronchiectasis (dilated bronchi).

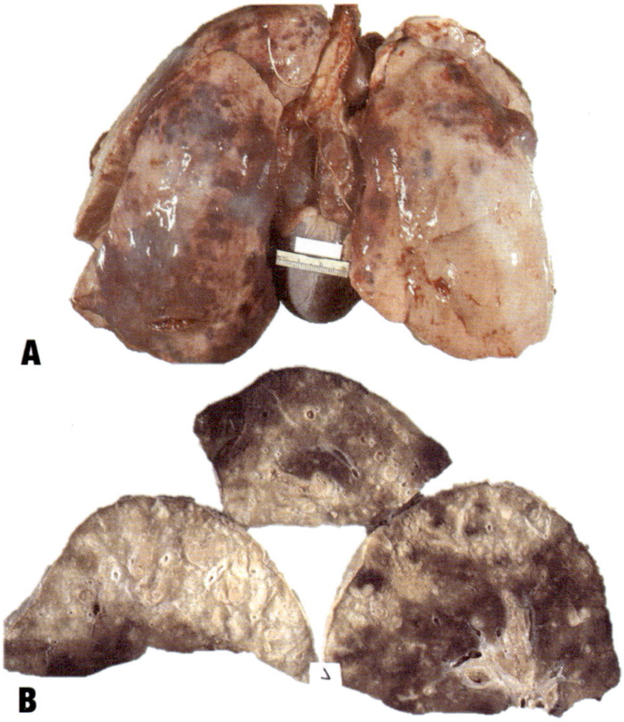

FIGURE 17.88. These images show further complications of cystic fibrosis. Image (A) shows liver cirrhosis in which dehydrated bile plugged liver-bile ducts and caused biliary cirrhosis. Image (B) shows a mucoid pancreas. Image (C) shows pancreatic cystosis due to cystic fibrosis. In rare cases, the pancreas is entirely replaced by multiple mucus-filled cysts.

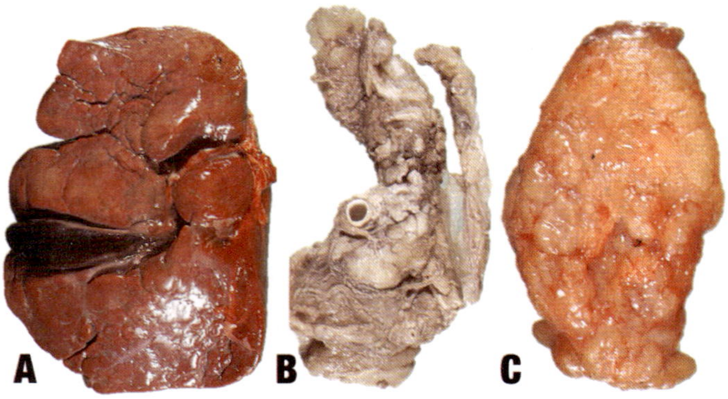

Iatrogenic complications

SYMPTOMATIC THROMBOEMBOLIC DISEASE

Critically ill neonates, both term and preterm, are at great risk for developing symptomatic thromboembolic disease. Important risk factors include catheterization, asphyxia, sepsis, prematurity, disseminated intravascular coagulation (DIC), impaired liver function, fluctuations in cardiac output, and congenital heart disease.

FIGURE 17.89. This image shows aortic thrombosis from catheterization.

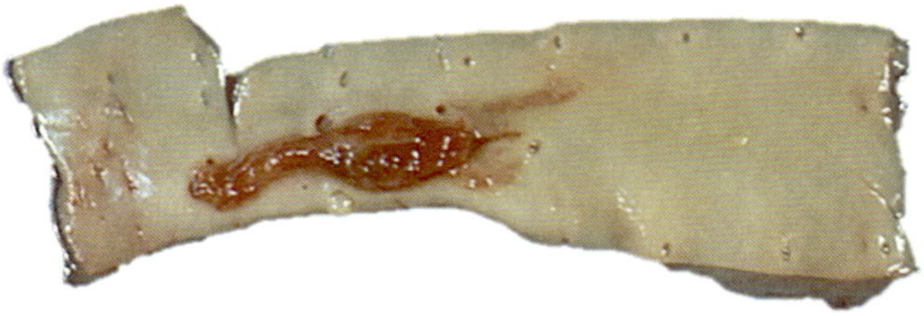

PULMONARY INTERSTITIAL EMPHYSEMA

Pulmonary interstitial emphysema is a complication from resuscitation efforts involving high-pressure ventilation.

FIGURE 17.90. This image shows a specimen demonstrating pulmonary interstitial emphysema.

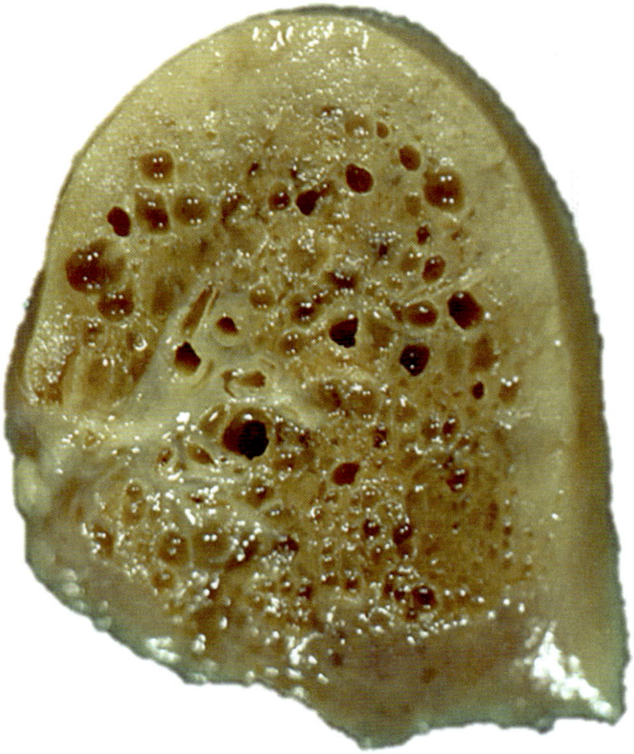

HEMORRHAGIC TRACHEITIS

Hemorrhagic tracheitis may result from trauma, infection (e.g., herpesvirus), or certain medications (e.g., mucolytic agents used to treat cystic fibrosis).

FIGURE 17.91. This image shows an intensely red, inflamed tracheal mucosa with hemorrhage.

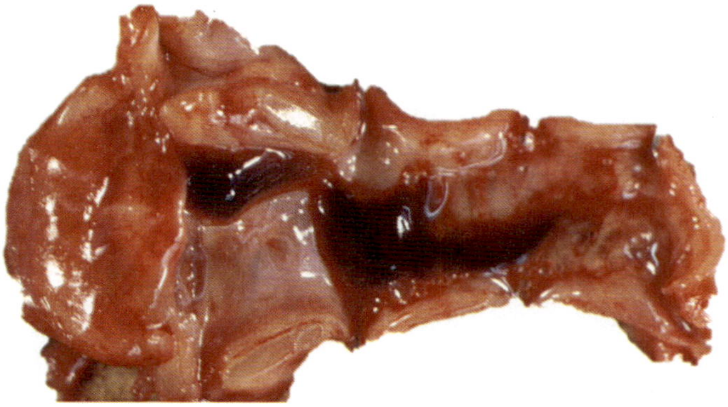

HEMOTHORAX

Hemothorax (presence of blood in the pleural space) is commonly due to trauma. Rarely, it may result from neoplasia, blood dyscrasia, infections, vascular malformation, or other causes.

FIGURE 17.92. This image shows an example of hemothorax.

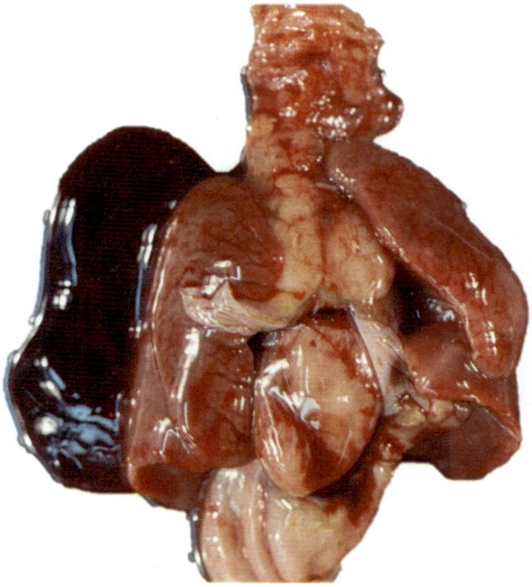

Periventricular hemorrhage–intraventricular hemorrhage (PVH-IVH)

PVH-IVH is an important cause of morbidity and mortality in premature infants. It is classified into 4 grades according to the extent of bleeding: subependymal PVH-IVH; PVH-IVH of the lateral ventricles with enlargement; PVH-IVH of the lateral ventricles without enlargement; and intraparenchymal PVH-IVH. The initial hemorrhage occurs in the fragile capillary network supplying the subependymal germinal matrix in the developing fetus. Cerebral perfusion change in the immature cerebral vasculature causes the hemorrhage. Complications include cerebral palsy, seizures, and developmental delay. The risk of the condition is increased with the severity of prematurity.

FIGURE 17.93. Image (A) shows a periventricular hemorrhage (arrow). Image (B) shows an intraventricular hemorrhage with extension into the third and fourth ventricles.

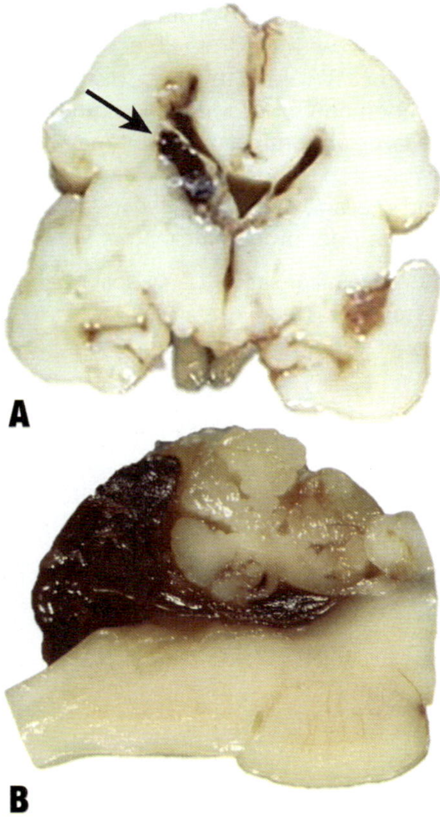

Necrotizing enterocolitis

Necrotizing enterocolitis occurs in 1 per 10 very low birth weight infants (< 1500 g). Any part of the small or large intestine can be involved with distension, congestion, frank gangrene, or perforation.

FIGURE 17.94. This image shows a dilated and congested bowel segment. A gas bubble within the intestinal wall (pneumatosis intestinalis) is present (arrow).

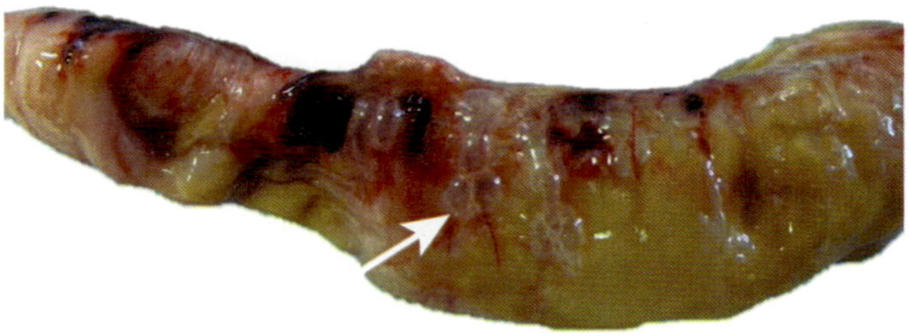

Pediatric Tumors

Wilms tumor (nephroblastoma)

Wilms tumor, or nephroblastoma, is the most common pediatric renal tumor. It occurs in 1 per 8000 to 10 000 children, with most cases diagnosed before age 6 years. Most Wilms tumors are sporadic, but they also have well-known associations with syndromes such as Wilms tumor–aniridia syndrome (WAGR), Denys–Drash syndrome, and Beckwith–Wiedemann syndrome. Wilms tumor usually presents as a large abdominal mass, but may sometimes present as a ruptured tumor or even as metastatic lung disease. Large size, age more than 2 years, advanced stage, and anaplasia are poor prognostic factors.

FIGURE 17.95. This image shows a large, solitary, well-circumscribed renal mass of yellow-tan color with a lobular pattern and some areas of hemorrhage and necrosis.

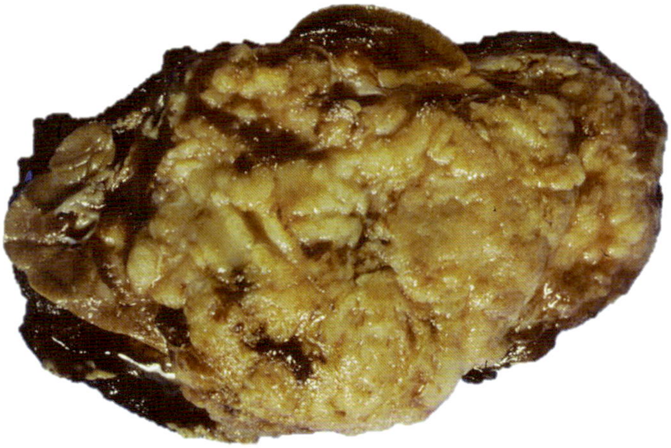

BLASTEMAL WILMS TUMOR

Classic Wilms tumor is triphasic, composed of differentiated epithelial cells, undifferentiated blastemal cells, and stromal cells. Sometimes 1 component predominates.

FIGURE 17.96. The CT image in (A) shows a large, heterogeneous, low density, solid, soft tissue mass with an intralesional hypodense component. This mass measures 114 mm × 96 mm × 133 mm and appears to arise from the upper pole of the left kidney parenchyma. The "claw sign" is visible (arrow). In (B), a nephrectomy specimen shows a large, soft, friable tumor at the upper and middle portion of the kidney. The nonneoplastic kidney corresponds to the "claw" on the CT image. The arrow illustrates an area of hemorrhage that tracks along the edge of the kidney. On histology, tumor tracking was confirmed.

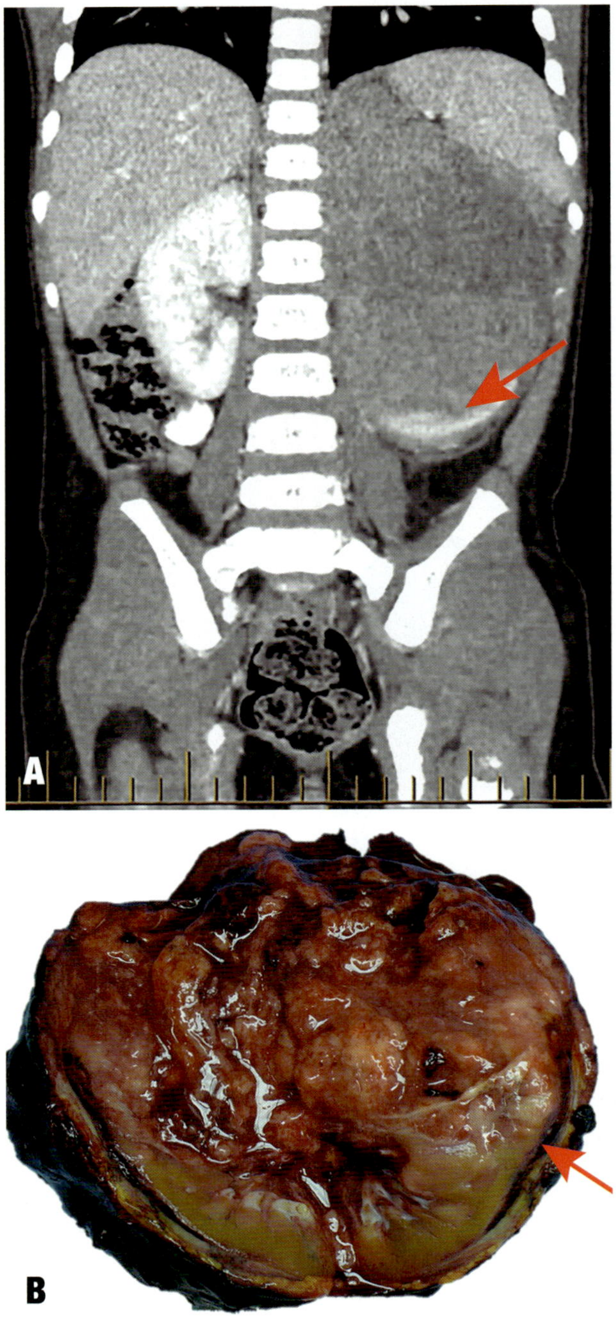

Courtesy of Dr. Van Hung Nguyen

Neuroblastoma

Neuroblastoma is a malignant tumor of neuroectodermal origin that affects young children (peak age 0 to 4 years). It can occur in the adrenal gland or anywhere along the sympathetic chain. Its presentation varies according to tumor location and extent; most commonly, it presents as an abdominal mass. Increasing age, N-Myc amplification, and 1p36 deletion are among the poor prognostic factors. Grossly, neuroblastomas are circumscribed ovoid-to-multilobulated masses, often with hemorrhagic areas.

FIGURE 17.97. Note the large retrorenal tumor mass.

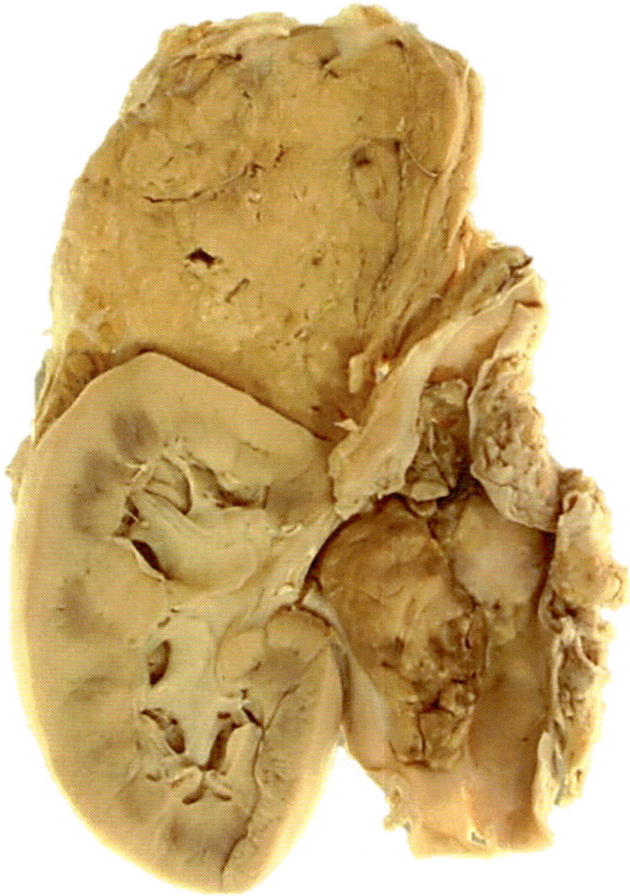

Retinoblastoma

Retinoblastoma is the most common pediatric intraocular tumor; it occurs in 1 per 20 000 live births. Forty percent of retinoblastomas are familial with autosomal dominant inheritance of germ-line mutation in the *RB* gene at 13q14. Familial tumors are more often bilateral and associated with sarcomas. Poor prognostic factors include invasion of the optic nerve, uveal tract, or sclera; vitreous seeding; anterior segment involvement; and extensive necrosis. Grossly, this tumor is creamy white, with yellow necrotic areas and calcifications that often appear chalky.

FIGURE 17.98. This retinoblastoma shows endophytic growth.

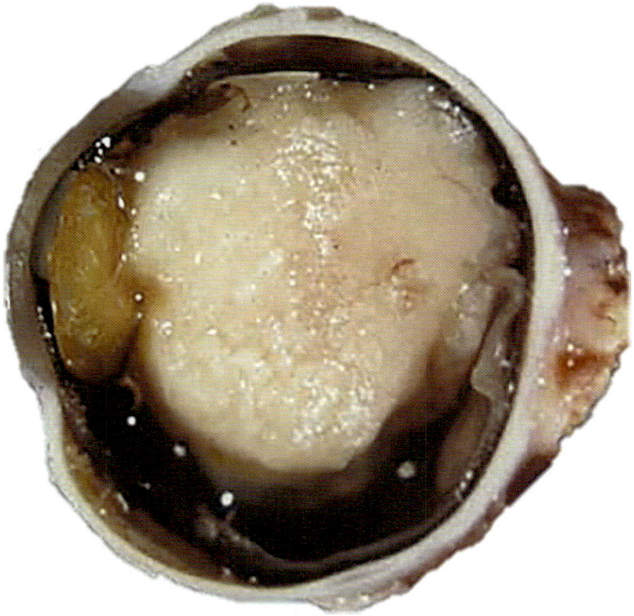

Sacrococcygeal teratoma

Sacrococcygeal teratoma is the most common germ cell tumor of childhood, and is most prevalent in females. The incidence of a malignant element increases proportionately with age.

FIGURE 17.99. Image (A) shows a bulky midline mass at the coccyx. The cut surface in (B) shows a nonencapsulated, solid tumor with mature elements (arrow).

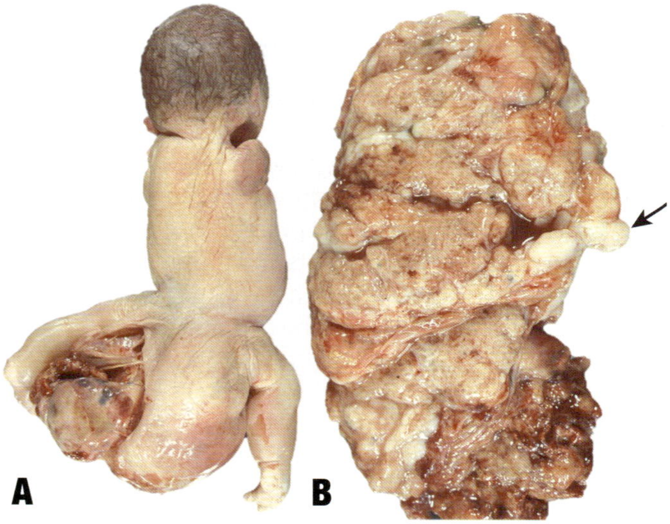

Liver hemangioma

Liver hemangioma is a benign neoplasm of blood vessels that is usually found incidentally. Rarely, when large, it can rupture and cause bleeding, necessitating resection.

FIGURE 17.100. This image shows a solitary, subcapsular, well-circumscribed, red, and soft mass (arrow).

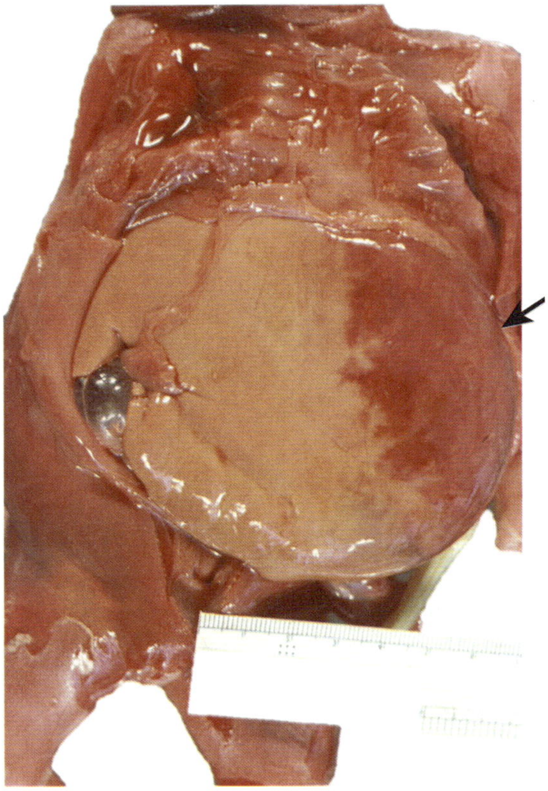

Hepatic mesenchymal hamartoma

Hepatic mesenchymal hamartoma is a rare liver tumor. Most patients are younger than 1 year. The tumor preferentially affects the right lobe. Classic hepatic mesenchymal hamartoma is a solitary, well-circumscribed, myxoid mass with fluid-filled cysts, but its appearance can vary depending on the number of cysts and the amounts of mesenchymal and fibrous tissue. It has a known association with mesenchymal dysplasia of the placenta.

FIGURE 17.101. This image shows a large circumscribed red mass.

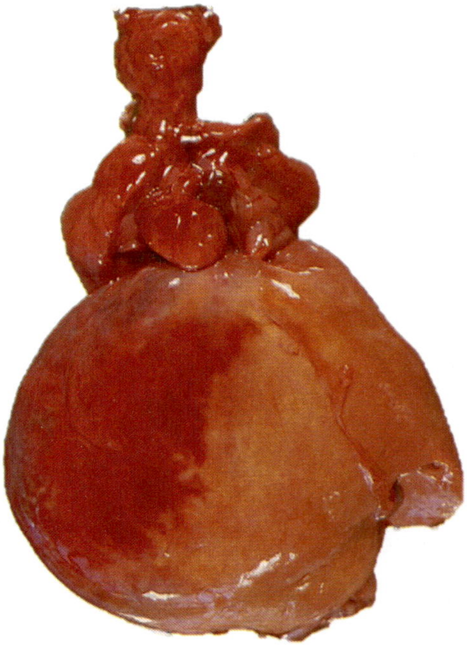

REFERENCES

Francis B, Hallam L, Kecskes Z, Ellwood D, Croaker D, Kent A. Placental mesenchymal dysplasia associated with hepatic mesenchymal hamartoma in the newborn. Pediatr Dev Pathol. 2007;10(1):50–54. https://doi.org/10.2350/06-03-0066.1. Medline:17378624

Genetics home reference [U.S. National Library of Medicine Website]. 2016 Apr 26 [accessed 2016 Apr 30]. Available from: http://ghr.nlm.nih.gov.

Gilbert-Barness E, Kapur RP, Oligny LL, Siebert JR. *Potter's pathology of the fetus, infant and child*. 2nd ed. Philadelphia: Mosby/Elsevier; 2007.

Hamid-Sowinska A, Ropacka-Lesiak M, Breborowicz GH. Congenital high airway obstruction syndrome. Neuro Endocrinol Lett. 2011;32(5):623–626. Medline:22167132

Husain AN, Stocker JT. *Color atlas of pediatric pathology*. New York: Demos Medical Publishing; 2011.

Kumar V, Abbas AK, Aster JC. *Robbins and Cotran pathologic basis of disease*. Philadelphia: Saunders/ Elsevier; 2015.

MacSweeney F, Papagiannopoulos K, Goldstraw P, Sheppard MN, Corrin B, Nicholson AG. An assessment of the expanded classification of congenital cystic adenomatoid malformations and their relationship to malignant transformation. Am J Surg Pathol. 2003;27(8):1139–1146. https://doi.org/10.1097/00000478-200308000-00012. Medline:12883247

Rare disease information [National Organization for Rare Disorders Website]. 2003 [accessed 2016 Mar 20]. Available from: http://rarediseases.org/for-patients-and-families/information-resources/rare-disease-information/.

Abbreviations

AAA abdominal aortic aneurysm
AAH atypical adenomatous hyperplasia
ABC aneurysmal bone cyst
ACC adenoid cystic carcinoma
ACTH adrenocorticotropic hormone
AD Alzheimer disease
ADPKD autosomal dominant polycystic kidney disease
AFH angiomatoid fibrous histiocytoma
AFLD alcoholic fatty liver disease
AFP alpha fetal protein
AIH autoimmune hepatitis
AJCC American Joint Committee on Cancer
AL light-chain amyloid
ALT atypical lipomatous tumor
AMD age-related macular degeneration
AML acute myeloid leukemia
ANA antinuclear antibody
APR abdominoperineal resection
AS aortic stenosis
ASA acetylsalicylic acid
AS ankylosing spondylitis
AV aortic valve
AVM arteriovenous malformation
BCC basal cell carcinoma
BE Barrett esophagus
BPH benign prostate hyperplasia
CA 19-9 cancer antigen 19-9
CABG coronary artery bypass graft
c-ANCA cytoplasmic antineutrophil cytoplasmic antibody
CCAM congenital cystic adenomatoid malformation
CCC clear cell carcinoma
CCS clear cell sarcoma
CEA carcinoembryonic antigen
CHAOS congenital high airway obstruction syndrome
ChRCC chromophobe renal cell carcinoma
CK creatine kinase
CNS central nervous system
COPD chronic obstructive pulmonary disease
CPAM congenital pulmonary airway malformation
CRC colorectal cancer
CS chondrosarcoma
CSF cerebrospinal fluid
CVST cerebral venous sinus thrombosis
CW the circle of Willis
DCIS ductal carcinoma in situ
DCM dilated cardiomyopathy
DF desmoplastic fibroma
DFSP dermatofibrosarcoma protuberans
DIC disseminated intravascular coagulation
DLBLCL diffuse large B-cell lymphoma
EBV Epstein–Barr virus
ECMO extracorporeal membrane oxygenation
EDH epidural hemorrhage
EHE epithelioid hemangioendothelioma
EIN endometrial intraepithelial neoplasia
EMC epithelial-myoepithelial carcinoma
EMR endoscopic mucosa resection
EoE eosinophilic esophagitis
ER estrogen receptor
ES Ewing sarcoma
ESMC extraskeletal myxoid chondrosarcoma
ESN endometrial stromal nodule
EVAR endovascular aneurysm repair
FAP familial adenomatous polyposis
FGFR3 FGF receptor 3
FIGO International Federation of Gynecology and Obstetrics
FNH focal nodular hyperplasia
FTLD frontotemporal lobar degeneration
GAVE gastric antral vascular ectasia
GCT giant cell tumor
GCT granulosa cell tumor
GERD gastroesophageal reflux disease
GI gastrointestinal
GIST gastrointestinal stromal tumor
GNET gastrointestinal neuroectodermal tumor
GPA granulomatosis with polyangiitis
GVHD graft versus host disease
H&E hematoxylin and eosin stain
HCA hepatocellular adenoma
HCC hepatocellular carcinoma
HCM hypertrophic cardiomyopathy
HDGC hereditary diffuse gastric cancer
HGESS high-grade endometrial stromal sarcoma
HGSC high-grade serous carcinoma
HLA human leukocyte antigen
HMB human melanoma black
HPF high power field
HPV human papilloma virus
HSIL high-grade squamous intraepithelial lesion
IBD inflammatory bowel disease
IE infective endocarditis
IgG immunoglobulin G
IMT inflammatory myofibroblastic tumor
IUD intrauterine device
IUGR intrauterine growth restriction
IVH intraventricular hemorrhage
KSHV Kaposi sarcoma–associated herpesvirus
LAD left anterior descending
LAM lymphangioleiomyomatosis
LAMN low-grade appendiceal mucinous neoplasm
LAR lower anterior resection
LCA left coronary artery
LCH Langerhans cell histiocytosis
LCIS lobular carcinoma in situ
LCNEC large cell neuroendocrine carcinoma

LDH	lactic dehydrogenase
LEF-1	lymphoid enhancer binding factor 1
LES	lower esophageal sphincter
LGESS	low-grade endometrial stromal sarcoma
LKM	liver–kidney microsomal antibody
LP	liver–pancreas antigen
LPF	low-power field
LV	left ventricle
LVH	left ventricular hypertrophy
MALT	mucosal-associated lymphoid tissue
MART-1	melanoma antigen recognized by T cells 1
MCA	middle cerebral artery
MEC	mucoepidermoid carcinoma
MEN	multiple endocrine neoplasia
MI	myocardial infarction
MIFS	myxoinflammatory fibroblastic sarcoma
MPNST	malignant peripheral nerve sheath tumor
MS	multiple sclerosis
NASH	nonalcoholic steatohepatitis
NBTE	nonbacterial thrombotic endocarditis
NET	neuroendocrine tumor
NF1	neurofibromatosis type 1
NF2	neurofibromatosis type 2
NG	nasogastric
NHL	non-Hodgkin lymphoma
NSAID	nonsteroidal antiinflammatory drug
NST	no special type
NTD	neural tube defect
OA	osteoarthritis
OI	osteogenesis imperfecta
OS	osteosarcoma
PAS	periodic acid–Schiff
PBC	primary biliary cholangitis
PDC	pyruvate dehydrogenase complex
PEC	perivascular epithelioid cell
PEComa	perivascular epithelial cell neoplasm
PET	positron emission tomography
PJS	Peutz–Jeghers syndrome
PKD	polycystic kidney disease
PMP	pseudomyxoma peritonei
PPI	proton pump inhibitor
PR	progesterone receptor
PSC	primary sclerosing cholangitis
PVH-IVH	periventricular hemorrhage–intraventricular hemorrhage
RCA	right coronary artery
RPE	retinal pigmented epithelium
RV	right ventricle
SAH	subarachnoid hemorrhage
SCC	squamous cell carcinoma
SCLC	small cell lung carcinoma
SDH	subdural hemorrhage
SEH	subependymal hemorrhage
SFT	solitary fibrous tumor
SIL	squamous intraepithelial lesion
SIN	salpingitis isthmica nodosa
SLA	anti–soluble liver antigen
SMA	anti–smooth muscle antibody
SS	synovial sarcoma
SSA/P	sessile serrated adenoma/polyp
STIC	serous tubal intraepithelial carcinoma
STUMP	smooth muscle tumor of uncertain malignant potential
TB	tuberculosis
TERT	telomerase reverse transcriptase
TIA	transient ischemic attack
TME	total mesorectal excision
TORCH	toxoplasmosis, other infections, rubella, cytomegalovirus, herpes simplex
TS	tuberous sclerosis
TTF-1	thyroid transcription factor 1
TV	tricuspid valve
UC	ulcerative colitis
UES	undifferentiated endometrial sarcoma
UPS	undifferentiated pleomorphic sarcoma
UUS	undifferentiated uterine sarcoma
VIN	vulvar intraepithelial neoplasia
VKH	Vogt-Koyanagi-Harada disease
VSD	ventricular septal defect
WAGR	Wilms tumor–aniridia syndrome
WHO	World Health Organization
YST	yolk sac tumor

Contributing Authors

Oluyomi E. Kabiawu Ajise, MD, FACP
Assistant professor, Department of Pathology
McGill University
Montreal, QC

Amal A. Al-Odaini, MBBS, MSc, FRCPC
Assistant professor, Department of Pathology and Laboratory Medicine, College of Medicine
Imam Abdulrahman Bin Faisal University
King Fahad Hospital of the University
Alkhobar, KSA

Sabrina Bergeron, PhD
Postdoctoral fellow, MUHC-McGill University Ocular Pathology and Translational Research Laboratory
Montreal, QC

Fadi Brimo, MD, FRCPC
Associate professor, Department of Pathology
McGill University
Montreal, QC

Miguel N. Burnier Jr. MD, MSc, PhD, FRCSC
Professor, Department of Pathology, Ophthalmology, Oncology, Medicine
Surgery director, MUHC-McGill University Ocular Pathology Laboratory
McGill University
Montreal, QC

Derin Caglar, MD
Assistant professor, Department of Pathology
McGill University
Montreal, QC

Sophie Camilleri-Broët, MD, PhD (Paris)
Associate professor, Department of Pathology
McGill University
Montreal, QC

Sonia Corredor Casas, MD
Instituto Mexicano de Oftalmologia Universidad Nacional Autonoma de México Queretaro
Queretaro, Mexico

Moy Fong Chen, MB, BS, FRCPC
Associate professor, Department of Pathology
McGill University
Montreal, QC

Wenqian Chen, MD
Endocrine, head, and neck pathology fellow, Department of Pathology, Yale School of Medicine
New Haven, CT USA

Martin Chevrier, MD
Resident physician, Department of Pathology
University of Sherbrooke
Sherbrooke, QC

Zari Dastani, MD, PhD
Resident physician, Department of Pathology
McGill University
Montreal, QC

Lisa M. DiFrancesco, MD, FRCPC, FCAP
Associate professor, Department of Pathology and Laboratory Medicine
University of Calgary and Calgary Laboratory Services
Calgary, AB

Linnea Duke, MD
Resident physician, Department of Pathology
McGill University
Montreal, QC

Evangelina Esposito, MD
Postdoctoral fellow, MUHC-McGill University
Ocular Pathology Laboratory McGill University
Montreal, QC

Pierre-Olivier Fiset, MD, PhD
Assistant professor, Department of Pathology
McGill University
Montreal, QC

Livia Florianova, MD
Resident physician, Department of Pathology
McGill University
Montreal, QC

Zu-hua Gao, MD, PhD, FRCPC
Professor and chair, Department of Pathology
McGill University
Montreal, QC

Lifeng Gu, MD
Resident physician, Department of Pathology
University of Sherbrooke
Sherbrooke, QC

Julie Guilmette, MD
Resident physician, Department of Pathology
University of Montreal
Montreal, QC

Jeffery T. Joseph, MD, PhD
Professor, Department of Pathology and Laboratory Medicine
University of Calgary and Calgary Laboratory Services
Calgary, AB

Sungmi Jung, MD
Assistant professor, Department of Pathology
McGill University
Montreal, QC

Jason Karamchandani, MD
Associate professor, Department of Pathology
McGill University
Montreal, QC

Katherine Lach, MD, CM (McG)
Resident physician, Department of Pathology
McGill University
Montreal, QC

Aimilios Lallas, MD
Dermatologist, First Department of Dermatology
Aristotle University
Thessaloniki, Greece

Patrick Logan, PhD
Postdoctoral fellow, MUHC-McGill University Ocular Pathology Laboratory
McGill University
Montreal, QC

Victoria Marcus, MD, FRCPC
Associate professor, Department of Pathology
McGill University
Montreal, QC

Jennifer Merrimen, MD, FRCPC
Associate professor, Department of Pathology and Urology
Dalhousie University
Halifax, NS

René P. Michel, MD, CM (McG), FRCPC
Professor, Department of Pathology
McGill University
Montreal, QC

Erik Nohr, MD
Pediatric pathology fellow, Department of Pathology and Laboratory Medicine
University of Calgary and Calgary Laboratory Services
Calgary, AB

Elizabeth O'Brien, MD, FRCPC
Associate professor, Department of Medicine Division of Dermatology
McGill University Health Centre
Montreal, QC

Alexandre Odashiro, MD, PhD
Staff pathologist, Département de biologie moléculaire, biochimie médicale et pathologie Centre Hospitalier Universitaire de Québec
Québec, QC

Manuela Pelmus MD, PhD, FRCPC
Associate professor, Department of Pathology Jewish General Hospital
McGill University
Montreal, QC

Sarah-Jeanne Pilon, MD
Resident physician, Department of Pathology
McGill University
Montreal, QC

Margaret Redpath, MD, PhD, FRCPC
Assistant professor, Department of Pathology
McGill University
Montreal, QC

Lara Richer, MD, CM (McG)
Resident physician, Department of Pathology
McGill University
Montreal, QC

Yu Shi, MD, PhD, FACP
Assistant professor, Department of Pathology
Dalhousie University
Staff pathologist, Dr. Everett Chalmers Regional Hospital, Horizon Health Network
Fredericton, NB

Gurdip Singh Tamber, MD
Resident physician, Department of Pathology
McGill University
Montreal, QC

Duc-Vinh Thai, MD
Resident physician, Department of Pathology
McGill University
Montreal, QC

Tuyet Nhung Ton Nu, MSc, MD, FRCPC
Assistant professor, Department of Pathology
McGill University
Montreal, QC

John P. Veinot, MD, FRCPC
Professor and head, Department of Pathology and Laboratory Medicine
University of Ottawa
Ottawa, ON

Judy Wang, MD, MSc
Elective student, Department of Pathology
McGill University
Montreal, QC

Hangjun Wang, MD
Assistant professor, Department of Pathology Jewish General Hospital
McGill University
Montreal, QC

Hui Jun Wang, MD
Resident physician, Department of Pathology
McGill University
Montreal, QC

Hua Yang, MD, FRCP
Clinical associate professor, Department of Pathology and Laboratory Medicine
University of Calgary and Calgary Laboratory Services
Calgary, AB

Pylyp Zolotarov, MD
Resident physician, Department of Pathology
McGill University
Montreal, QC

Pablo Zoroquiain, MD
Postdoctoral fellow, MUHC-McGill University Ocular Pathology Laboratory
McGill University
Montreal, QC

Index

A

B

C

D

E

F

G

K

L

M

N

O

P

R

S

T

U

V

W

X

Y

Z